ATTENTION-DEFICIT HYPERACTIVITY DISORDER

Attention-Deficit Hyperactivity Disorder

Third Edition

A HANDBOOK FOR DIAGNOSIS AND TREATMENT

RUSSELL A. BARKLEY

THE GUILFORD PRESS
New York   London

©2006 The Guilford Press
A Division of Guilford Publications, Inc.
72 Spring Street, New York, NY 10012
www.guilford.com

Printed in the United States of America

This book is printed on acid-free paper.

Last digit is print number: 9 8 7 6 5 4 3 2 1

Library of Congress Cataloging-in-Publication Data

Barkley, Russell A., 1949–
    Attention-deficit hyperactivity disorder : a handbook for diagnosis and treatment / Russell A. Barkley.—3rd ed.
       p. cm.
    Includes bibliographical references and index.
    ISBN 1-59385-210-X (hardcover: alk. paper)
    1. Attention-deficit hyperactivity disorder—Handbooks, manuals, etc.   2. Attention-deficit hyperactivity disorder—Treatment—Handbooks, manuals, etc.   3. Behavior therapy for children—Handbooks, manuals, etc.   I. Title.
    [DNLM: 1. Attention Deficit Disorder with Hyperactivity—diagnosis.   2. Attention Deficit Disorder with Hyperactivity—therapy.   3. Attention Deficit Disorder with Hyperactivity—etiology.   WS 350.8.A8 B256a 2006]
    RJ496.A86B37 2006
    618.92′8589—dc22
                                                                                2005016986

To my mother,
Mildred Terbush Barkley,
with love and gratitude
for instilling in me her insatiable curiosity and love of learning,
among many of her remarkable attributes

About the Author

Russell A. Barkley, PhD, is Research Professor of Psychiatry at the State University of New York (SUNY) Upstate Medical University at Syracuse. In 1978, he founded the Neuropsychology Service at the Medical College of Wisconsin and Milwaukee Children's Hospital, and served as its Chief until 1985. He then moved to the University of Massachusetts Medical School, where he served as Director of Psychology from 1985 to 2000 and established the research clinics for both child and adult Attention-Deficit/Hyperactivity Disorder (ADHD). In 2003, he relocated to a position as Professor in the Department of Psychiatry at the Medical University of South Carolina. He joined the faculty of the SUNY Upstate Medical University in 2005. Dr. Barkley has published 15 books, more than 200 scientific articles and book chapters, and 7 videos on ADHD and related disorders, including childhood defiance, and is editor of the newsletter *The ADHD Report*. A frequent conference presenter and speaker who is widely cited in the national media, he is past president of the Section on Clinical Child Psychology, Division 12 of the American Psychological Association, and of the International Society for Research in Child and Adolescent Psychopathology. His distinguished research contributions have been recognized with awards from the American Association of Applied and Preventive Psychology, the American Academy of Pediatrics, the Section on Clinical Child Psychology of the American Psychological Association, and the Society for a Science of Clinical Psychology.

Contributors

Arthur D. Anastopoulos, PhD, Professor, Department of Psychology, University of North Carolina at Greensboro, Greensboro, North Carolina

Russell A. Barkley, PhD, Research Professor, Department of Psychiatry, State University of New York Upstate Medical University, Syracuse, New York; Adjunct Professor, Department of Psychiatry, Medical University of South Carolina, Charleston, South Carolina

Joseph Biederman, MD, Director, Joint Program in Pediatric Psychopharmacology, McLean General Hospital and Massachusetts General Hospital; Professor, Department of Psychiatry, Harvard Medical School; Pediatric Psychopharmacology Unit, Massachusetts General Hospital and Harvard Medical School, Boston, Massachusetts

Daniel F. Connor, MD, Professor, Department of Psychiatry, and Director, Pediatric Psychopharmacology Clinic, University of Massachusetts Medical School, Worcester, Massachusetts

Charles E. Cunningham, PhD, Professor, Department of Psychiatry and Behavioural Neurosciences, Jack Laidlaw Chair in Patient Centered Health Care, Faculty of Health Sciences, McMaster University, Hamilton, Ontario, Canada

Lesley J. Cunningham, MSW, Hamilton–Wentworth District School Board, Hamilton, Ontario, Canada

Jodi K. Dooling-Litfin, PhD, Developmental Disability Consultants, P.C., Denver, Colorado

George J. DuPaul, PhD, Professor, Department of Counseling Psychology, School Psychology, and Special Education, Lehigh University, Bethlehem, Pennsylvania

Gwenyth Edwards, PhD, Private Practice, Delta Consultants, Wakefield, Rhode Island

Suzanne E. Farley, MA, Graduate Student, Department of Psychology, University of North Carolina at Greensboro, Greensboro, North Carolina

Michael Gordon, PhD, Professor, Chief Child Psychologist, and Director of Outpatient Services, Department of Psychiatry, State University of New York Upstate Medical University, Syracuse, New York

William L. Hathaway, PhD, Program Director, Doctoral Program in Clinical Psychology, Regent University, Virginia Beach, Virginia

Benjamin J. Lovett, MA, Psychology Intern, Department of Psychiatry, State University of New York Upstate Medical University, Syracuse, New York

Kevin R. Murphy, PhD, Director, Adult ADHD Clinic of Central Massachusetts, Northboro, Massachusetts

Linda J. Pfiffner, PhD, Associate Professor, Department of Psychiatry, Children's Center at Langley Porter, University of California at San Francisco, San Francisco, California

Jefferson B. Prince, MD, Director, Department of Child Psychiatry, North Shore Medical Center, Salem, Massachusetts; Staff, Department of Child Psychiatry, Massachusetts General Hospital; Instructor, Department of Psychiatry, Harvard Medical School, Boston, Massachusetts

Laura Hennis Rhoads, MA, Graduate Student, Department of Psychology, University of North Carolina at Greensboro, Greensboro, North Carolina

Arthur L. Robin, PhD, Professor of Psychiatry and Behavioral Neurosciences, Wayne State University School of Medicine, Detroit, Michigan.

Cheri J. Shapiro, PhD, Research Assistant Professor, Department of Psychology, University of South Carolina, Columbia, South Carolina

Bradley H. Smith, PhD, Associate Professor, Department of Psychology, University of South Carolina, Columbia, South Carolina

Thomas J. Spencer, MD, Assistant Director, Pediatric Psychopharmacology Clinic, Massachusetts General Hospital; Associate Professor, Department of Psychiatry, Harvard Medical School, Boston, Massachusetts

Timothy E. Wilens, MD, Director of Substance Abuse Services, Pediatric Psychopharmacology Clinic, Massachusetts General Hospital; Associate Professor, Department of Psychiatry, Harvard Medical School, Boston, Massachusetts

Preface

This book remains true to its original purpose, dating back to its initial version, *Hyperactive Children: A Handbook for Diagnosis and Treatment* (Barkley, 1981). That purpose is to extract from the mine of available scientific literature those nuggets of clinically important information regarding the nature, assessment, diagnosis, and management of Attention-Deficit/Hyperactivity Disorder (ADHD). The task of doing so has increased substantially since the preceding edition (Barkley, 1998), given the enormous expansion of the scientific literature. Several hundred studies are published in scientific journals every year; in fact, nearly 1,000 new studies on ADHD have been published since the 1998 edition was published. So formidable an undertaking requires the assistance of many individuals, for it is clear that no single individual can be an expert any longer in all facets of this disorder and its management.

To help me with this endeavor, I have invited back all of the principal authors of chapters from the 1998 edition, each expert in his or her own area of the ADHD literature. All were charged with updating their information; eliminating what had grown outdated or was no longer relevant or acceptable; incorporating new findings from studies published in the interim; and especially rendering any new conclusions and clinical recommendations from the available research and related publications. I am truly grateful that all chose to return and assist with this edition. New to this edition are colleagues Bradley H. Smith and Cheri J. Shapiro, who assisted me with reviewing the growing literature on combination treatments for ADHD (Chapter 20), and in particular the historic Multimodal Treatment Study of ADHD (MTA). Conducted under the auspices of the National Institute of Mental Health, the MTA took place at six sites in the United States and Canada, and involved more than 570 children with ADHD (Combined Type). As it is among the largest studies ever undertaken to evaluate treatments for ADHD, and surely the largest examining combined therapies, the MTA project is of great relevance to clinicians.

Besides new coverage of the research on combination therapies, other changes to this edition include expanded coverage of virtually every chapter and its topics to include not only hundreds of new studies on the history, nature, comorbidity, prevalence, etiology, assessment, and management of childhood ADHD, but also the growing awareness of and scientific literature on adult ADHD. And most chapters now conclude with a checklist of "Key Clinical Points" to aid the reader in summarizing the major conclusions and recommendations discussed in that chapter. Several bodies of literature have grown disproportionately since the 1998 edition, and these have received much greater coverage here, including genetics, neuroimaging, neuropsychology, follow-up studies, disorders likely to be comorbid with ADHD, health risks and costs, and research on ADHD in clinic-referred adults. Older treatments have been reevaluated and clarified, and new treatments are now covered that did not exist at the time of the 1998 edition. These include the new once-daily sustained delivery systems for stimulant medications, and the new medication atomoxetine, as well as numerous recommendations for home, classroom, and community management of the disorder.

From time to time, media flare-ups have centered around ADHD, sometimes challenging its very existence. Taken in its totality, this book is a complete and stunning refutation of such assertions. It shows that ADHD is as valid a mental disorder as we are likely to find, with massive evidence that it represents a serious deficiency in one or more psychological adaptations that produce harm to the individuals so afflicted. To assist readers with addressing these occasional misrepresentations of ADHD and its treatment in the popular media, the International Consensus Statement on ADHD is provided as an Appendix to Chapter 1. Signed by more than 80 of the world's leading clinical researchers on ADHD, it is a beautifully concise statement of the nature and validity of ADHD; it effectively undercuts social critics, politically motivated groups, and biased reporters who have tried to claim that ADHD is a fraud or that the use of medications as part of a total treatment package is scandalous and reprehensible.

As in previous editions, I once again thank Seymour Weingarten and Robert Matloff at The Guilford Press for supporting this book and providing a home for this and my other books. I also wish to thank Carolyn Graham, Marie Sprayberry, and Anna Nelson at Guilford for helping to shepherd this book through the publication process in a professional and expeditious manner. My debt to them and the rest of Guilford's superbly capable staff is incalculable for having assisted me over more than 24 years of publishing, and I express my deep appreciation to all members of the Guilford "family" here. I am also exceptionally appreciative of my wife, Patricia, who has stood by me for more than 36 years and provided a loving home for me and our two sons, Ken and Steve, and a sense of family in which we could flourish. In such homes can creative works as this be achieved.

RUSSELL A. BARKLEY, PhD
Charleston, South Carolina

REFERENCES

Barkley, R. A. (1981). *Hyperactive children: A handbook for diagnosis and treatment.* New York: Guilford Press.

Barkley, R. A. (1998). *Attention-deficit hyperactivity disorder: A handbook for diagnosis and treatment* (2nd ed.). New York: Guilford Press.

Contents

III. TREATMENT

PART **I**

THE NATURE OF ADHD

History

RUSSELL A. BARKLEY

Attention-Deficit/Hyperactivity Disorder (ADHD) is the current diagnostic label for children presenting with significant problems with attention, and typically with impulsiveness and excessive activity as well. Children with ADHD represent a rather heterogeneous population who display considerable variation in the degree of their symptoms, in the age of onset, in the cross-situational pervasiveness of those symptoms, and in the extent to which other disorders occur in association with ADHD. The disorder represents one of the most common reasons children are referred for behavioral problems to medical and mental health practitioners in the United States and is one of the most prevalent childhood psychiatric disorders. This chapter presents an overview of ADHD's history—a history that spans nearly a century of clinical and scientific publications on the disorder. Given that the history of ADHD through 1997 has not changed since the preceding edition of this text (Barkley, 1998), little has been done to update those sections of this chapter. Developments as the new century begins are described at the end of this chapter, however, and so readers familiar with the earlier edition may wish to skip to that discussion (p. 32).

In the history of ADHD reside the nascent concepts that serve as the foundation for the current conceptualization of the disorder as largely involving poor inhibition and self-regulation. Here also can be seen the emergence of current notions about its treatment. Such a history remains important for any serious student of ADHD, for it shows that many contemporary themes concerning its nature arose long ago and recurred throughout the 20th century as clinical scientists strove for a clearer, more accurate understanding of the very essence of this condition. Readers are directed to other sources for additional discussions of the history of this disorder (Accardo & Blondis, 2000; Goldstein & Goldstein, 1998; Kessler, 1980; Ross & Ross, 1976, 1982; Schachar, 1986; Werry, 1992).

THE ORIGINS OF ADHD

Still's Description

One of the first references to a child with hyperactivity or ADHD ("Fidgety Phil") was in the poetry of the German physician Heinrich Hoffman in 1865, who penned poems about many of the childhood maladies he saw in his medical practice (Stewart, 1970). But scientific credit is typically awarded to George Still and Alfred Tredgold for being the first authors to focus serious clinical attention on the behavioral condition in children that most closely approximates what is today known as ADHD.

In a series of three published lectures to the Royal College of Physicians, Still (1902) described 43 children in his clinical practice who had serious problems with sustained attention; he agreed with William James (1890/1950) that such attention may be an important element in the "moral control of behavior." Most were also quite overactive. Many were often aggressive, defiant, resistant to discipline, and excessively emotional or "passionate." These children showed little "inhibitory volition" over their behavior, and they also manifested "lawlessness," spitefulness, cruelty, and dishonesty. Still proposed that the immediate gratification of the self was the "keynote" quality of these and other attributes of the children. And among all of them, passion (or heightened emotionality) was the most commonly observed attribute and the most noteworthy. Still noted further that an insensitivity to punishment characterized many of these children, for they would be punished (even physically), yet would engage in the same infraction within a matter of hours.

Still believed that these children displayed a major "defect in moral control" in their behavior that was relatively chronic in most cases. He believed that in some cases, these children had acquired the defect secondary to an acute brain disease, and it might remit on recovery from the disease. He noted a higher risk for criminal acts in later development in some of the chronic cases, though not all. Although this defect could be associated with intellectual retardation, as it was in 23 of the cases, it could also arise in children of near-normal intelligence, as it seemed to do in the remaining 20.

To Still, the moral control of behavior meant "the control of action in conformity with the idea of the good of all" (p. 1008). Moral control was thought to arise out of a cognitive or conscious comparison of the individual's volitional activity with that of the good of all—a comparison he termed "moral consciousness." For purposes that will become evident later, it is important to realize here that to make such a comparison inherently involves the capacity to understand the consequences of one's actions over time and to hold in mind forms of information about oneself and one's actions, along with information on their context. Those forms of information involve the action being proposed by the individual, the context, and

the moral principle or rule against which it must be compared. This notion may link Still's views with the contemporary concepts of self-awareness, working memory, and rule-governed behavior discussed later in this text. Still did not specifically identify these inherent aspects of the comparative process, but they are clearly implied in the manner in which he used the term "conscious" in describing this process. He stipulated that this process of comparison of proposed action to a rule concerning the greater good involved the critical element of the conscious or cognitive relation of individuals to their environment, or self-awareness. Intellect was recognized as playing a part in moral consciousness, but equally or more important was the notion of volition or will. The latter is where Still believed the impairment arose in many of those with defective moral control who suffered no intellectual delay. Volition was viewed as being primarily inhibitory in nature, that a stimulus to act must be overpowered by the stimulus of the idea of the greater good of all.

Both volitional inhibition and the moral regulation of behavior founded on it were believed to develop gradually in children; therefore, younger children would find it more difficult to resist the stimulus to act on impulse than would older children. Thus, judging a child to be defective in volitional inhibition and moral control of behavior meant making a comparison to same-age normal children and taking into account the degree of appeal of the stimulus. Even at the same age, inhibition and moral control varied across children—in part because of environmental factors, but also, Still proposed, because of innate differences in these capacities. Still concluded that a defect in moral control could arise as a function of three distinct impairments: "(1) defect of cognitive relation to the environment; (2) defect of moral consciousness; and (3) defect in inhibitory volition" (p. 1011). He placed these impairments in a hierarchical relation to each other in the order shown, arguing that impairments at a lower level would affect those levels above it and ultimately the moral control of behavior.

Much as researchers do today, Still noted a greater proportion of males than females (3:1) in his sample, and he observed that the disorder appeared to arise in most cases before 8 years of age (typically in early childhood). Many of Still's cases displayed a higher incidence of minor anomalies in their physical appearance, or "stigmata of degeneration," such as abnormally large head size, malformed palate, or increased epicanthal fold. A proneness to accidental injuries was reported in these children—an observation corroborated by numerous subsequent studies reviewed in a later chapter. And Still saw these youngsters as posing an increased threat to the safety of other children because of their aggressive or violent behavior. Alcoholism, criminality, and affective disorders such as depression and suicide were noted to be more common among their biological relatives—an observation once again buttressed by numerous studies published in recent years. Some of the children displayed a history of significant brain damage or convulsions, while others did not. A few had associated tic disorders, or "microkinesia"; this was perhaps the first time tic disorders and ADHD were noted to be comorbid conditions. We now recognize that as many as 50–70% of children with tic disorders and Tourette syndrome have associated ADHD (Barkley, 1988b; Pliszka, 1998).

Although many children were reported to have a chaotic family life, others came from households with seemingly adequate upbringing. In fact, Still believed that when poor child rearing was clearly involved, the children should be exempt from the category of lack of moral control; he reserved it instead only for children who displayed a morbid (organic) failure of moral control despite adequate training. He proposed a biological predisposition to this behavioral condition that was probably hereditary in some children but the result of pre- or postnatal injury in others. In keeping with the theorizing of William James (1890/1950), Still hypothesized that the deficits in inhibitory volition, moral control, and sustained attention were causally related to each other and to the same underlying neurological deficiency. He cautiously speculated on the possibility of either a decreased threshold for inhibition of responding to stimuli or a cortical disconnection syndrome, where intellect was dissociated from "will" in a manner that might be due to neuronal cell modification. Any biologically compromising event that could cause significant brain damage ("cell modification") and retardation could, he conjectured, in its milder forms lead only to this defective moral control.

Later Tredgold (1908), and much later Pasamanick, Rogers, and Lilienfeld (1956), would use such a theory of early, mild, and undetected damage to account for these developmentally late-arising behavioral and learning deficiencies. Foreshadowing current views of treatment, both Still and Tredgold found that temporary improvements in conduct might be achieved by alterations in the environment or by medications, but they stressed the relative permanence of the defect even in these cases. The need for special educational environments for these children was strongly emphasized. We see here the origins of many later and even current notions about children with ADHD and Oppositional Defiant Disorder (ODD), although it would take almost 70 years to return to many of them—owing in part to the ascendance in the interim of psychoanalytic, psychodynamic, and behavioral views, which overemphasized child rearing as largely causing such behavioral disorders in children. The children whom Still and Tredgold described would probably now be diagnosed as having not only ADHD but also ODD or Conduct Disorder (CD), and most likely a learning disability as well (see Chapters 4 and 6, this volume, for discussions of ADHD's comorbidity with these disorders).

THE PERIOD 1920 TO 1950

The history of interest in ADHD in North America can be traced to the outbreak of an encephalitis epidemic in 1917–1918, when clinicians were presented with a number of children who survived this brain infection but were left with significant behavioral and cognitive sequelae (Cantwell, 1981; Kessler, 1980; Stewart, 1970). Numerous papers reported these sequelae (Ebaugh, 1923; Strecker & Ebaugh, 1924; Stryker, 1925), and they included many of the characteristics we now incorporate into the concept of ADHD. Such children were described as being impaired in their attention, regulation of activity, and impulsivity, as well as in other cognitive abilities, including memory; they were often noted to be socially disruptive as well. Symptoms of what would now be called ODD, as well as delinquency and CD, also arose in some cases. "Postencephalitic behavior disorder," as it was called, was clearly the result of brain damage. The large number of children affected resulted in significant professional and educational interest in this behavioral disorder. Its severity was such that many children were recommended for care and education outside the home and away from normal educational facilities. Despite a rather pessimistic view of the prognosis of these children, some facilities reported significant success in their treatment with simple behavior modification programs and increased supervision (Bender, 1942; Bond & Appel, 1931).

The Origins of a Brain Damage Syndrome

This association of a brain disease with behavioral pathology apparently led early investigators to study other potential causes of brain injury in children and their behavioral manifestations. Birth trauma (Shirley, 1939); other infections besides encephalitis, such as measles (Meyer & Byers, 1952); lead toxicity (Byers & Lord, 1943); epilepsy (Levin, 1938); and head injury (Blau, 1936; Werner & Strauss, 1941) were all studied in children and were found to be associated with numerous cognitive and behavioral impairments, including the triad of ADHD symptoms noted earlier. Other terms introduced during this era for children displaying these behavioral characteristics were "organic driveness" (Kahn & Cohen, 1934) and "restlessness" syndrome (Childers, 1935; Levin, 1938). Many of the children seen in these samples also had mental retardation or more serious behavioral disorders than what is today called ADHD. It would be several decades before investigators would attempt to parse out the separate contributions of intellectual delay, learning disabilities, or other neuropsychological deficits from those of the behavioral deficits to the maladjustment of these children. Even so, scientists at this time would discover that activity level was often inversely related to intelligence in children, increasing as intelligence declined in a sample—a finding supported in many subsequent studies (Rutter, 1989). It should also be noted that a large number of children in these older studies did in fact have brain damage or signs of such damage (epilepsy, hemiplegias, etc.).

Notable during this era was also the recognition of the striking similarity between hyperactivity in children and the behavioral sequelae of frontal lobe lesions in primates (Blau, 1936; Levin, 1938). Frontal lobe ablation studies of monkeys had been done more than 60 years earlier (Ferrier, 1876), and the lesions were known to result in excessive restlessness, poor ability to sustain interest in activities, aimless wandering, and excessive appetite, among other behavioral changes. Several investigators, such as Levin (1938), would use these similarities to postulate that severe restlessness in children might well be the result of pathological defects in the forebrain structures, although gross evidence of such was not always apparent in many of these children. Later investigators (e.g., Barkley, 1997b; Chelune, Ferguson, Koon, & Dickey, 1986; Lou, Henriksen, & Bruh, 1984; Lou, Henriksen, Bruhn, Borner, & Nielsen, 1989; Mattes, 1980) would return to this notion, but with greater evidence to substantiate their claims. Milder forms of hyperactivity, in contrast, were attributed in this era to psychological causes, such as "spoiled" child-rearing practices or delinquent family environments. This idea that poor or disrupted parenting causes ADHD would also be resurrected in the 1970s and continues even today among many laypeople and critics of ADHD.

Over the next decade, it became fashionable to consider most children hospitalized in psychiatric facilities with this symptom picture to have suffered from some type of brain damage (such as encephalitis or pre-/perinatal trauma), whether or not the clinical history of the case contained evidence of such. The concept of the "brain-injured child" was to be born in this era (Strauss & Lehtinen, 1947) and applied to children with these behavioral characteristics, many of whom had insufficient or no evidence of brain pathology. In fact, Strauss and Lehtinen argued that the psychological disturbances alone were de facto evidence of brain injury as the etiology. Owing in part to the absence of such evidence of brain damage, this term would later evolve into the concept of "minimal brain damage" and eventually "minimal brain dysfunction" (MBD) by the 1950s and 1960s. Even so, a few early investigators, such as Childers (1935), would raise serious questions about the notion of brain damage in these children when no historical documentation of damage existed. Substantial recommendations for educating these "brain-damaged" children were made in the classic text by Strauss and Lehtinen (1947), which served as a forerunner to special educational services adopted much later in U.S. public schools. These recommendations included placing these children in smaller, more carefully regulated classrooms and reducing the amount of distracting stimulation in the environment. Strikingly austere classrooms were developed, in which teachers could not wear jewelry or brightly colored clothing, and few pictures could adorn the walls so as not to interfere unnecessarily with the education of these highly distractible students.

Although the population served by the Pennsylvania center in which Strauss, Werner, and Lehtinen worked principally contained children with mental retardation, the work of Cruickshank and his students (Dolphin & Cruickshank, 1951a, 1951b, 1951c) later extended these neuropsychological findings to children with cerebral palsy but near-normal or normal intelligence. This extension resulted in the extrapolation of the educational recommendations of Strauss to children without mental retardation who manifested behavioral or perceptual disturbances (Cruickshank & Dolphin, 1951; Strauss & Lehtinen, 1947). Echoes of these recommendations are still commonplace today in most educational plans for children with ADHD or learning disabilities, despite the utter lack of scientific support for their efficacy (Kessler, 1980; Routh, 1978; Zentall, 1985). These classrooms are historically significant, as they were the predecessors as well as instigators of the types of educational resources that would be incorporated into the initial Education for All Handicapped Children Act of 1975 (Public Law 94-142) mandating the special education of children with learning disabilities and behavioral disorders, and its later reauthorization, the Individuals with Disabilities Education Act of 1990 (IDEA; Public Law 101-476).

The Beginnings of Child Psychopharmacology for ADHD

Another significant series of papers on the treatment of hyperactive children appeared in 1937–1941. These papers were to mark the beginnings of medication therapy (particularly stimulants) for behaviorally disordered children in particular as well as the field of child psychopharmacology in general (Bradley, 1937; Bradley & Bowen, 1940; Molitch & Eccles, 1937). Initiated originally to treat the headaches that resulted from conducting pneumoencephalograms during research studies of these disruptive youth, the administration of amphetamine resulted in a noticeable improvement in their behavioral problems and academic performance. Later studies would also confirm such a positive drug response in half or more of hyperactive hospitalized children

(Laufer, Denhoff, & Solomons, 1957). As a result, by the 1970s, stimulant medications were gradually becoming the treatment of choice for the behavioral symptoms now associated with ADHD. And so they remain today (see Chapter 17, this volume).

The Emergence of a Hyperkinetic Impulse Syndrome

In the 1950s, researchers began a number of investigations into the neurological mechanisms underlying these behavioral symptoms, the most famous of which was probably that by Laufer et al. (1957). These writers referred to children with ADHD as having "hyperkinetic impulse disorder," and reasoned that the central nervous system (CNS) deficit occurred in the thalamic area. Here, poor filtering of stimulation occurred, allowing an excess of stimulation to reach the brain. The evidence was based on a study of the effects of the "photo-Metrozol" method, in which the drug metronidazole (Metrozol) is administered while flashes of light are presented to a child. The amount of drug required to induce a muscle jerk of the forearms, along with a spike wave pattern on the electroencephalogram (EEG), serves as the measure of interest. Laufer et al. (1957) found that inpatient children with hyperactivity required less Metrozol than those without hyperactivity to induce this pattern of response. This finding suggested that the hyperactive children had a lower threshold for stimulation, possibly in the thalamic area. No attempts to replicate this study have been done, and it is unlikely that such research would pass today's standards of ethical conduct in research required by institutional review boards on research with human subjects. Nevertheless, it remains a milestone in the history of the disorder for its delineation of a more specific mechanism that might give rise to hyperactivity (low cortical thresholds or overstimulation). Others at the time also conjectured that an imbalance between cortical and subcortical areas existed. There was believed to be diminished control of subcortical areas responsible for sensory filtering that permitted excess stimulation to reach the cortex (Knobel, Wolman, & Mason, 1959).

By the end of this era, it seemed well accepted that hyperactivity was a brain damage syndrome, even when evidence of damage was lacking. The disorder was thought to be best treated through educational classrooms characterized by reduced stimulation or through residential centers. Its prognosis was considered fair to poor. The possibility that a relatively new class of medications, the stimulants, might hold promise for its treatment was beginning to be appreciated.

THE PERIOD 1960 TO 1969
The Decline of MBD

In the late 1950s and early 1960s, critical reviews began appearing questioning the concept of a unitary syndrome of brain damage in children. They also pointed out the logical fallacy that if brain damage resulted in some of these behavioral symptoms, these symptoms could be pathognomonic of brain damage without any other corroborating evidence of CNS lesions. Chief among these critical reviews were those of Birch (1964), Herbert (1964), and Rapin (1964), who questioned the validity of applying the concept of brain damage to children who had only equivocal signs of neurological involvement, not necessarily damage. A plethora of research followed on children with MBD (see Rie & Rie, 1980, for reviews); in addition, a task force by the National Institute of Neurological Diseases and Blindness (Clements, 1966) recognized at least 99 symptoms for this disorder. The concept of MBD would die a slow death as it eventually became recognized as vague, overinclusive, of little or no prescriptive value, and without much neurological evidence (Kirk, 1963). Its value remained in its emphasis on neurological mechanisms over the often excessive, pedantic, and convoluted environmental mechanisms proposed at that time—particularly those etiological hypotheses stemming from psychoanalytical theory, which blamed parental and family factors entirely for these problems (Hertzig, Bortner, & Birch, 1969; Kessler, 1980; Taylor, 1983). The term "MBD" would eventually be replaced by more specific labels applying to somewhat more homogeneous cognitive, learning, and behavioral disorders, such as "dyslexia," "language disorders," "learning disabilities," and "hyperactivity." These new labels were based on children's observable and descriptive deficits, rather than on some underlying unobservable etiological mechanism in the brain.

The Hyperactivity Syndrome

As dissatisfaction with the term "MBD" was occurring, clinical investigators shifted their emphasis to the behavioral symptom thought to most characterize the disorder—that of hyperactivity. And so the concept of a hyperactivity syndrome arose, described in the classic papers by Laufer and Denhoff (1957) and Chess (1960) and other reports of this era (Burks, 1960; Ounsted, 1955; Prechtl & Stemmer, 1962). Chess defined "hyperactivity" as follows: "The hyperactive child is one who carries out activities at a higher than normal rate of speed than the average child, or who is constantly in motion, or both" (p. 239). Chess's article was historically significant for several reasons: (1) It emphasized activity as the defining feature of the disorder, rather than speculative underlying neurological causes, as other scientists of the time would also do; (2) it stressed the need to consider objective evidence of the symptom beyond the subjective reports of parents or teachers; (3) it took the blame for the child's problems away from the parents; and (4) it separated the syndrome of hyperactivity from the concept of a brain damage syndrome. Other scientists of this era would emphasize similar points (Werry & Sprague, 1970). It would now be recognized that hyperactivity was a behavioral syndrome that could arise from organic pathology, but could also occur in its absence. Even so, it would continue to be viewed as the result of some biological difficulty, rather than due solely to environmental causes.

Chess described the characteristics of 36 children diagnosed with "physiological hyperactivity" from a total of 881 children seen in a private practice. The ratio of males to females was approximately 4:1, and many children were referred prior to 6 years of age, intimating a relatively earlier age of onset than that for other childhood behavioral disorders. Educational difficulties were common in this group, particularly scholastic underachievement, and many displayed oppositional defiant behavior and poor peer relationships. Impulsive and aggressive behaviors, as well as poor attention span, were commonly associated characteristics. Chess believed that the hyperactivity could also be associated with mental retardation, organic brain damage, or serious mental illness (e.g., schizophrenia). Similar findings in later research would lead others to question the specificity and hence the utility of this symptom for the diagnosis of ADHD (Douglas, 1972). As in many of today's prescriptions, a multimodal treatment approach incorporating parent counseling, behavior modification, psychotherapy, medication, and special education was recommended. Unlike Still, Chess and others writing in this era stressed the relatively benign nature of hyperactivity's symptoms and claimed that in most cases they resolved by puberty (Laufer & Denhoff, 1957; Solomons, 1965). Here then were the beginnings of a belief that would be widely held among clinicians well into the 1980s—that hyperactivity (ADHD) was outgrown by adolescence.

Also noteworthy in this era was the definition of hyperactivity given in the official diagnostic nomenclature at the time, the second edition of the *Diagnostic and Statistical Manual of Mental Disorders* (DSM-II; American Psychiatric Association, 1968). It employed only a single sentence describing the Hyperkinetic Reaction of Childhood disorder and, following the lead of Chess, stressed the view that the disorder was developmentally benign: "The disorder is characterized by overactivity, restlessness, distractibility, and short attention span, especially in young children; the behavior usually diminishes by adolescence" (p. 50).

Europe and North America Part Company

It is likely that during this period (or even earlier), the perspective on hyperactivity in North America began to diverge from that in Europe, particularly Great Britain. In North America, hyperactivity would become a behavioral syndrome recognized chiefly by greater-than-normal levels of activity; would be viewed as a relatively common disturbance of childhood; would not necessarily be associated with demonstrable brain pathology or mental retardation; and would be regarded as more of an extreme degree in the normal variation of temperament in children. In Great Britain, the earlier and narrower view of a brain damage syndrome would continue into the 1970s: Hyperactivity or hyperkinesis was seen as an extreme state of excessive activity of an almost driven quality; was viewed as highly uncommon; and was usually thought to occur in conjunction with other signs of brain damage (such as epilepsy, hemiplegias, or mental retar-

dation) or a clearer history of brain insult (such as trauma or infection) (Taylor, 1988). The divergence in views would lead to large discrepancies between North Americans and Europeans in their estimations of the prevalence of the disorder, their diagnostic criteria, and their preferred treatment modalities. A rapprochement between these views would not occur until well into the 1980s (Rutter, 1988, 1989; Taylor, 1986, 1988).

The Prevailing View by 1969

As Ross and Ross (1976) noted in their exhaustive and scholarly review of the era, the perspective on hyperactivity in the 1960s was that it remained a brain dysfunction syndrome, although of a milder magnitude than previously believed. The disorder was no longer ascribed to brain damage; instead, a focus on brain mechanisms prevailed. The disorder was also viewed as having a predominant and relatively homogeneous set of symptoms, chief among which was excessive activity level or hyperactivity. Its prognosis was now felt to be relatively benign, as it was believed to be often outgrown by puberty. The recommended treatments now consisted of short-term treatment with stimulant medication and psychotherapy, in addition to the minimum-stimulation types of classrooms recommended in earlier years.

THE PERIOD 1970 TO 1979

Research in the 1970s took a quantum leap forward, with more than 2,000 published studies existing by the time the decade ended (Weiss & Hechtman, 1979). Numerous clinical and scientific textbooks (Cantwell, 1975; Safer & Allen, 1976; Trites, 1979; Wender, 1971) appeared, along with a most thorough and scholarly review of the literature by Ross and Ross (1976). Special journal issues were devoted to the topic (Douglas, 1976; Barkley, 1978), along with numerous scientific gatherings (Knights & Bakker, 1976, 1980). Clearly, hyperactivity had become a subject of serious professional, scientific, and popular attention.

By the early 1970s, the defining features of hyperactivity or hyperkinesis were broadened to include what investigators previously felt to be only associated characteristics, including impulsivity, short attention span, low frustration tolerance, distractibility, and aggressiveness (Marwitt & Stenner, 1972; Safer & Allen, 1976). Others (Wender, 1971, 1973) persisted with the excessively inclusive concept of MBD, in which even more features (such as motor clumsiness, cognitive impairments, and parent–child conflict) were viewed as hallmarks of the syndrome, and in which hyperactivity was unnecessary for the diagnosis. As noted earlier, the diagnostic term "MBD" would fade from clinical and scientific usage by the end of this decade—the result in no small part of the scholarly tome by Rie and Rie (1980) and critical reviews by Rutter (1977, 1982). These writings emphasized the lack of evidence for such a broad syndrome. The symptoms were not well defined, did not correlate significantly among themselves, had no well-specified etiology, and displayed no common course and outcome. The heterogeneity of the disorder was overwhelming, and more than a few commentators took note of the apparent hypocrisy in defining an MBD syndrome with statements that there was often little or no evidence of neurological abnormality (Wender, 1971). Moreover, even in cases of well-established cerebral damage, the behavioral sequelae were not uniform across cases, and hyperactivity was seen in only a minority. Hence, contrary to 25 years of theorizing to this point, hyperactivity was not a common sequela of brain damage; children with true brain damage did not display a uniform pattern of behavioral deficits; and children with hyperactivity rarely had substantiated evidence of neurological damage (Rutter, 1989).

Wender's Theory of MBD

This decade was notable for two different models of the nature of ADHD (see also Barkley, 1998): Wender's theory of MBD (outlined here) and Douglas's model of attention and impulse control in hyperactive children (discussed in a later section). At the start of the decade, Wender (1971) described the essential psychological characteristics of children with MBD as consisting of six clusters of symptoms: problems in (1) motor behavior, (2) attentional and perceptual–cognitive functioning, (3) learning, (4) impulse control, (5) interpersonal relations, and (6) emotion. Many of the characteristics first reported by Still were echoed by Wender within these six domains of functioning.

1. Within the realm of motor behavior, the essential features were noted to be hyperactivity and poor motor coordination. Excessive speech, colic, and sleeping difficulties were thought to be related to the hyperactivity. Foreshadowing the later official designation of a group of children with attentional problems but without hyperactivity (American Psychiatric Association, 1980), Wender expressed the opinion that some of these children were hypoactive and listless while still demonstrating attention disturbances. Such cases might now be considered to have the Predominantly Inattentive Type of ADHD. He argued that they should be viewed as having this syndrome because of their manifestation of many of the other difficulties thought to characterize it.

2. Short attention span and poor concentration were described as the most striking deficit in the domain of attention and perceptual–cognitive functioning. Distractibility and daydreaming were also included with these attention disturbances, as was poor organization of ideas or percepts.

3. Learning difficulties were the third domain of dysfunction, with most of these children observed to be doing poorly in their academic performance. A large percentage were described as having specific difficulties with learning to read, with handwriting, and with reading comprehension and arithmetic.

4. Impulse control problems, or a decreased ability to inhibit behavior, were identified as a fourth characteristic of most children with MBD. Within this general category, Wender included low frustration tolerance; an inability to delay gratification; antisocial behavior; lack of planning, forethought, or judgment; and poor sphincter control, leading to enuresis and encopresis. Disorderliness or lack of organization and recklessness (particularly with regard to bodily safety) were also listed within this domain of dysfunction.

5. In the area of interpersonal relations, Wender singled out the unresponsiveness of these children to social demands as the most serious. Extroversion, excessive independence, obstinence, stubbornness, negativism, disobedience, noncompliance, sassiness, and imperviousness to discipline were some of the characteristics that instantiated the problem with interpersonal relations.

6. Finally, within the domain of emotional difficulties, Wender included increased lability

of mood, altered reactivity, increased anger, aggressiveness, and temper outbursts, as well as dysphoria. The dysphoria of these children involved the specific difficulties of anhedonia, depression, low self-esteem, and anxiety. A diminished sensitivity to both pain and punishment was also felt to typify this area of dysfunction in children with MBD. All these symptoms bear a striking resemblance to the case descriptions Still (1902) had provided in his lectures to support his contention that a defect in moral control and volitional inhibition could exist in children apart from intellectual delay.

Wender theorized that these six domains of dysfunction could be best accounted for by three primary deficits: (1) a decreased experience of pleasure and pain, (2) a generally high and poorly modulated level of activation, and (3) extroversion. A consequence of the first deficit was that children with MBD would prove less sensitive to both rewards and punishments, making them less susceptible to social influence. The generally high and poorly modulated level of activation was thought to be an aspect of poor inhibition. Hyperactivity, of course, was the consummate demonstration of this high level of activation. The problems with poor sustained attention and distractibility were conjectured to be secondary aspects of high activation. Emotional overreactivity, low frustration tolerance, quickness to anger, and temper outbursts resulted from the poor modulation of activation. These three primary deficits, then, created a cascading of effects into the larger social ecology of these children, resulting in numerous interpersonal problems and academic performance difficulties.

Like Still (1902), Wender gave a prominent role to the construct of poor inhibition. He believed it to explain both the activation difficulties and the attention problems stemming from these, as well as the excessive emotionality, low frustration tolerance, and hot-temperedness of these children. It is therefore quite puzzling why deficient inhibition was not made a primary symptom in this theory, in place of high activation and poor modulation of activation.

Unlike Still's attempt at a theory, however, Wender did not say much about normal developmental processes with respect to the three primary areas of deficit, and thus did not clarify more precisely what might be going awry in

them to give rise to these characteristics of MBD. The exception was his discussion of a diminished sensitivity to the reasonably well-understood processes of reinforcement and punishment. A higher-than-normal threshold for pleasure and pain, as noted earlier, was thought to create these insensitivities to behavioral consequences.

From a present-day perspective, Wender's theory is also unclear about a number of issues. For instance, how would the three primary deficits account for the difficulties with motor coordination that occurred alongside hyperactivity in his category of motor control problems? It is doubtful that the high level of activation that was said to cause the hyperactivity would also cause these motor deficits. Nor is it clear just how the academic achievement deficits in reading, math, and handwriting could arise from the three primary deficits in the model. It is also unclear why the construct of extroversion needed to be proposed at all, if what Wender meant by it was reduced social inhibition. This model might be just as parsimoniously explained by the deficit in behavioral inhibition already posited. And the meaning of the term "activation" as used by Wender is not very clearly specified. Did it refer to excessive behavior, in which case hyperactivity would have sufficed? Or did it refer to level of CNS arousal, in which case ample subsequent evidence has not found this to be the case (Hastings & Barkley, 1978; Rosenthal & Allen, 1978)? To his credit, Wender recognized the abstract nature of the term "activation" as he employed it in this theory, but he retained it because he felt it could be used to incorporate both hyperactivity and hypoactivity in children. It is never made clear just how this could be the case, however. Finally, Wender failed to distinguish symptoms from their consequences (impairments). The former would be the behavioral manifestations directly associated with or stemming from the disorder itself, such as impulsiveness, inattention, distractibility, and hyperactivity. The latter would be the effects of these behaviors on the social environment, such as interpersonal conflict within the family, poor educational performance, peer rejection, and accident proneness, to name just a few.

From the advantage of hindsight and subsequent research over the decades since the formulation of this theory, it is also evident that

Wender was combining the symptoms of ODD (and even CD) with those of ADHD to form a single disorder. Still (1902) did very much the same thing. This was understandable, given that clinic-referred cases were the starting point for both theories, and many clinic-referred cases are comorbid for both disorders (ADHD and ODD). Sufficient evidence has subsequently accumulated, however, to show that ADHD and ODD are not the same disorder (August & Stewart, 1983; Hinshaw, 1987; Stewart, deBlois, & Cummings, 1980).

The Emergence of Attention Deficits

At this time, disenchantment developed over the exclusive focus on hyperactivity as the sine qua non of this disorder (Werry & Sprague, 1970). Significant at this historical juncture would be the presidential address of Virginia Douglas to the Canadian Psychological Association (Douglas, 1972). She argued that deficits in sustained attention and impulse control were more likely than just hyperactivity to account for the difficulties seen in these children. These other symptoms were also seen as the major areas on which the stimulant medications used to treat the disorder had their impact. Douglas's paper was historically significant in other ways as well. Her extensive and thorough battery of objective measures of various behavioral and cognitive domains, heretofore unused in research on ADHD, allowed her to rule in or out various characteristics felt to be typical for these children in earlier clinical and scientific lore. For instance, Douglas found that hyperactive children did not necessarily and uniformly have more reading or other learning disabilities than other children, did not perseverate on concept-learning tasks, did not manifest auditory or right–left discrimination problems, and had no difficulties with short-term memory. Most important, she and Susan Campbell demonstrated that children with hyperactivity were not always more distractible than children without it, and that the sustained attention problems could emerge in conditions in which no significant distractions existed.

The McGill University research team headed by Douglas repeatedly demonstrated that hyperactive children had some of their greatest difficulties on tasks assessing vigilance or sustained attention, such as the continuous-performance test (CPT). These findings would be repeatedly reconfirmed over the next 30 years of research using CPTs (Corkum & Siegel, 1993; Frazier, Demaree, & Youngstrom, 2004). Variations of this test would eventually be standardized and commercially marketed for diagnosis of the disorder (Conners, 1995; Gordon, 1983; Greenberg & Waldman, 1992). Douglas remarked on the extreme degree of variability demonstrated during task performances by these children—a characteristic that would later be advanced as one of the defining features of the disorder. The McGill team (Freibergs, 1965; Freibergs & Douglas, 1969; Parry & Douglas, 1976) also found that hyperactive children could perform at normal or near-normal levels of sustained attention under conditions of continuous and immediate reinforcement, but that their performance deteriorated dramatically when partial reinforcement was introduced, particularly at schedules below 50% reinforcement. Campbell, Douglas, and Morgenstern (1971) further demonstrated substantial problems with impulse control and field dependence in the cognitive styles of hyperactive children. Like George Still 70 years earlier, Douglas commented on the probable association between deficits in attention/impulse control and deficiencies in moral development that were plaguing her subjects, particularly in their adolescent years. The research of the McGill team showed dramatic improvements in these attention deficiencies during stimulant medication treatment, as did the research at other laboratories at the time (Conners & Rothschild, 1968; Sprague, Barnes, & Werry, 1970).

Finally, of substantial significance were the observations of Douglas's colleague, Gabrielle Weiss, from her follow-up studies (see Weiss & Hechtman, 1986) that although the hyperactivity of these children often diminished by adolescence, their problems with poor sustained attention and impulsivity persisted. This persistence of the disabilities and the risk for greater academic and social maladjustment would be identified by other research teams from their own follow-up investigations (Mendelson, Johnson, & Stewart, 1971), and would be better substantiated by more rigorous studies in the next two decades (see Barkley, Fischer, Edelbrock, & Smallish, 1990; Barkley, Fischer, Smallish, & Fletcher, 2002; Brown & Borden, 1986; Gittelman, Mannuzza, Shenker, & Bonagura, 1985).

Douglas's Model of Attention Deficits

Douglas (1980a, 1980b, 1983; Douglas & Peters, 1979) later elaborated, refined, and further substantiated her model of hyperactivity. Her model culminated in the view that four major deficits could account for symptoms of ADHD: (1) the investment, organization, and maintenance of attention and effort; (2) the inhibition of impulsive responding; (3) the modulation of arousal levels to meet situational demands; and (4) an unusually strong inclination to seek immediate reinforcement. This perspective initiated or guided a substantial amount of research over the next 15 years, including my own early studies (Barkley, 1977, 1989b; Barkley & Ullman, 1975). It constituted a model as close to a scientific paradigm as the field of hyperactivity was likely to have in its history to that point. Yet, over the next 10 years results emerged that were somewhat at odds with this perspective. Scientists began to seriously question the adequacy of an attention model in accounting for the varied behavioral deficits seen in children with ADHD, as well as for the effects of stimulant medications on them (Barkley, 1981, 1984; Draeger, Prior, & Sanson, 1986; Haenlein & Caul, 1987; van der Meere & Sergeant, 1988a, 1988b). It also deserves mention that such a description of deficiencies constitutes a pattern and not a theory, given that it stipulates no conditional relations among its parts or how they orchestrate to create the problems seen in the disorder. That is, it makes no testable or falsifiable predictions apart from those contained in the pattern so described.

Douglas's paper and the subsequent research published by her team were so influential that they were probably the major reasons the disorder was renamed Attention Deficit Disorder (ADD) in 1980 with the publication of DSM-III (American Psychiatric Association, 1980). In this revised official taxonomy, deficits in sustained attention and impulse control were formally recognized as of greater significance in the diagnosis than hyperactivity. The shift to attention deficits rather than hyperactivity as the major difficulty of these children was useful, at least for a time, because of the growing evidence (1) that hyperactivity was not specific to this particular condition, but could be noted in other psychiatric disorders (anxiety, mania, autism, etc.); (2) that there was no clear delineation between "normal" and "abnormal" levels of activity; (3) that activity was in fact a multidimensional construct; and (4) that the symptoms of hyperactivity were quite situational in nature in many children (Rutter, 1989). But this approach only corrected the problem of definition for little over a decade before these same concerns also began to be raised about the construct of attention (multidimensional, situationally variable, etc.). Yet some research would show that at least deficits in vigilance or sustained attention could be used to discriminate this disorder from other psychiatric disorders (Werry, 1988).

Other Historical Developments

A number of other historical developments during this period deserve mention.

The Rise of Medication Therapy

One of these developments was the rapidly increasing use of stimulant medication with school-age hyperactive children. This use was no doubt spawned by the significant increase in research showing that stimulants often had dramatic effects on these children's hyperactive and inattentive behavior. A second development was the use of much more rigorous scientific methodology in drug studies. This was due in large measure to the early studies by C. Keith Conners (then working with Leon Eisenberg at Harvard University), and somewhat later to the research of Robert Sprague at the University of Illinois, Virginia Douglas at McGill University, and John Werry in New Zealand. This body of literature became voluminous (see Barkley, 1977; Ross & Ross, 1976), with more than 120 studies published through 1976 and more than twice this number by 1995 (Swanson, McBurnett, Christian, & Wigal, 1995), making this treatment approach the most well-studied therapy in child psychiatry.

Despite the proven efficacy of stimulant medication, public and professional misgivings about its increasingly widespread use with children emerged. For example, one news account (Maynard, 1970) reported that in Omaha, Nebraska, as many as 5–10% of the children in grade schools were receiving behavior-modifying drugs. This estimate of drug treatment would later be shown to be grossly exaggerated by as much as 10-fold, due to a misplaced decimal point in the story. And this would certainly not be the last instance of the mass media's penchant for hyperbole, sensation, and scandal in their accounts of stimulant medication treatments for ADHD—a penchant that seems only to have increased over subsequent years. Yet the public interest that was generated by the initial reports led to a congressional review of the use of psychotropic medications for school children. At this same time, the claim was being advanced that hyperactivity was a "myth" arising from intolerant teachers and parents and an inadequate educational system (Conrad, 1975; Schrag & Divoky, 1975).

Environment as Etiology

Almost simultaneous with this backlash against "drugging" school children for behavior problems came another significant development in this decade: a growing belief that hyperactivity was a result of environmental causes. It is not just coincidental that this development occurred at the same time that the United States was experiencing a popular interest in natural foods, health consciousness, the extension of life expectancy via environmental manipulations, psychoanalytic theory, and behaviorism. An extremely popular view was that allergic or toxic reactions to food additives, such as dyes, preservatives, and salicylates (Feingold, 1975), caused hyperactive behavior. It was claimed that more than half of all hyperactive children had developed their difficulties because of their diet. Effective treatment could be had if families of these children would buy or make foods that did not contain the offending substances. This view became so widespread that organized parent groups or "Feingold associations," composed mainly of parents advocating Feingold's diet, were established in almost every U.S. state, and legislation was introduced (although not passed) in California requiring that all school cafeteria foods be prepared without these substances. A sizable number of research investigations were undertaken (see Conners, 1980, for a review), the more rigorous of which found these substances to have little if any effect on children's behavior. A National Advisory Committee on Hyperkinesis and Food Additives (1980) was convened to review this literature and concluded more strongly than Conners that the available evidence clearly refuted Feingold's claims. Nevertheless, it would be more than 10

years before this notion receded in popularity, to be replaced by the equally unsupported hypothesis that refined sugar was more to blame for hyperactivity than were food additives (for reviews, see Milich, Wolraich, & Lindgren, 1986; Wolraich, Wilson, & White, 1995).

The emphasis on environmental causes, however, spread to possible sources other than diet. Block (1977) advanced the rather vague notion that technological development and more rapid cultural change would result in an increasing societal "tempo," causing growing excitation or environmental stimulation. This excitation or stimulation would interact with a predisposition in some children toward hyperactivity, making it manifest. It was felt that this theory explained the apparently increasing incidence of hyperactivity in developed cultures. Ross and Ross (1982) provided an excellent critique of the theory and concluded that there was insufficient evidence in support of it and some that would contradict it. Little evidence suggested that hyperactivity was increasing in its incidence, though its identification among children may well have been. Nor was there evidence that its prevalence varied as a function of societal development. Instead, Ross and Ross proposed that cultural effects on hyperactivity have more to do with whether important institutions of enculturation are consistent or inconsistent in the demands made and standards set for child behavior and development. These cultural views were said to determine the threshold for deviance that will be tolerated in children, as well as to exaggerate a predisposition to hyperactivity in some children. Consistent cultures will have fewer children diagnosed with hyperactivity, as they minimize individual differences among children and provide clear and consistent expectations and consequences for behavior that conforms to the expected norms. Inconsistent cultures, by contrast, will have more children diagnosed with hyperactivity, as they maximize or stress individual differences and provide ambiguous expectations and consequences to children regarding appropriate conduct. This intriguing hypothesis remains unstudied. However, on these grounds, an equally compelling case could be made for the opposite effects of cultural influences: In highly consistent, highly conforming cultures, hyperactive behavior may be considerably more obvious in children as they are unable to conform to these societal expectations, whereas inconsistent and low-conforming cultures may tolerate deviant behavior to a greater degree as part of the wider range of behavioral expression they encourage.

A different environmental view—that poor child rearing generally and poor child behavior management specifically lead to hyperactivity—was advanced by schools of psychology/psychiatry at diametrically opposite poles. Both psychoanalysts (Bettelheim, 1973; Harticollis, 1968) and behaviorists (Willis & Lovaas, 1977) promulgated this view, though for very different reasons. The psychoanalysts claimed that parents lacking tolerance for negative or hyperactive temperament in their infants would react with excessively negative, demanding parental responses giving rise to clinical levels of hyperactivity. The behaviorists stressed poor conditioning of children to stimulus control by commands and instructions that would give rise to noncompliant and hyperactive behavior. Both groups singled out mothers as especially etiologically important in this causal connection, and both could derive some support from studies that found negative mother–child interactions in the preschool years to be associated with the continuation of hyperactivity into the late childhood (Campbell, 1987) and adolescent (Barkley, Fischer, et al., 1990) years.

However, such correlational data cannot prove a cause. They do not prove that poor child rearing or negative parent–child interactions cause hyperactivity; they only show that such factors are associated with its persistence. It could just as easily be that the severity of hyperactivity elicits greater maternal negative reactions, and that this severity is related to persistence of the disorder over time. Supporting this interpretation are the studies of stimulant drug effects on the interactions of mothers and their hyperactive children, which show that mothers' negative and directive behavior is greatly reduced when stimulant medication is used to reduce the hyperactivity in their children (Barkley, 1989b; Barkley & Cunningham, 1979; Barkley, Karlsson, Pollard, & Murphy, 1985; Danforth, Barkley, & Stokes, 1991). Moreover, follow-up studies show that the degree of hyperactivity in childhood is predictive of its own persistence into later childhood and adolescence, apart from its association with maternal behavior (Barkley, Fischer, et al., 1990; Campbell & Ewing, 1990). And given the dramatic hereditary contribution to ADHD, it is also just as likely that the more

negative, impulsive, emotional, and inattentive behavior of mothers with their hyperactive children stems in part from the mothers' own ADHD—a factor that has never been taken into account in the analysis of such data or in interpreting findings in this area. Nevertheless, family context would still prove to be important in predicting the outcome of hyperactive children, even though the mechanism of its action was not yet specified (Weiss & Hechtman, 1986). Parent training in child behavior management, furthermore, would be increasingly recommended as an important therapy in its own right (Dubey & Kaufman, 1978; Pelham, 1977), despite a paucity of studies concerning its actual efficacy at the time (Barkley, 1989a).

The Passage of Public Law 94-142

Another highly significant development was the passage of Public Law 94-142 in 1975, mandating special educational services for physical, learning, and behavioral disabilities of children, in addition to those services already available for mental retardation (see Henker & Whalen, 1980, for a review of the legal precedents leading up to this law). Although many of its recommendations were foreshadowed by Section 504 of the Rehabilitation Act of 1973 (Public Law 93-112), it was the financial incentives for the states associated with the adoption of Public Law 94-142 that probably encouraged its immediate and widespread implementation by them all. Programs for learning disabilities, behavioral–emotional disturbance, language disorders, physical handicaps, and motor disabilities, among others, were now required to be provided to all eligible children in all public schools in the United States.

The full impact of these widely available educational treatment programs on hyperactive children has not yet been completely appreciated, for several reasons. First, hyperactivity, by itself, was overlooked in the initial criteria set forth for behavioral and learning disabilities warranting eligibility for these special classes. Children with such disabilities typically also had to have another condition, such as a learning disability, language delay, or emotional disorder, to receive exceptional educational services. The effects of special educational resources on the outcome of hyperactivity are difficult to assess, given this confounding of multiple disorders. It was only after the passage of IDEA in 1990 and a subsequent 1991 memorandum) that the U.S. Department of Education and its Office of Special Education chose to reinterpret these regulations, thereby allowing children with ADHD to receive special educational services for ADHD per se under the "Other Health Impaired" category of IDEA. And, second, the mandated services had been in existence for only a little more than a decade when the long-term outcome studies begun in the late 1970s began to be reported. Those studies (e.g., Barkley, Fischer, et al., 1990) suggested that over 35% of children with ADHD received some type of special educational placement. Although the availability of these services seems to have reduced the percentage of children with ADHD who were retained in grade for their academic problems, compared to earlier follow-up studies, the rates of school suspensions and expulsions did not decline appreciably from pre-1977 rates. A more careful analysis of the effects of Public Law 94-142, and especially of its more recent reauthorization as the IDEA, is in order before its efficacy for children with ADHD can be judged.

The Rise of Behavior Modification

This growing emphasis on educational intervention for children with behavioral and learning disorders was accompanied by a plethora of research on the use of behavior modification techniques in the management of disruptive classroom behavior, particularly as an alternative to stimulant medication (Allyon, Layman, & Kandel, 1975; O'Leary, Pelham, Rosenbaum, & Price, 1976). Supported in large part by their successful use for children with mental retardation, behavioral technologies were now being extended to a myriad of childhood disorders—not only as potential treatments of their symptoms, but also as theoretical statements of their origins. Although the studies demonstrated considerable efficacy of these techniques in the management of inattentive and hyperactive behavior, they were not found to achieve the same degree of behavioral improvement as the stimulants (Gittelman-Klein et al., 1976), and so did not replace them as a treatment of choice. Nevertheless, opinion was growing that the stimulant drugs should never be used as a sole intervention, but should be combined with parent training and behavioral interventions in the classroom to provide the most comprehensive management approach for the disorder.

Developments in Assessment

Another hallmark of this era was the widespread adoption of the parent and teacher rating scales developed by C. Keith Conners (1969) for the assessment of symptoms of hyperactivity, particularly during trials on stimulant medication. For at least 20 years, these simply constructed ratings of behavioral items would be the "gold standard" for rating children's hyperactivity for both research purposes and treatment with medication. The scales would also come to be used for monitoring treatment responses during clinical trials. Large-scale normative data were collected, particularly for the teacher scale, and epidemiological studies throughout the world relied on both scales for assessing the prevalence of hyperactivity in their populations. Their use moved the practice of diagnosis and the assessment of treatment effects from that of clinical impression alone to one in which at least some structured, semiobjective, and quantitative measure of behavioral deviance was employed. These scales would later be criticized for their confounding of hyperactivity with aggression. This confounding called into question whether the findings of research that relied on the scales were the result of oppositional, defiant, and hostile (aggressive) features of the population or of their hyperactivity (Ullmann, Sleator, & Sprague, 1984). Nevertheless, the widespread adoption of these rating scales in this era marks a historical turning point toward the use of quantitative assessment methods that can be empirically tested and can assist in determining developmental patterns and deviance from norms.

Also significant during this decade was the effort to study the social-ecological impact of hyperactive/inattentive behavior. This line of research set about evaluating the effects produced on family interactions by a child with hyperactivity. Originally initiated by Campbell (1973, 1975), this line of inquiry dominated my own research over the next decade (Barkley & Cunningham, 1979; Cunningham & Barkley, 1978, 1979; Danforth et al., 1991), particularly evaluations of the effects of stimulant medication on these social exchanges. These studies showed that children with hyperactivity were much less compliant and more oppositional during parent–child exchanges than children without it, and that their mothers were more directive, commanding, and negative than mothers of nonhyperactive children. These difficulties would increase substantially when the situation changed from free play to task-oriented demands. Studies also demonstrated that stimulant medication resulted in significant improvements in child compliance and decreases in maternal control and directiveness. Simultaneously, Humphries, Kinsbourne, and Swanson (1978) reported similar effects of stimulant medication, all of which suggested that much of parents' controlling and negative behavior toward hyperactive children was the result rather than the cause of the children's poor self-control and inattention. At the same time, Carol Whalen and Barbara Henker at the University of California–Irvine demonstrated similar interaction conflicts between hyperactive children and their teachers and peers, as well as similar effects of stimulant medication on these social interactions (Whalen & Henker, 1980; Whalen, Henker, & Dotemoto, 1980). This line of research would increase substantially in the next decade, and would be expanded by Charles Cunningham and others to include studies of peer interactions and the effects of stimulants on them (Cunningham, Siegel, & Offord, 1985).

A Focus on Psychophysiology

The decade of the 1970s was also noteworthy for a marked increase in the number of research studies on the psychophysiology of hyperactivity in children. Numerous studies were published measuring galvanic skin response, heart rate acceleration and deceleration, various parameters of the EEG, electropupillography, averaged evoked responses, and other aspects of electrophysiology. Many researchers were investigating the evidence for theories of over- or underarousal of the CNS in hyperactivity–theories that grew out of the speculations in the 1950s on cortical overstimulation and the ideas of both Wender and Douglas (see above) regarding abnormal arousal in the disorder. Most of these studies were seriously methodologically flawed, difficult to interpret, and often contradictory in their findings. Two influential reviews at the time (Hastings & Barkley, 1978; Rosenthal & Allen, 1978) were highly critical of most investigations, but concluded that if there was any consistency across findings, it might be that hyperactive children showed a sluggish or underreactive electrophysiological response to stimulation. These

reviews laid to rest the belief in an overstimulated cerebral cortex as the cause of the symptoms in hyperactivity, but did little to suggest a specific neurophysiological mechanism for the observed underreactivity. Further advances in the contributions of psychophysiology to understanding hyperactivity would await further refinements in instrumentation and in definition and diagnosis of the disorder, along with advances in computer-assisted analysis of electrophysiological measures.

An Emerging Interest in Adult MBD/Hyperactivity

Finally, the 1970s should be credited with the emergence of clinical and research interests in the existence of MBD or hyperactivity in adult clinical patients. Initial interest in adult MBD can be traced back to the latter part of the 1960s, seemingly arising as a result of two events. The first of these was the publication of several early follow-up studies demonstrating persistence of symptoms of hyperactivity/MBD into adulthood in many cases (Mendelson et al., 1971; Menkes, Rowe, & Menkes, 1967). The second was the publication by Harticollis (1968) of the results of neuropsychological and psychiatric assessments of 15 adolescent and young adult patients (ages 15–25) seen at the Menninger Clinic. The neuropsychological performance of these patients suggested evidence of moderate brain damage. Their behavioral profile suggested many of the symptoms that Still (1902) initially identified in the children he studied, particularly impulsiveness, overactivity, concreteness, mood lability, and proneness to aggressive behavior and depression. Some of the patients appeared to have demonstrated this behavior uniformly since childhood. Using psychoanalytic theory, Harticollis speculated that this condition arose from an early and possibly congenital defect in the ego apparatus, in interaction with busy, action-oriented, successful parents.

The following year, Quitkin and Klein (1969) reported on two behavioral syndromes in adults that might be related to MBD. The authors studied 105 patients at the Hillside Hospital in Glen Oaks, New York, for behavioral signs of "organicity" (brain damage); behavioral syndromes that might be considered neurological "soft signs" of CNS impairment; and any EEG findings, psychological testing results, or aspects of clinical presentation and history that might differentiate these patients from patients with other types of adult psychopathology. From the initial group of 105 patients, the authors selected those having a childhood history that suggested CNS damage, including early hyperactive and impulsive behavior. These subjects were further sorted into three groups based on current behavioral profiles: those having socially awkward and withdrawn behavior (*n* = 12), those having impulsive and destructive behavior (*n* = 19), and a "borderline" group that did not fit neatly into these other two groups (*n* = 11). The results indicated that nearly twice as many of the patients in these three "organic" groups as in the control group had EEG abnormalities and impairments on psychological testing indicating organicity. Furthermore, early history of hyperactive–impulsive–inattentive behavior was highly predictive of placement in the adult impulsive–destructive group, implying a persistent course of this behavioral pattern from childhood to adulthood. Of the 19 patients in the impulsive–destructive group, 17 had received clinical diagnoses of character disorders (primarily emotionally unstable types), as compared to only 5 in the socially awkward group (who received diagnoses of the schizoid and passive dependent types).

The results were interpreted as being in conflict with the beliefs widely held at the time that hyperactive–impulsive behavior tends to wane in adolescence. Instead, the authors argued that some of these children continued into young adulthood with this specific behavioral syndrome. Quitkin and Klein (1969) also took issue with Harticollis's psychoanalytic hypothesis that demanding and perfectionistic child rearing by parents was causal of or contributory to this syndrome, given that their impulsive–destructive patients did not uniformly experience such an upbringing. In keeping with Still's original belief that family environment could not account for this syndrome, these authors hypothesized "that such parents would intensify the difficulty, but are not necessary to the formation of the impulsive–destructive syndrome" (p. 140) and that the "illness shaping role of the psycho-social environment may have been over-emphasized by other authors" (p. 141). Treatment with a well-structured set of demands and educational procedures, as well as with phenothiazine medication, was thought to be indicated.

Later in this decade, Morrison and Minkoff (1975) similarly argued that explosive personality disorder or episodic dyscontrol syndrome in adulthood might well be the adult sequel to the hyperactivity syndrome in childhood. They also suggested that antidepressant medications might be useful in their management; this echoed a suggestion made earlier by Huessy (1974) in a letter to the editor of a journal that both antidepressants and stimulants might be the most useful medications for the treatment of adults with hyperkinesis or MBD. But the first truly scientific evaluation of the efficacy of stimulants for adults with MBD must be credited to Wood, Reimherr, Wender, and Johnson (1976). They used a double-blind, placebo-controlled method to assess response to methylphenidate in 11 of 15 adults with MBD, followed by an open trial of pemoline (another stimulant) and the antidepressants imipramine and amitriptyline. The authors found that 8 of the 11 tested on methylphenidate had a favorable response, whereas 10 of the 15 tested in the open trial showed a positive response to either the stimulants or the antidepressants. Others in the 1970s and into the 1980s would also make the case for the existence of an adult equivalent of childhood hyperkinesis or MBD and the efficacy of using stimulants and antidepressants for its management (Gomez, Janowsky, Zetin, Huey, & Clopton, 1981; Mann & Greenspan, 1976; Packer, 1978; Pontius, 1973; Rybak, 1977; Shelley & Riester, 1972). Yet it would not be until the 1990s that both the lay public and the professional field of adult psychiatry would begin to seriously recognize the adult equivalent of childhood ADHD on a more widespread basis and to recommend stimulant or antidepressant treatment in these cases (Spencer et al., 1995; Wender, 1995) and even then the view was not without its critics (Shaffer, 1994).

The work of Pontius (1973) in this decade is historically notable for her proposition that many cases of MBD in adults demonstrating hyperactive and impulsive behavior may arise from frontal lobe and caudate dysfunction. Such dysfunction would lead to "an inability to construct plans of action ahead of the act, to sketch out a goal of action, to keep it in mind for some time (as an overriding idea) and to follow it through in actions under the constructive guidance of such planning" (p. 286). Moreover, if adult MBD arises from dysfunction in this frontal–caudate network, it should also be associated with an inability "to re-program an ongoing activity and to shift within *principles* of action whenever necessary" (p. 286, emphasis in original). Pontius went on to show that indeed adults with MBD demonstrated deficits indicative of dysfunction in this brain network. Such observations would prove quite prophetic over 20 years later, when research demonstrated reduced size in the prefrontal–caudate network in children with ADHD (Castellanos et al., 1996; Filipek et al., 1997), and when theories of ADHD argued that the neuropsychological deficits associated with it involved the executive functions, such as planning, the control of behavior by mentally represented information, rule-governed behavior, and response fluency and flexibility, among others (Barkley, 1997a, 1997b).

The Prevailing View by 1979

The 1970s closed with the prevailing view that hyperactivity was not the only or most important behavioral deficit seen in hyperactive children, but that poor attention span and impulse control were equally (if not more) important in explaining their problems. Brain damage was relegated to an extremely minor role as a cause of the disorder, at least in the realm of childhood hyperactivity/MBD; however, other brain mechanisms, such as underarousal or underreactivity, brain neurotransmitter deficiencies (Wender, 1971), or neurological immaturity (Kinsbourne, 1977), were viewed as promising. Greater speculation about potential environmental causes or irritants emerged, particularly diet and child rearing. Thus the most frequently recommended therapies for hyperactivity were not only stimulant medication, but widely available special education programs, classroom behavior modification, dietary management, and parent training in child management skills. A greater appreciation for the effects of hyperactive children on their immediate social ecology, and for the impact of stimulant medication in altering these social conflicts, was beginning to emerge.

However, the sizable discrepancy between North American and European views of the disorder remained: North American professionals continued to recognize the disorder as more common, in need of medication, and more likely to be an attention deficit, while those in Europe continued to view it as uncommon, defined by severe overactivity, and associated with brain damage. Those children in North America being diagnosed as having hyperactivity or attention deficits would be likely to be diagnosed as having CD in Europe, where treatment would be psychotherapy, family therapy, and parent training in child management. Medication would be disparaged and little used. Nevertheless, the view that attention deficits were as important in the disorder as hyperactivity was beginning to make its way into European taxonomies (e.g., the *International Classification of Diseases*, ninth revision [ICD-9]; World Health Organization, 1978). Finally, some recognition occurred in the 1970s that there were adult equivalents of childhood hyperactivity or MBD, that they might be indicative of frontal–caudate dysfunction, and that these cases responded to the same medication treatments that had earlier been suggested for childhood ADHD (the stimulants and antidepressants).

THE PERIOD 1980 TO 1989

The exponential increase in research on hyperactivity characteristic of the 1970s continued unabated into the 1980s, making hyperactivity the most well-studied childhood psychiatric disorder in existence. More books were written, conferences convened, and scientific papers presented during this decade than in any previous historical period. This decade would become known for its emphasis on attempts to develop more specific diagnostic criteria; the differential conceptualization and diagnosis of hyperactivity versus other psychiatric disorders; and, later in the decade, critical attacks on the notion that inability to sustain attention was the core behavioral deficit in ADHD.

The Creation of an ADD Syndrome

Marking the beginning of this decade was the publication of DSM-III (American Psychiatric Association, 1980) and its radical reconceptualization (from that in DSM-II) of the Hyperkinetic Reaction of Childhood diagnosis to that of ADD (with or without Hyperactivity). The criteria for ADD are set forth in Table 1.1. The new diagnostic criteria were noteworthy not only for their greater emphasis on inattention and impulsivity as defining features of the disorder, but also for their creation of much more specific symptom lists, an explicit numerical

TABLE 1.1. DSM-III Diagnostic Criteria for Attention Deficit Disorder with and without Hyperactivity

The child displays, for his or her mental and chronological age, signs of developmentally inappropriate inattention, impulsivity, and hyperactivity. The signs must be reported by adults in the child's environment, such as parents and teachers. Because the symptoms are typically variable, they may not be observed directly by the clinician. When the reports of teachers and parents conflict, primary consideration should be given to the teacher reports because of greater familiarity with age-appropriate norms. Symptoms typically worsen in situations that require self-application, as in the classroom. Signs of the disorder may be absent when the child is in a new or a one-to-one situation.

The number of symptoms specified is for children between the ages of eight and ten, the peak age for referral. In younger children, more severe forms of the symptoms and a greater number of symptoms are usually present. The opposite is true of older children.

A. **Inattention.** At least three of the following:

    (1) often fails to finish things he or she starts
    (2) often doesn't seem to listen
    (3) easily distracted
    (4) has difficulty concentrating on schoolwork or other tasks requiring sustained attention
    (5) has difficulty sticking to a play activity

B. **Impulsivity.** At least three of the following:

    (1) often acts before thinking
    (2) shifts excessively from one activity to another
    (3) has difficulty organizing work (this not being due to cognitive impairment).
    (4) needs a lot of supervision
    (5) frequently calls out in class
    (6) has difficulty awaiting turn in games or group situations

C. **Hyperactivity.** At least two of the following:

    (1) runs about or climbs on things excessively
    (2) has difficulty sitting still or fidgets excessively
    (3) has difficulty staying seated
    (4) moves about excessively during sleep
    (5) is always "on the go" or acts as if "driven by a motor"

D. Onset before the age of seven.

E. Duration of at least six months.

F. Not due to Schizophrenia, Affective Disorder, or Severe or Profound Mental Retardation.

Note. The criteria as presented above are for Attention Deficit Disorder with Hyperactivity. All of the features of Attention Deficit Disorder without Hyperactivity are the same except for the absence of hyperactivity (Criterion C). From American Psychiatric Association (1980). Copyright 1980 by the American Psychiatric Association. Reprinted by permission.

cutoff score for symptoms, specific guidelines for age of onset and duration of symptoms, and the requirement of exclusion of other childhood psychiatric conditions as better explanations of the presenting symptoms. This was also a radical departure from the ICD-9 criteria set forth by the World Health Organization (1978) in its own taxonomy of child psychiatric disorders, which continued to emphasize pervasive hyperactivity as a hallmark of this disorder.

Even more controversial was the creation of subtypes of ADD, based on the presence or absence of hyperactivity (+ H/– H), in the DSM-III criteria. Little, if any, empirical research on this issue existed at the time these subtypes were formulated. Their creation in the official nomenclature of psychiatric disorders would, by the end of the 1980s, initiate numerous research studies into their existence, validity, and utility, along with a search for other potentially useful ways of subtyping ADD (situational pervasiveness, presence of aggression, stimulant drug response, etc.). Although the findings were at times conflicting, the trend in these studies was that children with ADD – H differed from those with ADD + H in some important domains of current adjustment. Those with ADD – H were characterized as more daydreamy, hypoactive, lethargic, and disabled in academic achievement, but as substantially less aggressive and less rejected by their peers (Barkley, Grodzinsky, & DuPaul, 1992; Carlson, 1986; Goodyear & Hynd, 1992; Lahey & Carlson, 1992). Unfortunately, this research came too late to be considered in the subsequent revision of DSM-III.

In that revision (DSM-III-R; American Psychiatric Association, 1987), the criteria for which are shown in Table 1.2, only the diagnostic criteria for ADD + H (now renamed ADHD; see "ADD Becomes ADHD," below) were stipulated. ADD – H was no longer officially recognized as a subtype of ADD, but was relegated to a minimally defined category, Undifferentiated ADD. This reorganization was associated with an admonition that far more research on the utility of this subtyping approach was necessary before its place in this taxonomy could be identified. Despite the controversy that arose over the demotion of ADD – H in this fashion, it was actually a prudent gesture on the part of the committee asked to formulate these criteria. At the time, the committee (on which I served) had little available research to guide its deliberations in

---

TABLE 1.2. DSM-III-R Diagnostic Criteria for Attention-Deficit Hyperactivity Disorder

A. A disturbance of at least six months during which at least eight of the following are present:
  (1) often fidgets with hands or feet or squirms in seat (in adolescents, may be limited to subjective feelings of restlessness)
  (2) has difficulty remaining seated when required to do so
  (3) is easily distracted by extraneous stimuli
  (4) has difficulty awaiting turn in games or group situations
  (5) often blurts out answers to questions before they have been completed
  (6) has difficulty following through on instructions from others (not due to oppositional behavior or failure of comprehension), e.g., fails to finish chores
  (7) has difficulty sustaining attention in tasks or play activities
  (8) often shifts from one uncompleted activity to another
  (9) has difficulty playing quietly
  (10) often talks excessively
  (11) often interrupts or intrudes on others, e.g., butts into other children's games
  (12) often does not seem to listen to what is being said to him or her
  (13) often loses things necessary for tasks or activities at school or at home (e.g., toys, pencils, books, assignments)
  (14) often engages in physically dangerous activities without considering possible consequences (not for the purpose of thrillseeking), e.g., runs into street without looking

Note: The above items are listed in descending order of discriminating power based on the data from a national field trial of the DSM-III-R criteria for Disruptive Behavior Disorders.

B. Onset before the age of seven.

C. Does not meet the criteria for a Pervasive Developmental Disorder.

Criteria for severity of Attention-Deficit Hyperactivity Disorder:

Mild: Few if any, symptoms in excess of those required to make the diagnosis **and** only minimal or no impairment in school and social functioning.

Moderate: Symptoms or functional impairment intermediate between "mild" and "severe."

Severe: Many symptoms in excess of those required to make the diagnosis **and** pervasive impairment in functioning at home and school and with peers.

Note. From American Psychiatric Association (1987). Copyright 1987 by the American Psychiatric Association. Reprinted by permission.

this matter. There was simply no indication whether ADD – H had a similar or qualitatively different type of attention deficit, which would make it a separate childhood psychiatric disorder in its own right. Rather than continue merely to conjecture about the nature of the subtype and how it should be diagnosed, the committee essentially placed the concept in abeyance until more research was available to its successor committee to guide its definition. Notable in the construction of DSM-III-R was its emphasis on the empirical validation of its diagnostic criteria through a field trial, which guided the selection of items for the symptom list and the recommended cutoff score on that list (Spitzer, Davies, & Barkley, 1990).

The Development of Research Diagnostic Criteria

At the same time that the DSM-III criteria for ADD + H and ADD – H were gaining in recognition, others attempted to specify research diagnostic criteria (Barkley, 1982; Loney, 1983). My own efforts in this endeavor were motivated by the rather idiosyncratic and highly variable approach to diagnosis being used in clinical practice up to that time, the vague or often unspecified criteria used in published research studies, and the lack of specificity in current theoretical writings on the disorder up to 1980. There was also the more pragmatic consideration that, as a young scientist attempting to select hyperactive children for research studies, I had no operational or consensus-based criteria available for doing so. Therefore, I set forth a more operational definition of hyperactivity, or ADD + H. This definition not only required the usual parent and/or teacher complaints of inattention, impulsivity, and overactivity, but also stipulated that these symptoms had to (1) be deviant for the child's mental age, as measured by well-standardized child behavior rating scales; (2) be relatively pervasive within the jurisdiction of the major caregivers in the child's life (parent/home and teacher/school); (3) have developed by 6 years of age; and (4) have lasted at least 12 months (Barkley, 1982).

Concurrently, Loney (1983) and her colleagues had been engaged in a series of historically important studies that would differentiate the symptoms of hyperactivity or ADD + H from those of aggression or conduct problems (Loney, Langhorne, & Paternite, 1978; Loney & Milich, 1982). Following an empirical/statistical approach to developing research diagnostic criteria, Loney demonstrated that a relatively short list of symptoms of hyperactivity could be empirically separated from a similarly short list of aggression symptoms. Empirically derived cutoff scores on these symptom ratings by teachers could create these two semi-independent constructs. These constructs would prove highly useful in accounting for much of the heterogeneity and disagreement across studies. Among other things, it would become well established that many of the negative outcomes of hyperactivity in adolescence and young adulthood were actually due to the presence and degree of aggression coexisting with the hyperactivity. Purely hyperactive children would be shown to display substantial cognitive problems with attention and overactivity, whereas purely aggressive children would not. Previous findings of greater family psychopathology in hyperactive children would also be shown to be primarily a function of the degree of coexisting aggression or CD in the children (August & Stewart, 1983; Lahey et al., 1988). Furthermore, hyperactivity would be found to be associated with signs of developmental and neurological delay or immaturity, whereas aggression was more likely to be associated with environmental disadvantage and family dysfunction (Hinshaw, 1987; Milich & Loney, 1979; Paternite & Loney, 1980; Rutter, 1989; Werry, 1988; Weiss & Hechtman, 1986). The need for future studies to clearly specify the makeup of their samples along these two dimensions was now obvious. And the raging debate as to whether hyperactivity was separate from or merely synonymous with conduct problems would be settled by the important research discovery of the semi-independence of these two behavioral dimensions and their differing correlates (Ross & Ross, 1982). These findings would also lead to the demise of the commonplace use of the Conners 10-item Hyperactivity Index to select children as hyperactive. It would now be shown that many of these items actually assessed aggression rather than hyperactivity, resulting in samples of children with mixed disorders (Ullmann et al., 1984).

The laudable drive toward greater clarity, specificity, and operational defining of diagnostic criteria would continue throughout this decade. Pressure would now be exerted from experts within the field (Quay, 1988a; Rutter, 1983, 1989; Werry, 1988) to demonstrate that the symptoms of ADHD could distinguish it from other childhood psychiatric disorders—a crucial test for the validity of a diagnostic entity—rather than continuing simply to demonstrate differences from nondisordered populations. The challenge would not be easily met. Eric Taylor (1986) and colleagues in Great Britain made notable advances in further refining the criteria and their measurement along more empirical lines. Taylor's (1989) statistical approach to studying clusters of behavioral disorders resulted in the recommendation that a syndrome of hyperactivity could be valid and distinctive from other disorders, particularly conduct problems. This distinction required that the symptoms of hyperactivity and inattention be excessive and handicapping to the children; occur in two of three broadly defined settings (e.g., home, school, and clinic); be objectively measured, rather than subjectively rated by parents and teachers; develop before age 6; last at least 6 months; and exclude children with autism, psychosis, anxiety, or affective/mood disorders (depression, mania, etc.).

Efforts to develop research diagnostic criteria for ADHD eventually led to an international symposium on the subject (Sergeant, 1988) and a general consensus that subjects selected for research on ADHD should at least meet the following criteria: (1) reports of problems with activity and attention by adults in at least two independent settings (home, school, clinic); (2) endorsement of at least three of four difficulties with activity and three of four with attention; (3) onset before 7 years of age; (4) duration of 2 years; (5) significantly elevated scores on parent/teacher ratings of these ADHD symptoms; and (6) exclusion of autism and psychosis. These proposed criteria were quite similar to others developed earlier in the decade (Barkley, 1982), but provided for greater specificity of symptoms of overactivity and inattention and a longer duration of symptoms.

Subtyping of ADD

Also important in this era was the attempt to identify useful approaches to subtyping other than those just based on the degree of hyperactivity (+ H/– H) or aggression associated with ADD. A significant though underappreciated line of research by Roscoe Dykman and Peggy Ackerman at the University of Arkansas distinguished between ADD with and ADD without learning disabilities, particularly reading impairments. Their research (Ackerman,

Dykman, & Oglesby, 1983; Dykman, Ackerman, & Holcomb, 1985) and that of others (McGee, Williams, Moffit, & Anderson, 1989) showed that some of the cognitive deficits (verbal memory, intelligence, etc.) formerly attributed to ADHD were actually more a function of the presence and degree of language/reading difficulties than of ADHD. And, although some studies showed that ADHD with reading disabilities is not a distinct subtype of ADHD (Halperin, Gittelman, Klein, & Rudel, 1984), the differential contributions of reading disorders to the cognitive test performance of children with ADHD required that subsequent researchers carefully select subjects with pure ADHD not associated with reading disability. If they did not, then they at least should identify the degree to which reading disorders exist in the sample and partial out the effects of these disorders on the cognitive test results.

Others in this era attempted to distinguish between "pervasive" and "situational" hyperactivity; the former was determined by the presence of hyperactivity at home and school, and the latter referred to hyperactivity in only one of these settings (Schachar, Rutter, & Smith, 1981). It would be shown that children with pervasive hyperactivity were likely to have more severe behavioral symptoms, greater aggression and peer relationship problems, and poor academic achievement. The DSM-III-R (American Psychiatric Association, 1987) incorporated this concept into an index of severity of ADHD (see the last portion of Table 1.2). British scientists even viewed pervasiveness as an essential criterion for the diagnosis of a distinct syndrome of hyperactivity (as noted earlier). However, research appearing at the end of the decade (Costello, Loeber, & Stouthamer-Loeber, 1991) demonstrated that such group differences were more likely to be the results of differences in the source of the information used to classify the children (parents vs. teachers) than of actual behavioral differences between the situational and pervasive subgroups. This did not mean that symptom pervasiveness might not be a useful means of subtyping or diagnosing ADHD, but that more objective means of establishing it were needed than just comparing parent and teacher ratings on a questionnaire.

A different and relatively understudied approach to subtyping was created by the presence or absence of significant anxiety or affective disturbance. Several studies demonstrated that children with both ADHD and significant problems with anxiety or affective disturbance were likely to show poor or adverse responses to stimulant medication (Taylor, 1983; Voelker, Lachar, & Gdowski, 1983) and would perhaps respond better to antidepressant medications (Pliszka, 1987). The utility of this latter subtyping approach would be investigated and supported further in the next decade (DuPaul, Barkley, & McMurray, 1994; Tannock, 2000).

ADD Becomes ADHD

Later in the 1980s, in an effort to further improve the criteria for defining this disorder, the DSM was revised (American Psychiatric Association, 1987) as noted above, resulting in the renaming of the disorder to ADHD. These revised diagnostic criteria are shown in Table 1.2. The revisions were significant in several respects. First, a single item list of symptoms and a single cutoff score replaced the three separate lists (inattention, impulsivity, and hyperactivity) and cutoff score in DSM-III. Second, the item list was now based more on empirically derived dimensions of child behavior from behavior rating scales, and the items and cutoff score underwent a large field trial to determine their sensitivity, specificity, and power to distinguish ADHD from other psychiatric disorders and from the absence of disorder (Spitzer et al., 1990). Third, the need was stressed that one had to establish the symptoms as developmentally inappropriate for the child's mental age. Fourth, the coexistence of mood disorders with ADHD no longer excluded the diagnosis of ADHD. And, more controversially, the subtype of ADD – H was removed as a subtype and relegated to a vaguely defined category, Undifferentiated ADD, which was in need of greater research on its merits. ADHD was now classified with two other behavioral disorders (ODD and CD) in a supraordinate family or category known as the disruptive behavior disorders, in view of their substantial overlap or comorbidity in clinic-referred populations of children.

ADHD as a Motivation Deficit Disorder

One of the more interesting conceptual developments in this decade only began to emerge in its latter half. This was the nascent and almost heretical view that ADHD was not actually a disorder of attention. Doubt about the central importance of attention to the disorder crept in late in the 1970s, as some researchers more fully plumbed the depths of the attention construct with objective measures, while others took note of the striking situational variability of the symptoms (Douglas & Peters, 1979; Rosenthal & Allen, 1978; Routh, 1978; Sroufe, 1975). As more rigorous and technical studies of attention in children with ADHD appeared in the 1980s, an increasing number failed to find evidence of problems with attention under some experimental conditions while observing them under others (see Douglas, 1983, 1988, for reviews; Barkley, 1984; Draeger et al., 1986; Sergeant, 1988; Sergeant & van der Meere, 1989; van der Meere & Sergeant, 1988a, 1988b). Moreover, if attention was conceptualized as involving the perception, filtering, and processing of information, no substantial evidence could be found in these studies for any such deficits. These findings, coupled with the realization that both instructional and motivational factors in an experiment played a strong role in determining the presence and degree of ADHD symptoms, led some investigators to hypothesize that deficits in motivation might be a better model for explaining the symptoms seen in ADHD (Glow & Glow, 1979; Rosenthal & Allen, 1978; Sroufe, 1975). Following this line of reasoning, others pursued a behavioral or functional analysis of these symptoms, resulting in hypothesized deficits in the stimulus control over behavior, particularly by rules and instructions. I argued that such deficits arose from neurological factors (Barkley, 1988a), whereas others argued that they arose from poor training of the child by parents (Willis & Lovaas, 1977).

I initially raised the possibility that rule-governed behavior might account for many of the deficits in ADHD, but later amended this view to include the strong probability that response to behavioral consequences might also be impaired and could conceivably account for the problems with following rules (Barkley, 1981, 1984, 1990). Others independently advanced the notion that a deficit in responding to behavioral consequences, not attention, might be the difficulty in ADHD (Benninger, 1989; Haenlein & Caul, 1987; Quay, 1988b; Sagvolden, Wultz, Moser, Moser, & Morkrid, 1989; Sergeant, 1988; van der Meere & Sergeant, 1988b). That is, ADHD might arise out of an insensitivity to consequences (reinforcement, punishment, or both). This insensitivity was viewed as being neurological in origin. Yet this idea was not new, having been advanced some 10–20 years earlier by investigators in Australia (Glow & Glow, 1979), by those studying children with conduct problems (see Patterson, 1982, for a review), and by Wender (1971) in his classic text on MBD (see above). What was original in these more recent ideas was a greater specificity of their hypotheses and increasing evidence supporting them. Others continued to argue against the merits of a Skinnerian or functional analysis of the deficits in ADHD (Douglas, 1989), and for the continued explanatory value of cognitive models of attention in accounting for the deficits in ADHD.

The appeal of the motivational model came from several different sources: (1) its greater explanatory value in accounting for the more recent research findings on situational variability in attention in ADHD; (2) its consistency with neuroanatomical studies suggesting decreased activation of brain reward centers and their cortical–limbic regulating circuits (Lou et al., 1984, 1989); (3) its consistency with studies of the functions of dopamine pathways in regulating locomotor behavior and incentive or operant learning (Benninger, 1989); and (4) its greater prescriptive power in suggesting potential treatments for the ADHD symptoms. Whether or not ADHD would be labeled a motivational deficit, there was little doubt that these new theories based on the construct of motivation required altering the way in which this disorder was to be conceptualized. From here on, any attempts at theory construction would need to incorporate some components and processes dealing with motivation or effort.

Other Historical Developments of the Era

The Increasing Importance of Social Ecology

The 1980s also witnessed considerably greater research into the social-ecological impact of ADHD symptoms on the children, their parents (Barkley, 1989b; Barkley, Karlsson, & Pollard, 1985; Mash & Johnston, 1982), teachers (Whalen et al., 1980; Whalen, Henker, & Dotemoto, 1981), siblings (Mash & Johnston, 1983), and peers (Cunningham et al., 1985; Henker & Whalen, 1980). These investigations further explored the effects of stimulant medications on these social systems; they buttressed

the conclusion that children with ADHD elicit significant negative, controlling, and hostile or rejecting interactions from others, which can be greatly reduced by stimulant medication. From these studies emerged the view that the disabilities associated with ADHD do not rest solely in a child, but in the interface between the child's capabilities and the environmental demands made within the social-ecological context in which that child must perform (Whalen & Henker, 1980). Changing the attitudes, behaviors, and expectations of caregivers, as well as the demands they make on children with ADHD in their care, should result in changes in the degree to which such children are disabled by their behavioral deficits.

Theoretical Advances

During this decade, Herbert Quay adopted Jeffrey Gray's neuropsychological model of anxiety (Gray, 1982, 1987, 1994) to explain the origin of the poor inhibition evident in ADHD (Quay, 1988a, 1988b, 1997). Gray identified both a behavioral inhibition system (BIS) and a behavioral activation system (BAS) as being critical to understanding emotion. He also stipulated mechanisms for basic nonspecific arousal and for the appraisal of incoming information that must be critical elements of any attempt to model the emotional functions of the brain. According to this theory, signals of reward serve to increase activity in the BAS, thus giving rise to approach behavior and the maintenance of such behavior. Active avoidance and escape from aversive consequences (negative reinforcement) likewise activate this system. Signals of impending punishment (particularly conditioned punishment) as well as frustrative nonreward (an absence of previously predictable reward) increase activity in the BIS. Another system is the fight–flight system, which reacts to unconditioned punitive stimuli.

Quay's use of this model for ADHD stated that the impulsiveness characterizing the disorder could arise from diminished activity in the brain's BIS. This model predicted that those with ADHD should prove less sensitive to such signals, particularly in passive avoidance paradigms (Quay, 1988a). The theory also specifies predictions that can be used to test and even falsify the model as it applies to ADHD. For instance, Quay (1988a, 1988b) predicted that there should be greater resistance to extinction following periods of continuous reinforcement in those with ADHD, but less resistance when training conditions involve partial reward. They should also demonstrate a decreased ability to inhibit behavior in passive avoidance paradigms when avoidance of the punishment is achieved through the inhibition of responding. And those with ADHD should also demonstrate diminished inhibition to signals of pain and novelty, as well as to conditioned signals of punishment. Finally, Quay predicted increased rates of responding by those with ADHD under fixed-interval or fixed-ratio schedules of consequences. Some of these predictions were supported by subsequent research; others either remained to be investigated more fully and rigorously, or have not been completely supported by the available evidence (see Milich, Hartung, Martin, & Haigler, 1994; Quay, 1997). Nevertheless, the theory remains a viable one for explaining the origin of the inhibitory deficits in ADHD and continues to deserve further research.

Further Developments in Nature, Etiology, and Course

Another noteworthy development in this decade was the greater sophistication of research designs attempting to explore the unique features of ADHD relative to other psychiatric conditions, rather than just in comparison to the absence of disorder. As Rutter (1983, 1989) noted repeatedly, the true test of the validity of a syndrome of ADHD is the ability to differentiate its features from other psychiatric disorders of children, such as mood or anxiety disorders, learning disorders, and particularly CD. Those studies that undertook such comparisons indicated that situational hyperactivity was not consistent in discriminating among psychiatric populations, but that difficulties with attention and pervasive (home and school) hyperactivity were more reliable in doing so and were often associated with patterns of neuropsychological immaturity (Firestone & Martin, 1979; Gittelman, 1988; McGee, Williams, & Silva, 1984a, 1984b; Rutter, 1989; Taylor, 1988; Werry, 1988).

The emerging interest in comparing children with ADD + H to those with ADD − H furthered this line of inquiry by demonstrating relatively unique features of each group in contrast to each other (see Chapter 3) and to groups of children with learning disabilities and no disability (Barkley, DuPaul, & McMurray, 1990, 1991). Further strengthening the position of ADHD as a psychiatric syndrome was evidence from family aggregation studies that relatives of children with ADHD had a different pattern of psychiatric disturbance from those of children with CD or mixed ADHD and CD (Biederman, Munir, & Knee, 1987; Lahey et al., 1988). Children with pure ADHD were more likely to have relatives with ADHD, academic achievement problems, and dysthymia, whereas those children with CD had a greater prevalence of relatives with CD, antisocial behavior, substance abuse, depression, and marital dysfunction. This finding led to speculation that ADHD had a different etiology from CD. The former was said to arise out of a biologically based disorder of temperament or a neuropsychological delay; the latter from inconsistent, coercive, and dysfunctional child rearing and management, which was frequently associated with parental psychiatric impairment (Hinshaw, 1987; Loeber, 1990; Patterson, 1982, 1986).

Equally elegant research was done on potential etiologies of ADHD. Several studies on cerebral blood flow revealed patterns of underactivity in the prefrontal areas of the CNS and their rich connections to the limbic system via the striatum (Lou et al., 1984, 1989). Other studies (Hunt, Cohen, Anderson, & Minderaa, 1988; Rapoport & Zametkin, 1988; Shaywitz, Shaywitz, Cohen, & Young, 1983; Shekim, Glaser, Horwitz, Javaid, & Dylund, 1988; Zametkin & Rapoport, 1986) on brain neurotransmitters provided further evidence that deficiencies in dopamine, norepinephrine, or both may be involved in explaining these patterns of brain underactivity—patterns arising in precisely those brain areas in which dopamine and norepinephrine are most involved. Drawing these lines of evidence together even further was the fact that these brain areas are critically involved in response inhibition, motivational learning, and response to reinforcement. More rigorous studies on the hereditary transmission of ADHD were published (Goodman & Stevenson, 1989), indicating a strong heritability for ADHD symptoms.

Follow-up studies appearing in this decade were also more methodologically sophisticated, and hence more revealing not only of widespread maladjustment in children with ADHD as they reached adolescence and adulthood, but of potential mechanisms involved in the differential courses shown within this population (Barkley, Fischer, et al., 1990; Barkley, Fischer, Edelbrock, & Smallish, 1991; Fischer, Barkley, Edelbrock, & Smallish, 1990; Gittelman et al., 1985; Lambert, 1988; Weiss & Hechtman, 1993). These findings are discussed in Chapter 4. Again, neuropsychological delays, the presence and pervasiveness of early aggression, and mother–child conflict were associated with a different, and more negative, outcome in later childhood and adolescence than was ADHD alone (Campbell, 1987; Paternite & Loney, 1980).

There was also a movement during this decade away from the strict reliance on clinic-referred samples of children with ADHD to the use of community-derived samples. This change was prompted by the widely acknowledged bias that occurs among clinic-referred samples of children with ADHD as a result of the process of referral itself. It is well known that children who are referred are often more (though not always the most) impaired, have more numerous comorbid conditions, are likely to have associated family difficulties, and are skewed toward those socioeconomic classes that value the utilization of mental health care resources. Such biases can create findings that are not representative of the nature of the disorder in its natural state. For instance, it has been shown that the ratio of boys to girls within clinic-referred samples of children with ADHD may range from 5:1 to 9:1, and that girls with ADHD within these samples are as likely to be aggressive or oppositional as boys (see Chapter 2). By contrast, in samples of children with ADHD derived from community- or school-based samples, the ratio of boys to girls is only 2.5:1, and girls with ADHD are considerably less likely to be aggressive than boys. For these and other reasons, a greater emphasis on studying epidemiological samples of children and the rates and nature of ADHD within them (Offord et al., 1987) arose toward the latter half of the 1980s.

Developments in Assessment

The 1980s also witnessed some advances in the tools of assessment, in addition to those for treatment. The Child Behavior Checklist (CBCL; Achenbach & Edelbrock, 1983, 1986) emerged as a more comprehensive, more rigorously developed, and better-normed alternative to the Conners rating scales (Barkley, 1988a). It

would become widely adopted in research on child psychopathology in general, not just in ADHD, by the end of this decade. Other rating scales more specific to ADHD were also developed, such as the ADD-H Comprehensive Teacher Rating Scale (ACTeRS; Ullmann et al., 1984), the Home and School Situations Questionnaires (Barkley & Edelbrock, 1987; DuPaul & Barkley, 1992), the Child Attention Profile (see Barkley, 1988a), and the ADHD Rating Scale (DuPaul, 1991).

Gordon (1983) developed, normed, and commercially marketed a small, portable, computerized device that administered two tests believed to be sensitive to the deficits in ADHD. One was a CPT measuring vigilance and impulsivity, and the other was a direct reinforcement of low rates (DRL) test assessing impulse control. This device became the first commercially available objective means of assessment for children with ADHD. Although the DRL test showed some promise in early research (Gordon, 1979), it was subsequently shown to be insensitive to stimulant medication effects (Barkley, Fischer, Newby, & Breen, 1988) and was eventually deemphasized as useful in the diagnosis in ADHD. The CPT, by contrast, showed satisfactory discrimination of children with ADHD from nondisabled groups and was sensitive to medication effects (Barkley et al., 1988; Gordon & Mettelman, 1988). Although cautionary statements would be made that more research evidence was needed to evaluate the utility of the instrument (Milich, Pelham, & Hinshaw, 1985), and that its false-negative rate (misses of children with legitimate ADHD) might be greater than that desired in a diagnostic tool, the device and others like it (Conners, 1995; Greenberg & Waldman, 1992) found a wide clinical following by the next decade.

Greater emphasis was also given to developing direct behavioral observation measures of ADHD symptoms that could be taken in the classroom or clinic, and that would be more objective and useful adjuncts to the parent and teacher rating scales in the diagnostic process. Abikoff, Gittelman-Klein, and Klein (1977) and O'Leary (1981) developed classroom observation codes with some promise for discriminating children with ADHD from children with other or no disabilities (Gittelman, 1988). Roberts (1979), drawing on the earlier work of Routh and Schroeder (1976) and Kalverboer (1988), refined a laboratory playroom observation procedure that would be found to discriminate children with ADHD not only from non-disabled children, but also from children with aggression or mixed aggression and ADHD. This coding system had excellent 2-year stability coefficients. Somewhat later I streamlined the system (Barkley, 1988c) for more convenient clinical or classroom use and found it to be sensitive to stimulant medication effects (Barkley et al., 1988), to differentiate between children with ADD + H and ADD − H (Barkley, DuPaul, & McMurray, 1991), and to correlate well with parent and teacher ratings of ADHD symptoms (Barkley, 1991). Nevertheless, problems with developing normative data and the practical implementation of such a procedure in busy clinic practices remained hindrances to its widespread adoption.

Developments in Therapy

Developments also continued in the realm of treatments for ADHD. Comparisons of single versus combined treatments were more common during the decade (Barkley, 1989c), as was the use of more sophisticated experimental designs (Hinshaw, Henker, & Whalen, 1984; Pelham, Schnedler, Bologna, & Contreras, 1980) and mixed interventions (Satterfield, Satterfield, & Cantwell, 1981). Several of these developments in treatment require historical mention. The first was the emergence of a new approach to the treatment of ADHD: cognitive-behavioral therapy, or CBT (Camp, 1980; Douglas, 1980a; Kendall & Braswell, 1985; Meichenbaum, 1988). Founded on the work of Russian neuropsychologists (Vygotsky and Luria), North American developmental and cognitive psychologists (Flavell, Beach, & Chinsky, 1966), and early cognitive-behavioral theories (Meichenbaum, 1977), the CBT approach stressed the need to develop self-directed speech in impulsive children to guide their definition of and attention to immediate problem situations, to generate solutions to these problems, and to guide their behavior as the solutions were performed (see Chapter 15). Self-evaluation, self-correction, and self-directed use of consequences were also viewed as important (Douglas, 1980a, 1980b). Although the first reports of the efficacy of this approach appeared in the late 1960s and the 1970s (Bornstein & Quevillon, 1976; Meichenbaum & Goodman, 1971), it was not until the 1980s that the initial claims of success with nonclinical populations of impulsive chil-dren were more fully tested in clinical populations of children with ADHD. The initial results were disappointing (Abikoff, 1987; Gittelman & Abikoff, 1989). Generally, they indicated some degree of improvement in impulsiveness on cognitive laboratory tasks; however, the improvement was insufficient to be detected in teacher or parent ratings of school and home ADHD behaviors, and CBT was certainly not as effective as stimulant medication (Brown, Wynne, & Medenis, 1985). Many continued to see some promise in these techniques (Barkley, 1981, 1989b; Meichenbaum, 1988; Whalen, Henker, & Hinshaw, 1985), particularly when they were implemented in natural environments by important caregivers (parents and teachers); others ended the decade with a challenge to those who persisted in their support of the CBT approach to provide further evidence for its efficacy (Gittelman & Abikoff, 1989). Such evidence would not be forthcoming (see Chapter 15). Later, even the conceptual basis for the treatment came under attack as being inconsistent with Vygotsky's theory of the internalization of language (Diaz & Berk, 1995).

A second development in treatment was the publication of a specific parent training format for families of children with ADHD and oppositional behavior. A specific set of steps for training parents of children with ADHD in child behavior management skills was developed (Barkley, 1981) and refined (Barkley, 1997c). The approach was founded on a substantial research literature (Barkley, 1997c; Forehand & McMahon, 1981; Patterson, 1982) demonstrating the efficacy of differential attention and time-out procedures for treating oppositional behavior in children—a behavior frequently associated with ADHD. These two procedures were coupled with additional components based on a theoretical formulation of ADHD as a developmental disorder that is typically chronic and associated with decreased rule-governed behavior and an insensitivity to certain consequences, particularly mild or social reinforcement. These components included counseling parents to conceptualize ADHD as a developmentally disabling condition; implementing more powerful home token economies to reinforce behavior, rather than relying on attention alone; using shaping techniques to develop nondisruptive, independent play; and training parents in cognitive-behavioral skills to teach their children during daily management encounters, particularly in managing disruptive behavior in public places (Anastopoulos & Barkley, 1990; see Chapter 12 for a detailed description of this program). Because of the demonstrated impact of parental and family dysfunction on the severity of children's ADHD symptoms, on the children's risk for developing ODD and CD, and on the parents' responsiveness to treatments for the children, clinicians began to pay closer attention to intervening in family systems rather than just in child management skills. Noteworthy among these attempts were the modifications to the previously described parent training program by Charles Cunningham at McMaster University Medical Center (Cunningham, 1990; see Chapter 13 for a detailed description of this approach). Arthur Robin at Wayne State University and the Children's Hospital of Michigan, and Sharon Foster at West Virginia University (Robin & Foster, 1989), also emphasized the need for work on family systems as well as on problem-solving and communication skills in treating the parent–adolescent conflicts so common in families of teenagers with ADHD (see Chapter 14 for a discussion of this approach).

A similar increase in more sophisticated approaches to the classroom management of children with ADHD occurred in this era (Barkley, Copeland, & Sivage, 1980; Pelham et al., 1980; Pfiffner & O'Leary, 1987; Whalen & Henker, 1980). These developments were based on earlier promising studies in the 1970s with contingency management methods in hyperactive children (Allyon et al., 1975; see Chapter 15 for the details of such an approach). Although these methods may not produce the degree of behavioral change seen with the stimulant medications (Gittelman et al., 1980), they provide a more socially desirable intervention that can be a useful alternative when children have mild ADHD and cannot take stimulants or their parents decline the prescription. More often, these methods serve as an adjunct to medication therapy to further enhance academic achievement.

The fourth area of treatment development was in social skills training for children with ADHD (see Chapter 15). Hinshaw et al. (1984) developed a program for training children with ADHD in anger control techniques. This program demonstrated some initial short-term effectiveness in assisting these children to deal with this common deficit in their social skills

and emotional control (Barkley et al., 2000). Related approaches to social skills training for children with ADHD also showed initially promising results (Pfiffner & McBurnett, 1997), but subsequent research did not bear out this promise and suggested that some children with ADHD may even become more aggressive after participation in such group training formats (see Chapter 15).

Finally, medication treatments for children with ADHD expanded to include the use of the tricyclic antidepressants, particularly for those children with characteristics that contraindicated using a stimulant medication (e.g., Tourette syndrome or other tic disorders) or for those with anxiety/depression (Pliszka, 1987). The work of Joseph Biederman and his colleagues at Massachusetts General Hospital (Biederman, Gastfriend, & Jellinek, 1986; Biederman, Baldessarini, Wright, Knee, & Harmatz, 1989) on the safety and efficacy of the tricyclic antidepressants encouraged the rapid adoption of these drugs by many practitioners (see Ryan, 1990), particularly when the stimulants, such as methylphenidate (Ritalin) were receiving such negative publicity in the popular media (see the next section). Simultaneously, initially positive research reports appeared on the use of the antihypertensive drug clonidine in the treatment of children with ADHD, particularly those with very high levels of hyperactive–impulsive behavior and aggression (Hunt, Caper, & O'Connell, 1990; Hunt, Minderaa, & Cohen, 1985) (see Chapter 18).

Developments in Public Awareness

Several noteworthy developments also occurred in the public forum during this decade. Chief and most constructive among these was the blossoming of numerous parent support associations for families with ADHD. Although less than a handful existed in the early 1980s, within 9 years there would be well over 100 such associations throughout the United States alone. By the end of the decade, these would begin to organize into national networks and political action organizations known as CHADD (originally Children with ADD, now Children and Adults with ADHD) and the Attention Deficit Disorder Association (ADDA). With this greater public/parent activism, initiatives were taken to have state and federal laws reevaluated and, it was hoped, changed to include ADHD as an educational disability in need of special educational services in public schools.

When Public Law 94-142 was passed in 1975, it included the concept of MBD under the category of learning disabilities that would be eligible for special educational services. But it did not include hyperactivity, ADD, or ADHD in its description of learning or behavioral disorders eligible for mandated special services in public school. This oversight would lead many public schools to deny access for children with ADD/ADHD to such services, and would cause much parental and teacher exasperation in trying to get educational recognition and assistance for this clearly academically disabling disorder. Other parents would initiate lawsuits against private schools for learning-disabled students for educational malpractice in failing to provide special services for children with ADHD (Skinner, 1988). By the early 1990s, these lobbying efforts would be partially successful in getting the U.S. Department of Education to reinterpret Public Law 94-142—and its 1990 reauthorization as IDEA—as including children with ADHD under the category of "Other Health Impaired" because of their difficulties in alertness and attention. Upon this reinterpretation, children with ADHD could now be considered eligible for special educational services, provided that the ADHD resulted in a significant impairment in academic performance. Such efforts to obtain special educational resources for ADHD in children and adolescents stemmed from their tremendous risk for academic underachievement, failure, retention, suspension, and expulsion, not to mention negative social and occupational outcomes (Barkley, Fischer, et al., 1990, 1991; Cantwell & Satterfield, 1978; Weiss & Hechtman, 1986).

The Church of Scientology Campaign

Yet with this increased public activism also came a tremendously destructive trend in the United States, primarily fueled by the Church of Scientology and its Citizens Commission on Human Rights (CCHR). This campaign capitalized on the mass media's general tendency to uncritically publish alarming or sensational anecdotes, as well as on the public's gullibility for such anecdotes. Drawing on evidence of an increase in stimulant medication use with school children as well as on the extant public concern

over drug abuse, members of CCHR effectively linked these events together to play on the public's general concern about using behavior-modifying drugs with children. In a campaign reminiscent of the gross overstatement seen in the earlier "reefer madness" campaign by the U.S. government against marijuana, members of CCHR selectively focused on the rare cases of adverse reactions to stimulants and greatly exaggerated both the number and degree of them to persuade the public that these reactions were commonplace. They also argued that massive overprescribing was posing a serious threat to schoolchildren, though actual evidence of such overprescribing was never presented. By picketing scientific and public conferences on ADHD, actively distributing leaflets to parents and students in many North American cities, seeking out appearances on many national television talk shows, and placing numerous letters to newspapers decrying the evils of Ritalin and the myth of ADHD (Bass, 1988; CCHR, 1987; Cowart, 1988; Dockx, 1988), CCHR members and others took this propaganda directly to the public. Ritalin, they claimed, was a dangerous and addictive drug often used by intolerant educators and parents and by money-hungry psychiatrists as a chemical straitjacket to subdue normally exuberant children (Clark, 1988; CCHR, 1987; Dockx, 1988). Dramatic, exaggerated, or unfounded claims were made that Ritalin could frequently result in violence or murder, suicide, Tourette syndrome, permanent brain damage or emotional disturbance, seizures, high blood pressure, confusion, agitation, and depression (CCHR, 1987; Clark, 1988; Dockx, 1988; Laccetti, 1988; "Ritalin Linked," 1988; Toufexis, 1989; Williams, 1988). It was also claimed that the increasing production and prescription of Ritalin were leading to increased abuse of these drugs by the general public (Associated Press, 1988; Cowart, 1988; "Rise in Ritalin Use," 1987). Great controversy was said to exist among the scientific and professional practice communities on this disorder and the use of medication. No evidence was presented in these articles, however, that demonstrated a rise in Ritalin abuse or linked it with the increased prescribing of the medication. Moreover, close inspection of professional journals and conferences revealed that no major or widespread controversy ever existed within the professional or scientific fields over the nature of the disorder or the effectiveness of stimulant medication. Yet lawsuits were threatened, initiated, or assisted by the CCHR against practitioners for medical negligence and malpractice, and against schools for complicity in "pressuring" parents to have their children placed on these medicines (Bass, 1988; Cowart, 1988; Henig, 1988; *Nightline*, 1988; Twyman, 1988). A major lawsuit ($125 million) was also filed by the CCHR against the American Psychiatric Association for fraud in developing the criteria for ADHD (Henig, 1988; "Psychiatrist Sued," 1987), though the suit would later be dismissed.

So effective was this national campaign by the CCHR, so widespread were newspaper and television stories on adverse Ritalin reactions, and so easily could public sentiment be misled about a disorder and its treatment by a fringe political–religious group and overzealous, scandal-mongering journalists that within 1 year the public attitude toward Ritalin was dramatically altered. Ritalin was seen as a dangerous and overprescribed drug, and the public believed that there was tremendous professional controversy over its use. The minor benefits to come out of this distorted reporting were that some practitioners would become more rigorous in their assessments and more cautious in their prescribing of medication. Schools also became highly sensitized to the percentage of their enrollment receiving stimulant medication, and in some cases encouraged exploration of alternative behavioral means of managing children.

Yet even the few modestly positive effects of this campaign were greatly outweighed by the damaging effects on parents and children. Many parents were scared into unilaterally discontinuing the medication with their children without consulting their treating physicians. Others rigidly refused to consider the treatment as one part of their child's treatment plan if recommended, or were harassed into such refusal by well-meaning relatives misled by the distorted church propaganda and media reports. Some adolescents with ADHD began refusing the treatment, even if it had been beneficial to them, after being alarmed by these stories. Some physicians stopped prescribing the medications altogether out of concern for the threats of litigation, thereby depriving many children within their care of the clear benefits of this treatment approach. Most frustrating to watch was the unnecessary anguish created for parents whose children were already on the

medication or who were contemplating its use. The psychological damage done to those children whose lives could have been improved by this treatment was incalculable. The meager, poorly organized, and sporadically disseminated response of the mental health professions was primarily defensive in nature (Weiner, 1988) and (as usual) too little, too late to change the tide of public opinion. It would take years to even partially reverse this regression in public opinion toward ADHD and its treatment by medication, as well as the chilling effect all this had on physicians' prescribing of the medication. Public suspicion and concern over medication use for ADHD remains even today.

The Prevailing View at the End of the 1980s

This decade closed with the professional view of ADHD as a developmentally disabling condition with a generally chronic nature, a strong biological or hereditary predisposition, and a significant negative impact on academic and social outcomes for many children. However, its severity, comorbidity, and outcome were viewed as significantly affected by environmental (particularly familial) factors. Growing doubts about the central role of attention deficits in the disorder arose late in the decade, while increasing interest focused on possible motivational factors or reinforcement mechanisms as the core difficulty in ADHD. Effective treatment was now viewed as requiring multiple methods and professional disciplines working in concert over longer time intervals, with periodic reintervention as required, to improve the long-term prognosis for ADHD. The view that environmental causes were involved in the genesis of the disorder was weakened by increasing evidence for the heritability of the condition and its neuroanatomical localization. Even so, evidence that familial/environmental factors were associated with outcome was further strengthened. Developments in treatment would expand the focus of interventions to parental disturbances and family dysfunction, as well as to the children's anger control and social skills. A potentially effective role for the use of tricyclic antidepressants and antihypertensive medications was also demonstrated, expanding the armamentarium of symptomatic interventions for helping children with ADHD.

Despite these tremendous developments in the scientific and professional fields, the general public became overly sensitized to and excessively alarmed by the increasing use of stimulant medication as a treatment for this disorder. Fortunately, the explosive growth of parent support/political action associations for ADHD arose almost simultaneously with this public controversy over Ritalin and held the promise of partially counteracting its effects, as well as of making the education of children with ADHD a national political priority at the start of the 1990s. These associations also offered the best hope that the general public could be provided with a more accurate depiction of ADHD and its treatment. Perhaps now the public could be made to understand that hyperactive, disruptive child behaviors could arise out of a biologically based disability that could be diminished or amplified by the social environment, rather than being entirely due to bad parenting and diet, as the simplistic yet pervasive societal view would maintain.

THE PERIOD 1990 TO 1999

During the 1990s, a number of noteworthy developments occurred in the history of ADHD, chief among them being the increase in research on the neurological and genetic basis of the disorder and on ADHD as it occurs in clinic-referred adults.

Neuroimaging Research

Researchers had long suspected that ADHD was associated in some way with abnormalities or developmental delays in brain functioning. Supporting such an interpretation in the 1990s were numerous neuropsychological studies showing deficits in performance by children with ADHD on tests that were presumed to assess frontal lobe or executive functions (for reviews, see Barkley, 1997b; Barkley et al., 1992; Goodyear & Hynd, 1992). Moreover, psychophysiological research in earlier decades had suggested brain underactivity, particularly in functioning related to the frontal lobes (Hastings & Barkley, 1978; Klorman, 1992). And thus there was good reason to suspect that delayed or disturbed functioning in the brain, and particularly the frontal lobes, might be involved in this disorder.

In 1990, Alan Zametkin and his colleagues at the National Institute of Mental Health (NIMH) published a landmark study (Zametkin et al., 1990). The authors evaluated brain metabolic activity in 25 adults with ADHD who had a childhood history of the disorder and who also had children with the disorder. The authors used positron emission tomography (PET), an exceptionally sensitive technique for detecting states of brain activity and its localization within the cerebral hemispheres. The results of this study indicated significantly reduced brain metabolic activity in adults with ADHD relative to a control group, primarily in frontal and striatal regions. Such results were certainly consistent in many, though not all, respects with the earlier demonstrations of reduced cerebral blood flow in the frontal and striatal regions in children with ADHD (Lou et al., 1984, 1989). Significant in the Zametkin et al. (1990) study, however, was its use of a much better-defined sample of patients with ADHD and its focus on adults with ADHD. Although later attempts by this research team to replicate their original results with teenagers were consistent with these initial results for girls with ADHD, no differences were found in boys with ADHD (see Ernst, 1996, for a review). Sample sizes in these studies were quite small, however, almost ensuring some difficulties with the reliable demonstration of the original findings. Despite these difficulties, the original report stands out as one of the clearest demonstrations to date of reduced brain activity, particularly in the frontal regions, in ADHD.

At the same time as the NIMH research using PET scans was appearing, other researchers were employing magnetic resonance imaging (MRI) to evaluate brain structures in children with ADHD. Hynd and his colleagues were the first to use this method, and they focused on the total brain volume as well as specific regions in the anterior and posterior brain sections. Children with ADHD were found to have abnormally smaller anterior cortical regions, especially on the right side, and they lacked the normal right–left frontal asymmetry (Hynd, Semrud-Clikeman, Lorys, Novey, & Eliopulos, 1990). Subsequent research by this team focused on the size of the corpus callosum, finding that both the anterior and posterior portions were smaller in children with ADHD (Hynd et al., 1991); however, in a later study, only the posterior region was found to be significantly smaller (Semrud-Clikeman et al., 1994). Additional studies were reported by Hynd et al. (1993), who found a smaller left caudate region in children with ADHD, and Giedd et al., (1994), who found smaller anterior regions of the corpus callosum (rostrum and rostral body).

More recently, two research teams published studies using MRI with considerably larger samples of children with ADHD (Castellanos et al., 1994, 1996; Filipek et al., 1997). These studies documented significantly smaller right prefrontal lobe and striatal regions in these children. Castellanos et al. (1996) also found smaller right-sided regions of structures in the basal ganglia, such as the striatum, as well as the right cerebellum. Filipek et al. (1997) observed the left striatal region to be smaller than the right. Despite some inconsistencies across these studies, most have implicated the prefrontal–striatal network as being smaller in children with ADHD, with the right prefrontal region being smaller than the left. Such studies have placed on a considerably firmer foundation the view that ADHD does indeed involve impairments in the development of the brain, particularly in the prefrontal–striatal regions, and that these impairments are likely to have originated in embryological development (Castellanos et al., 1996). Advances in neuroimaging technology continue to provide exciting and revealing new developments in the search for the structural differences in the brain that underlie this disorder (see Chapter 6). For instance, the advent of functional MRI (fMRI), with its greater sensitivity for localization of activity, has already resulted in a number of newly initiated investigations into possible impairments in these brain regions in children and adults with ADHD.

Genetic Research

Since the 1970s, studies have indicated that children with hyperactivity, ADD, or ADHD seem to have parents with a greater frequency of psychiatric disorders, including ADHD. Cantwell (1975) and Morrison and Stewart (1973) both reported higher rates of hyperactivity in the biological parents of hyperactive children than in adoptive parents of such children. Yet both studies were retrospective, and both failed to study the biological parents of the adopted hyperactive children as a comparison group (Pauls, 1991). In the 1990s, a number of studies, particularly those by Biederman and colleagues, clarified and strengthened this evidence of the familial nature of ADHD. Be-

tween 10% and 35% of the immediate family members of children with ADHD were found to have the disorder, with the risk to siblings of these children being approximately 32% (Biederman, Faraone, & Lapey, 1992; Biederman, Keenan, & Faraone, 1990; Pauls, 1991; Welner, Welner, Stewart, Palkes, & Wish, 1977). Even more striking, research has shown that if a parent has ADHD, the risk to the offspring is 57% (Biederman et al., 1995). Thus family aggregation studies find that ADHD clusters among biological relatives of children or adults with the disorder, strongly implying a hereditary basis to this condition.

At the same time that these studies were appearing, several studies of twins were focusing on the heritability of the dimensions of behavior underlying ADHD (i.e., hyperactive–impulsive and inattentive) behavior, or on the clinical diagnosis of ADHD itself. Large-scale twin studies on this issue have been quite consistent in their findings of a high heritability for ADHD symptoms or for the clinical diagnosis, with minimal or no contribution made by the shared environment (Edelbrock, Rende, Plomin, & Thompson, 1995; Levy & Hay, 1992). For instance, Gilger, Pennington, and DeFries (1992) found that if one twin was diagnosed as having ADHD, the concordance for the disorder was 81% in monozygotic twins and 29% in dizygotic twins. Stevenson (1994) summarized the status of twin studies on symptoms of ADHD by stating that the average heritability is .80 for symptoms of this disorder (range .50–.98). More recent large-scale twin studies are remarkably consistent with this conclusion, demonstrating that the majority of variance (70–90%) in the trait of hyperactivity–impulsivity is due to genetic factors (averaging approximately 80%), and that such a genetic contribution may increase as scores for this trait become more extreme, although this latter point is debatable (Faraone, 1996; Gjone, Stevenson, & Sundet, 1996; Gjone, Stevenson, Sundet, & Eilertsen, 1996; Rhee, Waldman, Hay, & Levy, 1995; Silberg et al., 1996; Thapar, Hervas, & McGuffin, 1995; van den Oord, Verhulst, & Boomsma, 1996). Thus twin studies added substantially more evidence to that already found in family aggregation studies supporting a strong genetic basis to ADHD and its behavioral symptoms. More recent twin studies have still further buttressed the strong genetic contribution to ADHD (see Chapter 5). Equally important is the evidence consistently appearing in such research that whatever environmental contributions may be made to ADHD symptoms fall more within the realm of unique (nonshared) environmental effects than within that of common or shared effects.

Also in this decade, a few studies began using molecular genetic techniques to analyze DNA taken from children with ADHD and their family members to identify genes that may be associated with the disorder. The initial focus of this research was on the dopamine Type 2 gene, given findings of its increased association with alcoholism, Tourette syndrome, and ADHD (Blum, Cull, Braverman, & Comings, 1996; Comings et al., 1991), but others failed to replicate this finding (Gelernter et al., 1991; Kelsoe et al., 1989). More recently, the dopamine transporter gene was implicated in ADHD (Cook et al., 1995; Cook, Stein, & Leventhal, 1997). Another gene related to dopamine, the D4RD (repeater gene) was found to be overrepresented in the seven-repetition form of the gene in children with ADHD (LaHoste et al., 1996). The latter finding has been replicated in a number of additional studies (see Chapter 5) and indicates that the presence of this allele increases the risk for ADHD by 1.5. Clearly, research into the molecular genetics involved in the transmission of ADHD across generations continues to be an exciting and fruitful area of research endeavor. Such research offers promise for the eventual development not only of genetic tests for ADHD and subtyping of ADHD into potentially more homogeneous and useful genotypes, but also of more specific pharmacological agents for treating ADHD.

ADHD in Adults

Although papers dealing with the adult equivalents of childhood hyperactivity/MBD date back to the late 1960s and the 1970s (see above), they did not initiate widespread acceptance of these adult equivalents in the field of adult psychiatry and clinical psychology. It was not until the 1990s that the professional fields and the general public recognized ADHD in adults as a legitimate disorder. This was due in large part to a best-selling book by Edward Hallowell and John Ratey (1994), *Driven to Distraction*, which brought the disorder to the public's attention. More serious and more rigorous scientific research was also conducted on

adults with ADHD across this decade. In addition, at this time the greater clinical professional community began to consider the disorder a legitimate clinical condition worthy of differential diagnosis and treatment (Goldstein, 1997; Nadeau, 1995; Wender, 1995).

This broadening acceptance of ADHD in adults continues to the present time and is likely to increase further in the decades ahead. It seems to have been strengthened in some part by the repeated publications throughout the 1990s of follow-up studies that documented the persistence of the disorder into adolescence in up to 70% and into adulthood in up to as many as 66% of childhood cases (Barkley et al., 1990, 2002; Mannuzza, Gittelman-Klein, Bessler, Malloy, & LaPadula, 1993; Weiss & Hechtman, 1993). And it can be attributed as well to published studies on clinically referred adults diagnosed with the disorder (Biederman et al., 1993; Murphy & Barkley, 1996; Shekim, Asarnow, Hess, Zaucha, & Wheeler, 1990; Spencer, Biederman, Wilens, & Faraone, 1994). But it also probably resulted in part from pressure from the general public, which was made more cognizant of this disorder in adults through various media. These media included the publication of other best-selling popular books on the subject (Kelly & Ramundo, 1992; Murphy & LeVert, 1994; Weiss, 1992); numerous media accounts of the condition in adults; the efforts of large-scale parent support groups discussed earlier, such as CHADD, to promote greater public awareness of this issue; and the advent of Internet chat rooms, web pages, and bulletin boards devoted to this topic (Gordon, 1997). Adults who obtain such information and seek out evaluation and treatment for their condition are simply not satisfied any longer with outdated opinions from adult mental health specialists that the disorder does not exist in adults and is commonly outgrown by adolescence, as was the widespread belief in the 1960s.

Also notable in the 1990s was the publication of more rigorous studies demonstrating the efficacy of the stimulants (Spencer et al., 1995) and the antidepressants (Wilens et al., 1996) in the management of adult ADHD. Such studies confirmed the initial clinical speculations in the 1970s, as well as the conclusions from earlier, smaller studies by Paul Wender and his colleagues in the 1970s and 1980s (described earlier), that such medications were efficacious for this disorder in adults (Wender, Reimherr, & Wood, 1981; Wender, Reimherr, Wood, & Ward, 1985). Thus the adult form of ADHD was found not only to share many patterns of symptoms and comorbid disorders with the childhood form, but also to respond just as well to the same medications that proved themselves so useful in the management of childhood ADHD (see Chapter 22).

Other Developments

The 1990s were marked by other significant developments in the field of ADHD. In 1994, new diagnostic criteria for the disorder were set forth in DSM-IV (American Psychiatric Association, 1994). These criteria contained several improvements over those in the earlier DSM-III-R. These criteria are discussed critically in the next chapter (see Table 2.1), but suffice it to say here that they reintroduced criteria for the diagnosis of a purely inattentive form of ADHD, similar to ADD – H in DSM-III. The diagnostic criteria also now require evidence of symptoms' pervasiveness across settings, as well as the demonstration of impairment in a major domain of life functioning (home, school, work). Based on a much larger field trial than any of their predecessors, the DSM-IV criteria for ADHD are the most empirically based in the history of this disorder (see Chapter 2).

A further development during this decade was the undertaking by the NIMH of a multisite study of ADHD that focused on various combinations of long-term treatments (Arnold et al., 1997; MTA Cooperative Group, 1999; see Chapter 20). This study (the Multimodal Treatment Study of ADHD, or MTA) determined what combinations of treatments were most effective for what subgroups of ADHD, based on those treatment strategies with the greatest empirical support in the prior treatment literature. Another long-term treatment study reported findings of great significance to the field: The Swedish government commissioned the longest treatment study of stimulant medication ever undertaken, the results of which indicated that amphetamine treatment remained effective for the entire 15 months of the investigation (see Gillberg et al., 1997). More sobering was the report that an intensive, year-long treatment program using primarily CBT strategies produced no substantial treatment effects, either at posttreatment or at follow-up (Braswell et al., 1997). Similarly, a year-long intensive early intervention program for hyperactive–aggressive children found no significant impact of parent training either at posttreatment or at 2-year follow-up (Barkley et al., 2000, 2002); the school-based portion of this multimethod program produced some immediate treatment gains, but by 2-year follow-up these had dissipated (Shelton et al., 2000). Finally, a multisite study of stimulant medication with and without intensive behavioral and psychosocial interventions was reported to have found that the psychosocial interventions added little or nothing to treatment outcome beyond that achieved by stimulant medication alone (Abikoff & Hechtman, 1995). Its final results were not reported until 2004 (see Chapter 20), but were in keeping with the findings of the MTA that the combination of the treatments was generally no better than medication treatment alone. Although these studies do not entirely undermine the earlier studies on the effectiveness of behavioral interventions for children with ADHD, they do suggest that some of those interventions produce minimal or no improvement when used on a large-scale basis; that the extent of improvement is difficult to detect when adjunctive stimulant medication is also used; and that treatment effects may not be maintained over time following treatment termination.

The 1990s also witnessed the emergence of trends that were to be further developed over the next decade. These trends included a renewed interest in theory development related to ADHD (Barkley, 1997a, 1997b; Quay, 1988b, 1997; Sergeant & van der Meere, 1994), as well as an expanding recognition and treatment of the disorder in countries outside the United States and Canada (Fonseca et al., 1995; Shalev, Hartman, Stavsky, & Sergeant, 1995; Toone & van der Linden, 1997; Vermeersch & Fombonne, 1995). A new stimulant combination, Adderall, appeared on the market in this decade that showed promise as being as effective for ADHD as the other stimulants (Swanson et al., 1998), and at least three new nonstimulant medications and an additional stimulant were in development or in Phase II clinical trials by several pharmaceutical companies during this decade. There also appeared to be an increasing interest in the use of peers as treatment agents in several new behavioral intervention programs for academic performance and peer conflict in school settings (DuPaul & Henningson, 1993; see Chapters 15 and 16, this volume).

The Prevailing View at the End of the 1990s

It seems clear that there was a shift during the 1990s back toward viewing ADHD as far more influenced by neurological and genetic factors than by social or environmental ones. Clearly, the interaction of these sources of influence is generally well accepted by professionals at this time, but greater emphasis is now being placed on the former than on the latter in understanding the potential causation of the disorder. Moreover, evidence began accruing that the influence of the environment on the symptoms of the disorder fall chiefly in the realm of unique or nonshared factors, rather than among the more oft-considered but now weakly supported common or shared family factors.

There was also a discernible shift over this decade toward the recognition that a deficit in behavioral inhibition may be the characteristic of ADHD that distinguishes it most clearly from other mental and developmental disorders (Barkley, 1997b; Nigg, 2001; Pennington & Ozonoff, 1996; Schachar, Tannock, & Logan, 1993), and that this deficit is associated with a significant disruption in the development of typical self-regulation. It is also noteworthy that the subtype of ADHD comprising chiefly inattention without hyperactive–impulsive behavior may possibly be a qualitatively distinct disorder from the subtype with hyperactive–impulsive behavior or the subtype with combined behavior (Barkley et al., 1992; Goodyear & Hynd, 1992; Lahey & Carlson, 1992). The issue of comorbidity became an increasingly important one in subgrouping children with ADHD, leading to greater understanding in the manner in which disorders coexisting with ADHD may influence family functioning, academic success, developmental course and outcome, and even treatment response. In contrast to the attitudes apparent in the middle of the 20th century, the view of ADHD at the close of this century was a less developmentally benign one, owing in large part to multiple follow-up studies that documented the pervasiveness of difficulties with adaptive functioning in the adult lives of many (though by no means all) persons clinically diagnosed with ADHD in childhood.

And there is little doubt that the use of pharmacology in the management of the disorder continued its dramatic rise in popularity, owing in no small part to the repeated demonstration of the efficacy of stimulants in the treatment of the disorder; the greater recognition of subtypes of ADHD, as well as girls and adults with ADHD; and the rather sobering results of multimethod intensive psychosocial intervention programs. Even so, combinations of medication with psychosocial and educational treatment programs remained the norm in recommendations for the management of the disorder across the 1990s, much as they were in the 1980s.

The expansion, solidification, and increased political activity and power of the patient and family support organizations, such as CHADD, across this decade were indeed a marvel to behold. They clearly led to far wider public recognition of the disorder, as well as to controversies over its existence, definition, and treatment with stimulant medications; still, the general trend toward greater public acceptance of ADHD as a developmental disability remained a largely optimistic one. Moreover, such political activity resulted in increased eligibility of those with ADHD for entitlements, under the IDEA, and legal protections, under the Americans with Disabilities Act of 1990 (Public Law 101-336).

THE PERIOD 2000 TO THE PRESENT

At this writing we are just 6 years into the new century, but already many exciting and important developments in the field of ADHD have occurred. Since they are covered in detail elsewhere throughout this volume, they receive only brief topical mention here for their importance to the history of the disorder. Trends from the 1990s have certainly continued into the 21st century, with far more research on heredity, molecular genetics, and neuroimaging being published, along with some initial efforts to link these fields together (see Chapter 5). Not only has the hereditary basis of ADHD become firmly established by many recent studies, but several recent papers may have discovered additional candidate genes for the disorder (DBH Taq I allele) and new chromosomal regions deserving of greater investigation (e.g., 16p13). Although no new theories of ADHD have been proposed, the existing theories, along with advances in neuroimaging of the disorder, have driven even more research on the neuropsychology of ADHD; the results have been an explosion in the size of this literature, and the publication of meta-analyses of various segments of it (Frazier et al., 2004; Hervey, Epstein, & Curry, 2004; see Chapter 3). Indeed, no segment of the literature on ADHD has grown as impressively as that of neuropsychology. This literature continues to support the view that ADHD comprises a problem with behavioral (executive) inhibition (Nigg, 2001), while suggesting that the attention problems associated with the disorder are likely to represent deficits in a broader neuropsychological domain of executive functioning, especially working memory. Combining neuropsychological measures with functional neuroimaging methods such as PET and fMRI offers greater promise in further revealing the neurological basis for the symptoms of the disorder and the nature of medication responses.

Efforts at subtyping ADHD have also received far more research since 2000 (see Chapter 4; see also Milich, Ballentine, & Lynam, 2001, and associated commentaries), leading to the possibility that a qualitatively new subtype if not a new disorder may have been substantiated. Known as "sluggish cognitive tempo," or SCT, this subset accounts for approximately 30–50% of those children now diagnosed as having the Predominantly Inattentive Type of ADHD. They are characterized by a cognitive sluggishness and social passivity, in sharp contrast to the distractible, impulsive, overactive, and emotional difficulties so characteristic of those with the Combined Type of the disorder. With advances in molecular genetics has also come the possibility of genetically subtyping samples of individuals with ADHD into those who do and do not possess a particular candidate allele, so as to study the impact of the allele over time on the psychological and social phenotype of the disorder and its developmental course. Such longitudinal studies are now underway, including in my own research team.

Further work has also occurred on comorbid disorders and the impact they may have on risk for impairments, life course, and even treatment response in ADHD (see Chapter 4; see also Angold, Costello, & Erkanli, 1999). It now appears that the overlap of ADHD with the learning disorders (reading, spelling, math) may stem from separate etiologies of each that arise together in particular cases, in contrast to the earlier, more simplistic view that one type

of disorder may be causing the other. For now, existing evidence suggests that the two sets of disorders are not genetically linked to each other. ADHD, however, may be a direct contributor to a progressive increase in problems with reading (and even story and video) comprehension, perhaps through its detrimental effects on working memory. The case for Major Depressive Disorder gives us fairly substantial evidence that ADHD may create a genetic susceptibility to this disorder, albeit one that may require exposure to stress, social disruption, or traumatic events to become fully manifest. By contrast, the link to anxiety disorders is significantly weaker and perhaps driven in part by referral bias (how samples are obtained) rather than by ADHD's carrying a substantial risk for anxiety, though some associated risk remains present (odds ratio of 1.3). The overlap of ADHD with Bipolar I Disorder remains controversial as of this writing, owing in large part to definitional and diagnostic ambiguity about how childhood Bipolar I Disorder is to be recognized, in contrast with the more well-established criteria for adult-onset manic–depression; challenges include the absence or minimal importance of mania in childhood cases, and its chronic rather than episodic course. What exists suggests a one-way comorbidity in which Bipolar I disorder carries a very high risk for comorbid ADHD, even though ADHD carries a low risk for Bipolar I Disorder. And the link of ADHD to ODD and CD continues to be well established by ongoing research.

The domain of treatment has seen several advances, not the least of which has been the continued reporting of findings from the MTA (see Chapter 20), although controversy exists as to how they should be interpreted. No one doubts that this monumental study found that medication treatment was superior to psychosocial treatment or community care as usual in the initial results. Disagreement appears to continue over whether the combination of medication with psychosocial components resulted in important benefits that were not as evident in the medication-only condition. Although my coauthors and I in Chapter 20 continue to adhere to the view that many cases require combined therapy and that it offers advantages for especially comorbid cases, the point is certainly conceded that some cases may do sufficiently well on medications as to require little additional psychosocial care.

Another advance in treatment was the development of sustained-release delivery systems for the previously extant stimulant medications (see Chapter 17). These new delivery systems are chemical engineering marvels (sustained-release pellets, osmotic pumps, etc.); within the few years of their initial introduction to the marketplace, they have become the standard of care for medication management, at least in the United States. Such delivery systems allow single doses of medication to manage ADHD symptoms effectively for periods of 8–12 hours. This eliminates the need for school dosing and its numerous associated problems, not the least of which was stigmatizion of children who required midday doses.

And no recording of the history of ADHD for the current decade would be complete without mentioning the development of the first new medication for management of ADHD symptoms, the norepinephrine reuptake inhibitor atomoxetine (Strattera). First approved for use in the United States in January 2003 by the U.S. Food and Drug Administration, atomoxetine was the first drug approved for management of ADHD in adults, along with use in children and teens. Over the next several years, the drug is slated for approval for use in numerous other countries. Attractive to many is the fact that this medication has no abuse potential and therefore is not a scheduled drug in the United States, making it far easier to prescribe than stimulants, which are Schedule II. As one of the most successful medications ever launched for a neuroscience indication, atomoxetine had captured 19% of the U.S. market share for ADHD drugs at this writing, making it nearly as widely used as the sustained-release delivery system of methylphenidate (Concerta) or that for amphetamine (Adderall XR). Other nonstimulant medications are now being studied for their potential effectiveness in managing ADHD.

The international recognition of ADHD has grown sharply since 2000, owing to the development of parent support groups in many countries, and efforts by CHADD to assist them in doing so. But substantial credit must also be given to the increasing access to the Internet and the information on ADHD that it can bring nearly instantaneously into any home connected to it by personal computer. As I remarked recently while lecturing to nearly 1,000 mental health professionals and parents in Rome, Italy (Barkley, 2004), there was a time when each country had its own view of mental

disorders, their causes, and their management. Hence the United States might view ADHD in one way, Sweden in another, and Italy, France, Germany, or Spain each in its own different way. Such walls between different countries' understandings of ADHD are now figuratively crashing down, with the democratizing spread of the Internet and the scientific (and non-scientific!) information it can bring to any user. This means that there is no longer going to be an Italian view of ADHD or a U.S. view, but an international view, founded on the most recent scientific advances as they become available on the Internet. Italian professionals, for instance, many of whom still practice a psychoanalytic view of childhood disorders as arising from early upbringing, can no longer count on this view's going unchallenged by parents of children in their practices. These parents can readily discover on the Internet that such views have no scientific credibility; that long-term, analytically focused psychotherapy is not effective for ADHD; and that medications and more empirically based psychosocial accommodations are the cutting edge treatments. If they cannot obtain them in their country, they can quickly locate a neighboring one that is better informed and where such therapies may be accessible. We should expect to see more such developments on the international scene in the coming years.

But so, too, can we expect the same sort of media sensationalizing and misrepresentation, baseless social criticism, and even Church of Scientology-like active counterpropaganda as this expanding international recognition unfolds. This leads to the mention of another landmark historical development since 2000: the creation in 2002 of an International Consensus Statement on ADHD, signed by more than 80 of the world's leading scientists specializing in the disorder. I organized this consensus group out of my own growing frustration and my sense that many other professionals have had the same experiences as my colleagues and I have had in dealing with superficial, biased, or sensational media accounts of ADHD. This is not to say that some journalists have not done admirable work in presenting the science of ADHD to their readers. Many have done so. But every signer has personally experienced as well the opposite circumstance—conflicting views of ADHD described as if they were some sporting event, with two sides being presented on the issues as if there was nothing but controversy in the professional community over the existence of ADHD, its causes, or its treatment with medication, when nothing could be further from the truth. The International Consensus Statement, appearing as Appendix A to this chapter, confronts such misrepresentations head on by showing that conclusions about the nature, causes, and management of ADHD, like those represented in this volume, are science-based and shared widely by the clinical scientific community researching ADHD. They are not just one person's perspective that can be contrasted against the opposing views of some nonexpert professional, ignorant social critic, or intentionally biased fringe political organization, as if both points of view have merit. Readers are encouraged to make copies of Appendix A and provide it to media representatives when they are contacted about potential stories on ADHD.

ADHD has undoubtedly become a mature disorder and topic of scientific study, widely accepted throughout the mental health and pediatric profession as a legitimate developmental disability. At this time, it is unmistakably one of the most well-studied childhood disorders; it is also the object of healthy, sustained research initiatives into its adult counterparts, which should eventually lead to as widespread an acceptance of adult ADHD as has occurred for the childhood version of the disorder. Further discoveries concerning its nature, causes, and developmental course promise tremendous advances in our insight not only into this disorder, but also into the very nature and development of human self-regulation more generally and its rather substantial neurological, genetic, and unique environmental underpinnings. Along with these advances will undoubtedly come new treatments and combinations of treatments. These, let us hope, will greatly limit the impairments experienced by many who suffer from ADHD across their lifespan.

KEY CLINICAL POINTS

✓ ADHD has a long and exceptionally rich history of clinical and scientific publications, numbering in the thousands since the initial descriptions of clinical patients by George Still in 1902.

✓ Early conceptualizations of ADHD focused on defective moral control of behavior and deficits in behavioral inhibition. Later views emphasized its association with brain damage, particularly to the frontal lobes, followed by an emphasis on brain dysfunction and then hyperactivity. The focus has broadened more recently to include inattention and impulsive behavior.

✓ Advances in developing diagnostic criteria have resulted in more precise specification of symptoms, along with two symptom lists; an emphasis on childhood onset of the disorder in most cases; and a requirement for both cross-setting pervasiveness of symptoms, and evidence of impairment in one or more major life activities.

✓ More recent theories of ADHD have viewed behavioral inhibition as central to the disorder, while also suggesting that deficits in executive functioning and self-regulation are likely to account for part or all of the inattentive symptoms associated with the disorder.

✓ Recent efforts at subtyping have identified a Predominantly Inattentive Type of the disorder that may be distinct from the more classical Hyperactive–Impulsive Type or Combined Type. This is particularly so for a subset of inattentive children manifesting sluggish cognitive tempo, social passivity, and other distinguishing clinical features.

✓ Research using neuroimaging techniques has served to isolate particular brain regions (especially the frontal–striatal–cerebellar network, and possibly other regions) as underlying the disorder, and particularly as involved in the difficulties with inhibition and executive functioning.

✓ Increasing research on heredity and genetics has clearly shown a striking hereditary basis to ADHD, along with the identification of several candidate genes that hold some promise in explaining some aspects of the disorder.

✓ Research into the neuropsychology of ADHD has increased substantially as well in the past decade; it supports the view of ADHD (primarily the Combined Type) as not only an inhibitory disorder, but one associated with deficits in executive functioning.

✓ Further research, especially on prenatal neurological hazards and postnatal injuries and environmental toxins, suggests that some cases of ADHD may arise from brain injury rather than genetics.

✓ Numerous longitudinal studies now support the conclusion that ADHD is a relatively chronic disorder affecting many domains of major life activities from childhood through adolescence and into adulthood.

✓ Within the past decade, new medications and delivery systems have been developed that broaden the range of treatment options for managing the heterogeneity of clinical cases, as well as for sustaining medication effects for longer periods across the day (with less need for in-school dosing).

✓ Advances in psychosocial treatment research have revealed specific subsets of individuals with ADHD who may be more or less likely to benefit from these empirically proven interventions. They have also revealed the limitations of these approaches for generalization and maintenance of treatment effects if they are not specifically programmed into the treatment protocol.

✓ ADHD is now recognized as a universal disorder, with an ever-growing international acceptance of both its existence and its status as a chronic disabling condition, for which combinations of medications and psychosocial treatments and accommodations may offer the most effective approach to management.

REFERENCES

Abikoff, E. (1987). An evaluation of cognitive behavior therapy for hyperactive children. In B. Lahey & A. Kazdin (Eds.), *Advances in clinical child psychology* (Vol. 10, pp. 171–216). New York: Plenum Press.

Abikoff, H., Gittelman-Klein, R., & Klein, D. (1977). Validation of a classroom observation code for hyperactive children. *Journal of Consulting and Clinical Psychology, 45*, 772–783.

Abikoff, H., & Hechtman, L. (1995, June). *Multimodal treatment study of children with attention deficit hyperactivity disorder.* Paper presented at the meeting of the International Society for Research in Child and Adolescent Psychopathology, London.

Accardo, P. J., & Blondis, T. A. (2000). The Strauss syndrome, minimal brain dysfunction, and the hyperactive child: A historical introduction to attention deficit-hyperactivity disorder. In P. J. Accardo, T. A. Blondis, B. Y. Whitman, & M. A. Stein (Eds.), *Attention deficits and hyperactivity in children and adults:* *Diagnosis, treatment, management* (pp. 1–12). New York: Dekker.

Achenbach, T. M., & Edelbrock, C. S. (1983). *Manual for the Child Behavior Profile and Child Behavior Checklist.* Burlington, VT: Authors.

Achenbach, T. M., & Edelbrock, C. S. (1986). Empirically based assessment of the behavioral/emotional problems of 2- and 3-year-old children. *Journal of Abnormal Child Psychology, 15*, 629–650.

Ackerman, P. T., Dykman, R. A., & Oglesby, D. M. (1983). Sex and group differences in reading and attention disordered children with and without hyperkinesis. *Journal of Learning Disabilities, 16*, 407–415.

Allyon, T., Layman, D., & Kandel, H. (1975). A behavioral–educational alternative to drug control of hyperactive children. *Journal of Applied Behavior Analysis, 8*, 137–146.

American Psychiatric Association. (1968). *Diagnostic and statistical manual of mental disorders* (2nd ed.). Washington, DC: Author.

American Psychiatric Association. (1980). *Diagnostic and statistical manual of mental disorders* (3rd ed.). Washington, DC: Author.

American Psychiatric Association. (1987). *Diagnostic and statistical manual of mental disorders* (3rd ed., rev.). Washington, DC: Author.

American Psychiatric Association. (1994). *Diagnostic and statistical manual of mental disorders* (4th ed.). Washington, DC: Author.

Anastopoulos, A. D., & Barkley, R. A. (1990). Counseling and parent training. In R. A. Barkley, *Attention-deficit hyperactivity disorder: A handbook for diagnosis and treatment* (pp. 397–431). New York: Guilford Press.

Angold, A., Costello, E. J., & Erkanli, A. (1999). Comorbidity. *Journal of Child Psychology and Psychiatry, 40*, 57–88.

Arnold, L. E., Abikoff, H. B., Cantwell, D. P., Connors, C. K., Elliott, G., Greenhill, L. L., et al. (1997). National Institute of Mental Health collaborative multimodal treatment study of children with ADHD (the MTA). *Archives of General Psychiatry, 54*, 865–870.

Associated Press. (1988, January). To many, Ritalin is a "chemical billy club." *Worcester Telegram and Gazette* [Worcester, MA].

August, G. J., & Stewart, M. A. (1983). Family subtypes of childhood hyperactivity. *Journal of Nervous and Mental Disease, 171*, 362–368.

Barkley, R. A. (1977). A review of stimulant drug research with hyperactive children. *Journal of Child Psychology and Psychiatry, 18*, 137–165.

Barkley, R. A. (Ed.). (1978). Special issue on hyperactivity. *Journal of Pediatric Psychology, 3*.

Barkley, R. A. (1981). *Hyperactive children: A handbook for diagnosis and treatment.* New York: Guilford Press.

Barkley, R. A. (1982). Guidelines for defining hyperactivity in children (attention deficit disorder with hyperactivity). In B. Lahey & A. Kazdin (Eds.), *Ad-*

vances in clinical child psychology (Vol. 5, pp. 137–180). New York: Plenum Press.

Barkley, R. A. (1984). *Do as we say, not as we do: The problem of stimulus control and rule-governed behavior in attention deficit disorder with hyperactivity.* Paper presented at the Highpoint Hospital Conference on Attention Deficit and Conduct Disorders, Toronto.

Barkley, R. A. (1988a). Child behavior rating scales and checklists. In M. Rutter, A. H. Tuma, & I. Lann (Eds.), *Assessment and diagnosis in child psychopathology* (pp. 113–155). New York: Guilford Press.

Barkley, R. A. (1988b). Tic disorders and Gilles de la Tourette syndrome. In E. J. Mash & L. G. Terdal (Eds.), *Behavioral assessment of childhood disorders* (2nd ed., pp. 552–585). New York: Guilford Press.

Barkley, R. A. (1988c). Attention deficit disorder with hyperactivity. In E. J. Mash & L. G. Terdal (Eds.), *Behavioral assessment of childhood disorders* (2nd ed., pp. 69–104). New York: Guilford Press.

Barkley, R. A. (1989a). The problem of stimulus control and rule-governed behavior in children with attention deficit disorder with hyperactivity. In L. M. Bloomingdale & J. M. Swanson (Eds.), *Attention deficit disorder* (Vol. 4, pp. 203–234). New York: Pergamon Press.

Barkley, R. A. (1989b). Hyperactive girls and boys: Stimulant drug effects on mother–child interactions. *Journal of Child Psychology and Psychiatry, 30,* 379–390.

Barkley, R. A. (1989c). Attention-deficit hyperactivity disorder. In E. J. Mash & R. A. Barkley (Eds.), *Treatment of childhood disorders* (pp. 39–72). New York: Guilford Press.

Barkley, R. A. (1990). *Attention-deficit hyperactivity disorder: A handbook for diagnosis and treatment.* New York: Guilford Press.

Barkley, R. A. (1991). The ecological validity of laboratory and analogue assessments of ADHD symptoms. *Journal of Abnormal Child Psychology, 19,* 149–178.

Barkley, R. A. (1997a). Inhibition, sustained attention, and executive functions: Constructing a unifying theory of ADHD. *Psychological Bulletin, 121,* 65–94.

Barkley, R. A. (1997b). *ADHD and the nature of self-control.* New York: Guilford Press.

Barkley, R. A. (1997c). *Defiant children: A clinician's manual for assessment and parent training* (2nd ed.). New York: Guilford Press.

Barkley, R. A. (1998). *Attention-deficit hyperactivity disorder: A handbook for diagnosis and treatment* (2nd ed.). New York: Guilford Press.

Barkley, R. A. (2004, November). *Attention-deficit hyperactivity disorder in children.* Workshop presented in Rome, Italy.

Barkley, R. A., Copeland, A., & Sivage, C. (1980). A self-control classroom for hyperactive children. *Journal of Autism and Developmental Disorders, 10,* 75–89.

Barkley, R. A., & Cunningham, C. E. (1979). The effects of methylphenidate on the mother–child interactions of hyperactive children. *Archives of General Psychiatry, 36,* 201–208.

Barkley, R. A., DuPaul, G. J., & McMurray, M. B. (1990). A comprehensive evaluation of attention deficit disorder with and without hyperactivity. *Journal of Consulting and Clinical Psychology, 58,* 775–789.

Barkley, R. A., DuPaul, G. J., & McMurray, M. B. (1991). Attention deficit disorder with and without hyperactivity: Clinical response to three doses of methylphenidate. *Pediatrics, 87,* 519–531.

Barkley, R. A., & Edelbrock, C. S. (1987). Assessing situational variation in children's behavior problems: The Home and School Situations Questionnaires. In R. Prinz (Ed.), *Advances in behavioral assessment of children and families* (Vol. 3, pp. 157–176). Greenwich, CT: JAI Press.

Barkley, R. A., Fischer, M., Edelbrock, C. S., & Smallish, L. (1990). The adolescent outcome of hyperactive children diagnosed by research criteria: I. An 8-year prospective followup study. *Journal of the American Academy of Child and Adolescent Psychiatry, 29,* 546–557.

Barkley, R. A., Fischer, M., Edelbrock, C. S., & Smallish, L. (1991). The adolescent outcome of hyperactive children diagnosed by research criteria: III. Mother–child interactions, family conflicts, and maternal psychopathology. *Journal of Child Psychology and Psychiatry, 32,* 233–256.

Barkley, R. A., Fischer, M., Newby, R., & Breen, M. (1988). Development of a multi-method clinical protocol for assessing stimulant drug responses in ADHD children. *Journal of Clinical Child Psychology, 17,* 14–24.

Barkley, R. A., Fischer, M., Smallish, L., & Fletcher, K. (2002). The persistence of attention-deficit/hyperactivity disorder into young adulthood as a function of reporting source and definition of disorder. *Journal of Abnormal Psychology, 111,* 279–289.

Barkley, R. A., Grodzinsky, G., & DuPaul, G. (1992). Frontal lobe functions in attention deficit disorder with and without hyperactivity: A review and research report. *Journal of Abnormal Child Psychology, 20,* 163–188.

Barkley, R. A., Karlsson, J., & Pollard, S. (1985). Effects of age on the mother–child interactions of hyperactive children. *Journal of Abnormal Child Psychology, 13,* 631–638.

Barkley, R. A., Karlsson, J., Pollard, S., & Murphy, J. V. (1985). Developmental changes in the mother–child interactions of hyperactive boys: Effects of two dose levels of Ritalin. *Journal of Child Psychology and Psychiatry, 26,* 705–715.

Barkley, R. A., Shelton, T. L., Crosswait, C., Moorehouse, M., Fletcher, K., Barrett, S., et al. (2000). Early psycho-educational intervention for children with disruptive behavior: Preliminary post-treatment outcome. *Journal of Child Psychology and Psychiatry, 41,* 319–332.

Barkley, R. A., & Ullman, D. G. (1975). A comparison

of objective measures of activity level and distractibility in hyperactive and nonhyperactive children. *Journal of Abnormal Child Psychology, 3,* 213–244.

Bass, A. (1988, March 28). Debate over Ritalin is heating up: Experts say critics are lashing out for all the wrong reasons. *Boston Globe,* pp. 36–38.

Bender, L. (1942). Postencephalitic behavior disorders in children. In J. B. Neal (Ed.), *Encephalitis: A clinical study.* New York: Grune & Stratton.

Benninger, R. J. (1989). Dopamine and learning: Implications for attention deficit disorder and hyperkinetic syndrome. In T. Sagvolden & T. Archer (Eds.), *Attention deficit disorder: Clinical and basic research* (pp. 323–338). Hillsdale, NJ: Erlbaum.

Bettelheim, B. (1973). Bringing up children. *Ladies' Home Journal,* p. 23.

Biederman, J., Baldessarini, R. J., Wright, V., Knee, D., & Harmatz, J. S. (1989). A double-blind placebo controlled study of desipramine in the treatment of ADD: I. Efficacy. *Journal of the American Academy of Child and Adolescent Psychiatry, 28,* 777–784.

Biederman, J., Faraone, S. V., & Lapey, K. (1992). Comorbidity of diagnosis in attention-deficit hyperactivity disorder. *Child and Adolescent Psychiatric Clinics of North America, 1,* 335–360.

Biederman, J., Faraone, S. V., Mick, E., Spencer, T., Wilens, T., Kiely, K., et al. (1995). High risk for attention deficit hyperactivity disorder among children of parents with childhood onset of the disorder: A pilot study. *American Journal of Psychiatry, 152,* 431–435.

Biederman, J., Faraone, S. V., Spencer, T., Wilens, T., Norman, D., Lapey, K. A., et al. (1993). Patterns of psychiatric comorbidity, cognition, and psychosocial functioning in adults with attention deficit hyperactivity disorder. *American Journal of Psychiatry, 150,* 1792–1798.

Biederman, J., Gastfriend, D. R., & Jellinek, M. S. (1986). Desipramine in the treatment of children with attention deficit disorder. *Journal of Clinical Psychopharmacology, 6,* 359–363.

Biederman, J., Keenan, K., & Faraone, S. V. (1990). Parent-based diagnosis of attention deficit disorder predicts a diagnosis based on teacher report. *American Journal of Child and Adolescent Psychiatry, 29,* 698–701.

Biederman, J., Munir, K., & Knee, D. (1987). Conduct and oppositional defiant disorder in clinically referred children with attention deficit disorder: A controlled family study. *Journal of the American Academy of Child and Adolescent Psychiatry, 26,* 724–727.

Birch, H. G. (1964). *Brain damage in children: The biological and social aspects.* Baltimore: Williams & Wilkins.

Blau, A. (1936). Mental changes following head trauma in children. *Archives of Neurology and Psychiatry, 35,* 722–769.

Block, G. H. (1977). Hyperactivity: A cultural perspective. *Journal of Learning Disabilities, 110,* 236–240.

Blum, K., Cull, J. G., Braverman, E. R., & Comings, D. E. (1996). Reward deficiency syndrome. *American Scientist, 84,* 132–145.

Bond, E. D., & Appel, K. E. (1931). *The treatment of behavior disorders following encephalitis.* New York: Commonwealth Fund.

Bornstein, P. H., & Quevillon, R. P. (1976). The effects of a self-instructional package on overactive preschool boys. *Journal of Applied Behavior Analysis, 9,* 179–188.

Bradley, W. (1937). The behavior of children receiving benzedrine. *American Journal of Psychiatry, 94,* 577–585.

Bradley, W., & Bowen, C. (1940). School performance of children receiving amphetamine (benzedrine) sulfate. *American Journal of Orthopsychiatry, 10,* 782–788.

Braswell, L., August, G. J., Bloomquist, M. L., Realmuto, G. M., Skare, S. S., & Crosby, R. D. (1997). School-based secondary prevention for children with disruptive behavior: Initial outcomes. *Journal of Abnormal Child Psychology, 25,* 197–208.

Brown, R. T., Wynne, M. E., & Medenis, R. (1985). Methylphenidate and cognitive therapy: A comparison of treatment approaches with hyperactive boys. *Journal of Abnormal Child Psychology, 13,* 69–88.

Burks, H. (1960). The hyperkinetic child. *Exceptional Children, 27,* 18.

Byers, R. K., & Lord, E. E. (1943). Late effects of lead poisoning on mental development. *American Journal of Diseases of Children, 66,* 471–494.

Camp, B. W. (1980). Two psychoeducational treatment programs for young aggressive boys. In C. Whalen & B. Henker (Eds.), *Hyperactive children: The social ecology of identification and treatment* (pp. 191–220). New York: Academic Press.

Campbell, S. B. (1973). Mother–child interaction in reflective, impulsive, and hyperacative children. *Developmental Psychology, 8,* 341–349.

Campbell, S. B. (1975). Mother-child interactions: A comparison of hyperactive, learning disabled, and normal boys. *American Journal of Orthopsychiatry, 45,* 51–57.

Campbell, S. B. (1987). Parent-referred problem three-year olds: Developmental changes in symptoms. *Journal of Child Psychology and Psychiatry, 28,* 835–846.

Campbell, S. B., Douglas, V. I., & Morganstern, G. (1971). Cognitive styles in hyperactive children and the effect of methylphenidate. *Journal of Child Psychology and Psychiatry, 12,* 55–67.

Campbell, S. B., & Ewing, L. J. (1990). Follow-up of hard-to-manage preschoolers: Adjustment at age nine years and predictors of continuing symptoms. *Journal of Child Psychology and Psychiatry, 31,* 891–910.

Cantwell, D. P. (1975). *The hyperactive child.* New York: Spectrum.

Cantwell, D. P. (1981). Foreword. In R. A. Barkley, *Hyperactive children: A handbook for diagnosis and treatment. New York: Guilford Press.

Cantwell, D. P., & Satterfield, J. H. (1978). The prevalence of academic underachievement in hyperactive children. Journal of Pediatric Psychology, 3, 168–171.

Carlson, C. (1986). Attention deficit disorder without hyperactivity: A review of preliminary experimental evidence. In B. Lahey & A. Kazdin (Eds.), Advances in clinical child psychology (Vol. 9, pp. 153–176). New York: Plenum Press.

Castellanos, F. X., Giedd, J. N., Eckburg, P., Marsh, W. L., Vaituzis, C., Kaysen, D., et al. (1994). Quantitative morphology of the caudate nucleus in attention deficit hyperactivity disorder. American Journal of Psychiatry, 151, 1791–1796.

Castellanos, F. X., Giedd, J. N., Marsh, W. L., Hamburger, S. D., Vaituzis, A. C., Dickstein, D. P., et al. (1996). Quantitative brain magnetic resonance imaging in attention-deficit hyperactivity disorder. Archives of General Psychiatry, 53, 607–616.

Chelune, G. J., Ferguson, W., Koon, R., & Dickey, T. O. (1986). Frontal lobe disinhibition in attention deficit disorder. Child Psychiatry and Human Development, 16, 221–234.

Chess, S. (1960). Diagnosis and treatment of the hyperactive child. New York State Journal of Medicine, 60, 2379–2385.

Childers, A. T. (1935). Hyper-activity in children having behavior disorders. American Journal of Orthopsychiatry, 5, 227–243.

Citizens Commission on Human Rights (CCHR). (1987). Ritalin: A warning to parents. Los Angeles: Church of Scientology.

Clark, D. (1988, January). [Guest on the syndicated television show Sally Jessy Raphael]. New York: Multimedia Entertainment.

Clements, S. D. (1966). Task Force One: Minimal brain dysfunction in children (National Institute of Neurological Diseases and Blindness, Monograph No. 3). Rockville, MD: U.S. Department of Health, Education and Welfare.

Comings, D. E., Comings, B. G., Muhleman, D., Dietz, G., Shahbahrami, B., Tast, D., et al. (1991). The dopamine D2 receptor locus as a modifying gene in neuropsychiatric disorders. Journal of the American Medical Association, 266, 1793–1800.

Conners, C. K. (1969). A teacher rating scale for use in drug studies with children. American Journal of Psychiatry, 126, 884–888.

Conners, C. K. (1980). Food additives and hyperactive children. New York: Plenum Press.

Conners, C. K. (1995). The Conners Continuous Performance Test. North Tonawanda, NY: Multi-Health Systems.

Conners, C. K., & Rothschild, G. H. (1968). Drugs and learning in children. In J. Hellmuth (Ed.), Learning disorders (Vol. 3, pp. 191–223). Seattle, WA: Special Child.

Conrad, P. (1975). The discovery of hyperkinesis: Notes on the medicalization of deviant behavior. Social Problems, 23, 12–21.

Cook, E. H., Stein, M. A., Krasowski, M. D., Cox, N. J., Olkon, D. M., Kieffer, J. E., et al. (1995). Association of attention deficit disorder and the dopamine transporter gene. American Journal of Human Genetics, 56, 993–998.

Cook, E. H., Stein, M. A., & Leventhal, D. L. (1997). Family-based association of attention-deficit/hyperactivity disorder and the dopamine transporter. In K. Blum & E. P. Noble (Eds.), Handbook of psychiatric genetics (pp. 297–310). Boca Raton, FL: CRC Press.

Corkum, P. V., & Siegel, L. S. (1993). Is the continuous performance task a valuable research tool for use with children with attention-deficit–hyperactivity disorder? Journal of Child Psychology and Psychiatry, 34, 1217–1239.

Costello, E. J., Loeber, R., & Stouthamer-Loeber, M. (1991). Pervasive and situational hyperactivity—Confounding effect of informant: A research note. Journal of Child Psychology and Psychiatry, 32, 367–376.

Cowart, V. S. (1988). The Ritalin controversy: What's made this drug's opponents hyperactive? Journal of the American Medical Association, 259, 2521–2523.

Cruickshank, W. M., & Dolphin, J. E. (1951). The educational implications of psychological studies of cerebral palsied children. Exceptional Children, 18, 3–11.

Cunningham, C. E. (1990). A family systems approach to parent training. In R. A. Barkley, Attention-deficit hyperactivity disorder: A handbook for diagnosis and treatment (pp. 432–461). New York: Guilford Press.

Cunningham, C. E., & Barkley, R. A. (1978). The effects of Ritalin on the mother–child interactions of hyperkinetic twin boys. Developmental Medicine and Child Neurology, 20, 634–642.

Cunningham, C. E., & Barkley, R. A. (1979). The interactions of hyperactive and normal children with their mothers during free play and structured task. Child Development, 50, 217–224.

Cunningham, C. E., Siegel, L. S., & Offord, D. R. (1985). A developmental dose response analysis of the effects of methylphenirtate on the peer interactions of attention deficit disordered boys. Journal of Child Psychology and Psychiatry, 26, 955–971.

Danforth, J. S., Barkley, R. A., & Stokes, T. F. (1991). Observations of parent–child interactions with hyperactive children: Research and clinical implications. Clinical Psychology Review, 11, 703–727.

Diaz, R. M., & Berk, L. E. (1995). A Vygotskian critique of self-instructional training. Development and Psychopathology, 7, 369–392.

Dockx, P. (1988, January 11). Are schoolchildren getting unnecessary drugs? Woonsocket Sun Chronicle [Woonsocket, RI], p. 15.

Dolphin, J. E., & Cruickshank, W. M. (1951a). The figure background relationship in children with cerebral palsy. Journal of Clinical Psychology, 7, 228–231.

Dolphin, J. E., & Cruickshank, W. M. (1951b). Pathology of concept formation in children with cerebral palsy. *American Journal of Mental Deficiency, 56,* 386–392.

Dolphin, J. E., & Cruickshank, W. M. (1951c). Visuomotor perception of children with cerebral palsy. *Quarterly Journal of Child Behavior, 3,* 189–209.

Douglas, V. I. (1972). Stop, look, and listen: The problem of sustained attention and impulse control in hyperactive and normal children. *Canadian Journal of Behavioural Science, 4,* 259–282.

Douglas, V. I. (Ed.). (1976). Special issue on hyperactivity. *Journal of Abnormal Child Psychology, 4.*

Douglas, V. I. (1980a). Higher mental processes in hyperactive children: Implications for training. In R. Knights & D. Bakker (Eds.), *Treatment of hyperactive and learning disordered children* (pp. 65–92). Baltimore: University Park Press.

Douglas, V. I. (1980b). Treatment and training approaches to hyperactivity: Establishing internal or external control. In C. Whalen & B. Henker (Eds.), *Hyperactive children: The social ecology of identification and treatment* (pp. 283–318). New York: Academic Press.

Douglas, V. I. (1983). Attention and cognitive problems. In M. Rutter (Ed.), *Developmental neuropsychiatry* (pp. 280–329). New York: Guilford Press.

Douglas, V. I. (1988). Cognitive deficits in children with attention deficit disorder with hyperactivity. In L. M. Bloomingdale & J. A. Sergeant (Eds.), *Attention deficit disorder: Criteria, cognition, intervention* (pp. 65–82). New York: Pergamon Press.

Douglas, V. I. (1989). Can Skinnerian psychology account for the deficits in attention deficit disorder?: A reply to Barkley. In L. M. Bloomingdale & J. M. Swanson (Eds.), *Attention deficit disorder* (Vol. 4, pp. 235–253). New York: Pergamon Press.

Douglas, V. I., & Peters, K. G. (1979). Toward a clearer definition of the attentional deficit of hyperactive children. In G. A. Hale & M. Lewis (Eds.), *Attention and the developments of cognitive skills* (pp. 173–248). New York: Plenum Press.

Draeger, S., Prior, M., & Sanson, A. (1986). Visual and auditory attention performance in hyperactive children: Competence or compliance. *Journal of Abnormal Child Psychology, 14,* 411–424.

Dubey, D. R., & Kaufman, K. F. (1978). Home management of hyperkinetic children. *Journal of Pediatrics, 93,* 141–146.

DuPaul, G. J. (1991). Parent and teacher ratings of ADHD symptoms: Psychometric properties in a community-based sample. *Journal of Clinical Child Psychology, 20,* 242–253.

DuPaul, G. J., & Barkley, R. A. (1992). Situational variability of attention problems: Psychometric properties of the Revised Home and School Situations Questionnaires. *Journal of Clinical Child Psychology, 21,* 178–188.

DuPaul, G. J., Barkley, R. A., & McMurray, M. B. (1994). Response of children with ADHD to methylphenidate: Interaction with internalizing symptoms. *Journal of the American Academy of Child and Adolescent Psychiatry, 93,* 894–903.

DuPaul, G. J., & Henningson, P. N. (1993). Peer tutoring effects on the classroom performance of children with attention-deficit hyperactivity disorder. *School Psychology Review, 22,* 134–143.

Dykman, R. A., Ackerman, P. T., & Holcomb, P. J. (1985). Reading disabled and ADD children: Similarities and differences. In D. B. Gray & J. F. Kavanagh (Eds.), *Biobehavioral measures of dyslexia* (pp. 47–62). Parkton, MD: York Press.

Ebaugh, F. G. (1923). Neuropsychiatric sequelae of acute epidemic encephalitis in children. *American Journal of Diseases of Children, 25,* 89–97.

Edelbrock, C. S., Rende, R., Plomin, R., & Thompson, L. (1995). A twin study of competence and problem behavior in childhood and early adolescence. *Journal of Child Psychology and Psychiatry, 36,* 775–786.

Ernst, M. (1996). Neuroimaging in attention-deficit/hyperactivity disorder. In G. R. Lyon & J. M. Rumsey (Eds.), *Neuroimaging: A window to the neurological foundations of learning and behavior in children* (pp. 95–118). Baltimore: Brookes.

Faraone, S. V. (1996). Discussion of "Genetic influence on parent-reported attention-related problems in a Norwegian general population twin sample." *Journal of the American Academy of Child and Adolescent Psychiatry, 35,* 596–598.

Feingold, B. (1975). *Why your child is hyperactive.* New York: Random House.

Ferrier, D. (1876). *The functions of the brain.* New York: Putnam.

Filipek, P. A., Semrud-Clikeman, M., Steingard, R. J., Renshaw, P. F., Kennedy, D. N., & Biederman, J. (1997). Volumetric MRI analysis comparing subjects having attention-deficit hyperactivity disorder with normal controls. *Neurology, 48,* 589–601.

Firestone, P., & Martin, J. E. (1979). An analysis of the hyperactive syndrome: A comparison of hyperactive, behavior problem, asthmatic, and normal children, *Journal of Abnormal Child Psychology, 7,* 261–273.

Fischer, M., Barkley, R. A., Edelbrock, C. S., & Smallish, L. (1990). The adolescent outcome of hyperactive children diagnosed by research criteria: II. Academic, attentional, and neuropsychological status. *Journal of Consulting and Clinical Psychology, 58,* 580–588.

Flavell, J. H., Beach, D. R., & Chinsky, J. M. (1966). Spontaneous verbal rehearsal in a memory task as a function of age. *Child Development, 37,* 283–299.

Fonseca, A. C., Simones, A., Rebelo, J. A., Ferreira, J. A., Cardoso, F., & Temudo, P. (1995). Hyperactivity and conduct disorder among Portuguese children and adolescents: Data from parents' and teachers' reports. In J. Sergeant (Ed.), *Eunethydis: European approaches to hyperkinetic disorder* (pp. 115–129). Amsterdam: University of Amsterdam.

Forehand, R., & McMahon, R. (1981). *Helping the noncompliant child.* New York: Guilford Press.

Frazier, T. W., Demaree, H. A., & Youngstrom, E. A. (2004). Meta-analysis of intellectual and neuropsychological test performance in attention-deficit/hyperactivity disorder. *Neuropsychology, 18,* 543–555.

Freibergs, V. (1965). *Concept learning in hyperactive and normal children.* Unpublished doctoral dissertation, McGill University.

Freibergs, V., & Douglas, V. I. (1969). Concept learning in hyperactive and normal children. *Journal of Abnormal Psychology, 74,* 388–395.

Gelernter, J. O., O'Malley, S., Risch, N., Kranzler, H. R., Krystal, J., Merikangas, K., et al. (1991). No association between an allele at the D2 dopamine receptor gene (DRD2) and alcoholism. *Journal of the American Medical Association, 266,* 1801–1807.

Giedd, J. N., Castellanos, F. X., Casey, B. J., Kozuch, P., King, A. C., Hamburger, S. D., et al. (1994). Quantitative morphology of the corpus callosum in attention deficit hyperactivity disorder. *American Journal of Psychiatry, 151,* 665–669.

Gilger, J. W., Pennington, B. F., & DeFries, J. C. (1992). A twin study of the etiology of comorbidity: Attention-deficit hyperactivity disorder and dyslexia. *Journal of the American Academy of Child and Adolescent Psychiatry, 31,* 343–348.

Gillberg, C., Melander, H., von Knorring, A.-L., Janols, L.-O., Thernlund, G., Hagglof, B., et al. (1997). Long-term stimulant treatment of children with attention-deficit hyperactivity disorder symptoms: A randomized, double-blind, placebo-controlled trial. *Archives of General Psychiatry, 54,* 857–864.

Gittelman, R. (1988). The assessment of hyperactivity: The DSM-III approach. In L. M. Bloomingdale & J. Sergeant (Eds.), *Attention deficit disorder: Criteria, cognition, intervention* (pp. 9–28). New York: Pergamon Press.

Gittelman, R., & Abikoff, H. (1989). The role of psychostimulants and psychosocial treatments in hyperkinesis. In T. Sagvolden & T. Archer (Eds.), *Attention deficit disorder: Clinical and basic research* (pp. 167–180). Hillsdale, NJ: Erlbaum.

Gittelman, R., Abikoff, H., Pollack, E., Klein, D., Katz, S., & Mattes, J. (1980). A controlled trial of behavior modification and methylphenidate in hyperactive children. In C. Whalen & B. Henker (Eds.), *Hyperactive children: The social ecology of identification and treatment* (pp. 221–246). New York: Academic Press.

Gittelman-Klein, R., Klein, D. F., Abikoff, H., Katz, S., Gloisten, C., & Kates, W. (1976). Relative efficacy of methylphenidate and behavior modification in hyperkinetic children: An interim report. *Journal of Abnormal Child Psychology, 4,* 261–279.

Gittelman, R., Mannuzza, S., Shenker, R., & Bonagura, N. (1985). Hyperactive boys almost grown up: I. Psychiatric status. *Archives of General Psychiatry, 42,* 937–947.

Gjone, H., Stevenson, J., & Sundet, J. M. (1996). Genetic influence on parent-reported attention-related problems in a Norwegian general population twin sample. *Journal of the American Academy of Child and Adolescent Psychiatry, 35,* 588–596.

Gjone, H., Stevenson, J., Sundet, J. M., & Eilertsen, D. E. (1996). Changes in heritability across increasing levels of behavior problems in young twins. *Behavior Genetics, 26,* 419–426.

Glow, P. H., & Glow, R. A. (1979). Hyperkinetic impulse disorder: A developmental defect of motivation. *Genetic Psychological Monographs, 100,* 159–231.

Goldstein, S. (1997). *Managing attention and learning disorders in late adolescence and adulthood.* New York: Wiley.

Goldstein, S., & Goldstein, M. (1998). *Managing attention deficit hyperactivity disorder in children: A guide for practitioners.* New York: Wiley.

Gomez, R. L., Janowsky, D., Zetin, M., Huey, L., & Clopton, P. L. (1981). Adult psychiatric diagnosis and symptoms compatible with the hyperactive syndrome: A retrospective study. *Journal of Clinical Psychiatry, 42,* 389–394.

Goodman, J. R., & Stevenson, J. (1989). A twin study of hyperactivity: II. The aetiological role of genes, family relationships, and perinatal adversity. *Journal of Child Psychology and Psychiatry, 30,* 691–709.

Goodyear, P., & Hynd, G. (1992). Attention deficit disorder with (ADD/H) and without (ADD/WO) hyperactivity: Behavioral and neuropsychological differentiation. *Journal of Clinical Child Psychology, 21,* 273–304.

Gordon, M. (1979). The assessment of impulsivity and mediating behaviors in hyperactive and non-hyperactive children. *Journal of Abnormal Child Psychology, 7,* 317–326.

Gordon, M. (1983). *The Gordon Diagnostic System.* DeWitt, NY: Gordon Systems.

Gordon, M. (1997). ADHD in cyberspace. *ADHD Report, 5*(4), 4–6.

Gordon, M., & Mettelman, B. B. (1988). The assessment of attention: I. Standardization and reliability of a behavior based measure. *Journal of Clinical Psychology, 44,* 682–690.

Gray, J. A. (1982). *The neuropsychology of anxiety.* New York: Oxford University Press.

Gray, J. A. (1987). *The psychology of fear and stress* (2nd ed.). Cambridge, UK: Cambridge University Press.

Gray, J. A. (1994). Three fundamental emotional systems. In P. Ekman & R. J. Davidson (Eds.), *The nature of emotion: Fundamental questions* (pp. 243–247). New York: Oxford University Press.

Greenberg, L. M., & Waldman, I. D. (1992). *Developmental normative data on the Test of Variables of Attention (T.O.V.A.).* Minneapolis: Department of Psychiatry, University of Minnesota Medical School.

Haenlein, M., & Caul, W. F. (1987). Attention deficit disorder with hyperactivity: A specific hypothesis of reward dysfunction. *Journal of the American Academy of Child and Adolescent Psychiatry, 26,* 356–362.

Hallowell, E. M., & Ratey, J. J. (1994). *Driven to distraction.* New York: Pantheon.

Halperin, J. M., Gittelman, R., Klein, D. F., & Rudel, R. G. (1984). Reading-disabled hyperactive children: A distinct subgroup of attention deficit disorder with hyperactivity? *Journal of Abnormal Child Psychology, 12,* 1–14.

Harticollis, P. (1968). The syndrome of minimal brain dysfunction in young adult patients. *Bulletin of the Menninger Clinic, 32,* 102–114.

Hastings, J., & Barkley, R. A. (1978). A review of psychophysiological research with hyperactive children. *Journal of Abnormal Child Psychology, 7,* 413–447.

Henig, R. M. (1988, March 15). Courts enter the hyperactivity fray: The drug Ritalin helps control behavior, but is it prescribed needlessly? *The Washington Post,* p. 8.

Henker, B., & Whalen, C. (1980). The changing faces of hyperactivity: Retrospect and prospect. In C. Whalen & B. Henker (Eds.), *Hyperactive children: The social ecology of identification and treatment* (pp. 321–364). New York: Academic Press.

Herbert, M. (1964). The concept and testing of brain damage in children: A review. *Journal of Child Psychology and Psychiatry, 5,* 197–217.

Hertzig, M. E., Bortner, M., & Birch, H. G. (1969). Neurologic findings in children educationally designated as "brain damaged." *American Journal of Orthopsychiatry, 39,* 437–447.

Hervey, A. S., Epstein, J. N., & Curry, J. F. (2004). Neuropsychology of adults with attention-deficit/hyperactivity disorder: A meta-analytic review. *Neuropsychology, 18,* 495–503.

Hinshaw, S. P. (1987). On the distinction between attentional deficits/hyperactivity and conduct problems/aggression in child psychopathology. *Psychological Bulletin, 101,* 443–447.

Hinshaw, S. P., Henker, B., & Whalen, C. K. (1984). Cognitive-behavioral and pharmacologic interventions for hyperactive boys: Comparative and combined effects. *Journal of Consulting and Clinical Psychology, 52,* 739–749.

Hoffman, H. (1865). Die Geschichte vom Zappel-Philipp. In H. Hoffman, *Der Struwwelpeter.* Erlangen, Germany: Pestalozzi-Verlag.

Huessy, H. J. (1974). The adult hyperkinetic [Letter to the editor]. *American Journal of Psychiatry, 131,* 724–725.

Humphries, T., Kinsbourne, M., & Swanson, J. (1978). Stimulant effects on cooperation and social interaction between hyperactive children and their mothers. *Journal of Child Psychology and Psychiatry, 19,* 13–22.

Hunt, R. D., Caper, L., & O'Connell, P. (1990). Clonidine in child and adolescent psychiatry. *Journal of Child and Adolescent Psychopharmacology, 1,* 87–102.

Hunt, R. D., Cohen, D. J., Anderson, G., & Minderaa, R. B. (1988). Noradrenergic mechanisms in ADD + H. In L. M. Bloomingdale (Ed.), *Attention deficit disorder: Vol. 3: New research in attention, treatment, and psychopharmacology* (pp. 129–148). New York: Pergamon Press.

Hunt, R. D., Minderaa, R., & Cohen, D. J. (1985). Clonidine benefits children with attention deficit disorder and hyperactivity: Report of a double-blind placebo crossover therapeutic trial. *Journal of the American Academy of Child and Adolescent Psychiatry, 24,* 617–629.

Hynd, G. W., Hern, K. L., Novey, E. S., Eliopulos, D., Marshall, R., Gonzalez, J. J., et al. (1993). Attention-deficit hyperactivity disorder and asymmetry of the caudate nucleus. *Journal of Child Neurology, 8,* 339–347.

Hynd, G. W., Semrud-Clikeman, M., Lorys, A. R., Novey, E. S., & Eliopulos, D. (1990). Brain morphology in developmental dyslexia and attention deficit disorder/hyperactivity. *Archives of Neurology, 47,* 919–926.

Hynd, G. W., Semrud-Clikeman, M., Lorys, A. R., Novey, E. S., Eliopulos, D., & Lyytinen, H. (1991). Corpus callosum morphology in attention deficit-hyperactivity disorder: Morphometric analysis of MRI. *Journal of Learning Disabilities, 24,* 141–146.

James, W. (1950). *The principles of psychology.* New York: Dover. (Original work published 1890)

Kahn, E., & Cohen, L. H. (1934). Organic driveness: A brain stem syndrome and an experience. *New England Journal of Medicine, 210,* 748–756.

Kalverboer, A. F. (1988). Hyperactivity and observational studies. In L. M. Bloomingdale & J. Sergeant (Eds.), *Attention deficit disorder: Criteria, cognition, intervention* (pp. 29–42). New York: Pergamon Press.

Kelly, K., & Ramundo, P. (1992). *You mean I'm not lazy, stupid, or crazy?* Cincinnati, OH: Tyrell & Jerem.

Kelsoe, J. R., Ginns, E. I., Egeland, J. A., Gerhard, D. S., Goldstein, A. M., Bale, S. J., et al. (1989). Re-evaluation of the linkage relationship between chromosome 11p loci and the gene for bipolar affective disorder in the Old Order Amish. *Nature, 342,* 238–243.

Kendall, P. C., & Braswell, L. (1985). *Cognitive-behavioral therapy for impulsive children.* New York: Guilford Press.

Kessler, J. W. (1980). History of minimal brain dysfunction. In H. Rie & E. Rie (Eds.), *Handbook of minimal brain dysfunctions: A critical view* (pp. 18–52). New York: Wiley.

Kinsbourne, M. (1977). The mechanism of hyperactivity. In M. Blau, I. Rapin, & M. Kinsbourne (Eds.), *Topics in child neurology* (pp. 289–306). New York: Spectrum.

Kirk, S. A. (1963). Behavioral diagnoses and remediation of learning disabilities. In *Proceedings of the annual meeting: Conference on exploration into the problems of the perceptually handicapped child* (Vol. 1, pp. 1–7). Evanston, IL.

Klorman, R. (1992). Cognitive event-related potentials

in attention deficit disorder. In S. E. Shaywitz & B. A. Shaywitz (Eds.), *Attention deficit disorder comes of age: Toward the twenty-first century* (pp. 221–244). Austin, TX: PRO-ED.

Knights, R. M., & Bakker, D. (Eds.). (1976). *The neuropsychology of learning disorders*. Baltimore: University Park Press.

Knights, R. M., & Bakker, D. (Eds.). (1980). *Treatment of hyperactive and learning disordered children*. Baltimore: University Park Press.

Knobel, M., Wolman, M. B., & Mason, E. (1959). Hyperkinesis and organicity in children. *Archives of General Psychiatry, 1*, 310–321.

Laccetti, S. (1988, August 13). Parents who blame son's suicide on Ritalin use will join protest. *The Atlanta Journal*, pp. B1, B7.

Lahey, B. B., & Carlson, C. L. (1992). Validity of the diagnostic category of attention deficit disorder without hyperactivity: A review of the literature. In S. E. Shaywitz & B. A. Shaywitz (Eds.), *Attention deficit disorder comes of age: Toward the twenty-first century* (pp. 119–144). Austin, TX: PRO-ED.

Lahey, B. B., Pelham, W. E., Schaughency, E. A., Atkins, M. S., Murphy, H. A., Hynd, G. W., et al. (1988). Dimensions and types of attention deficit disorder with hyperactivity in children: A factor and cluster-analytic approach. *Journal of the American Academy of Child and Adolescent Psychiatry, 27*, 330–335.

LaHoste, G. J., Swanson, J. M., Wigal, S. B., Glabe, C., Wigal, T., King, N., et al. (1996). Dopamine D4 receptor gene polymorphism is associated with attention deficit hyperactivity disorder. *Molecular Psychiatry, 1*, 121–124.

Lambert, N. M. (1988). Adolescent outcomes for hyperactive children. *American Psychologist, 43*, 786–799.

Laufer, M., & Denhoff, E. (1957). Hyperkinetic behavior syndrome in children. *Journal of Pediatrics, 50*, 463–474.

Laufer, M., Denhoff, E., & Solomons, G. (1957). Hyperkinetic impulse disorder in children's behavior problems. *Psychosomatic Medicine, 19*, 38–49.

Levin, P. M. (1938). Restlessness in children. *Archives of Neurology and Psychiatry, 39*, 764–770.

Levy, F., & Hay, D. (1992, February). *ADHD in twins and their siblings*. Paper presented at the meeting of the International Society for Research in Child and Adolescent Psychopathology, Sarasota, FL.

Loeber, R. (1990). Development and risk factors of juvenile antisocial behavior and delinquency. *Clinical Psychology Review, 10*, 1–42.

Loney, J. (1983). Research diagnostic criteria for childhood hyperactivity. In S. B. Guze, F. J. Earls, & J. E. Barrett (Eds.), *Childhood psychopathology and development* (pp. 109–137). New York: Raven Press.

Loney, J., Langhorne, J., & Paternite, C. (1978). An empirical basis for subgrouping the hyperkinetic/minimal brain dysfunction syndrome. *Journal of Abnormal Psychology, 87*, 431–444.

Loney, J., & Milich, R. (1982). Hyperactivity, inatten-

tion, and aggression in clinical practice. In D. Routh & M. Wolraich (Eds.), *Advances in developmental and behavioral pediatrics* (Vol. 3, pp. 113–147). Greenwich, CT: JAI Press.

Lou, H. C., Henriksen, L., & Bruhn, P. (1984). Focal cerebral hypoperfusion in children with dysphasia and/or attention deficit disorder. *Archives of Neurology, 41*, 825–829.

Lou, H. C., Henriksen, L., Bruhn, P., Borner, H., & Nielsen, J. B. (1989). Striatal dysfunction in attention deficit and hyperkinetic disorder. *Archives of Neurology, 46*, 48–52.

Mann, H. B., & Greenspan, S. I. (1976). The identification and treatment of adult brain dysfunction. *American Journal of Psychiatry, 133*, 1013–1017.

Mannuzza, S., Gittelman-Klein, R., Bessler, A., Malloy, P., & LaPadula, M. (1993). Adult outcome of hyperactive boys: Educational achievement, occupational rank, and psychiatric status. *Archives of General Psychiatry, 50*, 565–576.

Marwitt, S. J., & Stenner, A. J. (1972). Hyperkinesis: Delineation of two patterns. *Exceptional Children, 38*, 401–406.

Mash, E. J., & Johnston, C. (1982). A comparison of mother–child interactions of younger and older hyperactive and normal children. *Child Development, 53*, 1371–1381.

Mash, E. J., & Johnston, C. (1983). Sibling interactions of hyperactive and normal children and their relationship to reports of maternal stress and self-esteem. *Journal of Clinical Child Psychology, 12*, 91–99.

Mattes, J. A. (1980). The role of frontal lobe dysfunction in childhood hyperkinesis. *Comprehensive Psychiatry, 21*, 358–369.

Maynard, R. (1970, June 29). Omaha pupils given "behavior" drugs. *The Washington Post*.

McGee, R., Williams, S., Moffitt, T., & Anderson, J. (1989). A comparison of 13-year old boys with attention deficit and/or reading disorder on neuropsychological measures. *Journal of Abnormal Child Psychology, 17*, 37–53.

McGee, R., Williams, S., & Silva, P. A. (1984a). Behavioral and developmental characteristics of aggressive, hyperactive, and aggressive–hyperactive boys. *Journal of the American Academy of Child Psychiatry, 23*, 270–279.

McGee, R., Williams, S., & Silva, P. A. (1984b). Background characteristics of aggressive, hyperactive, and aggressive–hyperactive boys. *Journal of the American Academy of Child Psychiatry, 23*, 280–284.

Meichenbaum, D. (1977). *Cognitive behavior modification: An integrative approach*. New York: Plenum Press.

Meichenbaum, D. (1988). Cognitive behavioral modification with attention deficit hyperactive children. In L. M. Bloomingdale & J. Sergeant (Eds.), *Attention deficit disorder: Criteria, cognition, intervention* (pp. 127–140). New York: Pergamon Press.

Meichenbaum, D., & Goodman, J. (1971). Training impulsive children to talk to themselves: A means of developing self-control. *Journal of Abnormal Psychology, 77,* 115–126.

Mendelson, W., Johnson, N., & Stewart, M. A. (1971). Hyperactive children as teenagers: A follow-up study. *Journal of Nervous and Mental Disease, 153,* 273–279.

Menkes, M., Rowe, J., & Menkes, J. (1967). A five-year follow-up study on the hyperactive child with minimal brain dysfunction. *Pediatrics, 39,* 393–399.

Meyer, E., & Byers, R. K. (1952). Measles encephalitis: A follow-up study of sixteen patients. *American Journal of Diseases of Children, 84,* 543–579.

Milich, R., Ballentine, A. C., & Lynam, D. R. (2001). ADHD/combined type and ADHD/predominantly inattentive type are distinct and unrelated disorders. *Clinical Psychology: Science and Practice, 8,* 463–488.

Milich, R., Hartung, C. M., Martin, C. A., & Haigler, E. D. (1994). Behavioral disinhibition and underlying processes in adolescents with disruptive behavior disorders. In D. K. Routh (Ed.), *Disruptive behavior disorders in childhood* (pp. 109–138). New York: Plenum Press.

Milich, R., & Loney, J. (1979). The role of hyperactive and aggressive symptomatology in predicting adolescent outcome among hyperactive children. *Journal of Pediatric Psychology, 4,* 93–112.

Milich, R., Pelham, W., & Hinshaw, S. (1985). Issues in the diagnosis of attention deficit disorder: A cautionary note. *Psychopharmacology Bulletin, 22,* 1101–1104.

Milich, R., Wolraich, M., & Lindgren, S. (1986). Sugar and hyperactivity: A critical review of empirical findings. *Clinical Psychology Review, 6,* 493–513.

Molitch, M., & Eccles, A. K. (1937). Effect of benzedrine sulphate on intelligence scores of children. *American Journal of Psychiatry, 94,* 587–590.

Morrison, J. R., & Minkoff, K. (1975). Explosive personality as a sequel to the hyperactive child syndrome. *Comprehensive Psychiatry, 16,* 343–348.

Morrison, J. R., & Stewart, M. (1973). The psychiatric status of the legal families of adopted hyperactive children. *Archives of General Psychiatry, 28,* 888–891.

MTA Cooperative Group. (1999). A 14-month randomized clinical trial of treatment strategies for attention-deficit/hyperactivity disorder. *Archives of General Psychiatry, 56,* 1073–1086.

Murphy, K. R., & Barkley, R. A. (1996). Attention deficit hyperactivity disorder in adults. *Comprehensive Psychiatry, 37,* 393–401.

Murphy, K. R., & LeVert, S. (1994). *Out of the fog.* New York: Hyperion.

Nadeau, K. (1995). *A comprehensive guide to adults with attention deficit hyperactivity disorder.* New York: Brunner/Mazel.

National Advisory Committee on Hyperkinesis and Food Additives. (1980). [Report]. New York: Nutrition Foundation.

Nigg, J. T. (2001). Is ADHD an inhibitory disorder? *Psychological Bulletin, 125,* 571–596.

Nightline. (1988). [Segment on Ritalin controversy]. New York: American Broadcasting Company.

Offord, D. R., Boyle, M. H., Szatmari, P., Rae-Grant, N., Links, P. S., Cadman, D. T., et al. (1987). Ontario Child Health Study: Six month prevalence of disorder and rates of service utilization. *Archives of General Psychiatry, 44,* 832–836.

O'Leary, K. D. (1981). Assessment of hyperactivity: Observational and rating scale methodologies. In S. A. Miller (Ed.), *Nutrition and behavior* (pp. 291–298). Philadelphia: Franklin Institute Press.

O'Leary, K. D., Pelham, W. E., Rosenbaum., A., &, Price, G. H. (1976). Behavioral treatment of hyperkinetic children: An experimental evaluation of its usefulness. *Clinical Pediatrics, 15,* 510–515.

Ounsted, C. (1955). The hyperkinetic syndrome in epileptic children. *Lancet, 53,* 303–311.

Packer, S. (1978). Treatment of minimal brain dysfunction in a young adult. *Canadian Psychiatric Association Journal, 23,* 501–502.

Parry, P. A., & Douglas, V. I. (1976). *The effects of reward on the performance of hyperactive children.* Unpublished doctoral dissertation, McGill University.

Pasamanick, B., Rogers, M., & Lilienfeld, A. M. (1956). Pregnancy experience and the development of behavior disorder in children. *American Journal of Psychiatry, 112,* 613–617.

Paternite, C., & Loney, J. (1980). Childhood hyperkinesis: Relationships between symptomatology and home environment. In C. K. Whalen & B. Henker (Eds.), *Hyperactive children: The social ecology of identification and treatment* (pp. 105–141). New York: Academic Press.

Patterson, G. R. (1982). *Coercive family process.* Eugene, OR: Castalia.

Patterson, G. R. (1986). Performance models for antisocial boys. *American Psychologist, 41,* 432–444.

Pauls, D. L. (1991). Genetic factors in the expression of attention-deficit hyperactivity disorder. *Journal of Child and Adolescent Psychopharmacology, 1,* 353–360.

Pelham, W. E. (1977). Withdrawal of a stimulant drug and concurrent behavior intervention in the treatment of a hyperactive child. *Behavior Therapy, 8,* 473–479.

Pelham, W. E., Schnedler, R., Bologna, N., & Contreras, A. (1980). Behavioral and stimulant treatment of hyperactive children: A therapy study with methylphenidate probes in a within subject design. *Journal of Applied Behavior Analysis, 13,* 221–236.

Pennington, B. F., & Ozonoff, S. (1996). Executive functions and developmental psychopathology. *Journal of Child Psychology and Psychiatry, 37,* 51–87.

Pfiffner, L. J., & McBurnett, K. (1997). Social skills training with parent generalization: Treatment effects for children with attention deficit disorder. *Journal of Consulting and Clinical Psychology, 65,* 749–757.

Pfiffner, L. J., & O'Leary, S. G. (1987). The efficacy of all-positive management as a function of the prior use of negative consequences. *Journal of Applied Behavior Analysis, 20,* 265–271.

Pliszka, S. R. (1987). Tricyclic antidepressants in the treatment of children with attention deficit disorder. *Journal of the American Academy of Child and Adolescent Psychiatry, 26,* 127–132.

Pliszka, S. R. (1998). Comorbidity of attention-deficit/hyperactivity disorder with psychiatric disorder: an overview. *Journal of Clinical Psychiatry, 59*(Suppl. 7), 50–58.

Pontius, A. A. (1973). Dysfunction patterns analogous to frontal lobe system and caudate nucleus syndromes in some groups of minimal brain dysfunction. *Journal of the American Medical Women's Association, 26,* 285–292.

Prechtl, H., & Stemmer, C. (1962). The choreiform syndrome in children. *Developmental Medicine and Child Neurology, 8,* 149–159.

Psychiatrist sued over attention span drug. (1987, November 10). *Investors' Daily,* p. 26.

Quay, H. C. (1988a). The behavioral reward and inhibition systems in childhood behavior disorder. In L. M. Bloomingdale (Ed.), *Attention deficit disorder: Vol. 3. New research in treatment, psychopharmacology, and attention* (pp. 176–186). New York: Pergamon Press.

Quay, H. C. (1988b). Attention deficit disorder and the behavioral inhibition system: The relevance of the neuropsychological theory of Jeffrey A. Gray. In L. M. Bloomingdale & J. Sergeant (Eds.), *Attention deficit disorder: Criteria, cognition, intervention* (pp. 117–126). New York: Pergamon Press.

Quay, H. F. (1997). Inhibition and attention deficit hyperactivity disorder. *Journal of Abnormal Child Psychology, 25,* 7–14.

Quitkin, F., & Klein, D. F. (1969). Two behavioral syndromes in young adults related to possible minimal brain dysfunction. *Journal of Psychiatric Research, 7,* 131–142.

Rapin, I. (1964). Brain damage in children. In J. Brennemann (Ed.), *Practice of pediatrics* (Vol. 4). Hagerstown, MD: Prior.

Rapoport, J. L., & Zametkin, A. (1988). Drug treatment of attention deficit disorder. In L. M. Bloomingdale & J. Sergeant (Eds.), *Attention deficit disorder: Criteria, cognition, intervention* (pp. 161–182). New York: Pergamon Press.

Rhee, S. H., Waldman, I. D., Hay, D. A., & Levy, F. (1995). Sex differences in genetic and environmental influences on DSM-III-R attention-deficit hyperactivity disorder (ADHD). *Behavior Genetics, 25,* 285.

Rie, H. E., & Rie, E. D. (Eds.). (1980). *Handbook of minimal brain dysfunction: A critical review.* New York: Wiley.

Rise in Ritalin use could mean drug abuse. (1987, December 6). *Worcester Telegram and Gazette* [Worcester, MA].

Ritalin linked to bludgeoning death of teenager. (1988, March 8). *The Call* [Woonsocket, RI], p. 3.

Roberts, M. A. (1979). *A manual for the Restricted Academic Playroom Situation.* Iowa City, IA: Author.

Robin, A., & Foster, S. (1989). *Negotiating parent–adolescent conflict.* New York: Guilford Press.

Rosenthal, R. H., & Allen, T. W. (1978). An examination of attention, arousal, and learning dysfunctions of hyperkinetic children. *Psychological Bulletin, 85,* 689–715.

Ross, D. M., & Ross, S. A. (1976). *Hyperactivity: Research, theory, and action.* New York: Wiley.

Ross, D. M., & Ross, S. A. (1982). *Hyperactivity: Current issues, research, and theory.* New York: Wiley.

Routh, D. K. (1978). Hyperactivity. In P. Magrab (Ed.), *Psychological management of pediatric problems* (pp. 3–48). Baltimore: University Park Press.

Routh, D. K., & Schroeder, C. S. (1976). Standardized playroom measures as indices of hyperactivity. *Journal of Abnormal Child Psychology, 4,* 199–207.

Rutter, M. (1977). Brain damage syndromes in childhood: Concepts and findings. *Journal of Child Psychology and Psychiatry, 18,* 1–21.

Rutter, M. (1982). Syndromes attributable to "minimal brain dysfunction" in childhood. *American Journal of Psychiatry, 139,* 21–33.

Rutter, M. (1983). Introduction: Concepts of brain dysfunction syndromes. In M. Rutter (Ed.), *Developmental neuropsychiatry* (pp. 1–14). New York: Guilford Press.

Rutter, M. (1988). DSM-III-R: A postscript. In M. Rutter, A. H. Tuma, & I. S. Lann (Eds.), *Assessment and diagnosis in child psychopathology* (pp. 453–464). New York: Guilford Press.

Rutter, M. (1989). Attention deficit disorder/hyperkinetic syndrome: Conceptual and research issues regarding diagnosis and classification. In T. Sagvolden & T. Archer (Eds.), *Attention deficit disorder: Clinical and basic research* (pp. 1–24). Hillsdale, NJ: Erlbaum.

Ryan, N. D. (1990). Heterocyclic antidepressants in children and adolescents. *Journal of Child and Adolescent Psychopharmacology, 1,* 21–32.

Rybak, W. S. (1977). More adult minimal brain dysfunction. *American Journal of Psychiatry, 134,* 96–97.

Safer, D. J., & Allen, R. (1976). *Hyperactive children.* Baltimore: University Park Press.

Sagvolden, T., Wultz, B., Moser, E. I., Moser, M., & Morkrid, L. (1989). Results from a comparative neuropsychological research program indicate altered reinforcement mechanisms in children with ADD. In T. Sagvolden & T. Archer (Eds.), *Attention deficit disorder: Clinical and basic research* (pp. 261–286). Hillsdale, NJ: Erlbaum.

Satterfield, J. H., Satterfield, B. T., & Cantwell, D. P. (1981). Three-year multimodality treatment study of 100 hyperactive boys. *Journal of Pediatrics, 98,* 650–655.

Schachar, R. J. (1986). Hyperkinetic syndrome: Historical development of the concept. In E. A. Taylor (Ed.), *The overactive child* (pp. 19–40). Philadelphia: Lippincott.

Schachar, R. J., Rutter, M., & Smith, A. (1981). The characteristics of situationally and pervasively hyperactive children: Implications for syndrome definition. *Journal of Child Psychology and Psychiatry, 22,* 375–392.

Schachar, R. J., Tannock, R., & Logan, G. (1993). Inhibitory control, impulsiveness, and attention deficit hyperactivity disorder. *Clinical Psychology Review, 13,* 721–739.

Schrag, P., & Divoky, D. (1975). *The myth of the hyperactive child.* New York: Pantheon.

Semrud-Clikeman, M., Filipek, P. A., Biederman, J., Steingard, R., Kennedy, D., Renshaw, P., et al. (1994). Attention-deficit hyperactivity disorder: Magnetic resonance imaging morphometric analysis of the corpus callosum. *Journal of the American Academy of Child and Adolescent Psychiatry, 33,* 875–881.

Sergeant, J. (1988). From DSM-III attentional deficit disorder to functional defects. In L. M. Bloomingdale & J. Sergeant (Eds.), *Attention deficit disorder: Criteria, cognition, intervention* (pp. 183–198). New York: Pergamon Press.

Sergeant, J., & van der Meere, J. J. (1989). The diagnostic significance of attentional processing: Its significance for ADD + H classification—A future DSM. In T. Sagvolden & T. Archer (Eds.), *Attention deficit disorder: Clinical and basic research* (pp. 151–166). Hillsdale, NJ: Erlbaum.

Sergeant, J., & van der Meere, J. J. (1994). Toward an empirical child psychopathology. In D. K. Routh (Ed.), *Disruptive behavior disorders in children* (pp. 59–86). New York: Plenum Press.

Shaffer, D. (1994). Attention deficit hyperactivity disorder in adults. *American Journal of Psychiatry, 151,* 633–638.

Shalev, R. S., Hartman, C. A., Stavsky, M., & Sergeant, J. A. (1995). Conners Rating Scales of Israeli children. In J. Sergeant (Ed.), *Eunethydis: European approaches to hyperkinetic disorder* (pp. 131–147). Amsterdam: University of Amsterdam.

Shaywitz, S. E., Shaywitz, B. A., Cohen, D. J., & Young, J. G. (1983). Monoaminergic mechanisms in hyperactivity. In M. Rutter (Ed.), *Developmental neuropsychiatry* (pp. 330–347). New York: Guilford Press.

Shekim, W. O., Asarnow, R. F., Hess, E., Zaucha, K., & Wheeler, N. (1990). A clinical and demographic profile of a sample of adults with attention deficit hyperactivity disorder, residual state. *Comprehensive Psychiatry, 31,* 416–425.

Shekim, W. O., Glaser, E., Horwitz, E., Javaid, J., & Dylund, D. B. (1988). Psychoeducational correlates of catecholamine metabolites in hyperactive children. In L. M. Bloomingdale (Ed.), *Attention deficit disorder: New research in attention, treatment, and psychopharmacology* (Vol. 3, pp. 149–150). New York: Pergamon Press.

Shelley, E. M., & Riester, A. (1972). Syndrome of minimal brain damage in young adults. *Diseases of the Nervous System, 33,* 335–339.

Shelton, T. L., Barkley, R. A., Crosswait, C., Moorehouse, M., Fletcher, K., Barrett, S., et al. (2000). Multimethod psychoeducational intervention for preschool children with disruptive behavior: Two-year post-treatment follow-up. *Journal of Abnormal Child Psychology, 28,* 253–266.

Shirley, M. (1939). A behavior syndrome characterizing prematurely born children. *Child Development, 10,* 115–128.

Silberg, J., Rutter, M., Meyer, J., Maes, H., Hewitt, J., Simonoff, E., et al. (1996). Genetic and environmental influences on the covariation between hyperactivity and conduct disturbance in juvenile twins. *Journal of Child Psychology and Psychiatry, 37,* 803–816.

Skinner, N. (1988, June 22). Dyslexic boy's parents sue school. *Roanoke Gazette* [Roanoke, VA].

Solomons, G. (1965). The hyperactive child. *Journal of the Iowa Medical Society, 55,* 464–469.

Spencer, T., Biederman, J., Wilens, T., & Faraone, S. V. (1994). Is attention-deficit hyperactivity disorder in adults a valid disorder? *Harvard Review of Psychiatry, 1,* 326–335.

Spencer, T., Wilens, T., Biederman, J., Faraone, S. V., Ablon, S., & Lapey, K. (1995). A double-blind, crossover comparison of methylphenidate and placebo in adults with childhood onset attention-deficit hyperactivity disorder. *Archives of General Psychiatry, 52,* 434–443.

Spitzer, R. L., Davies, M., & Barkley, R. A. (1990). The DSM-III-R field trial for the disruptive behavior disorders. *Journal of the American Academy of Child and Adolescent Psychiatry, 29,* 690–697.

Sprague, R. L., Barnes, K. R., & Werry, J. S. (1970). Methylphenidate and thioridazine: Learning, activity, and behavior in emotionally disturbed boys. *American Journal of Orthopsychiatry, 40,* 613–628.

Sroufe, L. A. (1975). Drug treatment of children with behavior problems. In F. Horowitz (Ed.), *Review of child development research* (Vol. 4, pp. 347–408). Chicago: University of Chicago Press.

Stevenson, J. (1994, June). *Genetics of ADHD.* Paper presented at the Professional Group for ADD and Related Disorders, London.

Stewart, M. A., deBlois, S., & Cummings, C. (1980). Psychiatric disorder in the parents of hyperactive boys and those with conduct disorder. *Journal of Child Psychology and Psychiatry, 21,* 283–292.

Stewart, M. A. (1970). Hyperactive children. *Scientific American, 222,* 94–98.

Still, G. F. (1902). Some abnormal psychical conditions in children. *Lancet, i,* 1008–1012, 1077–1082, 1163–1168.

Strauss, A. A., & Lehtinen, L. E. (1947). *Psychopathology and education of the brain-injured child.* New York: Grune & Stratton.

Strecker, E., & Ebaugh, F. (1924). Neuropsychiatric

sequelae of cerebral trauma in children. *Archives of Neurology and Psychiatry, 12,* 443–453.

Stryker, S. (1925). Encephalitis lethargica: The behavior residuals. *Training School Bulletin, 22,* 152–157.

Swanson, J. M., McBurnett, K., Christian, D. L., & Wigal, T. (1995). Stimulant medications and the treatment of children with ADHD. In T. H. Ollendick & R. J. Prinz (Eds.), *Advances in clinical child psychology* (Vol. 17, pp. 265–322). New York: Plenum Press.

Swanson, J. M., Wigal, S., Greenhill, L., Browne, R., Waslick, B., Lerner, M., et al. (1998). Analog classroom assessment of Adderall in children with ADHD. *Journal of the American Academy of Child and Adolescent Psychiatry, 37,* 519–526.

Tannock, R. (2000). Attention-deficit/hyperactivity disorder with anxiety disorders. In T. E. Brown (Ed.), *Attention deficit disorders and comorbidities in children, adolescents, and adults* (pp. 125–170). Washington, DC: American Psychiatric Press.

Taylor, E. A. (1983). Drug response and diagnostic validation. In M. Rutter (Ed.), *Developmental neuropsychiatry* (pp. 348–368). New York: Guilford Press.

Taylor, E. A. (Ed.). (1986). *The overactive child.* Philadelphia: Lippincott.

Taylor, E. A. (1988). Diagnosis of hyperactivity: A British perspective. In L. M. Bloomingdale & J. Sergeant (Eds.), *Attention deficit disorder: Criteria, cognition, intervention* (pp. 141–160). New York: Pergamon Press.

Taylor, E. A. (1989). On the epidemiology of hyperactivity. In T. Sagvolden & T. Archer (Eds.), *Attention deficit disorder: Clinical and basic research* (pp. 31–52). Hillsdale, NJ: Erlbaum.

Thapar, A., Hervas, A., & McGuffin, P. (1995). Childhood hyperactivity scores are highly heritable and show sibling competition effects: Twin study evidence. *Behavior Genetics, 25,* 537–544.

Toone, B. K., & van der Linden, J. H. (1997). Attention deficit hyperactivity disorder or hyperkinetic disorder in adults. *British Journal of Psychiatry, 170,* 489–491.

Toufexis, A. (1989, January 16). Worries about overactive kids: Are too many youngsters being misdiagnosed and medicated? *Time,* p. 65.

Tredgold, A. F. (1908). *Mental deficiency (amentia).* New York: Wood.

Trites, R. L. (1979). *Hyperactivity in children: Etiology, measurement, and treatment implications.* Baltimore: University Park Press.

Twyman, A. S. (1988, May 4). Use of drug prompts suit. *Newton Graphic* [Newton, MA], p. 28.

Ullmann, R. K., Sleator, E. K., & Sprague, R. (1984). A new rating scale for diagnosis and monitoring of ADD children. *Psychopharmacology Bulletin, 20,* 160–164.

van den Oord, E. J. C. G., Verhulst, F. C., & Boomsma, D. I. (1996). A genetic study of maternal and paternal ratings of problem behaviors in 3-year-old twins. *Journal of Abnormal Psychology, 105,* 349–357.

van der Meere, J., & Sergeant, J. (1988a). Focused attention in pervasively hyperactive children. *Journal of Abnormal Child Psychology, 16,* 627–640.

van der Meere, J., & Sergeant, J. (1988b). Controlled processing and vigilance in hyperactivity: Time will tell. *Journal of Abnormal Child Psychology, 16,* 641–656.

Vermeersch, S., & Fombonne, E. (1995). Attention and aggressive problems among French school-aged children. In J. Sergeant (Ed.), *Eunethydis: European approaches to hyperkinetic disorder* (pp. 37–49). Amsterdam: University of Amsterdam.

Voelker, S. L., Lachar, D., & Gdowski, C. L. (1983). The Personality Inventory for Children and response to methylphenidate: Preliminary evidence for predictive validity. *Journal of Pediatric Psychology, 8,* 161–169.

Weiner, J. (1988, May 14). Diagnosis, treatment of ADHD requires skill. *Worcester Telegram and Gazette* [Worcester, MA], p. 14.

Weiss, G., & Hechtman, L. (1979). The hyperactive child syndrome. *Science, 205,* 1348–1354.

Weiss, G., & Hechtman, L. (1986). *Hyperactive children grown up.* New York: Guilford Press.

Weiss, G., & Hechtman, L. (1993). *Hyperactive children grown up* (2nd ed.). New York: Guilford Press.

Weiss, L. (1992). *ADD in adults.* Dallas, TX: Taylor.

Welner, Z., Welner, A., Stewart, M., Palkes, H., & Wish, E. (1977). A controlled study of siblings of hyperactive children. *Journal of Nervous and Mental Disease, 165,* 110–117.

Wender, P. H. (1971). *Minimal brain dysfunction.* New York: Wiley.

Wender, P. H. (1973). Minimal brain dysfunction in children. *Pediatric Clinics of North America, 20,* 187–202.

Wender, P. H. (1995). *Attention-deficit hyperactivity disorder in adults.* New York: Oxford University Press.

Wender, P. H., Reimherr, F. W., & Wood, D. R. (1981). Attention deficit disorder ("minimal brain dysfunction") in adults. *Archives of General Psychiatry, 38,* 449–456.

Wender, P. H., Reimherr, F. W., Wood, D. R., & Ward, M. (1985). A controlled study of methylphenidate in the treatment of attention deficit disorder, residual type, in adults. *American Journal of Psychiatry, 142,* 547–552.

Werner, H., & Strauss, A. A. (1941). Pathology of figure–ground relation in the child. *Journal of Abnormal and Social Psychology, 36,* 236–248.

Werry, J. S. (1988). Differential diagnosis of attention deficits and conduct disorders. In L. M. Bloomingdale & J. A. Sergeant (Eds.), *Attention deficit disorder: Criteria, cognition, intervention* (pp. 83–96). New York: Pergamon Press.

Werry, J. S. (1992). History, terminology, and manifestations at different ages. *Child and Adolescent Psychiatric Clinics of North America, 1,* 297–310.

Werry, J. S., & Sprague, R. (1970). Hyperactivity. In C.

G. Costello (Ed.), *Symptoms of psychopathology* (pp. 397–417). New York: Wiley.

Whalen, C. K., & Henker, B. (1980). *Hyperactive children: The social ecology of identification and treatment.* New York: Academic Press.

Whalen, C. K., Henker, B., & Dotemoto, S. (1980). Methylphenidate and hyperactivity: Effects on teacher behaviors. *Science, 208,* 1280–1282.

Whalen, C. K., Henker, B., & Dotemoto, S. (1981). Teacher response to methylphenidate (Ritalin) versus placebo status of hyperactive boys in the classroom. *Child Development, 52,* 1005–1014.

Whalen, C. K., Henker, B., & Hinshaw, S. (1985). Cognitive behavioral therapies for hyperactive children: Premises, problems, and prospects. *Journal of Abnormal Child Psychology, 13,* 391–410.

Wilens, T., Biederman, J., Prince, J., Spencer, T. J., Faraone, S. V., Warburton, R., et al. (1996). Six-week, double-blind, placebo-controlled study of desipramine for adult attention deficit hyperactivity disorder. *American Journal of Psychiatry, 153,* 1147–1153.

Williams, L. (1988, January 15). Parents and doctors fear growing misuse of drug used to treat hyperactive kids. *The Wall Street Journal,* p. 10.

Willis, T. J., & Lovaas, I. (1977). A behavioral approach to treating hyperactive children: The parent's role. In J. B. Millichap (Ed.), *Learning disabilities and related disorders* (pp. 119–140). Chicago: Year Book Medical.

Wolraich, M. L., Wilson, D. B., & White, J. W. (1995). The effect of sugar on behavior or cognition in children: A meta-analysis. *Journal of the American Medical Association, 274,* 1617–1621.

Wood, D. R., Reimherr, F. W., Wender, P. H., & Johnson, G. E. (1976). Diagnosis and treatment of minimal brain dysfunction in adults: A preliminary report. *Archives of General Psychiatry, 33,* 1453–1460.

World Health Organization. (1978). *International classification of diseases* (9th rev.). Geneva, Switzerland: Author.

Zametkin, A. J., Nordahl, T. E., Gross, M., King, A. C., Semple, W. E., Rumsey, J., et al. (1990). Cerebral glucose metabolism in adults with hyperactivity of childhood onset. *New England Journal of Medicine, 323,* 1361–1366.

Zametkin, A., & Rapoport, J. L. (1986). The pathophysiology of attention deficit disorder with hyperactivity: A review. In B. Lahey & A. Kazdin (Eds.), *Advances in clinical child psychology* (Vol. 9, pp. 177–216). New York: Plenum Press.

Zentall, S. S. (1985). A context for hyperactivity. In K. D. Gadow & I. Bialer (Eds.), *Advances in learning and behavioral disabilities* (Vol. 4, pp. 273–343). Greenwich, CT: JAI Press.

APPENDIX A.
International Consensus Statement on ADHD

We, the undersigned consortium of international scientists, are deeply concerned about the periodic inaccurate portrayal of attention deficit hyperactivity disorder (ADHD) in media reports. This is a disorder with which we are all very familiar and toward which many of us have dedicated scientific studies if not entire careers. We fear that inaccurate stories rendering ADHD as myth, fraud, or benign condition may cause thousands of sufferers not to seek treatment for their disorder. It also leaves the public with a general sense that this disorder is not valid or real or consists of a rather trivial affliction.

We have created this consensus statement on ADHD as a reference on the status of the scientific findings concerning this disorder, its validity, and its adverse impact on the lives of those diagnosed with the disorder as of this writing (January 2002).

Occasional coverage of the disorder casts the story in the form of a sporting event with evenly matched competitors. The views of a handful of nonexpert doctors that ADHD does not exist are contrasted against mainstream scientific views that it does, as if both views had equal merit. Such attempts at balance give the public the impression that there is substantial scientific disagreement over whether ADHD is a real medical condition. In fact, there is no such disagreement—at least no more so than there is over whether smoking causes cancer, for example, or whether a virus causes HIV/AIDS.

The U.S. Surgeon General, the American Medical Association, the American Psychiatric Association, the American Academy of Child and Adolescent Psychiatry, the American Psychological Association, and the American Academy of Pediatrics, among others, all recognize ADHD as a valid disorder. Although some of these organizations have issued guidelines for evaluation and management of the disorder for their membership, this is the first consensus statement issued by an independent consortium of leading scientists concerning the status of the disorder. Among scientists who have devoted years, if not entire careers, to the study of this disorder there is no controversy regarding its existence.

ADHD and Science

We cannot overemphasize the point that, as a matter of science, the notion that ADHD does not exist is simply wrong. All of the major medical associations and government health agencies recognize ADHD as a genuine disorder because the scientific evidence indicating it is so overwhelming.

Various approaches have been used to establish whether a condition rises to the level of a valid medical or psychiatric disorder. A very useful one stipulates that there must be scientifically established evidence that those suffering the condition have a serious deficiency in or failure of a physical or psychological mechanism that is universal to humans. That is, all humans normally would be expected, regardless of culture, to have developed that mental ability.

And there must be equally incontrovertible scientific evidence that this serious deficiency leads to harm to the individual. Harm is established through evidence of increased mortality, morbidity, or impairment in the major life activities required of one's developmental stage in life. Major life ctivities are those domains of functioning such as education, social relationships, family functioning, independence and self-sufficiency, and occupational functioning that all humans of that developmental level are expected to perform.

As attested to by the numerous scientists signing this document, there is no question among the world's leading clinical researchers that ADHD involves a serious deficiency in a set of psychological abilities and that these deficiencies pose serious harm to most individuals possessing the disorder. Current evidence indicates that deficits in behavioral inhibition and sustained attention are central to this

Address all correspondence to Russell A. Barkley, PhD, Department of Psychiatry and Neurology, University of Massachusetts Medical School, 55 Lake Avenue North, Worcester, Massachusetts 01655; e-mail: barkleyr@ummhc.org.

From *Clinical Child and Family Psychology Review*, 2002, 5(2), 89–111. Copyright 2002 by Kluwer Academic Publishers B. V. (now Springer Science + Business Media B. V.). Reprinted with permission of the author (R. A. Barkley) and publisher.

disorder—facts demonstrated through hundreds of scientific studies. And there is no doubt that ADHD leads to impairments in major life activities, including social relations, education, family functioning, occupational functioning, self-sufficiency, and adherence to social rules, norms, and laws. Evidence also indicates that those with ADHD are more prone to physical injury and accidental poisonings. This is why no professional medical, psychological, or scientific organization doubts the existence of ADHD as a legitimate disorder.

The central psychological deficits in those with ADHD have now been linked through numerous studies using various scientific methods to several specific brain regions (the frontal lobe, its connections to the basal ganglia, and their relationship to the central aspects of the cerebellum). Most neurological studies find that as a group those with ADHD have less brain electrical activity and show less reactivity to stimulation in one or more of these regions. And neuro-imaging studies of groups of those with ADHD also demonstrate relatively smaller areas of brain matter and less metabolic activity of this brain matter than is the case in control groups used in these studies.

These same psychological deficits in inhibition and attention have been found in numerous studies of identical and fraternal twins conducted across various countries (US, Great Britain, Norway, Australia, etc.) to be primarily inherited. The genetic contribution to these traits is routinely found to be among the highest for any psychiatric disorder (70–95% of trait variation in the population), nearly approaching the genetic contribution to human height. One gene has recently been reliably demonstrated to be associated with this disorder and the search for more is underway by more than 12 different scientific teams worldwide at this time.

Numerous studies of twins demonstrate that family environment makes no significant separate contribution to these traits. This is not to say that the home environment, parental management abilities, stressful life events, or deviant peer relationships are unimportant or have no influence on individuals having this disorder, as they certainly do. Genetic tendencies are expressed in interaction with the environment. Also, those having ADHD often have other associated disorders and problems, some of which are clearly related to their social environments. But it is to say that the underlying psychological deficits that comprise ADHD itself are not solely or primarily the result of these environmental factors.

This is why leading international scientists, such as the signers below, recognize the mounting evidence of neurological and genetic contributions to this disorder. This evidence, coupled with countless studies on the harm posed by the disorder and hundreds of studies on the effectiveness of medication, buttresses the need in many, though by no means all, cases for management of the disorder with multiple therapies. These include medication combined with educational, family, and other social accommodations. This is in striking contrast to the wholly unscientific views of some social critics in periodic media accounts that ADHD constitutes a fraud, that medicating those afflicted is questionable if not reprehensible, and that any behavior problems associated with ADHD are merely the result of problems in the home, excessive viewing of TV or playing of video games, diet, lack of love and attention, or teacher/school intolerance.

ADHD is not a benign disorder. For those it afflicts, ADHD can cause devastating problems. Follow-up studies of clinical samples suggest that sufferers are far more likely than normal people to drop out of school (32–40%), to rarely complete college (5–10%), to have few or no friends (50–70%), to underperform at work (70–80%), to engage in antisocial activities (40–50%), and to use tobacco or illicit drugs more than normal. Moreover, children growing up with ADHD are more likely to experience teen pregnancy (40%) and sexually transmitted diseases (16%), to speed excessively and have multiple car accidents, to experience depression (20–30%) and personality disorders (18–25%) as adults, and in hundreds of other ways mismanage and endanger their lives.

Yet despite these serious consequences, studies indicate that less than half of those with the disorder are receiving treatment. The media can help substantially to improve these circumstances. It can do so by portraying ADHD and the science about it as accurately and responsibly as possible while not purveying the propaganda of some social critics and fringe doctors whose political agenda would have you and the public believe there is no real disorder here. To publish stories that ADHD is a fictitious disorder or merely a conflict between today's Huckleberry Finns and their caregivers is tantamount to declaring the earth flat, the laws of gravity debatable, and the periodic table in chemistry a fraud. ADHD should be depicted in the media as realistically and accurately as it is depicted in science—as a valid disorder having varied and substantial adverse impact on those who may suffer from it through no fault of their own or their parents and teachers.

Sincerely,

Russell A. Barkley, PhD
Professor
Departments of Psychiatry and Neurology
University of Massachusetts Medical School
55 Lake Avenue North
Worcester, MA 01655

Edwin H. Cook, Jr, MD
Professor
Departments of Psychiatry and Pediatrics
University of Chicago
5841 S. Maryland Avenue
Chicago, IL

Adele Diamond, PhD
Professor of Psychiatry
Director, Center for Developmental Cognitive
    Neuroscience
University of Massachusetts Medical School
Shriver Center, Trapelo Road
Waltham, MA

Alan Zametkin, MD
Child Psychiatrist
Kensington, MD

Anita Thapar, MB BCh, MRCPsych, PhD
Professor, Child and Adolescent Psychiatry
    Section
Department of Psychological Medicine
University of Wales College of Medicine
Heath Park, Cardiff CF14 4XN, United Kingdom

Ann Teeter, EdD
Director of Training, School of Psychology
University of Wisconsin – Milwaukee
Milwaukee, WI 53201

Arthur D. Anastopoulos, PhD
Professor, Co-Director of Clinical Training
Department of Psychology
University of North Carolina at Greensboro
P. O. Box 26164
Greensboro, NC 27402-6164

Avi Sadeh, DSc
Director, Clinical Child Psychology Graduate
    Program
Director, The Laboratory for Children's Sleep
    Disorders
Department of Psychology
Tel-Aviv University
Ramat Aviv, Tel Aviv 69978
Israel

Bennett L. Leventhal, MD
Irving B. Harris
Professor of Child and Adolescent Psychiatry
Director, Child and Adolescent Psychiatry
Vice Chairman, Department of Psychiatry
The University of Chicago
5841 S. Maryland Ave.
Chicago, IL 60637

Betsy Hoza, PhD
Associate Professor
Department of Psychology, #1364
Purdue University
West Lafayette, IN 47907-1364

Blythe Corbett, PhD
M.I.N.D. Institute
University of California, Davis
4860 Y Street, Suite 3020
Sacramento, CA 95817

Brooke Molina, PhD
Assistant Professor of Psychiatry and Psychology
Western Psychiatric Institute and Clinic
University of Pittsburgh School of Medicine
3811 O'Hara Street
Pittsburgh, PA 15213

Bruce Pennington, PhD
Professor
Department of Psychology
University of Denver
2155 South Race Street
Denver, CO 80208

Carl E. Paternite, PhD
Professor of Psychology
Miami University
Oxford, OH 45056

Carol Whalen, PhD
Professor
Department of Psychology and Social Behavior
University of California at Irvine
3340 Social Ecology II
Irvine, CA 02215

Caryn Carlson, PhD
Professor
Department of Psychology
University of Texas at Austin
Mezes 330
Austin, TX 78712

Charlotte Johnston, PhD
Professor
Department of Psychology
University of British Columbia
2136 West Mall
Vancouver, BC, Canada V6T 1Z4

Christopher Gillberg, MD
Professor
Department of Child and Adolescent Psychiatry
University of Gothenburg
Gothenburg, Sweden

Cynthia Hartung, PhD
Assistant Professor
Oklahoma State University
215 North Murray
Stillwater, OK 74078

Daniel A. Waschbusch, PhD
Assistant Professor of Psychology
Director, Child Behaviour Program
Department of Psychology
Dalhousie University
Halifax, Canada NS, B3H 4R1

Daniel F. Connor, MD
Associate Professor
Department of Psychiatry
University of Massachusetts Medical School
55 Lake Avenue North
Worcester, MA 01655

Deborah L. Anderson, PhD
Assistant Professor
Department Pediatrics
Medical University of South Carolina
Charleston, SC 29425

Donald R. Lynam, PhD
Associate Professor
Department of Psychology
University of Kentucky
125 Kastle Hall
Lexington, KY 40506-0044

Eric J. Mash, PhD
Professor
Department of Psychology
University of Calgary
2500 University Drive N.W.
Calgary, Alberta T2N 1N4

Eric Taylor
Professor of Psychiatry
Institute of Psychiatry
London, England

Erik Willcutt, PhD
Assistant Professor
Department of Psychology
Muenzinger Hall D-338
345 UCB
University of Colorado
Boulder, CO 80309

Florence Levy, MD
Associate Professor, School of Psychiatry
University of New South Wales
Avoca Clinic
Joynton Avenue
Zetland, NSW 2017, Australia

Gabrielle Carlson, MD
Professor and Director
Division of Child and Adolescent Psychiatry
State University of New York at Stony Brook
Putnam Hall
Stony Brook, NY 11794

George J. DuPaul, PhD
Professor of School Psychology
Lehigh University
111 Research Drive, Hilltop Campus
Bethlehem, PA 18015

Harold S. Koplewicz, MD
Arnold and Debbie Simon Professor of Child and
    Adolescent
Psychiatry and Director of the NYU Child Study
    Center, New York 10016

Hector R. Bird, MD
Professor of Clinical Psychiatry
Columbia University
College of Physicians and Surgeons
1051 Riverside Drive (Unit 78)
New York, NY 10032

Herbert Quay, PhD
Professor Emeritus
University of Miami
2525 Gulf of Mexico Drive, #5C
Long Boat Key, FL 34228

Howard Abikoff, PhD
Pevaroff Cohn Professor of Child and Adolescent
    Psychiatry, NYU School of Medicine
Director of Research, NYU Child Study Center
550 First Avenue
New York, NY 10016

J. Bart Hodgens, PhD
Clinical Assistant Professor of Psychology and
    Pediatrics
Civitan International Research Center
University of Alabama at Birmingham
Birmingham, AL 35914

James J. McGough, MD
Associate Professor of Clinical Psychiatry
UCLA School of Medicine
760 Westwood Plaza
Los Angeles, CA 90024

Jan Loney, PhD
Professor Emeritus
State University of New York at Stony Brook
Lodge Associates (Box 9)
Mayslick, KY 41055

Jeffrey Halperin, PhD
Professor, Department of Psychology
Queens College, CUNY
65-30 Kissena Avenue
Flushing, NY 11367

John Piacentini, PhD
Associate Professor
Department of Psychiatry
UCLA Neuropsychiatric Institute
760 Westwood Plaza
Los Angeles, CA 90024-1759

John S. Werry, MD
Professor Emeritus
Department of Psychiatry
University of Auckland
Auckland, New Zealand

Jose J. Bauermeister, PhD
Professor, Department of Psychology
University of Puerto Rico
San Juan, PR 00927

Joseph Biederman, MD
Professor and Chief
Joint Program in Pediatric Psychopharmacology
Massachusetts General Hospital and Harvard
    Medical School
15 Parkman Street, WACC725
Boston, MA 02114

Joseph Sergeant, PhD
Chair of Clinical Neuropsychology
Free University
Van der Boecharst Straat 1
De Boelenlaan 1109
1018 BT Amsterdam, The Netherlands

Keith McBurnett, PhD
Associate Professor, Department of Psychiatry
University of California at San Francisco
Children's Center at Langley Porter
401 Parnassus Avenue, Box 0984
San Francisco, CA 94143

Ken C. Winters, PhD
Associate Professor and Director, Center for
    Adolescent Substance Abuse Research
Department of Psychiatry
University of Minnesota
F282/2A West, 2450 Riverside Avenue
Minneapolis, MN 55454

Kevin R. Murphy, PhD
Associate Professor
Department of Psychiatry
University of Massachusetts Medical School
55 Lake Avenue North
Worcester, MA 01655

Laurence Greenhill, MD
Professor of Clinical Psychiatry
Columbia University
Director, Research Unit on Pediatric
    Psychopharmacology
New York State Psychiatric Institute
1051 Riverside Drive
New York, NY 10032

Lawrence Lewandowski, PhD
Meredith Professor of Teaching Excellence
Department of Psychology
Syracuse University
Syracuse, NY

Lily Hechtman MD, FRCP
Professor of Psychiatry and Pediatrics, and Director
  of Research, Division of Child Psychiatry
McGill University and Montreal Children's Hospital
4018 St. Catherine St. West
Montreal, Quebec, Canada H3Z-1P2

Linda Pfiffner, PhD
Associate Professor, Department of Psychiatry
University of California at San Francisco
Children's Center at Langley Porter
401 Parnassus Avenue, Box 0984
San Francisco, CA 94143

Lisa L. Weyandt, PhD
Professor, Department of Psychology
Central Washington University
400 East 8th Avenue
Ellensburg, WA 98926-7575

Marc Atkins, PhD
Associate Professor
Department of Psychiatry
Institute for Juvenile Research
University of Illinois at Chicago
840 South Wood Street, Suite 130
Chicago, IL 60612-7347

Margot Prior, PhD
Professor
Department of Psychology
Royal Children's Hospital
Parkville, 3052 VIC
Australia

Mark A. Stein, PhD
Chair of Psychology
Children's National Medical Center
Professor of Psychiatry and Pediatrics
George Washington University Medical School
111 Michigan Avenue NW
Washington, DC 20010

Mark D. Rapport, PhD
Professor and Director of Clinical Training
Department of Psychology
University of Central Florida
P. O. Box 161390
Orlando, Florida 32816-1390

Mariellen Fischer, PhD
Professor, Department of Neurology
Medical College of Wisconsin
9200 W. Wisconsin Avenue
Milwaukee, WI 53226

Mary A. Fristad, PhD, ABPP
Professor, Psychiatry and Psychology
Director, Research and Psychological Services
Division of Child and Adolescent Psychiatry
The Ohio State University
1670 Upham Drive Suite 460G
Columbus, OH 43210–1250

Mary Solanto-Gardner, PhD
Associate Professor
Division of Child and Adolescent Psychiatry
The Mt. Sinai Medical Center
One Gustave L. Levy Place
New York, NY 10029–6574

Michael Aman, PhD
Professor of Psychology and Psychiatry
The Nisonger Center
Ohio State University
1581 Dodd Drive
Columbus, OH

Michael Gordon, PhD
Professor of Psychiatry
Director, Child & Adolescent Psychiatric Services,
  and Director, ADHD Program
SUNY Upstate Medical University
750 East Adams Street
Syracuse, NY 13210

Michelle DeKlyen, PhD
Office of Population Research
Princeton University
286 Wallace
Princeton, NJ 08544

Mina Dulcan, MD
Professor
Department of Child and Adolescent Psychiatry
2300 Children's Plaza #10
Children's Memorial Hospital
Chicago, IL 60614

Oscar Bukstein, MD
Associate Professor
Department of Psychiatry
Western Psychiatric Institute and Clinic
3811 O'Hara Street
Pittsburgh, PA 15213

Patrick H. Tolan, PhD
Director, Institute for Juvenile Research
Professor, Department of Psychiatry
University of Illinois at Chicago
840 S. Wood Street
Chicago, IL 60612

Philip Firestone, PhD
Professor
Departments of Psychology and Psychiatry
University of Ottawa
120 University Priv.
Ottawa, Canada K1N 6N5

Richard Milich, PhD
Professor of Psychology
Department of Psychology
University of Kentucky
Lexington, KY 40506-0044

Rob McGee, PhD
Associate Professor
Department of Preventive and Social Medicine
University of Otago Medical School
Box 913 Dunedin
New Zealand

Ronald T. Brown, PhD
Associate Dean, College of Health Professions
Professor of Pediatrics
Medical University of South Carolina
19 Hagood Avenue, P. O. Box 250822
Charleston, SC 29425

Rosemary Tannock, PhD
Brain and Behavior Research
Hospital for Sick Children
55 University Avenue
Toronto, Ontario, Canada M5G 1X8

Russell Schachar, MD
Professor of Psychiatry
Hospital for Sick Children
555 University Avenue
Toronto, Ontario
Canada M5G 1X8

Salvatore Mannuzza, MD
Research Professor of Psychiatry
New York University School of Medicine
550 First Avenue
New York, NY 10016

Sandra K. Loo, PhD
Research Psychologist
University of California, Los Angeles
Neuropsychiatric Institute
760 Westwood Plaza, Rm 47-406
Los Angeles, CA 90024

Sheila Eyberg, PhD, ABPP
Professor of Clinical & Health Psychology
University of Florida
Box 100165
600 SW Archer Blvd.
Gainesville, FL 32610

Stephen Houghton, PhD
Professor of Psychology
Director, Centre for Attention and Related
    Disorders
The University of Western Australia
Perth, Australia

Stephen P. Hinshaw, PhD
Professor
Department of Psychology, #1650
University of California at Berkeley
3210 Tolman Hall
Berkeley, CA 94720-1650

Stephen Shapiro, PhD
Department of Psychology
Auburn University
226 Thach
Auburn, AL 36849-5214

Stephen V. Faraone, PhD
Associate Professor of Psychology
Harvard University
750 Washington Street, Suite 255
South Easton, MA 02375

Steven R. Pliszka, MD
Associate Professor and Chief
Division of Child and Adolescent Psychiatry
University of Texas Health Sciences Center
7703 Floyd Curl Drive
San Antonio, TX 78229-3900

Steven W. Evans, PhD
Associate Professor of Psychology
MSC 1902
James Madison University
Harrisonburg, VA 22807

Susan Campbell, PhD
Professor
Department of Psychology
4015 O'Hara Street
University of Pittsburgh
Pittsburgh, PA 15260

Terje Sagvolden, PhD
Professor
Department of Physiology
University of Oslo
N-0316 Oslo, Norway

Terri L. Shelton, PhD
Director
Center for the Study of Social Issues
University of North Carolina – Greensboro
Greensboro, NC 27402

Thomas E. Brown, PhD
Assistant Professor
Department of Psychiatry
Yale University School of Medicine
New Haven, CT

Thomas Joiner, PhD
The Bright–Burton Professor of Psychology
Florida State University
Tallahassee, FL 32306-1270

Thomas M. Lock, MD
Associate Professor of Clinical Pediatrics
Acting Chief, Division of Developmental Pediatrics
    and Rehabilitation
Acting Director, Robert Warner Rehabilitation
    Center
State University of New York at Buffalo School of
    Medicine and Biomedical Sciences
936 Delaware Ave.
Buffalo, NY 14209

Thomas Spencer, MD
Associate Professor and Assistant Director,
    Pediatric Psychopharmacology
Harvard Medical School and Massachusetts General
    Hospital
15 Parkman Street, WACC725
Boston, MA 02114

William Pelham, Jr, PhD
Professor of Psychology
Center for Children and Families
State University of New York at Buffalo
318 Diefendorf Hall, 3435 Main Street, Building 20
Buffalo, NY 14214

CONSENSUS STATEMENT—SUPPORTING REFERENCES

Accardo, P. J., Blondis, T. A., Whitman, B. Y., & Stein, M. A. (2000). *Attention deficits and hyperactivity in children and adults.* New York: Marcel Dekker.

Achenbach, T. M. (1991). *Manual for the revised child behavior profile and child behavior checklist.* Burlington, VT: Author.

Achenbach, T. M., & Edelbrock, C. S. (1983). *Manual for the child behavior profile and child behavior checklist.* Burlington, VT: Achenbach (author).

Achenbach, T. M., & Edelbrock, C. S. (1987). Empirically based assessment of the behavioral/emotional problems of 2- and 3-year-old children. *Journal of Abnormal Child Psychology, 15,* 629–650.

Achenbach, T. M., McConaughy, S. H., & Howell, C. T. (1987). Child/adolescent behavioral and emotional problems: Implications of cross-informant correlations for situational specificity. *Psychological Bulletin, 101,* 213–232.

Altepeter, T. S., & Breen, M. J. (1992). Situational variation in problem behavior at home and school in attention deficit disorder with hyperactivity: A factor analytic study. *Journal of Child Psychology and Psychiatry, 33,* 741–748.

American Psychiatric Association. (1968). *Diagnostic and statistical manual of mental disorders* (2nd ed.). Washington, DC: Author.

American Psychiatric Association. (1980). *Diagnostic and statistical manual of mental disorders* (3rd ed.). Washington, DC: Author.

American Psychiatric Association. (1987). *Diagnostic and statistical manual of mental disorders* (3rd ed., Rev.). Washington, DC: Author.

American Psychiatric Association. (1994). *Diagnostic and statistical manual of mental disorders* (4th ed.). Washington, DC: Author.

Anderson, C. A., Hinshaw, S. P., & Simmel, C. (1994). Mother–child interactions in ADHD and comparison boys: Relationships with overt and covert externalizing behavior. *Journal of Abnormal Child Psychology, 22,* 247–265.

Angold, A., Costello, E. J., & Erkanli, A. (1999). Comorbidity. *Journal of Child Psychology and Psychiatry, 40,* 57–88.

Antrop, I., Roeyers, H., Van Oost, P., & Buysse, A. (2000). Stimulant seeking and hyperactivity in children with ADHD. *Journal of Child Psychology and Psychiatry, 41,* 225–231.

Applegate, B., Lahey, B. B., Hart, E. L., Waldman, I., Biederman, J., Hynd, G. W., et al. (1997). Validity of the age-of-onset criterion for ADHD: A report of the DSM-IV field trials. *Journal of American Academy of Child and Adolescent Psychiatry, 36,* 1211–1221.

Aronen, E. T., Paavonen, J., Fjallberg, M., Soininen, M., Torronen, J. (2000). Sleep and psychiatric symptoms in school-age children. *Journal of the American Academy of Child and Adolescent Psychiatry, 39,* 502–508.

August, G. J., & Stewart, M. A. (1983). Family subtypes of childhood hyperactivity. *Journal of Nervous and Mental Disease, 171,* 362–368.

August, G. J., Stewart, M. A., & Holmes, C. S. (1983). A four-year follow-up of hyperactive boys with and without conduct disorder. *British Journal of Psychiatry, 143,* 192–198.

Aylward, E. H., Reiss, A. L., Reader, M. J., Singer, H. S., Brown, J. E., & Denckla, M. B. (1996). Basal ganglia volumes in children with attention-deficit hyperactivity disorder. *Journal of Child Neurology, 11,* 112–115.

Ball, J. D., & Koloian, B. (1995). Sleep patterns among ADHD children. *Clinical Psychology Review, 15,* 681–691.

Ball, J. D., Tiernan, M., Janusz, J., & Furr, A. (1997). Sleep patterns among children with attention-deficit hyperactivity disorder: A reexamination of parent perceptions. *Journal of Pediatric Psychology, 22,* 389–398.

Baloh, R., Sturm, R., Green, B., & Gleser, G. (1975). Neuropsychological effects of chronic asymptomatic increased lead absorption. *Archives of Neurology, 32,* 326–330.

Barkley, R. A. (1985). The social interactions of hyperactive children: Developmental changes, drug effects, and situational variation. In R. McMahon & R. Peters (Eds.), *Childhood* disorders: Behavioral–developmental approaches (pp. 218–243). New York: Brunner/Mazel.

Barkley, R. A. (1988). The effects of methylphenidate on the interactions of preschool ADHD children with their mothers. Journal of the American Academy of Child and Adolescent Psychiatry, 27, 336–341.

Barkley, R. A. (1989a). The problem of stimulus control and rule-governed behavior in children with attention deficit disorder with hyperactivity. In J. Swanson & L. Bloomingdale (Eds.), Attention deficit disorders (pp. 203–234). New York: Pergamon.

Barkley, R. A. (1989b). Hyperactive girls and boys: Stimulant drug effects on mother–child interactions. Journal of Child Psychology and Psychiatry, 30, 379–390.

Barkley, R. A. (1990). Attention-deficit hyperactivity disorder: A handbook for diagnosis and treatment. New York: Guilford.

Barkley, R. A. (1994). Impaired delayed responding: A unified theory of attention deficit hyperactivity disorder. In D. K. Routh (Ed.), Disruptive behavior disorders: Essays in honor of Herbert Quay (pp. 11–57). New York: Plenum.

Barkley, R. A. (1997a). Behavioral inhibition sustained, attention, and executive functions: Constructing a unifying theory of ADHD. Psychological Bulletin, 121, 65–94.

Barkley, R. A. (1997b). ADHD and the nature of self-control. New York: Guilford.

Barkley, R. A. (1998). Attention-deficit hyperactivity disorder: A handbook for diagnosis and treatment (2nd ed.). New York: Guilford.

Barkley, R. A. (1999a). Response inhibition in attention deficit hyperactivity disorder. Mental Retardation and Developmental Disabilities Research Reviews, 5, 177–184.

Barkley, R. A. (1999b). Theories of attention-deficit/hyperactivity disorder. In H. Quay & A. Hogan (Eds.), Handbook of disruptive behavior disorders (pp. 295–316). New York: Plenum.

Barkley, R. A. (2001a). The inattentive type of ADHD as a distinct disorder: What remains to be done. Clinical Psychology: Science and Practice, 8, 489–493.

Barkley, R. A. (2001b). Genetics of childhood disorders: XVII. ADHD, Part I: The executive functions and ADHD. Journal of the American Academy of Child and Adolescent Psychiatry, 39, 1064–1068.

Barkley, R. A. (2001c). The executive functions and self-regulation: An evolutionary neuropsychological perspective. Neuropsychology Review, 11, 1–29.

Barkley, R. A., Anastopoulos, A. D., Guevremont, D. G., & Fletcher, K. F. (1991). Adolescents with attention deficit hyperactivity disorder: Patterns of behavioral adjustment, academic functioning, and treatment utilization. Journal of the American Academy of Child and Adolescent Psychiatry, 30, 752–761.

Barkley, R. A., Anastopoulos, A. D., Guevremont, D. G., & Fletcher, K. F. (1992). Adolescents with attention deficit hyperactivity disorder: Mother–adolescent interactions, family beliefs and conflicts, and maternal psychopathology. Journal of Abnormal Child Psychology, 20, 263–288.

Barkley, R. A., & Biederman, J. (1997). Towards a broader definition of the age of onset criterion for attention deficit hyperactivity disorder. Journal of the American Academy of Child and Adolescent Psychiatry, 36, 1204–1210.

Barkley, R. A., & Cunningham, C. E. (1979a). Stimulant drugs and activity level in hyperactive children. American Journal of Orthopsychiatry, 49, 491–499.

Barkley, R. A., & Cunningham, C. E. (1979b). The effects of methylphenidate on the mother–child interactions of hyperactive children. Archives of General Psychiatry, 36, 201–208.

Barkley, R., Cunningham, C., & Karlsson, J. (1983). The speech of hyperactive children and their mothers: Comparisons with normal children and stimulant drug effects. Journal of Learning Disabilities, 16, 105–110.

Barkley, R. A., DuPaul, G. J., & McMurray, M. B. (1990). A comprehensive evaluation of attention deficit disorder with and without hyperactivity. Journal of Consulting and Clinical Psychology, 58, 775–789.

Barkley, R. A., & Edelbrock, C. S. (1987). Assessing situational variation in children's behavior problems: The Home and School Situations Questionnaires. In R. Prinz (Ed.), Advances in behavioral assessment of children and families (Vol. 3, pp. 157–176). Greenwich, CT: JAI Press.

Barkley, R. A., Edwards, G., Laneri, M., Fletcher, K., & Metevia, L. (2001). Executive functioning, temporal discounting, and sense of time in adolescents with attention deficit hyperactivity disorder and oppositional defiant disorder. Journal of Abnormal Child Psychology, 29, 541–556.

Barkley, R. A., Fischer, M., Edelbrock, C. S., & Smallish, L. (1990). The adolescent outcome of hyperactive children diagnosed by research criteria: I. An 8 year prospective follow-up study. Journal of the American Academy of Child and Adolescent Psychiatry, 29, 546–557.

Barkley, R. A., Fischer, M., Edelbrock, C. S., & Smallish, L. (1991). The adolescent outcome of hyperactive children diagnosed by research criteria: III. Mother–child interactions, family conflicts, and maternal psychopathology. Journal of Child Psychology and Psychiatry, 32, 233–256.

Barkley, R. A., Fischer, M., Fletcher, K., & Smallish, L. (in press). Persistence of attention deficit hyperactivity disorder into adulthood as a function of reporting source and definition of disorder. Journal of Abnormal Psychology.

Barkley, R. A., Fischer, M., Smallish, L., & Fletcher, K. (in press). Does the treatment of ADHD with stimulant medication contribute to illicit drug use and abuse in adulthood? Results from a 15-year prospective study. Pediatrics.

Barkley, R. A., Grodzinsky, G., & DuPaul, G. (1992). Frontal lobe functions in attention deficit disorder with and without hyperactivity: A review and research report. Journal of Abnormal Child Psychology, 20, 163–188.

Barkley, R. A., Guevremont, D. G., Anastopoulos, A. D., DuPaul, G. J., & Shelton, T. L. (1993). Driving-related risks and outcomes of attention deficit hyperactivity disorder in adolescents and young adults: A 3–5 year follow-up survey. Pediatrics, 92, 212–218.

Barkley, R. A., Karlsson, J., & Pollard, S. (1985). Effects of age on the mother–child interactions of hyperactive children. Journal of Abnormal Child Psychology, 13, 631–638.

Barkley, R. A., Karlsson, J., Pollard, S., & Murphy, J. V. (1985). Developmental changes in the mother–child interactions of hyperactive boys: Effects of two dose levels of Ritalin. Journal of Child Psychology and Psychiatry and Allied Disciplines, 26, 705–715.

Barkley, R. A., Licho, R., McGough, J. J., Tuite, P., Feifel, D., Mishkin, F., et al. (2002). Excessive dopamine transporter density in adults with attention deficit hyperactivity disorder assessed by SPECT with [^{123} I] altropane. University of Massachusetts Medical School, Worcester, MA.

Barkley, R. A., Murphy, K. R., & Bush, T. (2001). Time perception and reproduction in young adults with attention deficit hyperactivity disorder (ADHD). Neuropsychology, 15, 351–360.

Barkley, R. A., Murphy, K. R., DuPaul, G. R., & Bush, T. (in press). Driving in young adults with attention deficit hyperactivity disorder: Knowledge, performance, adverse outcomes and the role of executive functions. Journal of the International Neuropsychological Society.

Barkley, R. A., Murphy, K. R., & Kwasnik, D. (1996a). Psychological functioning and adaptive impairments in young adults with ADHD. Journal of Attention Disorders, 1, 41–54.

Barkley, R. A., Murphy, K. R., & Kwasnik, D. (1996b). Motor vehicle driving competencies and risks in teens and young adults with attention deficit hyperactivity disorder. Pediatrics, 98, 1089–1095.

Barkley, R. A., Shelton, T. L., Crosswait, C., Moorehouse, M., Fletcher, K., Barrett, S., et al. (in press). Preschool children with high levels of disruptive behavior: Three-year outcomes as a function of adaptive disability. *Development and Psychopathology, 14,* 45–68.

Bate, A. J., Mathias, J. L., & Crawford, J. R. (2001). Performance of the Test of Everyday Attention and standard tests of attention following severe traumatic brain injury. *The Clinical Neuropsychologist, 15,* 405–422.

Baumgaertel, A., Wolraich, M. L., & Dietrich, M. (1995). Comparison of diagnostic criteria for attention deficit disorders in a German elementary school sample. *Journal of the American Academy of Child and Adolescent Psychiatry, 34,* 629–638.

Baving, L., Laucht, M., & Schmidt, M. H. (1999). A typical frontal brain activation in ADHD: Preschool and elementary school boys and girls. *Journal of the American Academy of Child and Adolescent Psychiatry, 38,* 1363–1371.

Bayliss, D. M., & Roodenrys, S. (2000). Executive processing and attention deficit hyperactivity disorder: An application of the supervisory attentional system. *Developmental Neuropsychology, 17,* 161–180.

Beauchaine, T. P., Katkin, E. S., Strassberg, Z., & Snarr, J. (2001). Disinhibitory psychopathology in male adolescents: Discriminating conduct disorder from attention-deficit/hyperactivity disorder through concurrent assessment of multiple autonomic states. *Journal of Abnormal Psychology, 110,* 610–624.

Befera, M., & Barkley, R. A. (1984). Hyperactive and normal girls and boys: Mother–child interactions, parent psychiatric status, and child psychopathology. *Journal of Child Psychology and Psychiatry, 26,* 439–452.

Beiser, M., Dion, R., & Gotowiec, A. (2000). The structure of attention-deficit and hyperactivity symptoms among native and non-native elementary school children. *Journal of Abnormal Child Psychology, 28,* 425–537.

Beitchman, J. H., Wekerle, C., & Hood, J. (1987). Diagnostic continuity from preschool to middle childhood. *Journal of the American Academy of Child and Adolescent Psychiatry, 26,* 694–699.

Bennett, L. A., Wolin, S. J., & Reiss, D. (1988). Cognitive, behavioral, and emotional problems among school-age children of alcoholic parents. *American Journal of Psychiatry, 145,* 185–190.

Benton, A. (1991). Prefrontal injury and behavior in children. *Developmental Neuropsychology, 7,* 275–282.

Berk, L. E., & Potts, M. K. (1991). Development and functional significance of private speech among attention-deficit hyperactivity disorder and normal boys. *Journal of Abnormal Child Psychology, 19,* 357–377.

Bhatia, M. S., Nigam, V. R., Bohra, N., & Malik, S. C. (1991). Attention deficit disorder with hyperactivity among paediatric outpatients. *Journal of Child Psychology and Psychiatry, 32,* 297–306.

Biederman, J., Faraone, S. V., Keenan, K., & Tsuang, M. T. (1991). Evidence of a familial association between attention deficit disorder and major affective disorders. *Archives of General Psychiatry, 48,* 633–642.

Biederman, J., Faraone, S. V., & Lapey, K. (1992). Comorbidity of diagnosis in attention-deficit hyperactivity disorder. In G. Weiss (Ed.), *Child and adolescent psychiatric clinics of North America: Attention-deficit hyperactivity disorder* (pp. 335–360). Philadelphia: Saunders.

Biederman, J., Faraone, S. V., Mick, E., Spencer, T., Wilens, T., Kiely, K., et al. (1995). High risk for attention deficit hyperactivity disorder among children of parents with childhood onset of the disorder: A pilot study. *American Journal of Psychiatry, 152,* 431–435.

Biederman, J., Faraone, S. V., Mick, E., Williamson, S., Wilens, T. E., Spencer, T. J., et al. (1999). Clinical correlates of ADHD in females: Findings from a large group of girls ascertained from pediatric and psychiatric referral sources. *Journal of the American Academy of Child and Adolescent Psychiatry, 38,* 966–975.

Biederman, J., Faraone, S., Milberger, S., Curtis, S., Chen, L., Marrs, A., et al. (1996). Predictors of persistence and remission of ADHD into adolescence: Results from a four-year prospective follow-up study. *Journal of the American Academy of Child and Adolescent Psychiatry, 35,* 343–351.

Biederman, J., Keenan, K., & Faraone, S. V. (1990). Parent-based diagnosis of attention deficit disorder predicts a diagnosis based on teacher report. *American Journal of Child and Adolescent Psychiatry, 29,* 698–701.

Biederman, J., Milberger, S., Faraone, S. V., Guite, J., & Warburton, R. (1994). Associations between childhood asthma and ADHD: Issues of psychiatric comorbidity and familiality. *Journal of the American Academy of Child and Adolescent Psychiatry, 33,* 842–848.

Biederman, J., Newcorn, J., & Sprich, S. (1991). Comorbidity of attention deficit hyperactivity disorder with conduct, depressive, anxiety, and other disorders. *American Journal of Psychiatry, 148,* 564–577.

Biederman, J., Wilens, T., Mick, E., Spencer, T., & Faraone, S. V. (1999). Pharmacotherapy of attention-deficit/hyperactivity disorder reduces risk for substance use disorder. *Pediatrics,* 104–109.

Biederman, J., Wozniak, J., Kiely, K., Ablon, S., Faraone, S., Mick, E., et al. (1995). CBCL clinical scales discriminate prepubertal children with structured-interview-derived diagnosis of mania from those with ADHD. *Journal of the American Academy of Child and Adolescent Psychiatry, 34,* 464–471.

Bijur, P., Golding, J., Haslum, M., & Kurzon, M. (1988). Behavioral predictors of injury in school-age children. *American Journal of Diseases of Children, 142,* 1307–1312.

Borger, N., & van der Meere, J. (2000). Visual behaviour of ADHD children during an attention test: An almost forgotten variable. *Journal of Child Psychology and Psychiatry, 41,* 525–532.

Braaten, E. B., & Rosen, L. A. (2000). Self-regulation of affect in attention deficit hyperactivity disorder (ADHD) and non-ADHD boys: Differences in empathic responding. *Journal of Consulting and Clinical Psychology, 68,* 313–321.

Breen, M. J. (1989). Cognitive and behavioral differences in ADHD boys and girls. *Journal of Child Psychology and Psychiatry, 30,* 711–716.

Breslau, N., Brown, G. G., DelDotto, J. E., Kumar, S., Exhuthachan, S., Andreski, P., et al. (1996). Psychiatric sequelae of low birth weight at 6 years of age. *Journal of Abnormal Child Psychology, 24,* 385–400.

Breton, J., Bergeron, L., Valla, J. P., Berthiaume, C., Gaudet, N., Lambert, J., et al. (1999). Quebec children mental health survey: Prevalence of DSM-III-R mental health disorders. *Journal of Child Psychology and Psychiatry, 40,* 375–384.

Briggs-Gowan, M. J., Horwitz, S. M., Schwab-Stone, M. E., Leventhal, J. M., & Leaf, P. J. (2000). Mental health in pediatric settings: Distribution of disorders and factors related to service use. *Journal of the American Academy of Child and Adolescent Psychiatry, 39,* 841–849.

Bu-Haroon, A., Eapen, V., & Bener, A. (1999). The prevalence of hyperactivity symptoms in the United Arab Emirates. *Nordic Journal of Psychiatry, 53,* 439–442.

Buhrmester, D., Camparo, L., Christensen, A., Gonzalez, L. S., & Hinshaw, S. P. (1992). Mothers and fathers interacting in dyads and triads with normal and hyperactive sons. *Developmental Psychology, 28,* 500–509.

Burke, J. D., Loeber, R., & Lahey, B. B. (2001). Which aspects of ADHD are associated with tobacco use in early adolescence? *Journal of Child Psychology and Psychiatry, 42,* 493–502.

Burks, H. (1960). The hyperkinetic child. *Exceptional Children, 27,* 18.

Burns, G. L., Boe, B., Walsh, J. A., Sommers-Flannagan, R., & Teegarden, L. A. (2001). A confirmatory factor analysis on the DSM-IV ADHD and ODD symptoms: What is the best model for the organization of tehse symptoms? *Journal of Abnormal Child Psychology, 29,* 339–349.

Burns, G. L., & Walsh, J. A. (in press). The influence of ADHD-hyperactivity/impulsivity symptoms on the development of oppositional defiant disorder symptoms in a two-year longitudinal study. *Journal of Abnormal Child Psychology.*

Burt, S. A., Krueger, R. F., McGue, M., & Iacono, W. G. (2001). Sources of covariation among attention-deficit hyperactivity disorder, oppositional defiant disorder, and conduct disorder: The importance of shared environment. *Journal of Abnormal Psychology, 110,* 516–525.

Cadesky, E. B., Mota, V. L., & Schachar, R. J. (2000). Beyond words: How do children with ADHD and/or conduct problems process nonverbal information about affect? *Journal of the American Academy of Child and Adolescent Psychiatry, 39,* 1160–1167.

Cadoret, R. J., & Stewart, M. A. (1991). An adoption study of attention deficit/hyperactivity/aggression and their relationship to adult antisocial personality. *Comprehensive Psychiatry, 32,* 73–82.

Campbell, S. B. (1990). *Behavior problems in preschool children.* New York: Guilford.

Campbell, S. B., March, C. L., Pierce, E. W., Ewing, L. J., & Szumowski, E. K. (1991). Hard-to-manage preschool boys: Family context and the stability of externalizing behavior. *Journal of Abnormal Child Psychology, 19,* 301–318.

Campbell, S. B., Schleifer, M., & Weiss, G. (1978). Continuities in maternal reports and child behaviors over time in hyperactive and comparison groups. *Journal of Abnormal Child Psychology, 6,* 33–45.

Campbell, S. B., Szumowski, E. K., Ewing, L. J., Gluck, D. S., & Breaux, A. M. (1982). A multidimensional assessment of parent-identified behavior problem toddlers. *Journal of Abnormal Child Psychology, 10,* 569–592.

Cantwell, D. (1975). *The hyperactive child.* New York: Spectrum.

Cantwell, D. P., & Baker, L. (1992). Association between attention deficit-hyperactivity disorder and learning disorders. In S. E. Shaywitz & B. A. Shaywitz (Eds.), *Attention deficit disorder comes of age: Toward the twenty-first century* (pp. 145–164). Austin, TX: Pro-ed.

Carlson, C. L., Lahey, B. B., & Neeper, R. (1986). Direct assessment of the cognitive correlates of attention deficit disorders with and without hyperactivity. *Journal of Behavioral Assessment and Psychopathology, 8,* 69–86.

Carlson, C. L., & Mann, M. (in press). *Sluggish cognitive tempo predicts a different pattern of impairment in the Attention Deficit Hyperactivity Disorder, Predominantly Inattentive Type.* University of Texas at Austin.

Carlson, C. L., & Tamm, L. (2000). Responsiveness of children with attention deficit hyperactivity disorder to reward and response cost: Differential impact on performance and motivation. *Journal of Consulting and Clinical Psychology, 68,* 73–83.

Carlson, C. L., Tamm, L., & Gaub, M. (1997). Gender differences in children with ADHD, ODD, and co-occurring ADHD/ODD identified in a school population. *Journal of the American Academy of Child and Adolescent Psychiatry, 36,* 1706–1714.

Carlson, E. A., Jacobvitz, D., & Sroufe, L. A. (1995). A developmental investigation of inattentiveness and hyperactivity. *Child Development, 66,* 37–54.

Carlson, G. A. (1990). Child and adolescent mania—diagnostic considerations. *Journal of Child Psychology and Psychiatry, 31,* 331–342.

Carte, E. T., Nigg, J. T., & Hinshaw, S. P. (1996). Neuropsychological functioning, motor speed, and language processing in boys with and without ADHD. *Journal of Abnormal Child Psychology, 24,* 481–498.

Casey, B. J., Castellanos, F. X., Giedd, J. N., Marsh, W. L., Hamburger, S. D., Schubert, A. B., et al. (1997). Implication of right frontstriatal circuitry in response inhibition and attention-deficit/hyperactivity disorder. *Journal of the American Academy of Child and Adolescent Psychiatry, 36,* 374–383.

Casey, J. E., Rourke, B. P., & Del Dotto, J. E. (1996). Learning disabilities in children with attention deficit disorder with and without hyperactivity. *Child Neuropsychology, 2,* 83–98.

Casey, R. J. (1996). Emotional competence in children with externalizing and internalizing disorders. In M. Lewis & M. W. Sullivan (Eds.), *Emotional development in atypical children* (pp. 161–183). Mahwah, NJ: Erlbaum.

Castellanos, F. X., Giedd, J. N., Eckburg, P., Marsh, W. L., Vaituzis, C., Kaysen, D., et al. (1994). Quantitative morphology of the caudate nucleus in attention deficit hyperactivity disorder. *American Journal of Psychiatry, 151,* 1791–1796.

Castellanos, F. X., Giedd, J. N., Marsh, W. L., Hamburger, S. D., Vaituzis, A. C., Dickstein, D. P., et al. (1996). Quantitative brain magnetic resonance imaging in attention-deficit hyperactivity disorder. *Archives of General Psychiatry, 53,* 607–616.

Castellanos, F. X., Marvasti, F. F., Ducharme, J. L., Walter, J. M., Israel, M. E., Krain, A., et al. (2000). Executive function oculomotor tasks in girls with ADHD. *Journal of the American Academy of Child and Adolescent Psychiatry, 39,* 644–650.

Chadwick, O., Taylor, E., Taylor, A., Heptinstall, E., & Danckaerts, M. (1999). Hyperactivity and reading disability: A longitudinal study of the nature of the association. *Journal of Child Psychology and Psychiatry, 40,* 1039–1050.

Chang, H. T., Klorman, R., Shaywitz, S. E., Fletcher, J. M., Marchione, K. E., Holahan, J. M., et al. (1999). Paired-associate learning in attention-deficit/hyperactivity disorder as a function of hyperactivity-impulsivity and oppositional defiant disorder. *Journal of Abnormal Child Psychology, 27,* 237–245.

Chess, S. (1960). Diagnosis and treatment of the hyperactive child. *New York State Journal of Medicine, 60,* 2379–2385.

Chilcoat, H. D., & Breslau, N. (1999). Pathways from ADHD to early drug use. *Journal of the American Academy of Child and Adolescent Psychiatry, 38,* 1347–1354.

Chabot, R. J., & Serfontein, G. (1996). Quantitative electroencephalographic profiles of children with attention deficit disorder. *Biological Psychiatry, 40,* 951–963.

Chelune, G. J., Ferguson, W., Koon, R., & Dickey, T. O. (1986). Frontal lobe disinhibition in attention deficit disorder. *Child Psychiatry and Human Development, 16,* 221–234.

Clark, C., Prior, M., & Kinsella, G. J. (2000). Do executive function deficits differentiate between adolescents with ADHD and oppositional defiant/conduct disorder? A neuropsychological study using the Six Elements Test and Hayling Sentence Completion Test. *Journal of Abnormal Child Psychology, 28,* 405–414.

Clark, M. L., Cheyne, J. A., Cunningham, C. E., & Siegel, L. S. (1988). Dyadic peer interaction and task orientation in attention-deficit-disordered children. *Journal of Abnormal Child Psychology, 16,* 1–15.

Claude, D., & Firestone, P. (1995). The development of ADHD boys: A 12-year follow-up. *Canadian Journal of Behavioural Science, 27,* 226–249.

Cohen, N. J., & Minde, K. (1983). The "hyperactive syndrome" in kindergarten children: Comparison of children with pervasive and situational symptoms. *Journal of Child Psychology and Psychiatry, 24,* 443–455.

Cohen, N. J., Sullivan, J., Minde, K., Novak, C., & Keens, S. (1983). Mother–child interaction in hyperactive and normal kindergarten-aged children and the effect of treatment. *Child Psychiatry and Human Development, 13,* 213–224.

Cohen, N. J., Vallance, D. D., Barwick, M., Im, N., Menna, R., Horodezky, N. B., et al. (2000). The interface between

ADHD and language impairment: An examination of language, achievement, and cognitive processing. *Journal of Child Psychology and Psychiatry, 41,* 353–362.

Comings, D. E. (2000). Attention deficit hyperactivity disorder with Tourette Syndrome. In T. E. Brown (Ed.), *Attention-deficit disorders and comorbidities in children, adolescents, and adults* (pp. 363–392). Washington, DC: American Psychiatric Press.

Comings, D. E., Comings, B. G., Muhleman, D., Dietz, G., Shahbahrami, B., Tast, D., et al. (1991). The dopamine D_2 receptor locus as a modifying gene in neuropsychiatric disorders. *Journal of the American Medical Association, 266,* 1793–1800.

Conners, C. K., & Wells, K. (1986). *Hyperactive children: A neuropsychological approach.* Beverly Hills, CA: Sage.

Conners, D. K. (1998). Other medications in the treatment of child and adolescent ADHD. In R. A. Barkley (Ed.), *Attention deficit hyperactivity disorder: A handbook for diagnosis and treatment* (pp. 564–581). New York: Guilford.

Cook, E. H., Stein, M. A., Krasowski, M. D., Cox, N. J., Olkon, D. M., Kieffer, J. E., & Leventhal, B. L. (1995). Association of attention deficit disorder and the dopamine transporter gene. *American Journal of Human Genetics, 56,* 993–998.

Cook, E. H., Stein, M. A., & Leventhal, D. L. (1997). Family-based association of attention-deficit/hyperactivity disorder and the dopamine transporter. In K. Blum (Ed.), *Handbook of Psychitric Genetics* (pp. 297–310). New York: CRC Press.

Coolidge, F. L., Thede, L. L., & Young, S. E. (2000). Heritability and the comorbidity of attention deficit hyperactivity disorder with behavioral disorders and executive function deficits: A preliminary investigation. *Developmental Neuropsychology, 17,* 273–287.

Corkum, P., Moldofsky, H., Hogg-Johnson, S., Humphries, T., & Tannock, R. (1999). Sleep problems in children with attention-deficit/hyperactivity disorder: Impact of subtype, comorbidity, and stimulant medication. *Journal of the American Academy of Child and Adolescent Psychiatry, 38,* 1285–1293.

Costello, E. J., Loeber, R., & Stouthamer-Loeber, M. (1991). Pervasive and situational hyperactivity—Confounding effect of informant: A research note. *Journal of Child Psychology and Psychiatry, 32,* 367–376.

Cruickshank, B. M., Eliason, M., & Merrifield, B. (1988). Long-term sequelae of water near-drowning. *Journal of Pediatric Psychology, 13,* 379–388.

Crystal, D. S., Ostrander, R., Chen, R. S., & August, G. J. (2001). Multimethod assessment of psychopathology among DSM-IV subtypes of children with attention deficit/hyperactivity disorder: Self-, parent, and teacher reports. *Journal of Abnormal Child Psychology, 29,* 189–205.

Cuffe, S. P., McKeown, R. E., Jackson, K. L., Addy, C. L., Abramson, R., & Garrison, C. Z. (2001). Prevalence of attention-deficit/hyperactivity disorder in a community sample of older adolescents. *Journal of the American Academy of Child and Adolescent Psychiatry, 40,* 1037–1044.

Cunningham, C. E., Benness, B. B., & Siegel, L. S. (1988). Family functioning, time allocation, and parental depression in the families of normal and ADDH children. *Journal of Clinical Child Psychology, 17,* 169–177.

Cunningham, C. E., & Siegel, L. S. (1987). Peer interactions of normal and attention-deficit disordered boys during free-play, cooperative task, and simulated classroom situations. *Journal of Abnormal Child Psychology, 15,* 247–268.

Cunningham, C. E., Siegel, L. S., & Offord, D. R. (1985). A developmental dose response analysis of the effects of methylphenidate on the peer interactions of attention deficit disordered boys. *Journal of Child Psychology and Psychiatry, 26,* 955–971.

Dane, A. V., Schachar, R. J., & Tannock, R. (2000). Does actigraphy differentiate ADHD subtypes in a clinical research setting? *Journal of the American Academy of Child and Adolescent Psychiatry, 39,* 752–760.

Danforth, J. S., Barkley, R. A., & Stokes, T. F. (1991). Observations of parent–child interactions with hyperactive children: Research and clinical implications. *Clinical Psychology Review, 11,* 703–727.

Daugherty, T. K., & Quay, H. C. (1991). Response perseveration and delayed responding in childhood behavior disorders. *Journal of Child Psychology and Psychiatry, 32,* 453–461.

David, O. J. (1974). Association between lower level lead concentrations and hyperactivity. *Environmental Health Perspective, 7,* 17–25.

de la Burde, B., & Choate, M. (1972). Does asymptomatic lead exposure in children have latent sequelae? *Journal of Pediatrics, 81,* 1088–1091.

de la Burde, B., & Choate, M. (1974). Early asymptomatic lead exposure and development at school age. *Journal of Pediatrics, 87,* 638–642.

Demaray, M. K., & Elliot, S. N. (2001). Perceived social support by children with characteristics of attention-deficit/hyperactivity disorder. *School Psychology Quarterly, 16,* 68–90.

Demb, H. B. (1991). Use of Ritalin in the treatment of children with mental retardation. In L. L. Greenhill & B. B. Osmon (Eds.), *Ritalin: Theory and patient management* (pp. 155–170). New York: Mary Ann Liebert.

Denckla, M. B. (1994). Measurement of executive function. In G. R. Lyon (Ed.), *Frames of reference for the assessment of learning disabilities: New views on measurement issues* (pp. 117–142). Baltimore: Brookes.

Denckla, M. B., & Rudel, R. G. (1978). Anomalies of motor development in hyperactive boys. *Annals of Neurology, 3,* 231–233.

Denckla, M. B., Rudel, R. G., Chapman, C., & Krieger, J. (1985). Motor proficiency in dyslexic children with and without attentional disorders. *Archives of Neurology, 42,* 228–231.

Denson, R., Nanson, J. L., & McWatters, M. A. (1975). Hyperkinesis and maternal smoking. *Canadian Psychiatric Association Journal, 20,* 183–187.

Dolphin, J. E., & Cruickshank, W. M. (1951). Pathology of concept formation in children with cerebral palsy. *American Journal of Mental Deficiency, 56,* 386–392.

Douglas, V. I. (1972). Stop, look, and listen: The problem of sustained attention and impulse control in hyperactive and normal children. *Canadian Journal of Behavioural Science, 4,* 259–282.

Douglas, V. I. (1980). Higher mental processes in hyperactive children: Implications for training. In R. Knights & D. Bakker (Eds.), *Treatment of hyperactive and learning disordered children* (pp. 65–92). Baltimore: University Park Press.

Douglas, V. I. (1983). Attention and cognitive problems. In M. Rutter (Ed.), *Developmental neuropsychiatry* (pp. 280–329). New York: Guilford.

Douglas, V. I. (1999). Cognitive control processes in attention-deficit/hyperactivity disorder. In H. C. Quay & A. Horgan (Eds.), *Handbook of disruptive behavior disorders* (pp. 105–138). New York: Plenum.

Douglas, V. I., & Parry, P. A. (1983). Effects of reward on delayed reaction time task performance of hyperactive children. *Journal of Abnormal Child Psychology, 11,* 313–326.

Douglas, V. I., & Parry, P. A. (1994). Effects of reward and nonreward on attention and frustration in attention deficit disorder. *Journal of Abnormal Child Psychology, 22,* 281–302.

Douglas, V. I., & Peters, K. G. (1978). Toward a clearer definition of the attentional deficit of hyperactive children. In G. A. Hale & M. Lewis (Eds.), *Attention and the development of cognitive skills* (pp. 173–248). New York: Plenum.

Dougherty, D. D., Bonab, A. A., Spencer, T. J., Rauch, S. L., Madras, B. K., & Fischman, A. J. (1999). Dopamine transporter density in patients with attention deficit hyperactivity disorder. *Lancet, 354,* 2132–2133.

Doyle, A. E., Faraone, S. V., DuPre, E. P., & Biederman, J. (2001). Separating attention deficit hyperactivity disorder and learning disabilities in girls: A familial risk analysis. *American Journal of Psychiatry, 158,* 1666–1672.

Draeger, S., Prior, M., & Sanson, A. (1986). Visual and auditory attention performance in hyperactive children: Competence or compliance. *Journal of Abnormal Child Psychology, 14,* 411–424.

DuPaul, G. J. (1991). Parent and teacher ratings of ADHD symptoms: Psychometric properties in a community-based sample. *Journal of Clinical Child Psychology, 20,* 245–253.

DuPaul, G. J., & Barkley, R. A. (1992). Situational variability of attention problems: Psychometric properties of the Revised Home and School Situations Questionnaires. *Journal of Clinical Child Psychology, 21,* 178–188.

DuPaul, G. J., Barkley, R. A., & Connor, D. F. (1998). Stimulants. In R. A. Barkley (Ed.), *Attention deficit hyperactivity disorder: A handbook for diagnosis and treatment* (pp. 510–551). New York: Guilford.

DuPaul, G. J., McGoey, K. E., Eckert, T. L., & VanBrakle, J. (2001). Preschool children with attention-deficit/hyperactivity disorder: Impairments in behavioral, social, and school functioning. *Journal of the American Academy of Child and Adolescent Psychiatry, 40,* 508–515.

DuPaul, G. J., Power, T. J., Anastopoulos, A. D., & Reid, R. (1999). *The ADHD Rating Scale-IV: Checklists, norms, and clinical interpretation.* New York: Guilford.

Ebaugh, F. G. (1923). Neuropsychiatric sequelae of acute epidemic encephalitis in children. *American Journal of Diseases of Children, 25,* 89–97.

Edelbrock, C. S., Costello, A., & Kessler, M. D. (1984). Empirical corroboration of attention deficit disorder. *Journal of the American Academy of Child and Adolescent Psychiatry, 23,* 285–290.

Edwards, F., Barkley, R., Laneri, M., Fletcher, K., & Metevia, L. (2001). Parent–adolescent conflict in teenagers with ADHD and ODD. *Journal of Abnormal Child Psychology, 29,* 557–572.

Elia, J., Gullotta, C., Rose, J. R., et al. (1994). Thyroid function in attention deficit hyperactivity disorder. *Journal of the American Academy of Child and Adolescent Psychiatry, 33,* 169–172.

Epstein, J. N., Goldberg, N. A., Conners, C. K., & March, J. S. (1997). The effects of anxiety on continuous performance test functioning in an ADHD clinic sample. *Journal of Attention Disorders, 2,* 45–52.

Erhardt, D., & Hinshaw, S. P. (1994). Initial sociometric impressions of attention-deficit hyperactivity disorder and comparison boys: Predictions from social behaviors and from nonbehavioral variables. *Journal of Consulting and Clinical Psychology, 62,* 833–842.

Ernst, M., Cohen, R. M., Liebenauer, L. L., Jons, P. H., & Zametkin, A. J. (1997). Cerebral glucose metabolism in adolescent girls with attention-deficit/hyperactivity disorder. *Journal of the American Acdemy of Child and Adolescent Psychiatry, 36,* 1399–1406.

Ernst, M., Liebenauer, L. L., King, A. C., Fitzgerald, G. A., Cohen, R. M., & Zametkin, A. J. (1994). Reduced brain metabolism in hyperactive girls. *Journal of the American Academy of Child and Adolescent Psychiatry, 33,* 858–868.

Ernst, M., Zametkin, A. J., Matochik, J. A., Pascualvaca, D., Jons, P. H., & Cohen, R. M. (1999). High midbrain [^{18}F]DOPA accumulation in children with attention deficit hyperactivity disorder. *American Journal of Psychiatry, 156,* 1209–1215.

Fallone, G., Acebo, C., Arnedt, J. T., Seifer, R., Carskadon, M. A. (2001). Effects of acute sleep restriction on behavior, sustained attention, and response inhibition in children. *Perceptual and Motor Skills, 93,* 213–229.

Faraone, S. V., & Biederman, J. (1997). Do attention deficit hyperactivity disorder and major depression share familial risk

factors? *Journal of Nervous and Mental Disease, 185,* 533–541.

Faraone, S. V., Biederman, J., Chen, W. J., Krifcher, B., Keenan, K., Moore, C., et al. (1992). Segregation analysis of attention deficit hyperactivity disorder. *Psychiatric Genetics, 2,* 257–275.

Faraone, S. V., Biederman, J., Lehman, B., Keenan, K., Norman, D., Seidman, L. J., et al. (1993). Evidence for the independent familial transmission of attention deficit hyperactivity disorder and learning disabilities: Results from a family genetic study. *American Journal of Psychiatry, 150,* 891–895.

Faraone, S. V., Biederman, J., Mennin, D., Russell, R., & Tsuang, M. T. (1998). Familial subtypes of attention deficit hyperactivity disorder: A 4-year follow-up study of children from antisocial-ADHD families. *Journal of Child Psychology and Psychiatry, 39,* 1045–1053.

Faraone, S. V., Biederman, J., Mick, E., Williamson, S., Wilens, T., Spencer, T., et al. (2000). Family study of girls with attention deficit hyperactivity disorder. *American Journal of Psychiatry, 157,* 1077–1083.

Faraone, S. V., Biederman, J., & Monuteaux, M. C. (2001). Attention deficit hyperactivity disorder and bipolar disorder in girls: Further evidence for a familial subtype? *Journal of Affective Disorders, 64,* 19–26.

Faraone, S. V., Biederman, J., Weber, W., & Russell, R. L. (1998). Psychiatric, neuropsychological, and psychosocial features of DSM-IV subtypes of attention-deficit/hyperactivity disorder: Results from a clinically referred sample. *Journal of the American Academy of Child and Adolescent Psychiatry, 37,* 185–193.

Faraone, S. V., Biederman, J., Weiffenbach, B., Keith, T., Chu, M. P., Weaver, A., et al. (1999). Dopamine D4 gene 7-repeat allele and attention deficit hyperactivity disorder. *American Journal of Psychiatry, 156,* 768–770.

Faraone, S. V., Biederman, J., Wozniak, J., Mundy, E., Mennin, D., & O'Donnell, D. (1997). Is comorbidity with ADHD a marker for juvenile-onset mania? *Journal of the American Academy of Child and Adolescent Psychiatry, 36,* 1046–1055.

Fergusson, D. M., Fergusson, I. E., Horwood, L. J., & Kinzett, N. G. (1988). A longitudinal study of dentine lead levels, intelligence, school performance, and behaviour. *Journal of Child Psychology and Psychiatry, 29,* 811–824.

Filipek, P. A., Semrud-Clikeman, M., Steingard, R. J., Renshaw, P. F., Kennedy, D. N., & Biederman, J. (1997). Volumetric MRI analysis comparing subjects having attention-deficit hyperactivity disorder with normal controls. *Neurology, 48,* 589–601.

Fischer, M. (1990). Parenting stress and the child with attention deficit hyperactivity disorder. *Journal of Clinical Child Psychology, 19,* 337–346.

Fischer, M., Barkley, R. A., Edelbrock, C. S., & Smallish, L. (1990). The adolescent outcome of hyperactive children diagnosed by research criteria: II. Academic, attentional, and neuropsychological status. *Journal of Consulting and Clinical Psychology, 58,* 580–588.

Fischer, M., Barkley, R. A., Fletcher, K., & Smallish, L. (1993a). The stability of dimensions of behavior in ADHD and normal children over an 8 year period. *Journal of Abnormal Child Psychology, 21,* 315–337.

Fischer, M., Barkley, R. A., Fletcher, K., & Smallish, L. (1993b). The adolescent outcome of hyperactive children diagnosed by research criteria: V. Predictors of outcome. *Journal of the American Academy of Child and Adolescent Psychiatry, 32,* 324–332.

Fischer, M., Barkley, R. A., Smallish, L., & Fletcher, K. R. (in press). Hyperactive children as young adults: Deficits in attention, inhibition, and response perseveration and their relationship to severity of childhood and current ADHD and conduct disorder. *Journal of Abnormal Psychology.*

Fischer, M., Barkley, R. A., Smallish, L., & Fletcher, K. R. (in press). Young adult outcome of hyperactive children as a function of severity of childhood conduct problems: Comorbid psychiatric disorders and interim mental health treatment. *Journal of Abnormal Child Psychology*.

Fletcher, K., Fischer, M., Barkley, R. A., & Smallish, L. (1996). A sequential analysis of the mother–adolescent interactions of ADHD, ADHD/ODD, and normal teenagers during neutral and conflict discussions. *Journal of Abnormal Child Psychology*, *24*, 271–298.

Frank, Y., & Ben-Nun, Y. (1988). Toward a clinical subgrouping of hyperactive and nonhyperactive attention deficit disorder: Results of a comprehensive neurological and neuropsychological assessment. *American Journal of Diseases of Children*, *142*, 153–155.

Frank, Y., Lazar, J. W., & Seiden, J. A. (1992). Cognitive event-related potentials in learning-disabled children with or without attention-deficit hyperactivity disorder [Abstract]. *Annals of Neurology*, *32*, 478.

Frick, P. J., Kamphaus, R. W., Lahey, B. B., Loeber, R., Christ, M. A. G., Hart, E. L., et al. (1991). Academic underachievement and the disruptive behavior disorders. *Journal of Consulting and Clinical Psychology*, *59*, 289–294.

Gadow, K. D., Nolan, E. E., Litcher, L., Carlson, G. A., Panina, N., Golovakha, E., et al. (2000). Comparison of attention-deficit/hyperactivity disorder symptom subtypes in Ukrainian schoolchildren. *Journal of the American Academy of Child and Adolescent Psychiatry*, *39*, 1520–1527.

Garcia-Sanchez, C., Estevez-Gonzalez, A., Suarez-Romero, E., & Junque, C. (1997). Right hemisphere dysfunction in subjects with attention-deficit disorder with and without hyperactivity. *Journal of Child Neurology*, *12*, 107–115.

Gaub, M., & Carlson, C. L. (1997). Gender differences in ADHD: A meta-analysis and critical review. *Journal of the American Academy of Child and Adolescent Psychiatry*, *36*, 1036–1045.

Geller, B., & Luby, J. (1997). Child and adolescent bipolar disorder: A review of the past 10 years. *Journal of the American Academy of Child and Adolescent Psychiatry*, *36*, 1168–1176.

Giedd, J. N., Castellanos, F. X., Casey, B. J., Kozuch, P., King, A. C., Hamburger, S. D., et al. (1994). Quantitative morphology of the corpus callosum in attention deficit hyperactivity disorder. *American Journal of Psychiatry*, *151*, 665–669.

Giedd, J. N., Snell, J. W., Lange, N., Rajapakse, J. C., Casey, B. J., Kozuch, P. L., et al. (1996). Quantitative magnetic resonance imaging of human brain development: Ages 4–18. *Cerebral Cortex*, *6*, 551–560.

Gilger, J. W., Pennington, B. F., & DeFries, J. C. (1992). A twin study of the etiology of comorbidity: Attention-deficit hyperactivity disorder and dyslexia. *Journal of the American Academy of Child and Adolescent Psychiatry*, *31*, 343–348.

Gill, M., Daly, G., Heron, S., Hawi, Z., & Fitzgerald, M. (1997). Confirmation of association between attention deficit hyperactivity disorder and a dopamine transporter polymorphism. *Molecular Psychiatry*, *2*, 311–313.

Gillberg, C., Carlström, G., & Rasmussen, P. (1983). Hyperkinetic disorders in seven-year-old children with perceptual, motor and attentional deficits. *Journal of Child Psychology and Psychiatry*, *24*(2), 233–246.

Gillberg, C. (1983). Perceptual, motor and attentional deficits in Swedish primary school children. Some child psychiatric aspects. *Journal of Child Psychology and Psychiatry*, *24*(3), 377–403.

Gillberg, I. C., & Gillberg, C. (1988). Generalized hyperkinesis: Follow-up study from age 7 to 13 years. *Journal of the American Academy of Child and Adolescent Psychiatry*, *27*(1), 55–59.

Gillberg, C., Melander, H., von Knorring, A.-L., Janols, L.-O., Thernlund, G., Hägglöf, B., et al. (1997). Long-term stimulant treatment of children with attention-deficit hyperactivity disorder symptoms. A randomized, double-blind, placebo-controlled trial. *Archives of General Psychiatry*, *54*(9), 857–864.

Gillis, J. J., Gilger, J. W., Pennington, B. F., & Defries, J. C. (1992). Attention deficit disorder in reading-disabled twins: Evidence for a genetic etiology. *Journal of Abnormal Child Psychology*, *20*, 303–315.

Gittelman, R., & Eskinazi, B. (1983). Lead and hyperactivity revisited. *Archives of General Psychiatry*, *40*, 827–833.

Gittelman, R., Mannuzza, S., Shenker, R., & Bonagura, N. (1985). Hyperactive boys almost grown up: I. Psychiatric status. *Archives of General Psychiatry*, *42*, 937–947.

Gjone, H., Stevenson, J., & Sundet, J. M. (1996). Genetic influence on parent-reported attention-related problems in a Norwegian general population twin sample. *Journal of the American Academy of Child and Adolescent Psychiatry*, *35*, 588–596.

Gjone, H., Stevenson, J., Sundet, J. M., & Eilertsen, D. E. (1996). Changes in heritability across increasing levels of behavior problems in young twins. *Behavior Genetics*, *26*, 419–426.

Glow, P. H., & Glow, R. A. (1979). Hyperkinetic impulse disorder: A developmental defect of motivation. *Genetic Psychological Monographs*, *100*, 159–231.

Gomez, R., & Sanson, A. V. (1994). Mother–child interactions and noncompliance in hyperactive boys with and without conduct problems. *Journal of Child Psychology and Psychiatry*, *35*, 477–490.

Goodman, J. R., & Stevenson, J. (1989). A twin study of hyperactivity: II. The aetiological role of genes, family relationships, and perinatal adversity. *Journal of Child Psychology and Psychiatry*, *30*, 691–709.

Grattan, L. M., & Eslinger, P. J. (1991). Frontal lobe damage in children and adults: A comparative review. *Developmental Neuropsychology*, *7*, 283–326.

Grenell, M. M., Glass, C. R., & Katz, K. S. (1987). Hyperactive children and peer interaction: Knowledge and performance of social skills. *Journal of Abnormal Child Psychology*, *15*, 1–13.

Gresham, F. M., MacMillan, D. L., Bocian, K. M., Ward, S. L., & Forness, S. R. (1998). Comorbidity of hyperactivity-impulsivity-inattention and conduct problems: Risk factors in social, affective, and academic domains. *Journal of Abnormal Child Psychology*, *26*, 393–406.

Grodzinsky, G. M., & Diamond, R. (1992). Frontal lobe functioning in boys with attention-deficit hyperactivity disorder. *Developmental Neuropsychology*, *8*, 427–445.

Gross-Tsur, V., Shalev, R. S., & Amir, N. (1991). Attention deficit disorder: Association with familial–genetic factors. *Pediatric Neurology*, *7*, 258–261.

Gruber, R., Sadeh, A., & Raviv, A. (2000). Instability of sleep patterns in children with attention-deficit/hyperactivity disorder. *Journal of the American Academy of Child and Adolescent Psychiatry*, *39*, 495–501.

Gustafsson, P., Thernlund, G., Ryding, E., Rosen, I., & Cederblad, M. (2000). Associations between cerebral blood-flow measured by single photon emission computed tomography (SPECT), electro-encephalogram (EEG), behavior symptoms, cognition and neurological soft signs in children with attention-deficit hyperactivity disorder (ADHD). *Acta Paediatrica*, *89*, 830–835.

Haenlein, M., & Caul, W. F. (1987). Attention deficit disorder with hyperactivity: A specific hypothesis of reward dysfunction. *Journal of the American Academy of Child and Adolescent Psychiatry*, *26*, 356–362.

Halperin, J. M., & Gittelman, R. (1982). Do hyperactive children and their siblings differ in IQ and academic achievement? *Psychiatry Research*, *6*, 253–258.

Halperin, J. M., Newcorn, J. H., Koda, V. H., Pick, L., McKay, K. E., & Knott, P. (1997). Nonadrenergic mechanisms in ADHD children with and without reading disabilities: A replication and extension. *Journal of the American Academy of Child and Adolescent Psychiatry, 36,* 1688–1697.

Hamlett, K. W., Pellegrini, D. S., & Conners, C. K. (1987). An investigation of executive processes in the problem solving of attention deficit disorder–hyperactive children. *Journal of Pediatric Psychology, 12,* 227–240.

Hart, E. L., Lahey, B. B., Loeber, R., Applegate, B., & Frick, P. J. (1995). Developmental changes in attention-deficit hyperactivity disorder in boys: A four-year longitudinal study. *Journal of Abnormal Child Psychology, 23,* 729–750.

Hartsough, C. S., & Lambert, N. M. (1985). Medical factors in hyperactive and normal children: Prenatal, developmental, and health history findings. *American Journal of Orthopsychiatry, 55,* 190–210.

Harvey, W. J., & Reid, G. (1997). Motor performance of children with attention-deficit hyperactivity disorder: A preliminary investigation. *Adapted Physical Activity Quarterly, 14,* 189–202.

Hastings, J., & Barkley, R. A. (1978). A review of psychophysiological research with hyperactive children. *Journal of Abnormal Child Psychology, 7,* 337–413.

Hauser, P., Zametkin, A. J., Martinez, P., Vitiello, B., Matochik, J., Mixson, A., & Weintraub, B. (1993). Attention deficit hyperactivity disorder in people with generalized resistance to thyroid hormone. *New England Journal of Medicine, 328,* 997–1001.

Heffron, W. A., Martin, C. A., & Welsh, R. J. (1984). Attention deficit disorder in three pairs of monozygotic twins: A case report. *Journal of the American Academy of Child Psychiatry, 23,* 299–301.

Heilman, K. M., Voeller, K. K. S., & Nadeau, S. E. (1991). A possible pathophysiological substrate of attention deficit hyperactivity disorder. *Journal of Child Neurology, 6,* 74–79.

Hendren, R. L., De Backer, I., & Pandina, G. J. (2000). Review of neuroimaging studies of child and adolescent psychiatric disorders from the past 10 years. *Journal of the American Academy of Child and Adolescent Psychiatry, 39,* 815–828.

Herpertz, S. C., Wenning, B., Mueller, B., Qunaibi, M., Sass, H., & Herpetz-Dahlmann, B. (2001). Psychological responses in ADHD boys with and without conduct disorder: Implications for adult antisocial behavior. *Journal of the American Academy of Child and Adolescent Psychiatry, 40,* 1222–1230.

Hinshaw, S. P. (1987). On the distinction between attentional deficits/hyperactivity and conduct problems/aggression in child psychopathology. *Psychological Bulletin, 101,* 443–447.

Hinshaw, S. P. (1992). Externalizing behavior problems and academic underachievement in childhood and adolescence: Causal relationships and underlying mechanisms. *Psychological Bulletin, 111,* 127–155.

Hinshaw, S. P. (1994). *Attention deficits and hyperactivity in children.* Thousand Oaks, CA: Sage.

Hinshaw, S. P. (2001). Is the inattentive type of ADHD a separate disorder? *Clinical Psychology: Science and Practice, 8,* 498–501.

Hinshaw, S. P., Buhrmeister, D., & Heller, T. (1989). Anger control in response to verbal provocation: Effects of stimulant medication for boys with ADHD. *Journal of Abnormal Child Psychology, 17,* 393–408.

Hinshaw, S. P., Heller, T., & McHale, J. P. (1992). Covert antisocial behavior in boys with attention-deficit hyperactivity disorder: External validation and effects of methyl-phenidate. *Journal of Consulting and Clinical Psychology, 60,* 274–281.

Hinshaw, S. P., & Melnick, S. M. (1995). Peer relationships in boys with attention-deficit hyperactivity disorder with and without comorbid aggression. *Development and Psychopathology, 7,* 627–647.

Hinshaw, S. P., Morrison, D. C., Carte, E. T., & Cornsweet, C. (1987). Factorial dimensions of the Revised Behavior Problem Checklist: Replication and validation within a kindergarten sample. *Journal of Abnormal Child Psychology, 15,* 309–327.

Hodgens, J. B., Cole, J., & Boldizar, J. (2000). Peer-based differences among boys with ADHD. *Journal of Clinical Child Psychology, 29,* 443–452.

Hohman, L. B. (1922). Post-encephalitic behavior disorders in children. *Johns Hopkins Hospital Bulletin, 33,* 372–375.

Holdsworth, L., & Whitmore, K. (1974). A study of children with epilepsy attending ordinary schools: I. Their seizure patterns, progress, and behaviour in school. *Developmental Medicine and Child Neurology, 16,* 746–758.

Hoy, E., Weiss, G., Minde, K., & Cohen, N. (1978). The hyperactive child at adolescence: Cognitive, emotional, and social functioning. *Journal of Abnormal Child Psychology, 6,* 311–324.

Hoza, B., Pelham, W. E., Waschbusch, D. A., Kipp, H., & Owens, J. S. (2001). Academic task performance of normally achieving ADHD and control boys: Performance, self-evaluations, and attributions. *Journal of Consulting and Clinical Psychology, 69,* 271–283.

Humphries, T., Kinsbourne, M., & Swanson, J. (1978). Stimulant effects on cooperation and social interaction between hyperactive children and their mothers. *Journal of Child Psychology and Psychiatry, 19,* 13–22.

Humphries, T., Koltun, H., Malone, M., & Roberts, W. (1994). Teacher-identified oral language difficulties among boys with attention problems. *Developmental and Behavioral Pediatrics, 15,* 92–98.

Hynd, G. W., Hern, K. L., Novey, E. S., Eliopulos, D., Marshall, R., Gonzalez, J. J., et al. (1993). Attention-deficit hyperactivity disorder and asymmetry of the caudate nucleus. *Journal of Child Neurology, 8,* 339–347.

Hynd, G. W., Lorys, A. R., Semrud-Clikeman, M., Nieves, N., Huettner, M. I. S., & Lahey, B. B. (1991). Attention deficit disorder without hyperactivity: A distinct behavioral and neurocognitive syndrome. *Journal of Child Neurology, 6,* S37–S43.

Hynd, G. W., Semrud-Clikeman, M., Lorys, A. R., Novey, E. S., & Eliopulos, D. (1990). Brain morphology in developmental dyslexia and attention deficit disorder/hyperactivity. *Archives of Neurology, 47,* 919–926.

Hynd, G. W., Semrud-Clikeman, M., Lorys, A. R., Novey, E. S., Eliopulos, D., & Lyytinen, H. (1991). Corpus callosum morphology in attention deficit-hyperactivity disorder: Morphometric analysis of MRI. *Journal of Learning Disabilities, 24,* 141–146.

Jacobvitz, D., & Sroufe, L. A. (1987). The early caregiver-child relationship and attention-deficit disorder with hyperactivity in kindergarten: A prospective study. *Child Development, 58,* 1488–1495.

Jensen, P. S., Martin, D., & Cantwell, D. P. (1997). Comorbidity in ADHD: Implications for research, practice, and DSM-V. *Journal of the American Academy of Child and Adolescent Psychiatry, 36,* 1065–1079.

Jensen, P. S., Shervette, R. E., Xenakis, S. N., & Bain, M. W. (1988). Psychosocial and medical histories of stimulant-treated children. *Journal of the American Academy of Child and Adolescent Psychiatry, 27,* 798–801.

Jensen, P. S., Shervette, R. E., III, Xenakis, S. N., & Richters, J. (1993). Anxiety and depressive disorders in attention deficit disorder with hyperactivity: New Findings. *American Journal of Psychiatry, 150,* 1203–1209.

Jensen, P. S., Watanabe, H. K., Richters, J. E., Cortes, R., Roper, M., & Liu, S. (1995). Prevalence of mental disorder in military children and adolescents: Findings from a two-stage community survey. *Journal of the American Academy of Child and Adolescent Psychiatry, 34,* 1514–1524.

Johnson, B. D., Altmaier, E. M., & Richman, L. C. (1999). Attention deficits and reading disabilities: Are immediate memory defects additive? *Developmental Neuropsychology, 15,* 213–226.

Johnson, J. G., Cohen, P., Kasen, S., Smailes, E., & Brook, J. S. (2001). Association of maladaptive parental behavior with psychiatric disorder among parents and their offspring. *Archives of General Psychiatry, 58,* 453–460.

Johnson, R. C., & Rosen, L. A. (2000). Sports behavior of ADHD children. *Journal of Attention Disorders, 4,* 150–160.

Johnston, C. (1996). Parent characteristics and parent-child interactions in families of nonproblem children and ADHD children with higher and lower levels of oppositional-defiant disorder. *Journal of Abnormal Child Psychology, 24,* 85–104.

Johnston, C., & Mash, E. J. (2001). Families of children with attention-deficit/hyperactivity disorder: Review and recommendations for future research. *Clinical Child and Family Psychology Review, 4,* 183–207.

Johnstone, S. J., Barry, R. J., & Anderson, J. W. (2001). Topographic distribution and developmental timecourse of auditory event-related potentials in two subtypes of attention-deficit hyperactivity disorder. *International Journal of Psychophysiology, 42,* 73–94.

Kadesjö, B., & Gillberg, C. (1998). Attention deficits and clumsiness in Swedish 7-year-old children. *Developmental Medicine and Child Neurology, 40,* 796–811.

Kadesjö, C., Kadesjö, B., Hägglöf, B., & Gillberg, C. (2001). ADHD in Swedish 3-7-year-old children. *Journal of the American Academy of Child and Adolescent Psychiatry, 40*(9), 1021–1028.

Kadesjo, B., & Gillberg, C. (2001). The comorbidity of ADHD in the general population of Swedish school-age children. *Journal of Child Psychology and Psychiatry, 42,* 487–492.

Kanbayashi, Y., Nakata, Y., Fujii, K., Kita, M., & Wada, K. (1994). ADHD-related behavior among non-referred children: Parents' ratings of DSM-III-R symptoms. *Child Psychiatry and Human Development, 25,* 13–29.

Kaplan, B. J., McNichol, J., Conte, R. A., & Moghadam, H. K. (1987). Sleep disturbance in preschool-aged hyperactive and nonhyperactive children. *Pediatrics, 80,* 839–844.

Keenan, K. (2000). Emotion dysregulation as a risk factor for child psychopathology. *Clinical Psychology: Science and Practice, 7,* 418–434.

Kessler, J. W. (1980). History of minimal brain dysfunction. In H. Rie & E. Rie (Eds.), *Handbook of minimal brain dysfunctions: A critical view* (pp. 18–52). New York: Wiley.

Klorman, R. (1992). Cognitive event-related potentials in attention deficit disorder. In S. E. Shaywitz & B. A. Shaywitz (Eds.), *Attention deficit disorder comes of age: Toward the twenty-first century* (pp. 221–244). Austin, TX: Pro-ed.

Klorman, R., Salzman, L. F., & Borgstedt, A. D. (1988). Brain event-related potentials in evaluation of cognitive deficits in attention deficit disorder and outcome of stimulant therapy. In L. Bloomingdale (Ed.), *Attention deficit disorder* (Vol. 3, pp. 49–80). New York: Pergamon.

Klorman, R., Hazel-Fernandez, H., Shaywitz, S. E., Fletcher, J. M., Marchione, K. E., Holahan, J. M., et al. (1999). Executive functioning deficits in attention-deficit/hyperactivity disorder are independent of oppositional defiant or reading disorder. *Journal of the American Academy of Child and Adolescent Psychiatry, 38,* 1148–1155.

Knobel, M., Wolman, M. B., & Mason, E. (1959). Hyperkinesis and organicity in children. *Archives of General Psychiatry, 1,* 310–321.

Krause, K., Dresel, S. H., Krause, J., Kung, H. F., & Tatsch, K. (2000). Increased striatal dopamine transporter in adult patients with attention deficit hyperactivity disorder: Effects of methylphenidate as measured by single photon emission computed tomography. *Neuroscience Letters, 285,* 107–110.

Kroes, M., Kalff, A. C., Kessels, A. G. H., Steyaert, J., Feron, F., van Someren, A., et al. (2001). Child psychiatric diagnoses in a population of Dutch schoolchildren aged 6 to 8 years. *Journal of the American Academy of Child and Adolescent Psychiatry, 40,* 1401–1409.

Kuntsi, J., Oosterlaan, J., & Stevenson, J. (2001). Psychological mechanisms in hyperactivity: I. Response inhibition deficit, working memory impairment, delay aversion, or something else? *Journal of Child Psychology and Psychiatry, 42,* 199–210.

Kuperman, S., Johnson, B., Arndt, S., Lindgren, S., & Wolraich, M. (1996). Quantitative EEG differences in a nonclinical sample of children with ADHD and undifferentiated ADD. *Journal of the American Academy of Child and Adolescent Psychiatry, 35,* 1009–1017.

Lahey, B. B. (2001). Should the combined and predominantly inattentive types of ADHD be considered distinct and unrelated disorders? Not now, at least. *Clinical Psychology: Science and Practice, 8,* 494–497.

Lahey, B. B., Applegate, B., McBurnett, K., Biederman, J., Greenhill, L., et al. (1994). DSM-IV field trials for attention deficit/hyperactivity disorder in children and adolescents. *American Journal of Psychiatry, 151,* 1673–1685.

Lahey, B. B., & Carlson, C. L. (1992). Validity of the diagnostic category of attention deficit disorder without hyperactivity: A review of the literature. In S. E. Shaywitz & B. A. Shaywitz (Eds.), *Attention deficit disorder comes of age: Toward the twenty-first century* (pp. 119–144). Austin, TX: Pro-ed.

Lahey, B. B., McBurnett, K., & Loeber, R. (2000). Are attention-deficit/hyperactivity disorder and oppositional defiant disorder developmental precursors to conduct disorder? In A. J. Sameroff, M. Lewis, & S. M. Miller (Eds.), *Handbook of developmental psychopathology* (2nd ed., pp. 431–446.). New York: Plenum.

Lahey, B. B., Pelham, W. E., Schaughency, E. A., Atkins, M. S., Murphy, H. A., Hynd, G. W., et al. (1988). Dimensions and types of attention deficit disorder with hyperactivity in children: A factor and cluster-analytic approach. *Journal of the American Academy of Child and Adolescent Psychiatry, 27,* 330–335.

Lahey, B. B., Schaughency, E., Hynd, G., Carlson, C., & Nieves, N. (1987). Attention deficit disorder with and without hyperactivity: Comparison of behavioral characteristics of clinic-referred children. *Journal of the American Academy of Child Psychiatry, 26,* 718–723.

Lahey, B. B., Schaughency, E., Strauss, C., & Frame, C. (1984). Are attention deficit disorders with and without hyperactivity similar or dissimilar disorders? *Journal of the American Academy of Child Psychiatry, 23,* 302–309.

Lahoste, G. J., Swanson, J. M., Wigal, S. B., Glabe, C., Wigal, T., King, N., et al. (1996). Dopamine D4 receptor gene polymorphism is associated with attention deficit hyperactivity disorder. *Molecular Psychiatry, 1,* 121–124.

Lambert, N. M. (1988). Adolescent outcomes for hyperactive children. *American Psychologist, 43,* 786–799.

Lambert, N. M., & Hartsough, C. S. (1998). Prospective study of tobacco smoking and substance dependencies among samples of ADHD and non-ADHD participants. *Journal of Learning Disabilities, 31,* 533–544.

Lambert, N. M. (in press). Stimulant treatment as a risk factor for nicotine use and substance abuse. In P. S. Jensen & J. R. Cooper (Eds.), *Diagnosis and treatment of attention deficit hyperactivity disorder: An evidence-based approach.* New York: American Medical Association Press.

Lambert, N. M., Sandoval, J., & Sassone, D. (1978). Prevalence of hyperactivity in elementary school children as a function of social system definers. *American Journal of Orthopsychiatry, 48,* 446–463.

Lamminmaki, T., Ahonen, T., Narhi, V., Lyytinent, H., & de Barra, H. T. (1995). Attention deficit hyperactivity disorder subtypes: Are there differences in academic problems? *Developmental Neuropsychology, 11,* 297–310.

Langsdorf, R., Anderson, R. F., Walchter, D., Madrigal, J. F., & Juarez, L. J. (1979). Ethnicity, social class, and perception of hyperactivity. *Psychology in the Schools, 16,* 293–298.

Lapouse, R., & Monk, M. (1958). An epidemiological study of behavior characteristics in children. *American Journal of Public Health, 48,* 1134–1144.

Last, C. G., Hersen, M., Kazdin, A., Orvaschel, H., & Perrin, S. (1991). Anxiety disorders in children and their families. *Archives of General Psychiatry, 48,* 928–934.

Laufer, M., Denhoff, E., & Solomons, G. (1957). Hyperkinetic impulse disorder in children's behavior problems. *Psychosomatic Medicine, 19,* 38–49.

Lavigne, J. V., Gibbons, R. D., Christoffel, K., Arend, R., Rosenbaum, D., Binns, H., et al. (1996). Prevalence rates and correlates of psychiatric disorders among preschool children. *Journal of the American Academy of Child and Adolescent Psychiatry, 35,* 204–214.

Lecendreux, M., Konofal, E., Bouvard, M., Falissard, B., Simeoni, M. M. (2000). Sleep and alertness in children with ADHD. *Journal of Child Psychology and Psychiatry, 41,* 803–812.

Lerner, J. A., Inui, T. S., Trupin, E. W., & Douglas, E. (1985). Preschool behavior can predict future psychiatric disorders. *Journal of the American Academy of Child Psychiatry, 24,* 42–48.

Levin, P. M. (1938). Restlessness in children. *Archives of Neurology and Psychiatry, 39,* 764–770.

Levy, F., & Hay, D. (2001). *Attention, genes, and ADHD.* Philadelphia, PA: Brunner-Routledge.

Levy, F., Hay, D. A., McStephen, M., Wood, C., & Waldman, I. (1997). Attention-deficit hyperactivity disorder: A category or a continuum? Genetic analysis of a large-scale twin study. *Journal of the American Academy of Child and Adolescent Psychiatry, 36,* 737–744.

Levy, F., & Hobbes, G. (1989). Reading, spelling, and vigilance in attention deficit and conduct disorder. *Journal of Abnormal Child Psychology, 17,* 291–298.

Lewinsohn, P. M., Hops, H., Roberts, R. E., Seeley, J. R., & Andrews, J. A. (1993). Adolescent psychopathology: I. Prevalence and incidence of depression and other DSM-III-R disorders in high school students. *Journal of Abnormal Psychology, 102,* 133–144.

Liu, X., Kurita, H., Guo, C., Tachimori, H., Ze, J., & Okawa, M. (2000). Behavioral and emotional problems in Chinese children: Teacher reports for ages 6 to 11. *Journal of Child Psychology and Psychiatry, 41,* 253–260.

Loeber, R., Burke, J. D., Lahey, B. B., Winters, A., & Zera, M. (2000). Oppositional defiant and conduct disorder: A review of the past 10 years, Part I. *Journal of the American Academy of Child and Adolescent Psychiatry, 39,* 1468–1484.

Loeber, R., Green, S. M., Lahey, B. B., Christ, M. A. G., & Frick, P. J. (1992). Developmental sequences in the age of onset of disruptive child behaviors. *Journal of Child and Family Studies, 1,* 21–41.

Loney, J., Kramer, J., & Milich, R. (1981). The hyperkinetic child grows up: Predictors of symptoms, delinquency, and achievement at follow-up. In K. Gadow & J. Loney (Eds.), *Psychosocial aspects of drug treatment for hyperactivity.* Boulder, CO: Westview Press.

Loney, J., Kramer, J. R., & Salisbury, H. (in press). Medicated versus unmedicated ADHD children: Adult involvement with legal and illegal drugs. In P. S. Jensen & J. R. Cooper (Eds.), *Diagnosis and treatment of attention deficit hyperactivity disorder: An evidence-based approach.* New York: American Medical Association Press.

Lorch, E. P., Milich, M., Sanchez, R. P., van den Broek, P., Baer, S., Hooks, K., et al. (2000). Comprehension of televised stories in bos with attention deficit/hyperactivity disorder and nonreferred boys. *Journal of Abnormal Psychology, 109,* 321–330.

Lou, H. C., Henriksen, L., & Bruhn, P. (1984). Focal cerebral hypoperfusion in children with dysphasia and/or attention deficit disorder. *Archives of Neurology, 41,* 825–829.

Lou, H. C., Henriksen, L., Bruhn, P., Borner, H., & Nielsen, J. B. (1989). Striatal dysfunction in attention deficit and hyperkinetic disorder. *Archives of Neurology, 46,* 48–52.

Luk, S. (1985). Direct observations studies of hyperactive behaviors. *Journal of the American Academy of Child and Adolescent Psychiatry, 24,* 338–344.

Lynam, D., Moffitt, T., & Stouthamer-Loeber, M. (1993). Explaining the relation between IQ and deliquency: Class, race, test motivation, school failure, or self-control? *Journal of Abnormal Psychology, 102,* 187–196.

Madan-Swain, A., & Zentall, S. S. (1990). Behavioral comparisons of liked and disliked hyperactive children in play contexts and the behavioral accommodations by teir classmates. *Journal of Consulting and Clinical Psychology, 58,* 197–209.

Maedgen, J. W., & Carlson, C. L. (2000). Social functioning and emotional regulation in the attention deficit hyperactivity disorder subtypes. *Journal of Clinical Child Psychology, 29,* 30–42.

Malone, M. A., & Swanson, J. M. (1993). Effects of methylphenidate on impulsive responding in children with attention deficit hyperactivity disorder. *Journal of Child Neurology, 8,* 157–163.

Mannuzza, S., & Gittelman, R. (1986). Informant variance in the diagnostic assessment of hyperactive children as young adults. In J. E. Barrett & R. M. Rose (Eds.), *Mental disorders in the Community* (pp. 243–254). New York: Guilford.

Mannuzza, S., Klein, R., Bessler, A., Malloy, P., & LaPadula, M. (1993). Adult outcome of hyperactive boys: Educational achievement, occupational rank, and psychiatric status. *Archives of General Psychiatry, 50,* 565–576.

Mannuzza, S., Klein, R., Bessler, A., Malloy, P., & LaPadula, M. (1998). Adult psychiatric status of hyperactive boys grown up. *American Journal of Psychiatry, 155,* 493–498.

Mannuzza, S., Klein, R. G., Bonagura, N., Malloy, P., Giampino, H., & Addalli, K. A. (1991). Hyperactive boys almost grown up: Replication of psychiatric status. *Archives of General Psychiatry, 48,* 77–83.

Mannuzza, S., & Klein, R. (1992). Predictors of outcome of children with attention-deficit hyperactivity disorder. In G. Weiss (Ed.), *Child and adolescent psychiatric clinics of North America: Attention-deficit hyperactivity disorder* (pp. 567–578). Philadelphia: Saunders.

Marcotte, A. C., & Stern, C. (1997). Qualitative analysis of graphomotor output in children with attentional disorders. *Child Neuropsychology, 3,* 147–153.

Mariani, M., & Barkley, R. A. (1997). Neuropsychological and academic functioning in preschool children with attention deficit hyperactivity disorder. *Developmental Neuropsychology, 13,* 111–129.

Marshall, R. M., Hynd, G. W., Handwerk, M. J., & Hall, J. (1997). Academic underachievement in ADHD subtypes. *Journal of Learning Disabilities, 30,* 635–642.

Mash, E. J., & Johnston, C. (1982). A comparison of mother–child interactions of younger and older hyperactive and normal children. *Child Development, 53,* 1371–1381.

Mash, E. J., & Johnston, C. (1983a). Sibling interactions of hyperactive and normal children and their relationship to reports of maternal stress and self-esteem. *Journal of Clinical Child Psychology, 12,* 91–99.

Mash, E. J., & Johnston, C. (1983b). The prediction of mothers' behavior with their hyperactive children during play and task situations. *Child and Family Behavior Therapy, 5,* 1–14.

Mash, E. J., & Johnston, C. (1990). Determinants of parenting stress: Illustrations from families of hyperactive children and families of physically abused children. *Journal of Clinical Child Psychology, 19,* 313–328.

Mattes, J. A. (1980). The role of frontal lobe dysfunction in childhood hyperkinesis. *Comprehensive Psychiatry, 21,* 358–369.

Matthys, W., Cuperus, J. M., & Van Engeland, H. (1999). Deficient social problem-solving in boys with ODD/CD, with ADHD, and with both disorders. *Journal of the American Academy of Child and Adolescent Psychiatry, 38,* 311–321.

Matthys, W., van Goozen, S. H. M., de Vries, H., Cohen-Kettenis, P. T., & van Engeland, H. (1998). The dominance of behavioral activation over behavioural inhibition in conduct disordered boys with or without attention deficit hyperactivity disorder. *Journal of Child Psychology and Psychiatry, 39,* 643–651.

McArdle, P., O'Brien, G., & Kolvin, I. (1995). Hyperactivity: Prevalence and relationship with conduct disorder. *Journal of Child Psychology and Psychiatry, 36,* 279–303.

McBurnett, K., Pfiffner, L. J., Willcutt, E., Tamm, L., Lerner, M., Ottolini, Y. L., et al. (1999). Experimental cross-validation of DSM-IV types of attention deficit/hyperactivity disorder. *Journal of the American Academy of Child and Adolescent Psychiatry, 38,* 17–24.

McBurnett, K., Pfiffner, L. J., & Frick, P. J. (2001). Symptom properties as a function of ADHD type: An argument for continued study of sluggish cognitive tempo. *Journal of Abnormal Child Psychology, 29,* 207–213.

McGee, R., Feehan, M., Williams, S., Partridge, F., Silva, P. A., & Kelly, J. (1990). DSM-III disorders in a large sample of adolescents. *Journal of the American Academy of Child and Adolescent Psychiatry, 29,* 611–619.

McGee, R., Stanton, W. R., & Sears, M. R. (1993). Allergic disorders and attention deficit disorder in children. *Journal of Abnormal Child Psychology, 21,* 79–88.

McGee, R., Williams, S., & Feehan, M. (1992). Attention deficit disorder and age of onset of problem behaviors. *Journal of Abnormal Child Psychology, 20,* 487–502.

McGee, R., Williams, S., & Silva, P. A. (1984). Behavioral and developmental characteristics of aggressive, hyperactive, and aggressive–hyperactive boys. *Journal of the American Academy of Child Psychiatry, 23,* 270–279.

McMohan, S. A., & Greenberg, L. M. (1977). Serial neurologic examination of hyperactive children. *Pediatrics, 59,* 584–587.

Melnick, S. M., & Hinshaw, S. P. (1996). What they want and what they get: The social goals of boys with ADHD and comparison boys. *Journal of Abnormal Child Psychology, 24,* 169–185.

Melnick, S. M., & Hinshaw, S. P. (2000). Emotion regulation and parenting in AD/HD and comparison boys: Linkages with social behaviors and peer preference. *Journal of Abnormal Child Psychology, 28,* 73–86.

Mick, E., Biederman, J., & Faraone, S. V. (1996). Is season of birth a risk factor for attention-deficit hyperactivity disorder? *Journal of the American Academy of Child and Adolescent Psychiatry, 35,* 1470–1476.

Milberger, S., Biederman, J., Faraone, S. V., Chen, L., & Jones, J. (1996a). Is maternal smoking during pregnancy a risk factor for attention deficit hyperactivity disorder in children? *American Journal of Psychiatry, 153,* 1138–1142.

Milberger, S., Biederman, J., Faraone, S. V., Chen, L., & Jones, J. (1996b). ADHD is associated with early initiation of cigarette smoking in children and adolescents. *Journal of the American Academy of Child and Adolescent Psychiatry, 36,* 37–44.

Milich, R., Hartung, C. M., Matrin, C. A., & Haigler, E. D. (1994). Behavioral disinhibition and underlying processes in adolescents with disruptive behavior disorders. In D. K. Routh (Ed.), *Disruptive behavior disorders in childhood* (pp. 109–138). New York: Plenum Press.

Milich, R., Lynam, D., & Ballentine, A. C. (2001). ADHD Combined Type and ADHD Predominantly Inattentive Type are distinct and unrelated disorders. *Clinical Psychology: Science and Practice, 8,* 463–488.

Minde, K., Webb, G., & Sykes, D. (1968). Studies on the hyperactive child: VI. Prenatal and perinatal factors associated with hyperactivity. *Developmental Medicine and Child Neurology, 10,* 355–363.

Mitchell, E. A., Aman, M. G., Turbott, S. H., & Manku, M. (1987). Clinical characteristics and serum essential fatty acid levels in hyperactive children. *Clinical Pediatrics, 26,* 406–411.

Mitsis, E. M., McKay, K. E., Schulz, K. P., Newcorn, J. H., & Halperin, J. M. (2000). Parent–teacher concordance in DSM-IV attention-deficit/hyperactivity disorder in a clinic-referred sample. *Journal of the American Academy of Child and Adolescent Psychiatry, 39,* 308–313.

Moffitt, T. E. (1990). Juvenile delinquency and attention deficit disorder: Boys' developmental trajectories from age 3 to 15. *Child Development, 61,* 893–910.

Molina, B. S. G., & Pelham, W. E. (2001). Substance use, substance abuse, and LD among adolescents with a childhood history of ADHD. *Journal of Learning Disabilities, 34,* 333–342.

Molina, B. S. G., Smith, B. H., & Pelham, W. E. (1999). Interactive effects of attention deficit hyperactivity disorder and conduct disorder on early adolescent substance use. *Psychology of Addictive Behavior, 13,* 348-358.

Monastra, V. J., Lubar, J. F., & Linden, M. (2001). The development of quantitative a electroencephalographic scanning process for attention deficit/hyperactivity disorder: Reliability and validity studies. *Neuropsychology, 15,* 136–144.

Mori, L., & Peterson, L. (1995). Knowledge of safety of high and low active-impulsive boys: Implications for child injury prevention. *Journal of Clinical Child Psychology, 24,* 370–376.

Morgan, A. E., Hynd, G. W., Riccio, C. A., & Hall, J. (1996). Validity of DSM-IV predominantly inattentive and combined types: Relationship to previous DSM diagnoses/subtype differences. *Journal of the American Academy of Child and Adolescent Psychiatry, 35,* 325–333.

Morrison, J., & Stewart, M. (1973). The psychiatric status of the legal families of adopted hyperactive children. *Archives of General Psychiatry, 28,* 888–891.

Murphy, K. R., & Barkley, R. A. (1996a). Prevalence of DSM-IV symptoms of ADHD in adult licensed drivers: Implications for clinical diagnosis. *Journal of Attention Disorders, 1,* 147–161.

Murphy, K. R., & Barkley, R. A. (1996b). Attention deficit hyperactivity disorder in adults: Comorbidities and adaptive impairments. *Comprehensive Psychiatry, 37,* 393–401.

Murphy, K. R., Barkley, R. A., & Bush, T. (2001). Executive functioning and olfactory identification in young adults with attention deficit hyperactivity disorder. *Neuropsychology, 15,* 211–220.

Nada-Raja, S., Langley, J. D., McGee, R., Williams, S. M., Begg, D. J., & Reeder, A. I. (1997). Inattentive and hyperactive behaviors and driving offenses in adolescence. *Journal of the American Academy of Child and Adolescent Psychiatry, 36,* 515–522.

Needleman, H. L., Gunnoe, C., Leviton, A., Reed, R., Peresie, H., & Maher, C., et al. (1979). Deficits in psychologic and classroom performance of children with elevated dentine lead levels. *New England Journal of Medicine, 300,* 689–695.

Needleman, H. L., Schell, A., Bellinger, D. C., Leviton, L., & Alfred, E. D. (1990). The long-term effects of exposure to low doses of lead in childhood: An 11-year follow-up report. *New England Journal of Medicine, 322,* 83–88.

Newcorn, J. H., Halperin, J. M., Jensen, P. S., Abikoff, H. B., Arnold, L. E., Cantwell, D. P., et al. (2001). Symptom profiles in children with ADHD: Comorbidity and gender. *Journal of the American Academy of Child and Adolescent Psychiatry, 40,* 137–146.

Nichols, P. L., & Chen, T. C. (1981). *Minimal brain dysfunction: A prospective study.* Hillsdale, NJ: Erlbaum.

Nigg, J. T. (1999). The ADHD response-inhibition deficit as measured by the stop task: Replication with DSM-IV Combined Type, extension, and qualification. *Journal of Abnormal Child Psychology, 27,* 393–402.

Nigg, J. T. (2000). On inhibition/disinhibition in developmental psychopathology: Views from cognitive and personality psychology and a working inhibition taxonomy. *Psychological Bulletin, 126,* 220–246.

Nigg, J. T. (2001). Is ADHD an inhibitory disorder? *Psychological Bulletin, 125,* 571–596.

Nigg, J. T., Blaskey, L. G., Huang-Pollock, C. L., & Rappley, M. D. (2002). Neuropsychological executive functions in DSM-IV ADHD subtypes. *Journal of the American Academy of Child and Adolescent Psychiatry, 41,* 59–66.

Nucci, L. P., & Herman, S. (1982). Behavioral disordered children's conceptions of moral, conventional, and personal issues. *Journal of Abnormal Child Psychology, 10,* 411–426.

Nigg, J. T., Hinshaw, S. P., Carte, E. T., & Treuting, J. J. (1998). Neuropsychological correlates of childhood attention-deficit/hyperactivity disorder: Explainable by comorbid disruptive behavior or reading problems? *Journal of Abnormal Psychology, 107,* 468–480.

Nolan, E. E., Gadow, K. D., & Sprafkin, J. (2001). Teacher reports of DSM-IV ADHD, ODD, and CD symptoms in schoolchildren. *Journal of the American Academy of Child and Adolescent Psychiatry, 40,* 241–249.

O'Connor, M., Foch, T., Sherry, T., & Plomin, R. (1980). A twin study of specific behavioral problems of socialization as viewed by parents. *Journal of Abnormal Child Psychology, 8,* 189–199.

O'Dougherty, M., Nuechterlein, K. H., & Drew, B. (1984). Hyperactive and hypoxic children: Signal detection, sustained attention, and behavior. *Journal of Abnormal Psychology, 93,* 178–191.

O'Leary, K. D., Vivian, D., & Nisi, A. (1985). Hyperactivity in Italy. *Journal of Abnormal Child Psychology, 13,* 485–500.

Olson, S. L., Bates, J. E., Sandy, J. M., & Lanthier, R. (2000). Early developmental precursors of externalizing behavior in middle childhood and adolescence. *Journal of Abnormal Child Psychology, 28,* 119–133.

Olson, S. L., Schilling, E. M., & Bates, J. E. (1999). Measurement of impulsivity: Construct coherence, longitudinal stability, and relationship with externalizing problems in middle childhood and adolescence. *Journal of Abnormal Child Psychology, 27,* 151–165.

Oosterlaan, J., Logan, G. D., & Sergeant, J. A. (1998). Response inhibition in AD/HD, CD, comorbid AD/HD+CD, anxious, and control children: A meta-analysis of studies with the Stop Task. *Journal of Child Psychology and Psychiatry, 39,* 411–425.

Oosterlaan, J., Scheres, A., & Sergeant, J. A. (in press). Verbal fluency, working memory, and planning in children with ADHD, ODD/CD, and comorbid ADHD+ODD/CD: Specificity of executive functioning deficits. *Journal of Abnormal Psychology.*

Palfrey, J. S., Levine, M. D., Walker, D. K., & Sullivan, M. (1985). The emergence of attention deficits in early childhood: A prospective study. *Developmental and Behavioral Pediatrics, 6,* 339–348.

Parry, P. A., & Douglas, V. I. (1983). Effects of reinforcement on concept identification in hyperactive children. *Journal of Abnormal Child Psychology, 11,* 327–340.

Patterson, G. R., Degarmo, D. S., & Knutson, N. (2000). Hyperactive and antisocial behaviors: Comorbid or two points in the same process. *Development and Psychopathology, 12,* 91–106.

Pauls, D. L. (1991). Genetic factors in the expression of attention-deficit hyperactivity disorder. *Journal of Child and Adolescent Psychopharmacology, 1,* 353–360.

Pauls, D. L., Hurst, C. R., Kidd, K. K., Kruger, S. D., Leckman, J. F., & Cohen, D. J. (1986). Tourette syndrome and attention deficit disorder: Evidence against a genetic relationship. *Archives of General Psychiatry, 43,* 1177–1179.

Pelham, W. E., Jr. (2001). Are ADHD/I and ADHD/C the same or different? Does it matter? *Clinical Psychology: Science and Practice, 8,* 502–506.

Pelham, W. E., Gnagy, E. M., Greenslade, K. E., & Milich, R. (1992). Teacher ratings of DSM-III-R symptoms for the disruptive behavior disorders. *Journal of the American Academy of Child and Adolescent Psychiatry, 31,* 210–218.

Pelham, W. E., & Lang, A. R. (1993). Parental alcohol consumption and deviant child behavior: Laboratory studies of reciprocal effects. *Clinical Psychology Review, 13,* 763–784.

Pennington, B. F., & Ozonoff, S. (1996). Executive functions and developmental psychopathology. *Journal of Child Psychology and Psychiatry, 37,* 51–87.

Peterson, B. S., Pine, D. S., Cohen, P., & Brook, J. S. (2001). Prospective, longitudinal study of tic, obsessive-compulsive, and attention-deficit/hyperactivity disorders in an epidemiological sample. *Journal of the American Academy of Child and Adolescent Psychiatry, 40,* 685–695.

Pfiffner, L. J., McBurnett, K., & Rathouz, P. J. (2001). Father absence and familial antisocial characteristics. *Journal of Abnormal Child Psychology, 29,* 357–367.

Pike, A., & Plomin, R. (1996). Importance of nonshared environmental factors for childhood and adolescent psychopathology. *Journal of the American Academy of Child and Adolescent Psychiatry, 35,* 560–570.

Pillow, D. R., Pelham, W. E., Jr., Hoza, B., Molina, B. S. G., & Stultz, C. H. (1998). Confirmatory factor analyses examining attention deficit hyperactivity disorder symptoms and other childhood disruptive behaviors. *Journal of Abnormal Child Psychology, 26,* 293–309.

Pineda, D., Ardila, A., Rosselli, M., Arias, B. E., Henao, G. C., Gomex, L. F., et al. (1999). Prevalence of attention-deficit/hyperactivity disorder symptoms in 4- to 17-year old children in the general population. *Journal of Abnormal Child Psychology, 27,* 455–462.

Pliszka, S. R. (1992). Comorbidity of attention-deficit hyperactivity disorder and overanxious disorder. *Journal of the American Academy of Child and Adolescent Psychiatry, 31,* 197–203.

Pliszka, S. R., Liotti, M., & Woldorff, M. G. (2000). Inhibitory control in children with attention-deficit/hyperactivity disorder: Event-related potentials identify the processing component and timing of an impaired right-frontal response-inhibition mechanism. *Biological Psychiatry, 48,* 238–246.

Pliszka, S. R., McCracken, J. T., & Mass, J. W. (1996). Catecholamines in attention deficit hyperactivity disorder: Current perspectives. *Journal of the American Academy of Child and Adolescent Psychiatry, 35,* 264–272.

Plomin, R. (1995). Genetics and children's experiences in the family. *Journal of Child Psychology and Psychiatry, 36,* 33–68.

Porrino, L. J., Rapoport, J. L., Behar, D., Sceery, W., Ismond, D. R., & Bunney, W. E., Jr. (1983). A naturalistic assessment of the motor activity of hyperactive boys. *Archives of General Psychiatry, 40,* 681–687.

Quay, H. C. (1997). Inhibition and attention deficit hyperactivity disorder. *Journal of Abnormal Child Psychology, 25,* 7–13.

Rabiner, D., Coie, J. D., and the Conduct Problems Prevention Research Group. (2000). Early attention problems and children's reading achievement: A longitudinal investigation. *Journal of the American Academy of Child and Adolescent Psychiatry, 39,* 859–867.

Rapoport, J. L., Buchsbaum, M. S., Zahn, T. P., Weingarten, H., Ludlow, C., & Mikkelsen, E. J. (1978). Destroamphetamine: Cognitive and behavioral effects in normal prepubertal boys. *Science, 199,* 560–563.

Rapoport, J. L., Donnelly, M., Zametkin, A., & Carrougher, J. (1986). "Situational hyperactivity" in a U.S. clinical setting. *Journal of Child Psychology and Psychiatry, 27,* 639–646.

Rapport, M. D., Scanlan, S. W., & Denney, C. B. (1999). Attention–deficit/hyperactivity disorder and scholastic achievement: A model of dual developmental pathways. *Journal of Child Psychology and Psychiatry, 40,* 1169–1183.

Rapport, M. D., Tucker, S. B., DuPaul, G. J., Merlo, M., & Stoner, G. (1986). Hyperactivity and frustration: The influence of control over and size of rewards in delaying gratification. *Journal of Abnormal Child Psychology, 14,* 181–204.

Raskin, L. A. Shaywitz, S. E., Shaywitz, B. A., Anderson, G. M., & Cohen, D. J. (1984). Neurochemical correlates of attention deficit disorder. *Pediatric Clinics of North America, 31,* 387–396.

Rasmussen, P., & Gillberg, C. (2001). Natural outcome of ADHD with developmental coordination disorder at age 22 years: A controlled, longitudinal, community-based study. *Journal of the American Academy of Child and Adolescent Psychiatry, 39,* 1424–1431.

Rhee, S. H., Waldman, I. D., Hay, D. A., & Levy, F. (1995). Sex differences in genetic and environmental influences on DSM-III-R attention-deficit hyperactivity disorder (ADHD). *Behavior Genetics, 25,* 285.

Richman, N., Stevenson, J., & Graham, P. (1982). *Preschool to school: A behavioural study.* New York: Academic Press.

Roberts, M. A. (1990). A behavioral observation method for differentiating hyperactive and aggressive boys. *Journal of Abnormal Child Psychology, 18,* 131–142.

Rohde, L. A., Biederman, J., Busnello, E. A., Zimmermann, H., Schmitz, M., Martins, S., et al. (1999). ADHD in a school sample of Brazilian adolescents: A study of prevalence, comorbid conditions, and impairments. *Journal of the American Academy of Child and Adolescent Psychiatry, 38,* 716–722.

Roizen, N. J., Blondis, T. A., Irwin, M., & Stein, M. (1994). Adaptive functioning in children with attention-deficit hyperactivity disorder. *Archives of Pediatric and Adolescent Medicine, 148,* 1137–1142.

Romano, E., Tremblay, R. E., Vitaro, F., Zoccolillo, M., and Pagani, L. (2001). Prevalence of psychiatric diagnoses and the role of perceived impairment: Findings from and adolescent community sample. *Journal of Child Psychology and Psychiatry, 42,* 451–462.

Roth, N., Beyreiss, J., Schlenzka, K., & Beyer, H. (1991). Coincidence of attention deficit disorder and atopic disorders in children: Empirical findings and hypothetical background. *Journal of Abnormal Child Psychology, 19,* 1–13.

Rothenberger, A. (1995). Electrical brain activity in children with hyperkinetic syndrome: Evidence of a frontal cortical dysfunction. In J. A. Sergeant (Ed.), *Eunethydis: European approaches to hyperkinetic disorder* (pp. 255–270). Amsterdam: Author.

Routh, D. K., & Schroeder, C. S. (1976). Standardized playroom measures as indices of hyperactivity. *Journal of Abnormal Child Psychology, 4,* 199–207.

Rubia, K., Overmeyer, S., Taylor, E., Brammer, M., Williams, S. C. R., Simmons, A., & Bullmore, E. T. (1999). Hypofrontality in attention deficit hyperactivity disorder during higher-order motor control: A study with functional MRI. *American Journal of Psychiatry, 156,* 891–896.

Rucklidge, J. J., & Tannock, R. (2001). Psychiatric, psychosocial, and cognitive functioning of female adolescents with ADHD. *Journal of the American Academy of Child and Adolescent Psychiatry, 40,* 530–540.

Russo, M. F., & Beidel, D. C. (1994). Comorbidity of childhood anxiety and externalizing disorders: Prevalence, associated characteristics, and validation issues. *Clinical Psychology Review, 14,* 199–221.

Rutter, M. (1977). Brain damage syndromes in childhood: Concepts and findings. *Journal of Child Psychology and Psychiatry, 18,* 1–21.

Sachs, G. S., Baldassano, C. F., Truman, C. J., & Guille, C. (2000). Comorbidity of attention deficit hyperactivity disorder with early- and late-onset bipolar disorder. *American Journal of Psychiatry, 157,* 466–468.

Samuel, V. J., George, P., Thornell, A., Curtis, S., Taylor, A., Brome, D., et al. (1999). A pilot controlled family study of DSM-III-R and DSM-IV ADHD in African-American children. *Journal of the American Academy of Child and Adolescent Psychiatry, 38,* 34–39.

Sanchez, R. P., Lorch, E. P., Milich, R., & Welsh, R. (1999). Comprehension of televised stories in preschool children with ADHD. *Journal of Clinical Child Psychology, 28,* 376–385.

Satterfield, J. H., Hoppe, C. M., & Schell, A. M. (1982). A prospective study of delinquency in 110 adolescent boys with attention deficit disorder and 88 normal adolescent boys. *American Journal of Psychiatry, 139,* 795–798.

Schachar, R. J., & Logan, G. D. (1990). Impulsivity and inhibitory control in normal development and childhood psychopathology. *Developmental Psychology, 26,* 710–720.

Schachar, R., Rutter, M., & Smith, A. (1981). The characteristics of situationally and pervasively hyperactive children: Implications for syndrome definition. *Journal of Child Psychology and Psychiatry, 22,* 375–392.

Schachar, R. J., Tannock, R., & Logan, G. (1993). Inhibitory control, impulsiveness, and attention deficit hyperactivity disorder. *Clinical Psychology Review, 13,* 721–740.

Schachar, R., Taylor, E., Weiselberg, M., Thorley, G., & Rutter, M. (1987). Changes in family function and relationships in children who respond to methylphenidate. *Journal of the American Academy of Child and Adolescent Psychiatry, 26,* 728–732.

Scheres, A., Oosterlaan, J., & Sergeant, J. A. (2001). Response execution and inhibition in children with AD/HD and other disruptive disorders: The role of behavioural activation. *Journal of Child Psychology and Psychiatry, 42,* 347–357.

Schleifer, M., Weiss, G., Cohen, N. J., Elman, M., Cvejic, H., & Kruger, E. (1975). Hyperactivity in preschoolers and the effect of methylphenidate. *American Journal of Orthopsychiatry, 45,* 38–50.

Schothorst, P. F., & van Engeland, H. (1996). Long-term behavioral sequelae of prematurity. *Journal of the American Academy of Child and Adolescent Psychiatry, 35,* 175–183.

Schweitzer, J. B., Faber, T. L., Grafton, S. T., Tune, L. E., Hoffman, J. M., Kilts, C. D. (2000). Alterations in the functional anatomy of working memory in adult attention deficit hyperactivity disorder. *American Journal of Psychiatry, 157,* 278–280.

Seidman, L. J., Benedict, K. B., Biederman, J., Bernstein, J. H., Seiverd, K., Milberger, S., et al. (1995). Performance of children with ADHD on the Rey-Osterrieth Complex Figure: A pilot neuropsychological study. *Journal of Child Psychology and Psychiatry, 36,* 1459–1473.

Seidman, L. J., Biederman, J., Faraone, S. V., Milberger, S., Norman, D., Seiverd, K., et al. (1995). Effects of family history and comorbidity on the neuropsychological performance of children with ADHD: Preliminary findings. *Journal of the American Academy of Child and Adolescent Psychiatry, 34,* 1015–1024.

Seidman, L. J., Biederman, J., Faraone, S. V., Weber, W., & Ouellette, C. (1997). Toward defining a neuropsychology of attention deficit-hyperactivity disorder: Performance of children and adolescence from a large clinically referred sample. *Journal of Consulting and Clinical Psychology, 65,* 150–160.

Seguin, J. R., Boulerice, B., Harden, P. W., Tremblay, R. E., & Pihl, R. O. (1999). Executive functions and physical aggression after controlling for attention deficit hyperactivity disorder, general memory, and IQ. *Journal of Child Psychology and Psychiatry, 40,* 1197–1208.

Semrud-Clikeman, M., Biederman, J., Sprich-Buckminster, S., Lehman, B. K., Faraone, S. V., & Norman, D. (1992). Comorbidity between ADDH and learning disability: A review and report in a clinically referred sample. *Journal of the American Academy of Child and Adolescent Psychiatry, 31,* 439–448.

Semrud-Clikeman, M., Filipek, P. A., Biederman, J., Steingard, R., Kennedy, D., Renshaw, P., et al. (1994). Attention-deficit hyperactivity disorder: Magnetic resonance imaging morphometric analysis of the corpus callosum. *Journal of the American Academy of Child and Adolescent Psychiatry, 33,* 875–881.

Semrud-Clikeman, M., Steingard, R. J., Filipek, P., Biederman, J., Bekken, K., & Renshaw, P. F. (2000). Using MRI to examine brain-behavior relationships in males with attention deficit disorder with hyperactivity. *Journal of the American Academy of Child and Adolescent Psychiatry, 39,* 477–484.

Sergeant, J. (1988). From DSM-III attentional deficit disorder to functional defects. In L. Bloomingdale & J. Sergeant (Eds.), *Attention deficit disorder: Criteria, cognition, and intervention* (pp. 183–198). New York: Pergamon.

Sergeant, J., & van der Meere, J. P. (1994). Toward an empirical child psychopathology. In D. K. Routh (Ed.), *Disruptive behavior disorders in children* (pp. 59–86). New York: Plenum.

Shaywitz, S. E., Cohen, D. J., & Shaywitz, B. E. (1980). Behavior and learning difficulties in children of normal intelligence born to alcoholic mothers. *Journal of Pediatrics, 96,* 978–982.

Shaywitz, S. E., Shaywitz, B. A., Cohen, D. J., & Young, J. G. (1983). Monoaminergic mechanisms in hyperactivity. In M. Rutter (Ed.), *Developmental neuropsychiatry* (pp. 330–347). New York: Guilford.

Shaywitz, S. E., Shaywitz, B. A., Jatlow, P. R., Sebrechts, M., Anderson, G. M., & Cohen, D. J. (1986). Biological differentiation of attention deficit disorder with and without hyperactivity. A preliminary report. *Annals of Neurology, 21,* 363.

Shelton, T. L., Barkley, R. A., Crosswait, C., Moorehouse, M., Fletcher, K., Barrett, S., et al. (1998). Psychiatric and psychological morbidity as a function of adaptive disability in preschool children with high levels of aggressive and hyperactive-impulsive-inattentive behavior. *Journal of Abnormal Child Psychology, 26,* 475–494.

Sherman, D. K., Iacono, W. G., & McGue M. K. (1997). Attention-deficit hyperactivity disorder dimensions: A twin study of inattention and impulsivity-hyperactivity. *Journal of the American Academy of Child and Adolescent Psychiatry, 36,* 745–753.

Sherman, D. K., McGue, M. K., & Iacono, W. G. (1997). Twin concordance for attention deficit hyperactivity disorder: A comparison of teachers' and mothers' reports. *American Journal of Psychiatry, 154,* 532–535.

Silberg, J., Rutter, M., Meyer, J., Maes, H., Hewitt, J., Simonoff, E., et al. (1996). Genetic and environmental influences on the covariation between hyperactivity and conduct disturbance in juvenile twins. *Journal of Child Psychology and Psychiatry, 37,* 803–816.

Silva, P. A., Hughes, P., Williams, S., & Faed, J. M. (1988). Blood lead, intelligence, reading attainment, and behaviour in eleven year old children in Dunedin, New Zealand. *Journal of Child Psychology and Psychiatry, 29,* 43–52.

Singer, H. S., Reiss, A. L., Brown, J. E., Aylward, E. H., Shih, B., Chee, E., et al. (1993). Volumetric MRI changes in basal ganglia of children with Tourette's syndrome. *Neurology, 43,* 950–956.

Slusarek, M., Velling, S., Bunk, D., & Eggers, C. (2001). Motivational effects on inhibitory control in children with ADHD. *Journal of the American Academy of Child and Adolescent Psychiatry, 40,* 355–363.

Smalley, S. L., McGough, J. J., Del'Homme, M., NewDelman, J., Gordon, E., Kim, T., et al. (2000). Familial clustering of symptoms and disruptive behaviors in multiplex families with attention-deficit/hyperactivity disorder. *Journal of the American Academy of Child and Adolescent Psychiatry, 39,* 1135–1143.

Sonuga-Barke, E. J., Lamparelli, M., Stevenson, J., Thompson, M., & Henry, A. (1994). Behaviour problems and pre-school intellectual attainment: The associations of hyperactivity and conduct problems. *Journal of Child Psychology and Psychiatry, 35,* 949–960.

Sonuga-Barke, E. J. S., Taylor, E., & Hepinstall, E. (1992). Hyperactivity and delay aversion: II. The effect of self versus externally imposed stimulus presentation periods on memory. *Journal of Child Psychology and Psychiatry, 33,* 399–409.

Solanto, M. V., Abikoff, H., Sonuga-Barke, E., Schachar, R., Logan, G. D., Wigal, T., et al. (2001). The ecological validity of delay aversion and response inhibition as measures of impulsivity in AD/HD: A supplement to the NIMH Multimodal Treatment Study of ADHD. *Journal of Abnormal Child Psychology, 29,* 215–228.

Southam-Gerow, M. A., & Kendall, P. C. (2002). Emotion regulation and understanding: Impliations for child psychopathology and therapy. *Clinical Psychology Review, 22,* 189–222.

Spencer, T. J., Biederman, J., Faraone, S., Mick, E., Coffey, B., Geller, D., et al. (2001). Impact of tic disorders on ADHD outcome across the life cycle: Findings from a large group of adults with and without ADHD. *American Journal of Psychiatry, 158,* 611–617.

Spencer, T. J., Biederman, J., Harding, M., O'Donnell, D., Faraone, S. V., & Wilens, T. E. (1996). Growth deficits in ADHD children revisited: Evidence for disorder-associated growth delays? *Journal of the American Academy of Child and Adolescent Psychiatry, 35,* 1460–1469.

Spencer, T., Wilens, T., Biederman, J., Wozniak, J., & Harding-Crawford, M. (2000). Attention-deficit/hyperactivity disorder with mood disorders. In T. E. Brown (Ed.), *Attention deficit disorders and comorbidities in children, adolescents, and adults* (pp. 79–124). Washington, DC: American PsychiatricPress.

Sprich, S., Biederman, J., Crawford, M. H., Mundy, E., & Faraone, S. V. (2000). Adoptive and biological families of children and adolescents with ADHD. *Journal of the American Academy of Child and Adolesent Psychiatry, 39,* 1432–1437.

Stein, M. A. (1999). Unravelling sleep problems in treated and untreated children with ADHD. *Journal of Child and Adolescent Psychopharmacology, 9,* 157–168.

Stein, M. A., Szumowski, E., Blondis, T. A., & Roizen, N. J. (1995). Adaptive skills dysfunction in ADD and ADHD children. *Journal of Child Psychology and Psychiatry, 36,* 663–670.

Stein, M. A., Weiss, R. E., & Refetoff, S. (1995). Neurocognitive characteristics of individuals with resistance to thyroid hormone: Comparisons with individuals with attention-deficit hyperactivity disorder. *Journal of Developmental and Behavioral Pediatrics, 16,* 406–411.

Stevenson, J., Pennington, B. F., Gilger, J. W., DeFries, J. C., & Gilies, J. J. (1993). Hyperactivity and spelling disability: Testing for shared genetic aetiology. *Journal of Child Psychology and Psychiatry, 34,* 1137–1152.

Stewart, M. A. (1970). Hyperactive children. *Scientific American, 222,* 94–98.

Stewart, M. A., Pitts, F. N., Craig, A. G., & Dieruf, W. (1966). The hyperactive child syndrome. *American Journal of Orthopsychiatry, 36,* 861–867.

Stewart, M. A., Thach, B. T., & Friedin, M. R. (1970). Accidental poisoning and the hyperactive child syndrome. *Disease of the Nervous System, 31,* 403–407.

Still, G. F. (1902). Some abnormal psychical conditions in children. *Lancet, 1,* 1008–1012, 1077–1082, 1163–1168.

Strauss, A. A., & Kephardt, N. C. (1955). *Psychopathology and education of the brain-injured child: Vol. 2. Progress in theory and clinic.* New York: Grune & Stratton.

Strauss, A. A., & Lehtinen, L. E. (1947). *Psychopathology and education of the brain-injured child.* New York: Grune & Stratton.

Strauss, M. E., Thompson, P., Adams, N. L., Redline, S., & Burant, C. (2000). Evaluation of a model of attention with confirmatory factor analysis. *Neuropsychology, 14,* 201–208.

Streissguth, A. P., Bookstein, F. L., Sampson, P. D., & Barr, H. M. (1995). Attention: Prenatal alcohol and continuities of vigilance and attentional problems from 4 through 14 years. *Development and Psychopathology, 7,* 419–446.

Streissguth, A. P., Martin, D. C., Barr, H. M., Sandman, B. M., Kirchner, G. L., & Darby, B. L. (1984). Intrauterine alcohol and nicotine exposure: Attention and reaction time in 4-year-old children. *Developmental Psychology, 20,* 533–541.

Stryker, S. (1925). Encephalitis lethargica—The behavior residuals. *Training School Bulletin, 22,* 152–157.

Swaab-Barneveld, H., DeSonneville, L., Cohen-Kettenis, P., Gielen, A., Buitelaar, J., & van Engeland, H. (2000). Visual sustained attention in a child psychiatric population. *Journal of the American Academy of Child and Adolescent Psychiatry, 39,* 651–659.

Sykes, D. H., Hoy, E. A., Bill, J. M., McClure, B. G., Halliday, H. L., & Reid, M. M. (1997). Behavioural adjustment in school of very low birthweight children. *Journal of Child Psychology and Psychiatry, 38,* 315–325.

Szatmari, P. (1992). The epidemiology of attention-deficit hyperactivity disorders. In G. Weiss (Ed.), *Child and adolescent psychiatric clinics of North America: Attention-deficit hyperactivity disorder* (pp. 361–372). Philadelphia: Saunders.

Szatmari, P., Offord, D. R., & Boyle, M. H. (1989). Correlates, associated impairments, and patterns of service utilization of children with attention deficit disorders: Findings from the Ontario Child Health Study. *Journal of Child Psychology and Psychiatry, 30,* 205–217.

Szatmari, P., Saigal, S., Rosenbaum, P., & Campbell, D. (1993). Psychopathology and adaptive functioning among extremely low birthweight children at eight years of age. *Development and Psychopathology, 5,* 345–357.

Tallmadge, J., & Barkley, R. A. (1983). The interactions of hyperactive and normal boys with their mothers and fathers. *Journal of Abnormal Child Psychology, 11,* 565–579.

Tannock, R. (1998). Attention deficit hyperactivity disorder: Advances in cognitive, neurobiological, and genetic research. *Journal of Child Psychology and Psychiatry, 39,* 65–100.

Tannock, R. (2000). Attention–deficit/hyperactivity disorder with anxiety disorders. In T. E. Brown (Ed.), *Attention deficit disorders and comorbidities in children, adolescents, and adults* (pp. 125–170). Washington, DC: American Psychiatric Press.

Tannock, R., & Brown, T. E. (2000). Attention-deficit disorders with learning disorders in children and adolescents. In T. E. Brown (Ed.), *Attention deficit disorders and comorbidities in children, adolescents, and adults* (pp. 231–296). Washington, DC: American Psychiatric Press.

Tannock, R., Martinussen, R., & Frijters, J. (2000). Naming speed performance and stimulant effects indicate effortful, semantic processing deficits in attention-deficit/hyperactivity disorder. *Journal of Abnormal Child Psychology, 28,* 237–252.

Tarver-Behring, S., Barkley, R. A., & Karlsson, J. (1985). The mother–child interactions of hyperactive boys and their normal siblings. *American Journal of Orthopsychiatry, 55,* 202–209.

Taylor, E. (1999). Developmental neuropsychology of attention deficit and impulsiveness. *Development and Psychopathology, 11,* 607–628.

Taylor, E., Sandberg, S., Thorley, G., & Giles, S. (1991). *The epidemiology of childhood hyperactivity.* Oxford, UK: Oxford University Press.

Teicher, M. H., Anderson, C. M., Polcari, A., Glod, C. A., Maas, L. C., & Renshaw, P. F. (2000). Functional deficits in basal ganglia of children with attention-deficit/hyperactivity disorder shown with functional magnetic resonance imaging relaxometry. *Nature Medicine, 6,* 470–473.

Thapar, A. J. (1999). Genetic basis of attention deficit and hyperactivity. *Briisht Journal of Psychiatry, 174,* 105–111.

Thapar, A., Hervas, A., & McGuffin, P. (1995). Childhood hyperactivity scores are highly heritable and show sibling competition effects: Twin study evidence. *Behavior Genetics, 25,* 537–544.

Torgesen, J. K. (1994). Issues in the assessment of executive function: An information-processing perspective. In G. R. Lyon (Ed.), *Frames of reference for the assessment of learning disabilities: New views on measurement issues* (pp. 143–162). Baltimore: Brookes.

Tripp, G., & Alsop, B. (1999). Sensitivity to reward frequency in boys with attention deficit hyperactivity disorder. *Journal of Clinical Child Psychology, 28,* 366–375.

Tripp, G., & Alsop, B. (2001). Sensitivity to reward delay in children with attention deficit hyperactivity disorder (ADHD). *Journal of Child Psychology and Psychiatry, 42,* 691–698.

Trites, R. L. (1979). *Hyperactivity in children: Etiology, measurement, and treatment implications.* Baltimore: University Park Press.

Trites, R. L., Dugas, F., Lynch, G., & Ferguson, B. (1979). Incidence of hyperactivity. *Journal of Pediatric Psychology, 4,* 179–188.

Trommer, B. L., Hoeppner, J. B., Rosenberg, R. S., Armstrong, K. J., & Rothstein, J. A. (1988). Sleep disturbances in children with attention deficit disorder. *Annals of Neurology, 24,* 325.

Ullman, D. G., Barkley, R. A., & Brown, H. W. (1978). The behavioral symptoms of hyperkinetic children who successfully responded to stimulant drug treatment. *American Journal of Orthopsychiatry, 48,* 425–437.

Vaidya, C. J., Austin, G., Kirkorian, G., Ridlehuber, H. W., Desmond, J. E., Glover, G. H., et al. (1998). Selective effects of methylphenidate in attention deficit hyperactivity disorder: A functional magnetic resonance study. *Proceedings of the national Academy of Science, 95,* 14494–14499.

van den Oord, E. J. C. G., Boomsma, D. I., & Verhulst, F. C. (1994). A study of problem behaviors in 10- to 15-year-old biologically related and unrelated international adoptees. *Behavior Genetics, 24,* 193–205.

van den Oord, E. J. C., & Rowe, D. C. (1997). Continuity and change in children's social maladjustment: A developmental behavior genetic study. *Developmental Psychology, 33,* 319–332.

Velez, C. N., Johnson, J., & Cohen, P. (1989). A longitudinal analysis of selected risk factors for childhood psychopathology. *Journal of the American Academy of Child and Adolescent Psychiatry, 28,* 861–864.

Velting, O. N., & Whitehurst, G. J. (1997). Inattention-hyperactivity and reading achievement in children from low-income families: A longitudinal model. *Journal of Abnormal Child Psychology, 25,* 321–331.

Voelker, S. L., Carter, R. A., Sprague, D. J., Gdowski, C. L., & Lachar, D. (1989). Developmental trends in memory and metamemory in children with attention deficit disorder. *Journal of Pediatric Psychology, 14,* 75–88.

Volkow, N. D., Wang, G. J., Fowler, J. S., Logan, J., Gerasimov, M., Maynard, L., et al. (2001). Therapeutic doses of oral methylphenidate significantly increase extracellur dopamine in the human brain. *The journal of Neuroscience, 21,* 1–5.

Wakefield, J. C. (1999). Evolutionary versus prototype analyses of the concept of disorder. *Journal of Abnormal Psychology, 108,* 374–399.

Wallander, J. L., Schroeder, S. R., Michelli, J. A., & Gualtieri, C. T. (1987). Classroom social interactions of attention deficit disorder with hyperactivity children as a function of stimulant medication. *Journal of Pediatric Psychology, 12,* 61–76.

Weiss, G., & Hechtman, L. (1993). *Hyperactive children grown up* (2nd ed.). New York: Guilford.

Weiss, G., & Hechtman, L. (in press). *Hyperactive children grown up* (3rd ed.). New York: Guilford.

Weiss, R. E., Stein, M. A., Trommer, B., & Refetoff, S. (1993). Attention-deficit hyperactivity disorder and thyroid function. *Journal of Pediatrics, 123,* 539–545.

Welner, Z., Welner, A., Stewart, M., Palkes, H., & Wish, E. (1977). A controlled study of siblings of hyperactive children. *Journal of Nervous and Mental Disease, 165,* 110–117.

Welsh, M. C., & Pennington, B. F. (1988). Assessing frontal lobe functioning in children: Views from developmental psychology. *Developmental Neuropsychology, 4,* 199–230.

Werner, E. E., Bierman, J. M., French, F. W., Simonian, K., Connor, A., Smith, R. S., et al. (1971). Reproductive and environmental casualties: A report on the 10-year follow-up of the children of the Kauai pregnancy study. *Pediatrics, 42,* 112–127.

Werry, J. S., Elkind, G. S., & Reeves, J. S. (1987). Attention deficit, conduct, oppositional, and anxiety disorders in children: III. Laboratory differences. *Journal of Abnormal Child Psychology, 15,* 409–428.

Werry, J. S., & Quay, H. C. (1971). The prevalence of behavior symptoms in younger elementary school children. *American Journal of Orthopsychiatry, 41,* 136–143.

Whalen, C. K., & Henker, B. (1992). The social profile of attention-deficit hyperactivity disorder: Five fundamental facets. In G. Weiss (Ed.), *Child and adolescent psychiatric clinics of North America: Attention-deficit hyperactivity disorder* (pp. 395–410). Philadelphia: Saunders.

Whalen, C. K., Henker, B., Collins, B. E., McAuliffe, S., & Vaux, A. (1979). Peer interaction in structured communication task: Comparisons of normal and hyperactive boys and of methylphenidate (Ritalin) and placebo effects. *Child Development, 50,* 388–401.

Whalen, C. K., Henker, B., & Dotemoto, S. (1980). Methylphenidate and hyperactivity: Effects on teacher behaviors. *Science, 208,* 1280–1282.

Whalen, C. K., Henker, B., Swanson, J. M., Granger, D., Kliewer, W., & Spencer, J. (1987). Natural social behaviors in hyperactive children: Dose effects of methylphenidate. *Journal of Consulting and Clinical Psychology, 55,* 187–193.

White, H. R., Xie, M., Thompson, W., Loeber, R., & Stouthamer-Loeber, M. (in press). Psychopathology as a predictor of adolescent drug use trajectories. *Psychology of Addictive Behavior.*

Whittaker, A. H., Van Rossem, R., Feldman, J. F., Schonfeld, I. S., Pinto-Martin, J. A., Torre, C., et al. (1997). Psychiatric outcomes in low-birth-weight children at age 6 years: Relation to neonatal cranial ultrasound abnormalities. *Archives of General Psychiatry, 54,* 847–856.

Wiers, R. W., Gunning, W. B., & Sergeant, J. A. (1998). Is a mild deficit in executive functions in boys related to childhood ADHD or to parental multigenerational alcoholism. *Journal of Abnormal Child Psychology, 26,* 415–430.

Wilens, T. E., Biederman, J., & Spencer, T. (1994). Clonidine for sleep disturbances associated with attention-deficit hyperactivity disorder. *Journal of the American Academy of Child and Adolescent Psychiatry, 33,* 424–426.

Willcutt, E. G., Pennington, B. F., Boada, R., Ogline, J. S., Tunick, R. A., Chhabildas, N. A., et al. (2001). A comparison of the cognitive deficits in reading disability and attention-deficit/hyperactivity disorder. *Journal of Abnormal Psychology, 110,* 157–172.

Willcutt, E. G., Pennington, B. F., Chhabildas, N. A., Friedman, M. C., & Alexander, J. (1999). Psychiatric comorbidity associated with DSM-IV ADHD in a nonreferred sample of twins. *Journal of the American Academy of Child and Adolescent Psychiatry, 38,* 1355–1362.

Willerman, L. (1973). Activity level and hyperactivity in twins. *Child Development, 44,* 288–293.

Willis, T. J., & Lovaas, I. (1977). A behavioral approach to treating hyperactive children: The parent's role. In J. B. Millichap (Ed.), *Learning disabilities and related disorders* (pp. 119–140). Chicago: Yearbook Medical Publications.

Winsler, A. (1998). Parent-child interaction and private speech in boys with ADHD. *Applied Developmental Science, 2,* 17–39.

Winsler, A., Diaz, R. M., Atencio, D. J., McCarthy, E. M., & Chabay, L. A. (2000). Verbal self-regulation over time in preschool children at risk for attention and behavior problems. *Journal of Child Psychology and Psychiatry, 41,* 875–886.

Wolraich, M. L., Hannah, J. N., Baumgaertel, A., & Feurer, I. D. (1998). Examination of DSM-IV criteria for attention deficit/hyperactivity disorder in a county-wide sample. *Journal of Developmental and Behavioral Pediatrics, 19,* 162–168.

Wolraich, M. L., Hannah, J. N., Pinnock, T. Y., Baumgaertel, A., & Brown, J. (1996). Comparison of diagnostic criteria for attention-deficit hyperactivity disorder in a countrywide sample. *Journal of the American Academy of Child and Adolescent Psychiatry, 35,* 319–324.

Wood, F. B., & Felton, R. H. (1994). Separate linguistic and attentional factors in the development of reading. *Topics in language disorders, 14,* 52–57.

Woodward, L. J., Fergusson, D. M., & Horwood, L. J. (2000). Driving outcomes of young people with attentional difficulties in adolescence. *Journal of the American Academy of Child and Adolescent Psychiatry, 39,* 627–634.

World Health Organization. (1993). *The ICD-10 classification of mental and behavioral disorders: Diagnostic criteria for research.* Geneva, Switzerland: Author.

Wozniak, J., Biederman, J., Kiely, K., Ablon, S., Faraone, S. V., Mundy, E., et al. (1995). Mania-like symptoms suggestive of childhood-onset bipolar disorder in clinically referred children. *Journal of the American Academy of Child and Adolescent Psychiatry, 34,* 867–876.

Zagar, R., & Bowers, N. D. (1983). The effect of time of day on problem-solving and classroom behavior. *Psychology in the Schools, 20,* 337–345.

Zametkin, A. J., Liebenauer, L. L., Fitzgerald, G. A., King, A. C., Minkunas, D. V., Herscovitch, P., et al. (1993). Brain metabolism in teenagers with attention-deficit hyperactivity disorder. *Archives of General Psychiatry, 50,* 333–340.

Zametkin, A. J., Nordahl, T. E., Gross, M., King, A. C., Semple, W. E., Rumsey, J., et al. (1990). Cerebral glucose metabolism in adults with hyperactivity of childhood onset. *New England Journal of Medicine, 323,* 1361–1366.

Zametkin, A. J., & Rapoport, J. L. (1986). The pathophysiology of attention deficit disorder with hyperactivity: A review. In B. B. Lahey & A. E. Kazdin (Eds.), *Advances in clinical child psychology* (Vol. 9, pp. 177–216). New York: Plenum.

Zentall, S. S. (1985). A context for hyperactivity. In K. Gadow & I. Bialer (Eds.), *Advances in learning and behavioral disabilities* (Vol. 4, pp. 273–343). Greenwich, CT: JAI Press.

Zentall, S. S. (1988). Production deficiencies in elicited language but not in the spontaneous verbalizations of hyperactive children. *Journal of Abnormal Child Psychology, 16,* 657–673.

Zentall, S. S., & Smith, Y. S. (1993). Mathematical performance and behavior of children with hyperactivity with and without coexisting aggression. *Behavior Research and Therapy, 31,* 701–710.

Primary Symptoms, Diagnostic Criteria, Prevalence, and Gender Differences

RUSSELL A. BARKLEY

A tremendous amount of research has been published on children with Attention-Deficit/ Hyperactivity Disorder (ADHD) and their primary characteristics and related problems, as well as on the situational variability of these problems, their prevalence, and their etiologies. It was estimated by 1979 that more than 2,000 studies existed on this disorder (Weiss & Hechtman, 1979), and this figure has surely tripled since then. In this edition, I have attempted to cull from a substantial fund of research the information I believe is most useful for clinical work with these children and adults. Yet it is surely not the intent of this chapter, or of this book, to provide a critical review of the scientific literature. Instead, it is to glean from that literature whatever has a direct bearing on the clinical understanding, diagnosis, assessment, and management of ADHD. This chapter reviews the clinically useful findings on the primary symptoms of this condition as they occur in both children and adults, along with information pertaining to the situational variability and pervasiveness of those symptoms. This chapter also discusses the prevalence of ADHD, as well as gender differences that may exist in its expression.

Throughout this chapter and the remainder of this book, the term "ADHD" is used, although the research on which this discussion is based may have employed the related diagnoses of "hyperactivity," "Hyperkinetic Reaction of Childhood," "minimal brain dysfunction," or "Attention Deficit Disorder (ADD) with or without Hyperactivity." I realize that these terms and the diagnostic criteria used for them in this research are not perfectly equivalent. However, I believe that the clinical descriptions of the children studied under these terms and the criteria used to select them for study are sufficiently similar to those now used for ADHD Combined Type (ADHD-C) to permit some clinical generalities to be drawn about this literature. To gain a general impression of the disorder, and for the clinical purposes of this text, the minor differences that may exist among these groups because of these somewhat different terms and selection criteria do not seem (at least to me) sufficiently important to justify qualifying each and every conclusion to be discussed here by the manner in which the particular cases were selected and diagnosed. If reassurance of this position is needed, consider the fact that in my own research, children selected as having "hyperactivity" in my longitudinal study with Mariellen Fischer in the late 1970s would easily meet today's diagnostic criteria for ADHD-C in the *Diagnostic and Statistical Manual of Mental Disorders* (DSM), with 70–80% of them continuing to do so 8–10 years later when evaluated as adolescents, and 45–66% of them continuing to do so 13–15 years later in young adulthood (Barkley, Fischer, Edelbrock, & Smallish, 1990; Barkley, Fischer, Smallish, & Fletcher, 2002). This text will certainly distinguish those children having the newly recognized ADHD, Predominantly Inattentive Type (ADHD-PI), especially that subset manifesting "sluggish cognitive tempo" (SCT; Milich, Ballentine, & Lynam, 2001), given the many quantitative and qualitative differences that seem to be accumulating for this subset of inattentive children.

PRIMARY SYMPTOMS

An important distinction should be made at the outset. The term "symptom" as used here refers to a behavior (e.g., skipping from one uncompleted activity to another) or to a response class of behaviors that significantly covary together (e.g., inattention) and are believed to represent a dimension of a mental disorder. The term "symptom" must be distinguished from that of "impairment," as the two are often confused in clinical discussions of disorders. "Impairments" are the consequences or outcomes of symptoms or symptom classes, such as retention in grade, failure to graduate from high school, vehicular crashes, license suspensions, teen pregnancy, or criminal arrests. Here I describe the major symptom dimensions of ADHD. In Chapters 3 and 6 of this volume, I describe many of the impairments associated with the disorder.

Little has changed in the symptoms and their lists or dimensions believed to characterize ADHD in children and adults since the preceding edition of this book (Barkley, 1998). Those with ADHD are commonly observed by others as having chronic difficulties with inattention and/or impulsivity–hyperactivity. They are believed to display these characteristics early, to a degree that is excessive and inappropriate for their age or developmental level, and across a variety of situations that tax their capacity to pay attention, restrain their movement, inhibit their impulses, and regulate their own behavior

relative to rules, time, and the future. As noted in Chapter 1, definitions have varied considerably throughout the history of this disorder, as have the recommended criteria for obtaining a diagnosis. The currently recommended criteria are set forth later in this chapter, and these too have not changed since the 1998 edition. More has been learned about special adjustments to these criteria that may apply to specific subsets of those with ADHD, however. I first review the nature of the major symptom constructs that form the essential nature of this disorder as they are expressed in children and adults. I then proceed to a discussion of diagnostic criteria, followed by information on prevalence and gender differences.

Inattention

By definition, children and adults who have ADHD, particularly ADHD-C, are said to display difficulties with attention relative to nondisabled children or other control groups of the same age and gender. Parents and teachers often describe these attention problems in terms such as "Doesn't seem to listen," "Fails to finish assigned tasks," "Daydreams," "Often loses things," "Can't concentrate," "Easily distracted," "Can't work independently of supervision," "Requires more redirection," "Shifts from one uncompleted activity to another," and "Confused or seems to be in a fog" (Barkley, DuPaul, & McMurray, 1990; Stewart, Pitts, Craig, & Dieruf, 1966). Many of these terms are the most frequently endorsed items from rating scales completed by the caregivers of these children (DuPaul, Power, Anastopoulos, & Reid, 1998; Mahone et al., 2002). Lest critics of ADHD believe that these are just subjective opinions having no anchor to reality, studies using direct observations of child behavior find that off-task behavior or not paying attention to work is recorded substantially more often for children and adolescents with ADHD than for those with learning disabilities or no disabilities (Abikoff, Gittelman-Klein, & Klein, 1977; Barkley, DuPaul, & McMurray, 1990; Borger & van der Meere, 2000; Luk, 1985 [a review]; Fischer, Barkley, Edelbrock, & Smallish, 1990; Barkley & Cunningham, 1979; Sawyer, Taylor, & Chadwick, 2001; Ullman, Barkley, & Brown, 1978).

Two dimensions of behavior are almost uniformly found when the symptoms of ADHD as rated by parents and teachers are factor-analyzed (Burns, Boe, Walsh, Sommers-Flanagan, & Teegarden, 2001; DuPaul et al., 1998; Gioia, Isquith, Guy, & Kenworthy, 2000; Lahey et al., 1994). These are used to create and diagnose the disorder and construct its subtypes, at least within the DSM. One of these reflects a dimension termed "inattention" and largely comprises the symptoms noted above. These dimensions are found across ethnic and cultural groups (Puerto Ricans: Baumeister, 1992; Native Americans: Beiser, Dion, & Gotowiec, 2000; several U.S. ethnic groups: DuPaul et al., 1998; Australia: Gomez, Harvey, Quick, Scharer, & Harris, 1999; Brazilians: Rasmussen et al., 2002; Spanish, German, and U.S. children: Wolraich et al., 2003). It is this dimension of inattention after which the disorder is named. The second dimension, to be discussed below, comprises symptoms of impulsive, hyperactive, and talkative behavior.

However, clinicians should recognize that the construct of attention as studied in neuropsychology is multidimensional and can refer to alertness, arousal, selectivity or focus–execution, encoding, sustained attention, distractibility, or span of apprehension, among others (Barkley, 1988, 1994; Hale & Lewis, 1979; Mirsky, 1996; Strauss, Thompson, Adams, Redline, & Burant, 2000). The number of distinct components identified in neuropsychological batteries remains unclear, however (Strauss et al., 2000). Research shows that those with ADHD do not have significant difficulties with automatic orienting to visual information, which may be mediated by posterior brain attention circuits (Huang-Pollock & Nigg, 2003). Instead, they have their greatest difficulties with aspects of attention related to persistence of effort, or sustaining their attention (responding) to tasks; this is sometimes called "vigilance" (Douglas, 1983; Newcorn et al., 2001; Swaab-Barneveld et al., 2000) and is believed to be mediated through frontal brain attention circuits (Huang-Pollack & Nigg, 2003). These difficulties with persistence are sometimes apparent in free-play settings, as evidenced by shorter durations of play with each toy and frequent shifts in play across various toys (Barkley & Ullman, 1975; Routh & Schroeder, 1976; Zentall, 1985). However, they are seen most dramatically in situations requiring a child to sustain attention to dull, boring, repetitive tasks (Barkley, DuPaul, & McMurray, 1990; Fischer, Barkley, Smallish, &

Fletcher, 2004; Luk, 1985; Newcorn et al., 2001; Shelton et al., 2000; Milich, Landau, Kilby, & Whitten, 1982; Ullman, Barkley, & Brown, 1978; see Zentall, 1985, for a review), such as independent schoolwork (Hoza, Pelham, Waschbusch, Kipp, & Owens, 2001), homework or chores (Danforth, Barkley, & Stokes, 1991), or experimental lab tasks (Newcorn et al., 2001; Sawyer et al., 2001; Swaab-Barneveld et al., 2000).

Another problem is distractibility, or the likelihood that a child will respond to the occurrence of extraneous events unrelated to the task. Parent and teacher ratings often rate this symptom as significantly elevated among children with ADHD. Laboratory research on the matter is somewhat contradictory. Some early studies found children with ADHD to be no more distractible than nondisabled children to extratask stimulation (Campbell, Douglas, & Morgenstern, 1971; Cohen, Weiss, & Minde, 1972; Rosenthal & Allen, 1980; Steinkamp, 1980). The findings for such distracting irrelevant stimulation, however, appear to be a function of whether the distractors are contained within the task or outside of the task materials. Some studies have found that such stimulation, when embedded in the task materials, worsens the performance of children with ADHD (Barkley, Koplowitz, Anderson, & McMurray, 1997; Brodeur & Pond, 2001; Marzocchi, Lucangeli, De Meo, Fini, & Cornoldi, 2002; Rosenthal & Allen, 1980). This appears to be the case even with video games (Lawrence et al., 2002). Others find no such effect when studying teens with ADHD (Fischer, Barkley, Fletcher, & Smallish, 1993b), suggesting an age-related improvement in this specific problem (Brodeur & Pond, 2001). One study found an enhancing effect on attention from intratask stimulation (Zentall, Falkenberg, & Smith, 1985). The weight of the evidence appears to suggest that distractors within the task will prove more disruptive than those outside the task. It is more than likely that the problem with distractibility depends on the cognitive loading or difficulty of the task (demands for working memory) and its demands for the protection of executive actions (thinking) through interference control. And the salience of the distracting events will also determine the extent to which extraneous events disrupt the task. For instance, Lawrence et al. (2002) observed children with ADHD while they were playing a video game of varying cognitive load and distracting information, and also observed them at a local zoo while they were required to accomplish certain instructions in that setting. The children with ADHD had significantly more difficulties inhibiting responses to distracting events, both in the game and at the zoo, and therefore took more time to complete their assignments than did control children.

The attention problem in the more common ADHD-C appears consistently to be one of diminished persistence of effort or sustained responding to tasks that have little intrinsic appeal or minimal immediate consequences for completion (Barkley, 1989a, 1997a). Children with ADHD also spend much more time engaged in off-task behavior instead of attending to their assigned tasks (Sawyer et al., 2001), which could give others the impression that they are distractible when they are merely unable to persist as well as others (Hoza et al., 2001).

The clinical picture may be different, however, when alternative or competing activities are available that promise immediate reinforcement or gratification, in contrast to the weaker reinforcement or consequences associated with the assigned task. In such cases, a child with ADHD may appear distracted, and in fact is likely to shift off task to engage in the highly rewarding competing activity. For example, Landau, Lorch, and Milich (1992) showed that children with ADHD spend significantly less time observing a television program when toys are available for play than do nondisabled children. It is not clear whether this shift represents true distraction as described previously (orienting to extraneous stimuli), lack of effort or motivation to attend (Hoza et al., 2001), or behavioral disinhibition (failing to follow rules or instructions when provided with competing, highly rewarding activities).

Some new findings from direct behavioral observations of inattention in adults with ADHD now parallel the previously cited research in children in finding greater off-task behavior during task performance, including driving (Fischer et al., 2004). Most studies document greater difficulties with attention on continuous-performance tests (CPTs) or vigilance tests (Barkley, Murphy, & Kwasnik, 1996; Murphy, Barkley, & Bush, 2001; Seidman, Biederman, Faraone, Weber, & Ouellette, 1997), though one did not (Holdnack, Moberg, Arnold, Gur, & Gur, 1995). Yet even the Holdnack et al. study found adults with ADHD to have slower reaction times, which previously have been interpreted by oth-

ers as reflecting lapses in attention to the task (Barkley, 1988).

Adults with ADHD are also highly likely to self-report many of the same symptoms of inattention from the DSM symptom list that are reported by parents of children with ADHD. One study (Murphy & Barkley, 1996a) found that 83% of adults diagnosed with ADHD reported having difficulties with sustaining attention (vs. 68% of a clinical control group and 10% of a nondisabled sample); 94% reported being easily distracted (vs. 86% and 19%, respectively); 90% claimed that they often did not listen to others (vs. 57% and 6%, respectively); 91% reported that they often failed to follow through on tasks or activities (vs. 78% and 6%, respectively); and 86% reported that they frequently shifted from one uncompleted activity to another (vs. 75% and 12%, respectively). These self-reports were corroborated by others who knew the subjects well, such as spouses ($r = .64$) or parents ($r = .75$), as was the recall by these adults of similar symptoms during their childhood years ($r = .74$ with parent reports) (Murphy & Barkley, 1996a). Thus there is ample justification for believing that adults with ADHD suffer from many of the same attention problems as do children who have the disorder.

Notwithstanding all of the points made above, research since the preceding edition of this text has clearly shown that another construct or dimension of inattention symptoms exists among clinically referred children. Those symptoms are not represented in the current DSM inattention list; indeed, they were eliminated from it as a result of the field trial, which showed them to have low or weak association with the other inattention symptoms (see Lahey et al., 1994). Yet this subset of symptoms is becoming useful at identifying another subtype of inattentive children, and possibly adults. As noted earlier, children with these symptoms are now described as having SCT, and are rated by parents and teachers as being more sluggish, passive, hypoactive, daydreamy, slow-moving, staring, confused, and "in a fog" than are children with no disability or with ADHD-C (see Milich et al., 2001, for a review; see also McBurnett, Pfiffner, & Frick, 2001, for the predictive power of SCT symptoms). Indeed, some of these symptoms are the very antithesis of ADHD (e.g., hypoactivity).

Growing evidence indicates that children with ADHD-PI therefore may be rather heterogeneous. A subset may simply have milder, barely subthreshold versions of the ADHD-C (four or five symptoms of hyperactivity–impulsivity and six or more symptoms of inattention) (Milich et al., 2001). They would differ only slightly in degree from children with full-fledged ADHD-C, as the review by Milich et al. (2001) and subsequent commentaries appear to suggest. But another subset of children with ADHD-PI manifest SCT (e.g., hypoactivity, lethargy, daydreaming), and thus may be qualitatively different from those with ADHD-C (and from others with ADHD-PI) in many important respects (Milich et al., 2001; McBurnett et al., 2001) that are deserving of greater research (see Chapter 4). For instance, children with SCT have fewer externalizing symptoms; more internalizing symptoms of unhappiness, anxiety, depression, and social withdrawal; and more information-processing deficits than children with ADHD-C (Carlson & Mann, 2000; Milich et al., 2001). Such differences have led some to argue that the SCT subtype of ADHD-PI may constitute a distinct disorder from ADHD, or at least a qualitatively distinct subtype of ADHD (Barkley, 1998, 2001a; Hinshaw, 2001; Lahey, 2001; McBurnett et al., 2001; Milich et al., 2001). Lab studies suggest that children with SCT may manifest significantly more errors with information processing, set shifting, focused attention, and possibly memory retrieval that are not evident in ADHD-C (Milich et al., 2001).

To date, then, evidence suggests that clinicians need to recognize two distinct dimensions of inattention. The first is the well-known and overwhelmingly established set of inattentive symptoms set forth in the DSM and in many child behavior rating scales. These symptoms can be thought of as primarily reflecting distractibility. The second dimension reflects a more daydreamy quality that is more passive and lethargic in form, and that has been described as SCT. Research may eventually reveal these to represent two distinct disorders of attention. If so, then it would be clinically possible (and likely) that these disorders can be found both separately and even jointly in cases of ADHD, in contrast to the current DSM view of such subtypes as mutually exclusive.

Impulsivity (Behavioral Disinhibition) and Hyperactivity

The second dimension of symptoms that emerges from factor analyses of symptom ratings in both children and adults is that of poor inhibition and associated hyperactivity (Burns et al., 2001; DuPaul et al., 1998; Gioia et al., 2000; Lahey et al., 1994; Murphy & Barkley, 1996a). Clinically, those with ADHD are often noted to respond quickly to situations without waiting for instructions to be completed or adequately appreciating what is required in the setting. Heedless or careless errors are often the results. These individuals may also fail to consider the potentially negative, destructive, or even dangerous consequences that may be associated with particular situations or behaviors. Thus they seem to engage in frequent, unnecessary risk taking. Taking chances on a dare or whim, especially from a peer, may occur more often than is typical. Consequently, accidental poisonings and injuries are not uncommon in children with ADHD (see Chapter 3, this volume). They may carelessly damage or destroy others' property considerably more frequently than do children without ADHD.

Waiting for their turn in a game or in a group lineup before going to an activity is often problematic for children with ADHD; indeed, waiting in general may be problematic for all ages of the disorder. When faced with tasks or situations in which they are encouraged to delay seeking gratification and to work toward a longer-term goal and larger reward, they often opt for the immediate, smaller reward that requires less work to achieve. They are notorious for taking "shortcuts" in their work performance, applying the least amount of effort and taking the least amount of time in performing tasks they find boring or aversive. When they desire something to which others control access and they must wait a while to obtain it, as in a parent's promise to eventually take them shopping or to a movie, they may badger the parent excessively during the waiting interval, appearing to others as incessantly demanding and self-centered. Situations or games that involve sharing, cooperation, and restraint with peers are particularly problematic for these impulsive children. Verbally, they often say things indiscreetly, without regard for the feelings of others or for the social consequences to themselves. Blurting out answers to questions prematurely and interrupting the conversations of others are commonplace. The layperson's impression of these children, therefore, is often one of poor self-control, verbosity, irresponsibility, immaturity or childishness, laziness, and outright rudeness. Little wonder that these children experience more punishment, criticism, censure, and ostracism by adults and their peers than do children without ADHD. There is some suggestive evidence from one factor-analytic study of ADHD symptoms in adults that the verbal impulsivity reflected in the DSM symptom list may actually come to form a separate, albeit less robust, dimension of impulse control by adulthood (Murphy & Barkley, 1996a).

Impulsivity

Like attention, impulsivity is multidimensional in nature (Kindlon, Mezzacappa, & Earls, 1995; Milich & Kramer, 1985; Nigg, 2000, 2001). These often involve constructs of executive control, delay of gratification, effort, and even compliance (Olson, Schilling, & Bates, 1999). Others reorganize inhibition into executive (volitional), motivational (precipitated by fear or anxiety), and automatic attentional inhibitory processes (Nigg, 2000). Those forms of impulsivity often associated with ADHD involve the undercontrol of behavior (poor executive functioning), poor sustained inhibition, the inability to delay a response or defer gratification, or the inability to inhibit dominant or prepotent responses (Barkley, 1985, 1997a; Campbell, 1987; Gordon, 1979; Kendall & Wilcox, 1979; Kindlon et al., 1995; Neef, Bicard, & Endo, 2001; Newcorn et al., 2001; Nigg, 1999, 2000, 2001; Rapport, Tucker, DuPaul, Merlo, & Stoner, 1986; Scheres et al., 2004). But there is also evidence that children with ADHD have an equal or greater problem with delay aversion: They find waiting to be aversive, and therefore act impulsively to terminate the delay more quickly (Sonuga-Barke, Taylor, & Hepinstall, 1992; Solanto et al., 2001). Interestingly, young children who manifest such inhibitory problems in laboratory tasks are more likely to be described later in development as having higher levels of ADHD symptoms (Olson et al., 1999).

Evidence that behavioral disinhibition, or poor effortful regulation and inhibition of behavior, is in fact the hallmark of this disorder is so substantial that it can be considered a fact (for reviews, see Barkley, 1997a; Nigg, 2001; Nigg, Goldsmith, & Sachek, 2004; Pennington & Ozonoff, 1996). First, studies typically show that inattention does not distinguish children with ADHD from those with other clinical disorders or no disorders as much as their hyperactive, impulsive, disinhibited, and poorly regulated behaviors do (Barkley, Grodzinsky, &

DuPaul, 1992; Frazier, Demaree, & Youngstrom, 2004; Halperin, Matier, Bedi, Sharma, & Newcorn, 1992; Newcorn et al., 2001; Nigg, 1999, 2001; Rubia, Taylor, Oksannen, Overmeyer, & Newman, 2001; Schachar, Mota, Logan, Tannock, & Klim, 2000; Sergeant, Geurts, & Oosterlaan, 2002; Swaab-Barneveld et al., 2000). Second, when objective measures of the three sets of symptoms of ADHD are subjected to a discriminant-function analysis (a statistical method of examining the variables that contribute most to group discrimination), it is routinely the symptoms of impulsive errors, typically on vigilance tasks or those assessing response inhibition, and excessive activity level that best discriminate children with ADHD from those without ADHD (Barkley, DuPaul, & McMurray, 1990; Corkum & Siegel, 1993; Grodzinsky & Diamond, 1992; Losier, McGrath, & Klein, 1996). A third source of evidence is derived from the field trial of the DSM-III-R symptom list (Spitzer, Davies, & Barkley, 1990), which tested these symptoms' sensitivity and specificity (see Chapter 1, Table 1.2, this volume, for this symptom list). These descriptors were rank-ordered by their discriminating power and presented in DSM-III-R in descending order. Careful inspection of this rank ordering revealed that, again, symptoms characteristic of disinhibition, such as poorly regulated activity and impulsivity, were more likely to discriminate children with ADHD from those with other psychiatric disorders or no disorder. For these reasons, the evidence available is sufficient for the conclusion that it is not inattention as much as behavioral disinhibition that is the hallmark of ADHD. In fact, this disinhibition or poor inhibitory regulation of behavior may result in some of the attention problems often noted in these children, such as their heightened distractibility. That is, some of the attention problems may be secondary to a disorder of behavioral regulation and inhibition, rather than being a primary and distinct deficit apart from such disinhibition. The theory of ADHD presented in Chapter 7 of this volume further develops this idea.

A recent meta-analysis of studies using CPTs demonstrated more errors of commission or impulsiveness in adults with ADHD than in control groups (Hervey, Epstein, & Curry, 2004). Adults diagnosed with ADHD, in comparison to clinical and nondisabled control groups, often self-report symptoms of poor impulse control, such as difficulty awaiting turns (67% vs. 39% of a control group and 18% of a nondisabled sample), blurting out answers (57% vs. 46% vs. 16%, respectively), and interrupting or intruding on others (57% vs. 39% vs. 9%, respectively) (Murphy & Barkley, 1996a). These symptoms are often thought of as the hallmarks of the poor impulse control seen in clinically diagnosed children with ADHD. These adults are also highly likely to report difficulties with their driving associated with poor impulse control (e.g., excessive speeding) and to make more impulsive errors on a driving simulator (Barkley, 2004a). Impulsive comments to others, difficulties in inhibiting the impulsive spending of money, and poor inhibition in their emotional reactions to others are often described by patients in our clinic for adults with ADHD. Thus, once again, it appears that the symptoms characterizing childhood ADHD are likely to be associated with its adult equivalent.

Recent studies have also suggested that among children with ADHD who have significant problems with inhibition on laboratory tasks, there is a higher incidence of ADHD among their biological relatives (Crosbie & Schachar, 2001). Also, the siblings of children with ADHD, though not expressing the disorder, may also show greater difficulties on measures of inhibition (Slaats-Willemse, Swaab-Barneveld, Sonneville, van der Meulen, & Buitelaar, 2003). Both of these findings imply that poor behavioral inhibition may represent a cognitive endophenotype of ADHD that appears in children with ADHD and even in their unaffected relatives. "Endophenotypes" are latent traits that are related indirectly to the more classic symptoms of a disorder, such as ADHD, and may be more closely linked to underlying genetic or neurological factors than is the symptom complex of the disorder itself (Slaats-Willemse et al., 2003).

Hyperactivity

Related to the difficulties with impulse control in those with ADHD are symptoms of excessive or developmentally inappropriate levels of activity, whether motor or vocal. Restlessness, fidgeting, and generally unnecessary gross bodily movements are commonplace, both in the complaints received from parents and teachers and in objective measures (Barkley & Cunningham, 1979; Dane, Schachar, &

Tannock, 2000; Luk, 1985; Stewart et al., 1966; Still, 1902). These movements are often irrelevant to the task or situation, and at times seem purposeless. A parent often describes such a child as "always up and on the go," "acts as if driven by a motor," "climbs excessively," "can't sit still," "talks excessively," "often hums or makes odd noises," and "is squirmy" (DuPaul et al., 1998). Observations of such children at school or while working on independent tasks find them out of their seats, moving around the classroom without permission, restlessly moving their arms and legs while working, playing with objects not related to the task, talking out of turn to others, and making unusual vocal noises (Abikoff et al., 1977; Barkley, DuPaul, & McMurray, 1990; Cammann & Miehlke, 1989; Fischer et al., 1990; Luk, 1985). The restlessness is likely to be more problematic in boring or low-stimulation situations than in ones where greater stimulation is available (Antrop, Roeyers, Van Oost, & Buysse, 2000). Making running commentaries on the activities around them or about others' behavior is not unusual. Direct observations of their social interactions with others, as well as of their self-speech during play and work performance, also indicate generally excessive speech and commentary (Barkley, Cunningham, & Karlsson, 1983; Berk & Potts, 1991; Copeland, 1979; Zentall, 1988).

Numerous scientific studies using objective measures of activity level therefore attest to complaints that children with ADHD are more active, restless, and fidgety than nondisabled children throughout the day and even during sleep (Barkley & Cunningham, 1979; Porrino et al., 1983; Teicher, Ito, Glod, & Barber, 1996). Their activity levels in early morning hours may not be different from those of nondisabled children, but may become so by the afternoon (Dane et al., 2000). As with poor sustained attention, however, there are many different types of activity (Barkley & Ullman, 1975; Cromwell, Baumeister, & Hawkins, 1963), and it is not always clear exactly which types are the most deviant for children with ADHD. Measures of ankle movement and locomotion seem to differentiate them most reliably from nondisabled children (Barkley & Cunningham, 1979), but even some studies of wrist activity and total body motion found them to be different as well (Barkley & Ullman, 1975; Porrino et al., 1983; Teicher et al.,

1996). And objective measurement of their activity level during tasks demanding sustained attention reveals them to move their heads and bodies more than others, to move further about from their chairs than others, to cover a greater spatial area in doing so, and to show more simplified or less complex movement patterns in doing so (Teicher et al., 1996). There are also significant situational fluctuations in this symptom (Jacob, O'Leary, & Rosenblad, 1978; Luk, 1985; Porrino et al., 1983), implying that the failure to regulate activity level to setting or task demands may be what is so socially problematic in ADHD (Routh, 1978), in addition to just a greater-than-normal absolute level of movement. There is some compelling evidence that some hyperactivity is a form of stimulation seeking, in that these symptoms (as noted above) increase in frequency in boring or understimulating environments and decrease when stimulation is added to the setting (Antrop et al., 2000; Zentall, 1985).

Some research suggests that the pervasiveness of the hyperactivity across settings (home and school) may be what separates ADHD from these other diagnostic categories (Taylor, 1986). Indeed, some earlier investigators have gone so far as to advocate that the clinical syndrome or disorder be restricted only to those children having such pervasiveness of symptoms (Schachar, Rutter, & Smith, 1981). As discussed later, this distinction may have more to do with the sources of information (parents vs. teachers) than with real differences in the nature of children with situational versus pervasive ADHD (Costello, Loeber, & Stouthamer-Loeber, 1991; Mitsis, McKay, Schulz, Newcorn, & Halperin, 2000; Rapoport, Donnelly, Zametkin, & Carrougher, 1986).

As noted previously for impulsivity, it is difficult in studies of objective measures or behavior ratings of hyperactivity to find that hyperactivity forms a separate factor or dimension apart from impulsivity. Typically, studies that factor-analyze behavioral ratings often find that items of restlessness or other types of overactivity load on a factor constituting impulsive or disinhibited behavior (Achenbach & Edelbrock, 1983; DuPaul, 1991; DuPaul et al., 1998; Lahey et al., 1994; Milich & Kramer, 1985). Objective measures of inhibition are also likely to be related to measures of hyperactivity (Berlin & Bohlin, 2002). These findings mean that overactivity is not a separate dimension of behavioral impairment apart from poor inhibition in these children. As noted earlier, it is this latter factor, rather than inattention, that best distinguishes ADHD from other clinical conditions and from no disorder. Hence, in ranking the importance of these primary symptoms for clinical diagnosis, greater weight should probably be given to the behavioral class of impulsive–hyperactive characteristics than to inattention in conceptualizing this disorder and in its clinical delineation. Once again, the poor self-regulation and inhibition of behavior are what seem to be distinctive in this disorder.

In adults with ADHD, symptoms of hyperactive or restless behavior are often present but appear to involve more difficulties with fidgeting, a more subjective sense of restlessness, and excessive speech than the more gross motor overactivity characteristic of young children with ADHD. We (Murphy & Barkley, 1996a) found that nearly 74% of adults with ADHD reported often fidgeting with their hands or feet, versus 57% of a clinical control group and only 20% of a nondisabled sample of adults. Nearly 66% of adults clinically diagnosed with ADHD complained of often having difficulties remaining seated, versus 32% of the clinical control group and only 6% of the nondisabled sample. Like children with ADHD, adults with the disorder often verbalize more than others, with nearly 60% complaining that they often talked excessively. Although this complaint did not distinguish them from the clinical control group (60% of whom also reported excessive speech), both of these groups reported speaking more often than did the nondisabled sample of adults (only 22% of whom reported such a difficulty). Again, further research into the symptoms of ADHD in adults is in order. No direct observational studies of these adults have been conducted to corroborate these self-reports of symptoms of hyperactivity.

CONSENSUS DIAGNOSTIC CRITERIA FOR ADHD

At present, the primary characteristics of ADHD and the diagnostic criteria officially developed for clinical use are set forth in the fourth edition of the DSM (DSM-IV; American Psychiatric Association, 1994) and its text revision (DSM-IV-TR; American Psychiatric Association, 2000), which are used primarily in the United States. The DSM definition is similar, though not identical, to the definition of the disorder in the 10th revision of the *International Classification of Diseases* (ICD-10; World Health Organization, 1994), which is used mainly in Europe. Table 2.1 presents the DSM-IV-TR criteria.

The DSM-IV(-TR) criteria stipulate that individuals must have had their symptoms of ADHD for at least 6 months, that these symptoms must occur to a degree that is developmentally deviant, and that symptoms producing impairment must have developed by 7 years of age. From the inattention item list, six of nine items must be endorsed as developmentally inappropriate. From the combined hyperactivity and impulsivity item lists, six of nine items must be endorsed as deviant. The type of ADHD to be diagnosed depends on whether criteria are met for inattention, hyperactivity–impulsivity, or both: the Predominantly Inattentive Type (ADHD-PI), the Predominantly Hyperactive–Impulsive Type (ADHD-PHI), or the Combined Type (ADHD-C).

Merits of DSM-IV(-TR)

The DSM-IV(-TR) diagnostic criteria are some of the most rigorous and most empirically derived criteria ever available in the history of ADHD. They were derived from a process in which (1) a committee of some of the leading experts in the field met to discuss its development; (2) a literature review of ADHD symptoms was conducted; (3) a survey of rating scales assessing the behavioral dimensions related to ADHD, along with their factor structure and psychometric properties, was undertaken; and (4) a field trial of the subsequently developed item pool was conducted with 380 children from 10 different sites in North America (Applegate et al., 1997; Lahey et al., 1994). The criteria are a considerable improvement over those provided in the earlier versions of DSM (American Psychiatric Association, 1968, 1980, 1987) in many respects:

1. The items used to make the diagnosis were selected primarily from factor analyses of items from parent and teacher rating scales in which the items already showed high intercorrelations with each other and the underlying dimension, as well as validity in distinguishing children with ADHD from other groups of children (Lahey et al., 1994; Spitzer et al., 1990).

2. The DSM-IV(-TR) clusters items underneath two main constructs (i.e., inattention and hyperactivity–impulsivity), based on empirical information that supports these constructs (a factor analysis of the items) (Lahey et al., 1994), and consistent with the two dimensions often found in other studies of parent and teacher ratings having similar item content (DuPaul, 1991; DuPaul et al., 1998; Goyette, Conners, & Ulrich, 1978).

3. Unlike the earlier versions of DSM and ICD, the cutoff points for the number of symptoms necessary for a diagnosis (six) were determined in a field trial (Lahey et al., 1994) as having the greatest interjudge reliability and discrimination of children with ADHD from those without ADHD. Thus they have some empirical basis for their selection. Although the DSM-III-R also used a field trial for much the same purpose (Spitzer et al., 1990), it was not of the same degree of rigor or magnitude as the DSM-IV field trial.

4. The specification of guidelines in DSM-IV(-TR) for establishing the degree of situational pervasiveness of the symptoms seems important to many researchers in the field, in view of findings that the pervasiveness of symptoms across home and school settings may be an important marker for at least the more severe cases of the disorder, if not for the clinical syndrome itself (Goodman & Stevenson, 1989; Schachar et al., 1981). Nevertheless, clinicians should keep in mind that this means of determining pervasiveness may confound the source of information (parent vs. teacher) with the settings across which one is attempting to determine pervasiveness (Mitsis et al., 2000). Thus any differences between these groups may simply be artifacts of the source (Costello et al., 1991; Rapoport et al., 1986). Perhaps it would be more useful or clinically prudent to establish that *a history* of symptoms exists across the home and school settings, rather than requiring current parent–teacher agreement on symptoms to establish the presence of the disorder. Research suggests that when agreement across parent, teacher, and clinician is a requirement for diagnosis, it severely reduces the diagnosis (particularly for the ADHD-PI and ADHD-PHI subtypes) within the childhood population (Lambert, Sandoval, & Sassone, 1978; Mitsis et al., 2000; Szatmari, Offord, & Boyle, 1989).

TABLE 2.1. DSM-IV-TR Criteria for ADHD

A. Either (1) or (2):

 (1) six (or more) of the following symptoms of **inattention** have persisted for at least 6 months to a degree that is maladaptive and inconsistent with developmental level:

 Inattention
 (a) often fails to give close attention to details or makes careless mistakes in schoolwork, work, or other activities
 (b) often has difficulty sustaining attention in tasks or play activities
 (c) often does not seem to listen when spoken to directly
 (d) often does not follow through on instructions and fails to finish schoolwork, chores, or duties in the workplace (not due to oppositional behavior or failure to understand instructions)
 (e) often has difficulty organizing tasks and activities
 (f) often avoids, dislikes, or is reluctant to engage in tasks that require sustained mental effort (such as schoolwork or homework)
 (g) often loses things necessary for tasks or activities (e.g., toys, school assignments, pencils, books, or tools)
 (h) is often easily distracted by extraneous stimuli
 (i) is often forgetful in daily activities

 (2) six (or more) of the following symptoms of **hyperactivity–impulsivity** have persisted for at least 6 months to a degree that is maladaptive and inconsistent with developmental level:

 Hyperactivity
 (a) often fidgets with hands or feet or squirms in seat
 (b) often leaves seat in classroom or in other situations in which remaining seated is expected
 (c) often runs about or climbs excessively in situations in which it is inappropriate (in adolescents or adults, may be limited to subjective feelings of restlessness)
 (d) often has difficulty playing or engaging in leisure activities quietly
 (e) is often "on the go" or often acts as if "driven by a motor"
 (f) often talks excessively

 Impulsivity
 (g) often blurts out answers before questions have been completed
 (h) often has difficulty awaiting turn
 (i) often interrupts or intrudes on others (e.g., butts into conversations or games)

B. Some hyperactive–impulsive or inattentive symptoms that caused impairment were present before age 7 years.

C. Some impairment from the symptoms is present in two or more settings (e.g., at school [or work] and at home).

D. There must be clear evidence of clinically significant impairment in social, academic, or occupational functioning.

E. The symptoms do not occur exclusively during the course of a Pervasive Developmental Disorder, Schizophrenia, or other Psychotic Disorder, and are not better accounted for by another mental disorder (e.g., Mood Disorder, Anxiety Disorder, Dissociative Disorder, or a Personality Disorder).

(continued)

TABLE 2.1. *(continued)*

Code based on type:

314.01 Attention-Deficit/Hyperactivity Disorder, Combined Type: if both Criteria A1 and A2 are met for the past 6 months

314.00 Attention-Deficit/Hyperactivity Disorder, Predominantly Inattentive Type: if Criterion A1 is met but Criterion A2 is not met for the past 6 months

314.01 Attention-Deficit/Hyperactivity Disorder, Predominantly Hyperactive–Impulsive Type: if Criterion A2 is met but Criterion A1 is not met for the past 6 months

Coding note: For individuals (especially adolescents and adults) who currently have symptoms that no longer meet full criteria, "In Partial Remission" should be specified.

Note. From American Psychiatric Association (2000). Copyright 2000 by the American Psychiatric Association. Reprinted by permission.

5. DSM-IV(-TR) has returned to the subtyping of ADD with and without Hyperactivity as first presented in DSM-III. There are differences, however, between the earlier and later versions of this subtype. ADD without Hyperactivity is now ADHD-PI, but the symptoms of impulsivity are no longer included as they were in ADD without Hyperactivity, where both inattention and impulsivity items could count toward the subtyping classification. And of course the number of symptoms required to meet this subtyping approach has changed to six or more inattention symptoms. This subtyping certainly permits clinicians the opportunity to diagnose clinic-referred children who have significant attention dysfunction but no significant disinhibition. Yet, as noted later, it has not been established in research that this subtype is actually a true subtype of ADHD having the same problems with inattention as ADHD-C, or whether, as suggested above, the ADHD-PI is a qualitatively different disorder entirely, with a different attention disturbance from that seen in ADHD-C.

6. The addition of a requirement of impairment as a criterion for diagnosis of a mental disorder is crucial, and its importance cannot be overemphasized. Efforts to define the nature of a mental disorder typically incorporate such a requirement, to distinguish a mental disorder from the wide range of normal human behavior and problems in living that do not necessarily lead to a harmful dysfunction or impairment (Wakefield, 1997). Simply because a child or adult may show a higher frequency or severity of symptoms related to ADHD than is typical of others does not, by itself, warrant a diagnosis of ADHD (a mental disorder). This more

extreme degree of symptoms must also lead to increased mortality, increased morbidity, or significant interference or disruption in one or more of the major domains of life activities associated with that age group (typically home, school, or work).

Issues Requiring Further Consideration in the DSM-IV(-TR) View of ADHD

This discussion of the merits of DSM-IV(-TR) does not imply that its criteria cannot be improved. Science is a self-correcting process, and to the extent that the DSM is based on empirically derived information, it will continue to be refined as new scientific findings are used to inform the DSM process. Recent research on the disorder suggests that the following issues may need to be considered, so as to further improve the rigor or sensitivity of these criteria in distinguishing ADHD from no disorder and from other clinical disorders.

1. *Individuals with ADHD-PI are a heterogeneous group, a subset of whom may not actually have a subtype of ADHD, but may share a common attention deficit with the other types.* This issue is discussed further in Chapter 3. Suffice it to say here that a number of qualitative differences between individuals with the SCT subset of ADHD-PI and those with the ADHD-C are emerging in research, suggesting that these groups do not have the same impairment in attention. Recall from the earlier discussion on inattention symptoms that a subset of perhaps 30–50% of children diagnosed with ADHD-PI have more problems in focused/selective attention and sluggish information pro-

cessing, whereas ADHD-C is associated more with problems of persistence of effort and distractibility. Should these group differences continue to be confirmed in additional research, it would indicate that the subset of individuals with SCT diagnosed with ADHD-PI should be said to have made a separate, distinct, and independent disorder, or at least an independent subtype of ADHD.

This would also mean that clinicians and researchers will need to take greater care in their classification of cases of ADHD in adolescents and adults into these subtypes. Problems arise because the hyperactivity symptoms in DSM-IV(-TR) decline more steeply over development than do the symptoms of inattention (Hart, Lahey, Loeber, Applegate, & Frick, 1995; Loeber, Green, Lahey, Christ, & Frick, 1992). Thus there will be many individuals who are initially diagnosed with ADHD-C, but who by adolescence or young adulthood no longer have sufficient symptoms of hyperactivity to qualify for an ADHD-C diagnosis according to DSM decision rules. If the DSM criteria were strictly followed, these individuals must now be rediagnosed as having ADHD-PI. Yet conceptually they will retain many of the features of ADHD-C and will not be similar to that subgroup of patients who have been diagnosed with ADHD-PI since childhood and who have never had significant symptoms of hyperactivity or disinhibition. Clinicians and researchers would do well to continue to conceptualize the former group as still having classic ADHD-C, even though they no longer have sufficient hyperactive symptoms to qualify for a formal diagnosis. This is because the sine qua non of ADHD-C is actually disinhibition. As long as members of this group present clinically with inhibitory difficulties, despite a decline in gross motor overactivity with age, those members should remain conceptualized as having the disinhibitory form of the disorder (ADHD-C). As noted above, those adolescents or adults who have always been diagnosed with ADHD-PI since childhood, who present with SCT symptoms (see above), and who have no significant difficulties with disinhibition (either currently or earlier in childhood) should be thought of as having a qualitatively different condition.

To summarize, children and adults with ADHD-PI are a mixed group. Some of them (perhaps 30–50%) have an SCT form of attention disturbance, which may constitute a quali-

tatively unique disorder from the attention disturbance in ADHD-C. Others are older children and adults who used to be diagnosed as having ADHD-C, but have shown a decrease in the number and severity of their symptoms of hyperactivity with age, such that they now fall below the critical number of six such symptoms required for the ADHD-C diagnosis. The DSM decision rules would reclassify these individuals as having ADHD-PI, whereas I recommend that clinicians continue conceptualizing and treating them as having ADHD-C. Finally, the remaining children and adults have had some symptoms of hyperactive–impulsive behavior, but never enough to qualify for an ADHD-C diagnosis, though they have inattentive symptoms as well. These individuals probably just have mild, subthreshold, or borderline cases of ADHD-C.

2. Individuals with ADHD-PHI are also a heterogeneous group. Some such individuals really do not have a separate type of ADHD from ADHD-C, but simply an earlier developmental stage of it. The field trial found that those with ADHD-PHI were primarily preschool-age children, whereas those with ADHD-C were primarily school-age children. As noted earlier, this is what one would expect to find, given that previous research found hyperactive–impulsive symptoms to appear first in development, followed within a few years by those of inattention (Hart et al., 1995; Loeber et al., 1992). If inattention symptoms are required to be part of the diagnostic criteria, then ADHD-C will of necessity have a later age of onset than ADHD-PHI, which seems to be the case (Applegate et al., 1997). Thus it seems that some cases of ADHD-PHI may actually merely represent an earlier developmental stage of ADHD-C. Other cases, however, will simply be milder, borderline, or subthreshold cases of ADHD-C, simply because they are one or two symptoms shy of meeting the six required on the inattention list to qualify for the ADHD-C diagnosis. There does appear to be, however, a subset of ADHD-C cases that are simply preschool instances of Oppositional Defiant Disorder (ODD). Parents more readily confuse symptoms of ODD with symptoms of ADHD, and thus may tend to rate young children with ODD as having ADHD symptoms when they do not. Given that cases where ODD occurs alone have a high remission rate (50% remitting every 2 years; Barkley, 1997b), such cases of ADHD-PHI may remit with age, and such children probably never really had ADHD-PHI at all.

3. *Should significant inattention be a requirement to diagnose ADHD?* This may sound like diagnostic heresy to some, given that the very name "ADHD" signifies that inattention must be present in this disorder. But inattention characterizes many psychiatric disorders, making it of limited value in differential diagnosis. And given that many children with ADHD-PHI are likely to move eventually into ADHD-C or to remain simply with a milder form of ADHD-C, does the added requirement of significant inattention for the group with hyperactive–impulsive symptoms provide any greater power in predicting additional impairments not already achieved by the hyperactive–impulsive symptoms alone? Apparently they do not add much, according to the results of the field trial (Lahey et al., 1994). Significant levels of inattention were found mainly to predict additional problems with completing homework, which were not as well predicted by the hyperactive–impulsive behaviors. Otherwise, the latter behaviors predicted most of the other areas of impairment studied in this field trial. This study is consistent with the findings in follow-up studies that childhood symptoms of hyperactivity are related to adolescent negative outcomes, whereas those of inattention are much less so (if at all), and when they are predictive of outcome, are mainly limited to academic outcome (Fischer, Barkley, Fletcher, & Smallish, 1993a; Fergusson, Lynskey, & Horwood, 1997; Weiss & Hechtman, 1993).

The status of inattention for the diagnosis (primary, secondary?) is not settled and certainly causes conceptual confusion. Is ADHD at its core a disorder of behavioral inhibition, as current theorists have argued (Barkley, 1997a; Quay, 1997; Nigg, 2001)? If so, then the problems with inattention (impersistence, distractibility, etc.) may be distinct but secondary to this core problem, or may just be associated symptoms of it. After all, research finds the two dimensions representing ADHD (inattention, inhibition) to be highly correlated, at least until much of their overlap is then removed by the factor rotation method chosen in the analysis (Beiser et al., 2000; DuPaul et al., 1998; Lahey et al., 1994). Or is ADHD at its core both an inhibitory *and* an attention disorder? And to confuse matters even further, are the symptoms of inattention actually inattention, or do they represent deficits in executive functioning instead (particularly working memory), as will be discussed in Chapters 3 and 7? Much theoretical work remains to be done. Critics of ADHD should not take this to mean that the disorder is a myth or that clinical scientists have no idea what the disorder represents. Those are not the issues raised here, and any critic taking solace in them would be sorely mistaken, if not intentionally misrepresenting the status of the science on ADHD. What clinical science is deliberating here is the priority that should be given to these symptom dimensions and how they relate to each other in conceptualizing the disorder (theory building), not whether or not they exist as clinical symptoms or whether there is any disorder here.

4. *Can the diagnostic thresholds for the two sets of symptoms (inattention and hyperactivity–impulsivity) be applied to age groups outside those used in the field trial?* Those ages were 4–16 years. This concern arises out of the well-known findings that the behavioral items constituting these sets of symptoms decline significantly with age, particularly the items for hyperactivity–impulsivity (Hart et al., 1995). Applying the same threshold across such a declining developmental slope could produce a diminishing sensitivity to disorder: a situation in which a larger percentage of young preschool-age children (ages 2–3) would be inappropriately diagnosed as having ADHD (false positives), while a smaller-than-expected percentage of adults would meet the criteria (false negatives). A study (Murphy & Barkley, 1996b) that collected norms for the DSM-IV item sets on a large sample of adults ages 17–84 years suggested just such a problem with using these criteria for adults. The threshold needed to place an individual at the 93rd percentile for his or her age group declined to four of nine inattention items and five of nine hyperactivity–impulsivity items for ages 17–29 years, then to four of nine in each set for the 30- to 49-year age group, then to three of nine in each set for those 50 years and older. Studies of the applicability of the diagnostic thresholds to preschool children remain to be done. This shows that adhering to a single symptom cutoff score, regardless of age, could result in increasingly fewer individuals with the disorder meeting that threshold with age. They would outgrow the diagnostic criteria while not actually outgrowing their disorder, as was suggested in my own longitudinal study (Barkley et al., 2002). Until more research is done, it seems

prudent to utilize the recommended thresholds for each symptom set only for children ages 4–16 years, while using lower thresholds for adults. Better yet, the use of well-standardized rating scales of ADHD symptoms for adults (as recommended in Chapter 11) would give a clearer indication of their true deviance from nondisabled individuals of their age group than would just using the DSM criteria alone.

5. *Are the item sets appropriate for different developmental periods?* History shows that the items used to construct the DSM symptom lists were based almost entirely on research on children. Inspection of the three item lists suggests that the items for inattention may have a wider developmental applicability across the school-age ranges of childhood and possibly into adolescence and young adulthood. Those for hyperactivity, in contrast, seem much more applicable to young children and less appropriate or not at all applicable to older teens and adults. The items for impulsivity are few and may or may not be as applicable to teens and adults as much as to children. Consider the items that pertain to climbing on things, not playing quietly, or acting as if driven by a motor. And, as discussed in more detail in Chapter 7, disinhibition may be the central feature of the disorder; if so, this means that symptoms of this core deficit are grossly underrepresented on this list. Recall the observations (Hart et al., 1995) that the symptoms of inattention remain stable across middle childhood into early adolescence, while those for hyperactive behavior decline significantly over this same course. Although this may represent a true developmental decline in the severity of the latter symptoms with maturation, and possibly in the severity and prevalence of ADHD itself, it could also represent an illusory developmental trend. That is, it might be an artifact of the developmental restrictedness of some items (hyperactivity) more than others (inattention), and of the minimal sampling of impulsive behavior appropriate for the various developmental periods.

An analogy using mental retardation illustrates the issue. Consider the following items that might be chosen to assess developmental level in preschool-age children: being toilet-trained, recognizing primary colors, counting to 10, repeating five digits, being able to use buttons or snaps on clothing, recognizing and drawing simple geometric shapes, and using a vocabulary repertoire of at least 100 words.

This is a fixed item set, like that of the DSM. Evaluating whether or not children are able to do these things may prove to be very useful in distinguishing preschoolers with from those without mental retardation. However, if we continued to use this same item set to assess mentally retarded children as they grew older, we would find an illusory decline in the severity of retardation with age in these children as they achieved progressively more items with maturation. We would also find that the prevalence of mental retardation declined with age, as many children formerly diagnosed with it outgrew this diagnostic threshold. But we know these findings are illusory, because mental retardation represents a *developmentally relative deficit* in the achievement of these and other mental and adaptive milestones. All that is happening with age is that the symptom list is increasingly less sensitive to disorder, and children with mental retardation are simply outgrowing the symptom list, not the disorder.

To return to the diagnosis of ADHD, if we apply the same fixed item sets developed on children throughout development, with no attempt to adjust either the thresholds or (just as important) the types of items developmentally appropriate for different age periods, we might see the same results as with the analogy to mental retardation. The fact that similar results to this analogy do occur with ADHD (i.e., sensitivity to disorder does seem to diminish with age) should give us pause before we interpret the observed decline in symptom severity (and even the observed decline in apparent prevalence) as being accurate (e.g., see Barkley et al., 2002). Developmentally sensitive sets of items for inattention and disinhibition–hyperactivity need to be created and tested for different age groups to more accurately capture the nature of ADHD and the fact that it, like mental retardation, probably represents a developmentally relative deficit. As it now stands, ADHD is defined mainly by items reflecting its status in childhood. It is also diagnosed by one of its earliest developmental manifestations (hyperactivity) and one of its later (school-age) sequelae (inattention or goal-directed impersistence), and only minimally by its central feature (disinhibition).

The issue is not just speculative. In research that has followed children with ADHD into their adulthood, my colleagues and I have demonstrated the chronicity of impairments created by the disorder, despite an *apparent* decline in the percentage of cases continuing to meet DSM diagnostic criteria and an *apparent* decline in the severity of the symptoms used in these criteria (Barkley, Fischer, et al., 1990; Barkley et al., 2002; Fischer et al., 1993b; Fischer et al., 2004). Making developmentally referenced adjustments to the diagnostic thresholds at the adolescent follow-up resulted in a larger number of adolescents' continuing to meet criteria for the disorder (71–84%). And at the young adult follow-up, the disparity in diagnosed cases was even greater (46% with DSM criteria vs. 66% with developmentally referenced criteria; Barkley et al., 2002). Such adjustments, however, did not correct for the potentially increasing inappropriateness of the items themselves for this aging sample; thus it is difficult to say how many of those not meeting these adjusted criteria may still have had the disorder.

6. *Should the criteria be adjusted for the sex of the clinic-referred individual?* Research evaluating these and similar item sets demonstrates that male children in the general population display more of these items and to a more severe degree than do females (Achenbach, 1991; DuPaul, 1991; DuPaul et al., 1998; Goyette et al., 1978). If so, should the same threshold for diagnosis be applied to both genders? Doing so would seem to result in females' having to meet a higher threshold relative to other females to be diagnosed as ADHD than do males relative to other males. The problem is further accentuated by the fact that the majority of individuals in the DSM field trial were males, making the DSM criteria primarily male-referenced. Adjusting the cutoff scores for each gender separately might well result in nullifying the finding that ADHD is more common in males than females by a ratio of roughly 3:1 (see later discussion). A conference held at the National Institute of Mental Health in November 1994 to discuss gender differences in ADHD did not recommend that this be done as yet (Arnold, 1997). But a consensus emerged that sufficient evidence existed to warrant further study. Whether gender-based thresholds for diagnosis are necessary thus remains an open issue.

7. *Should the criterion that the age of onset for ADHD symptoms must be before 7 years be abandoned?* This criterion was challenged by the results of its own field trial (Applegate et al., 1997), as well as by other longitudinal studies (McGee, Williams, & Feehan, 1992). The age-of-onset criterion suggests that there

may be qualitative differences between those who meet this precise criterion (onset before age 7) and those who do not (later onset). Some results do indicate that those with an onset before age 6 may have more severe and persistent conditions, and more problems with reading and school performance more generally (McGee et al., 1992). But these were matters of degree and not of kind in this study. The DSM-IV field trial also was not able to show any clear discontinuities in degree of ADHD or in the types of impairments it examined between those meeting and not meeting the 7-year age-of-onset criterion. In short, no qualitative differences emerged, nor was there a sharp demarcation in symptoms, between cases with onset before age 7 and those with onset after age 7. It remains unclear at this time just how specific an age of onset may need to be for distinguishing valid cases of ADHD from other disorders. Meanwhile, Joseph Biederman and I have argued (Barkley & Biederman, 1997) that the age-of-onset criterion be generously broadened to include onset of symptoms during childhood, in keeping with the conceptualization of this disorder as having a childhood onset, while not restricting it with a wholly indefensible and highly specific onset of 7 years of age. This argument would have the added advantage of making the DSM-IV(-TR) criteria more suitable for use with adults, who would have less difficulty recalling an onset of their symptoms sometime in childhood than one prior to 7 years of age specifically.

8. *Is there a lower-bound age group below which no diagnosis should be made?* Just how young can the diagnosis of ADHD be reliably and validly made? This question is important, because research on preschool children shows that a separate dimension of hyperactive–impulsive behavior is not distinguishable from one of aggression or defiant behavior until about 3 years of age (Achenbach, 2001; Achenbach & Edelbrock, 1987; Campbell, 1990). Below this age, these behaviors cluster together to form "behavioral immaturity," or an undercontrolled pattern of temperament or conduct. All this implies that the symptoms of ADHD may be difficult to distinguish from other early behavioral disorders or extremes of temperament until at least 3 years of age; thus this age might serve as a lower bound for diagnostic applications.

9. *Is there a lower bound of IQ below which the diagnosis should not be given?* For

instance, Rutter and colleagues (Rutter, Bolton, et al., 1990; Rutter, Macdonald, et al., 1990) concluded that children who fall below an IQ of 50 may have a qualitatively different form of mental retardation. This conclusion is inferred from findings that this group is overrepresented for its position along a normal distribution, and from findings that genetic defects contribute more heavily to mental retardation in this subgroup. Given this shift in the prevalence and causes of mental retardation below this level of IQ, a similar state of affairs might exist for the form of ADHD associated with it, necessitating its distinction from the type of ADHD that occurs in individuals above this IQ level. Consistent with such a view are findings that the percentage of positive response to stimulant medication in those with ADHD falls off sharply below this threshold of IQ (Demb, 1991).

10. *Is the duration requirement of 6 months for symptom presence enough?* This number was chosen mainly in keeping with the criteria set forth in earlier DSMs and for consistency with criteria used for other disorders; there is little or no research support for selecting this particular length of time for symptom presence in the case of ADHD. It is undoubtedly important that the symptoms be relatively persistent if we are to view this disorder as arising from intraindividual sources (genetics, neurology), rather than arising purely from context or out of a transient, normal developmental stage. Yet specifying a precise duration is difficult in the absence of research to guide the issue. Research on preschool-age children might prove helpful here, however. Such research shows that many children age 3 years or younger may have parents or preschool teachers who report concerns about the activity level or attention of the children, but that these concerns have a high likelihood of remission within 12 months (Beitchman, Wekerle, & Hood, 1987; Campbell, 1990; Lerner, Inui, Trupin, & Douglas, 1985; Palfrey, Levine, Walker, & Sullivan, 1985). It would seem for preschoolers, then, that the 6-month duration specified in DSM-IV(-TR) may be too brief, resulting in the possibility of overidentification of ADHD in children at this age (false positives). However, this same body of research found that for those children whose problems lasted at least 12 months or beyond age 4 years, a persistent pattern of behavior was established that was highly predictive of its continuance into the

school-age range. The finding suggests that the duration of symptoms might be better set at 12 months or longer, to improve the rigor of diagnosis in detecting true cases of disorder.

11. *Is symptom pervasiveness across two or more settings important for accurate diagnosis?* The requirement that the symptoms be demonstrated in at least two of three environments to establish pervasiveness of symptoms is new to DSM-IV(-TR) and potentially problematic. By stipulating that the symptoms must be present in at least two of three contexts (home, school, work, in the case of DSM-IV (-TR); home, school, clinic, in the case of ICD-10), the criteria now confound settings with sources of information (parent, teacher, employer, clinician), as noted earlier. Research shows that the degree of agreement between parents and teachers, for instance, is modest for any dimension of psychological development; it often ranges between .30 and .50, depending on the behavioral dimension being rated (Achenbach, McConaughy, & Howell, 1987; Mitsis et al., 2000). This low degree of agreement sets an upper limit on the extent to which parents and teachers can agree on the severity of ADHD symptoms, and thus on whether or not a child has the disorder. Such disagreements among sources certainly reflect in part real differences in the child's behavior in these different settings, probably as a function of true differences in situational demands. School, after all, is quite different from the home environment in its expectations, tasks, social context, and general demands for public self-regulation. But the disagreements may also reflect differences in the attitudes, experiences, and judgments of different people. And so there is no scientific reason at this time to side with one person's view or the other; instead, these views should be considered as providing information on the child *in that particular context* and nothing more, rather than as evidence at some diagnostic trial as to whether or not the child really has the disorder. More importantly, the crux of the issue of clinical diagnosis is whether or not impairment exists in children identified by parent-only or teacher-only report as having clinical symptoms of ADHD. If impairment is believed to be present, it is to be treated even if the diagnosis is less than certain, because this is a major cornerstone to the existence of mental health professions—the relief of suffering! Diagnosis, it should be remem-

bered, is a means to this end, not the end in itself.

Insisting on such agreement on diagnostic criteria also may reduce the application of the diagnosis to some children unfairly, simply as a result of such well-established differences between parents' and teachers' opinions. It may also create a confounding of ADHD with comorbid ODD (Costello et al., 1991). Parent-only-identified children with ADHD may have predominantly ODD with relatively milder ADHD, whereas teacher-only-identified children with ADHD may have chiefly ADHD and minimal or no ODD symptoms. Children identified by both parents and teachers as having ADHD, therefore, not only may have ADHD but may also carry a higher likelihood of ODD. They may also simply have a more severe form of ADHD than do home- or school-only-identified children—a form that is different in degree, rather than in kind (Tripp & Luk, 1997). Research is clearly conflicting on the matter of whether pervasiveness of symptoms defines a valid syndrome (Cohen & Minde, 1983; Rapoport et al., 1986; Schachar et al., 1981; Taylor, Sandberg, Thorley, & Giles, 1991; Tripp & Luk, 1997), and the issue has received scant attention since the preceding edition of this text. One follow-up study found that children with pervasively defined ADHD (home and school) were more likely to have Antisocial Personality Disorder as adults than were children with ADHD identified only at home (Mannuzza, Klein, & Moulton, 2002). The results attest mainly to the validity of teacher reports in identifying a group of children with ADHD at higher risk for adult Antisocial Personality Disorder. Considering that teacher information on children is not always obtainable or convenient to obtain, and that diagnosis based on parents' reports will lead to a diagnosis based on teacher reports 90% of the time (Biederman, Keenan, & Faraone, 1990), parent reports may suffice for diagnostic purposes for now. Until more research is done to address this issue, the requirement of pervasiveness should probably be interpreted to mean *a history* of symptoms in multiple settings, rather than current agreement between parents and teachers on number and severity of symptoms. Clinicians need to keep in mind that the DSM definition of ADHD was constructed by blending the reports of parents and teachers, and they should do likewise. The number of different symptoms reported by one source was tallied and then the number of additional symptoms identified by the other source was then added to it, giving a sum total of the number of different items endorsed across both sources.

12. *Can the diagnostic criteria be more precise in specifying how developmental inappropriateness is to be established?* A final point for further improvement pertains to the stipulation in DSM-IV(-TR) that symptoms must be developmentally inappropriate. That is all well and good, but how many symptoms must an individual have, and how severe must they be, to be considered "developmentally inappropriate?" To borrow another analogy from the disorder of mental retardation, a specific degree of general cognitive delay is specified in the criteria: an IQ score below 70. In contrast, for ADHD, no guidance is given as to just what constitutes developmental inappropriateness or how to assess it. The ubiquity of well-normed behavior rating scales assessing ADHD symptoms generally, and now DSM-IV(-TR) ADHD symptoms specifically, argues for the use of such instruments to determine the extent of developmental deviance in a particular case (see Chapter 8, for a discussion of such scales). Although not wholly objective, such instruments do provide a means of quantifying parent and teacher opinions in the case of children, and adult self-reports and other-reports of symptoms in the case of adults, being evaluated for ADHD. Moreover, national norms are now available for the parent and teacher versions of these instruments (DuPaul, Power, et al., 1997; DuPaul et al., 1998), and for adults (Conners, Erhardt, & Sparrow, 2000). The use of such scales automatically provides a means for establishing deviance relative to both age and gender membership of an individual, given that norms are provided separately for males and females by age groups. With such norms available, we must then specify a recommended threshold that is considered "inappropriate." It would seem prudent to establish a cutoff score on these scales of at least the 90th percentile, and preferably the 93rd percentile, as the demarcation for clinical significance, given that the 93rd percentile (+1.5 standard deviations above the mean) is a traditionally employed cutoff point for this purpose (Achenbach, 2001). Such a threshold is not to be intended as religious dogma, but as a guideline for determining developmental deviance. As with mental retardation, cases falling near but not quite over the deviance threshold would be considered

borderline or subthreshold cases, while those falling just across the threshold would be mild cases, with more pronounced cases being identified as moderate or severe.

I previously (Barkley, 1990) suggested that mental age be taken into consideration in the use of such norms on rating scales, given the low but significant negative correlation between symptoms of ADHD and IQ (see Barkley, 1997a). Research in the interim suggests that using a chronological-age comparison group is sufficient for making determinations of developmental inappropriateness of symptoms, and that adjusting for mental age is actually unnecessary (Pearson & Aman, 1994). I therefore stand corrected.

Despite these numerous problematic issues for the DSM-IV(-TR) approach to diagnosis, the criteria are actually the best ever advanced to date for the disorder and represent a vast improvement over the state of affairs that existed prior to 1980. The various editions of DSM have also spawned a large amount of research into ADHD—its symptoms, subtypes, criteria, and even etiologies—that probably would not have occurred had such criteria not been set forth for professional consumption and criticism. The most recent criteria provide clinicians with guidelines that are more specific, reliable, empirically based or justifiable (valid), and closer to the scientific literature on ADHD than those of earlier editions, and thus deserve to be adopted in clinical practice. In fact, they have now become the standard of care within the mental health professions. Yet the issues raised here suggest that such adoption should not become diagnostic dogma, but instead must be done with some clinical judgment and awareness of these problematic issues as applied in individual cases.

IS ADHD A MENTAL DISORDER?

Social critics (Kohn, 1989; McGinnis, 1997; Schrag & Divoky, 1975), some nonexpert professionals (Timimi, 2004), and fringe political–religious groups (the Church of Scientology and affiliated groups) charge that ADHD is a myth—or, more specifically, that professionals have been too quick to label energetic and exuberant children as having a mental disorder, and that educators also may be using these labels as an excuse for simply poor educational environments. In other words, children diagnosed with hyperactivity or ADHD are actually normal, but are being labeled "mentally disordered" because of parent and teacher intolerance (Kohn, 1989), parental and cultural anxiety surrounding child rearing (Timimi, 2004), or some unspecified and undocumented conspiracy between the mental health community and pharmaceutical companies (Timimi, 2004).

If this claim of ADHD as myth were actually true, and not just the propaganda it often turns out to represent, we should find no differences of any cognitive, behavioral, or social significance between children with and without the ADHD label. We should also find that being diagnosed with ADHD is not associated with any significant later risks in development for maladjustment within any domains of adaptive functioning or social or school performance. Furthermore, research on potential etiologies for the disorder should likewise come up empty-handed. This is hardly the case. The first six chapters of this textbook constitute a direct and monumental refutation of such claims. Differences between children with and without ADHD are numerous. And, as shown later, numerous developmental risks await the children meeting clinical diagnostic criteria for the disorder. Moreover, certain potential etiological factors are becoming consistently noted in the research literature as being associated with ADHD. Therefore, any claims that ADHD is a myth reflect either a stunning level of scientific illiteracy or outright attempts to misrepresent the science of ADHD so as to mislead the public with propaganda (Barkley, 2004b).

The fact that ADHD is all too real, however, does not automatically entitle it to be placed within the realm of mental disorders. Determining whether or not ADHD is a valid disorder requires that some standards for defining "disorder" be available. Jerome Wakefield (1992, 1997) has provided the field with the best available criteria to date for doing so. He has argued that mental disorders must meet two criteria to be viewed as such: (1) They must involve the dysfunction of universal mental mechanisms (adaptations) that have been selected in an evolutionary sense (have survival value); and (2) they must engender substantial harm to the individual (mortality, morbidity, or impaired major life activities). It should become clear from the totality of information on

ADHD presented in this text that the disorder handily meets both criteria. Those with ADHD, as described previously, have significant deficits in behavioral inhibition and (as shown here and in Chapters 3 and 7) in several of the executive functions that are critical for effective self-regulation. It has been argued that these functions are universal adaptations selected for in evolution to assist individuals with organizing their behavior relative to time and the social future, and thereby to help them maximize long-term over short-term social consequences (Barkley, 1997a, 1997c, 2001b; Fuster, 1997). And those with ADHD experience significant and numerous risks for harm to themselves over the course of their development (see Chapter 4). Thus we can readily conclude that ADHD is a valid mental disorder, because it produces a harmful dysfunction in a set of mental mechanisms evolved to have a survival advantage.

IS ADHD A CLINICAL SYNDROME?

A previously troublesome issue for attempts to define a disorder or syndrome is the frequent finding that objective measures of ADHD symptoms do not correlate well with each other (Barkley, 1991; Barkley & Ullman, 1975; Routh & Roberts, 1972; Ullman et al., 1978). Typically, for a disorder to be viewed as a syndrome, its major features should be related: The more deviant an individual is on one symptom, the more the individual should be on the other major symptoms. The relatively weak or insignificant correlations among laboratory measures of activity, attention, and impulsivity are a smoke-screen often used as evidence against the existence of ADHD as a disorder or syndrome by social critics (Kohn, 1989; Schrag & Divoky, 1975). However, these weak relationships may have more to do with the methods used in such assessments and the manner in which we define the attention deficits or overactivity problems in children with ADHD (Barkley, 1991; Rutter, 1989). How long a child looks at a classroom lecturer may be a very different type of attention process from that required to search out important from unimportant features in a picture (Barkley, 1988; Ullman et al., 1978). Similarly, taking adequate time to examine a picture before choosing one identical to it from a number of similar pictures may be a different type of impulsivity from that

seen when a child is asked to draw a line slowly, or is asked whether he or she wishes to work a little for a small reward now or do more work for a large reward later (Milich & Kramer, 1985; Rapport et al., 1986). It is small wonder, then, that these types of measures do not correlate well with each other.

In contrast, studies that factor-analyze parent or teacher ratings of ADHD symptoms often find that they are highly interrelated (Achenbach, 2001; DuPaul et al., 1998; Hinshaw, 1987; Lahey et al., 1994) and comprise two dimensions (Inattention–Restlessness and Impulsivity–Hyperactivity). Similarly, when measures of attention and impulsivity are taken within the same task, as in scores for omission and commission errors on a CPT, they are highly related to each other (Barkley, 1991; Gordon, 1983). This finding suggests that the frequent failure to find relationships among various lab measures of ADHD symptoms has more to do with the source or types of measures chosen; their highly limited sampling of behavior (typically 20 minutes or less per task); and their sampling of quite diverse aspects of attention, impulsivity, or activity than to a lack of relationships among the natural behaviors of these children.

Furthermore, even if the symptoms may not occur to a uniform degree in the same children, this does not rule out the value of considering ADHD a syndrome. As Rutter (1977, 1989) has noted, a disorder need not show such uniform variation to be clinically useful as a syndrome. If such children show a relatively similar course and outcome, if their symptoms predict differential responses to certain treatments relative to other disorders, or if they tend to share a common etiology or set of etiologies, it may still be valuable to consider children with such characteristics as having a syndrome of ADHD. Other researchers (Douglas, 1983; Rutter, 1989; Taylor, 1986; Taylor et al., 1991) and I believe that the evidence supports such an interpretation of ADHD.

More problematic for the concept of a syndrome, however, is whether the defining features of ADHD can discriminate ADHD from other types of psychiatric disturbance in children. The evidence here was certainly conflicting and less compelling (Reeves, Werry, Elkind, & Zametkin, 1987; Werry, Elkind, & Reeves, 1987) until the end of the 1980s. Children with mental retardation, autism, psychosis, depression, Conduct Disorder (CD), anxiety, and learning disabilities were all thought to show deficits in attention, suggesting that inattention was a rather nonspecific symptom. When early studies compared such groups, they often found few differences among them on measures of ADHD characteristics (see Werry, 1988, for a review). However, such studies often did not take into account the comorbidity of many of these disorders with each other. "Comorbidity" means that children with one disorder may have a high likelihood of having a second. Some children may have only one of these disorders, some may have another, and many have both. This is often noted with ADHD, ODD, CD, and the learning disabilities. Many studies on this issue have not taken care to choose subjects with only one of these disorders to compare against those with "pure" cases of the other disorders. As a result, they compare mixed cases of ADHD with mixed cases of other disorders, which greatly weakens the likelihood that differences among the groups will emerge. When this has been done, differences between pure ADHD and other disorders are more significant and numerous (August & Stewart, 1983; Barkley, DuPaul, & McMurray, 1990, 1991; Barkley, Fischer, et al., 1990; McGee, Williams, & Silva, 1984a, 1984b; Pennington & Ozonoff, 1996) (see the earlier discussions of inattention and impulsivity). Moreover, it appears that deficits in response inhibition are reasonably specific to ADHD (Barkley, 1997a; Nigg, 1999, 2001; Pennington & Ozonoff, 1996).

Certainly, differences in the approaches that were previously taken to define ADHD also contributed to the difficulties in evaluating ADHD as a distinct clinical syndrome. Research in the 1960s and 1970s was characterized by poorly specified and often subjective criteria for deciding on which subjects would be described as having hyperactivity or ADHD, with tremendous discrepancies across studies in these selection criteria (Barkley, 1982; Sergeant, 1988). Such criteria guaranteed not only that the studies would differ greatly in their findings, but also that many would employ subjects with various types of comorbidity, ensuring a conflicting pattern of results across the literature. With the development of consensus criteria for clinical diagnosis in DSM-IV, and with greater attention to the study of pure cases of the disorder, better, more critical tests of the notion of ADHD as a distinct disorder have been undertaken. These support the independent existence of ADHD versus other disorders.

IS ADHD A DIMENSION OR A CATEGORY?

One debate in the scientific literature during the 1980s and 1990s was whether or not ADHD represents a category or a dimension of behavior. The notion of applying categories for psychopathologies of children seems to derive from the medical model, where such categories constitute disease states (Edelbrock & Costello, 1984). From this perspective, an individual either has a disorder or does not. The DSM, in one sense, uses this categorical approach (all or none) by requiring that a person meet certain thresholds to be diagnosed with ADHD. The view of psychopathologies as representing dimensions of behavior, or even typologies (profiles) of these dimensions, arises from the perspective of developmental psychopathology (Achenbach & Edelbrock, 1983). In this view, ADHD constitutes the extreme end of a dimension, or dimensions, of behavior that falls along a continuum with the behavior of typical children. The dimensional view (more or less) does not necessarily see ADHD as a disease entity, but as a matter of degree in what is otherwise a characteristic of typical children.

The debate as it pertains to ADHD has ceased for several reasons, some of which relate to the construction of DSM-IV. The answer to the question posed in this heading, then, is that ADHD is both a category and a dimension. First, and not widely known, is the fact that the DSM-III-R and DSM-IV committees relied on several of the most commonly used behavior rating scales (the Conners scales, the Child Behavior Checklist [CBCL], the Behavior Problem Checklist) sources in selecting items to be included in the symptom list(s) and to be tested out in the field trials (Spitzer et al., 1990). These scales and their item pools are dimensional. Second, the casting of these symptoms into lists along which a threshold of severity is placed for granting a diagnosis tacitly represents the disorder as a dimension. Third, the ICD-10 criteria for this disorder, as well as the American Academy of Pediatrics (2001) and the American Academy of Child and Adolescent Psychiatry (1997), formally recommend the use of standardized dimensional measures to assess the individual's degree of deviancy in determining the presence of the disorder—a further acknowledgment of the dimensional nature of ADHD. A fourth line of evidence supporting the dimensional view comes from demonstrations that the majority of cases placed at extreme ends of dimensions of behavior related to ADHD on rating scales will receive the diagnosis when structured interviews using the diagnostic criteria are given (Chen, Faraone, Biederman, & Tsuang, 1994; Edelbrock & Costello, 1984). Of course, this is not surprising, given the previous three points bearing on this issue. Finally, genetic studies support the notion that ADHD represents a dimensional condition rather than a pathological category (Levy, Hay, McStephen, Wood, & Waldman, 1997; Sherman, McGee, & Iacono, 1997). The dimensional approach to ADHD seems most consistent with the available evidence, whereas the categorical approach remains one of convenience, parsimony, and tradition (Hinshaw, 1994). Moreover, dimensions can be carved into categories when the purpose of decision making necessitates dichotomous choices (whether or not to grant special education, whether or not to use medication, etc.).

SITUATIONAL AND TEMPORAL VARIATION

As already noted, all the primary symptoms of ADHD show significant fluctuations across various settings and caregivers (Barkley, 1981; Zentall, 1985). When children are playing alone, when they are washing and bathing, and when the father is at home are a few of the situations that are less troublesome for children with ADHD, whereas instances when children are asked to do chores, when parents are on the telephone, when visitors are in the home, or when children are in public places may be times of their disorder's peak severity (Barkley, 1990; Porrino et al., 1983). Significant fluctuations in activity are evident across these different contexts for both children with ADHD and nondisabled children, with the differences between them becoming most evident during school classes in reading and math. Despite these situational fluctuations, children with ADHD appear to be more deviant in their primary symptoms than typical children in most settings; yet these differences can be exaggerated greatly as a function of several factors related to the settings and the tasks children are given to perform in them (Luk, 1985; Zentall, 1985).

DEGREE OF ENVIRONMENTAL DEMANDS FOR INHIBITION

Some of the factors determining this variation have been delineated. One of these—the extent to which caregivers make demands on children with ADHD to restrict behavior—appears to affect the degree of deviance of these children's behavior from that of nondisabled children. In free-play or low-demand settings, children with ADHD are less distinguishable from typical children than in highly restrictive ones (Barkley, 1985; Jacob et al., 1978; Luk, 1985; Routh & Schroeder, 1976). Related to this issue of setting demands is the effect of task complexity on children with ADHD. The more complicated a task, and hence its greater demands for planning, organization, and executive regulation of behavior, the greater the likelihood that children with ADHD will perform more poorly on the task than nondisabled children (Douglas, 1983; Luk, 1985; Lawrence et al., 2002; Marzocchi et al., 2002). Clearly, the symptoms of ADHD are most disabling when the demands of the environment or task exceed a child's capacity to sustain attention, resist distractions, regulate activity, and restrain impulses. In environments that place little or no demands on these behavioral faculties, children with ADHD will appear less deviant and certainly be viewed by others as less troublesome than in settings or tasks that place high demands on these abilities. As Zentall (1985) rightly noted in her comprehensive review of setting factors in the expression of ADHD symptoms, we must look closely at the nature of the stimuli in the task and at the setting to which the children are being required to respond, to gain a better understanding of why these children have so much trouble in some settings and with some tasks than others.

BEHAVIOR WITH FATHERS COMPARED TO MOTHERS

Children who have ADHD appear to be more compliant and less disruptive with their fathers than with their mothers (Tallmadge & Barkley, 1983). They are certainly rated routinely as manifesting lower levels of symptoms by their fathers than by their mothers (DuPaul et al., 1998). There are several possible reasons for this. For one, mothers are still the primary custodians of children within the family, even when they are employed outside the home, and may therefore be the ones who are most likely to tax or exceed the children's limitations in the areas of persistence of attention, activity regulation, impulse control, and rule-governed behavior. Getting children to do chores and schoolwork, perform self-care routines, and control their behavior in public remain predominantly maternal responsibilities; thus mothers may be more likely to witness ADHD symptoms than fathers may be. It would be interesting to examine families of children with ADHD in which these roles were reversed, to see whether fathers were the ones reporting more deviance of the children's behavior.

Another reason may be that mothers and fathers tend to view and hence respond to inappropriate child behavior somewhat differently. Mothers may be more likely to reason with children, to repeat their instructions, and to use affection as a means of governing child compliance. Fathers seem to repeat their commands less, to reason less, and to be quicker to discipline children for misconduct or noncompliance. The larger size of fathers and their consequently greater strength, among other characteristics, may also be perceived as more threatening by children and hence more likely to elicit compliance to commands given by fathers. For whatever reason, the greater obedience of children with ADHD to their fathers than to their mothers is now well established. It should not necessarily be construed as a sign either that a child does not actually have ADHD or that the child's problems are entirely the result of maternal mismanagement.

Repetition of Instructions

On tasks in which instructions are repeated frequently to children with ADHD, problems with sustained responding are lessened (Douglas, 1980, 1983). Research has shown that when directions for a laboratory task or psychological test are repeated by the examiner, better performance is derived from these children. However, it is not clear whether this is specific to these laboratory tasks and the novel examiner, or whether it can be generalized to activities done with routine caregivers. I raise this doubt because, as noted earlier, parents and teachers frequently complain that repeating their commands and instructions to children with ADHD produces little change in compliance (Danforth et al., 1991).

Novelty and Task Stimulation

Children with ADHD display fewer behavioral problems in novel or unfamiliar surroundings or when tasks are unusually novel, but increase their level of deviant behavior as familiarity with the setting increases (Barkley, 1977; Zentall, 1985). It would not be unexpected to find that these children are rated as far better in their behavior at the beginning of the academic year, when they are presented with new teachers, classmates, classrooms, and sometimes even school facilities. Their behavioral control, however, should deteriorate over the initial weeks of school. Similarly, when children with ADHD visit grandparents whom they have not seen frequently, who are likely to provide them with considerable one-to-one attention, and who are unlikely to make numerous demands on their self-control, it seems likely that such children would be at their best levels of behavioral control.

The degree of stimulation in the task also seems to be a factor in the performance of children with ADHD. Research suggests that colorful or highly stimulating educational materials are more likely to improve the attention of these children than relatively low-stimulation or uncolored materials (Zentall, 1985). Interestingly, such differences may not affect the attention of nondisabled children as much or may even worsen it. One might assume that video games or television offer children with ADHD more stimulation than would many other activities. This assumption leads many to suggest that children with ADHD should show less difficulties with attention or hyperactivity during these activities. Yet studies do show that children with ADHD look away from these activities more than do typical children and, in the case of video games, may have more problems with their performance than do typical children (Barkley & Ullman, 1975; Landau et al., 1992; Lawrence et al., 2002; Tannock, 1997).

Timing and Magnitude of Consequences

Settings or tasks that involve a high rate of immediate reinforcement or punishment for compliance to instructions result in significant reductions in, or in some cases amelioration of, attention deficits (Barkley, 1997b; Barkley, Copeland, & Sivage, 1980; Douglas, 1983; Douglas & Parry, 1983). Differences in activity level between groups with and without hyper-activity while watching television may be less than in other activities, whereas such differences are substantially evident during reading and math classes at school (Porrino et al., 1983). It seems that when children with ADHD are engaged in highly reinforcing activities, they may even perform at levels close to those of typical children. Indeed, children with ADHD seem to prefer immediate to delayed rewards (Barkley, Edwards, Laneri, Fletcher, & Metevia; 2001; Neef et al., 2001). However, when the schedule and magnitude of reinforcement are decreased, the behavior of these children may become readily distinguishable from that of typical children (Barkley et al., 1980). Such dramatic changes in the degree of deviance of behavior as a function of motivational parameters in the setting have led several scientists to suggest that ADHD involves a problem in the manner in which behavior is regulated by rules and by motivational factors in the task (Barkley, 1989a, 1997c; Draeger, Prior, & Sanson, 1986; Glow & Glow, 1979; Haenlein & Caul, 1987; Prior, Wallace, & Milton, 1984).

A situational factor related to motivation appears to involve the degree of individualized attention being provided to the children with ADHD. During one-to-one situations, these children may appear less active, inattentive, and impulsive, whereas in group situations, where there is little such attention, the children may appear at their worst. Some studies, for instance, found that whether an experimenter sits in the room with a child or not greatly determines whether differences between children with ADHD and control children are found on visual or auditory attention tasks or on attention to arithmetic work (Draeger et al., 1986; Steinkamp, 1980). Both of these factors (response consequences and individualized attention) are often incorporated as treatment recommendations into home and school management programs (see Chapters 12–16).

Fatigue

Fatigue or time of day (or both) may have an impact on the degree of deviance of ADHD symptoms. Zagar and Bowers (1983) studied children with ADHD in their classrooms and found them to perform significantly better on various problem-solving tasks in the mornings, whereas their classroom behavior was signifi-

cantly worse in the afternoons. These changes in behavior with time of day did not appear to be a function of boredom or fatigue with the task, as efforts were made to counterbalance the order of administration of the tests across mornings and afternoons. Performance in the afternoon was routinely worse, whether it was the first or second administration of the task. However, general fatigue (defined simply as time since the last resting or sleeping period) might still explain these results. Similar time-of-day effects were noted in the study by Porrino et al. (1983), which monitored 24-hour activity levels across school days and weekends separately.

This is not to say that differences between children with and without hyperactivity do not exist in early mornings but emerge only as time of day advances, for this is not the case (Porrino et al., 1983). Nonhyperactive children show similar time-of-day effects on their behavior, and thus hyperactive children appear to be more active and inattentive than these children, regardless of time of day. It is to say, however, that relatively better performances on tasks and in classrooms by children with ADHD may be obtained at some times of the day than at others. The findings so far suggest that educators would do well to schedule overlearned, repetitive, or difficult tasks that require the greatest powers of attention and behavioral restraint for morning periods, while placing recreational, entertaining, or physical activities in the afternoons (Zagar & Bowers, 1983). Such findings certainly raise serious doubts about the adequacy of the practice of scheduling homework periods for children with ADHD in late afternoons or early evenings.

PREVALENCE AND GENDER RATIO

The current consensus of expert opinion is that approximately 3–7% of the childhood population has ADHD (American Psychiatric Association, 2000). On what is this based? A number of prevalence studies have now been published. The figures chosen for prevalence depend greatly, however, on the methods chosen to define and measure ADHD; the population studied; the geographic locale of the survey; and even the degree of agreement required between parents, teachers, and professionals in the diagnosis itself (Lambert et al., 1978). Early estimates varied between 1% and 20% (DuPaul, 1991; Ross & Ross, 1982; Szatmari et al., 1989).

There is no doubt that the individual symptoms of ADHD, at least in mild form, can be found in a large percentage of non-clinic-referred children and adolescents (Cuffe et al., 2001; DuPaul et al., 1998). For instance, Lapouse and Monk (1958) had teachers evaluate a large sample of school-age children for the presence of various behavior problems. Their findings revealed that 57% of the boys and 42% of the girls were rated as overactive. Similarly, 13 years later, Werry and Quay (1971) also surveyed a large population of school children and found that teachers rated 30% of the boys and 12% of the girls as overactive, 49% of the boys and 27% of the girls as restless, and 43% of the boys and 25% of the girls as having a short attention span. Being inattentive, active, and somewhat impulsive is obviously a normal aspect of childhood and probably reflects the progressive maturation of inhibition and self-regulation. The presence of symptoms alone, therefore, does not mean that a child has a disorder.

Defining Deviance

A problem, admittedly, in establishing prevalence has always been deciding what cutoff point is needed along the dimension or distribution of ADHD symptoms to determine that a child's behavior is "developmentally inappropriate." Some have used the criterion of 1.5 standard deviations above the mean for nondisabled children on parent or teacher rating scales of ADHD symptoms. However, surveys of large samples of children, such as that done by Trites, Dugas, Lynch, and Ferguson (1979) with 14,083 school children, have found that this cutoff score can identify an average of 14% of the population as hyperactive. Other researchers (see DuPaul et al., 1998; Szatmari et al., 1989; Taylor, 1986), using cutoff scores ranging from 1 to 2 standard deviations above the mean on either rating scales or structured psychiatric diagnostic interviews, have obtained estimates ranging from less than 1% to more than 22%. However, when investigators have applied the cutoff of 2 standard deviations above the mean and have used DSM-III-R symptoms, they have diagnosed a more acceptable range of 2–9% as having hyperactivity or ADHD (DuPaul, 1991).

Applying a more stringent statistical criterion, such as 2 standard deviations from the mean, is obviously somewhat arbitrary, but it is consistent with tradition in defining other conditions (e.g., learning disabilities and mental retardation) as deviant. It also ensures that an excessive number of children are not being given a psychiatric diagnosis and reserves the diagnosis for the most severely afflicted. When such a stringent criterion as the 97th percentile is applied (2 standard deviations above the mean), it does identify a group of children whose ADHD symptoms are not only seriously deviant but are also stable over as long a time as 8–10 years and highly predictive of later maladjustment, particularly in academic adjustment and attainment (Barkley, Fischer, et al., 1990; Barkley et al., 2002). Yet such a cutoff point can be overly stringent, excluding children who are both relatively deviant and, more importantly, impaired by their symptoms. Given that one should err in clinical practice on the side of over- rather than underidentification, it would seem prudent to employ a cutoff criterion somewhat below the 97th percentile, or 2 standard deviations; a cutoff of 1.5 standard deviations (the 93rd percentile) would seem to serve this purpose adequately and has been suggested by others as a useful demarcation of clinical significance (Achenbach, 2001; DuPaul et al., 1998).

The real issue, though, is the following: At what level of developmental deviance is impairment in one or more major life activities likely to be evident? In short, disorder begins where impairment begins. If all or nearly all of the children exceeding the 93rd percentile have evidence of impairment, we can rest assured that this cutoff score is diagnostically meaningful. If not, then the threshold needs to be set either higher or lower until we find a threshold that achieves this purpose. And so, while the actual number chosen as the diagnostic threshold may be a bit arbitrary, it is hardly meaningless. The further above this threshold a child or adult scores, the greater the likelihood that he or she will experience impairment in major life activities and the more such activities are likely to be impaired.

Prevalence Determined by Rating Scales

A rather common approach to establishing the prevalence of ADHD has been to employ a parent or teacher rating scale of the symptoms of the disorder and then to survey large populations of children. The percentage of children who exceed a predetermined threshold on the rating scale is taken as suggestive evidence of the upper-bound prevalence of the disorder. Because such an approach does not incorporate other important criteria relevant to a diagnosis, the prevalence figures it may yield are undoubtedly overestimates. Such scales are useful for screening for disorder and suggesting an upper limit to prevalence, but do not alone define the true prevalence of ADHD. For instance, using samples in the United States and using teacher ratings of DSM-III-R symptoms, Pelham, Nagy, Greenslade, and Milich (1992) found a prevalence of 7.1% among 931 boys (Pittsburgh area) in grades K–8. Similarly, Wolraich, Hannah, Pinnock, Baumgaertel, and Brown (1996), also using teacher ratings of DSM-III-R symptoms, reported a prevalence of 7.3% among 8,258 children (one school district in Tennessee) in grades K–5. Gadow and Sprafkin (1997), studying samples of children from New York, Missouri, and Wisconsin (a total of 1,441 children) and using DSM-IV items and recommended symptom thresholds, reported a prevalence of 7.7% for ADHD-PI, 2% for ADHD-PHI, and 2.9% for ADHD-C. These results are all quite similar to those of the much smaller community survey using DSM-III-R symptoms conducted by DuPaul (1991) in Worcester, Massachusetts. Wolraich et al. (1996) also examined teacher ratings of the DSM-IV symptom list in their Tennessee study and found a prevalence of 6% when ADHD-PI was excluded—a figure not too different from the 4.9% found by Gadow and Sprafkin (1997) and the 7% found by Pelham et al. (1992). Wolraich, Hannah, Baumgaertel, and Feurer (1998) evaluated 4,323 children in this same school district of Tennessee 1 year later, and found a prevalence of 2.6% for ADHD-PHI and 4.7% for ADHD-C. The rate for ADHD-PI ranged from 5.4% to 8.8% in these studies (Gadow & Sprafkin, 1997; Wolraich et al., 1996, 1998).

Findings clearly vary by age, gender, and source of ratings as well. For example, Nolan, Gadow, and Sprafkin (2001), using teacher reports, found a screening prevalence of 18.2% for ADHD (all types) among preschool children. The figure fell to 15.9% for elementary-age children and to 14.8% for secondary-age children. Among preschoolers, the percentage

was 21.5% for males versus 13.6% for females. In elementary-age children, these figures were 23.1% and 8.2%, while among secondary-age children, the percentages were 20.1% and 8.8%, respectively. Comparing just preschoolers, Gadow, Sprafkin, and Nolan (2001) found percentages of 8.1% for males by parent reports versus 22.4% by teacher reports, while for girls the percentages were 3.9% by parent reports and 12.9% by teacher reports. Prevalence is therefore highest among preschoolers and males, and when teacher reports are used.

Such estimates of prevalence are, of course, very high. They are good starting points for determining prevalence, but suffer from the fact that no diagnostic criteria for symptom duration, age of onset, or impairment from symptoms are imposed. Overidentification of cases is likely to occur in the absence of these additional diagnostic criteria. For instance, when Wolraich et al. (1998) imposed a requirement for evidence of impairment, the total prevalence of ADHD (all types) fell from 16.1% to 6.8%. The subtype prevalences were 3.2% for ADHD-PI, 0.6% for ADHD-PHI, and 2.9% for ADHD-C.

Prevalence based on rating scales also varies as a function of the country being surveyed. In Canada, Szatmari et al. (1989) reported the results of a survey of the entire province of Ontario, in which they found the prevalence of ADHD to be 9% in boys and 3.3% in girls. These rates varied somewhat by age for boys, with a prevalence of slightly more than 10% in the 4- to 11-year age group dropping to 7.3% in the 12- to 16-year age group. The prevalence for girls, however, did not vary significantly across these age groupings (3.3% vs. 3.4%, respectively). The study is difficult to compare with those conducted in the United States, because DSM symptom lists for ADHD were not used.

A study in a different country (Germany) obtained an even higher rate of prevalence. Using teacher ratings of DSM-III-R symptoms with 1,077 German schoolchildren, Baumgaertel, Wolraich, and Dietrich (1995) found a prevalence of 10.9%, which rose to 17.8% if DSM-IV symptoms and cutoff scores were employed and all three subtypes were considered. However, more than half of this prevalence figure (9%) was the result of including children with ADHD-PI, a group not typically considered in earlier studies of prevalence using rating scales. Excluding this group left a prevalence of 8.7%.

In Japan, Kanbayashi, Nakata, Fujii, Kita, and Wada (1994) employed parent ratings of DSM-III-R symptoms of ADHD with 1,022 children ages 4–12 and found a prevalence of 7.7%. The findings of this study are very close to those discussed previously for the United States when DSM III-R symptoms were employed. Overall, then, approximately 7–17% of children between 4 and 16 years of age are likely to have ADHD if only rating scales are used to establish prevalence. If ADHD-PI is considered separately, the rates of ADHD for the two remaining subtypes are roughly 4–10%. The prevalence of ADHD-PI appears to be between 5% and 9% when rating scales of inattentive symptoms are employed.

Liu et al. (2000) reported results for a Chinese population (2,936) ranging in age from 6 to 11 years in Shandong Province. Using the teacher version of the CBCL, these researchers found 7.8% of boys and 2.8% of girls to manifest clinical significant levels of attention problems on this scale. In a later study by Liu et al. (2001) using this same report form (CBCL) with 1,649 adolescents (12–16 years), the prevalence was 3.9% by parent reports and 1.1% by teacher reports, reflecting once again a decline in prevalence from childhood to adolescence.

In a study of DSM-IV symptoms as rated by parents and teachers in an Australian sample 1,275 (ages 5–11 years), Gomez et al. (1999) found prevalence rates of 1.6% for ADHD-PI, 0.2% for ADHD-PHI, and 0.6% for ADHD-C when parent and teacher agreement on symptoms was required for diagnosis. By parent reports only, the rates were 4.2%, 2.7%, and 2.9%, respectively (9.9% for all types); by teacher reports, these figures were 5.8%, 0.9%, and 2.1% (8.8% for all types). Boys were two to seven times more likely to receive the diagnosis than girls.

Bu-Haroon, Eapen, and Bener (1999), using the Conners Teacher Rating Scale, reported results for 31,764 children in the United Arab Emirates. The prevalence rates were 18.3% of males and 11.4% of females.

A study conducted in Colombia (Pineda et al., 1999) used DSM-IV ratings with 540 children randomly sampled from 80,000 and reported a prevalence of 5.1% for ADHD-PI, 9.9% for ADHD-PHI, and 4.8% for ADHD-C among boys and 3.4%, 7.1%, and 1.9%, respectively, among girls ages 4–18 years. Age

was a significant factor in prevalence, however, with rates being significantly lower in 12- to 18-year-olds than in 6- to 11-year-olds.

A more recent study in Ukraine based on 600 children ages 10–12 years used parent ratings of DSM-IV and found a prevalence of 19.8% (all types), with 7.2% ADHD-PI, 8.5% ADHD-PHI, and 4.2% ADHD-C (Gadow et al., 2000).

Prevalence Determined by Cases Identified to Schools

A somewhat different approach to establishing the prevalence of ADHD is to review school records to determine the percentage of children identified to schools as having a clinical diagnosis of ADHD. There are serious flaws in such an approach, not the least of which is that schools may not be told by either parents or professionals that children have received the diagnosis. It is also quite possible that a child may have the disorder but may never have been referred or diagnosed. In either scenario, the school records would miss detecting such cases. Despite these flaws, a few studies have used this method of ascertaining disorder, one of which has received substantial media coverage and so warrants some comment here. Some studies have found somewhat lower prevalence in school-based samples than in community samples, but higher prevalence rates also tend to emerge when the samples focus on elementary grades as in many of the studies cited above. Jensen et al. (1995) studied prevalence from school records across four communities and found rates varying from 1.6% to 9.4%, with an average of 5.8%.

But the study that gained widespread media coverage was that of LeFever, Dawson, and Morrow (1999). It reported prevalence rates of ADHD in two southeastern Virginia school districts that were two to three times higher than the DSM-IV cited average prevalence range of 3–5% (American Psychiatric Association, 1994). LeFever et al. examined school-identified cases to estimate prevalence of ADHD in grades 2–5. In addition to these rates higher than DSM-IV's, the researchers found a disproportionate percentage of white males (18–20%) to be diagnosed with ADHD in both districts. The results of the LeFever et al. (1999) study were touted by its authors and others (see Timimi, 2004) as evidence of ADHD "overdiagnosis" in the popular media and on many professional listservs. The LeFever et al. (1999) study was also used as evidence of overuse of psychostimulant medication to manage behavioral concerns (see Chapter 17). The researchers found a prevalence for stimulant treatment as identified in school records ranging from 7% to 10%, among the highest found anywhere in the United States.

A second study by Tjersland, Grabowski, Hathaway, and Holley (2005) was recently completed in an attempt to replicate and extend the work of LeFever et al. (1999). It also used cases of ADHD identified in school records to determine prevalence of disorder and of psychostimulant treatment in a school district adjoining the two studied by LeFever and her colleagues. This district is highly similar if not identical demographically to those used by LeFever et al. Several sources of information were reviewed, including student information cards that contained medical history and that listed ADHD as a known condition if applicable. Information was also collected from an inspection of physician forms authorizing medication treatment at school. A second phase of the data collection involved a review of student cumulative files. Record reviews of student files were conducted for students with Section 504 plans and for students receiving special education services for learning disabilities, emotional disturbances, developmental delays, or the "Other Health Impaired" category. As a consequence, this study was a more comprehensive review of school records than that undertaken by LeFever et al. (1999) and therefore should have identified as many if not more cases of ADHD and stimulant treatment than did LeFever et al.

The Tjersland et al. (2005) record reviews were completed (with school permission) by the first author, who was at the time an employee of the school district and a doctoral student in clinical psychology. Data from these sources were available for 67.3% of the students in the school district, representing a total sample of 25,575 drawn from 27 out of the 44 schools in the district. Record reviews did not occur for the remaining 33% of students, because their schools declined participation in the study. However, demographic data on the children in these schools were available, and comparison of the nonparticipating with participating districts revealed no significant differences in socioeconomic characteristics between children who were included in the sample and those who were not.

The results of this second study completely contradicted the LeFever et al. (1999) results. The study found a prevalence rate for ADHD of just 4.4%, closely matching the DSM-IV estimated prevalence, as well as the average of studies using clinical diagnosis (to be reviewed below). The study also found that 4% of the children were being treated for psychostimulant medication—well below the 7–10% figure cited by LeFever et al. (1999). Data on prevalence at each grade level from 1st through 12th indicated that the highest prevalence rates were evident in 4th (7.1%) and 5th (6.3%) grades. LeFever et al. (1999) have claimed that national averages obscure the "clear overdiagnosis" of ADHD in some groups. LeFever et al. (1999) suggest that one in every three white elementary boys is being diagnosed with the disorder in southeastern Virginia. The data from the Tjersland et al. (2005) study did not replicate this finding; it found that only 8.1% of white males received the ADHD diagnosis, based on the school records. The reasons for such a gross disparity of findings between studies conducted in the same region, using similar methodologies and comparable school districts, is at the very least puzzling and at the worst suspicious. Further scientific investigation of this disparity in findings is certainly warranted. In the meantime, however, any claims about the prevalence of ADHD or of stimulant use that are based on the outlier results of LeFever et al. (1999) should be viewed with great skepticism, if not dismissed outright, until the reasons for this gross disparity can be settled.

Prevalence Determined by Clinical Diagnostic Criteria

As noted earlier, the diagnostic criteria for a mental disorder should and do consist of more than simply establishing a level of statistical deviance on a rating scale. The DSM-IV(-TR) criteria also include an interview with caregivers, early onset of symptoms (before age 7), pervasiveness across settings, the exclusion of other disorders, and (most important) impairment in one or more major domains of life functioning. Imposing these additional diagnostic criteria will undoubtedly reduce the figures for prevalence of ADHD from those cited above. Given the use of more complete clinical diagnostic criteria, such studies as the ones reviewed in this section should give us a closer approximation to the true prevalence of the disorder than those cited above, which merely used rating scales for this purpose. A number of studies now exist that employed complete clinical diagnostic criteria through interviews with parents, children, and/or teachers. Table 2.2 shows the results for 24 studies. The studies are organized first by country and then, within country (as needed), by the version of the DSM or the *International Classification of Diseases* (ICD) that was used in the study.

United States

As Table 2.2 indicates, the prevalence of ADHD ranges from 2.2% to 12.0% of U.S. children when DSM-III criteria are utilized, with a mean of approximately 5%. When DSM-III-R criteria are utilized, the U.S. prevalence ranges from 1.4% to 13.3% with an average of 6.7% based on adult reports (and presence of impairment). Only one study used self-reports (with a considerably older adolescent and young adult sample), and it found a prevalence of 1.5%. This is in contrast to the 7.6% rate found by Peterson, Pine, Cohen, and Brook (2001), using combined parent and child interviews with 11- to 22-year-olds. One of the highest prevalence rates (12.2%) was obtained in the study by Jensen et al. (1995), employing children of military personnel. Peterson et al. (2001) also found a rate of 12% among early adolescents (mean age 13.7 years, range 9–20 years), using DSM-III-R criteria and parent/child interviews. The real outlier is the study by Velez, Johnson, and Cohen (1989) of children in upstate New York, which found a higher-than-average prevalence rate of 13.3%. It is not possible to determine from this study why its rate is so far above those found in the remaining studies (except for Jensen et al.'s study of military children) using DSM-III-R criteria, which ranged from 1.4% to 12.0% and had an average of 3.8%. Only two studies to date have reported U.S. prevalence rates when DSM-IV criteria are used, and these found figures of 7.4–9.9%. The fact that these figures are higher than the average for DSM-III-R studies is probably due to the inclusion of the new ADHD-PI and ADHD-PHI types of ADHD not recognized in DSM-III-R. Adding these subtypes, it would seem, nearly doubles the prevalence of the disorder in the United States.

Canada

Only two Canadian studies using DSM-based diagnostic interviews could be located, and both took place in the province of Québec. Both used DSM-III-R criteria and found very similar results when parent report and an impairment criterion were used (3.3% and 4.0%; mean = 3.65%). These rates are very similar to the U.S. average of 3.8% cited above for studies using the DSM-III-R (excluding the two outlier studies noted earlier). Note that the use of teacher reports resulted in a higher prevalence (8.9%), while the use of self-reports once again resulted in a lower prevalence (0.6–3.3%).

Australia

Only one study reported the prevalence of ADHD in Australia; it used DSM-IV criteria and a diagnostic interview, and its prevalence estimate of 7.5% (6.8% with impairment required) is comparable to those in U.S. studies using these same DSM-IV criteria.

New Zealand

Three studies have been reported from New Zealand, all of older children or adolescents (ages 11 and 15). Two used 15-year-olds, with the one using DSM-III finding a prevalence of 2% and that using DSM-III-R finding 3%. The study of older children, age 11 years, used DSM-III criteria and found a 6.7% prevalence. As noted earlier, lower figures would be expected for teenagers than for children, given the decline in the symptoms of the disorder with age. The average prevalence across studies would be 3.9%—very close to the U.S. prevalence of 3.8% and the Canadian prevalence of 3.65% in studies using comparable versions of the DSM (DSM-III or III-R).

The Netherlands

Two studies were conducted with Dutch children; one used DSM-III-R with teenagers (ages 13–18) and yielded a prevalence of 1.8%, while the other used DSM-IV with children (ages 6–8) and found 3.8%. Again, using DSM-IV relative to DSM-III-R would be expected to yield a higher prevalence, as would the use of children relative to teens. Even so, the figure for children is approximately half the

TABLE 2.2. Summary of Prevalence Studies of ADHD Employing DSM/ICD Criteria and Diagnostic Interviews

Country and study	Sample	Age[a]	Criteria	Prevalence	Comments
United States					
Kashani et al. (1989)	4,810	8, 12, and 17	DSM-III	3.3%	7.2% at age 8; 2.9% at age 12; 0.0% at age 17
Costello et al. (1988)	785	7–11	DSM-III	2.2%	Criteria employed were more severe than DSM-III requires
Bird et al. (1988) (Puerto Rico)	777	4–17	DSM-III	9.5%	With impairment
Velez et al. (1989)	776	9–18	DSM-III-R	13.3%	Average prevalence across ages 12–18
Lewinsohn et al. (1993)	1,710	High school	DSM-III-R	3.1%	1.8% girls; 4.5% boys
Siminoff et al. (1997)	2,762 (twins)	8–16	DSM-III-R	2.4% 1.4%	Without impairment With impairment
August et al. (1996)	7,231	Grades 1–4	DSM-III-R	2.8%	
Jensen et al. (1995) (U.S. military dependents)	294	6–17	DSM-III-R	11.9% 12.2%	With impairment Without impairment
Briggs-Gowan et al. (2000)	1,060	5–9	DSM-III-R	7.9%	Parent report
Cuffe et al. (2001)	3,419	16–22	DSM-III-R	1.5%	Self-report
Peterson et al. (2001)	976	9–20 11–22	DSM-III DSM-III-R	12% 7.6%	By parent or child report By parent or child report
Barbaresi et al. (2002)	5,718	5–19	DSM-IV	7.4%	Clinical diagnosis (2+ people)
Hudziak et al. (1998)	3,098 (female twins)	12–19	DSM-IV	9.9%	Clinical interview of parents
Canada (Québec)					
Romano et al. (2001)	1,201	14–17	DSM-III-R	1.1% 0.6% 3.7% 3.3%	Self-report (symptom criteria) Self-report (with impairment) Parent report (symptom criteria) Parent report (with impairment)
Breton et al. (1999)	2,400	6–14	DSM-III-R	5.0% 4.0% 8.9% 3.3%	Parent report (symptom criteria) Parent report (with impairment) Teacher report Self-report
Australia					
Graetz et al. (2001)	3,597	6–17	DSM-IV	7.5% 6.8%	Parent interview (symptoms) (with impairment required)

(continued)

TABLE 2.2. (continued)

Country and study	Sample	Age[a]	Criteria	Prevalence	Comments
New Zealand					
McGee et al. (1990)	943	15	DSM-III	2.0%	1% girls; 3% boys; male–female ratio of 2.5:1
Anderson et al. (1987)	792	11	DSM-III	6.7%	Male–female ratio of 5.1:1
Fergusson et al. (1993)	986	15	DSM-III-R	3.0% 2.8%	Parent report Self-report
Germany					
Esser et al. (1990)	216	8	ICD-9	4.2%	All diagnosed subjects were boys
The Netherlands					
Verhulst et al. (1997)	780	13–18	DSM-III-R	1.8%	Parent report
Kroes et al. (2001)	2,290	6–8	DSM-IV	3.8% 1.3%	Parent report Self-report
India					
Bhatia et al. (1991)	1,000	3–12	DSM-III	5.2–29%	Ages 3–4 to ages 11–12
China					
Leung et al. (1996)	3,069	School age	DSM-III DSM-III-R	6.1% 8.9%	
Brazil					
Rohde et al. (1999)	1,013	12–14	DSM-IV	5.8%	Clinical diagnosis

[a]Ages are given in years unless otherwise indicated.

rate found in the U.S. studies using DSM-IV criteria (7.4%).

Other Countries

One study in Germany, using the ICD-9 criteria, found a prevalence very similar to the averages for the United States, Canada, and New Zealand of 4.2% for 8-year-old children. The figures for China are considerably higher than the averages for other countries reviewed above in studies using comparable DSMs—for DSM-III, the Chinese rate was 6.1%, and for DSM-III-R, it was 8.9%. Why this should be so is unclear, but it could have resulted from prob-

lems with translation and meaning of the criteria, differences in cultural norms for child disruptive behavior (perceptions of deviance), or even differences in etiological factors known to be associated with ADHD (prenatal care, child medical care and disease prevention, exposure to toxins, etc.). The one study conducted in Brazil used the DSM-IV and yielded a prevalence of 5.8% for a young adolescent age group—a figure somewhat lower than the 7.4% in the U.S. studies using the DSM-IV. This could be due in part to the Brazilian study's use of early adolescents, for whom prevalence rates are usually lower than when children are the focus of the study. The major outlier among international studies is the extraordinarily high rate of disorder (29%) found in the oldest age group (11- to 12-year-olds) in the study of Indian children by Bhatia, Nigam, Bohra, and Malik (1991), using DSM-III criteria. As with the Chinese study described above, whether this reflects a true difference in prevalence (perhaps owing to socioeconomic and medical factors that differ significantly from those in Western countries), or a problem with translation and meaning of the DSM criteria in a different language, is not clear from the results.

As Table 2.2 also suggests, the use of an impairment criterion as a necessity in the diagnosis of the disorder reduces the prevalence of the disorder to some extent. The prevalence is also affected by age, with adolescent samples being likely to have lower prevalence rates than younger ones. The source of information is also important, with teachers reporting higher rates (8.9%) than parents, who in turn report higher rates (1.8–13.3%) than teens (0.6–3.3%). And DSM-IV criteria may result in the identification of somewhat more children as having ADHD than DSM-III or DSM-III-R criteria may. It should be recalled from Chapter 1 that the DSM-III criteria were not based on any field trial or empirical information, and that they subtyped ADD quite differently than DSM-IV subtypes ADHD. In contrast, DSM-III-R and DSM-IV were empirically evaluated, making their criteria somewhat more rigorously developed and empirically defensible, and hence preferable to the criteria of DSM-III. Consistent with the research of Baumgaertel et al. (1995) in Germany and Wolraich et al. (1996) in Tennessee using ratings of DSM-III, DSM-III-R, and DSM-IV criteria as discussed earlier, the DSM-IV criteria result in the identification of an even larger percentage of children as having ADHD than do previous DSMs. This is due largely to DSM-IV's inclusion of the new ADHD-PI and ADHD-PHI subtypes, which were not included in DSM-III-R and were poorly and unempirically defined in DSM-III.

One lesson from this review of prevalence rates is that there can be no doubt that ADHD is a worldwide phenomenon; it has been found in every country in which it has been studied.

Prevalence of Adult ADHD

At this writing, five studies could be located that attempted to determine the prevalence of

ADHD in an adult sample. The first (Murphy & Barkley, 1996b) surveyed a sample of 720 adults renewing their driver's licenses in central Massachusetts, and used a rating scale of DSM-IV symptoms (both current and childhood symptoms). This study found a prevalence of 4.7% for all subtypes of ADHD. The subtype prevalence rates were 0.9% for ADHD-C, 2.5% for ADHD-PHI, and 1.3% for ADHD-PI. In a sample of 700 college students from three geographically diverse sites around the United States, DuPaul, Weyandt, Schaughency, and Ota (1997) found almost precisely these same prevalence rates, using DSM-IV symptom lists and diagnostic thresholds: 0.6% for ADHD-C, 2.6% for ADHD-PHI, and 1.3% for ADHD-PI. Similarly, Heiligenstein, Conyers, Berns, and Smith (1997) collected self-reports of DSM-IV symptoms from 468 college students in Madison, Wisconsin. They reported a 4% prevalence for all subtypes, just slightly lower than the 4.5% found by DuPaul, Weyandt, et al. (1997) and the 4.7% found by Murphy and Barkley (1996b) for adults ages 17–83. The prevalence for each subtype in the Heiligenstein et al. study was 0.9% for ADHD-C, 0.9% for ADHD-PHI, and 2.2% for ADHD-PI. Weyandt, Linterman, and Rice (1995) also reported a study of college students in which 4% reported significantly elevated symptoms on an adult rating scale using DSM-III-R items. Although none of these studies of college students required that subjects meet symptom thresholds for childhood symptoms (assessed by recall of the subjects), as did the Murphy and Barkley (1996b) study, the estimates of both overall and subtype prevalence across these studies are strikingly similar. It should be kept in mind, however, that no criterion of impairment was imposed in any of these studies. In studies of children, when this is done, prevalence can drop considerably.

Factors Affecting Prevalence

Szatmari (1992; Szatmari et al., 1989) found that the prevalence of ADHD in a large sample of children from Ontario, Canada also varied as a function of age, male gender, chronic health problems, family dysfunction, low socioeconomic status (SES), presence of a developmental impairment, and urban living. More recently, Boyle and Lipman (2002) also found that family and neighborhood factors (in that order) affected rates of disorder in Ontario. Others found similar conditions associated with the risk for ADHD (Velez et al., 1989). Important, however, was the additional finding in the Szatmari et al. (1989) study that when comorbidity with other disorders (especially ODD and CD) was statistically controlled for in the analyses, gender, family dysfunction, and low SES were no longer significantly associated with occurrence of the disorder. Health problems, developmental impairment, young age, and urban living remained significantly associated with the occurrence of the disorder.

As already discussed above, apart from the source of information (parent, teacher, child self-reports), the DSM or ICD version being used, and the country in which the study is conducted, age and sex are clearly factors in the prevalence of ADHD: Rates decline from the elementary grade years to adolescence, and percentages are three to seven times greater among males than among females. As noted previously in the discussion of the DSM criteria, the declining prevalence of ADHD with age may be partly an artifact of the DSM items' being chiefly applicable to young children. These items may reflect the underlying constructs of ADHD very well at younger ages, but may be increasingly less applicable to ever older age groups. This could create a situation where individuals remain impaired in the constructs comprising ADHD as they mature while outgrowing the symptom lists for the disorder, resulting in an illusory decline in prevalence, as was noted in the earlier example of mental retardation. Until more age-appropriate symptoms are studied for adolescent and adult populations, this issue remains unresolved.

Few studies have examined the relation of ADHD to SES, and those that have are not especially consistent. Lambert et al. (1978) found only slight differences in the prevalence of hyperactivity across SES when a child's parent, teacher, and physician all agreed on the diagnosis. However, SES differences in prevalence did arise when only two of these three sources had to agree, with there generally being more children with ADHD from lower- than higher-SES backgrounds. For instance, when parent and teacher agreement (but not physician) was required, 18% of children identified as hyperactive were of high, 36% of middle, and 45% of low SES. When only teachers' opinion was used, the percentages were 17%, 41%, and 41%, respectively. Likewise, Trites (1979)

found the prevalence of hyperactivity, as defined by a threshold on a teacher rating scale, to vary as a function of neighborhood and SES. More recently, Boyle and Lipman (2002) also found that SES had a low but significant inverse relationship with rates of hyperactivity in a Canadian sample. Being male, coming from a single-parent family, coming from a smaller family with fewer children, and being in a disadvantaged neighborhood all significantly increased the likelihood of hyperactivity. As noted earlier, Szatmari (1992) found in his review that rates of ADHD tended to increase with lower SES as well. However, his own study (Szatmari et al., 1989) found that psychosocial variables, such as low SES, were no longer associated with rates of ADHD when other comorbid conditions, such as CD, were controlled. For now, it is clear that ADHD occurs across all SES levels. When differences in prevalence rates are found across SES levels, they may be artifacts of the source used to define the disorder or of the comorbidity of ADHD with other disorders known to be related to SES, such as aggression and CD. Certainly, no one has made the argument that the nature or qualitative aspects of ADHD differ across SES levels.

The Problem of Agreement among Caregivers

The prevalence of ADHD appears to differ significantly as a function of how many people must agree on the diagnosis. The study by Lambert et al. (1978) on this issue is the one most often cited. In this study, parents, teachers, and physicians of 5,000 children in elementary school were asked to identify the children they considered to be hyperactive. Approximately 5% of these children were defined as hyperactive when the opinion of only one of these caregivers (parent, teacher, physician) was required—a prevalence figure close to the average figure reported by the 22 studies in Table 2.2. However, this prevalence figure dropped to about 1% in the Lambert et al. study when agreement among all three sources was required. This finding should hardly be surprising, considering that no effort was made to provide these "social definers" with any criteria for making their judgments or any training in the actual symptoms believed to constitute this disorder. Research routinely finds agreements between people to be low to modest when they are judging the behavior of another, unless more specific and operational definitions of the behavior being judged and training in the application of the definitions are provided.

It is well established, for instance, that parent and teacher ratings of many different types of child behavioral problems are likely to have interrater agreement coefficients of less than .50 (Achenbach et al., 1987). Even fathers and mothers may have agreements of little more than .60 to .70. Certainly, the fact that children behave differently in different situations and with different adults can be a major factor contributing to this lack of agreement. The often subjective judgments required in determining whether a child's behavior occurs "often" or is "deviant" can be another. Undoubtedly, the fleeting or ephemeral nature of behavior, as well as the constant stream of children's new behaviors or actions, can create further confusion as to which of these actions should be considered in the judgment. Finally, the use of adult opinions to determine a diagnosis of hyperactivity/ADHD in a child will always be somewhat confounded by the characteristics and mental status of the adult informant, in addition to the child's actual behavior. As discussed in more detail in Chapter 8 (this volume) on behavior rating scales, psychological distress, depression, family discord, and social biases can affect the judgments adults make about children, and can therefore add to the lack of agreement among adults about the presence and degree of a child's ADHD. Hence the lack of agreement across caregivers, and the variations in the prevalence of ADHD that may arise as a result of it, are hardly indictments of the concept of ADHD as a disorder; they apply to many other types of human behavior and virtually all mental disorders.

Gender Differences in Prevalence

The prevalence of ADHD is also known to vary significantly as a function of gender of the children being studied, as has already been well documented above. The proportion of males versus females manifesting the disorder varies considerably across studies, from 2:1 to 10:1 (Ross & Ross, 1982), with an average of 6:1 most often cited for clinic-referred samples of children. However, epidemiological studies, as shown in Table 2.2, find the proportion ranging from 2.5:1 to 5.1:1, with an average of approximately 3.4:1 among non-clinic-referred children. The considerably higher rate of males in clinic-referred samples of children than in community surveys seems to be due to referral bias. Males are more likely than females to exhibit aggressive and antisocial behavior, and such behavior is more likely to get a child referred to a psychiatric center for treatment. Hence more males than females with ADHD will be referred to such centers. In support of this explanation are the findings (1) that aggression occurs far more frequently in clinic-referred children with ADHD than in those identified through epidemiological sampling (community surveys); (2) that hyperactive girls identified in community surveys are often less aggressive than hyperactive boys (see "Gender Differences in the Nature of ADHD," below); but (3) that girls who are seen in psychiatric clinics are likely to be as aggressive as boys with ADHD (Befera & Barkley, 1984; Breen & Barkley, 1988; Gaub & Carlson, 1997). Even so, males remain more likely to manifest ADHD than girls even in community-based samples, suggesting that there may be some gender-linked mechanism involved in the expression of the disorder.

GENDER DIFFERENCES IN THE NATURE OF ADHD

As already noted, boys are three times more likely to have ADHD than girls, and five to nine times more likely than girls to be seen with ADHD among clinic-referred children. Given these differences in prevalence, one might wonder whether there are differences in the expression of the disorder or its related features between boys and girls. One study (Brown, Abramowitz, Dadan-Swain, Eckstrand, & Dulcan, 1989) evaluated a sample of clinic-referred children diagnosed as having ADHD. They found that girls ($n = 18$) were more socially withdrawn and had more internalizing symptoms (anxiety, depression) than did boys ($n = 38$). Studies of school-identified hyperactive children tended to find that girls were rated as having fewer behavioral and conduct problems (e.g., aggressiveness) than boys, but usually were not different on any laboratory measures of their symptoms (deHaas, 1986; deHaas & Young, 1984; Pascaulvaca, Wolf, Healey, Tweedy, & Halperin, 1988). In contrast, two early studies using children referred to pediatric learning and developmental disability clinics suggested that hyperactive girls had lower Verbal IQ scores, were more likely to have language disabilities, had a greater prevalence of problems with mood and enuresis, and had a lower prevalence of conduct problems (Berry, Shaywitz, & Shaywitz, 1985). These studies may have been biased toward finding greater cognitive and developmental problems in their samples because of the source of referrals (clinics for those with learning disorders). Subsequent studies that used referrals to psychology or psychiatry clinics found virtually no differences between boys and girls with ADHD on measures of intelligence, academic achievement, peer relations, emotional problems, or behavioral disorders (Breen, 1989; Horn, Wagner, & Ialongo, 1989; McGee, Williams, & Silva, 1987; Sharp et al., 1997). The exception to this was the report by Taylor (1986, pp. 141–143) that girls referred to a child psychiatry service at Maudsley Hospital in London had a greater degree of intellectual deficits than boys, but were otherwise equivalent in the onset and severity of their hyperactive symptoms. Sharp et al. (1997) also found girls with ADHD to be more impaired in reading ability.

But individual studies can vary considerably, depending on the source of the samples (clinic or community), the source of information (parent, teacher, clinician, tests), and other sample characteristics (age, SES, etc.). Combining results across studies via meta-analysis is a better way of ascertaining what we may know about gender differences. Gaub and Carlson (1997) conducted a meta-analysis of past research on gender differences in samples of children with ADHD. They concluded that there were no gender differences in levels of impulsiveness, academic performance, social functioning, fine motor control, or family factors (e.g., parental education level or parental depression). Girls were found to be more impaired in their intelligence, less hyperactive, and less likely to demonstrate other externalizing symptoms (i.e., aggression, defiance, and conduct problems). These gender differences appeared to be related to whether the samples under investigation were derived from clinical or community-based samples. Within clinical samples, there were likely to be few gender differences apparent, but in community-derived samples, girls were likely to be less aggressive and to show less internalizing symptoms than boys. Many of the same findings were reported later in a study of

127 mostly clinic-referred children with ADHD (Hartung et al., 2002). The large Multimodal Treatment Study of ADHD (MTA; $n = 498$) likewise found that girls with ADHD received lower ratings on core symptoms and made fewer errors on CPTs than did boys with ADHD (Newcorn et al., 2001).

Gershon (2002) conducted a later meta-analysis of these same studies and additional ones published since the Gaub and Carlson (1997) paper. He also found that girls with ADHD had lower ratings of hyperactive, inattentive, and impulsive symptoms; had lower levels of other externalizing behaviors (aggression, delinquency); and experienced greater intellectual impairment—all in agreement with the Gaub and Carlson review. The Gershon review, however, also found that girls with ADHD manifested more internalizing symptoms (anxiety, depression, etc.) than did boys with ADHD, in contrast to the earlier meta-analysis by Gaub and Carlson (1997) and the two large studies by Hartung et al. (2002) and Newcorn et al. (2001). The studies by Biederman and colleagues (see below) did not find this to be the case, however, leaving open to question this aspect of Gershon's findings.

Problematic in these reviews is the fact that many of the studies they incorporated used very small samples of girls. In a study of gender differences in children with ADHD that employed a larger sample of girls, Biederman (1997) and colleagues (Faraone, 1997; Milberger, 1997) compared 130 girls with ADHD (ages 6–17) with 120 nondisabled control girls. In terms of their risk for comorbid psychiatric disorders, the girls with ADHD showed elevated rates of Major Depressive Disorder (17%), anxiety disorders (32%), and Bipolar I Disorder (10%), comparable to those found in past studies of boys by these same investigators. The only findings that differed from their earlier studies of boys were the rates of ODD and CD, which were found to be about half the rates found in boys with ADHD. Approximately 33% of the girls with ADHD had ODD, and 10% had CD. Although these girls with ADHD had somewhat lower intelligence, reading, and math scores than the control girls, they still fell within the average range on these measures and were comparable in this respect to boys with ADHD studied by this same research team. The same findings held true for the types of services these girls required, such as tutoring for school, special education, counseling, and medication treatment—all of which were elevated above those for the control girls, but were in the same range of frequency as those for the boys with ADHD. The levels of psychiatric disorders among the relatives and specifically the siblings of the girls with ADHD were likewise similar to those seen in boys with ADHD (Mick, 1997). Interestingly, the risks of comorbid disorders to siblings were entirely mediated by whether or not the siblings also had ADHD. Thus it would seem that the most reliable difference between girls and boys with ADHD is the lowered risk of girls for ODD and CD relative to boys.

A subsequent study by Biederman et al. (2002) evaluated 140 boys and 140 girls with ADHD, and compared them to each other and to 120 boys and 122 girls without ADHD. Girls were more likely to have ADHD-PI; were less likely to have learning disabilities; were less likely to manifest problems in school or in their spare time; and were less at risk for Major Depressive Disorder, CD, and ODD than were boys with ADHD. Again, the girls had slightly but significantly lower IQ scores than the boys with ADHD, but both sexes fell within the average range in their scores. Boys with ADHD were also more likely to have substance use disorders. Both of the studies by Biederman and colleagues thus appear to disagree with Gershon's (2002) conclusion that girls with ADHD may be more at risk for depression and anxiety disorders.

Slight differences have been found in mothers' treatment of boys with ADHD compared to girls with ADHD. Specifically, boys received greater praise and direction from their mothers, but boys were less compliant than girls with their mothers' commands (Barkley, 1989b; Befera & Barkley, 1984). No gender differences were noted in the effects of stimulant medication on these interactions (Barkley, 1989b) or in the clinical response of girls to stimulants more generally (Pelham, Walker, Sturgis, & Hoza, 1989; Sharp et al., 1997).

A study of a large sample of girls and boys with ADHD examined their classroom behavior relative to control girls and boys in the large MTA (see Chapter 20). There were numerous differences between the children with ADHD and the control children, as would be expected, but only a few that distinguished girls with ADHD from boys with ADHD. Girls with ADHD engaged in less rule breaking, less social interference, less gross motor activity, and lower levels of externalizing behavior than boys with ADHD (Abikoff et al., 2002).

Blachman and Hinshaw (2002) evaluated the social status of girls with and without ADHD in a 5-week summer camp program. The girls with ADHD had fewer mutual friends and were more likely to be friendless. They also had higher levels of conflict and relational aggression than did comparison girls and were less able to sustain relationships over time. More recently, Zalecki and Hinshaw (2004) further studied the social relationships of girls with ADHD (93 with ADHD-C and 47 with ADHD-PI) compared to control girls (88) in a similar summer camp environment. Girls with ADHD-C manifested significantly higher rates of relational and overt aggression than did girls with ADHD-PI, but even the latter girls showed more such aggression than did control girls. Peer relationships among the girls with ADHD were a function of their levels of both overt and relational aggression, though the former was a more powerful predictor than the latter. In sum, these two large-sample studies of girls with ADHD indicate significant problems in their social relationships—specifically, higher rates of overt aggression (as seen in boys with ADHD), but also more covert relational aggression.

KEY CLINICAL POINTS

✓ The primary symptoms of ADHD are in the realms of (1) behavioral disinhibition (impulsivity), and associated hyperactivity, and (2) inattention. These are well documented in research using parent and teacher reports, direct observations, and psychological tests of these behavioral domains.

✓ Individuals with the recently developed subtype of Predominantly Inattentive ADHD (ADHD-PI), which is discussed further in Chapter 3, are a heterogeneous group. A subset of these individuals manifest sluggish cognitive tempo (SCT) and may represent a qualitatively distinct group.

✓ The diagnostic criteria set forth in DSM-IV (-TR) for ADHD have been reviewed, and their many merits have been discussed.

✓ Nevertheless, a number of areas for improvement in these criteria have been discussed, and clinicians should heed these areas in an effort to make clinical diagnosis more rigorous until DSM-V is created.

✓ Evidence suggests that ADHD clearly qualifies as a mental disorder under the conditions specified by Wakefield (1997), in that it comprises a dysfunction in a cognitive evolutionary adaptation that leads to harm for the individual.

✓ ADHD can be considered a clinical syndrome based on the covariation among its symptoms, its distinction from other mental disorders in these regards, and its relatively chronic course.

✓ ADHD symptoms also may be affected by situational factors, such as time of day, fatigue, motivational factors (availability and timing of consequences), supervision, gender of parent, and others.

✓ A review of prevalence research suggests that the prevalence of the disorder is approximately 3.8% in U.S. studies using earlier versions of the DSM, and nearly double this (7.4%) in studies using DSM-IV. This rise in prevalence may result from the inclusion of two new subtypes (ADHD-PI and ADHD-PHI) not recognized in earlier DSMs. Similar prevalence estimates were found in Canada (Québec), New Zealand, Germany, and Brazil for comparable versions of the DSM.

✓ ADHD may occur more often in some subgroups of U.S. society (military dependents, Puerto Ricans) and in some other countries (China, India), while occurring less often in other countries (The Netherlands).

✓ ADHD occurs in boys approximately three times as often as in girls in community samples, and five to nine times more often in clinical samples.

✓ Studies suggest that girls and boys with ADHD are quite similar in their presenting symptoms, but that girls may manifest somewhat lower symptom levels and are considerably less likely to manifest aggressive behavior (though they will do so more often than control girls; this is true for both overt and relational aggression). Girls with ADHD may have a lower risk of ODD, CD, externalizing problems more generally, and possibly depression than boys with the disorder, but the girls may have somewhat lower levels of intelligence.

✓ ADHD is a valid mental disorder that is found universally across countries and that can be differentiated in its major symptoms both from the absence of disability and from other psychiatric disorders.

REFERENCES

Abikoff, H., Gittelman-Klein, R., & Klein, D. (1977). Validation of a classroom observation code for hyperactive children. *Journal of Consulting and Clinical Psychology, 45*, 772–783.

Abikoff, H., Jensen, P. S., Arnold, L. L., Hoza, B., Hechtman, L., Pollack, S., et al. (2002). Observed classroom behavior of children with ADHD: Relationship to gender and comorbidity. *Journal of Abnormal Child Psychology, 30*, 349–359.

Achenbach, T. M. (1991). *Child Behavior Checklist and Child Behavior Profile: Cross-Informant Version.* Burlington, VT: Author.

Achenbach, T. M., & Edelbrock, C. S. (1983). *Manual for the Child Behavior Profile and Child Behavior Checklist.* Burlington, VT: Author.

Achenbach, T. M., & Edelbrock, C. S. (1987). Empirically based assessment of the behavioral/emotional problems of 2- and 3-year-old children. *Journal of Abnormal Child Psychology, 15*, 629–650.

Achenbach, T. M., McConaughy, S. H., & Howell, C. T. (1987). Child/adolescent behavioral and emotional problems: Implications of cross informant correlations for situational specificity. *Psychological Bulletin, 101*, 213–232.

American Academy of Child and Adolescent Psychiatry. (1997). Practice parameters for the assessment and treatment of children, adolescents, and adults with attention-deficit/hyperactivity disorder. *Journal of the American Academy of Child and Adolescent Psychiatry, 36*(10, Suppl.), 085S–121S.

American Academy of Pediatrics. (2001). Clinical practice guideline: Treatment of the school-aged child with attention-deficit/hyperactivity disorder. *Pediatrics, 108*, 1033–1044.

American Psychiatric Association. (1968). *Diagnostic and statistical manual of mental disorders* (2nd ed.). Washington, DC: Author.

American Psychiatric Association. (1980). *Diagnostic and statistical manual of mental disorders* (3rd ed.). Washington, DC: Author.

American Psychiatric Association. (1987). *Diagnostic and statistical manual of mental disorders* (3rd ed., rev.). Washington, DC: Author.

American Psychiatric Association. (1994). *Diagnostic and statistical manual of mental disorders* (4th ed.). Washington, DC: Author.

American Psychiatric Association. (2000). *Diagnostic and statistical manual of mental disorders* (4th ed., text rev.). Washington, DC: Author.

Anderson, J. C., Williams, S., McGee, R., & Silva, P. A. (1987). DSM-III disorders in preadolescent children: Prevalence in a large sample from the general population. *Archives of General Psychiatry, 44*, 69–76.

Antrop, I., Roeyers, H., Van Oost, P., & Buysse, A.

(2000). Stimulant seeking and hyperactivity in children with ADHD. *Journal of Child Psychology and Psychiatry, 41*, 225–231.

Applegate, B., Lahey, B. B., Hart, E. L., Waldman, I., Biederman, J., Hynd, G. W., et al. (1997) . Validity of the age of onset criterion for ADHD: A report from the DSM-IV field trials. *Journal of the American Academy of Child and Adolescent Psychiatry, 36*, 1211–1221.

Arnold, L. E. (1997). Sex differences in ADHD: Conference summary. *Journal of Abnormal Child Psychology, 24*, 555–569.

August, G. J., Realmuto, G. M., MacDonald, A. W., Nugent, S. M., & Crosby, R. (1996). Prevalence of ADHD and comorbid disorders among elementary school children screened for disruptive behavior. *Journal of Abnormal Child Psychology, 24*, 571–595.

August, G. J., & Stewart, M. A. (1983). Family subtypes of childhood hyperactivity. *Journal of Nervous and Mental Disease, 171*, 362–368.

Barbaresi, W. J., Katusic, S. K., Colligan, R. C., Pankratz, S., Weaver, A. L., Weber, K. J., et al. (2002). How common is attention-deficit/hyperactivity disorder?: Incidence in a population-based birth cohort in Rochester, Minn. *Archives of Pediatric and Adolescent Medicine, 156*, 217–224.

Barkley, R. A. (1977). The effects of methylphenidate on various measures of activity level and attention in hyperkinetic children. *Journal of Abnormal Child Psychology, 5*, 351–369.

Barkley, R. A. (1981). Hyperactivity. In E. J. Mash & L. G. Terdal (Eds.), *Behavioral assessment of childhood disorders* (pp. 127–184). New York: Guilford Press.

Barkley, R. A. (1982). Guidelines for defining hyperactivity in children (attention-deficit disorder with hyperactivity). In B. Lahey & A. Kazdin (Eds.), *Advances in clinical child psychology* (Vol. 5, pp. 137–180). New York: Plenum Press.

Barkley, R. A. (1985). The social interactions of hyperactive children: Developmental changes, drug effects, and situational variation. In R. McMahon & R. Peters (Eds.), *Childhood disorders: Behavioral–developmental approaches* (pp. 218–243). New York: Brunner/Mazel.

Barkley, R. A. (1988). Attention. In M. Tramontana & S. Hooper (Eds.), *Assessment issues in child neuropsychology* (pp. 145–176). New York: Plenum Press.

Barkley, R. A. (1989a). The problem of stimulus control and rule-governed behavior in children with attention deficit disorder with hyperactivity. In L. M. Bloomingdale & J. M. Swanson (Eds.), *Attention deficit disorders* (Vol. 4, pp. 203–234). New York: Pergamon Press.

Barkley, R. A. (1989b). Hyperactive girls and boys: Stimulant drug effects on mother–child interactions. *Journal of Child Psychology and Psychiatry, 30*, 379–390.

Barkley, R. A. (1990). *Attention-deficit hyperactivity disorder: A handbook for diagnosis and treatment.* New York: Guilford Press.

Barkley, R. A. (1991). The ecological validity of laboratory and analogue assessments of ADHD symptoms. *Journal of Abnormal Child Psychology, 19*, 149–178.

Barkley, R. A. (1994). Impaired delayed responding: A unified theory of attention deficit hyperactivity disorder. In D. K. Routh (Ed.), *Disruptive behavior disorders: Essays in honor of Herbert Quay* (pp. 11–57). New York: Plenum Press.

Barkley, R. A. (1997a). *ADHD and the nature of self-control.* New York: Guilford Press.

Barkley, R. A. (1997b). ADHD, self-regulation, and time: Towards a more comprehensive theory of ADHD. *Journal of Developmental and Behavioral Pediatrics, 18*, 271–279.

Barkley, R. A. (1997c). Age dependent decline in ADHD: True recovery or statistical illusion? *ADHD Report, 5*(1), 1–5.

Barkley, R. A. (1998). *Attention-deficit hyperactivity disorder: A handbook for diagnosis and treatment* (2nd ed.). New York: Guilford Press.

Barkley, R. A. (2001a). The inattentive type of ADHD as a distinct disorder: What remains to be done. *Clinical Psychology: Science and Practice, 8*, 489–493.

Barkley, R. A. (2001b). The executive functions and self-regulation: An evolutionary neuropsychological perspective. *Neuropsychology Review, 11*, 1–29.

Barkley, R. A. (2004a). Driving impairments in teens and adults with attention-deficit/hyperactivity disorder. *Psychiatric Clinics of North America, 27*(2), 233–260.

Barkley, R. A. (2004b). Critique or misrepresentation?: A reply to Timimi et al. *Clinical Child and Family Psychology Review, 7*, 65–69.

Barkley, R. A., & Biederman, J. (1997). Towards a broader definition of the age of onset criterion for attention deficit hyperactivity disorder. *Journal of the American Academy of Child and Adolescent Psychiatry, 36*, 1204–1210.

Barkley, R. A., Copeland, A., & Sivage, C. (1980). A self-control classroom for hyperactive children. *Journal of Autism and Developmental Disorders, 10*, 75–89.

Barkley, R. A., & Cunningham, C. E. (1979). The effects of methylphenidate on the mother–child interactions of hyperactive children. *Archives of General Psychiatry, 36*, 201–208.

Barkley, R. A., Cunningham, C. E., & Karlsson, J. (1983). The speech of hyperactive children and their mothers: Comparisons with normal children and stimulant drug effects. *Journal of Learning Disabilities, 16*, 105–110.

Barkley, R. A., DuPaul, G. J., & McMurray, M. B. (1990). A comprehensive evaluation of attention deficit disorder with and without hyperactivity. *Journal of Consulting and Clinical Psychology, 58*, 775–789.

Barkley, R. A., DuPaul, G. J., & McMurray, M. B.

(1991). Attention deficit disorder with and without hyperactivity: Clinical response to three doses of methylphenidate. *Pediatrics, 87,* 519–531.

Barkley, R. A., Edwards, G., Laneri, M., Fletcher, K., & Metevia, L. (2001). Executive functioning, temporal discounting, and a sense of time in adolescents with attention deficit hyperactivity disorder and oppositional defiant disorder. *Journal of Abnormal Child Psychology, 29,* 541–556.

Barkley, R. A., Fischer, M., Edelbrock, C. S., & Smallish, L. (1990). The adolescent outcome of hyperactive children diagnosed by research criteria: I. An 8 year prospective follow-up study. *Journal of the American Academy of Child and Adolescent Psychiatry, 29,* 546–557.

Barkley, R. A., Fischer, M., Smallish, L., & Fletcher, K. (2002). The persistence of attention-deficit/hyperactivity disorder into young adulthood as a function of reporting source and definition of disorder. *Journal of Abnormal Psychology, 111,* 279–289.

Barkley, R. A., Grodzinsky, G., & DuPaul, G. (1992). Frontal lobe functions in attention deficit disorder with and without hyperactivity: A review and research report. *Journal of Abnormal Child Psychology, 20,* 163–188.

Barkley, R. A., Koplowitz, S., Anderson, T., & McMurray, M. B. (1997). Sense of time in children with ADHD: Effects of duration, distraction, and stimulant medication. *Journal of the International Neuropsychological Society, 3,* 359–369.

Barkley, R. A., Murphy, K. R., & Kwasnik, D. (1996). Psychological adjustment and adaptive impairments in young adults with ADHD. *Journal of Attention Disorders, 1,* 41–54.

Barkley, R. A., & Ullman, D. G. (1975). A comparison of objective measures of activity level and distractibility in hyperactive and nonhyperactive children. *Journal of Abnormal Child Psychology, 3,* 213–244.

Baumeister, J. J. (1992). Factor analysis of teacher rat ings of attention-deficit hyperactivity and oppositional defiant symptoms in children aged four through thirteen years. *Journal of Clinical Child Psychology, 21,* 27–34.

Baumgaertel, A., Wolraich, M. L., & Dietrich, M. (1995). Comparison of diagnostic criteria for attention deficit disorders in a German elementary school sample. *Journal of the American Academy of Child and Adolescent Psychiatry, 34,* 629–638.

Befera, M., & Barkley, R. A. (1984). Hyperactive and normal girls and boys: Mother–child interactions, parent psychiatric status, and child psychopathology. *Journal of Child Psychology and Psychiatry, 26,* 439–452.

Beiser, M., Dion, R., & Gotowiec, A. (2000). The structure of attention-deficit and hyperactivity symptoms among Native and non-Native elementary school children. *Journal of Abnormal Child Psychology, 28,* 425–537.

Beitchman, J. H., Wekerle, C., & Hood, J. (1987). Diag-nostic continuity from preschool to middle childhood. *Journal of the American Academy of Child and Adolescent Psychiatry, 26,* 694–699.

Berk, L. E., & Potts, M. K. (1991). Development and functional significance of private speech among at tention-deficit hyperactivity disorder and normal boys. *Journal of Abnormal Child Psychology, 19,* 357–377.

Berlin, L., & Bohlin, G. (2002). Response inhibition, hyperactivity, and conduct problems among preschool children. *Journal of Clinical Child Psychology, 31,* 242–251.

Berry, C. A., Shaywitz, S. E., & Shaywitz, B. A. (1985). Girls with attention deficit disorder: A silent majority? A report on behavioral and cognitive characteristics. *Pediatrics, 76,* 801–809.

Bhatia, M. S., Nigam, V. R., Bohra, N., & Malik, S. C. (1991). Attention deficit disorder with hyperactivity among paedritic outpatients. *Journal of Child Psychology and Psychiatry, 32,* 297–306.

Biederman, J. (1997, October). *Comorbidity in girls with ADHD.* Paper presented at the annual meeting of the American Academy of Child and Adolescent Psychiatry, Toronto.

Biederman, J., Keenan, K., & Faraone, S. V. (1990). Parent-based diagnosis of attention deficit disorder predicts a diagnosis based on teacher report. *American Journal of Child and Adolescent Psychiatry, 29,* 698–701.

Biederman, J., Mick, E., Faraone, S. V., Braaten, E., Doyle, A., Spencer, T., et al. (2002). Influence of gender on attention deficit hyperactivity disorder in children referred to a psychiatric clinic. *American Journal of Psychiatry, 159,* 36–42.

Bird, H. R., Canino, G., Rubio-Stipec, M., Gould, M. S., Ribera, J., Sesman, M., et al. (1988). Estimates of the prevalence of childhood maladjustment in a community survey in Puerto Rico. *Archives of General Psychiatry, 45,* 1120–1126.

Blachman, D. R., & Hinshaw, S. P. (2002). Patterns of friendship among girls with and without attention-deficit/hyperactivity disorder. *Journal of Abnormal Child Psychology, 30,* 625–640.

Borger, N., & van der Meere, J. (2000). Visual behaviour of ADHD children during an attention test: An almost forgotten variable. *Journal of Child Psychology and Psychiatry, 41,* 525–532.

Boyle, M. H., & Lipman, E. L. (2002). Do places matter?: Socioeconomic disadvantage and behavioral problems of children in Canada. *Journal of Consulting and Clinical Psychology, 70,* 378–389.

Breen, M. J. (1989). ADHD girls and boys: An analysis of attentional, emotional, cognitive, and family variables. *Journal of Child Psychology and Psychiatry, 30,* 711–716.

Breen, M. J., & Barkley, R. A. (1988). Parenting stress with ADDH girls and boys. *Journal of Pediatric Psychology, 13,* 265–280.

Breton, J., Bergeron, L., Valla, J. P., Berthiaume, C.,

Gaudet, N., Lambert, J., et al. (1999). Quebec children mental health survey: Prevalence of DSM-III-R mental health disorders. *Journal of Child Psychology and Psychiatry, 40*, 375–384.

Briggs-Gowan, M. J., Horwitz, S. M., Schwab-Stone, M. E., Leventhal, J. M., & Leaf, P. J. (2000). Mental health in pediatric settings: Distribution of disorders and factors related to service use. *Journal of the American Academy of Child and Adolescent Psychiatry, 39*, 841–849.

Brodeur, D. A., & Pond, M. (2001). The development of selective attention in children with attention deficit hyperactivity disorder. *Journal of Abnormal Child Psychology, 29*, 229–239.

Brown, R. T., Abramowitz, A. J., Madan-Swain, A., Eckstrand, D., & Dulcan, M. (1989, October). *ADHD gender differences in a clinic-referred sample.* Paper presented at the annual meeting of the American Academy of Child and Adolescent Psychiatry, New York.

Bu-Haroon, A., Eapen, V., & Bener, A. (1999). The prevalence of hyperactivity symptoms in the United Arab Emirates. *Nordic Journal of Psychiatry, 53*, 439–442.

Burns, G. L., Boe, B., Walsh, J. A., Sommers-Flannagan, R., & Teegarden, L. A. (2001). A confirmatory factor analysis on the DSM-IV ADHD and ODD symptoms: What is the best model for the organization of these symptoms? *Journal of Abnormal Child Psychology, 29*, 339–349.

Cammann, R., & Miehlke, A. (1989). Differentiation of motor activity of normally active and hyperactive boys in schools: Some preliminary results. *Journal of Child Psychology and Psychiatry, 30*, 899–906.

Campbell, S. B. (1987). Parent-referred problem three-year-olds: Developmental changes in symptoms. *Journal of Child Psychology and Psychiatry, 28*, 835–846.

Campbell, S. B. (1990). *Behavior problems in preschool children.* New York: Guilford Press.

Campbell, S. B., Douglas, V. I., & Morganstern, G. (1971). Cognitive styles in hyperactive children and the effect of methylphenidate. *Journal of Child Psychology and Psychiatry, 12*, 55–67.

Carlson, C. L., & Mann, M. (2000). Attention deficit hyperactivity disorder, predominantly inattentive subtype. *Child and Adolescent Psychiatric Clinics of North America, 9*, 499–510.

Chen, W. J., Faraone, S. V., Biederman, J., & Tsuang, M. T. (1994). Diagnostic accuracy of the Child Behavior Checklist scales for attention-deficit hyperactivity disorder: A receiver-operating characteristic analysis. *Journal of Consulting and Clinical Psychology, 62*, 1017–1025.

Cohen, N. J., & Minde, K. (1983). The "hyperactive syndrome" in kindergarten children: Comparison of children with pervasive and situational symptoms. *Journal of Child Psychology and Psychiatry, 24*, 443–455.

Cohen, N. J., Weiss, G., & Minde, K. (1972). Cognitive styles in adolescents previously diagnosed as hyperactive. *Journal of Child Psychology and Psychiatry, 13*, 203–209.

Conners, C. K., Erhardt, D., & Sparrow, E. (2000). *Conners Adult ADHD Rating Scales.* North Tonawanda, NY: Multi-Health Systems.

Copeland, A. P. (1979). Types of private speech produced by hyperactive and nonhyperactive boys. *Journal of Abnormal Child Psychology, 7*, 169–177.

Corkum, P. V., & Siegel, L. S. (1993). Is the continuous performance task a valuable research tool for use with children with attention-deficit-hyperactivity disorder? *Journal of Child Psychology and Psychiatry, 34*, 1217–1239.

Costello, E. J., Costello, A. J., & Edelbrock, C. S. (1988). Psychiatric disorders in pediatric primary care. *Archives of General Psychiatry, 45*, 1107–1116.

Costello, E. J., Loeber, R., & Stouthamer-Loeber, M. (1991). Pervasive and situational hyperactivity—Confounding effect of informant: A research note. *Journal of Child Psychology and Psychiatry, 32*, 367–376.

Cromwell, R. L., Baumeister, A., & Hawkins, W. F. (1963). Research in activity level. In N. R. Ellis (Ed.), *Handbook of mental deficiency.* New York: McGraw-Hill.

Crosbie, J., & Schachar, R. (2001). Deficient inhibition as a marker for familial ADHD. *American Journal of Psychiatry, 158*, 1884–1890.

Cuffe, S. P., McKeown, R. E., Jackson, K. L., Addy, C. L., Abramson, R., & Garrison, C. Z. (2001). Prevalence of attention-deficit/hyperactivity disorder in a community sample of older adolescents. *Journal of the American Academy of Child and Adolescent Psychiatry, 40*, 1037–1044.

Dane, A. V., Schachar, R. J., & Tannock, R. (2000). Does actigraphy differentiate ADHD subtypes in a clinical research setting? *Journal of the American Academy of Child and Adolescent Psychiatry, 39*, 752–760.

Danforth, J. S., Barkley, R. A., & Stokes, T. F. (1991). Observations of parent–child interactions with hyperactive children: Research and clinical implications. *Clinical Psychology Review, 11*, 703–727.

deHaas, P. A. (1986). Attention styles and peer relationships of hyperactive and normal boys and girls. *Journal of Abnormal Child Psychology, 14*, 457–467.

deHaas, P. A., & Young, R. D. (1984). Attention styles of hyperactive and normal girls. *Journal of Abnormal Child Psychology, 12*, 531–546.

Demb, H. B. (1991). Use of Ritalin in the treatment of children with mental retardation. In L. Greenhill & B. Osmon (Eds.), *Ritalin: Theory and patient management* (pp. 155–170). New York: Liebert.

Douglas, V. I. (1980). Higher mental processes in hyperactive children: Implications for training. In R. Knights & D. Bakker (Eds.), *Treatment of hyperactive and learning disordered children* (pp. 65–92). Baltimore: University Park Press.

Douglas, V. I. (1983). Attention and cognitive problems.

In M. Rutter (Ed.), *Developmental neuropsychiatry* (pp. 280–329). New York: Guilford Press.

Douglas, V. I., & Parry, P. A. (1983). Effects of reward on delayed reaction time task performance of hyperactive children. *Journal of Abnormal Child Psychology, 11*, 313–326.

Draeger, S., Prior, M., & Sanson, A. (1986). Visual and auditory attention performance in hyperactive children: competence or compliance. *Journal of Abnormal Child Psychology, 14*, 411–424.

DuPaul, G. J. (1991). Parent and teacher ratings of ADHD symptoms: Psychometric properties in a community-based sample. *Journal of Clinical Child Psychology, 20*, 242–253.

DuPaul, G. J., Power, T. J., Anastopoulos, A. D., & Reid, R. (1998). *The ADHD Rating Scale–IV: Checklists, norms, and clinical interpretation.* New York: Guilford Press.

DuPaul, G. J., Power, T. J., Anastopoulos, A. D., Reid, R., McGoey, K. E., & Ikeda, M. J. (1997). Teacher ratings of attention-deficit/hyperactivity disorder symptoms: Factor structure, normative data, and psychometric properties. *Psychological Assessment, 9*, 436–444.

DuPaul, G. J., Weyandt, L., Schaughency, L., & Ota, K. (1997). *Self-report of ADHD symptoms in U.S. college students: Factor structure and symptom prevalence.* Unpublished manuscript, Lehigh University, Bethlehem, PA.

Edelbrock, C. S., & Costello, A. (1984). Structured psychiatric interviews for children and adolescents. In G. Goldstein & M. Hersen (Eds.), *Handbook of psychological assessment* (pp. 276–290). New York: Pergamon Press.

Esser, G., Schmidt, M. H., & Woerner, W. (1990). Epidemiology and course of psychiatric disorders in school-age children: Results of a longitudinal study. *Journal of Child Psychology and Psychiatry, 31*, 243–263.

Faraone, S. V. (1997, October). *Familial aggregation of ADHD in families of girls with ADHD.* Paper presented at the annual meeting of the American Academy of Child and Adolescent Psychiatry, Toronto.

Fergusson, D. M., Horwood, L. J., & Lynskey, M. T. (1993). Prevalence and comorbidity of DSM-III-R diagnoses in a birth cohort of 15 year olds. *Journal of the American Academy of Child and Adolescent Psychiatry, 32*, 1127–1134.

Fergusson, D. M., Lynskey, M. T., & Horwood, L. J. (1997). Attentional difficulties in middle childhood and psychosocial outcomes in young adulthood. *Journal of Child Psychology and Psychiatry, 38*, 633–644.

Fischer, M., Barkley, R. A., Edelbrock, C. S., & Smallish, L. (1990). The adolescent outcome of hyperactive children diagnosed by research criteria: II. Academic, attentional, and neuropsychological status. *Journal of Consulting and Clinical Psychology, 58*, 580–588.

Fischer, M., Barkley, R. A., Fletcher, K. E., & Smallish, L. (1993a). The adolescent outcome of hyperactive children: Predictors of psychiatric, academic, social, and emotional adjustment. *Journal of the American Academy of Child and Adolescent Psychiatry, 32*, 324–332.

Fischer, M., Barkley, R. A., Fletcher, K. E., & Smallish, L. (1993b). The stability of dimensions of behavior in ADHD and normal children over an 8-year follow-up. *Journal of Abnormal Child Psychology, 21*, 315–337.

Fischer, M., Barkley, R. A., Smallish, L., & Fletcher, K. (2004). Hyperactive children as young adults: Deficits in inhibition, attention, and response perseveration and their relationship to severity of childhood and current ADHD and conduct disorder. *Developmental Neuropsychology, 27*, 107–133.

Frazier, T. W., Demaree, H. A., & Youngstrom, E. A. (2004). Meta-analysis of intellectual and neuropsychological test performance in attention-deficit/hyperactivity disorder. *Neuropsychology, 18*, 543–555.

Fuster, J. M. (1997). *The prefrontal cortex* (3rd ed.). New York: Raven Press.

Gadow, K. D., Nolan, E. E., Litcher, L., Carlson, G. A., Panina, N., Golovakha, E., et al. (2000). Comparison of attention-deficit/hyperactivity disorder symptom subtypes in Ukrainian schoolchildren. *Journal of the American Academy of Child and Adolescent Psychiatry, 39*, 1520–1527.

Gadow, K. D., & Sprafkin, J. (1997). *Child Symptom Inventory 4: Norms manual.* Stony Brook, NY: Checkmate Plus.

Gadow, K. D., Sprafkin, J., & Nolan, E. E. (2001). DSM-IV symptoms in community and clinic preschool children. *Journal of the American Academy of Child and Adolescent Psychiatry, 40*, 1383–1392.

Gaub, M., & Carlson, C. L. (1997). Gender differences in ADHD: A meta-analysis and critical review. *Journal of the American Academy of Child and Adolescent Psychiatry, 36*, 1036–1045.

Gershon, J. (2002). A meta-analytic review of gender differences in ADHD. *Journal of Attention Disorders, 5*, 143–154.

Gioia, G. A., Isquith, P. K., Guy, S. C., & Kenworthy, L. (2000). *Behavior Rating Inventory of Executive Functioning.* Lutz, FL: Psychological Assessment Resources.

Glow, P. H., & Glow, R. A. (1979). Hyperkinetic impulse disorder: A developmental defect of motivation. *Genetic Psychology Monographs, 100*, 159–231.

Gomez, R., Harvey, J., Quick, C., Scharer, I., & Harris, G. (1999). DSM-IV AD/HD: Confirmatory factor models, prevalence, and gender and age differences based on parent and teacher ratings of Australian primary school children. *Journal of Child Psychology and Psychiatry, 40*, 265–274.

Goodman, J. R., & Stevenson, J. (1989). A twin study of hyperactivity: II. The aetiological role of genes, family relationships, and perinatal adversity. *Journal of Child Psychology and Psychiatry, 30*, 691–709.

Gordon, M. (1979). The assessment of impulsivity and mediating behaviors in hyperactive and nonhyperactive children. *Journal of Abnormal Child Psychology, 7*, 317–326.

Gordon, M. (1983). *The Gordon Diagnostic System.* DeWitt, NY: Gordon Systems.

Goyette, C. H., Conners, C. K., & Ulrich, R. F. (1978). Normative data on revised Conners Parent and Teacher Rating Scales. *Journal of Abnormal Child Psychology, 6*, 221–236.

Graetz, B. W., Sawyer, M. G., Hazell, P. L., Arney, F., & Baghurst, P. (2001). Validity of DSM-IV ADHD subtypes in a nationally representative sample of Australian children and adolescents. *Journal of the American Academy of Child and Adolescent Psychiatry, 40*, 1410–1417.

Grodzinsky, G. M., & Diamond, R. (1992). Frontal lobe functioning in boys with attention-deficit hyperactivity disorder. *Developmental Neuropsychology, 8*, 427–445.

Haenlein, M., & Caul, W. F. (1987). Attention deficit disorder with hyperactivity: A specific hypothesis of reward dysfunction. *Journal of the American Academy of Child and Adolescent Psychiatry, 26*, 356–362.

Hale, G. A., & Lewis, M. (1979). *Attention and cognitive development.* New York: Plenum Press.

Halperin, J. M., Matier, K., Bedi, G., Sharma, V., & Newcorn, J. H. (1992). Specificity of inattention, impulsivity, and hyperactivity to the diagnosis of attention-deficit hyperactivity disorder. *Journal of the American Academy of Child and Adolescent Psychiatry, 31*, 190–196.

Hart, E. L., Lahey, B. B., Loeber, R., Applegate, B., & Frick, P. J. (1995). Developmental changes in attention-deficit hyperactivity disorder in boys: A four-year longitudinal study. *Journal of Abnormal Child Psychology, 23*, 729–750.

Hartung, C. M., Willcutt, E. G., Lahey, B. B., Pelham, W. E., Loney, J., Stein, M. A., et al. (2002). Sex differences in young children who meet criteria for attention deficit hyperactivity disorder. *Journal of Clinical Child and Adolescent Psychology, 31*, 453–464.

Heiligenstein, E., Conyers, L. M., Berns, A. R., & Smith, M. A. (1997). *Preliminary normative data on DSM-IV attention deficit hyperactivity disorder in college students.* Unpublished manuscript, University of Wisconsin, Madison, WI.

Hervey, A. S., Epstein, J. N., & Curry, J. F. (2004). Neuropsychology of adults with attention-deficit/hyperactivity disorder: A meta-analytic review. *Neuropsychology, 18*, 495–503.

Hinshaw, S. P. (1987). On the distinction between attentional deficits/hyperactivity and conduct problems/aggression in child psychopathology. *Psychological Bulletin, 101*, 443–447.

Hinshaw, S. P. (1994). *Attention deficits and hyperactivity in children.* Thousand Oaks, CA: Sage.

Hinshaw, S. P. (2001). Is the inattentive type of ADHD a separate disorder? *Clinical Psychology: Science and Practice, 8*, 498–501.

Holdnack, J. A., Moberg, P. J., Arnold, S. E., Gur, R. C., & Gur, R. E. (1995). Speed of processing and verbal learning deficits in adults diagnosed with attention deficit disorder. *Neuropsychiatry, Neuropsychology, and Behavioral Neurology, 8*, 282–292.

Horn, W. F., Wagner, A. E., & Ialongo, N. (1989). Sex differences in school-aged children with pervasive attention deficit hyperactivity disorder. *Journal of Abnormal Child Psychology, 17*, 109–125.

Hoza, B., Pelham, W. E., Waschbusch, D. A., Kipp, H., & Owens, J. S. (2001). Academic task performance of normally achieving ADHD and control boys: Performance, self-evaluations, and attributions. *Journal of Consulting and Clinical Psychology, 69*, 271–283.

Huang-Pollock, C. L., & Nigg, J. T. (2003). Searching for the attention deficit in attention deficit hyperactivity disorder: the case of visuospatial orienting. *Clinical Psychology Review, 23*, 801–830.

Hudziak, J. J., Heath, A. C., Madden, P. F., Reich, W., Bucholz, K. K., Slutske, W., et al. (1998). Latent class and factor analysis of DSM-IV ADHD: A twin study of female adolescents. *Journal of the American Academy of Child and Adolescent Psychiatry, 37*, 848–857.

Jacob, R. G., O'Leary, K. D., & Rosenblad, C. (1978). Formal and informal classroom settings: Effects on hyperactivity. *Journal of Abnormal Child Psychology, 6*, 47–59.

Jensen, P. S., Watanabe, H. K., Richters, J. E., Cortes, R., Roper, M., & Liu, S. (1995). Prevalence of mental disorder in military children and adolescents: Findings from a two-stage community survey. *Journal of the American Academy of Child and Adolescent Psychiatry, 34*, 1514–1524.

Kanbayashi, Y., Nakata, Y., Fujii, K., Kita, M., & Wada, K. (1994). ADHD-related behavior among non-referred children: Parents' ratings of DSM-III-R symptoms. *Child Psychiatry and Human Development, 25*, 13–29.

Kashani, J. H., Orvaschel, H., Ronsenberg, T. K., & Reid, J. C. (1989). Psychopathology in a community sample of children and adolescents: A developmental perspective. *Journal of the American Academy of Child and Adolescent Psychiatry, 28*, 701–706.

Kendall, P. C., & Wilcox, L. E. (1979). Self-control in children: Development of a rating scale. *Journal of Consulting and Clinical Psychology, 47*, 1020–1029.

Kindlon, D., Mezzacappa, E., & Earls, F. (1995). Psychometric properties of impulsivity measures: Temporal stability, validity and factor structure. *Journal of Child Psychology and Psychiatry, 36*, 645–661.

Kohn, A. (1989, November). Suffer the restless children. *Atlantic Monthly,* pp. 90–100.

Kroes, M., Kalff, A. C., Kessels, A. G. H., Steyaert, J., Feron, F., van Someren, A., et al. (2001). Child psychiatric diagnoses in a population of Dutch schoolchildren aged 6 to 8 years. *Journal of the American*

Academy of Child and Adolescent Psychiatry, 40, 1401–1409.

Lahey, B. B. (2001). Should the combined and predominantly inattentive types of ADHD be considered distinct and unrelated disorders?: Not now, at least. *Clinical Psychology: Science and Practice, 8,* 494–497.

Lahey, B. B., Applegate, B., McBurnett, K., Biederman, J., Greenhill, L., Hynd, G. W., et al. (1994). DSM-IV field trials for attention deficit/hyperactivity disorder in children and adolescents. *Journal of the American Academy of Child and Adolescent Psychiatry, 151,* 1673–1685.

Lambert, N. M., Sandoval, J., & Sassone, D. (1978). Prevalence of hyperactivity in elementary school children as a function of social system definers. *American Journal of Orthopsychiatry, 48,* 446–463.

Landau, S., Lorch, E. P., & Milich, R. (1992). Visual attention to and comprehension of television in attention deficit hyperactivity disordered and normal boys. *Child Development, 63,* 928–937.

Lapouse, R., & Monk, M. (1958). An epidemiological study of behavior characteristics in children. *American Journal of Public Health, 48,* 1134–1144.

Lawrence, V., Houghton, S., Tannock, R., Douglas, G., Durkin, K., & Whiting, K. (2002). ADHD outside the laboratory: Boys' executive function performance on tasks in videogame play and on a visit to the zoo. *Journal of Abnormal Child Psychology, 30,* 447–462.

LeFever, G. B., Dawson, K. V., & Morrow, A. L. (1999). The extent of drug therapy for attention deficit hyperactivity disorder among children in public schools. *American Journal of Public Health, 89,* 1359–1364.

Lerner, J. A., Inui, T. S., Trupin, E. W., & Douglas, E. (1985). Preschool behavior can predict future psychiatric disorders. *Journal of the American Academy of Child Psychiatry, 24,* 42–48.

Leung, P. W. L., Luk, S. L., Ho, T. P., Taylor, E., Mak, F. L., & Bacon-Shone, J. (1996). The diagnosis and prevalence of hyperactivity in Chinese schoolboys. *British Journal of Psychiatry, 168,* 486–496.

Levy, F., Hay, D. A., McStephen, M., Wood, C., & Waldman, I. (1997). Attention-deficit hyperactivity disorder: A category or a continuum? Genetic analysis of a large-scale twin study. *Journal of the American Academy of Child and Adolescent Psychiatry, 36,* 737–744.

Lewinsohn, P. M., Hops, H., Roberts, R. E., Seeley, J. R., & Andrews, J. A. (1993). Adolescent psychopathology: I. Prevalence and incidence of depression and other DSM-III-R disorders in high school students. *Journal of Abnormal Psychology, 102,* 133–144.

Liu, X., Kurita, H., Guo, C., Tachimori, H., Ze, J., & Okawa, M. (2000). Behavioral and emotional problems in Chinese children: Teacher reports for ages 6 to 11. *Journal of Child Psychology and Psychiatry, 41,* 253–260.

Liu, X., Sun, Z., Neiderhiser, J. M., Uchiyama, M., Okawa, M., & Rogan, W. (2001). Behavioral and emotional problems in Chinese adolescents: Parent and teacher reports. *Journal of the American Academy of Child Psychiatry, 40,* 828–836.

Loeber, R., Green, S. M., Lahey, B. B., Christ, M. A. G., & Frick, P. J. (1992). Developmental sequences in the age of onset of disruptive child behaviors. *Journal of Child and Family Studies, 1,* 21–41.

Losier, B. J., McGrath, P. J., & Klein, R. M. (1996). Error patterns on the continuous performance test in non-medication and medicated samples of children with and without ADHD: A meta-analysis. *Journal of Child Psychology and Psychiatry, 37,* 971–987.

Luk, S. (1985). Direct observations studies of hyperactive behaviors. *Journal of the American Academy of Child and Adolescent Psychiatry, 24,* 338–344.

Mahone, E. M., Cirino, P. T., Cutting, L. E., Cerrone, P. M., Hagelthron, K. M., Hiemenz, J. R., et al. (2002). Validity of the behavior rating inventory of executive function in children with ADHD and/or Tourette syndrome. *Archives of Clinical Neuropsychology, 17,* 643–662.

Mannuzza, S., Klein, R. G., & Moulton, J. L., III. (2002). Young adult outcome of children with "situational" hyperactivity: A prospective, controlled follow-up study. *Journal of Abnormal Child Psychology, 30,* 191–198.

Marzocchi, G. M., Lucangeli, D., De Meo, T., Fini, F., & Cornoldi, C. (2002). The disturbing effect of irrelevant information on arithmetic problem solving in inattentive children. *Developmental Neuropsychology, 21,* 73–92.

McBurnett, K., Pfiffner, L. J., & Frick, P. J. (2001). Symptom properties as a function of ADHD type: An argument for continued study of sluggish cognitive tempo. *Journal of Abnormal Child Psychology, 29,* 207–213.

McGee, R., Feehan, M., Williams, S., Partridge, F., Silva, P. A., & Kelly, J. (1990). DSM-III disorders in a large sample of adolescents. *Journal of the American Academy of Child and Adolescent Psychiatry, 29,* 611–619.

McGee, R., Williams, S., & Feehan, M. (1992). Attention deficit disorder and age of onset of problem behaviors. *Journal of Abnormal Child Psychology, 20,* 487–502.

McGee, R., Williams, S., & Silva, P. A. (1984a). Behavioral and developmental characteristics of aggressive, hyperactive, and aggressive–hyperactive boys. *Journal of the American Academy of Child Psychiatry, 23,* 270–279.

McGee, R., Williams, S., & Silva, P. A. (1984b). Background characteristics of aggressive, hyperactive, and aggressive–hyperactive boys. *Journal of the American Academy of Child and Adolescent Psychiatry, 23,* 280–284.

McGee, R., Williams, S., & Silva, P. A. (1987). A comparison of girls and boys with teacher-identified problems of attention. *Journal of the American Academy of Child and Adolescent Psychiatry, 26,* 711–717.

McGinnis, J. (1997, September). Attention deficit disaster. *The Wall Street Journal.*

Mick, E. J. (1997, October). *Psychiatric and social functioning in siblings of girls with ADHD.* Paper presented at the annual meeting of the American Academy of Child and Adolescent Psychiatry, Toronto.

Milberger, S. (1997, October). *Impact of adversity on functioning and comorbidity of girls with ADHD.* Paper presented at the annual meeting of the American Academy of Child and Adolescent Psychiatry, Toronto.

Milich, R., Ballentine, A. C., & Lynam, D. R. (2001). ADHD/combined type and ADHD/predominantly inattentive type are distinct and unrelated disorders. *Clinical Psychology: Science and Practice, 8,* 463–488.

Milich, R., & Kramer, J. (1985). Reflections on impulsivity: An empirical investigation of impulsivity as a construct. In K. Gadow & I. Bialer (Eds.), *Advances in learning and behavioral disabilities* (Vol. 3, pp. 57–94). Greenwich, CT: JAI Press.

Milich, R., Landau, S., Kilby, G., & Whitten, P. (1982). Preschool peer perceptions of the behavior of hyperactive and aggressive children. *Journal of Abnormal Child Psychology, 10,* 497–510.

Mirsky, A. F. (1996). Disorders of attention: A neuropsychological perspective. In R. G. Lyon & N. A. Krasnegor (Eds.), *Attention, memory, and executive function* (pp. 71–96). Baltimore: Brookes.

Mitsis, E. M., McKay, K. E., Schulz, K. P., Newcorn, J. H., & Halperin, J. M. (2000). Parent–teacher concordance for DSM-IV attention-deficit/hyperactivity disorder in a clinic-referred sample. *Journal of the American Academy of Child and Adolescent Psychiatry, 39,* 308–313.

Murphy, K., & Barkley, R. A. (1996a). Attention deficit hyperactivity disorder in adults. *Comprehensive Psychiatry, 37,* 393–401.

Murphy, K., & Barkley, R. A. (1996b). Prevalence of DSM-IV symptoms of ADHD in adult licensed drivers: Implications for clinical diagnosis. *Journal of Attention Disorders, 1,* 147–161.

Murphy, K. R., Barkley, R. A., & Bush, T. (2001). Executive functions in young adults with attention deficit hyperactivity disorder, *Neuropsychology, 15,* 211–220.

Neef, N. A., Bicard, D. F., & Endo, S. (2001). Assessment of impulsivity and the development of self-control in students with attention deficit hyperactivity disorder. *Journal of Applied Behavior Analysis, 34,* 397–408.

Newcorn, J. H., Halperin, J. M., Jensen, P., Abikoff, H. B., Arnold, E., Cantwell, D. P., et al. (2001). Symptom profiles in children with ADHD: Effects of comorbidity and gender. *Journal of the American Academy of Child and Adolescent Psychiatry, 40,* 137–146.

Nigg, J. T. (1999). The ADHD response-inhibition deficit as measured by the stop task: Replication with DSM-IV combined type, extension, and qualification. *Journal of Abnormal Child Psychology, 27,* 393–402.

Nigg, J. T. (2000). On inhibition/disinhibition in developmental psychopathology: Views from cognitive and personality psychology and a working inhibition taxonomy. *Psychological Bulletin, 126,* 220–246.

Nigg, J. T. (2001). Is ADHD an inhibitory disorder? *Psychological Bulletin, 125,* 571–596.

Nigg, J. T., Goldsmith, H. H., & Sacheck, J. (2004). Temperament and attention deficit hyperactivity disorder: The development of a multiple pathway model. *Journal of Clinical Child and Adolescent Psychology, 33,* 42–53.

Nolan, E. E., Gadow, K. D., & Sprafkin, J. (2001). Teacher reports of DSM-IV ADHD, ODD, and CD symptoms in schoolchildren. *Journal of the American Academy of Child and Adolescent Psychiatry, 40,* 241–249.

Olson, S. L., Schilling, E. M., & Bates, J. E. (1999). Measurement of impulsivity: Construct coherence, longitudinal stability, and relationship with externalizing problems in middle childhood and adolescence. *Journal of Abnormal Child Psychology, 27,* 151–165.

Palfrey, J. S., Levine, M. D., Walker, D. K., & Sullivan, M. (1985). The emergence of attention deficits in early childhood: A prospective study. *Journal of Developmental and Behavioral Pediatrics, 6,* 339–348.

Pascaulvaca, D. M., Wolf, L. E., Healey, J. M., Tweedy, J. R., & Halperin, J. M. (1988, January). *Sex differences in attention and behavior in school-aged children.* Paper presented at the 16th annual meeting of the International Neuropsychological Society, New Orleans, LA.

Pearson, D. A., & Aman, M. G. (1994). Ratings of hyperactivity and developmental indices: Should clinicians correct for developmental level? *Journal of Autism and Developmental Disorders, 24,* 395–411.

Pelham, W. E., Gnagy, E. M., Greenslade, K. E., & Milich, R. (1992). Teacher ratings of DSM-III-R symptoms for the disruptive behavior disorders. *Journal of the American Academy of Child and Adolescent Psychiatry, 31,* 210–218.

Pelham, W. E., Walker, J. L., Sturgis, J., & Hoza, J. (1989). Comparative effects of methylphenidate on ADD girls and ADD boys. *Journal of the American Academy of Child and Adolescent Psychiatry, 28,* 773–776.

Pennington, B. F., & Ozonoff, S. (1996). Executive functions and developmental psychopathology. *Journal of Child Psychology and Psychiatry, 37,* 51–87.

Peterson, B. S., Pine, D. S., Cohen, P., & Brook, J. S. (2001). Prospective, longitudinal study of tic, obsessive–compulsive, and attention-deficit/hyperactivity disorders in an epidemiological sample. *Journal of the American Academy of Child and Adolescent Psychiatry, 40,* 685–695.

Pineda, D., Ardila, A., Rosselli, M., Arias, B. E., Henao, G. C., Gomez, L. F., et al. (1999). Prevalence of attention-deficit/hyperactivity disorder symptoms in 4- to 17-year old children in the general population. *Journal of Abnormal Child Psychology, 27*, 455–462.

Porrino, L. J., Rapoport, J. L., Behar, D., Sceery, W., Ismond, D. R., & Bunney, W. E., Jr. (1983). A naturalistic assessment of the motor activity of hyperactive boys. *Archives of General Psychiatry, 40*, 681–687.

Prior, M., Wallace, M., & Milton, I. (1984). Schedule-induced behavior in hyperactive children. *Journal of Abnormal Child Psychology, 12*, 227–244.

Quay, H. C. (1997). Inhibition and attention deficit hyperactivity disorder. *Journal of Abnormal Child Psychology, 25*, 7–14.

Rapoport, J. L., Donnelly, M., Zametkin, A., & Carrougher, J. (1986). "Situational hyperactivity" in a U.S. clinical setting. *Journal of Child Psychology and Psychiatry, 27*, 639–646.

Rapport, M. D., Tucker, S. B., DuPaul, G. J., Merlo, M., & Stoner, G. (1986). Hyperactivity and frustration: The influence of control over and size of rewards in delaying gratification. *Journal of Abnormal Child Psychology, 14*, 181–204.

Rasmussen, E. R., Todd, R. D., Neuman, R. J., Heath, A. C., Reich, W., & Rohde, L. A. (2002). Comparison of male adolescent-report of attention-deficit/hyperactivity disorder (ADHD) symptoms across two cultures using latent class and principal components analysis. *Journal of Child Psychology and Psychiatry, 43*, 797–805.

Reeves, J. C., Werry, J., Elkind, G. S., & Zametkin, A. (1987). Attention deficit, conduct, oppositional, and anxiety disorders in children: II. Clinical characteristics. *Journal of the American Academy of Child and Adolescent Psychiatry, 26*, 133–143.

Rohde, L. A., Biederman, J., Busnello, E. A., Zimmermann, H., Schmitz, M., Martins, S., et al. (1999). ADHD in a school sample of Brazilian adolescents: A study of prevalence, comorbid conditions, and impairments. *Journal of the American Academy of Child and Adolescent Psychiatry, 38*, 716–722.

Romano, E., Tremblay, R. E., Vitaro, F., Zoccolillo, M., & Pagani, L. (2001). Prevalene of psychiatric diagnoses and the role of perceived impairment: Findings from an adolescent community · sample. *Journal of Child Psychology and Psychiatry, 42*, 451–462.

Rosenthal, R. H., & Allen, T. W. (1980). Intratask distractibility in hyperkinetic and nonhyperkinetic children. *Journal of Abnormal Child Psychology, 8*, 175–187.

Ross, D. M., & Ross, S. A. (1982). *Hyperactivity: Research, theory and action.* New York: Wiley.

Routh, D. K. (1978). Hyperactivity. In P. Magrab (Ed.), *Psychological management of pediatric problems* (pp. 3–48). Baltimore: University Park Press.

Routh, D. K., & Roberts, R. D. (1972). Minimal brain dysfunction in children: Failure to find evidence for a behavioral syndrome. *Psychological Reports, 31*, 307–314.

Routh, D. K., & Schroeder, C. S. (1976). Standardized playroom measures as indices of hyperactivity. *Journal of Abnormal Child Psychology, 4*, 199–207.

Rubia, K., Taylor, E., Smith, A. B., Oksannen, H., Overmeyer, S., & Newman, S. (2001). Neuropsychological analyses of impulsiveness in childhood hyperactivity. *British Journal of Psychiatry, 179*, 138–143.

Rutter, M. (1977). Brain damage syndromes in childhood: Concepts and findings. *Journal of Child Psychology and Psychiatry, 18*, 1–21.

Rutter, M. (1989). Attention deficit disorder/hyperkinetic syndrome: Conceptual and research issues regarding diagnosis and classification. In T. Sagvolden & T. Archer (Eds.), *Attention deficit disorder: Clinical and basic research* (pp. 1–24). Hillsdale, NJ: Erlbaum.

Rutter, M., Bolton, P., Harrington, R., LeCouteur, A., Macdonald, H., & Simonoff, E. (1990). Genetic factors in child psychiatric disorders: I. A review of research strategies. *Journal of Child Psychology and Psychiatry, 31*, 3–37.

Rutter, M., Macdonald, H., LeCouteur, A., Harrington, R., Bolton, P., & Bailey, P. (1990). Genetic factors in child psychiatric disorders: II. Empirical findings. *Journal of Child Psychology and Psychiatry, 31*, 39–83.

Sawyer, A. M., Taylor, E., & Chadwick, O. (2001). The effect of off-task behaviors on the task performance of hyperkinetic children. *Journal of Attention Disorders, 5*, 1–10.

Schachar, R., Mota, V. L., Logan, G. D., Tannock, R., & Klim, P. (2000). Confirmation of an inhibition control deficit in attention-deficit/hyperactivity disorder. *Journal of Abnormal Child Psychology, 28*, 227–235.

Schachar, R., Rutter, M., & Smith, A. (1981). The characteristics of situationally and pervasively hyperactive children: Implications for syndrome definition. *Journal of Child Psychology and Psychiatry, 22*, 375–392.

Scheres, A., Oosterlaan, J., Geurts, H., Morein-Zamir, S., Meiran, N., Schut, H., et al. (2004). Executive functioning in boys with ADHD primarily an inhibition deficit? *Archives of Clinical Neuropsychology, 19*, 569–594.

Schrag, P., & Divoky, D. (1975). *The myth of the hyperactive child.* New York: Pantheon.

Seidman, L. J., Biederman, J., Faraone, S. V., Weber, W., & Ouellette, C. (1997). Toward defining a neuropsychology of attention deficit–hyperactivity disorder: Performance of children and adolescence from a large clinically referred sample. *Journal of Consulting and Clinical Psychology, 65*, 150–160.

Sergeant, J. (1988). From DSM-III attentional deficit disorder to functional defects. In L. M. Bloomingdale & J. Sergeant (Eds.), *Attention deficit disorder: Criteria, cognition, intervention* (pp. 183–198). New York: Pergamon Press.

Sergeant, J. A., Geurts, H., & Oosterlaan, J. (2002). How specific is a deficit of executive functioning for attention-deficit/hyperactivity disorder? *Behavioural Brain Research, 130*, 3–28.

Sharp, W. S., Walter, J. M., Hamburger, S. D., Marsh, W. L., Rapoport, J. L., & Castellanos, F. X. (1997, October). *Comparison between girls and boys with ADHD: A controlled study.* Paper presented at the annual meeting of the American Academy of Child and Adolescent Psychiatry, Toronto.

Shelton, T. L., Barkley, R. A., Crosswait, C., Moorehouse, M., Fletcher, K., Barrett, S., et al. (2000). Multimethod psychoeducational intervention for preschool children with disruptive behavior: Two-year post-treatment follow-up. *Journal of Abnormal Child Psychology, 28*, 253–266.

Sherman, D. K., McGee, M. K., & Iacono, W. G. (1997). Twin concordance for attention deficit hyperactivity disorder: A comparison of teachers' and mothers' reports. *American Journal of Psychiatry, 154*, 532–535.

Siminoff, E., Pickles, A., Meyer, J. M., Silberg, J. L., Maes, H. H., Loeber, R., et al. (1997). The Virginia Twin Study of adolescent behavioral development. *Archives of General Psychiatry, 54*, 801–808.

Slaats-Willemse, D., Swaab-Barneveld, H., Sonneville, L., van der Meulen, E., & Buitelaar, J. (2003). Deficient response inhibition as a cognitive endophenotype of ADHD. *Journal of the American Academy of Child and Adolescent Psychiatry, 42*, 1242–1248.

Solanto, M. V., Abikoff, H., Sonuga-Barke, E., Schachar, R., Logan, G. D., Wigal, T., et al. (2001). The ecological validity of delay aversion and response inhibition as measures of impulsivity in AD/HD: A supplement to the NIMH Multimodal Treatment Study of ADHD. *Journal of Abnormal Child Psychology, 29*, 215–228.

Sonuga-Barke, E. J. S., Taylor, E., & Hepinstall, E. (1992). Hyperactivity and delay aversion: II. The effect of self versus externally imposed stimulus presentation periods on memory. *Journal of Child Psychology and Psychiatry, 33*, 399–409.

Spitzer, R. L., Davies, M., & Barkley, R. A. (1990). The DSM-III-R field trial for the disruptive behavior disorders. *Journal of the American Academy of Child and Adolescent Psychiatry, 29*, 690–697.

Steinkamp, M. W. (1980). Relationships between environmental distractions and task performance of hyperactive and normal children. *Journal of Learning Disabilities, 13*, 40–45.

Stewart, M. A., Pitts, F. N., Craig, A. G., & Dieruf, W. (1966). The hyperactive child syndrome. *American Journal of Orthopsychiatry, 36*, 861–867.

Still, G. F. (1902). Some abnormal psychical conditions in children. *Lancet, i*, 1008–1012, 1077–1082, 1163–1168.

Strauss, M. E., Thompson, P., Adams, N. L., Redline, S., & Burant, C. (2000). Evaluation of a model of attention with confirmatory factor analysis. *Neuropsychology, 14*, 201–208.

Swaab-Barneveld, H., DeSonneville, L., Cohen-Kettenis, P., Gielen, A., Buitelaar, J., & van Engeland, H. (2000). Visual sustained attention in a child psychiatric population. *Journal of the American Academy of Child and Adolescent Psychiatry, 39*, 651–659.

Szatmari, P. (1992). The epidemiology of attention-deficit hyperactivity disorders. *Child and Adolescent Psychiatry Clinics of North America, 1*, 361–372.

Szatmari, P., Offord, D. R., & Boyle, M. H. (1989). Correlates, associated impairments, and patterns of service utilization of children with attention deficit disorders: Findings from the Ontario Child Health Study. *Journal of Child Psychology and Psychiatry, 30*, 205–217.

Tallmadge, J., & Barkley, R. A. (1983). The interactions of hyperactive and normal boys with their mothers and fathers. *Journal of Abnormal Child Psychology, 11*, 565–579.

Tannock, R. (1997). Television, video games, and ADHD: Challenging a popular belief. *ADHD Report, 5*(3), 3–7.

Taylor, E. A. (Ed.). (1986). *The overactive child.* Philadelphia: Lippincott.

Taylor, E. A., Sandberg, S., Thorley, G., & Giles, S. (1991). *The epidemiology of childhood hyperactivity.* London: Oxford University Press.

Teicher, M. H., Ito, Y, Glod, C. A., & Barber, N. I. (1996). Objective measurement of hyperactivity and attentional problems in ADHD. *Journal of the American Academy of Child and Adolescent Psychiatry, 35*, 334–342.

Timimi, S. (2004). A critique of the International Consensus Statement on ADHD. *Clinical Child and Family Psychology Review, 7*, 59–63.

Tjersland, T. P., Grabowski, K. L., Hathaway, W. L., & Holley, T. (2005). *Is there an overabundance of ADHD in southeastern Virginia?* Unpublished manuscript, Regent University.

Tripp, G., & Luk, S. L. (1997). The identification of pervasive hyperactivity: Is clinic observation necessary? *Journal of Child Psychology and Psychiatry, 38*, 219–234.

Trites, R. L. (1979). *Hyperactivity in children: Etiology, measurement, and treatment implications.* Baltimore: University Park Press.

Trites, R. L., Dugas, F., Lynch, G., & Ferguson, B. (1979). Incidence of hyperactivity. *Journal of Pediatric Psychology, 4*, 179–188.

Ullman, D. G., Barkley, R. A., & Brown, H. W. (1978). The behavioral symptoms of hyperkinetic children who successfully responded to stimulant drug treatment. *American Journal of Orthopsychiatry, 48*, 425–437.

Velez, C. N., Johnson, J., & Cohen, P. (1989). A longitudinal analysis of selected risk factors for childhood psychopathology. *Journal of the American Academy of Child and Adolescent Psychiatry, 28*, 861–864.

Verhulst, F. C., van der Ende, J., Ferdinand, R. F., & Kasius, M. C. (1997). The prevalence of DSM-III-R diagnoses in a national sample of Dutch adolescents. *Archives of General Psychiatry, 54,* 329–336.

Wakefield, J. C. (1992). The concept of mental disorder: On the boundary between biological facts and social values. *American Psychologist, 47,* 373–388.

Wakefield, J. C. (1997). Normal inability versus pathological disability: Why Ossorio's definition of mental disorder is not sufficient. *Clinical Psychology: Science and Practice, 4,* 249–258.

Weiss, G., & Hechtman, L. (1979). The hyperactive child syndrome. *Science, 205,* 1348–1354.

Weiss, G., & Hechtman, L. (1993). *Hyperactive children grown up* (2nd ed.). New York: Guilford Press.

Werry, J. S. (1988). Differential diagnosis of attention deficits and conduct disorders. In. L. M. Bloomingdale & J. Sergeant (Eds.), *Attention deficit disorder: Criteria, cognition, intervention* (pp. 83–96). London: Pergamon Press.

Werry, J. S., Elkind, G. S., & Reeves, J. S. (1987). Attention deficit, conduct, oppositional, and anxiety disorders in children: III. Laboratory differences. *Journal of Abnormal Child Psychology, 15,* 409–428.

Werry, J. S., & Quay, H. C. (1971). The prevalence of behavior symptoms in younger elementary school children. *American Journal of Orthopsychiatry, 41,* 136–143.

Weyandt, L. L., Linterman, I., & Rice, J. A. (1995). Reported prevalence of attentional difficulties in a general sample of college students. *Journal of Psychopathology and Behavioral Assessment, 17,* 293–304.

Wolraich, M. L., Hannah, J. N., Baumgaertel, A., & Feurer, I. D. (1998). Examination of DSM-IV criteria for attention deficit/hyperactivity disorder in a county-wide sample. *Journal of Developmental and Behavioral Pediatrics, 19,* 162–168.

Wolraich, M. L., Hannah, J. N., Pinnock, T. Y., Baumgaertel, A., & Brown, J. (1996). Comparison of diagnostic criteria for attention-deficit hyperactivity disorder in a country-wide sample. *Journal of the American Academy of Child and Adolescent Psychiatry, 35,* 319–324.

Wolraich, M. L., Lambert, E. W., Baumgaertel, A., Garcia-Tornel, S., Feurer, I. D., Bickman, L., et al. (2003). Teachers' screening for attention deficit/hyperactivity disorder: comparing multinational samples on teacher ratings of ADHD. *Journal of Abnormal Child Psychology, 31,* 445–455.

World Health Organization. (1994). *International classification of diseases* (10th rev.). Geneva, Switzerland: Author.

Zagar, R., & Bowers, N. D. (1983). The effect of time of day on problem-solving and classroom behavior. *Psychology in the Schools, 20,* 337–345.

Zalecki, C. A., & Hinshaw, S. P. (2004). Overt and relational aggression in girls with attention deficit hyperactivity disorder. *Journal of Clinical Child and Adolescent Psychology, 33,* 125–137.

Zentall, S. S. (1985). A context for hyperactivity. In K. D. Gadow & I. Bialer (Eds.), *Advances in learning and behavioral disabilities* (Vol. 4, pp. 273–343). Greenwich, CT: JAI Press.

Zentall, S. S. (1988). Production deficiencies in elicited language but not in the spontaneous verbalizations of hyperactive children. *Journal of Abnormal Child Psychology, 16,* 657–673.

Zentall, S. S., Falkenberg, S. D., & Smith, L. B. (1985). Effects of color stimulation and information on the copying performance of attention-problem adolescents. *Journal of Abnormal Child Psychology, 13,* 501–511.

Associated Cognitive, Developmental, and Health Problems

RUSSELL A. BARKLEY

Besides their primary problems with inattention, impulsivity, and overactivity, children with Attention-Deficit/Hyperactivity Disorder (ADHD) may have a variety of other difficulties. Such children have a higher likelihood of having other cognitive, developmental, academic, and even medical or health-related difficulties. Not all children with ADHD display all these problems, but as a group they display them to a degree that is greater than expected in typical children. Because these difficulties are not considered to be the core or essence of the disorder, they are discussed here as associated features. They are not diagnostic of the disorder when present, nor do they rule out the diagnosis when absent. This chapter describes these frequently coexisting problems. Chapter 4 reviews the psychiatric disorders often associated with ADHD in children, along with their social difficulties; Chapter 6 describes these disorders in adults with ADHD.

INTELLECTUAL DEVELOPMENT

There is no longer any doubt that children with ADHD display lower levels of intellectual performance than either nondisabled children or their own siblings do (Frazier, Demaree, &

Youngstrom, 2004). The effect size difference between children with ADHD and nondisabled children averages 0.61 standard deviation (*SD*) (Frazier et al., 2004), for an average deficit of 9 points (range of 7–15 points) on standardized intelligence tests (Barkley, Karlsson, & Pollard, 1985; Faraone et al., 1993; Fischer, Barkley, Fletcher, & Smallish, 1990; Mariani & Barkley, 1997; McGee, Williams, & Feehan, 1992; McGee, Williams, Moffitt, & Anderson, 1989; Moffitt, 1990; Prior, Leonard, & Wood, 1983; Stewart, Pitts, Craig, & Dieruf, 1966; Tarver-Behring, Barkley, & Karlsson, 1985; Werry, Elkind, & Reeves, 1987). The effect size difference between adults with ADHD and control adults is somewhat smaller (an average of 0.39 *SD*, or 6 points) but still significant (Hervey, Epstein, & Curry, 2004). Some have suggested that the lower intelligence scores in the groups with ADHD could be related to coexisting learning disabilities (LDs) and not to the ADHD per se (Bohline, 1985). However, in a study of children with ADHD and children with LDs in our clinic, the children with LDs but not ADHD actually had IQ estimates even lower than those found in the group with both types of disorders, whose IQ estimates were still lower than those of the nondisabled control group (Barkley, DuPaul, & McMurray,

1990). Despite this mild deficit in intelligence, children with ADHD are likely to represent the entire spectrum of intellectual development: Some are gifted, while others have low intelligence, learn slowly, or have mild intellectual retardation.

As discussed in Chapter 7, the impairment in behavioral inhibition and in the executive functions seen in children with ADHD could be expected to result in a small but significant and negative relationship between ADHD and IQ. This is because IQ is related to the executive functions of working memory, internalized speech, and the eventual development of verbal thought, all of which are deficient in children with ADHD (see below) and in adults with ADHD (Hervey et al., 2004). Such cognitive deficits, among others, could partly explain the decrement in IQ evident in ADHD. Studies using both nondisabled samples (Hinshaw, Morrison, Carte, & Cornsweet, 1987; McGee, Williams, & Silva, 1984) and samples with behavioral problems (Sonuga-Barke, Lamparelli, Stevenson, Thompson, & Henry, 1994) found significant negative associations between degree of rated hyperactive–impulsive behavior and measures of intelligence. In contrast, associations between ratings of conduct problems and intelligence in children are often much smaller or even nonsignificant, particularly when hyperactive–impulsive behavior is partialed out of the relationship (Hinshaw et al., 1987; Lynam, Moffitt, & Stouthamer-Loeber, 1993; Sonuga-Barke et al., 1994). Such findings suggest that the relationship between IQ and disruptive behavior in children is relatively specific to the hyperactive–impulsive element of the disruptive behavior (see Hinshaw, 1992, for a review).

Differences in IQ have also been found between hyperactive boys and their nondisabled siblings (Halperin & Gittelman, 1982; Tarver-Behring et al., 1985; Welner, Welner, Stewart, Palkes, & Wish, 1977), suggesting that impulsive–hyperactive behavior generally, and ADHD specifically, has an inherent association with diminished IQ (Halperin & Gittelman, 1982; Hinshaw, 1992; McGee et al., 1992; Sonuga-Barke et al., 1994; Werry et al., 1987). This small but significant relationship implies that between 3% and 10% of the variance in IQ may be a function of symptoms of ADHD (hyperactive–impulsive behavior). It also implies that when differences in IQ between a group with ADHD and a control group are found in a study, they should not be statistically controlled for in the analyses, as this may remove some of the variation in the measures under study that is due to ADHD itself.

ADAPTIVE FUNCTIONING

"Adaptive functioning" refers to the "performance of the daily activities required for personal and social sufficiency" (Sparrow, Balla, & Cicchetti, 1984). It represents a child's actual performance of the typical demands of daily living in natural home and community settings. These often include self-help skills (i.e., dresses, bathes, and feeds self, etc.); independence (i.e., functions well about the home, yard, or community without supervision, respects property, etc.); self-knowledge (i.e., is aware of one's own body and its parts, age, address, phone number, and other aspects of personal identity); motor skills (i.e., sits up, walks, balances, runs, buttons, zips, cuts with scissors, uses eating and writing utensils, etc.); social knowledge (e.g., recognizes and uses time and monetary units, knows major community resources such as police and fire departments, etc.); and language/communication skills with others (i.e., identifies objects, obeys two-step commands, communicates using complete sentences, counts to 100, introduces self to others, etc.).

Several studies have consistently documented diminished overall adaptive functioning in children with ADHD relative to nondisabled or other control groups of children (Barkley, Fischer, Edelbrock, & Smallish, 1990; Greene et al., 1996; Roizen, Blondis, Irwin, & Stein, 1994; Stein, Szumowski, Blondis, & Roizen, 1995). These studies find that children with ADHD often function in the low-average to borderline range of adaptive functioning, despite having generally average intelligence. And although children with other psychiatric and developmental disorders often demonstrate low adaptive functioning, the discrepancy between adaptive functioning and IQ is often greater in children with ADHD than in these other groups (Stein et al., 1995). This discrepancy suggests that, apart from the lower levels of intelligence that may be associated with ADHD (see above), ADHD takes a specific toll on adaptive functioning.

For instance, Roizen et al. (1994) found that the deficits in adaptive functioning in children with ADHD were substantially below the children's levels of tested intelligence, often by as much as 1.5–2 *SD*s. In contrast, nondisabled children may show only a small disparity (averaging approximately 3 standard score points) between intelligence or general cognitive ability and daily adaptive functioning (Sparrow et al., 1984). Roizen et al. (1994) found that such disparities were not significantly affected by the presence of either comorbid LDs or other disruptive behavior disorders, but did increase as a function of age. The authors speculated that this disparity may actually be useful as a marker of functional impairment in children with ADHD. Such a disparity probably reflects a discrepancy between knowing and doing, or ability and performance, given that measures of adaptive behavior assess children's actual and typical performance in daily life situations rather than their factual knowledge or cognitive abilities.

To further evaluate this type of disparity as a marker of impairment in ADHD, Stein et al. (1995) computed the degree of disparity between measured intelligence and adaptive functioning, as assessed by the Vineland Adaptive Behavior Scales, in three groups of clinic-referred children: those with ADHD, those with Attention Deficit Disorder without Hyperactivity (ADD–H), and those with a pervasive developmental disorder (PDD) or mental retardation (MR). After controlling for degree of externalizing behaviors (symptoms of Oppositional Defiant Disorder [ODD] and Conduct Disorder [CD], ODD/CD), the authors found that both the children with ADHD and those with ADD–H demonstrated significantly lower adaptive functioning relative to their intelligence than did the group with PDD/MR in two of the three domains of adaptive functioning assessed by the Vineland: communication and daily living. No significant difference was found among the groups in their disparity between IQ and the socialization domain of adaptive functioning, once ODD/CD symptoms were statistically covaried; this finding implies that the presence of ODD/CD symptoms may be necessary to create disparity in that specific domain of adaptive functioning. The general level of adaptive functioning in the children with PDD/MR, like that of nondisabled children, was observed to be relatively consistent with their level of intelligence. Yet this was not the case for the children with ADHD/ADD–H, for whom significant adaptive disability, or disparity between IQ and adaptive functioning, was substantial.

A separate study compared adolescents with ADHD with and without ODD/CD to those with only ODD/CD and to a nondisabled control group on the Vineland Adaptive Behavior Inventory (Clark, Prior, & Kinsella, 2002). Poorer adaptive communication skills were specifically associated with ADHD relative to ODD/CD and no disability. As in the Stein et al. (1995) study, poor socialization was associated with both ADHD and ODD/CD again implying that it is mainly the association of ODD/CD with ADHD that results in much of the deficit in this domain of adaptive functioning. This study extends the findings of poor adaptive functioning in childhood ADHD to ADHD in adolescence. It also demonstrated that deficits in executive functioning, to be discussed later, were associated with deficits in adaptive functioning. This suggests that, as with the decrements in intelligence discussed above, deficits in executive functions may partially or wholly explain (or contribute to) the deficits found in adaptive functioning in ADHD.

Taking the concept of adaptive disability introduced by Stein et al. (1995) a step further, Greene et al. (1996) developed a psychometric formula for determining the presence of a significant IQ–functioning disparity, which was borrowed from the literature on definitions of LDs (Reynolds, 1984). However, instead of using an adaptive functioning measure, Greene et al. used one of social functioning (the Social Adjustment Inventory for Children and Adolescents). This measure of social functioning is not identical to a measure of adaptive functioning, concentrating as it does primarily on social skills and peer relations, though it may overlap somewhat with the socialization domain of measures like the Vineland. Based on the correlation of IQ with their social functioning measure, Greene et al. used intelligence scores to generate expected social functioning scores for children in their study. They then employed a threshold of 1.65 or greater on a standardized discrepancy score between observed and expected scores on the social functioning measure to define subjects with ADHD as having a social disability. The subjects with both ADHD and social disability had significantly higher rates of major depression, multiple anxiety disorders, and CD than did the children with ADHD but without social disability. The two groups did not differ in rates of ADHD among family members, but both differed substantially from control children in this respect. The group with both disabilities also had higher ratings on most scales of the parent version of the Child Behavior Checklist than did either the children with ADHD only or the control children, and this dually disabled group also differed from the control children in greater levels of impairment in family functioning. Using this same definition of social disability in a 4-year longitudinal study of children with ADHD, Greene, Biederman, Faraone, Sienna, and Garcia-Jetton (1997) found that social disability was strongly predictive of higher rates of mood, anxiety, disruptive, and substance use disorders at outcome.

Given the success of Greene et al. in using an IQ–social functioning discrepancy formula to identify social disability in children with ADHD, Barkley, Shelton, et al. (2002) hypothesized that this formula might be usefully extrapolated to identifying children having adaptive disability as discussed by Roizen et al. (1994) and later by Stein et al. (1995). In this case, a measure of adaptive functioning would be substituted into the Reynolds (1984) formula for that of social functioning, so as to further evaluate the utility of the adaptive disability concept. Children with high levels of aggressive, hyperactive, impulsive, and inattentive behavior (disruptive behavior, abbreviated as DB in this study; $n = 154$) were identified at kindergarten registration, along with a control group of 47 children without DB. The children with DB were further subdivided into those who did ($n = 38$) and did not ($n = 116$) have adaptive disability (DB ± AD), based on discrepancies between expected and actual adaptive functioning. Compared to children with DB – AD, children with DB + AD had (1) more CD; (2) greater inattention symptoms at home and school; (3) greater aggression and thought problems at home; (4) more social problems, less academic competence, and poorer self-control at school; (5) more severe and pervasive behavior problems across multiple home and school settings; (6) worse math achievement scores; and (7) poorer parental child management practices. Thus the concept of adaptive disability appears to have some utility as a marker for more severe and pervasive impairments in children with ADHD symptoms and associated disruptive behavior.

These children were then followed for 3 years and reevaluated. The children with DB + AD had more symptoms of ADHD and CD, more severe and pervasive behavior problems at home, more parent-rated externalizing and internalizing behaviors, and lower academic competence and more behavioral problems at school. Parents of these children also reported greater parenting stress than did parents in the other groups. A significant contribution of AD to adverse outcomes in the group with DB remained on some measures even after the investigators controlled for initial severity of DB. AD also contributed significantly to CD symptoms at follow-up even after controls for initial DB severity and initial CD symptoms. The results thus corroborated and extended the earlier findings of the utility of adaptive disability as a risk factor beyond that contributed by the severity of ADHD or disruptive behavior alone.

ACADEMIC PERFORMANCE

One area of tremendous difficulty for children with ADHD is in their academic performance (work productivity in the classroom) and achievement (the difficulty level of the material the children have mastered). Almost all clinic-referred children with ADHD are doing poorly at school; they are typically underperforming relative to their known levels of ability as determined by intelligence and academic achievement tests. Such performance is believed to be the result of their inattentive, impulsive, and restless behavior in the classroom. Evidence supporting this interpretation comes from numerous studies that demonstrate significant improvements in academic productivity and sometimes accuracy when children with ADHD are on stimulant medication (Barkley, 1977; Pelham, Bender, Caddell, Booth, & Moorer, 1985; Rapport, DuPaul, Stoner, & Jones, 1986; see Chapter 17, this volume). Even so, children with ADHD are also likely to show performances that are lower than their classmates' by as much as 10–30 standard score points on various standardized achievement tests, including tests of reading, spelling, math, and reading comprehension (Barkley, DuPaul, & McMurray, 1990; Brock & Knapp, 1996; Cantwell & Satterfield, 1978; Casey, Rourke, & Del Dotto, 1996; Dykman & Ackerman, 1992; Fischer et al., 1990; Semrud-Clikeman et al., 1992). These deficits may even be present in preacademic skills among preschoolers with ADHD (Mariani & Barkley, 1997).

When research on a subject becomes as voluminous as that on academic achievement in ADHD (especially when many studies have used small sample sizes), it helps to combine studies into a meta-analysis, as was recently done by Frazier et al. (2004). Of 24 studies examining reading, a weighted mean effect size of 0.64 (95% confidence interval [CI] of 0.53–0.75) was found reflecting the difference between ADHD and control groups as a proportion of an *SD*; for spelling, 15 studies were available, yielding a weighted mean effect size of 0.87 (95% CI = 0.72–1.02); 21 studies examined arithmetic, resulting in a weighted mean effect size of 0.89 (95% CI = 0.78–1.00). Hence it is safe to conclude that ADHD is associated with large decrements (effect sizes) in academic achievement skills.

Rapport, Scanlan, and Denney (1999) demonstrated that ADHD and its associated decrements in intelligence are what account for scholastic underachievement, rather than the conduct problems that are often seen in conjunction with ADHD. This finding replicated an earlier and similar demonstration by Fergusson and Horwood (1995).

Given these deficits in academic skills, it is not surprising to find that as many as 56% of children with ADHD may require academic tutoring, that approximately 30% may repeat a grade in school, and that 30–40% may be placed in one or more special education programs. As many as 46% may be suspended from school, and 10–35% may drop out entirely and fail to complete high school (Barkley, DuPaul, & McMurray, 1990; Barkley, Fischer, et al., 1990; Fischer, Barkley, Smallish, & Fletcher, in press; Brown & Borden, 1986; Faraone et al., 1993; Munir, Biederman, & Knee, 1987; Stewart et al., 1966; Szatmari, Offord, & Boyle, 1989; Weiss & Hechtman, 1993).

LEARNING DISABILITIES

At a certain point, deficits in academic achievement skills rise to the level of being considered specific LDs. Little additional research on LDs in children with ADHD has been conducted since the preceding edition of this text. In view of their deficits in academic achievement skills noted above, it is not surprising that children with ADHD are more likely than children without it to have LDs (Safer & Allen, 1976). An LD, however, is not simply failing to do one's work in school; it is typically defined as a significant discrepancy between one's intelligence, or general mental abilities, and academic achievement in some area, such as reading, math, spelling, handwriting, or language. The prevalence rates of LDs can vary greatly as a function of whether and how this significant discrepancy between IQ and achievement is defined.

Several different formulas can be applied to define an LD. For a review of previous research on LDs in children with ADHD using a variety of approaches, see the report by Semrud-Clikeman et al. (1992). One such formula used in past research with children having ADHD (Lambert & Sandoval, 1980) compared scores on intelligence tests with those on achievement tests for reading and math. An LD is defined as a significant discrepancy between these scores. Such a discrepancy can be based on an absolute amount (say, 20 points) or on the *SD* or error of the tests (say, 15 points or 1 *SD*, where both tests have a mean of 100 and *SD* of 15). A problem with this IQ–achievement discrepancy approach is that it tends to overestimate the prevalence of LDs, especially in children who are performing typically in school and those who are intellectually above average or gifted. For instance, when Dykman and Ackerman (1992) defined a reading disorder as a discrepancy between IQ and achievement of only 10 points, as well as a standard score on the reading test below 90, they found that 45% had such a disorder. Likewise, when Semrud-Clikeman et al. (1992) required only a 10-point discrepancy between IQ and achievement, 38% of their children with ADHD could be considered to have a reading disability and 55% a math disability (the rates for children without ADHD were 8% and 33%, respectively). Such children may be performing perfectly adequately in school and on achievement tests, but, because of higher-than-average levels of intelligence, they may have a significant discrepancy between their IQ and achievement test scores (e.g., IQ = 130 whereas reading standard score = 100). In an earlier edition of this text (Barkley, 1990), I reported on the prevalence of children with ADHD who had an LD by this relatively simple criterion (15-point IQ–achievement discrepancy), using the results of one of my studies (Barkley, DuPaul, & McMurray, 1990). The rates were 40% in reading, nearly 60% in spelling, and nearly 60% in math. However, the rates in the control group without ADHD were 20%, 38%, and

35%, respectively, who were defined as having an LD. Clearly, this is not a rigorous approach to defining an LD.

Using a somewhat larger discrepancy (20 points), Frick et al. (1991) estimated that 16% of children with ADHD had a reading disability, whereas 21% had a math disability. The corresponding prevalences in their control group without ADHD were 5% and 7%, respectively. Likewise, when Semrud-Clikeman et al. (1992) increased the required discrepancy to 20 points, 23% of the children with ADHD could be considered to have a reading disability and 30% a math disability, versus 2% and 22% of children without ADHD, respectively.

A second approach is to define an LD as a score falling below 1.5 SDs from the mean on an achievement test (7th percentile), regardless of the child's IQ. This approach makes more sense, given the close association of IQ and academic achievement, and is far less likely to diagnose typically performing children as having an LD. But it may diagnose children with borderline intellectual functioning or mild MR as such, because their achievement test scores would be consistent with their exceptionally low IQ scores and place them below this LD cutoff point. Using this approach (Barkley, 1990), I found the following prevalence of LDs in children with ADHD: 21% in reading, 26% in spelling, and over 28% in math. For children without ADHD, these rates were 0%, 2.9%, and 2.9%, respectively. None of the children in this particular study were in the borderline range of IQ or lower (MR), and thus the rate of misclassifying children with both ADHD and such low IQ scores cannot be determined from this study.

A more intricate approach to calculating a discrepancy formula involves first converting the standard scores on the IQ and achievement tests to z scores, and then estimating the expected achievement score with a regression equation that takes into consideration both the correlation between the IQ and achievement test and the standard error of estimate for the achievement test. To have an LD, a child must have a discrepancy that exceeds a z score of -1.65 (the $p < .05$ confidence level). Using this approach, Frick et al. (1991) reported a prevalence of 13% for reading disability and 14% for math disability (23% for either). Faraone et al. (1993) also used this approach to defining an LD, and found that 18% of their group with ADHD had a reading disability and 21% had a math disability.

A different approach being used in research is to combine several of the previously discussed methods. In this case, an LD is defined as both a score below some level on an achievement test (say, 1.5 SDs, or 7th percentile) on an achievement test, *and* a significant discrepancy between IQ and achievement on that test (say, 1.5 SDs, or 15 points). Requiring that children be at the 7th percentile on their achievement test and have at least a 15-point discrepancy between their IQ and achievement test resulted in the following rates of LDs in my sample of children with ADHD: 19% in reading, nearly 24% in spelling, and over 26% in math (Barkley, 1990). The rates among the control group were 0%, 0%, and nearly 3%, respectively. Similarly, August and Garfinkel (1990) defined an LD as a 15-point IQ–achievement discrepancy and a standard score below 85 (1 SD), on a reading test and found that 39% of their children with ADHD had a reading disability. Using the same formula, Semrud-Clikeman et al. (1992) found that 15% had a reading disability and 33% had a math disability (compared to none of the control group). Again, using this same formula, Casey et al. (1996) found that nearly 31% of children with ADD + H had a reading disorder, 27% had a spelling disorder, and nearly 13% had a math disorder. When Frick et al. (1991) required their children both to have a 20-point IQ–achievement discrepancy and to be below a standard score of 1 SD below the mean (84) on the achievement test, they found that 8% had a reading disability and 12% had a math disability (control group rates were 2% and 2%, respectively).

In conclusion, if the more rigorous approaches to defining an LD are employed (i.e., Frick et al.'s regression equation or the combined approach discussed previously), then approximately 8–39% of children with ADHD are likely to have a reading disability, 12–30% to have a math disability, and 12–27% to have a spelling disorder. It is worth noting here that Frick et al. (1991) found similar rates of LDs in a sample of children with CD, but this was entirely due to the presence of comorbid ADHD in those children. This finding underscores the point made earlier by Hinshaw (1987, 1992) that ADHD is more often associated with cognitive and achievement deficits than CD is. It is also consistent with Rapport et al.'s (1999) demonstration (see above) that academic deficits are a function of the severity of ADHD and associated low IQ, not of coexisting conduct problems. Where academic achievement is low among children having ADHD and conduct problems, then one can be confident that their ADHD is what is contributing to this problem. It also means that the possible presence of ADHD needs to be evaluated in children diagnosed with CD, as it is more likely to account for their academic and cognitive deficits than is their diagnosis of CD.

An important clinical issue is whether the presence of early learning difficulties or LDs can lead to the development of ADHD or vice versa. The available evidence has grown since the 1998 edition of this book, but is not substantial. When the topic was initially reviewed by McGee and Share (1988), the conclusion (albeit very tentative) was that longitudinal research did not indicate that ADHD could lead to later LDs, but that early learning difficulties might be associated with a rise in ADHD symptoms over development, even though this was not consistently shown across the studies reviewed. In their longitudinal study of children, Fergusson and Horwood (1992) reached the opposite conclusion, finding that early attention problems increased the risk for later reading difficulties, whereas reading difficulties did not increase the later risk for attention problems. Rabiner, Coie, and the Conduct Problems Prevention Research Group (2000) evaluated 387 children followed from kindergarten through fifth grade and found the same result: Early attention problems may be associated with concurrent and later reading problems, but not vice versa. Velting and Whitehurst (1997) found that it was specifically inattention–hyperactivity in first grade that was most closely associated with poorer reading skills. Chadwick, Taylor, Hepinstall, and Danckaerts (1999) followed four groups of children ages 7–8 over a 9-year period. These groups had hyperactivity, reading disability, both, or neither. The results found no evidence that reading disability led to hyperactivity at follow-up or vice versa. Thus, whereas early inattention at first grade may be predictive of lower reading ability later on, early hyperactivity is not likely to do so.

SPEECH AND LANGUAGE DEVELOPMENT

Although children with ADHD do not appear to have a high rate of serious or generalized language delays, they are more likely to have specific problems in their speech development than children without ADHD are. Using community-based samples, some studies have found children with ADHD to be somewhat more likely than typical children to have a delayed onset of talking in early childhood (6–35% vs. 2–5.5%) (Hartsough & Lambert, 1985; Stewart et al., 1966; Szatmari et al., 1989); other studies, using clinic-referred children, have found no differences in the risk for delayed speech development (Barkley, DuPaul, & McMurray, 1990). However, whether speech onset is delayed or not, studies do show that children with ADHD are more likely to have problems in expressive language than in receptive language, with 10–54% having speech problems compared to 2–25% of typical children (Barkley, DuPaul, & McMurray, 1990; Hartsough & Lambert, 1985; Munir et al., 1987; Szatmari et al., 1989). A few studies, however, have not found this relationship (Humphries, Koltun, Malone, & Roberts, 1994) when evaluating children who had simply higher than normal levels of inattention. Nevertheless, such inattentive children did have more difficulties with the organization and conversational pragmatics of their speech than did children with LDs or no disabilities.

Conversely, up to 64% of children with speech and language disorders are likely to have a psychiatric disorder, with the most common one being ADHD (16–46%) (Baker & Cantwell, 1987; Cohen et al., 1998). Given this significant overlap between these two disorders, it is essential to determine what deficits in speech and language are attributable to which of these disorders. Cohen et al. (2000) compared children having ADHD with and without language impairment (LI) to children having other psychiatric disorders either with or without LI. Children with LI showed the greatest difficulties with language tasks, regardless of comorbid diagnosis. Children with ADHD but without LI mainly had difficulties with story recall on these language measures. The group with LI also demonstrated greater deficits in several areas of academic achievement (primarily reading decoding, reading comprehension, and spelling), but not in math. So did children with ADHD but without LI, though not to the degree shown by children with LI. And the children with LI also showed significant problems with working memory, whether verbal, spatial, or combined, but not on other executive function measures (mazes, inhibition, motor control). The group with LI also had difficulties with visual–motor integration; yet so did the children with ADHD, regardless of LI status. The group with ADHD, regardless of LI status, was more likely to have difficulties with achievement and working memory tasks, but was not as impaired as the group with LI. Children with both ADHD and LI showed the greatest deficits but did not show a unique profile. Instead, their deficits were what would be expected from a combination of those deficits associated with each disorder. It appears, then, that ADHD is not associated with structural problems with language, but with difficulties in story recall and academic achievement. If LI coexists with ADHD, even greater difficulties in structural aspects of speech, language-based academic achievement skills, and working memory will be evident. ADHD is also associated with problems in the executive aspects of story narratives (organization and cohesion in story retelling) and probably with pragmatic aspects of speech (Tannock & Schachar, 1996).

As already noted, children with ADHD are likely to talk more than typical children, especially during spontaneous conversation (Barkley, Cunningham, & Karlsson, 1983; Zentall, 1988). However, when confronted with tasks in which they must organize and generate speech in response to specific task demands, they are likely to talk less; to be more dysfluent (e.g., to use pauses, fillers such as "uh," "er," and "um," and misarticulations); and to be less proficient in their organization of speech (Hamlett, Pelligrini, & Conners, 1987; Purvis & Tannock, 1997; Zentall, 1985). Because confrontational speech or explanatory speech is more difficult and requires more careful thought and organization than does spontaneous or descriptive speech, these speech difficulties of children with ADHD suggest that their problems are not so much in speech and language per se as in the higher-order cognitive processes involved in organizing and monitoring thinking and behavior, known as "executive fucntions."

Children with ADHD have been noted to perform more poorly on tests of simple verbal fluency (Carte, Nigg, & Hinshaw, 1996; Grodzinsky & Diamond, 1992; Reader, Harris, Schuerholz, & Denckla, 1994), although others have not documented such differences (Fischer et al., 1990; Loge, Staton, & Beatty, 1990; McGee et al., 1989; Weyandt & Willis, 1994). These tests evaluate the ability to generate a diversity of verbal responses (usually

words) within a short time period (usually 1 minute), sometimes called "generativity." The discrepancy in findings across studies may pertain in part to the type of fluency test used in the study. Tests in which children generate words within semantic categories (Weyandt & Willis, 1994), such as names for animals or fruits, are easier and thus not as likely to discriminate children with ADHD from control children as those using more subtle organizing cues, such as letters (Grodzinsky & Diamond, 1992; Reader et al., 1994). Age may also be a factor, given that older children with ADHD may have far fewer difficulties on such tests than younger children with the disorder (Grodzinsky & Diamond, 1992; Fischer et al., 1990). Low statistical power due to small samples, and the use of nonclinical samples of milder severity (Loge et al., 1990; McGee et al., 1989), could also contribute to failures to find differences between children with ADHD and control groups in these studies. One recent study did not find ADHD to be associated with problems with either semantic or letter fluency, though its sample of children with ADHD ($n = 20$) was also small (Hurks et al., 2004). However, it did find that those with ADHD exhibited a greater lag in generating words during the first 15 seconds of the task than was evident in children with other psychiatric disorders or nondisabled control children. Another recent study did find deficits in verbal fluency on this same task (Geurts, Verte, Oosterlaan, Roeyers, & Sergeant, 2004).

As noted earlier, the best means of evaluating a large body of literature such as this, in which many studies had small sample sizes and yielded conflicting results, is to conduct a meta-analysis. This was recently done by Frazier et al. (2004) and included 13 studies of letter fluency and 9 of category or semantic fluency. The mean effect size for category fluency was not significant (0.46), but it was for letter fluency (0.54) allowing us to conclude that ADHD is associated with such a deficit of moderate effect size. It appears, then, that simple word fluency, particularly on tasks using letters as the generative rule, may be diminished in children with ADHD. This deficit may decline or even dissipate with age, and may even result from or at least be associated with a lag in initiating automated responding to such verbal tasks.

Another task of verbal fluency is the Hayling Sentence Completion Test, which comprises two parts. In Part A, subjects complete the missing word at the end of a sentence, the word being highly suggested by the content of the sentence. In Part B, subjects complete the sentence with a word that is irrelevant or nonsensical in the context of that sentence. Two scores are obtained. The first is for thinking time and is obtained by subtracting response latency scores from Part A from those for Part B, reflecting the additional time it takes a person to generate a novel word. The second score is an error score across both parts. Clark, Prior, and Kinsella (2000) found adolescents with ADHD to perform more poorly on this task than did control adolescents or those with ODD/CD, implying that the deficit may be relatively specific to ADHD. Shallice et al. (2002) used a junior version of this test with younger children with ADHD and also found significant differences from control children. Scores on the task were also associated with level of adaptive functioning in the adolescents (Clark et al., 2002). Taken together with the results for letter fluency tasks, the results are reasonably consistent in showing a difficulty with verbal fluency in ADHD.

The ability to rapidly name items, such as objects, letters, numbers, or colors, was once thought to be a function of attention and so might be expected to be impaired in children with ADHD. Studies to date, however, have found this deficit to be primarily associated with reading disorders and not with ADHD (Felton, Wood, Brown, Campbell, & Harter 1987; Semrud-Clikeman, Guy, Griffin, & Hynd, 2000). Rucklidge and Tannock (2002), however, did find that problems in rapid naming of objects were associated with ADHD, whereas problems in rapid naming of colors and numbers were related more to reading disorders. Similarly, impaired perception of voice and tone onset and of phonemes is entirely associated with reading disorders and not with ADHD (Breier et al., 2001).

Studies of more complex language fluency and discourse organization are much more likely to reveal problems in children with ADHD. As noted previously, children with ADHD appear to produce less speech in response to confrontational questioning than do control children (Tannock, 1996; Tannock & Schachar, 1996; Ludlow, Rapoport, Brown, & Mikkelson, 1979). They are also less competent in verbal problem-solving tasks (Douglas, 1983; Hamlett et al., 1987); are less capable of communicating task-essential information to

peers in cooperative tasks (Whalen, Henker, Collins, McAuliffe, & Vaux, 1979); and produce less information and less organized information in their story narratives (Tannock & Schachar, 1996; Tannock, Purvis, & Schachar, 1992; Zentall, 1988) or in describing their own strategies used during task performance (Hamlett et al., 1987). When no goal or task is specified, the verbal discourse of children with ADHD does not appear to differ as much from that of nondisabled children (Barkley et al., 1983; Zentall, 1988).

Given that ADHD is associated with difficulties in the organization, expression, and cohesion of language, it is unclear to what extent such problems differ from those that are known to be associated with thought disorders, such as schizophrenia. Only one study has examined this issue (Caplan, Guthrie, Tang, Nuechterlein, & Asarnow, 2001). It compared the speech samples of 115 children with ADHD to 88 children with schizophrenia and 190 nondisabled children of comparable IQ (ages 8–15 years). Both the children with ADHD and those with schizophrenia showed evidence of thought disorder relative to the control group. The group with ADHD, however, showed a narrower range of less severe thought disorder than did the group with schizophrenia. Relative to the control children, the group with ADHD used more illogical thinking, fewer conjunctions, but more lexical cohesion. Compared to the group with schizophrenia, the group with ADHD had lower scores on illogical thinking, greater referential and lexical cohesion, and no loose associations. Schizophrenia is therefore associated with greater illogical thinking, less cohesion, and greater loose associations than are seen in ADHD, which is mainly associated with milder difficulties with logical thinking. Both groups had more significant thought disorder among their younger members than among older children, suggesting some potential improvement in thinking difficulties with age. Interestingly, evidence from this study showed that the thinking problems evident in the group with ADHD were associated with problems with executive functioning (working memory), inattention, and IQ, whereas this was not the case in the group with schizophrenia. It is therefore possible that the thought disorder evident in ADHD may be secondary to the difficulties ADHD creates in executive functioning.

The relationship of ADHD to the language

processing problem known as central auditory processing disorder (CAPD) is uncertain. Some researchers imply that they may not be separate disorders at all, given that teacher ratings of inattention in children with ADHD were significantly related to several tests of auditory processing (Gascon, Johnson, & Burd, 1986). The problem here is largely though not entirely due to problems in definition. CAPD has been generously defined as comprising deficits in the processing of audible signals that cannot be ascribed to peripheral hearing sensitivity or intellectual impairment—in essence, inattention in the auditory domain. The nub of the issue is that CAPD may involve distractibility and inattentiveness, as well as difficulties with memory, reading, spelling, and written language. As Riccio, Hynd, Cohen, Hall, and Molt (1994) note, it is this inclusion of inattention (albeit in the auditory domain) in the conceptualization of CAPD that is so problematic. It creates an automatic overlap with ADHD symptoms, the inattention of which is thought to be generalized or transmodal rather than limited to a single sense modality (audition). Children with ADHD often have difficulties with auditory vigilance or attention (Gascon et al., 1986; Keith & Engineer, 1991), and so they may automatically qualify for a diagnosis of CAPD on that basis alone. Some (Moss & Sheiffe, 1994) have more appropriately restricted the definition of CAPD to deficits in processing speech and language specifically, which would greatly assist with determining the degree of overlap with ADHD and would be likely to restrict it. If that is the case, then one would anticipate little or no conceptual overlap between disorders, given that (as noted above) difficulties with speech perception, phoneme awareness, and language processing generally are associated with LI and reading disorders, not with ADHD.

To study the overlap of these disorders, Riccio et al. (1994) studied children referred to a speech and language clinic and to a neuropsychology clinic who met diagnostic criteria for CAPD. These criteria included evidence of impairment on at least two of four auditory processing tasks involving both speech and nonspeech information. Of 30 children with CAPD, 50% met criteria for a diagnosis of ADHD according to the third revised edition of the *Diagnostic and Statistical Manual of Mental Disorders* (DSM-III-R; American Psychiatric Association, 1987). The authors also utilized the older DSM-III criteria, which permitted subtyping of the subjects into those having ADD + H and ADD – H. In this case, 33.3% of the subjects had ADHD, half of whom fell into each subtype. Although the prevalence of ADHD among children referred for and meeting diagnostic criteria for CAPD was higher than that expected of a typical population (i.e., 3–5%), it is similar to the rate of ADHD found among children referred to a speech and language clinic and diagnosed with such speech and language difficulties, up to 46% of whom have ADHD according to DSM-III criteria (Baker & Cantwell, 1987; Cohen et al., 2000). What is clear from this study is that CAPD and ADHD are not identical disorders if more rigorous definitions and criteria are used to determine the presence of CAPD, apart from merely clinical complaints of auditory inattentiveness. It remains uncertain whether CAPD should be considered a valid disorder apart from other already well-documented language disorders of children or whether it merely represents a more recent relabeling of those previously identified language disorders. It is interesting to note that among children with ADHD and evidence of CAPD, some researchers have found that their auditory processing deficits improve significantly with stimulant medication (Gascon et al., 1986; Keith & Engineer, 1991), suggesting that the inattention due to ADHD may have been mainly involved in the diagnosis of CAPD. Others have not found such medication effects, however (Dalebout, Nelson, Hleto, & Frentheway, 1991).

DEFICIENT RULE-GOVERNED BEHAVIOR

Although the idea is still not yet widely accepted, some investigators suggested since the 1980s that poor rule-governed behavior, or difficulties with adherence to rules and instructions, may also be a primary deficit or at least an associated condition of ADHD in children (American Psychiatric Association, 1987, 1994; Barkley, 1981, 1989, 1990; Kendall & Braswell, 1985). Care is taken here to exclude poor compliance that may stem from sensory handicaps (i.e., deafness); from impaired language development; or from refusal to obey, as in ODD. Rules and instructions, then, are hypothesized not to influence or guide behavior in children with ADHD as well as in typical children.

Rules are contingency-specifying stimuli; they specify a relationship among an event, a response, and the consequences likely to occur for that response. Language provides a substantial number of such stimuli. Skinner (1953) hypothesized that this influence of language over behavior occurs in three stages: (1) the control of behavior by the language of others; (2) the progressive control of behavior by self-directed and eventually private speech, as discussed earlier; and (3) the creation of new rules by the individual, which comes about through the use of self-directed questions (second-order rules). Rule-governed behavior appears to provide a means of sustaining behavior across large gaps in time among the units of a behavioral contingency (event–response–outcome). By formulating rules, the individual can construct novel, complex (hierarchically organized), and prolonged behavioral chains. These rules can then provide the template for creating the appropriate sequences of behavioral chains, guiding behavior toward the attainment of a future goal (Cerutti, 1989; Hayes, 1989; Skinner, 1969). By means of this process, the individual's behavior is no longer under the total control of the immediate surrounding context. Behavior is now shifted to control by internally represented information (in this case, covert verbal behavior [self-speech] and the rules it generates).

Do children with ADHD manifest a delay in rule-governed behavior or the ability to comply with or complete verbal instructions? Available evidence, though hardly definitive, is suggestive of such a problem. Children with ADHD have been observed to be less compliant with directions and commands given by their mothers than are nondisabled children (see Danforth, Barkley, & Stokes, 1991, for a review). The problem seems most acute, however, in the subgroup having ODD; this implies that although ADHD interferes with compliance, much of the difficulty in compliance may be attributable to the willful defiance characteristic of ODD. In addition, children with ADHD appear to be less able to restrict their behavior in accordance with experimenter instructions to do so during lab playroom observations when rewarding activities are available; the latter findings are not always consistently obtained, however (see Luk, 1985, for a review). What evidence there is suggests that when rules compete with prevailing reinforcement in a given situation, the rule is less likely to control behavior. And stud-

ies discussed in Chapter 2 (this volume) have found groups with ADHD to be much less able to resist forbidden temptations than same-age nondisabled peers. Such rule following seems to be particularly difficult for children with ADHD when the rules compete with rewards available for committing rule violations (Hinshaw, Heller, & McHale, 1992; Hinshaw, Simmel, & Heller, 1995). These results may indicate problems with the manner in which rules and instructions control behavior in children with ADHD, especially if the rule conflicts with rewards or other consequences that may be co-occurring in the same context.

Further evidence consistent with a developmental delay in rule-governed behavior comes from studies showing that children with ADHD are less adequate at problem solving (Douglas, 1983; Hamlett et al., 1987; Tant & Douglas, 1982), and are also less likely to use organizational rules and strategies in their performance of memory tasks (August, 1987; Butterbaugh et al., 1989; Douglas & Benezra, 1990; Voelker, Carter, Sprague, Gdowski, & Lachar, 1989). Problem solving and the discovery of strategies may be direct functions of rule-governed behavior and the self-questioning associated with it (Cerutti, 1989).

Hayes (1989) has set forth a number of features that would characterize rule-governed behavior. The features can be considered predictions about the types of deficiencies that may be evident in children with ADHD, if their behavior, is indeed less rule-governed. Some evidence does seem to exist for these predicted deficiencies in children with ADHD:

1. These children demonstrate significantly greater variability in patterns of responding to laboratory tasks, such as reaction time or continuous-performance tests (CPTs) (for reviews, see Frazier et al., 2004; Corkum & Siegel, 1993; Douglas, 1983; and Douglas & Peters, 1978; see also van der Meere & Sergeant, 1988a, 1988b; Zahn, Krusei, & Rapoport, 1991).

2. They perform better under conditions of immediate versus delayed rewards (Neef, Bicard, & Endo, 2001; for reviews of evidence for this item through item 5, see Barkley, 1989; Douglas, 1983; Haenlein & Caul, 1987; Sagvolden, Wultz, Moser, Moser, & Morkrid, 1989).

3. They have significantly greater problems

with task performance when delays are imposed within the task and as these delays increase in duration.

4. They display a greater and more rapid decline in task performance as contingencies of reinforcement move from being continuous to intermittent.

5. They show a greater disruption in task performance when noncontingent consequences occur during the task (Douglas & Parry, 1994; Freibergs & Douglas, 1969; Parry & Douglas, 1983; Schweitzer & Sulzer-Azaroff, 1995; Sonuga-Barke, Taylor, & Hepinstall, 1992; Sonuga-Barke, Taylor, Sembi, & Smith, 1992; Zahn et al., 1991).

6. They are less able to work for delayed rewards in delay-of-gratification tasks (Rapport, Tucker, DuPaul, Merlo, & Stoner, 1986) and show a steeper discounting of the value of the delayed reward than do control groups of children (Barkley, Edwards, Laneri, Fletcher, & Metevia, 2001).

However, others have not found evidence for item 4—namely, that partial reinforcement schedules are necessarily detrimental to the task performances of children with ADHD, relative to their performance under continuous reinforcement. Instead, the schedule of reinforcement appears to interact with task difficulty in determining the effect of reinforcement on performance by these children (Barber & Milich, 1989). It is also possible that differences in the delay periods between reinforcement contribute to these inconsistent findings; if delay intervals are sufficiently brief, no differences between children with ADHD and typical children under partial reinforcement should be noted. Thus studies of reinforcement schedules and children with ADHD cannot be interpreted in any straightforward fashion as supportive of the view that poor rule-governed behavior underlies any problem these children may have with partial reinforcement schedules. Barber, Milich, and Welsh (1996) have suggested that an inability to sustain effort over time may better explain these findings. Thus these results seem more suggestive of poor self-regulation of motivation than of just a problem with rule-governed behavior.

The problems with rule-governed behavior suggested here indicate that those with ADHD seem to have more trouble in doing what they know than in knowing what to do. Such a problem was evident in a study by Greve, Williams, and Dickens (1996), in which children with ADHD displayed deficiencies in sorting cards by a rule, even when the examiner gave them the rule they needed to do so. Children with ADHD have been shown to have more difficulty not only in spontaneously developing a strategy to organize material to be memorized (August, 1987), but also in following that rule over time (August, 1987). Conte and Regehr (1991) also found that hyperactive children were less likely to transfer the rules they had acquired on a prior task to a new task, consistent with this hypothesis.

Other evidence, albeit less direct, also suggests that ADHD is associated with a problem in poor governing of behavioral performance knowledge. Studies of hyperactive–impulsive children or those with ADHD find them to be more prone to accidents than are typical children (Barkley, 2001; Bijur, Golding, Haslum, & Kurzon, 1988; Methany & Fisher, 1984; Taylor, Sandberg, Thorley, & Giles, 1991; see "Accidental Injuries," below); yet they are not deficient in their knowledge of safety or accident prevention (Mori & Peterson, 1995). We (Barkley, Murphy, & Kwasnik, 1996b) have also found that teens and young adults with ADHD have significantly more motor vehicle accidents and other driving risks (see "Driving-Related Difficulties," below), but they demonstrate no deficiencies in their knowledge of driving, safety, and accident prevention (see also Barkley, 2004).

In any case, it is quite common clinically to hear these children described as not listening, failing to initiate compliance to instructions, being unable to maintain compliance to an instruction over time, and being poor at adhering to directions associated with a task. All these descriptors are problems in the regulation and inhibition of behavior, especially by rules. Their failure to develop adequately in ADHD speaks to serious problems with both behavioral inhibition and the extent to which rules may guide behavior in this disorder.

DELAYED INTERNALIZATION OF LANGUAGE

It is conceivable that the origin of the difficulties with rule-governed behavior in children with ADHD may reside in the delayed internalization of language consistently demonstrated in these children to date.

The Internalization of Language

Vygotsky's theory on the development of private speech remains the most widely accepted view on the topic at this time (Berk, 1992, 1994; Diaz & Berk, 1992; Vygotsky, 1978, 1987). Such speech is defined as "speech uttered aloud by children that is addressed either to the self or to no one in particular" (Berk & Potts, 1991, p. 358). In its earliest stages, it is thought spoken out loud that accompanies ongoing action. As it matures, it functions as a form of self-guidance and direction by assisting with the formulation of a plan that will eventually assist the child in controlling his or her own actions (Berk & Potts, 1991). Gradually, as speech becomes progressively more private or internalized and as behavior comes increasingly under its control, such speech is now internal, verbal thought that can exert a substantial controlling influence over behavior. This internalization of speech proceeds in an orderly fashion. It seems to evolve from more conversational, task-irrelevant, and possibly self-stimulating forms of speech to more descriptive, task-relevant forms, and then on to more prescriptive and self-guiding speech. It then progresses to more private, inaudible speech and finally to fully private, subvocal speech (Berk, 1992, 1994; Berk & Garvin, 1984; Berk & Potts, 1991; Bivens & Berk, 1990; Frauenglass & Diaz, 1985; Kohlberg, Yaeger, & Hjertholm, 1968). Ample research exists to show that overt private speech increases with the difficulty of the task being done and has more of an impact on performance in the next encounter with the same task than with current performance (Berk, 1992; Diaz & Berk, 1992). Private speech thus serves self-regulatory functions. It helps to guide behavior across time, to facilitate problem solving, and to generate rules and meta-rules (rules that lead to other rules).

Delays in the Internalization of Speech in ADHD

Studies of hyperactive children or those with ADHD have consistently found them are to be less mature in their self-speech and developmentally delayed in the sequence or progression from public to private self-speech (Rosenbaum & Baker, 1984; Berk & Potts, 1991; Copeland, 1979; Gordon, 1979). Among the early studies, the most rigorous were those of Berk and her colleagues (Berk & Potts, 1991; Berk & Landau, 1993; Landau, Berk, & Mangione, 1996). In their initial study (Berk & Potts, 1991), children with ADHD and nondisabled children were observed in their natural classroom settings. The occurrences of private (self-directed but publicly observable) speech were recorded while the children were engaged in math work at their desks. These observations were classified into one of three levels of private speech believed to reflect the maturational progression of such private speech as originally proposed by Vygotsky. Level I speech consisted of task-irrelevant utterances. Level II consisted of task-relevant externalized private speech, such as describing one's own actions and giving self-guiding comments; asking task-relevant, self-answered questions; reading aloud and sounding out words; and expressing task-relevant affect. Level III comprised task-relevant external manifestations of inner speech. These included inaudible muttering but mouthing of clear words related to the task, and lip and tongue movements associated with the task.

The results indicated that the overall amount of private speech was not significantly different between groups, but differences were observed in the levels of private speech employed by each group. The group with ADHD used significantly more Level II and significantly less Level III speech than did their matched control counterparts. In contrast, to the findings of Copeland (1979), who observed more task-irrelevant speech in her early study, the two groups in the Berk and Potts (1991) study did not differ in their use of Level I (task-irrelevant) speech. Berk and Potts (1991) analyzed their results as a function of age of the children in these groups and found significant differences in the developmental patterns. No significant effects related to age were evident in Level I speech or in total private speech. But children with ADHD at all ages engaged in more Level II speech than did control children. Both groups declined significantly in their use of this level of private speech with age. Regarding Level III speech, children with ADHD were found to increase markedly in this level of speech between ages 6–7 and 8–9, leveling off at ages 10–11. Control children, in contrast, remained high in their use of this form of speech across the two youngest ages (6–7, 8–9 years) and then declined in their use of this level of speech by the oldest age group (10–11 years). This decline in Level III speech was interpreted as being consistent with Vygotsky's theoretical position that speech by this age is moving to being fully internalized (covert) and so less observable. To summarize, children with and without ADHD show a similar pattern of development of private speech, but those with ADHD are considerably delayed in this process relative to control children.

It is important to demonstrate in such a study that the private speech of children serves a controlling or governing function over behavior. Berk and Potts (1991) correlated the private speech categories of these children with observations of the motor behavior associated with the task, as well as with their attention to the task. Children in both groups who were more likely to have difficulty sustaining attention were found to display more Level II forms of private speech. Both Level I and Level II speech were also negatively correlated with focused attention and were positively correlated with diversions from seatwork. Level II speech was also significantly and positively associated with the amount of task-facilitating behavior shown by the children. Greater degrees of Level III speech, thought to reflect greater maturity, were significantly correlated with degree of focused attention and were negatively associated with amount of task diversion (off-task behavior). Interestingly, only the boys with ADHD showed a significant positive association between Level III speech and self-stimulating forms of behavior. The authors interpreted such findings as indicative of a delay in speech's effects in gaining control over behavior as it proceeds to internalization.

Three additional studies further support this conclusion. Berk and Landau (1993) observed 56 children with LDs (some of whom had ADHD) and 56 nondisabled children in grades 3–6 while they performed their daily math and language assignments at their desks in their natural classroom settings. When the children with both ADHD and LDs were separated and contrasted with the other two groups (children with pure LDs and controls), the results showed that the first group displayed more than three times as much task-relevant, externalized (Level II) speech as did the second group and about four times as much as the control children. The children with ADHD and LDs also demonstrated significantly less Level III speech, which is the most mature stage of internalization measured in this study, than did the children with pure LDs or the control chil-

dren. These findings suggest that ADHD contributes more than LDs to a delay in the internalization of speech.

In a later study, Landau et al. (1996) compared the self-speech of impulsive and non-impulsive children during their performance of math problems. These children were not clinically diagnosed as having ADHD, but represented 55 regular school students in first through third grades who were rated as either most or least impulsive by their teachers. Impulsive children were found to be significantly more dependent on externalized private speech for problem solving than were the nonimpulsive children. However, as the level of difficulty of the problems rose to becoming very challenging, the private speech of nonimpulsive children increased, as predicted by Vygotsky and shown in other research (Berk, 1992), while it decreased for impulsive children. In general, impulsive children used more task-irrelevant, less mature speech as the math problems became more challenging; the nonimpulsive group did not use task-irrelevant speech at any level of difficulty, but increased their task-relevant speech as problem difficulty increased.

Subsequently, Winsler (1998) evaluated the self-speech of children with ADHD during a joint problem-solving task with their parents (mostly mothers) and also while the children were performing a task alone, and compared these results to those for control parent–child dyads. As shown in other studies (Danforth et al., 1991; see also Chapter 4), the parents of the children with ADHD used more negative verbal control strategies, used poorer-quality scaffolding of their speech (assistance with problem solving), and withdrew their control less over the collaborative task than did the parents of the control children. Also consistent with substantial prior research, the children with ADHD were more noncompliant and off-task than the control group. More to the point of this section, results indicated that the children with ADHD used more task-irrelevant speech, used less speech related to the ongoing task and activities, and showed a delay in the progression of speech through the levels discussed above.

In contrast to these findings, a later study by Winsler, Diaz, Atencio, McCarthy, and Chabay (2000) evaluated preschool children at high risk for attention and behavior problems at age 3 years and again over a 2-year follow-up period in their self-regulation, private speech, and speech–action coordination. Note that these children are not clinically referred or diagnosed as having ADHD. The at-risk children showed more spontaneous speech across all tasks, but no differences from control children in amounts of task-irrelevant speech or in speech–action coordination. Both groups showed increasing silence during the task with success over time. Developmental changes in private speech were associated with task performance, increasing speech–action coordination, and a measure of executive functioning (trail making). This study shows that private speech does serve a controlling function over behavior, increases such control with age, and is related to some extent to level of executive functioning. But it did not find that children at risk for behavioral problems were uniquely or qualitatively different in their private speech, or that they were delayed in this process—only that they verbalized more than control children. Given that the children in this study were not clinically diagnosed with ADHD, the study has less relevance to our purposes here, though it does provide support for other issues involved in the development of private speech.

All of the studies described above that used children with ADHD or impulsive children provide considerable support for the conclusion that ADHD and impulsiveness more generally are associated with a significant delay in the internalization of speech. Although behaviorally at-risk preschool children may not manifest such a delay, highly impulsive children as well as those with clinically diagnosed ADHD consistently do so.

GREATER VARIABILITY OF TASK PERFORMANCE

Another characteristic that some believe to be a primary deficit in children with ADHD is their excessive variability of task or work performance over time. Douglas (1972) first described this problem while observing children with ADHD performing reaction time tasks or serial problem solving. Many others have reported it since (see Kuntsi, Oosterlaan, & Stevenson, 2001; Rucklidge & Tannock, 2002). It is a finding repeatedly noted on other tasks as well. Researchers often find that these children's standard deviation of performance on multitrial tasks is considerably larger than

that seen in typical children. Both the number of problems or items they complete and the accuracy of their performance change substantially from moment to moment, trial to trial, or day to day in the same setting. Teachers often anecdotally report much greater variability in homework and test grades, as well as in-class performance, than is seen in typical children. An inspection of the teacher's grade book for a child with ADHD often reveals this pattern of performance. Similarly, parents may find that their children with ADHD perform certain chores swiftly and accurately on some occasions, yet sloppily if at all on other days.

MEMORY AND PLANNING DIFFICULTIES

Deficits in children with ADHD have not typically been found on traditional measures of memory, such as recall, long-term storage, and long-term retrieval (Barkley, DuPaul, & McMurray, 1990; Douglas, 1983). However, on tasks thought to assess working memory, a number of studies have documented deficits in this type of executive function (Barkley, 1997a, 1997b). "Working memory" has been defined as the capacity to hold information actively in mind that will be used to guide a subsequent response (Fuster, 1997; Goldman-Rakic, 1995). The construct has been assessed in neuropsychological research with a variety of tasks. Nonverbal working memory has been less studied than verbal working memory in general neuropsychological research (see Becker, 1994, for reviews). Tasks assessing nonverbal working memory typically involve delayed memory recall for objects and particularly for their spatial location. Measures assessing nonverbal planning ability are also considered to fall within this domain (Barkley, 1997b), though such measures rarely reflect pure assessments of nonverbal abilities. I review evidence relating to nonverbal working memory deficits associated with ADHD first, sparse as it is, before turning to the evidence pertaining to verbal working memory, which is far more substantial.

Nonverbal Working Memory

Nonverbal working memory can probably be usefully subdivided into visual–spatial working memory (e.g., memory for the spatial location of objects or for designs), sequential working memory (e.g., memory for event sequences), and the sense of time (e.g., memory for time durations).

Visual–Spatial Working Memory

Research on visual–spatial working memory in children with ADHD is very limited. Some evidence for deficits in this form of working memory comes from findings of impaired memory for spatial location (Mariani & Barkley, 1997) among preschool-age children with ADHD. However, Weyandt and Willis (1994) were unable to find such deficits associated with ADHD in an apparently related task requiring visual search of a display for a target item.

The use of visual–spatial working memory might seem to be involved in the organization and reproduction of complex designs, such as in the Rey–Osterrieth Complex Figure Drawing Test. Studies of children with ADHD identified organizational deficits on this task (Douglas & Benezra, 1990; Grodzinsky & Diamond, 1992; Sadeh, Ariel, & Inbar, 1996; Seidman, Benedict, et al., 1995). Yet two studies did not find such group differences (Moffitt & Silva, 1988; Reader et al., 1994), while another two found deficits only in children having both ADHD and reading disorders (McGee et al., 1989; Seidman, Biederman, Monuteaux, Doyle, & Faraone, 2001). Two of these studies reporting nonsignificant results employed samples drawn from community screenings of children, where the severity of ADHD would probably not be as great as among clinic-referred children. Most of the studies that found group differences used clinic-referred samples.

When studies are small and inconsistent as these clearly are, it pays (once again) to conduct a meta-analysis using all of their results. A recent meta-analysis (Frazier et al., 2004) of six studies using this task did not find a significant group difference (mean effect size) on accuracy scores for either the immediate-copy or delayed-recall portions of this task (effect sizes of 0.24 and 0.26, respectively), but organization of the children's drawings was not specifically examined in this analysis. Evidence to date therefore suggests that while accuracy of design copying may not be a problem for children with ADHD, the organization of their copies may be impaired, particularly in clinic-referred groups with ADHD.

Likewise, two studies of spatial working memory in children with ADHD by Karatekin (2004; Karatekin & Asarnow, 1998) produced conflicting results. Other negative studies have also been reported. Another spatial working memory task is self-ordered pointing, requiring children to point to a new or different design on a new card that had not appeared on previous cards. A recent study employing this task found no significant differences between c children with ADHD and a control group (Geurts et al., 2004). A study of preschool children using a nonverbal paired-associates learning task (associating pictures with noises) found that deficits in this task were not associated with severity of ADHD symptoms once IQ was controlled for (though, as noted earlier, this is a questionable procedure). Eye movement tasks have been used to examine spatial working memory; in such tasks, a person must remember a position of an object across a delay period and then, when cued, move his or her eyes toward that location. A study using this task reported girls with ADHD to be more impaired than control girls (Castellanos et al., 2000).

To summarize, research on visual–spatial working memory in ADHD is rather limited, characterized by a diversity of tasks believed to evaluate this construct, and plagued by conflicting results. What findings there are seem to be largely negative. For the moment, we must conclude that such a deficit may not be associated with ADHD. More evidence exists to show a difficulty with the organization of copying of spatial information (designs), at least among clinic-referred children with ADHD.

Sequential Working Memory

The capacity to hold a sequence of information in mind may comprise another aspect of nonverbal working memory. Such a capacity would seem to be involved in the ability to imitate the complex and lengthy behavioral sequences performed by others that may be novel to a child. Several studies employed rudimentary imitation tasks that could be taken to suggest a deficit in such imitative sequential behavior. These studies found that children with ADHD are less proficient at imitating increasingly lengthy and novel sequences of three simple motor gestures (fist, palm on side, palm down) like those required on the Kaufman Assessment Battery for Children Hand Movements Test than are typical children (Breen, 1989; Grodzinsky & Diamond, 1992; Mariani & Barkley, 1997). It is less clear whether this reflects a problem with memory or with motor coordination.

Another study used the "Simon game" as a measure of sequential working memory (Barkley, Edwards, et al., 2001). In this game, the subject uses a large plastic disk that contains four different-colored keys, each of which emits a musical note when pressed. The game generates increasingly longer note sequences that the participant must imitate or recreate by pressing the buttons in the proper melodic sequence. No differences were found between teens with ADHD ($n = 101$) and control teens ($n = 39$) on this task, even though two other studies found adults with ADHD to perform less well than control adults (Murphy, Barkley, & Bush, 2001).

A recent study found a deficit in sequential memory associated with ADHD on the Finger Windows subtest of the Wide Range Assessment of Memory and Learning. In this task, the examiner sticks a pencil through a sequence of holes in a card; the child must then replicate this sequence by sticking his or her finger through the same holes in the same sequential order. But the same deficit was also found in children with LI, with or without ADHD, implying that it is a characteristic of both ADHD and LI (McInnes, Humphries, Hogg-Johnson, & Tannock, 2003).

A commonly used task of sequencing ability that involves memory to a small extent is the Trail Making Test from the Halstead–Reitan Neuropsychological Test Battery. Part A simply has a child connect a series of numbered circles (1, 2, 3, etc.) in their proper sequence as quickly as possible, using a pencil. Part B is more difficult and requires the child to alternate number with letter sequences while connecting the circles (1, A, 2, B, 3, C, etc.). A recent meta-analysis of 14 studies (Frazier et al., 2004) found a weighted mean effect size for Part A of 0.40 (95% CI = 0.26–0.54) and for Part B of 0.59 (95% CI = 0.46–0.72), but, surprisingly, these were not statistically significant.

The evidence for a sequential working memory deficit is conflicting. Studies of hand movement sequences are the most consistent in finding such a deficit, while those involving trail-making sequences have not revealed such a deficit.

Sense of Time

The sense of time is in part a function of working memory, though it involves other neuropsychological systems as well. The psychological sense of time is multidimensional. Those dimensions most often studied are (1) time perception, (2) motor timing, (3) time estimation, (4) time production, (5) time reproduction, and (6) routine use of time and time management in natural settings (Zakay, 1990). The processing of temporal information at intervals greater than 100 milliseconds (ms) is effortful and does not appear to be automatic as part of normal encoding activities during processing of nontemporal information (Michon & Jackson, 1984). Intervals shorter than 100 ms are typically perceived as instantaneous, while those between roughly 100 ms and 5 seconds (s) are perceived as existing within the temporal now. Intervals of roughly 5–30 s require working memory for accurate recall (in adults, at least), while durations beyond 30 s may exceed working memory capacity and thus require reference to long-term memory (Mimura, Kinsbourne, & O'Connor, 2000; Zakay, 1990). Though inexact, these time parameters suggest that both the demand for memory and type of memory needed are functions of duration length (Mimura et al., 2000; Zakay, 1990). Most or all of these aspects of sense of time may be impaired in children with ADHD. Aspects of timing behavior are mediated largely, though not entirely, by the prefrontal cortex, basal ganglia, and cerebellum (Fuster, 1997). These are also the candidate regions likely to be associated with ADHD. Timing may be disrupted by disease or injury to the prefrontal cortex and its connections to the basal ganglia, as found in Parkinson disease (Pastor, Artieda, Jahanshahi, & Obeso, 1992) and frontal lobe lesions (Mimura et al., 2000). All this implies that ADHD may be associated with impaired components of the sense of time.

Time Perception. Time perception typically involves the presentation of pairs of relatively short-duration stimuli (often in milliseconds) to a participant, who then must make judgments about differences in the durations of these intervals (same or different). One study found children with ADHD to be impaired in this sort of time discrimination of very short intervals (between 1,000 and 1,300 ms); the paired stimuli needed to differ by at least 50 ms to be perceived as different by the group with ADHD (Smith, Taylor, Rogers, Newman, & Rubia, 2002). Another study did not find group differences at short durations (500–550 ms), but did find that children with ADHD made more errors of discrimination at a longer duration (4 s) (Radonovich & Mostofsky, 2003).

Motor Timing. Motor timing reflects the ability of the individual either to freely reproduce a repetitive motor response at a regular interval, or to synchronize (match) a repetitive motor response to a brief, repetitive stimulus (Rubia, Noorloos, Smith, Gunning, & Sergeant, 2003). In some cases, the participant must then sustain the timing of the repetitive response when the timing cues are removed (Harrington, Haaland, & Hermanowicz, 1998). For instance, a person may be asked to tap a finger repeatedly in a regular rhythm (free tapping) or to a regularly recurring stimulus (synchronized tapping). The measure is typically the average of the intervals (duration) between the subject's finger taps once the time cues are withdrawn, or it can be the average deviations between the sample timing duration and the subject's own tapping interval durations. Neuropsychologists have found this form of timing (< 1 s) to involve the basal ganglia (Harrington et al., 1998; Rao et al., 1997) and cerebellum (Mangels, Ivry, & Shimizu, 1998). Given that both of these structures have been implicated in ADHD (see Chapter 5), children with ADHD should be impaired in short-interval motor timing. Only one study has examined this sort of motor timing, and it found children with ADHD to show more variable motor responses only on the synchronized-tapping task (not on the free-tapping task) than were seen in control children (Rubia et al., 2003). This is a topic worthy of future research.

Time Estimation. Time estimation is the individual's ability to accurately perceive the duration of a temporal interval, typically lasting a few seconds or longer (Zakay, 1990). In "prospective" time estimation, the person is warned to pay attention to a sample duration that is then provided to the subject—for instance, by turning a light bulb on and off. The subject is then asked to verbally report the duration of the interval, usually in seconds. As noted earlier, the extent to which working memory and long-term memory are needed here is a function of the duration (> 5 s and >30 s, respectively). This form of timing is often facilitated by the individual's ability to refer to

some repetitive internal or external metric, such as verbally counting to him- or herself. As a result, it is not exclusively a nonverbal working memory task. The duration must then be translated into a standard clock metric (typically seconds). This component hinges directly on the amount of effortful attention allocated to processing the passage of time (Zakay, 1990, 1992). Before 5 years of age, typical children have considerable difficulty with this task, regardless of how short the durations. But by age 5, they begin to rely mainly on self-counting to assess the interval and convert it to standard time units (Zakay, 1992).

In "retrospective" time estimation, the individual is not warned to attend to time, but is simply asked at the end of an activity or event (or later) how long he or she believes the activity or event lasted. It does not depend on self-counting, but instead relies heavily on the individual's ability to extract any traces of temporal information after the fact from his or her memory for the event (Brown, 1985). It also depends on the extent to which the person may have been allocating attention to such temporal cues during that event. Forewarning the person to attend to temporal information, as in prospective estimation, often increases his or her accuracy on retrospective tasks.

I do not believe that ADHD should be associated with a basic problem in prospective time perception (estimation). Demands for inhibition and working memory seem less involved (though not entirely absent) in this type of task than in the other timing tasks below, given that the individual often merely counts as a metric for timing the interval. Thus only the current ongoing counting has to be held in mind, and that only briefly. For this reason, any deficits on this paradigm found in those with ADHD would be expected to be of a far lesser magnitude, if present at all, than in the time reproduction tasks discussed below. Several of my previous studies seem to bear out this prediction, in that a problem with prospective time estimation has not been found with ADHD in teens (Barkley, Edwards, et al., 2001) or in young adults (Barkley, Murphy, & Kwasnik, 1996a). A small deficit was evident in adults with ADHD at long intervals (Barkley, Murphy, & Bush, 2001). A more recent study also failed to find time estimation problems in ADHD (Smith et al., 2002), but it used only a single trial of a single duration (10 s). Rubia et al. (2003) also found greater errors and variability in their group with ADHD on a time estimation and discrimination task, in which children had to decide whether two stimuli (airplanes) presented on a computer screen in succession occurred for the same duration or a different duration. Evidence for a prospective time estimation deficit in ADHD is therefore somewhat conflicting.

However, two additional factors in the task may lead to impairment in prospective time estimation in those with ADHD where little or none would ordinarily exist. The first factor occurs when distractors are presented during the task. Distractors frequently result in greater errors of estimation in typical children (Zakay, 1992). Given the greater distractibility associated with ADHD (see Chapter 2 and the discussion below of TV viewing), time estimation may become more disrupted than usual by distracting events presented to children with ADHD. The second factor in the task that could lead to disrupted time estimation is the poor sustained attention (persistence) that is characteristic of these children. They may not be able to sustain their attention to relatively long sample time intervals to estimate the duration accurately. Longer time durations are also likely to be more taxing of working memory than shorter ones, at least up to 30 s for adults (Mimura et al., 2000). These reasons suggest that the accuracy of estimation should decline more markedly in those with ADHD than it does in nondisabled children as the duration of the sample intervals increase. This is what we found in adults with ADHD (Barkley, Murphy, & Bush, 2001). But it was not evident in our smaller study of adults with ADHD, perhaps due to low power (Barkley et al., 1996a).

Predictions for retrospective (remembered) time estimations among children with ADHD are less clear. Such estimations rely more heavily on long-term memory, the extent to which an individual can extract temporal information from memory, the degree to which the individual may have been attending to nontemporal versus temporal cues during the task or event to be estimated, level of arousal during the event, the delay between the event and the requested recall of that event, and several other factors (Block, 1990; Vitulli & Shepherd, 1996; Vitulli & Nemeth, 2001; Zakay, 1990; Zakay & Block, 1997). As a consequence, retrospective estimations are often less accurate and of shorter duration than prospective (forewarned or experienced) time estimations in typical children and adults. However, the longer the delay between event and recall of it, the longer the estimated duration becomes, often leading to overestimation of the actual duration if the delay in recall is long enough. Whether or not children with ADHD manifest problems with retrospective timing would seem to depend to a large degree on their long-term memory ability. Since this is not typically impaired in children with ADHD, retrospective time estimates should not be different in children with ADHD than in nondisabled children. Past results in this area for groups with ADHD are mixed. Teens with ADHD did show deficits in retrospective estimates but only under low-arousal conditions (Shaw & Brown, 1999), whereas children with ADHD showed no such deficits (Barkley, Koplowitz, Anderson, & McMurray, 1997). On a more complicated task, students with elevated ADHD symptoms retrospectively estimated that daily activities took less time than did students without ADHD, but not after group differences in IQ were controlled (Grskovic, Zentall, & Stormont-Spurgin, 1995). Children defined as impulsive gave less accurate retrospective time estimates than control children (Goldman & Everett, 1985), but these children did not have clinical cases of ADHD. Numerous limitations exist in the methods of these past studies, warranting a closer examination of time estimation in ADHD in future research.

Time Production. Time production reflects the ability to generate a verbally specified clock time interval (Zakay, 1992). In these tasks, participants may be asked to turn a flashlight on and off for a verbally defined interval, such as 5 or 10 s. Like time estimation, time production is thought to make less demand on working memory than reproduction tasks do (see below), as the individual may simply self-count the requested duration with little need to hold the duration online, in mind. I would predict that those with ADHD should have little or no impairment in time production except, again, as a consequence of the two factors noted earlier: distractors and unusually lengthy sample durations.

My colleagues and I have studied time production in only one prior, small study of young adults with ADHD (Barkley et al., 1996a). Partially consistent with this prediction, no group differences were evident, not even at longer durations (up to 60 s). The small sample size (n's = 25 children with ADHD and 23 controls), however, greatly limited the statistical power of the study to test for interactions of group with duration. Even so, the results are consistent with those of Mimura et al. (2000), who did not find time production problems in patients with frontal lobe lesions. However, Cappella, Gentile, and Juliano (1977) demonstrated time production deficits in two studies of hyperactive children. The first employed relatively long durations (15, 30, and 60 s). The second study used shorter ones (7, 15, and 30 s). Both studies found hyperactive children to produce longer estimates than controls; group differences were greatest at the longest durations. This research is problematic, however, as it did not use children with clinically diagnosed ADHD, but children rated by teachers as hyperactive and distractible. An attempt to replicate the research using just 6 hyperactive boys and 135 controls failed to do so, but the hyperactive group was so small that it provided very low power, and only a 30-s interval was tested (Senior, Towne, & Huessy, 1979). Walker (1982) compared 20 impulsive boys (defined as such by the Matching Familiar Figures Test) to 20 reflective boys and found no differences in production of six 12-s intervals. In sum, the studies are conflicting: One of hyperactive children found production problems, but two others using either hyperactive or impulsive children and one of adults with ADHD did not find this to be the case. Given the substantial and varied limitations of these studies, further work in ADHD is in order.

Time Reproduction. Time reproduction paradigms are typically the most difficult of the timing tasks and place heavy demands on working memory (Zakay, 1990). The individual is shown a sample duration (e.g., by turning a flashlight on and off), but is not told the actual length of the duration. The person must then reproduce the sample duration, typically using the same means by which the sample was presented (in this example, a flashlight). To do this task accurately, the individual must attend to the initial sample interval, hold that duration in mind, and then use it to generate an equivalent duration of response. It more closely evaluates the capacity of the individual to govern his or her own behavior relative to a mentally represented time interval (the sample duration) than do the other timing paradigms do, and it appears to be more taxing of working memory. For this reason, this task may also be more susceptible to any problems with distraction. Supporting this are findings that scores on this task correlate significantly with measures of impulsiveness, apparently more so than other timing tasks (Gerbing, Ahadi, & Patton, 1987). Logically, then, one would expect ADHD to produce impairments on this task, even in the absence of distracting events. All eight previous studies support this conclusion (Barkley et al., 1997; Barkley, Edwards, et al., 2001; Barkley, Murphy, & Bush, 2001; Bauermeister et al., 2005; Dooling-Litfin, 1998; Meaux & Chelonis, 2003; Smith et al., 2002; Walker, 1982). All found reproduction deficits in the samples with ADHD, making these deficits the most reliable timing problem associated with ADHD found to date. This pattern is typified in the results from our study with teenagers with ADHD (Barkley, Edwards, et al., 2001), shown in Figure 3.1. As this figure shows, teens with ADHD made greater errors on the time reproduction task, and these errors increased with the duration to be estimated (from 2 to 60 s). Relatively long time durations would be expected to worsen the impairment, which they did in all studies that used more than a single duration. Distractors would also be expected to worsen the deficit, which they did in the only study to test this issue (Barkley et al., 1997). That study had many methodological limitations, however. The time reproduction deficit in ADHD would seem to be well established.

Use of Time and Time Management in Natural Settings. Though they are not exactly measures of nonverbal temporal working memory, the use of time and time management in daily life may partly be functions of such memory, and so they are reviewed here. Only four previous studies have examined time use and management in daily life activities in children with ADHD. All found the groups with ADHD to be impaired when parent or teacher reports were used, but they were not consistent for the reports of children. We (Barkley et al., 1997) had parents rate their children on a scale of 25 items related to sense of and use of time (e.g., how often the children got ready for deadlines on time, did homework on time, completed chores on time, and talked about time and their past). The children with ADHD (n = 91) had significantly more problems than the control group (n = 36). Indeed, the distribu-

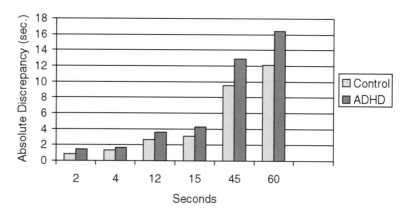

FIGURE 3.1. Mean errors (absolute discrepancy scores) for the control group and the group with ADHD across six time durations (2, 4, 12, 15, 45, and 60 s). From Barkley, Edwards, Laneri, Fletcher, and Metevia (2001). Copyright 2001 by Kluwer/Plenum. Reprinted by permission.

tions were almost nonoverlapping between the two groups. However, on the children's self-reports on this same rating scale, much smaller group differences emerged, though still significant. The finding was replicated for the parent scale with another small sample of children with ADHD and control children (*n*'s = 14) (Dooling-Litfin, 1998). One study with Puerto Rican children likewise found differences on this scale between children with ADHD and control children (Bauermeister et al., 2005). Shaw and Brown (1999) used a cursory survey (three items) of teacher reports of time use, as well as a brief eight-item self-report rating scale. Significant group differences were evident on the teacher ratings, but not in the self-reports provided by the teens. Sample sizes were small in these comparisons (*n*'s = 12), however, limiting power. Both studies suffered from additional methodological problems, including lack of explicit clinical diagnostic criteria in determining the groups with ADHD, no examination of the impact of comorbid disorders on the results, no inspection of the internal consistency of the scales or their reliability, and, in my (Barkley et al., 1997) study, the presence of a substantial subset of children with ADHD taking medication for their disorder at the time the ratings were collected. These and other limitations require that further, more rigorous research be done on the use of time and time management in children with ADHD before the finding of deficits in this area of functioning can be said to have much veracity.

Verbal Working Memory

In contrast to the literature on nonverbal working memory in ADHD, that on verbal working memory is abundant. Such tasks typically involve the retention and oral repetition of digit spans (especially in reverse order); mental computation or arithmetic, such as serial addition; and memory tasks that require the retention of verbal material across delay intervals. Often the latter tasks impose a demand for organizing the material in some way, so that individuals can more easily restate the material when called on to do so. Children with ADHD have been found to be significantly less proficient than control children in mental computation (Ackerman, Anhalt, & Dykman, 1986; Barkley, DuPaul, & McMurray, 1990; Mariani & Barkley, 1997; Zentall & Smith, 1993; Zentall, Smith, Lee, & Wieczorek, 1994). More recently, adolescents with ADHD have been shown to have a similar deficiency (MacLeod & Prior, 1996). A recent meta-analysis (Frazier et al., 2004) of nine studies using a mental arithmetic test reported a weighted average effect size of 0.70 (95% CI = 0.57–0.83) that was statistically significant. Thus verbal working memory as assessed by mental computation is reliably impaired in ADHD.

Both children and adults with ADHD have also shown more difficulties with digit span (particularly backwards) (Barkley et al., 1996b; Mariani & Barkley, 1997). The Freedom from Distractibility factor of the Wechsler Intelligence Scale for Children—Revised

(WISC-R) comprises tests of digit span, mental arithmetic, and coding (digit–symbol), and thus has been interpreted as reflecting executive processes, such as verbal working memory and resistance to distraction (Ownby & Matthews, 1985). Children with ADHD have been found to perform more poorly on this factor than do nondisabled children (Anastopoulos, Spisto, & Maher, 1994; Golden, 1996; Lufi, Cohen, & Parish-Plass, 1990; Milich & Loney, 1979; van der Meere, Gunning, & Stemerdink, 1996), but its utility in diagnosing or classifying cases of ADHD is questionable (Anastopoulos et al., 1994). The recent meta-analysis of 12 studies using this factor by Frazier et al. (2004) found a significant mean weighted effect size of 0.75 (94% CI = 0.62–0.88), indicating a reliable deficit in this factor associated with ADHD. By themselves, such findings might suggest a variety of problems besides working memory (deficient arithmetic knowledge, slow motor speed, etc.). However, Zentall and Smith (1993) were able to rule out some of these potential confounding factors in their study of mental computation in children with ADHD, thus giving greater weight to deficient verbal working memory as being associated with ADHD.

A recent meta-analysis (Frazier et al., 2004) involving 12 studies using the Digit Span subtest of the Wechsler scales reported a significant weighted mean effect size of 0.64 (95% CI = 0.52–0.76), indicating moderate deficits in this domain associated with ADHD. Subsequent studies using digit span, n-back (numbers that occur two positions back in an ongoing sequence), paired-associate learning, paced serial auditory addition, and sentence span have reported comparable results (Chang et al., 1999; Kuntsi et al., 2001; Shallice et al., 2002; Siklos & Kerns, 2004).

Nevertheless, the high comorbidity of LDs with ADHD argues for some caution in interpreting these findings as being necessarily specific or exclusive to ADHD. As noted earlier, the presence of LDs, particularly LI and reading disorders, often accounts for deficits on verbal tasks among children with ADHD or may worsen those that already exist. This has certainly been found in studies using verbal working memory tasks in samples with ADHD and with mixed ADHD and reading disorders (or LI) (McInnes et al., 2003; Ricklidge & Tannock, 2002; Seidman et al., 2001; Willcutt

et al., 1998). Thus, while there is abundant evidence that ADHD is associated with deficits in verbal working memory on a variety of tasks, the presence of a reading disorder or LI may be a contributing factor to some or all of these results.

As noted previously, the storage and recall of simple information on verbal memory tests has not been found to be impaired in those with ADHD (Barkley, DuPaul, & McMurray, 1990; Cahn & Marcotte, 1995; Douglas, 1983, 1988). Instead, it seems that when larger, and more complex amounts of verbal information must be held in mind, especially over a lengthy delay period, such deficits become evident (Douglas, 1983, 1988; Seidman, Biederman, et al., 1995; Seidman, Biederman, Faraone, Weber, & Oullette, 1997). Also, when strategies are required that assist with organizing material to respond to it or to remember it more effectively, those with ADHD are less proficient than control groups (Amin, Douglas, Mendelson, & Dufresne, 1993; August, 1987; Benezra & Douglas, 1988; Borcherding et al., 1988; Douglas, 1983; Douglas & Benezra, 1990; Felton et al., 1987; Frost, Moffitt, & McGee, 1989; Shapiro, Hughes, August, & Bloomquist, 1993). Not only is this true of children with ADHD, but it has more recently been demonstrated in adults with ADHD (Holdnack, Morberg, Arnold, Gur, & Gur, 1995).

One task that would seem to tax verbal working memory and the associated executive ability of organizing verbal information is story (listening, watching, or reading) comprehension. The topic has been studied extensively in children with ADHD by Elizabeth Lorch and her colleagues, using television programs (see Lorch et al., 2000, 2004). Both elementary-age and preschool-age children with ADHD demonstrated impaired recall of story information after watching televised stories. Particularly problematic was their recall of causal connections (Lorch et al., 1999, 2000, 2004; Sanchez, Lorch, Milich, & Welsh, 1999). Cued recall did not seem to be problematic, especially for simple details. But unassisted recall, particularly for deeper information such as knowledge of relations and causal connections, was more impaired by ADHD. An interesting finding (in keeping with the information on distractors discussed in Chapter 2) was that when toys were present during the television viewing, they produced a significantly greater detrimental impact on the group with ADHD than on the control group in regard to the recall of the structural (relational and causal connections) elements of the story, but not so much in regard to simple story details (Lorch et al., 1999, 2000; Sanchez et al., 1999). Assistance with studying appeared to produce a preferential benefit on story recall in the group with ADHD versus the control group, once level of prestudy recall was statistically controlled for (Lorch et al., 2004). Again, some research suggests that listening comprehension is also problematic in children with LI as well as those with ADHD, raising some questions about the Lorch research group's findings and their specificity to ADHD alone (McInnes et al., 2003). But, as Lorch et al.'s research implies, ADHD is certainly associated with higher-order problems in listening comprehension that have shown some association with other working memory tasks (McInnes et al., 2003), and with the presence of distractors during TV viewing.

HINDSIGHT, FORETHOUGHT, AND PLANNING

Working memory, or the capacity to hold information in mind across a delay in time to guide a subsequent response, has been thought to be composed of two temporally symmetrical functions: the "retrospective" and "prospective" functions. Both Fuster (1997) and Goldman-Rakic (1995) have described these functions; they have also been called "hindsight" and "forethought" (Bronowski, 1977). These constructs have not been well studied in those with ADHD, except as they are likely to pertain to measures of planning (e.g., in such tasks as the tower tests and maze performances, discussed just below). But if in its most elementary form "hindsight" can be taken to mean the ability to alter subsequent responses based on immediately past mistakes, then research findings imply a deficit in hindsight in ADHD. Children with ADHD, like adults with prefrontal lobe injuries, are less likely to adjust their subsequent responses based on an immediately past incorrect response in an information-processing task (Sergeant & van der Meere, 1988).

Research using complex reaction time tasks with warning stimuli and preparation intervals may be relevant to the construct of forethought. In such research, children with ADHD often failed to use the warning stimulus to prepare for the upcoming response trial

(Douglas, 1983), with longer preparatory intervals making the performance of children with ADHD worse than that of control children (Chee, Logan, Schachar, Lindsay, & Wachsmuth, 1989; van der Meere, Vreeling, & Sergeant, 1992; Zahn et al., 1991). The capacity to create and maintain an anticipatory set (preparation to act) for an impending event has also been shown to be impaired in ADHD (van der Meere et al., 1992).

Neuropsychological tasks believed to assess the construct of planning are a rather diverse group. The most commonly used among them are the tower tasks. The Tower of London (TOL) task places heavy emphasis on visual–spatial and sequential working memory and the manipulation of information being held in mind. This task requires the subject to construct a design using colored disks of different sizes and three upright pegs, to employ the fewest moves possible, and often to obey several constraints (e.g., a large disk cannot be stored on a small disk, etc.). Forethought and planning are felt to be instrumental to performance of this task. The task requires that individuals be able to mentally represent and test out various ways of removing and replacing disks on a set of pegs or spindles to match the design presented by the experimenter. This task involves substantial mental planning that must occur before and during the actual motor execution of the rearrangement. Five studies of ADHD using the TOL and a related task, the Tower of Hanoi (TOH), found children with ADHD to perform more poorly than nondisabled children (Brady & Denckla, 1994; Cornoldi, Barbieri, Gaiani, & Zocchi, 1999; Klorman et al., 1999; Pennington, Grossier, & Welsh, 1993; Weyandt & Willis, 1994) as did a study of adults with ADHD (see meta-analysis by Hervey et al., 2004). Two studies did not find significant group differences between children with ADHD and control children (Geurts et al., 2004; Wu, Anderson, & Castiello, 2002), nor did one other study of ADHD in adults (Riccio, Wolfe, Romine, Davis, & Sullivan, 2004). A study of a general sample of preschool children did not find an association of planning ability with severity of ADHD symptoms, but the study did not explore clinically diagnosed children with ADHD, and so its relevance to that disorder is less clear (Sonuga-Barke, Dalen, Daley, & Remington, 2002).

Like performance on the TOL and TOH, maze performance probably reflects aspects of planning ability, though perhaps not as much so. After all, the solution to the maze is obviously within the maze design that sits before the child but simply must be discovered, whereas the solution to the TOL design problem is not as readily apparent. Perhaps this explains why some studies found children with ADHD to perform poorly on maze tasks (Nigg, Hinshaw, Carte, & Treuting, 1998; Weyandt & Willis, 1994), but many others did not (Barkley, Grodzinsky, & DuPaul, 1992; Grodzinsky & Diamond, 1992; Mariani & Barkley, 1997; McGee et al., 1989; Milich & Kramer, 1985; Moffitt & Silva, 1988). The young age of the subjects may be a factor in some of the negative findings (Mariani & Barkley, 1997), as may be the version of the maze used (Porteus, WISC, etc.), as well as low power associated with the use of small samples ($n < 20$ per group) (Barkley et al., 1992; McGee et al., 1989; Moffitt & Silva, 1988). Nevertheless, the weight of the evidence (five negative studies vs. two affirmative) to date is against an association between a deficit in maze performance and ADHD.

Another measure of planning ability is the Six Elements Test. Children are given three different types of tasks (storytelling, math problems, and object naming), with two sets of problems being provided for each type of task. The children must work on the six tasks within 10 minutes, adhering to two rules: (1) They cannot do the second set of the same task after working on the first set, and (2) they must try to complete part of all six tasks. Planning, task scheduling, and performance monitoring are believed to be involved in this test. Adolescents with ADHD show more deficient performance on the test than do control teens or those with ODD/CD (Clark et al., 2000).

As already noted, the TOH and TOL tasks may better reflect the capacity to plan or "look ahead" (Pennington et al., 1993), and children with ADHD may perform poorly on these tasks, though evidence here is conflicting. Only one study has examined the Six Elements Test and found a deficit in teens with ADHD. Yet it is not clear how it relates to other planning tasks. The findings reviewed here are at least suggestive of some deficiencies in hindsight, forethought, and planning ability that depend on working memory. Far more research on the issue using larger samples seems in order, however, before definitive statements to this effect can be made. Certainly, a meta-analysis of existing studies using the TOL and TOH tasks is to be encouraged.

TEMPORAL DISCOUNTING

One domain of cognitive functioning that is related both to impulsiveness and to future planning is known as "temporal discounting." This reflects the extent to which an individual discounts the value of a future reward by the amount of the time delay until he or she can obtain that reward. Impulsive individuals are more likely to discount the value of a reward as a function of its delay than are nonimpulsive individuals. We tested this notion in our study of adolescents with ADHD (Barkley, Edwards, et al., 2001), in which teens were given a series of choices between varying amounts of money that they could have now ($1–100) or $100 later. The delay to the later reward was also varied from 1 month to 1, 5, and 10 years. We did the same task with a $1,000 delayed reward as well. Results are shown in Figure 3.2 and indicated that for the $100 task, teens with ADHD ($n = 101$) more steeply discounted or devalued the delayed reward than did control teens ($n = 39$), although both groups showed the classic finding of devaluing rewards progressively more as the delay increased. No differences were evident at the $1,000 delay—perhaps owing to the larger amount of money offered immediately in this task, which made both groups more likely to choose the immediate over the delayed amount.

COGNITIVE FLEXIBILITY AND PERSEVERATION

Another frequently described executive function is cognitive flexibility or its opposite, perseveration, which is often indexed by the Wisconsin Card Sort Test (WCST). Clinical descriptions of children with ADHD often suggest that they are more likely to respond with overlearned and automatic responses when faced with problem-solving situations or contexts that demand the thoughtful formation of strategies and the flexible shifting of thought. Such response flexibility, often called "set shifting," may be measured using certain scores from the WCST. A large number of studies have used the WCST with samples of children having ADHD. I reviewed a total of 20 such

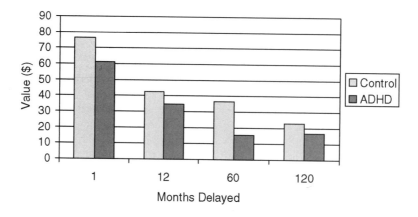

FIGURE 3.2. Mean values (in dollars) for the $100 delayed reward across four delay periods (1 month to 10 years) for the group with ADHD and the control group on the Reward Discount Task. From Barkley, Edwards, Laneri, Fletcher, and Metevia (2001). Copyright 2001 by Kluwer/Plenum. Reprinted with permission.

studies (Barkley, 1997b). In a meta-analysis of 25 studies, Frazier et al. (2004) found a mean weighted effect size of 0.35 for response perseveration scores (95% CI = 0.26–0.44), which was not significant. Effect sizes for the scores of number of categories achieved (strategy or rule detection) and set failure were 0.29 and 0.15, respectively, which were also nonsignificant. Several studies not included in that meta-analysis also used the WCST. One of these found a small but significant difference between ADHD and control groups, but only for perseverative errors (Seidman et al., 2001); another found that such errors were significant only in a comparison group of high-functioning autistic children, but not in children with ADHD (Geurts et al., 2004). Three more studies of adults with ADHD exist that used the WCST, and they did not find group differences on this measure (see the meta-analysis by Hervey et al., 2004). Problems with cognitive flexibility and set shifting therefore do not appear to be associated with ADHD, at least as indexed by this task.

Another task believed to assess rule discovery and set shifting is the Junior Brixton Rule Attainment Test, used by Shallice et al. (2002) in their study of two age groups of children with and without ADHD. Children with ADHD made more perseverative errors, used more guessing, and had fewer correct responses than control children. Although older children in both groups did better than younger children, there was no group × age interaction,

suggesting that the group differences remained across the ages studied here (7–12 years).

A study by Greve et al. (1996) is perhaps revealing of the specific problem that children with ADHD may have on such tasks. This study used a test similar to the WCST, known as the California Card Sorting Test, with children having ADHD and control children. Although subjects must sort cards based on rules, the test involves three different forms of administration. One includes telling the subject the rule to be used for sorting (Cued Sort); another involves the examiner's sorting the cards, but the child's stating the rule from the sorting pattern (Structured Sort); and the third involves the subject's both sorting the cards and stating the rule he or she is using (Free Sort). It was hypothesized that if children with ADHD have problems with concept formation, they will have difficulties with Free Sort and Structured Sort, both of which require a child to identify or formulate the rule in effect. They will have no difficulty on Cued Sort, because they have been explicitly told the rule to use for sorting. Conversely, if children with ADHD have difficulty with rule-governed behavior (the control of the rule over motor responding), then deficits will be apparent in Cued Sort as well as in the other sorting routines. In the other two sort procedures, however, they will be able to accurately describe the rule in use when they are correctly sorting. Their errors, then, in the latter two sorts will be evidence of poor rule execution not of rule formulation.

The results of this study indicated that children with ADHD differed on scores that implied a problem with rule execution. These results may indicate that any difficulties children with ADHD may have with the WCST or other rule discovery tasks is not so much that they cannot discover or formulate the new sorting rule as that they cannot adhere to it in response execution.

CREATIVITY

Elsewhere, I (Barkley, 1997a, 1997b; see also Chapter 7, this volume) have suggested that behavioral or verbal creativity (originality) may be impaired in those with ADHD as a consequence of their poor behavioral inhibition. Certainly, as noted above, there is an abundant literature showing that those with ADHD have difficulties with verbal fluency, or the generation of novel words on demand under timed fluency tests. This is a relatively simple form of verbal creativity that is consistent with such a prediction. But studies of other forms of creativity in ADHD are few in number. They are plagued, as is the field of creativity research itself, by problems in the very definition of "creativity" (Boden, 1994; Brown, 1989; Sternberg & Lubart, 1996). Creativity during free play (Alessandri, 1992) and performance of nonverbal, figural creativity tasks (Funk, Chessare, Weaver, & Exley, 1993) have been noted to be significantly below average in children with ADHD. This would seem to support the earlier prediction of such deficits' being associated with ADHD. However, Shaw and Brown (1990) did not find a deficit in creativity in a small sample of high-IQ children with ADHD. They did find that those with ADHD gathered and used more diverse, nonverbal, and poorly focused information and displayed higher figural creativity. Using so small a sample and only bright children, however, hardly poses a reasonable test of this prediction. More research on creativity in ADHD is clearly needed in testing this prediction of the model.

My colleagues and I studied two forms of creativity in teens with ADHD and in a control group (Barkley, Edwards, et al., 2001). One form of creativity, ideational fluency, is assessed by the Object Usage Test. The number of novel uses a child is able to describe for several common objects (brick, bucket, rope) represents the dependent measure. For each object, children are given 1 minute to describe as many different uses of the object as possible. We also assessed nonverbal creativity or fluency, in which children were given three common geometric shapes (square, circle, and triangle) and asked to create as many different combinations of these shapes into recognizable objects during a 2-minute period. Some verbal labeling ability was required, as the children had to tell the examiner what their shapes represented. Both tasks loaded on the same factor as verbal fluency, digit span, and the Simon game described earlier in the discussions of verbal working memory and language. The teens with ADHD did not differ from controls on this factor, implying no differences in creative ability, though scores for the individual creativity tasks were not analyzed separately. The same Object Usage Test was employed in another study in my lab (Murphy et al., 2001), which also revealed no significant differences between adults with ADHD and control adults. And, so while verbal fluency may be impaired in ADHD, ideational creativity appears not to be so. Tests of nonverbal, figural creativity have shown mixed results.

SELF-REGULATION OF EMOTION

Irritability, hostility, excitability, and a general emotional hyperresponsiveness toward others have been frequently described in the clinical literature on ADHD (see Barkley, 1990; Still, 1902). Douglas (1983, 1988) anecdotally observed and later objectively documented the tendency of children with ADHD to become overaroused and excitable in response to rewards, and to be more visibly frustrated when past rates of reinforcement declined (Douglas & Parry, 1994; Wigal et al., 1993). Rosenbaum and Baker (1984) also reported finding greater negative affect expressed by children with ADHD during a concept-learning task involving noncontingent negative feedback. And Cole, Zahn-Waxler, and Smith (1994) found that levels of negative affect were significantly and positively correlated with symptoms of and risk for ADHD, but only in boys. The opposite proved true for girls. These clinical observations and research studies intimate that emotional self-control may be problematic for children with ADHD, particularly concerning the expression of negative emotions.

Greater emotional reactivity has also been reported in the social interactions of children with ADHD. Eric Mash (personal communication, February 1993) found that such children displayed greater emotional intonation in their verbal interactions with their mothers. Studies of peer interactions have also found children with ADHD to be more negative and emotional in their social communications with peers. This greater level of expressed negative emotion is most salient in the subgroup of children with ADHD who have high levels of comorbid aggression (Hinshaw & Melnick, 1995). Consistent with such findings, Keltner, Moffitt, and Stouthamer-Loeber (1995) recorded the facial expressions of adolescent boys during a structured social interaction. Four groups of boys were created. One was rated as having high levels of externalizing symptoms (hyperactive–impulsive–inattentive–aggressive behavior); a second consisted of boys rated as having more internalizing symptoms (anxiety, depression, etc.); a third group consisted of boys having elevations on ratings of both types of symptoms; and the fourth group was composed of nondisordered adolescent boys. Boys showing high levels of externalizing symptoms were found to demonstrate significantly more facial expressions of anger than the other groups, which were low in externalizing symptoms. These results suggest the possibility that the commonly noted association of ADHD with defiant and hostile behavior (see Hinshaw, 1987, for a review) may, at least in part, stem from a deficiency in emotional self-regulation in those with ADHD. Again, however, these findings merely suggest rather than confirm a link between ADHD and emotional self-regulation, and they tend to imply that the poorest emotion modulation may be within the aggressive subgroup of children with ADHD.

Since the preceding edition of this text, additional studies have focused on this issue in children with ADHD. Walcott and Landau (2004), for instance, evaluated boys with ADHD during a frustrating peer competition task in which half of the boys in each group were instructed to try to hide their feelings if they became upset. Boys with ADHD were less effective at doing so than control boys. Melnick and Hinshaw (2000) observed children with ADHD during a family problem-solving task that elicited frustration. Only a highly aggressive subgroup of boys with ADHD demon-strated a less constructive pattern of emotional coping, compared to nonaggressive or control boys. The overall emotional self-regulation of these boys was found to be predictive of their noncompliance in a summer camp environment. Kitchens, Rosen, and Braaten (1999) found that both children with ADHD and their mothers rated the children as more angry and depressed than mothers of children, without ADHD rated their offspring; the higher depression ratings were more typical of males with ADHD than of females. In a subsequent study, Braaten and Rosen (2000) reported that boys with ADHD expressed lower levels of empathy and exhibited more sadness, anger, and guilt than control boys.

Despite these apparent difficulties with emotional self-control, children with ADHD have not been found to have any difficulties with the perception or recognition of others' emotions (Shapiro et al., 1993); such children were not observed to be significantly different from children in their processing of emotional information, except on two auditory tests that appeared to make demands on auditory–verbal working memory.

Research to date therefore seems to suggest that children with ADHD have difficulties with regulation of their emotional states, particularly in response to frustration; it also indicates that they appear to show higher levels of aggression, anger, and sadness or depression (mainly boys), and possibly lower levels of empathy, than control children. Not surprisingly, these problems with emotional self-control may be most apparent in the highly aggressive subset of children with ADHD.

SELF-AWARENESS

Clinical lore has long held that children with ADHD have low self-esteem and often think poorly of themselves and their performance of tasks. Since the preceding edition of this text, a number of studies have been conducted to evaluate this idea. Not only do these results of these studies not support this widely held view, but they actually find just the opposite—that children with ADHD have a positive illusory bias in their self-perceptions of their competence. It is helpful to distinguish among several levels of self-perceptions in understanding this literature (Harter, 1985; Hoza, Pelham, Dobbs, Owens, & Pillow, 2002). Harter (1985) argued for two different self-perception concepts. One consists of domain-specific self-perceptions (e.g., perceptions of social acceptance or scholastic competence); the second consists of global self-worth, which is not simply a summation of all domain-specific self-perceptions, but an independent construct. To these two concepts, Hoza et al. (2002) have added a third: task-specific self-perceptions of competence.

In their review of this literature, Hoza et al. (2002) found very conflicting evidence that children with ADHD express low self-evaluations of global self-worth or even domain-specific self-evaluations, except in the area of behavioral conduct. These authors suggested that where evidence exists for low self-evaluations in both constructs (domain-specific or global), it may have more to do with disorders that are comorbid with ADHD (aggression or CD, LDs, or depression). On task-specific self-perceptions, however, children with ADHD overestimate their competence. This is not to say that their self-perceptions are above those of nondisabled control children; rather, their self-perceptions are very similar to those given by control children, even though the performance of the group with ADHD on various tasks is often well below that of the control group. All children tend to overestimate their competence on tasks, viewing themselves as better than average. What the results would indicate is that children with ADHD show more limited awareness of their deficient areas of competence. It is the disparity between self-evaluation and task performance of competence that distinguishes children with ADHD from control children. Hoza and colleagues concluded that there is strong evidence for a positive illusory bias among children with ADHD in their self-perceptions of task-specific competence.

Hoza et al. (2002) then examined these issues further in their own research, and found boys with ADHD to show a positive illusory bias in their self-perceptions of domain-specific functioning (scholastic, social, and behavioral domains). These overestimates were most prominent in those domains in which subsets of children with ADHD may be the most impaired. For instance, boys with both aggression and ADHD demonstrated a greater illusory bias in the social and behavioral domains, whereas the boys doing poorly in academic competence were more biased toward seeing themselves as doing normally in the scholastic

domain. Global self-worth was likely to be low only in boys with ADHD who had coexisting depression. These findings were replicated using the much larger samples (n = 487 children with ADHD, 287 control children) from the National Institute of Mental Health Multimodal Treatment Study of ADHD (Hoza et al., 2004) in which children with ADHD showed the greatest disparity in self-perceptions in domains in which they were the most impaired. We (Knouse, Bagwell, Barkley, & Murphy, in press) recently found evidence for this same illusory bias among adults with ADHD in the domain of driving competence. Some evidence suggests that these biased self-perceptions are more likely to occur in the Combined Type of ADHD than in the Predominantly Inattentive Type, and that they are more strongly correlated with severity of impulsive–hyperactive behavior than with severity of inattention (Owens & Hoza, 2003).

Diener and Milich (1997) argued that such a positive illusory bias might be self-protective, allowing children with ADHD to cope better on a daily basis despite their failure experiences. The results of Hoza et al.'s work (Hoza, Waschbusch, Pelham, Molina, & Milich, 2000; Hoza et al., 2002, 2004) are consistent with such a view, in that the greater disparities between self-perceptions and actual functioning were in those domains that were the most impaired. But a study by Ohan and Johnston (2002) found that the self-protection hypothesis was supported only in biased self-perceptions of social competence, whereas it did not seem to account for the self-perceptions in the area of academic performance. Unresolved is whether this self-protection represents a conscious or willful attempt at self-protection, as it seems to be for the social domain of functioning (such as would be involved in actively attempting to present oneself always in a positive light), or whether it represents truly inaccurate self-perception (as it may be in the academic competence domain). The latter is certainly a possibility, given that ADHD is believed to arise from difficulties in frontal lobe functioning, and that self-awareness and evaluation are largely frontal lobe functions (see Barkley, 1997b; see also Chapter 5).

Children with ADHD have also been found to attribute much of their success on various tasks to luck or external, uncontrollable factors, and to do so more strongly than nondisabled children do. They are less likely than nondisabled children, however, to attribute their failures to lack of effort (Hoza et al., 2000; Hoza, Pelham, Waschbusch, Kipp, & Owens, 2001). All of this suggests that children with ADHD perceive the outcomes of their performance as being more out of their own control than do nondisabled children.

MOTIVATIONAL DIFFICULTIES

Impaired Persistence of Effort

Clinical descriptions of children and adults with ADHD are often rife with references to poor motivation in general and impaired persistence of effort in particular. As noted above, those with ADHD demonstrate a greater variability of task performance and discount the value of future rewards more steeply than control children as the delay to the reward increases. Researchers have also frequently commented on such difficulties in tasks requiring repetitive responding that involve little or no reinforcement (Barber et al., 1996; Barkley, 1990; Douglas, 1972, 1983, 1989). Written productivity in arithmetic tasks, in particular, may be taken as a measure of persistence; those with ADHD have been found to be less productive on such tasks than control children (Barkley, DuPaul, & McMurray, 1990). Multiple studies also have documented that children with ADHD show impaired persistence of effort in laboratory tasks (August, 1987; August & Garfinkel, 1990; Barber et al., 1996; Borcherding et al., 1988; Douglas & Benezra, 1990; Milich, in press; Ott & Lyman, 1993; Solanto, Wender, & Bartell, 1997; van der Meere, Shalev, Borger, & Gross-Tsur, 1995; Wilkison, Kircher, McMahon, & Sloane, 1995). For instance, Hoza et al. (2001) observed that children with ADHD simply quit working on laboratory tasks more often than did control children. Thus the evidence for difficulties in the self-regulation of motivation (particularly persistence of effort) in ADHD is impressive. Indeed, Paul Green (personal communication, April 2001) has informed me of results from his own research suggesting that 50% of the variance in performance on neuropsychological tests, such as those described earlier (WCST, fluency tasks, trails, etc.) is accounted for by the level of effort a person applies to the task. Degree of effort, he argues, can be readily assessed by using two simple lab tasks—a digit recognition task and a paired-word recognition task. If such effort is not measured and controlled in group comparisons, it may lead to erroneous conclusions about deficiencies on neuropsychological tests that are largely due to the more limited effort applied by those with ADHD to these tasks.

Some have suggested that children with ADHD have an apparent insensitivity to reinforcement (for reviews, see Barkley, 1989; Douglas, 1989; Haenlein & Caul, 1987; Luman, Oosterlaan, & Sergeant, 2005; Sagvolden et al., 1989). Studies using varying schedules of reinforcement typically find that children with ADHD and nondisabled children do not differ in their task performances under immediate and continuous reward (Barber et al., 1996; Cunningham & Knights, 1978; Douglas & Parry, 1983, 1994; Parry & Douglas, 1983), although children with ADHD seem to benefit from high-intensity reinforcement (Luman et al., 2005). In contrast, when partial or delayed reinforcement is introduced, the performance of children with ADHD may decline relative to that of nondisabled children (Parry & Douglas, 1983; Freibergs & Douglas, 1969). Just as many studies, however, have not found this decline (Barber et al., 1996; Pelham, Milich, & Walker, 1986; Stevens, Quittner, Zuckerman, & Moore, 2002) or have found that the difficulty of the task moderates the effect (Barber & Milich, 1989). In a similar vein, the performance of children with ADHD during relatively tedious tasks involving little or no reward is often enhanced by the addition of reinforcement; however, so is the performance of nondisabled children (Carlson & Alexander, 1993; Iaboni, Douglas, & Baker, 1995; Kupietz, Camp, & Weissman, 1976; Pelham et al., 1986; Solanto, 1990; van der Meere, Hughes, Borger, & Sallee, 1995; see the recent review by Luman et al., 2005). And the addition of reinforcement to the task does not seem to alter the significant deterioration in effort over time seen in children with ADHD on such tasks (Solanto et al., 1997). Although some interpreted the early findings in this area as suggesting that children with ADHD have a reduced sensitivity to reinforcement (Haenlein & Caul, 1987) or are dominated by immediate reinforcement (Douglas, 1983; Sagvolden et al., 1989), the similar enhancement of the performance of nondisabled children by reward in the studies noted above challenged this interpretation (Pelham et al., 1986; Solanto, 1990). Moreover, Douglas and her colleagues (Iaboni et al., 1995) did not find the reward dominance effect that she earlier hypothesized might be associated with ADHD (Douglas, 1989). Later studies have found a preference among children with ADHD for more immediate than delayed rewards (Barkley, Edwards, et al., 2001; Luman et al., 2005; Tripp & Alsop, 1999, 2001).

Elsewhere, I have suggested a possible explanation for these results (Barkley, 1997b; see also Chapter 7). It focuses on the observations that the performance of nondisabled children is superior to that of children with ADHD under conditions of little or no reward and may be less affected by reductions in schedules of reinforcement, depending on the task duration and its difficulty level. This effect may result from nondisabled children's developing the capacity to bridge temporal delays between the elements of behavioral contingencies via their better-developed working memory abilities and internalized language. Combined with working memory as well as self-directed speech and the rule-governed behavior it permits, this self-regulation of motivation may allow nondisabled children not only to retain the goal of their performance in mind and subvocally encourage themselves in their persistence, but in so doing to create the drive necessary for such persistence, as has been suggested by others (Berkowitz, 1982; Mischel, Shoda, & Peake, 1988). This line of reasoning would suggest that, across development, the behavior of those with ADHD remains more contingency-shaped, or under the control of the immediate and external sources of reward, than it does in nondisabled children. Therefore, it is not that children with ADHD are either less sensitive to reinforcement or, conversely, dominated by a tendency to seek immediate rewards. They instead have a diminished capacity to bridge delays in reinforcement and to permit the persistence of goal-directed acts. Their performance in the absence of reward or under relatively low-reward conditions is most likely to lead to impersistence and to discriminate them from nondisabled children.

Some evidence for this was reported by Carlson and Tamm (2000), who studied the task performance of children with ADHD and control children under conditions of reward, response cost, and noncontingent reward. The children with ADHD also performed better on a high- than a low-interest task. The control children showed little differences in performance across these conditions, in keeping with the explanation above. Children with ADHD, however, benefited from both the reward and the response cost conditions (particularly the latter), but the latter condition led to a reduction in self-rated motivation. Similarly, a study by Slusarek, Velling, Bunk, and Eggers (2001) found that children with ADHD did not differ from children with other psychiatric disorders or with no disorder under conditions of high incentives, but were less able to inhibit their behavior and had longer reaction times under the low-incentive condition while performing a laboratory stop signal task.

In conclusion, it seems that children with ADHD may demonstrate a greater preference for immediate over delayed reinforcement, may more steeply discount delayed rewards as a function of the time delay, and seem to show a lesser sensitivity to reinforcement on psychophysiological measures than do control children (Luman et al., 2005). It may be delayed reinforcement, more than partial reinforcement, that is detrimental to their task performance. The ability of nondisabled children to persist in task performance in the absence of reinforcement may have to do with their greater capacity to self-regulate intrinsic motivation by using self-directed language and other mental representations to bridge delays between performance and the reinforcement that may be available for it.

Response Perseveration

Children with high levels of externalizing behavior, like adults with psychopathy, have been found to demonstrate greater persistence of responding (perseveration) in pursuit of reward, despite punishment or changes in contingencies that indicate an increasing likelihood of punishment. Left unclear from earlier studies has been whether this problem is characteristic of those who specifically have ADHD or of individuals who are more likely to have CD or psychopathy.

Although ADHD and CD may often occur together, they are thought to represent at least semi-independent, albeit overlapping conditions (Hinshaw, 1987). As noted in this and other chapters of this volume, ADHD is often associated with neurodevelopmental immaturity, motor coordination difficulties, and cognitive impairments (particularly in attention and executive functioning), and shows exceptionally high heritability. CD, by contrast, is typically associated with social adversity, family disruption, poor parental management skills, diminished parental monitoring, affiliation with deviant peers, and low verbal intelligence, as well as a somewhat lower level of heritability (Burt, Krueger, McGue, & Iacono, 2001; Hinshaw & Lee, 2003; Loeber, 1990; Loeber, Burke, Lahey, Winters, & Zera, 2000). Even so, some genetic liability appears to be shared between the two disorders, at least in childhood, although separate genetic contributions may emerge by adolescence (Coolidge, Thede, & Young, 2000; Silberg et al., 1996). There may also be some shared genetic liability among these two disorders and impaired executive functioning (Coolidge et al., 2000). Where the disorders co-occur, all of these associated characteristics may be present.

Several theorists have argued that ADHD may comprise a deficiency in response inhibition (Barkley, 1997a, 1997b; Quay, 1988, 1997; Schachar, Tannock, & Logan, 1993), particularly in the aspect of inhibition that may be under executive or volitional control (Barkley, 1997a, 1997b; Nigg, 2001; Still, 1902). CD also has been conceptualized as involving a form of impulsivity, but of a different sort. That form is thought to arise from motivational disturbances, such as a heightened sensitivity to reward or a greater inclination toward reward-seeking behavior (Newman & Wallace, 1993; Nigg, 2001; Quay, 1988). Quay has argued that the two disorders may be distinguished in part by the nature of their inhibitory deficits. Both Quay and Newman based their original views of the inhibitory deficit found in CD largely on Gray's (1982, 1987) neuropsychological model of anxiety.

As I have described in Chapter 1 of this book, Gray proposed a neuropsychological theory of behavioral approach, inhibition, and motivation that incorporates two distinct behavioral systems. One is the behavioral inhibition system (BIS), which responds to signals of impending punishment or nonreward so as to result in passive avoidance behavior and extinction. The other system is the behavioral activation (reward) system (BAS), which responds to conditioned stimuli associated with reward or nonpunishment. Gray hypothesized that anxiety-prone individuals have a relatively more active or stronger BIS, while those with impulsive behavior have a relatively underactive BIS.

Using this model, Quay (1988) proposed that CD represents an overactive BAS relative to BIS, such that the behavior of those having CD can be characterized as reward-dominant or excessively sensitive to reinforcement. In contrast, Quay hypothesized ADHD to represent an underactive BIS relative to BAS, resulting in poor impulse control or response inhibition. To test this notion, Shapiro, Quay, Hogan, and Schwartz (1988) employed Newman's adaptation (Newman, Patterson, & Kosson, 1987) of Siegel's (1978) Card Playing Task. This task requires the participant to bet money on whether a face card will appear on a computer screen in each of a series of 100 trials. Each card is initially displayed face down, while the participant decides to bet whether or not a face card will appear when the card is uncovered. Early trials have a high rate of reinforcement (90%), while later trials decrease progressively to 0% by the end of the deck. Newman et al. (1987) and Siegel (1978) both found that adults with psychopathy perseverated in responding on this task, despite an increasing likelihood of punishment (lost bets) across the task. They therefore achieved fewer winnings than did control adults. Consistent with Quay's distinction between ADHD and CD, Shapiro et al. (1988) found that children with CD played significantly more cards in this task than did control children. Daugherty and Quay (1991) found much the same result, whereas children with ADHD did not show such perseveration.

A later study by Milich, Hartung, Martin, and Haigler (1994), however, did not find an association between level of CD symptoms and either perseverative responding or earnings on this task, contrary to Quay's predictions. In contrast, a more recent study by Seguin, Arseneault, Boulerice, Harden, and Tremblay (2002) tested 13-year-old boys chosen on the basis of childhood histories of physical aggression (stable, unstable, or nonaggressive). They found that physical aggression, regardless of its stability from childhood to adolescence, was associated with perseveration on this same task.

Mariellen Fischer and I recently reported a study of children with ADHD followed to adulthood, in which we tested them on the Card Playing Task and examined whether their performance was a function of their ADHD or of coexisting CD (Fischer, Barkley, Smallish, & Fletcher, 2004). Our results indicated that lifetime CD did not contribute to severity of inattention, inhibition, reaction time, or greater ADHD-related behavior during task performance, consistent with our hypothesis predicated on Quay's theory of CD. But CD was distinctly associated with response perseveration on the Card Playing Task, again in keeping with our hypothesis and Quay's theory. The subset of participants with ADHD who also qualified for lifetime CD played significantly more cards than those without CD. Severity of CD was also found in the regression analysis to contribute significantly to individual differences on this measure, even after we controlled for severity of childhood hyperactivity, current IQ, severity of current ADHD, and level of current anxiety and depression. These results support Quay's hypothesis that CD, not ADHD, is chiefly related to difficulties with perseveration, replicating earlier studies that also documented such a relationship (Daugherty & Quay, 1991; Shapiro et al., 1988; Seguin et al., 2002). Yet the results are just as consistent with Nigg's (2001) distinction between executive and motivational forms of poor inhibition. As noted earlier, difficulties with inhibiting behavior on command, as in a CPT, may have more to do with poor executive control (rule governance) of responding, whereas response perseveration may be more indicative of motivational problems (in this case, reward seeking) interfering with behavioral control. Our results cannot distinguish among these competing explanations. But as Seguin et al. (2002) noted, playing more cards on this task is not necessarily an index of perseverative behavior, given that playing early trials actually increases the reinforcement available to the participant and thus is a rational strategy. It is only when cards are played beyond that point where the ratio of rewards to punishments becomes equally likely or even increasingly punitive that perseveration can be said to exist. Our study demonstrated that when this stricter definition of perseveration was employed (playing either 34+ or 75+ cards), the association with CD remained evident.

These results may be viewed as supportive of Quay's view that overactivity in the BAS (reward system) may be uniquely associated with CD/psychopathy and not with ADHD. But they may also support Beauchaine's (Beauchaine, 2001; Beauchaine, Katkin, Strassberg, & Snarr, 2001) hypothesis that under activity in the BAS could lead to reward seeking behav-

ior as a form of stimulation seeking. Given that the Card Playing Task measures only a behavioral outcome, it cannot by itself index precisely whether over- or underactivity in the BAS mediates this behavior. Moreover, perseveration on this task could be a function not just of a heightened sensitivity to reward or a greater inclination to reward seeking, but also of a failure to attend adequately to peripheral information that would direct one to shift to a more effective strategy, as Seguin et al. (2002) and Newman and Wallace (1993) have asserted. Such a failure could arise either from heightened arousal to the consequences that interferes with processing such information or from a restriction of attention away from peripheral cues during goal-directed activities, as these authors discuss. Our study is unable to distinguish among these various interpretations, but encourages further research to do so, given our replicated association of CD with perseveration.

PROBLEMS WITH AROUSAL

Some evidence does exist for possible problems in the regulation of central and autonomic nervous system arousal to meet task demands in those with ADHD. Multiple reviews of the psychophysiological (Borger & van der Meere, 2000; Beauchaine et al., 2001; Brand & van der Vlugt, 1989; Hastings & Barkley, 1978; Herpertz et al., 2001; Klorman et al., 1988; Rosenthal & Allen, 1978; Rothenberger, 1995) and cognitive (Douglas, 1983, 1988) literatures have concluded that children with ADHD show greater variability in central and autonomic arousal patterns. They also seem to be underreactive to stimulation in evoked response paradigms, particularly in the later P300 features of the evoked response (Klorman et al., 1988; Klorman, 1992). These P300 characteristics have been shown to be associated with frontal lobe activation (Klorman et al., 1988; Klorman, 1992). Children with ADHD have also been shown to display less anticipatory electroencephalographic (EEG) activation in response to impending events within tasks (known as the contingent negative variation or "expectancy" wave) (Hastings & Barkley, 1978), and to have less recruiting of psychophysiological activity over the frontal regions when necessary for appropriate task performance (Brand & van der Vlugt, 1989;

Rothenberger, 1995), relative to control groups.

Far more consistent have been the results of quantitative EEG and evoked response potential measures, sometimes taken in conjunction with vigilance tests (Monastra et al., 1999; El-Sayed, Larsson, Persson, & Rydelius, 2002; see Loo & Barkley, 2005, for a review). The most consistent patterns for EEG research are increased slow-wave or theta activity, particularly in the frontal lobe, and excess beta activity—all indicative of a pattern of underarousal and underreactivity in ADHD (Monastra, Lubar, & Linden, 2001).

Studies using positron emission tomography as a means of measuring brain activity have also found diminished brain activity in adults as well as adolescent females with ADHD (Ernst et al., 1994; Zametkin et al., 1990). Results have not been as reliably obtained with adolescent males (Zametkin et al., 1993). Similarly, studies using cerebral blood flow as a means of measuring brain activity have found decreased perfusion of the frontal regions and striatum in those with ADHD (Lou, Henriksen, & Bruhn, 1984; Lou, Henriksen, Bruhn, Borner, & Neilsen, 1989; Sieg, Gaffney, Preston, & Hellings, 1995). All this implies that ADHD is associated with difficulties with phasic or reactive arousal and activation, particularly in response to environmental events.

SENSORY PROBLEMS

No evidence indicates that children with ADHD are any more likely than nondisabled children to have difficulties in the development of their peripheral hearing, although they may have more otitis media or middle-ear infections than typical children do (Mitchell, Aman, Turbott, & Manku, 1987). Some research suggests that children with ADHD may be more sensitive to auditory loudness, preferring lower levels of speech when asked to define what sound level is most comfortable and tolerable for them (Lucker, Geffner, & Koch, 1996). The precise meaning of this research is unclear at the moment, though it could imply a hypersensitivity to speech loudness associated with ADHD. Other research has also shown that children with ADHD may have difficulties with the accurate discrimination of the speech of others when either speech or nonspeech noise

occurs in the background (Geffner, Lucker, & Koch, 1996). If replicated, these results would suggest that teachers and parents should make an effort to reduce background noise when attempting to teach, instruct, or otherwise direct children with ADHD through verbal means. However, as noted in the earlier discussion of language problems, more recent research has not found these children to have problems with detection of voice or with tone onset unless ADHD co-occurs with reading disorders (Breier et al., 2001). It may be the large overlap of ADHD with reading disorders that has contributed to the findings described above, since reading disorders were not assessed or ruled out in the earlier studies.

Some have noted greater difficulties in vision for children with ADHD, particularly with strabismus (Hartsough & Lambert, 1985; Stewart et al., 1966), but these findings were based on children diagnosed before the development of the more rigorous DSM diagnostic criteria and did not attempt to control for the association of ADHD with other disorders that could account for such findings. Even so, the percentage of children in these studies with such visual problems was quite low (19–21%). Others (Barkley, DuPaul, & McMurray, 1990), however have not found any history of visual problems in children with ADHD diagnosed according to more recent DSM criteria. It is conceptually unlikely that ADHD would be associated with peripheral visual problems, given what is now known about its pathophysiology that does not implicate the primary visual system.

PROBLEMS WITH MOTOR DEVELOPMENT

Results are conflicting as to whether children with ADHD experience a greater risk of delays in walking, with some studies not finding any higher prevalence of this problem (Hartsough & Lambert, 1985) and others finding it (Mitchell et al., 1987; Szatmari et al., 1989). Some studies (Hartsough & Lambert, 1985) found children with ADHD to be somewhat more likely to have delays in the onset of crawling (6.5%) than nondisabled children (1.6%). Others found no greater risk for delays in any areas of motor milestones (Barkley, DuPaul, & McMurray, 1990). Nevertheless, although the onset of major motor milestones may not be definitively delayed for children with ADHD as a group, as many as 52% of such children compared to up to 35% of typical children are characterized as having poor motor coordination (Barkley, DuPaul, & McMurray, 1990; Gillberg & Kadesjo, 2000; Hartsough & Lambert, 1985; Stewart et al., 1966; Szatmari et al., 1989). Kadesjo and Gillberg (1999, 2001) have clearly documented that 47% of children with ADHD met DSM-IV criteria for Developmental Coordination Disorder (DCD), compared to 9% of control cases. They also found the inverse comorbidity when they conducted a longitudinal study of DCD in children in Sweden: Approximately half of the children with DCD had moderate to severe symptoms of ADHD, with 19% of such children meeting full criteria for a diagnosis of ADHD (see Gillberg & Kadesjo, 2000, for a review).

It is therefore not surprising that studies examining neurological "soft signs" related to motor coordination and motor overflow movements find children with ADHD to demonstrate more of such signs as well as generally sluggish gross motor movements than control children, including those with pure LDs (Carte et al., 1996; Denckla & Rudel, 1978; Denckla, Rudel, Chapman, & Krieger, 1985; McMahon & Greenberg, 1977; Shaywitz & Shaywitz, 1984; Werry et al., 1972). Motor overflow movements have also been documented and have been interpreted as indicators of delayed development of motor inhibition (Denckla et al., 1985).

Studies using tests of fine motor coordination, such as balance, fine motor gestures, electronic or paper-and-pencil mazes, and pursuit tracking, often find children with ADHD to be less coordinated in these actions (Hoy, Weiss, Minde, & Cohen, 1978; Mariani & Barkley, 1997; McMahon & Greenberg, 1977; Moffitt, 1990; Shaywitz & Shaywitz, 1984; Ullman, Barkley, & Brown, 1978). Simple motor speed, as measured by finger-tapping rate or grooved pegboard tests, does not seem to be as affected in ADHD as is the execution of complex, coordinated sequences of motor movements (Barkley et al., 1996a; Breen, 1989; Grodzinsky & Diamond, 1992; Mariani & Barkley, 1997; Seidman, Biederman, et al., 1995; Seidman et al., 1997). Therefore, the bulk of the available evidence supports the existence of deficits in motor control, particularly when motor sequences must be performed, in those with ADHD.

Compelling evidence for a motor control deficit in ADHD also comes from the substantial programmatic research of Sergeant and van der Meere (1990) and colleagues in the Netherlands. Employing an information-processing paradigm, these studies isolated the cognitive deficit in those with ADHD to the motor control stage rather than to an attentional or information-processing stage. Specifically, their research suggests that the deficit is not at the response choice stage, but at the motor presetting stage involved in motor preparedness to act (Oosterlaan & Sergeant, 1995; van der Meere et al., 1996). Both a greater sluggishness and greater variability in motor preparation seem evident. This program of research also identified an insensitivity to errors in the motor performance of children with ADHD (Oosterlaan & Sergeant, 1995; Sergeant & van der Meere, 1988). In agreement with these results, other investigators (Hall, Halperin, Schwartz, & Newcorn, 1997) have also shown that ADHD is associated with deficits in response decision making and response organization, particularly in children who may have comorbid reading disorders.

Handwriting has often been noted in the clinical literature to be less mature in those with ADHD (Sleator & Pelham, 1986), and was subsequently shown by more objective means to be significantly impaired in both the Combined and Predominantly Inattentive Types of ADHD, though more so in the former than the latter (Marcotte & Stern, 1997). Difficulties with drawing have likewise been found in children with ADHD (Hoy et al., 1978; McGee et al., 1992). As noted earlier in this chapter, one test which seems to capture a simpler form of motor sequencing is the Hand Movements Test from the Kaufman Assessment Battery for Children. Three studies used this task and all found the group with ADHD to be significantly less proficient (Breen, 1989; Grodzinsky & Diamond, 1992; Mariani & Barkley, 1997), suggesting a problem with temporal ordering of motor sequences (Kesner, Hopkins, & Fineman, 1994). The developers of the test battery also commented that hyperactive children performed poorly on this task during the clinical validation trials of the battery (Kaufman & Kaufman, 1983).

Harvey and Reid (2003) recently reviewed 49 studies of motor functioning, movement skill, and physical fitness in children with

ADHD. They concluded that these children are at significantly greater risk of movement skill difficulties; often have lower levels of physical fitness (greater body fat, less flexibility, poor stamina); show an elevated risk for DCD as a comorbid condition; and often have few interventions aimed expressly at these motor and fitness problems.

MINOR PHYSICAL ANOMALIES

It has been repeatedly shown that children with ADHD have more minor physical anomalies than do typical children (Firestone, Lewy, & Douglas, 1976; Lerer, 1977; Quinn & Rapoport, 1974; Still, 1902). "Minor physical anomalies" refer to slight deviations in a child's outward appearance, such as an index finger longer than the middle finger; a curved fifth finger; a third toe as long or longer than the second toe; adherent ear lobes; a single transverse palmar crease; furrowed tongue; greater-than-normal head circumference; low-seated or soft, fleshy ears; electric, fine hair; two whorls of hair on the back of the head; eyes placed slightly further apart than normal; and greater skin on the nasal side of the eyelid (among others). Studies of infants have shown that a higher number of minor anomalies in infancy may be significantly related to the development of behavioral problems and specifically hyperactivity at age 3 (Waldrop, Bell, McLaughlin, & Halverson, 1978). Others, however, have been unable to replicate these findings (Burg, Hart, Quinn, & Rapoport, 1978; Quinn, Renfield, Burg, & Rapoport, 1977; Rapoport, Pandoni, Renfield, Lake, & Ziegler, 1977). Still other studies have noted that minor anomalies are related to hyperactivity in boys, but to overly inhibited and hypoactive behavior in girls (Waldrop, Bell, & Goering, 1976). However, these findings were contradicted by a later study (Jacklin, Maccoby, & Halverson, 1980), and another found no relationship whatsoever between number of anomalies and behavior (LaVeck, Hammond, & LaVeck, 1980). Thus, although children with ADHD may display more of these anomalies, there is little if any consistent relationship between high numbers of minor anomalies and hyperactive behavior (Firestone et al., 1976; Krouse & Kauffman, 1982). The topic appears to have received little additional research attention since the preceding edition of this book.

GENERAL HEALTH AND SLEEP PROBLEMS

Some studies have noted a greater incidence of maternal health and pre- and perinatal complications, such as toxemia, preeclampsia, postmaturity, and fetal distress, in the pregnancies of children with ADHD compared to nondisabled children (Hartsough & Lambert, 1985). However, as many or more studies have not found this to be the case (Barkley, DuPaul, & McMurray, 1990; Stewart et al., 1966).

Several studies have found children with ADHD to have more problems with general health than typical children. Hartsough and Lambert (1985) found that 50.9% of children with hyperactivity were described as in poor health during infancy, whereas Stewart et al. (1966) found that 24% of their sample were so described. The figures for control children were 29.2 and 2.7%, respectively. Chronic health problems, such as recurring upper respiratory infections and allergies, were also noted more often in hyperactive than in control children (39–44% vs. 8–25%) (Hartsough & Lambert, 1985; Mitchell et al., 1987; Szatmari et al., 1989). Trites, Tryphonas, and Ferguson (1980) also noted more allergies among hyperactive than nonhyperactive children, and others have noted the inverse—that is, more ADHD symptoms among children with atopic (allergic) disorders (Roth, Beyreiss, Schlenzka, & Beyer, 1991). One study found that only children with hyperactivity not associated with conduct problems were more likely to have allergies (Blank & Remschmidt, 1993). But others have not found an association between ADHD and allergies (McGee, Stanton, & Sears, 1993; Mitchell et al., 1987), or any association between the specific allergy of atopic rhinitis (hay fever) and ADHD (Hart, Lahey, Hynd, Loeber, & McBurnett, 1995). Thus the nature of an association between ADHD and allergies remains unclear at this writing.

Several studies have examined whether children with ADHD are more likely to suffer from asthma. An initial report by Hartsough and Lambert (1985) suggested such an increased risk for asthma among children considered hyperactive. Yet several subsequent studies using large samples of children ($n = 140$) have not found this to be the case when clinical diagnostic criteria for ADHD were used to identify the children (Biederman, Milberger, Faraone, Guite, & Warburton, 1994; Biederman et al., 1995). Nevertheless, a more recent study involving a birth cohort of 4,119 children found that of those who met criteria for ADHD (about 7.5%), there was a significantly increased risk of asthma (22% vs. 13%) (Leibson, Katusic, Barbaresi, Ransom, & O'Brien, 2003). And so the relationship of ADHD to increased risk for asthma remains an open question.

One study examined a large sample of 124 children and adolescents with ADHD for the presence of growth deficits in height and weight (Spencer et al., 1996). The investigators found no evidence of weight deficits in children with ADHD, even though 89% of the sample had been treated with stimulant medications, which were previously thought to create reductions in weight. The children with ADHD showed small but significant deficits in height compared to their control group, but the adolescents with ADHD showed no such deficits. The children's deficits were not related to treatment with stimulant medications. The authors concluded that ADHD may be associated with temporary deficits in growth in childhood through midadolescence, but that these may no longer be evident by late adolescence.

Enuresis (particularly nighttime bedwetting) was noted in early studies to occur in as many as 43% of hyperactive children, compared to 28% of control children (Stewart et al., 1966). Two subsequent studies, however, did not find this to be the case (Barkley, DuPaul, & McMurray, 1990; Kaplan, McNichol, Conte, & Moghadam, 1988). Hartsough and Lambert (1985) reported that children with ADHD were more likely to have difficulties with bowel training than nondisabled children (10.1% vs. 4.5%), whereas Munir et al. (1987) found that 18% of their sample with ADHD had functional encopresis. We were unable to replicate either of these findings, however (Barkley, DuPaul, & McMurray, 1990). Thus it is not clear whether children with ADHD are more likely to have problems with enuresis or encopresis, but the evidence seems far from convincing to date.

A recent study employing a population-based case–control study of children in Iceland has demonstrated a significant association of ADHD with risk for epilepsy and unprovoked seizures (Hesdorffer et al., 2004). In this study, children with ADHD were 2.5 times more likely to develop epilepsy or unprovoked seizures, particularly if they had the Predominantly Inattentive Type of the disorder. The inverse relationship also held true: A history of ADHD (Predominantly Inattentive Type) was found to be 2.5 times more common among children with epilepsy or unprovoked seizures.

Several studies have found children with ADHD to have a higher likelihood of sleeping problems than nondisabled children. Difficulties with time taken to fall asleep may be seen in as many as 56% of children with ADHD compared to 23% of typical children, and up to 39% of those with ADHD may show problems with frequent night waking (see Corkum, Tannock, & Moldofsky, 1998, for a review; Greenhill, Anich, Goetz, Hanton, & Davies, 1983; Kaplan et al., 1987; Stein, 1999; Stewart et al., 1966; Trommer, Hoeppner, Rosenberg, Armstrong, & Rothstein, 1988). A study by Ball, Tiernan, Janusz, and Furr (1997) found that 53–64% of their group with ADHD had sleep problems as reported by parents, and that whether or not the children were taking stimulant medication did not seem to influence these results. This higher incidence of sleep difficulties may appear as early as babyhood (Stewart et al., 1966; Trommer et al., 1988), with as many as 52% of children with ADHD described as having disturbed sleep in infancy, compared to 21% of nondisabled children. Resistance to going to bed and fewer total sleep hours may be the most obvious sleep difficulties that children with ADHD experience as reported by parents (Stein, 1999; Wilens, Biederman, & Spencer, 1994). Difficulties with sleep onset and night waking are believed to characterize an unstable sleep pattern that has been shown to be significantly associated with ADHD (Gruber, Sadeh, & Raviv, 2000). More than 55% of these children have also been described by parents as tired on awakening, compared to 27% of nondisabled children (Trommer et al., 1988). And children with ADHD manifest more frequent episodes of sleepiness during the day (Lecendreux, Konofal, Bouvard, Falissard, & Mouren-Simeoni, 2000).

Yet studies using objective measures of sleep, such as polysomnograms of overnight sleep, have not documented any difficulties in the physiological nature of sleeping itself associated with ADHD (Ball & Koloian, 1995; Corkum et al., 1998; Lecendreaux et al., 2000). Sleep quality (objectively measured) does not seem to account for these daytime reports of tiredness and sleepiness.

Importantly, it appears that many of the behavioral difficulties surrounding children's bedtime are more a function of the disorders often comorbid with ADHD (ODD, anxiety disorders) than of ADHD itself (Corkum, Beig, Tannock, & Moldofsky, 1997; Corkum, Moldofsky, Hogg-Johnson, Humphries, & Tannock, 1999). Or they may be nonspecific to ADHD, in that they characterize other behavior problems or learning disorders as well (Gregory & O'Connor, 2002; Marcotte et al., 1998). Therefore, it is not clear yet that ADHD per se is associated with sleep problems or whether it is the frequently associated comorbid conditions, such as ODD, LDs, or anxiety depression (Corkum et al., 1999; Gregory & O'Connor, 2002; Marcotte et al., 1998), are contributing to these findings of greater sleep difficulties in groups with ADHD than in control groups. One characteristic of the sleep of children with ADHD may be greater movement during sleep (Corkum et al., 1999; Porrino et al., 1983; see Corkum et al., 1998 for a review).

Few studies have examined adolescents with ADHD, but one has found no greater frequency of sleep difficulties than in a control group (Stein et al., 2002). Only stimulant medication status was associated with elevated sleep difficulties in the group with ADHD. However, depression was significantly associated with sleeping difficulties in these adolescents; this finding is consistent with other results suggesting that with increasing age, depression is more predictive than ADHD of sleeping difficulties into adolescence and adulthood (Gregory & O'Connor, 2002).

The quantity of sleep a child gets is certainly associated with teacher ratings of externalizing behavioral problems, particularly inattention (Aronen, Paavonen, Fjallberg, Soininen, & Torronen, 2000). One study examined the relationship between different dimensions of children's psychopathology and different dimensions of sleeping problems (Stein, Mendelsohn, Obermeyer, Amromin, & Benca, 2001). Insomnia was the only sleep problem related to ratings of inattention, while noisy sleep was related to ratings of aggression, and parasomnias (sleepwalking, nightmares, night terrors, headbanging) were related to anxiety/depression, thought problems, and social problems. Some authors have argued that this means that sleep problems may be contributing to psychopathology in these children (Aronen et al., 2000). But the direction of effect in these studies is unclear, given the correlational nature of these findings. Is limited sleep (insomnia) a direct contributor to school behavioral problems and inattention, or is it that children more likely to misbehave and be inattentive are also more likely to have difficulties getting to sleep at night? These results simply cannot answer the question. One study, however, did manipulate sleep quantity while examining its impact on daytime behavior problems in typical, healthy children (Fallone, Acebo, Arnedt, Seifer, & Carskadon, 2001). Children whose sleep had been restricted to 4 hours on one occasion were found the next day to have increased inattention, but not increased hyperactive or impulsive behavior. Nor did they have impaired performance on a lab measure of inattention and impulsiveness. This study suggests that limited sleep may well increase inattentiveness in children, but the short duration of the sleep manipulation may have limited the study's ability to test this relationship between sleep and other behavioral indicators. Sadeh, Gruber, and Raviv (2003) restricted the sleep of nondisabled children by an hour over three consecutive nights and did find an effect on lab measures of neurobehavioral functioning (attention, inhibition, etc.). Also of interest is the recent finding that while reduced sleep may well be associated with inattentiveness in typical, healthy children, it is not related to the behavioral symptoms in children with ADHD (Gruber & Sadeh, 2004). These results suggest that the causal connection between sleep and inattention that may be evident in normal children does not arise from the same mechanism(s) as may exist between ADHD and its associated sleep problems.

ACCIDENTAL INJURIES

Children with ADHD are considerably more likely to experience injuries due to accidents than are nondisabled children (see Barkley, 2001, for a review), with up to 57% being described as accident-prone and 15% having had at least four or more serious accidental injuries, such as broken bones, lacerations, head injuries, severe bruises, lost teeth, or accidental poisonings (Hartsough & Lambert, 1985; Mitchell et al., 1987; Reebye, 1997; Stewart et al., 1966). Results for the comparison or nondisabled groups of children in these studies were 11% and 4.8%, respectively. Stewart, Thach, and Friedin (1970) found that 21% of hyperactive children had experienced at least one accidental poisoning, compared to 7.7% of typical children. In a much larger study of more than 2,600 children, Szatmari et al. (1989) found that 7.3% of children with ADHD had an accidental poisoning and that 23.2% had suffered bone fractures, compared to 2.6% and 15.1%, respectively, in the control group. In a study of all children living in British Columbia, children with disruptive behavior (identified through ADHD medication treatment records) were substantially more likely to have experienced an injury than control children, as well as to have suffered greater postoperative complications and more adverse effects of drug treatments. Leibson et al. (2003), using a large birth cohort, reported an elevated risk for major injuries among children with ADHD (59% vs. 49%). Consistent with this finding, Swensen, Birnbaum, et al. (2004) also found a higher incidence of accident claims among children with ADHD (28% vs. 18%) and adolescents with ADHD (32% vs. 23%) in a study examining medical claims for a large population of employees of national manufacturers. The injuries that children with ADHD sustain may also be more frequent and more severe. For instance, Mangus, Bergman, Zieger, and Coleman (2004) examined children admitted over a 7-year period to a regional pediatric burn unit and found that those having ADHD had a greater likelihood of a thermal rather than a flame burn, more extensive burn injuries, and a longer stay in the unit. Hoare and Beattie (2003) compared children with ADHD and control children who had attended an accident and emergency department in Edinburgh, Scotland; they noted that children with ADHD were more likely to attend because of injury, and that these children had a greater frequency of injury as well as different types of injuries (head, wound laceration, poisoning). It seems clear that children with ADHD have an elevated risk of physical injury, of more frequent injuries, and of more severe injuries than do nondisabled children.

Some retrospective and prospective studies generally find a relationship between the degree of aggressiveness (not the degree of overactivity) and the likelihood of accidental injury in preschoolers (Davidson, Hughes, & O'Connor, 1988; Langley, McGee, Silva, & Williams, 1983). Because children with ADHD are more likely to be aggressive or oppositional, it may be this characteristic that increases their accident proneness, rather than their higher rates of activity level or impulsivity (Langley et al., 1983; Manheimer & Mellinger, 1967). Yet a large population study of 10,394 British children found that both overactivity and aggression contributed independently to the prediction of accidents (Bijur et al., 1988). A later study (Lalloo, Sheiham, & Nazroo, 2003) examined 6,000 children in England and found that only hyperactivity was predictive of an increase in accidental injury, once demographic and socioeconomic factors were controlled for. Since the latter factors are more likely to be related to childhood aggressiveness, controlling for them may explain why aggressiveness itself was no longer predictive of accident risk in this study. And a recent study by Rowe, Maughan, and Goodman (2004) of injuries among more than 10,000 children in Britain found that ADHD was more likely to be related to fractures, while ODD was more closely related to burns and poisonings. Thus both ADHD and aggression or ODD may be linked to accidental injuries, but of different forms.

And what of the inverse question? Do children who experience more accidental injuries show an elevated level of ADHD? Research on children experiencing accidents suggests that they are more likely to be overactive, impulsive, and defiant (Cataldo et al., 1992; Rosen & Peterson, 1990; Stewart et al., 1970). Pless, Taylor, and Arsenault (1995) found that children injured as pedestrians or bicycle riders in traffic accidents performed more poorly on tests of vigilance and impulse control, and that they received higher parent and teacher ratings of hyperactive–aggressive behavior. This study suggests that among those experiencing such serious accidents, a higher percentage may have either ADHD per se or more ADHD symptoms than average.

Why do those with ADHD apparently have a greater risk for accidents, accidental injuries (other than head injuries), and accidental poisonings than those without the disorder? Obviously, the symptoms of the disorder would contribute to such risk. Parents report that their children with ADHD are inattentive while engaging in risky activities, are more heedless or thoughtless of the consequences of their actions, and thus place themselves in situations or engage in activities that are more likely than usual to result in physical harm. But there may be other reasons as well that deserve consideration, such as the following:

• *Motor incoordination.* As discussed above, children with ADHD demonstrate greater motor clumsiness, more awkwardness, and more rapid and ill-timed motor movements than other children. They also demonstrate slower reaction times than typical children. It is not hard to see how such clumsiness or even DCD might contribute to accident risk, particularly in an already impulsive group of children.

• *Comorbid ODD and CD.* Another, more important contributor may be comorbidity for ODD and CD. As has been repeatedly noted above, children experiencing accidents are frequently more aggressive, defiant, and oppositional than other children, or at least pose more discipline problems for parents. ODD and CD, as stated earlier, are far more common in children with ADHD, and such comorbidity may contribute to an even greater risk for accidents and injuries than would be the case in ADHD alone. Indeed, some have argued that this pattern of defiant and aggressive behavior is far more contributory to accident risk than is hyperactivity per se.

• *Poor parental supervision or monitoring of children's activities.* A few studies of children's accidents, particularly those taking place out of doors, suggest that parents of these children may supervise their children's play activities less than other parents do. Accident proneness is therefore moderated by certain parental characteristics such as degree of monitoring of child behavior and maternal neuroticism (Davidson et al., 1988; Davidson, Taylor, Sandberg, & Thorley, 1992). Parents of children described as hyperactive or injury-prone play less often with them, allow the children out of their homes for longer periods of time, and let them go to school alone more often than do parents of control children (see Chapter 4). Schwebel, Brezausek, Ramey, and Ramey (2004) found that among children at high risk for injury (males, those with hyperactivity, and those with families living in poverty), positive parenting and greater time available for parents to be with children were protective against risk for injuries. Though far more research remains to be done on the issue of parental supervision and its quality in relation to accident risk, present evidence suggests that parental monitoring may be either a risk factor (if low) or a protective factor (if high), and that such monitoring may be less adequate among parents of children with ADHD.

These and other factors are worth considering by clinicians in efforts to reduce the injury risk to children with ADHD.

DRIVING-RELATED DIFFICULTIES

Until a decade ago, one domain of major life activity for teens and adults that had not been well explored in research on ADHD was driving, or the independent operation of a motor vehicle. Driving is often an underappreciated domain of self-sufficiency and major life activity for adults. Yet it is one that facilitates most other adaptive domains, including employment; family care, responsibilities, and overall functioning; education; and social engagements, shopping, and entertainment. All these domains would suffer extreme curtailment if an adult were to be deprived of this privilege, especially in the United States. In these domains, driving permits greater independence from others, exposure to more numerous opportunities, and greater efficiency in accomplishing various goals. It also, however, opens up greater exposure to harm to oneself, to others, and to property by providing access to a 1- to 2-ton projectile that is often used at speeds in excess of 50–60 miles per hour. Thus any disorder that may have an adverse impact on driving would be expected to have a pervasive (albeit secondary) impact on many other domains of daily adaptive functioning in other major life activities, while simultaneously exposing the individual to greater liabilities for the various harms noted above. ADHD is just such a disorder that should have some impact on operation of a motor vehicle. What follows has been drawn from my recent review of this literature (Barkley, 2004).

An early longitudinal study of hyperactive children followed to adulthood suggested that the disorder might be associated with greater adverse outcomes associated with driving. Weiss, Hechtman, Perlman, Hopkins, and Wener (1979) found that as adolescents and as young adults, individuals with hyperactivity were more likely to be involved in traffic accidents as drivers than their nondisabled peers. They were also likely to incur greater damage to their vehicles relative to nondisabled controls (Hechtman, Weiss, Perlman, & Tuck, 1981). Interesting as the results were concerning a likely relationship of ADHD to poor driving, these risks were largely determined through self-reports and were not corroborated through the official driving records of the participants. Nor was the basis for these driving-related adverse outcomes evident in this early study. Was it the inattention associated with ADHD that led to such risks, the impulsivity, or both? Or were these risks the result of comorbid disorders, especially CD (in which case they would constitute one more manifestation of antisocial conduct)?

To pursue these various lines of reasoning, my colleagues and I undertook a series of studies on the driving problems associated with ADHD. Our first project involved a 3- to 5-year followup survey of nondisabled adolescents and adolescents with ADHD who had been recruited into an earlier study of teens with ADHD and their family functioning (Barkley, Guevremont, Anastopoulos, DuPaul, & Shelton, 1993). The survey asked parents about a variety of negative driving outcomes their teens might have experienced in the interim followup period since the teens began driving. The following findings were obtained:

- The teens and young adults with ADHD were more likely to have driven an automobile illegally prior to the time they became licensed drivers.
- They were less likely to be employing sound driving habits in their current driving performance, as reported by their parents.
- They were more likely to have had their licenses suspended or revoked.
- They were more likely to have received repeated traffic citations, most notably for speeding.
- Importantly, they were nearly four times more likely to have had an accident while driving a vehicle.
- Although the degree of current ADHD symptoms was significantly associated with driving risks, some risks were further associated with the degree of oppositional and conduct problems.

This led us to question adults with ADHD about their driving problems when they were recruited to participate in a separate study on clinical impairments associated with ADHD. That study used 171 adults diagnosed with ADHD and 30 adults seen in this same clinic but not diagnosed with ADHD (their diagnoses

were predominantly anxiety or mood disorders) (Murphy & Barkley, 1996). Similar results to those found above for teens with ADHD were evident. The adults with ADHD were more than three times as likely to have had automobile accidents, tended to have more such accidents ($p < .06$), and had more traffic citations for speeding than did the psychiatric control group.

About this time, Lambert (1995) provided an unpublished report to the U.S. Department of Transportation's National Highway Traffic Safety Administration, using data from her longitudinal study of hyperactive and control children. She found that, by age 25 years, those with severe ADHD in childhood had a significantly greater likelihood of traffic citations in their later driving histories than did control children or those with mild ADHD. They were also more likely to repeat the same traffic offenses than were the comparison groups. There was also a trend for the group with severe ADHD to have had more accidents but this was not statistically significant. At about this same time, an epidemiological study of adolescents followed in the Dunedin (New Zealand) longitudinal project also documented increased driving offenses and vehicular crashes in teens with significantly elevated symptoms of ADHD (Nada-Raja et al., 1997). A comparable study using the Christchurch longitudinal sample (also in New Zealand) found a similar association of attention difficulties with risk for accidents involving injury, driving without a license, and traffic violations, even after conduct problems, driving experience, and gender were controlled (Woodward, Fergusson, & Horwood, 2000).

We have subsequently conducted several studies exploring the impact of ADHD on driving at the operational level (skill in using a vehicle) and tactical level (maneuvering in the presence of other drivers). We have also examined driving knowledge in addition to operational skills. Strategic driving (the goals of the trip and use of the car to accomplish them), however, has not been evaluated in these studies, leaving open the issue of the impact of ADHD on driving at this level and suggesting an avenue for future research.

In our initial pilot study, our research team (Barkley et al., 1996b) compared 25 young adults with ADHD to 23 young adults from the community. Not only were the participants interviewed about their driving histories and their traffic offenses and crashes (adverse driving outcomes) as in past studies, but the study also obtained their official driving records from the state Department of Motor Vehicles (DMV). We also assessed the driving abilities of participants, using a computer-simulated driving test like that sometimes used by occupational therapists or clinical neuropsychologists to assess driving ability among elderly or neurologically impaired patients. The test was chosen as a means of determining the basis for the driving problems that seemed to be associated with ADHD. The testing device comprised a computer monitor placed on top of a small cabinet that also contained a small steering wheel and directional signal, both of which were connected to a computer. The apparatus also included gas and brake pedals on the floor, likewise connected to the computer hardware. A two-dimensional roadway, like a maze, moved vertically across the monitor, and the subject had to steer a small rectangle (the vehicle) through the roadway (maze) while following various instructions from the examiner. Finally, we evaluated driving knowledge and decision-making abilities, using a videotape test of actual driving situations. This commercially available videotape is used to screen applicants for positions with commercial transportation companies.

As in earlier studies, more of these young adults with ADHD had received speeding tickets (100% vs. 54%), had had their licenses suspended or revoked (32% vs. 4%), and had been involved in a crash as the driver (80% vs. 52%) than young adults in the control group. They also had received more speeding tickets (4.9 vs. 1.3) and experienced significantly more crashes (means = 2.7 vs. 1.6). In addition, more of the group with ADHD had been involved in crashes resulting in injuries (60% vs. 17%). DMV records corroborated many of these adverse outcomes. Furthermore, the young adults with ADHD rated themselves as employing poorer driving habits while operating their own motor vehicles, and were rated by others as using poorer driving habits, compared to the control group. No differences in driving knowledge were evident on the videotape test, suggesting that those with ADHD seemed to know as much about driving as the control group. But the group with ADHD showed significantly more erratic control of the simulated motor vehicle in the driving simulator and had

more scrapes and crashes in this test. This was the first study to demonstrate that ADHD may adversely affect individuals' tactical management of a motor vehicle beyond predisposing them toward more traffic offenses and vehicular crashes. Thus we were able to conclude that the tactical level of driving is problematic for those with ADHD, whereas problems with knowledge were not evident here. The study, however, did not explore the operational level concerning basic cognitive abilities that are essential for safe operation of the vehicle, though such deficits have been clearly established in earlier research on the disorder. Unfortunately, the small samples used in this study reduced its statistical power, such that it was able to detect only large effect sizes as significant. This factor may have accounted for its failure to find any group differences on the videotape test of driving knowledge and decision-making ability.

Nevertheless, this small study was sufficiently promising to warrant a much larger examination of driving in ADHD (Barkley, Murphy, DuPaul, & Bush, 2002). We did so by comparing large samples of teens and young adults with ADHD ($n = 105$) and community controls ($n = 64$). Like our pilot study, this one not only used self-reports of driving history and negative outcomes, but also obtained DMV records on all participants. It once again evaluated the actual driving behavior of participants through self-ratings and ratings by others who knew the participants' driving well. Unlike any prior studies of ADHD, however, this study also assessed the cognitive abilities necessary for safe driving (e.g., reaction time, visual discrimination, and rule-following ability). This provided for a multimethod, multi-informant, and multilevel evaluation of driving knowledge, competence, and adverse outcomes of the participants—an evaluation more comprehensive in scope than had been attempted in prior studies.

Again, this study found that young adults with ADHD experienced more adverse driving outcomes than control adults. This was evident both in the participants' own self-reported histories and in their official DMV records. Young adults with ADHD had received more than twice as many driving citations (means = 11.7 vs. 4.8), particularly for speeding (3.9 vs. 2.4), as the control group; they had also had more license suspensions/revocations in their relatively short driving careers to date (0.5 vs. 0.1). Moreover, the group with ADHD reported being involved in more vehicular crashes as the driver (1.9 vs. 1.2) over the average of 4.5 years they had been driving, being at fault in more such crashes (1.3 vs. 0.9), and having more severe crashes as reflected in dollar value of damage than did the control group ($4,221 vs. $1,665). With the exception of vehicular crashes, group differences on several of these adverse outcomes were further corroborated in the official DMV records. Such driving risks may have begun even earlier in adolescence in the ADHD than in the control group. As we found in a previous smaller study of teens, significantly more of the group with ADHD (64% vs. 40%) reported having driven a motor vehicle illegally as teenagers prior to being licensed to drive than did the control group. These findings clearly highlight the high risks that those with ADHD both experience and create in their daily driving activities.

Moreover, as noted above, this large-scale study extended earlier research by examining multiple levels of basic cognitive ability and driving performance beyond just assessing adverse outcomes from driving histories. Here, as well, the group with ADHD manifested some limitations in basic cognitive functions related to driving. On the CPT, the participants with ADHD were substantially less attentive during the task than the controls. They were not, however, more impulsive on that task (but were on a computerized CPT). The group with ADHD also performed comparably to the control group on basic visual discrimination and reaction time tasks, suggesting no perceptual impairments that might affect driving. In contrast, those with ADHD made significantly more errors when the instructions for this task were reversed, implying difficulties in rule-governed behavior under such circumstances. In other words, they were more governed by the events in the stimulus fields than by the rules in effect that competed with those stimuli. And they achieved significantly fewer correct responses in a visual scanning task, particularly when items were presented to the right visual field. Why this should be the case is unclear and is deserving of replication in future studies.

The difficulties with attentiveness, impulse control on a computerized CPT, and rule following evident here have been found in previous studies of cognitive functioning in ADHD children (see Chapter 2). They extend those deficits to the young adult age group with this disorder and may provide some hint as to one

reason for the greater frequency of accidents in those with ADHD. Driver inattentiveness was given by both participants with ADHD and control participants here as the single most frequent reason for their vehicular crashes (approximately 45%). These results clearly suggest that ADHD has an adverse impact on the operational or basic cognitive level necessary for driving, and that driver inattention, poor rule adherence, reduced inhibition, and deficient resistance to distraction may be mechanisms by which ADHD adversely affects driving.

Four areas of knowledge were assessed here. In three of these, the group with ADHD did not differ from the control group, suggesting equivalent knowledge in perceptual skills, traffic risk situations, and driving procedures. In contrast, general driving knowledge (driving laws and rules of the road) was significantly lower in the group with ADHD than in the control group. This is the first study to document that drivers having ADHD may be at a disadvantage in some areas of driving knowledge, compared to drivers without ADHD. It is not clear whether this represents a deficit in driving knowledge or in the rapid application of that knowledge during decision making.

Efforts were again made here to evaluate the tactical or operational driving performance of participants through the use of a computer-based driving simulation program previously used for screening elderly and head-injured adults. Our previous study of a smaller sample of young adults (Barkley et al., 1996b) found the group with ADHD to have more steering incoordination, more scrapes, and more crashes of the simulated vehicle while driving through the three different courses, as noted earlier. This study was unable to replicate these results. This occurred despite testing participants twice on the simulator to enhance the sensitivity of the measure to any potential impairment in the group with ADHD. It is possible that young adults with ADHD simply have no difficulties with the tactical operation of a motor vehicle in terms of negotiating driving courses. Or the previous results may have been due more to group differences in IQ than to ADHD, given that the effect of IQ level on simulator performance in that study was not examined.

It is also possible that an inexpensive, computer-based simulator such as the one used here is simply not sensitive enough to any subtle difficulties that young adults with ADHD may have in operating a motor vehicle. After all, a cabinet with a computer monitor and small steering wheel hardly approximates a real vehicle, nor does a two-dimensional black-and-white maze have much similarity to three-dimensional roadways with traffic. The results here may suggest that simple driving simulators are inadequate for evaluating the driving risks of young adults with ADHD. More modern virtual-reality driving simulation systems may be required to detect group differences (see below).

Although these simulator results might suggest that those with ADHD have no difficulties in the tactical level of driving, the ratings noted above concerning the actual use of safe driving habits while driving suggest otherwise. Both the drivers with ADHD and others who knew them well rated them as poorer in vehicle management and in other tactical aspects of safe driving behavior than was the case in the control group. This constitutes the third study to find such group differences on ratings of actual driving, and it clearly supports a problem with the safe tactical operation of a vehicle in those with ADHD. Given that such ratings have been shown to have a significant relation to accidents and traffic citations (Barkley et al., 1993), such poor ratings have some predictive validity.

This study made special efforts to examine what other factors than ADHD may have contributed to these group differences. Gender of the participants and ADHD subtype appeared to make no contribution. Nor did the initial group differences in IQ. Although several of the lab measures of basic cognitive abilities and driving knowledge and performance showed significant main effects for IQ level in this study, in no instance was there a significant interaction of group with IQ level. Comorbid ODD, depression, and anxiety, as well as frequency of alcohol use, drunkenness, and drug use, also did not account for the group differences reported here. It is still possible that these comorbid conditions may have contributed small effects to the measures collected here that went undetected, given the relatively modest sample sizes available for each comparison. Nevertheless, these results lend some support to the conclusion that the group differences evident here are largely, if not wholly, the result of ADHD.

In our most recent study (Barkley, Murphy, O'Connell, Anderson, & Connor, in press), we have explored the effects of two doses of alcohol on the driving performance of adults with ADHD. Our findings suggest that those with ADHD experience a more marked deterioration in their driving performance even at lower doses of alcohol than do control adults. This has led us to recommend that clinicians caution those with ADHD not to consume alcohol at all when they are about to operate a motor vehicle.

To summarize, ADHD clearly predisposes drivers to greater risks of adverse driving outcomes, such as more traffic citations, repeated vehicular crashes, more severe crashes, and ultimately a greater likelihood of license suspension or revocation. One basis for such elevated risks appears to consist of the underlying cognitive impairments inherent in the disorder—specifically, attention deficits, poor resistance to distraction, greater difficulties with response inhibition, and problems in executive functioning (such as rule adherence and working memory). ADHD therefore disrupts the operational level of driving. It remains likely that ADHD also contributes to difficulties at the tactical level of vehicular operation. Although this was evident in one study of ours using a relatively simple driving simulator, this result was not subsequently replicated. A more modern virtual-reality driving simulator, however, is showing some promise in detecting such tactical deficits in the driving of adults with ADHD in our lab. Even so, if behavior ratings of the use of safe driving habits in natural settings can be taken as an index of this level of driving, then all of our studies have found ADHD to be associated with such poor use of safe driving behavior.

The two studies examining the knowledge aspect of driving have not made a convincing case that ADHD disrupts this dimension or component of driving. Our initial small study found no differences in knowledge, while our larger subsequent study found a deficit mainly in knowledge of driving laws, but not in three other areas of driving knowledge. No studies to date have examined the strategic level of driving, much less the higher dimensions of driving identified in driving models—for instance, value judgments, the emotional/motivational aspects of driving, or how driving contributes to larger life goals and self-sufficiency. Nevertheless, it is abundantly evident that ADHD is likely to contribute directly to various driving performance problems and associated adverse outcomes. And use of alcohol apparently results in a greater impairment in driving performance among adults with ADHD than among control adults.

LIFE EXPECTANCY

The relationships between ADHD and increased (1) accident proneness in childhood; (2) speeding and auto accidents in adolescence and young adulthood; (3) crime (Satterfield, Hoppe, & Schell, 1982); (4) suicide attempts (Weiss & Hechtman, 1993); (5) use and abuse of substances (alcohol and tobacco, primarily) in adolescence and adulthood (Biederman et al., 1996); and (6) a general pattern of risk-taking behavior all intimate that ADHD might be expected to be associated with a reduced life expectancy. The diminished regard for the future consequences of one's behavior that characterizes many adolescents and adults with ADHD would also predict a reduced concern for health-conscious behavior, such as exercise, proper diet, and moderation in using legal substances (caffeine, tobacco, and alcohol) throughout life (Barkley, Fischer, et al., 1990; Milberger, Biederman, Faraone, Chen, & Jones, 1996).

No follow-up studies of children with hyperactivity or ADHD have lasted long enough to document such a reduction in life expectancy; the oldest subjects now appear to be entering their 40s (Weiss & Hechtman, 1993). Yet concern over life expectancy in ADHD is not unfounded. One study recently found that individuals with ADHD are more than twice as likely to die prematurely from their misadventures as are controls (Swensen, Allen, Kruesi, Buesching, & Goldberg, 2004).

Further cause for concern arises from the follow-up study of Terman's original sample of highly intelligent children. Most of those subjects are now in their 70s or older, and half of them are deceased (Friedman et al., 1995). The follow-up study of that group indicated that the most significant childhood personality traits predictive of reduced life expectancy by all causes were impulsive, undercontrolled personality characteristics. Individuals who were classified as having this set of characteristics lived an average of 8 years less than those who were not (73 vs. 81 years). Subjects in this study were defined as impulsive by virtue of falling within the lowest 25% of the sample in

impulse control. Given that subjects defined as having ADHD typically fall well below this threshold (i.e., in the lowest 5–7%), the risk for reduced longevity in those with ADHD would seem to be even greater than was found among Terman's subjects. That conclusion would seem to be further supported by the fact that Terman's subjects were intellectually gifted and came from families of above-average or higher economic backgrounds. Both of these factors probably would have conveyed a greater advantage toward longer life expectancy than would be the case for intellectually average children with ADHD, who tend to come from middle or lower economic backgrounds. Thus there is some reason to suspect that the implications of this model for reduced life expectancy as a function of ADHD are not without some merit—at least as an issue deserving of future research, if not as a well-supported conclusion at the moment.

UTILIZATION OF MEDICAL CARE

Early studies did not find children with ADHD to have any more hospitalizations, length of hospital stays, or surgeries than nondisabled children (Barkley, DuPaul, & McMurray, 1990; Hartsough & Lambert, 1985; Stewart et al., 1966). But in view of their clearly elevated risks for various injuries, children with ADHD probably should use more medical care and generate greater medical costs. This has been observed in more recent studies using larger samples. Children with ADHD have a significantly greater use of outpatient medical services and are especially more likely to utilize emergency department services (Leibson et al., 2003). This resulted in a significantly greater annual medical care cost for children with ADHD ($4,306 vs. $1,944) than for control children. Swensen et al. (2003) studied a large population sample (<100,000) and also found that annual medical care costs for children with ADHD were three times greater than in control cases ($1,574 vs. $571). But they also found that medical care cost claims were also greater among immediate family members (who did not have ADHD themselves) of the children with ADHD as well ($2,728 vs. $1,440). This finding is perhaps attributable to the greater risk of psychopathology, substance dependence and abuse, stress, and depression among these family members (see Chapter 4).

SUMMARY

This chapter has reviewed the myriad cognitive, academic, social, emotional, health, and developmental problems associated with ADHD. These problems are summarized in Table 3.1. They are clearly substantial and serious. At the very least, such findings ought to give considerable pause to anyone who would contend that ADHD is a phantom disorder (Kohn, 1989; McGinnis, 1997); that it is simply a label being used to give a psychiatric diagnosis to otherwise normally exuberant children who do not want to take responsibility for their own behavior; that it merely reflects parental or teacher intolerance for such childhood exuberance; or that it is an otherwise benign condition, with few or no developmental, psychiatric, educational, or social consequences. Henceforth, such claims ought to be dismissed as the scientifically illiterate statements they represent, rather than considered to reflect a true scientific debate over the validity and worth of the diagnosis of ADHD. This validity and utility have been well established by nearly a century of research and thousands of published studies on the distinguishing symptoms, associated impairments, and developmental risks that befall those children and adolescents unfortunate enough to receive a clinical diagnosis of this condition. Even more than the evidence presented in Chapter 2 of this volume, the evidence reviewed here overwhelmingly demonstrates that ADHD comprises a harmful dysfunction (Wakefield, 1992, 1997). It therefore deserves the status of a true mental disorder as much as, or more than, any other child psychiatric disorder currently known.

KEY CLINICAL POINTS

✓ ADHD is associated with numerous developmental, cognitive, academic, and health risks and impairments.

✓ In the cognitive and academic domains, ADHD is specifically associated with a modest reduction in intelligence; moderate or greater deficiencies in domains of adaptive functioning and academic achievement skills; and a considerably higher risk for LDs.

✓ ADHD is also associated with deficiencies in speech pragmatics, story recall, verbal flu-

TABLE 3.1. Summary of Impairments Likely to Be Associated with ADHD

Cognitive
- Mild deficits in intelligence (approximately 7–10 points)
- Deficient academic achievement skills (range of 10–30 standard score points)
- Learning disabilities: reading (8–39%), spelling (12–26%), math (12–33%), and handwriting (common 60%+)
- Poor use of time in daily time management; inaccurate time reproduction
- Decreased verbal working memory
- Impaired planning ability
- Reduced sensitivity to errors
- Delayed adaptive and social functioning (10–30 standard score points below average)

Language
- Delayed onset of language (up to 35%, but not consistent)
- Speech impairments, mostly expressive or pragmatic (10–54%)
- Excessive conversational speech (commonplace); reduced speech to confrontation
- Decreased verbal fluency
- Poor organization and inefficient and illogical expression of ideas
- Impaired verbal problem solving
- Poor rule-governed behavior
- Delayed internalization of speech (≥30% delay)
- Deficient listening comprehension, especially when distractions are present
- Diminished development of moral reasoning

Motor development
- Delayed motor coordination (up to 52%); Developmental Coordination Disorder
- More neurological "soft signs" related to motor coordination and overflow movements
- Sluggish gross motor movements
- Poor graphomotor (writing) ability

Emotion
- Poor self-regulation of emotion; greater emotional expression, especially anger and aggression
- Greater problems coping with frustration

(continued)

TABLE 3.1. *(continued)*

- Possibly reduced empathy
- Underreactive arousal to tasks and stimulation

School performance
- Disruptive classroom behavior (commonplace)
- Underperforming in school relative to ability (commonplace)
- Academic tutoring (up to 56%)
- Repetition of a grade (30% or more)
- Placement in one or more special education programs (30–40%)
- School suspensions (up to 46%)
- School expulsions (10–20%)
- Failure to graduate from high school (10–35%)

Task performance
- Poor persistence of effort/motivation (giving up on tasks easily)
- Greater variability in reaction time and in task performance
- Decreased performance/productivity under delayed rewards
- Greater problems when time delays are imposed within a task and as they increase in duration
- Decline in performance as reinforcement changes from being continuous to intermittent or delayed
- Greater disruption when noncontingent consequences occur during the task

Medical/health risks
- Greater proneness to accidental injuries of all types
- Greater medical care costs
- Possibly delayed growth during childhood
- Possibly greater risk of asthma
- Difficulties getting to bed; insomnia (up to 30–60%)
- Greater driving risks: vehicular crashes, speeding tickets, traffic citations, and license suspensions
- Greater deterioration of driving performance after alcohol consumption

ency, and verbal problem solving; poor rule-governed behavior; mild to moderate difficulties in verbal thinking (less logic, fewer conjunctions, poor organization); and a delay in the internalization or privatization of speech.

✓ There is little consistent evidence for problems in spatial or sequential forms of working memory in association with ADHD, but greater evidence of moderate difficulties with verbal working memory.

✓ Evidence is substantial that ADHD involves impairment in short-interval time discrimination, and especially the ability to attend to, hold in mind, and subsequently duplicate durations of time intervals. Complaints by parents and teachers of poor time management are also common.

✓ Research findings are also suggestive of deficiencies in planning ability in conjunction with ADHD.

✓ Perseverative responding on tasks of cognitive flexibility, set shifting, and rule learning is not routinely found in children with ADHD, but difficulties in adhering to the rules of the task are sometimes evident.

✓ No convincing evidence exists that ADHD is associated with either deficits in or enhanced capability of various forms of verbal, figural, and conceptual creativity.

✓ ADHD is strongly associated with difficulties with emotion regulation, particularly the management of frustration. Children with ADHD display higher levels of aggression, anger, and sadness, while possibly showing lower levels of empathy.

✓ The self-awareness of children with ADHD appears to be characterized by a positive illusory bias, in that their self-reports of their competence are less accurate (particularly in areas in which they are most deficient) than is the case in nondisabled children.

✓ Under conditions of little or no reinforcement, children with ADHD have considerably greater difficulties with sustaining their task performance than control children, and may be more improved in their task performance than control children by the introduction of immediate and consistent reinforcement.

✓ Reward-seeking behavior, or perseverative responding toward tasks that were previously reinforcing but have become increasingly punitive, is not an associated feature of ADHD but has been repeatedly linked to conduct problems, CD, and psychopathy.

✓ ADHD is associated with a reduced level of brain electrical arousal on EEG and a reduced reactivity to stimulation on evoked responses than is seen in control children.

✓ Primary sensory problems are not associated with ADHD.

✓ Difficulties in motor development are a common comorbidity (poorer motor coordination, reduced physical fitness, and a greater occurrence of DCD).

✓ The most commonly associated health problems seen in ADHD may be a greater risk of asthma (not consistently observed); a greater risk for unprovoked seizures or epilepsy; greater difficulties with sleep onset or insomnia (other sleep problems may be better explained by comorbid disorders, especially depression); and greater physical movement during sleep.

✓ Voluminous evidence attests that a greater risk of accidental injury is associated with ADHD, as well as more frequent and severe injuries.

✓ Children with ADHD and their family members show greater utilization of the medical care system and greater medical costs.

✓ An impressive and growing body of evidence also demonstrates more impaired driving performance and a greater risk of associated adverse outcomes (crashes, citations, license suspension, etc.) in the driving histories of teens and adults with ADHD.

✓ Concerns have begun to arise that ADHD may be associated with reduced life expectancy, given the risks for accidental injuries, the twofold risk for premature death from risk taking, and evidence that reduced life expectancy is predicted by low levels of childhood conscientiousness (impulsivity).

REFERENCES

Ackerman, P. T., Anhalt, J. M., & Dykman, R. A. (1986). Arithmetic automatization failure in children with attention and reading disorders: Associations and sequelae. *Journal of Learning Disabilities, 19,* 222–232.

Alessandri, S. M. (1992). Attention, play, and social behavior in ADHD preschoolers. *Journal of Abnormal Child Psychology, 20,* 289–302.

American Psychiatric Association. (1987). *Diagnostic and statistical manual of mental disorders* (3rd ed., rev.). Washington, DC: Author.

American Psychiatric Association. (1994). *Diagnostic and statistical manual of mental disorders* (4th ed.). Washington, DC: Author.

Amin, K., Douglas, V. I., Mendelson, M. J., & Dufresne, J. (1993). Separable/integral classification by hyperactive and normal children. *Development and Psychopathology, 5,* 415–431.

Anastopoulos, A. D., Spisto, M. A., & Maher, M. C. (1994). The WISC-III Freedom from Distractibility factor: Its utility in identifying children with attention deficit hyperactivity disorder. *Psychological Assessment, 6,* 368–371.

Aronen, E. T., Paavonen, E. J., Fjallberg, M., Soininen, M., & Torronen, J. (2000). Sleep and psychiatric symptoms in school-age children. *Journal of the American Academy of Child and Adolescent Psychiatry, 39,* 502–508.

August, G. J. (1987). Production deficiencies in free recall: A comparison of hyperactive, learning-disabled, and normal children. *Journal of Abnormal Child Psychology, 15,* 429–440.

August, G. J., & Garfinkel, B. D. (1990). Comorbidity of ADHD and reading disability among clinic-referred children. *Journal of Abnormal Child Psychology, 18,* 29–45.

Baker, L., & Cantwell, D. P. (1987). A prospective psychiatric follow-up of children with speech/language disorders. *Journal of the American Academy of Child and Adolescent Psychiatry, 26,* 545–553.

Ball, J. D., & Koloian, B. (1995). Sleep patterns among ADHD children. *Clinical Psychology Review, 15,* 681–691.

Ball, J. D., Tiernan, M., Janusz, J., & Furr, A. (1997). Sleep patterns among children with attention-deficit hyperactivity disorder: A reexamination of parent perceptions. *Journal of Pediatric Psychology, 22,* 389–398.

Barber, M. A., & Milich, R. (1989, February). *The effects of reinforcement schedule and task characteristics on the behavior of attention-deficit hyperactivity disordered boys.* Paper presented at the annual meeting of the Society for Research in Child and Adolescent Psychopathology, Miami, FL.

Barber, M. A., Milich, R., & Welsh, R. (1996). Effects of reinforcement schedule and task difficulty on the performance of attention deficit hyperactivity disordered and control boys. *Journal of Clinical Child Psychology, 25,* 66–76.

Barkley, R. A. (1977). A review of stimulant drug research with hyperactive children. *Journal of Child Psychology and Psychiatry, 18,* 137–165.

Barkley, R. A. (1981). *Hyperactive children: A handbook for diagnosis and treatment.* New York: Guilford Press.

Barkley, R. A. (1989). The problem of stimulus control

and rule-governed behavior in children with attention deficit disorder with hyperactivity. In L. M. Bloomingdale & J. M. Swanson (Eds.), *Attention deficit disorder* (Vol. 4, pp. 203–234). New York: Pergamon Press.

Barkley, R. A. (1990). *Attention-deficit hyperactivity disorder: A handbook for diagnosis and treatment.* New York: Guilford Press.

Barkley, R. A. (1997a). Behavioral inhibition, sustained attention, and executive functions: Constructing a unifying theory of ADHD. *Psychological Bulletin, 121,* 65–94.

Barkley, R. A. (1997b). *ADHD and the nature of self-control.* New York: Guilford Press.

Barkley, R. A. (2001). Accidents and ADHD. *The Economics of Neuroscience, 3,* 64–68.

Barkley, R. A. (2004). Driving impairments in teens and adults with attention-deficit/hyperactivity disorder. *Psychiatric Clinics of North America, 27*(2), 233–260.

Barkley, R. A., Cunningham, C., & Karlsson, J. (1983). The speech of hyperactive children and their mothers: Comparisons with normal children and stimulant drug effects. *Journal of Learning Disabilities, 16,* 105–110.

Barkley, R. A., DuPaul, G. J., & McMurray, M. B. (1990). A comprehensive evaluation of attention deficit disorder with and without hyperactivity. *Journal of Consulting and Clinical Psychology, 58,* 775–789.

Barkley, R. A., Edwards, G., Laneri, M., Fletcher, K., & Metevia, L. (2001). Executive functioning, temporal discounting, and sense of time in adolescents with attention deficit hyperactivity disorder and oppositional defiant disorder. *Journal of Abnormal Child Psychology, 29,* 541–556.

Barkley, R. A., Fischer, M., Edelbrock, C. S., & Smallish, L. (1990). The adolescent outcome of hyperactive children diagnosed by research criteria: I. An 8 year prospective follow-up study. *Journal of the American Academy of Child and Adolescent Psychiatry, 29,* 546–557.

Barkley, R. A., Grodzinsky, G., & DuPaul, G. (1992). Frontal lobe functions in attention deficit disorder with and without hyperactivity: A review and research report. *Journal of Abnormal Child Psychology, 20,* 163–188.

Barkley, R. A., Guevremont, D. C., Anastopoulos, A. D., DuPaul, G. J., & Shelton, T. L. (1993). Driving-related risks and outcomes of attention deficit hyperactivity disorder in adolescents and young adults: A 3–5-year follow-up survey. *Pediatrics, 92,* 212–218.

Barkley, R. A., Karlsson, J., & Pollard, S. (1985). Effects of age on the mother–child interactions of hyperactive children. *Journal of Abnormal Child Psychology, 13,* 631–638.

Barkley, R. A., Koplowicz, S., Anderson, T., & McMurray, M. B. (1997). Sense of time in children with ADHD: Effects of duration, distraction, and stimulant medication. *Journal of the International Neuropsychological Society, 3,* 359–369.

Barkley, R. A., Murphy, K. R., & Bush, T. (2001). Time perception and reproduction in young adults with attention deficit hyperactivity disorder. *Neuropsychology, 15,* 351–360.

Barkley, R. A., Murphy, K. R., DuPaul, G. J., & Bush, T. (2002). Driving in young adults with attention deficit hyperactivity disorder: Knowledge, performance, adverse outcomes, and the role of executive functioning. *Journal of the International Neuropsychological Society, 8,* 655–672.

Barkley, R. A., Murphy, K. R., & Kwasnik, D. (1996a). Psychological adjustment and adaptive impairments in young adults with ADHD. *Journal of Attention Disorders, 1,* 41–54.

Barkley, R. A., Murphy, K. R., & Kwasnik, D. (1996b). Motor vehicle driving competencies and risks in teens and young adults with ADHD. *Pediatrics, 98,* 1089–1095.

Barkley, R. A., Murphy, K. R., O'Connell, T., Anderson, D., & Connor, D. F. (in press). Effects of two doses of alcohol on simulator driving performance in adults with attention deficit hyperactivity disorder. *Neuropsychology.*

Barkley, R. A., Shelton, T. L., Crosswait, C., Moorehouse, M., Fletcher, K., Barrett, S., et al. (2002). Preschool children with high levels of disruptive behavior: Three-year outcomes as a function of adaptive disability. *Development and Psychopathology, 14,* 45–68.

Bauermeister, J. J., Barkley, R. A., Martinez, J. V., Cumba, E., Ramirez, R. R., Reina, G., et al. Time estimation and performance on reproduction tasks in subtypes of children with Attention-Deficit Hyperactivity Disorder. *Journal of Clinical Child and Adolescent Psychology, 34,* 151–162.

Beauchaine, T. P. (2001). Vagal tone, development, and Gray's motivational theory: Toward an integrated model of autonomic nervous system functioning in psychopathology. *Development and Psychopathology, 13,* 183–214.

Beauchaine, T. P., Katkin, E. S., Strassberg, Z., & Snarr, J. (2001). Disinhibitory psychopathology in male adolescents: Discriminating conduct disorder from attention-deficit/hyperactivity disorder through concurrent assessment of multiple autonomic states. *Journal of Abnormal Psychology, 110,* 610–624.

Becker, J. T. (Ed.). (1994). Special section: Working memory. *Neuropsychology, 8,* 483–562.

Benezra, E., & Douglas, V. I. (1988). Short-term serial recall in ADDH, normal, and reading-disabled boys. *Journal of Abnormal Child Psychology, 16,* 511–525.

Berk, L. E. (1992). Children's private speech: An overview of theory and the status of research. In R. M. Diaz & L. E. Berk (Eds.), *Private speech: From social interaction to self-regulation* (pp. 17–54). Hillsdale, NJ: Erlbaum.

Berk, L. E. (1994, November). Why children talk to themselves. *Scientific American,* pp. 78–83.

Berk, L. E., & Garvin, R. A. (1984). Development of

private speech among low-income Appalachian children. *Developmental Psychology, 20,* 271–286.

Berk, L. E., & Landau, S. (1993). Private speech of learning disabled and normally achieving children in classroom academic and laboratory contexts. *Child Development, 64,* 556–571.

Berk, L. E., & Potts, M. K. (1991). Development and functional significance of private speech among attention-deficit hyperactivity disorder and normal boys. *Journal of Abnormal Child Psychology, 19,* 357–377.

Berkowitz, M. W. (1982). Self-control development and relation to prosocial behavior: A response to Peterson. *Merrill–Palmer Quarterly, 28,* 223–236.

Biederman, J., Milberger, S., Faraone, S. V., Guite, J., & Warburton, R. (1994). Associations between childhood asthma and ADHD: Issues of psychiatric comorbidity and familiality. *Journal of the American Academy of Child and Adolescent Psychiatry, 33,* 842–848.

Biederman, J., Milberger, S., Faraone, S. V., Lapey, K. A., Reed, E. D., & Seidman, L. J. (1995). No confirmation of Geschwind's hypothesis of associations between reading disability, immune disorders, and motor preference in ADHD. *Journal of Abnormal Child Psychology, 23,* 545–552.

Biederman, J., Wilens, T., Mick, E., Faraone, S. V., Weber, W., Curtis, S., et al. (1996). Is ADHD a risk factor for psychoactive substance use disorders?: Findings from a four-year prospective follow-up study. *Journal of the American Academy of Child and Adolescent Psychiatry, 36,* 21–29.

Bijur, P., Golding, J., Haslum, M., & Kurzon, M. (1988). Behavioral predictors of injury in school-age children. *American Journal of Diseases of Children, 142,* 1307–1312.

Bivens, J. A., & Berk, L. E. (1990). A longitudinal study of the development of elementary school children's private speech. *Merrill–Palmer Quarterly, 36,* 443–463.

Blank, R., & Remschmidt, H. (1993). *Hyperkinetic syndrome: The role of allergy among psychological and neurological factors.* Unpublished manuscript, Kinderzentrum Munchen, Germany.

Block, R. A. (1990). Models of psychological time. In R. Block (Eds.), *Cognitive models of psychological time* (pp. 1–35). Hillsdale, NJ: Erlbaum.

Boden, M. A. (1994). Precis of *The creative mind: Myths and mechanisms. Behavioral and Brain Sciences, 17,* 519–570.

Bohline, D. S. (1985). Intellectual and effective characteristics of attention deficit disordered children. *Journal of Learning Disabilities, 18,* 604–608.

Borcherding, B., Thompson, K., Krusei, M., Bartko, J., Rapoport, J. L., & Weingartner, H. (1988). Automatic and effortful processing in attention deficit/hyperactivity disorder. *Journal of Abnormal Child Psychology, 16,* 333–345.

Borger, N., & van der Meere, J. (2000). Visual behaviour of ADHD children during an attention test: An almost forgotten variable. *Journal of Child Psychology and Psychiatry, 41,* 525–532.

Braaten, E. B., & Rosen, L. A. (2000). Self-regulation of affect in attention deficit-hyperactivity disorder (ADHD) and non-ADHD boys: Differences in empathic responding. *Journal of Consulting and Clinical Psychology, 68,* 315–321.

Brady, K. D., & Denckla, M. B. (1994). *Performance of children with attention deficit hyperactivity disorder on the Tower of Hanoi task.* Unpublished manuscript, Johns Hopkins University School of Medicine.

Brand, E., & van der Vlugt, H. (1989). Activation: Base-level and responsivity—A search for subtypes of ADDH children by means of electrocardiac, dermal, and respiratory measures. In T. Sagvolden & T. Archer (Eds.), *Attention deficit disorder: Clinical and basic research* (pp. 137–150). Hillsdale, NJ: Erlbaum.

Breen, M. J. (1989). ADHD girls and boys: An analysis of attentional, emotional, cognitive, and family variables. *Journal of Child Psychology and Psychiatry, 30,* 711–716.

Breier, J. I., Gray, L., Fletcher, J. M., Diehl, R. L., Klaas, P., Foorman, B. R., & Molis, M. R. (2001). Perception of voice and tone onset time continua in children with dyslexia with and without attention deficit/hyperactivity disorder. *Journal of Experimental Child Psychology, 80,* 245–270.

Brock, S. W., & Knapp, P. K. (1996). Reading comprehension abilities of children with attention-deficit/hyperactivity disorder. *Journal of Attention Disorders, 1,* 173–186.

Bronowski, J. (1977). Human and animal languages. In P. E. Ariotti (Ed.), *A sense of the future* (pp. 104–131). Cambridge, MA: MIT Press.

Brown, R. T. (1989). Creativity: What are we to measure? In J. A. Glover, R. R. Ronning, & C. R. Reynolds (Eds.), *Handbook of creativity* (pp. 3–32). New York: Plenum Press.

Brown, R. T., & Borden, K. A. (1986). Hyperactivity at adolescence: Some misconceptions and new directions. *Journal of Clinical Child Psychology, 15,* 194–209.

Brown, S. W. (1985). Time perception and attention: The effects of prospective versus retrospective paradigms and task demands on perceived duration. *Perception and Psychophysics, 38,* 115–124.

Burg, C., Hart, D., Quinn, P. O., & Rapoport, J. L. (1978). Clinical evaluation of one-year old infants: Possible predictors of risk for the "hyperactivity syndrome." *Journal of Pediatric Psychology, 3,* 164–167.

Burt, S. A., Krueger, R. F., McGue, M., & Iacono, W. G. (2001). Sources of covariation among attention-deficit hyperactivity disorder, oppositional defiant disorder, and conduct disorder: The importance of shared environment. *Journal of Abnormal Psychology, 110,* 516–525.

Butterbaugh, G., Giordani, B., Dillon, J., Alessi, N., Breen, M., & Berent, S. (1989, October). *Effortful learning in children with hyperactivity and/or depressive disorders*. Paper presented at the annual meeting of the American Academy of Child and Adolescent Psychiatry, New York.

Cahn, D. A., & Marcotte, A. C. (1995). Rates of forgetting in attention deficit hyperactivity disorder. *Child Neuropsychology, 1,* 158–163.

Cantwell, D. P., & Satterfield, J. H. (1978). The prevalence of academic underachievement in hyperactive children. *Journal of Pediatric Psychology, 3,* 168–171.

Caplan, R., Guthrie, D., Tang, B., Nuechterlein, K. H., & Asarnow, R. F. (2001). Thought disorder in attention-deficit hyperactivity disorder. *Journal of the American Academy of Child and Adolescent Psychiatry, 40,* 965–972.

Cappella, B., Gentile, J. R., & Juliano, D. B. (1977). Time estimation by hyperactive and normal children. *Perceptual and Motor Skills, 44,* 787–790.

Carlson, C. L., & Alexander, D. K. (1993, February). *Effects of variations in reinforcement and feedback strategies on the performance and intrinsic motivation of ADHD children.* Paper presented at the annual meeting of the Society for Research in Child and Adolescent Psychopathology, Santa Fe, NM.

Carlson, C. L., & Tamm, L. (2000). Responsiveness of children with attention deficit-hyperactivity disorder to reward and response cost: Differential impact on performance and motivation. *Journal of Consulting and Clinical Psychology, 68,* 73–83.

Carte, E. T., Nigg, J. T., & Hinshaw, S. P. (1996). Neuropsychological functioning, motor speed, and language processing in boys with and without ADHD. *Journal of Abnormal Child Psychology, 24,* 481–498.

Casey, J. E., Rourke, B. P., & Del Dotto, J. E. (1996). Learning disabilities in children with attention deficit disorder with and without hyperactivity. *Child Neuropsychology, 2,* 83–98.

Castellanos, F. X., Marvasti, F. F., Ducharme, J. L., Walter, J. M., Israel, M. E., Krain, A., et al. (2000). Executive function oculomotor tasks in girls with ADHD. *Journal of the American Academy of Child and Adolescent Psychiatry, 39,* 644–650.

Cataldo, M. F., Finney, J. W., Richman, G. S., Riley, A. W., Hook, R. J., Brophy, C. J., et al. (1992). Behavior of injured and uninjured children and their parents in a simulated hazardous setting. *Journal of Pediatric Psychology, 17,* 73–80.

Cerutti, D. T. (1989). Discrimination theory of rule-governed behavior. *Journal of the Experimental Analysis of Behavior, 51,* 259–276.

Chadwick, O., Taylor, E., Taylor, A., Hepinstall, E., & Danckaerts, M. (1999). Hyperactivity and reading disability: A longitudinal study of the nature of the association. *Journal of Child Psychology and Psychiatry, 40,* 1039–1050.

Chang, H. T., Klorman, R., Shaywitz, S. E., Fletcher, J. M., Marchione, K. E., Holahan, J. M., et al. (1999). Paired-associate learning in attention-deficit/hyperactivity disorder as a function of hyperactivity–impulsivity and oppositional defiant disorder. *Journal of Abnormal Child Psychology, 27,* 237–245.

Chee, P., Logan, G., Schachar, R., Lindsay, P., & Wachsmuth, R. (1989). Effects of event rate and display time on sustained attention in hyperactive, normal, and control children. *Journal of Abnormal Child Psychology, 17,* 371–391.

Clark, C., Prior, M., & Kinsella, G. J. (2000). Do executive function deficits differentiate between adolescents with ADHD and oppositional defiant/conduct disorder?: A neuropsychological study using the Six Elements Test and Hayling Sentence Completion Test. *Journal of Abnormal Child Psychology, 28,* 403–414.

Clark, C., Prior, M., & Kinsella, G. J. (2002). The relationship between executive function abilities, adaptive behaviour, and academic achievement in children with externalizing behaviour problems. *Journal of Child Psychology and Psychiatry, 43,* 785–796.

Cohen, N. J., Menna, R., Vallance, D. D., Barwick, M. A., Im, N., & Horodezky, N. (1998). Language, social cognitive processing, and behavioral characteristics of psychiatrically disturbed children with previously identified and unsuspected language impairments. *Journal of Child Psychology and Psychiatry, 39,* 853–864.

Cohen, N. J., Vallance, D. D., Barwick, M., Im, N., Menna, R., Horodezky, N. B., et al. (2000). The interface between ADHD and language impairment: An examination of language, achievement, and cognitive processing. *Journal of Child Psychology and Psychiatry, 41,* 353–363.

Cole, P. M., Zahn-Waxler, C., & Smith, D. (1994). Expressive control during a disappointment: Variations related to preschoolers' behavior problems. *Developmental Psychology, 30,* 835–846.

Conte, R., & Regehr, S. M. (1991). Learning and transfer of inductive reasoning rules in overactive children. *Cognitive Therapy and Research, 15,* 129–139.

Coolidge, F. L., Thede, L. L., & Young, S. E. (2000). Heritability of the comorbidity of attention deficit hyperactivity disorder with behavioral disorders and executive function deficits: A preliminary investigation. *Developmental Neuropsychology, 17,* 273–287.

Copeland, A. P. (1979). Types of private speech produced by hyperactive and nonhyperactive boys. *Journal of Abnormal Child Psychology, 7,* 169–177.

Corkum, P., Beig, S., Tannock, R., & Moldofsky, H. (1997, October). *Comorbidity: The potential link between attention-deficit/hyperactivity disorder and sleep problems.* Paper presented at the annual meeting of the American Academy of Child and Adolescent Psychiatry, Toronto.

Corkum, P., Moldofsky, H., Hogg-Johnson, S., Humphries, T., & Tannock, R. (1999). Sleep problems in children with attention-deficit/hyperactivity disorder: Impact of subtype, comorbidity, and stimulant medication. *Journal of the American Academy of Child and Adolescent Psychiatry, 38,* 1285–1293.

Corkum, P., & Siegel, L. S. (1993). Is the continuous performance task a valuable research tool for use with children with attention-deficit–hyperactivity disorder? *Journal of Child Psychology and Psychiatry, 34,* 1217–1239.

Corkum, P., Tannock, R., & Moldofsky, H. (1998). Sleep disturbances in children with attention-deficit/hyperactivity disorder. *Journal of the American Academy of Child and Adolescent Psychiatry, 37,* 637–646.

Cornoldi, C., Barbieri, D., Gaiani, C., & Zocchi, S. (1999). Strategic memory deficits in attention deficit disorder with hyperactivity participants: The role of executive processes. *Developmental Neuropsychology, 15,* 53–71.

Cunningham, S. J., & Knights, R. M. (1978). The performance of hyperactive and normal boys under differing reward and punishment schedules. *Journal of Pediatric Psychology, 3,* 195–201.

Dalebout, S. D., Nelson, N. W., Hleto, P. J., & Frentheway, B. (1991). Selective auditory attention and children with attention-deficit hyperactivity disorder: Effects of repeated measurement with and without methylphenidate. *Language, Speech, and Hearing Services in Schools, 22,* 219–227.

Danforth, J. S., Barkley, R. A., & Stokes, T. F. (1991). Observations of parent–child interactions with hyperactive children: Research and clinical implications. *Clinical Psychology Review, 11,* 703–727.

Daugherty, T. K., & Quay, H. C. (1991). Response perseveration and delayed responding in childhood behavior disorders. *Journal of Child Psychology and Psychiatry, 32,* 453–461.

Davidson, L. L., Hughes, S. J., & O'Connor, P. A. (1988). Preschool behavior problems and subsequent risk of injury. *Pediatrics, 82,* 644–651.

Davidson, L. L., Taylor, E. A., Sandberg, S. T., & Thorley, G. (1992). Hyperactivity in school-age boys and subsequent risk of injury. *Pediatrics, 90,* 697–702.

Denckla, M. B., & Rudel, R. G. (1978). Anomalies of motor development in hyperactive boys. *Annals of Neurology, 3,* 231–233.

Denckla, M. B., Rudel, R. G., Chapman, C., & Krieger, J. (1985). Motor proficiency in dyslexic children with and without attentional disorders. *Archives of Neurology, 42,* 228–231.

Diaz, R. M., & Berk, L. E. (Eds.). (1992). *Private speech: From social interaction to self-regulation.* Hillsdale, NJ: Erlbaum.

Diener, M. B., & Milich, R. (1997). Effects of positive feedback on the social interactions of boys with attention deficit hyperactivity disorder: A test of the self-protective hypothesis. *Journal of Clinical Child Psychology, 26,* 256–265.

Dooling-Litfin, J. (1997). Time perception in children with ADHD. *ADHD Report, 5*(5), 13–16.

Douglas, V. I. (1972). Stop, look, and listen: The problem of sustained attention and impulse control in hy-peractive and normal children. *Canadian Journal of Behavioural Science, 4,* 259–282.

Douglas, V. I. (1983). Attention and cognitive problems. In M. Rutter (Ed.), *Developmental neuropsychiatry* (pp. 280–329). New York: Guilford Press.

Douglas, V. I. (1988). Cognitive deficits in children with attention deficit disorder with hyperactivity. In L. M. Bloomingdale & J. A. Sergeant (Eds.), *Attention deficit disorder: Criteria, cognition, intervention* (pp. 65–82). London: Pergamon Press.

Douglas, V. I. (1989). Can Skinnerian psychology account for the deficits in attention deficit disorder?: A reply to Barkley. In L. M. Bloomingdale & J. M. Swanson (Eds.), *Attention deficit disorder* (Vol. 4, pp. 235–253). New York: Pergamon Press.

Douglas, V. I., & Benezra, E. (1990). Supraspan verbal memory in attention deficit disorder with hyperactivity, normal, and reading disabled boys. *Journal of Abnormal Child Psychology, 18,* 617–638.

Douglas, V. I., & Parry, P. A. (1983). Effects of reward on delayed reaction time task performance of hyperactive children. *Journal of Abnormal Child Psychology, 11,* 313–326.

Douglas, V. I., & Parry, P. A. (1994). Effects of reward and non-reward on attention and frustration in attention deficit disorder. *Journal of Abnormal Child Psychology, 22,* 281–302.

Douglas, V. I., & Peters, K. G. (1978). Toward a clearer definition of the attentional deficit of hyperactive children. In G. A. Hale & M. Lewis (Eds.), *Attention and the development of cognitive skills* (pp. 173–248). New York: Plenum Press.

Dykman, R. A., & Ackerman, P. T. (1992). Attention deficit disorder and specific reading disability: Separate but often overlapping disorders. In S. Shaywitz & B. A. Shaywitz (Eds.), *Attention deficit disorder comes of age: Toward the twenty-first century* (pp. 165–184). Austin, TX: PRO-ED.

El-Sayed, E., Larsson, J. O., Persson, H. E., & Rydelius, P. (2002). Altered cortical activity in children with attention-deficit/hyperactivity disorder during attentional load task. *Journal of the American Academy of Child and Adolescent Psychiatry, 41,* 811–819.

Ernst, M., Liebenauer, L. L., King, A. C., Fitzgerald, G. A., Cohen, R. M., & Zametkin, A. J. (1994). Reduced brain metabolism in hyperactive girls. *Journal of the American Academy of Child and Adolescent Psychiatry, 33,* 858–868.

Fallone, G., Acebo, C., Arnedt, J. T., Seifer, R., & Carskadon, M. A. (2001). Effects of acute sleep restriction on behavior, sustained attention, and response inhibition in children. *Perceptual and Motor Skills, 93,* 213–229.

Faraone, S. V., Biederman, J., Lehman, B., Keenan, K., Norman, D., Seidman, L. J., et al. (1993). Evidence for the independent familial transmission of attention deficit hyperactivity disorder and learning disabilities: Results from a family genetic study. *American Journal of Psychiatry, 150,* 891–895.

Felton, R. H., Wood, F. B., Brown, I. S., Campbell, S. K., & Harter, M. R. (1987). Separate verbal memory and naming deficits in attention deficit disorder and reading disability. *Brain and Language*, *31*, 171–184.

Fergusson, D. M., & Horwood, L. J. (1992). Attention deficit and reading achievement. *Journal of Child Psychology and Psychiatry*, *33*, 375–385.

Fergusson, D. M., & Horwood, L. J. (1995). Early disruptive behavior, IQ, and later school achievement and delinquent behavior. *Journal of Abnormal Child Psychology*, *23*, 183–199.

Firestone, P., Lewy, F., & Douglas, V. I. (1976). Hyperactivity and physical anomalies. *Canadian Psychiatric Association Journal*, *21*, 23–26.

Fischer, M., Barkley, R., Fletcher, K., & Smallish, L. (1990). The adolescent outcome of hyperactive children diagnosed by research criteria: II. Academic, attentional, and neuropsychological status. *Journal of Consulting and Clinical Psychology*, *58*, 580–588.

Fischer, M., Barkley, R. A., Smallish, L., & Fletcher, K. (2004). Hyperactive children as young adults: Deficits in inhibition, attention, and response perseveration and their relationship to severity of childhood and current ADHD and conduct disorder. *Developmental Neuropsychology*, *27*, 107–133.

Fischer, M., Barkley, R. A., Smallish, L., & Fletcher, K. (in press). Young adult follow-up of hyperactive children: Educational, occupational, social, sexual, and financial functioning. *Journal of the American Academy of Child and Adolescent Psychiatry*.

Frauenglass, M. H., & Diaz, R. M. (1985). Self-regulatory functions of children's private speech: A critical analysis and recent challenges to Vygotsky's theory. *Developmental Psychology*, *21*, 357–364.

Frazier, T. W., Demaree, H. A., & Youngstrom, E. A. (2004). Meta-analysis of intellectual and neuropsychological test performance in attention-deficit/hyperactivity disorder. *Neuropsychology*, *18*, 543–555.

Freibergs, V., & Douglas, V. I. (1969). Concept learning in hyperactive and normal children. *Journal of Abnormal Psychology*, *74*, 388–395.

Frick, P. J., Kamphaus, R. W., Lahey, B. B., Loeber, R., Christ, M. A. G., Hart, E. L., et al. (1991). Academic underachievement and the disruptive behavior disorders. *Journal of Consulting and Clinical Psychology*, *59*, 289–294.

Friedman, H. S., Tucker, J. S., Schwartz, J. E., Tomlinson-Keasey, C., Martin, L. R., Wingard, D. L., et al. (1995). Psychosocial and behavioral predictors of longevity: The aging and death of the "Termites." *American Psychologist*, *50*, 69–78.

Frost, L. A., Moffitt, T. E., & McGee, R. (1989). Neuropsychological correlates of psychopathology in an unselected cohort of young adolescents. *Journal of Abnormal Psychology*, *98*, 307–313.

Funk, J. B., Chessare, J. B., Weaver, M. T., & Exley, A. R. (1993). Attention deficit hyperactivity disorder, creativity, and the effects of methylphenidate. *Pediatrics*, *91*, 816–819.

Fuster, J. M. (1997). *The prefrontal cortex* (3rd ed.). New York: Raven Press.

Gascon, G. G., Johnson, R., & Burd, L. (1986). Central auditory processing and attention deficit disorders. *Journal of Child Neurology*, *1*, 27–33.

Geffner, D., Lucker, J. R., & Koch, W. (1996). Evaluation of auditory discrimination in children with ADD and without ADD. *Child Psychiatry and Human Development*, *26*, 169–180.

Gerbing, D. W., Ahadi, S. A., & Patton, J. H. (1987). Toward a conceptualization of impulsivity: Components across the behavioral and self-report domains. *Multivariate Behavioral Research*, *22*, 357–379.

Geurts, H. M., Verte, S., Oosterlaan, J., Roeyers, H., & Sergeant, J. A. (2004). How specific are executive functioning deficits in attention deficit hyperactivity disorder and autism? *Journal of Child Psychology and Psychiatry*, *45*, 836–854.

Gillberg, C., & Kadesjo, B. (2000). Attention-deficit/hyperactivity disorder and developmental coordination disorder. In T. E. Brown (Ed.), *Attention deficit disorders and comorbidities in children, adolescents, and adults* (pp. 393–406). Washington, DC: American Psychiatric Press.

Golden, J. (1996). Are tests of working memory and inattention diagnostically useful in children with ADHD? *ADHD Report*, *4*(5), 6–8.

Goldman, A., & Everett, F. (1985). Delay of gratification and time concept in reflective and impulsive children. *Child Study Journal*, *15*, 167–179.

Goldman-Rakic, P. S. (1995). Architecture of the prefrontal cortex and the central executive. *Annals of the New York Academy of Sciences*, *769*, 71–83.

Gordon, M. (1979). The assessment of impulsivity and mediating behaviors in hyperactive and nonhyperactive children. *Journal of Abnormal Child Psychology*, *7*, 317–326.

Gray, J. A. (1982). *The neuropsychology of anxiety: An enquiry into the functions of the septo-hippocampal system*. New York: Oxford University Press.

Gray, J. A. (1987). *The psychology of fear and stress*. Cambridge, UK: Cambridge University Press.

Greene, R. W., Biederman, J., Faraone, S. V., Ouellette, C. A., Penn, C., & Griffin, S. M. (1996). Toward a new psychometric definition of social disability in children with attention-deficit hyperactivity disorder. *Journal of the American Academy of Child and Adolescent Psychiatry*, *35*, 571–578.

Greene, R. W., Biederman, J., Faraone, S. V., Sienna, M., & Garcia-Jetton, J. (1997). Adolescent outcome of boys with attention-deficit/hyperactivity disorder and social disability: Results from a 4-year longitudinal follow-up study. *Journal of Consulting and Clinical Psychology*, *65*, 758–767.

Greenhill, L., Anich, J. P., Goetz, R., Hanton, C., & Davies, M. (1983). Sleep architecture and REM sleep measures in prepubertal children with attention deficit disorder with hyperactivity. *Sleep*, *6*, 91–101.

Gregory, A. M., & O'Connor, T. G. (2002). Sleep problems in childhood: A longitudinal study of developmental change and association with behavioral problems. *Journal of the American Academy of Child and Adolescent Psychiatry, 41,* 964–971.

Greve, K. W., Williams, M. C., & Dickens, T. J., Jr. (1996, February). *Concept formation in attention disordered children.* Poster presented at the meeting of the International Neuropsychological Society, Chicago.

Grodzinsky, G. M., & Diamond, R. (1992). Frontal lobe functioning in boys with attention-deficit hyperactivity disorder. *Developmental Neuropsychology, 8,* 427–445.

Grskovic, J. A., Zentall, S. S., & Stormont-Spurgin, M. (1995). Time estimation and planning abilities: Students with and without mild disabilities. *Behavioral Disorders, 20,* 197–203.

Gruber, R., & Sadeh, A. (2004). Sleep and neurobehavioral functioning in boys with attention-deficit/hyperactivity disorder and no reported breathing problems. *Sleep, 27,* 267–273.

Gruber, R., Sadeh, A., & Raviv, A. (2000). Instability of sleep patterns in children with attention-deficit/hyperactivity disorder. *Journal of the American Academy of Child and Adolescent Psychiatry, 39,* 495–501.

Haenlein, M., & Caul, W. F. (1987). Attention deficit disorder with hyperactivity: A specific hypothesis of reward dysfunction. *Journal of the American Academy of Child and Adolescent Psychiatry, 26,* 356–362.

Hall, S. J., Halperin, J. M., Schwartz, S. T., & Newcorn, J. H. (1997). Behavioral and executive functions in children with attention-deficit hyperactivity disorder and reading disability. *Journal of Attention Disorders, 1,* 235–247.

Halperin, J. M., & Gittelman, R. (1982). Do hyperactive children and their siblings differ in IQ and academic achievement? *Psychiatry Research, 6,* 253–258.

Hamlett, K. W., Pellegrini, D. S., & Conners, C. K. (1987). An investigation of executive processes in the problem-solving of attention deficit disorder–hyperactive children. *Journal of Pediatric Psychology, 12,* 227–240.

Harrington, D. L., Haaland, K. Y., & Hermanowicz, N. (1998). Temporal processing in the basal ganglia. *Neuropsychology, 12,* 3–12.

Hart, E. L., Lahey, B. B., Hynd, G. W., Loeber, R., & McBurnett, K. (1995). Association of chronic overanxious disorder with atopic rhinitis in boys: A four-year longitudinal study. *Journal of Clinical Child Psychology, 24,* 332–337.

Harter, S. (1985). *Manual for the Self-Perception Profile for Children.* Unpublished manuscript, University of Denver, Denver, CO.

Hartsough, C. S., & Lambert, N. M. (1985). Medical factors in hyperactive and normal children: Prenatal, developmental, and health history findings. *American Journal of Orthopsychiatry, 55,* 190–210.

Harvey, W. J., & Reid, G. (2003). Attention-deficit/hyperactivity disorder: A review of research on movement skill performance and physical fitness. *Adapted Physical Activity Quarterly, 20,* 1–25.

Hastings, J., & Barkley, R. A. (1978). A review of psychophysiological research with hyperactive children. *Journal of Abnormal Child Psychology, 7,* 413–337.

Hayes, S. (1989). *Rule-governed behavior.* New York: Plenum Press.

Hechtman, L., Weiss, G., Perlman, T., & Tuck, D. (1981). Hyperactives as young adults: Various clinical outcomes. *Adolescent Psychiatry, 9,* 295–306.

Herpertz, S. C., Wenning, B., Mueller, B., Qunaibi, M., Sass, H., & Herpetz-Dahlmann, B. (2001). Psychological responses in ADHD boys with and without conduct disorder: Implications for adult antisocial behavior. *Journal of the American Academy of Child and Adolescent Psychiatry, 40,* 1222–1230.

Hervey, A. S., Epstein, J. N., & Curry, J. F. (2004). Neuropsychology of adults with attention-deficit/hyperactivity disorder: A meta-analytic review. *Neuropsychology, 18,* 495–503.

Hesdorffer, D. C., Ludvigsson, P., Olafsson, E., Gudmundsson, G., Kjartansson, O., & Hauser, W. A. (2004). ADHD as a risk factor for incident unprovoked seizures and epilepsy in children. *Archives of General Psychiatry, 61,* 731–736.

Hinshaw, S. P. (1987). On the distinction between attentional deficits/hyperactivity and conduct problems/aggression in child psychopathology. *Psychological Bulletin, 101,* 443–447.

Hinshaw, S. P. (1992). Externalizing behavior problems and academic underachievement in childhood and adolescence: Causal relationships and underlying mechanisms. *Psychological Bulletin, 111,* 127–155.

Hinshaw, S. P., Heller, T., & McHale, J. P. (1992). Covert antisocial behavior in boys with attention-deficit hyperactivity disorder: External validation and effects of methylphenidate. *Journal of Consulting and Clinical Psychology, 60,* 274–281.

Hinshaw, S. P., & Lee, S. S. (2003). Conduct and oppositional defiant disorders. In E. J. Mash & R. A. Barkley (Eds.), *Child psychopathology* (2nd ed., pp. 144–198). New York: Guilford Press.

Hinshaw, S. P., & Melnick, S. M. (1995). Peer relationships in boys with attention-deficit hyperactivity disorder with and without comorbid aggression. *Development and Psychopathology, 7,* 627–647.

Hinshaw, S. P., Morrison, D. C., Carte, E. T., & Cornsweet, C. (1987). Factorial dimensions of the Revised Behavior Problem Checklist: Replication and validation within a kindergarten sample. *Journal of Abnormal Child Psychology, 15,* 309–327.

Hinshaw, S. P., Simmel, C., & Heller, T. L. (1995). Multimethod assessment of covert antisocial behavior in children: Laboratory observations, adult ratings, and child self-report. *Psychological Assessment, 7,* 209–219.

Hoare, P., & Beattie, T. (2003). Children with attention

deficit hyperactivity disorder and attendance at hospital. *European Journal of Emergency Medicine, 10,* 98–100.

Holdnack, J. A., Moberg, P. J., Arnold, S. E., Gur, R. C., & Gur, R. E. (1995). Speed of processing and verbal learning deficits in adults diagnosed with attention deficit disorder. *Neuropsychiatry, Neuropsychology, and Behavioral Neurology, 8,* 282–292.

Hoy, E., Weiss, G., Minde, K., & Cohen, N. (1978). The hyperactive child at adolescence: Cognitive, emotional, and social functioning. *Journal of Abnormal Child Psychology, 6,* 311–324.

Hoza, B., Gerdes, A. C., Hinshaw, S. P., Arnold, L. E., Pelham, W. E., Jr., Molina, B. S. G., et al. (2004). Self-perceptions of competence in children with ADHD and comparison children. *Journal of Consulting and Clinical Psychology, 72,* 382–391.

Hoza, B., Pelham, W. E., Dobbs, J., Owens, J. S., & Pillow, D. R. (2002). Do boys with attention-deficit/hyperactivity disorder have positive illusory self-concepts? *Journal of Abnormal Psychology, 111,* 268–278.

Hoza, B., Pelham, W. E., Waschbusch, D. A., Kipp, H., & Owens, J. S. (2001). Academic task persistence of normally achieving ADHD and control boys: Performance, self-evaluations, and attributions. *Journal of Consulting and Clinical Psychology, 69,* 281–283.

Hoza, B., Waschbusch, D. A., Pelham, W. E., Molina, B. S. G., & Milich, R. (2000). Attention-deficit/hyperactivity disordered and control boys' responses to social success and failure. *Child Development, 71,* 432–446.

Humphries, T., Koltun, H., Malone, M., & Roberts, W. (1994). Teacher-identified oral language difficulties among boys with attention problems. *Journal of Developmental and Behavioral Pediatrics, 15,* 92–98.

Hurks, P. P. M., Hendriksen, J. G. M., Vles, J. S. H., Kalff, A. C., Feron, F. J. M., Kroes, M., et al. (2004). Verbal fluency over time as a measure of automatic and controlled processing in children with ADHD. *Brain and Cognition, 55,* 415–435.

Iaboni, F., Douglas, V. I., & Baker, A. G. (1995). Effects of reward and response costs on inhibition in ADHD children. *Journal of Abnormal Psychology, 104,* 232–240.

Jacklin, C. G., Maccoby, E. E., & Halverson, C. F. Jr. (1980). Minor anomalies and preschool behavior. *Journal of Pediatric Psychology, 5,* 199–205.

Kadesjo, B., & Gillberg, C. (1999). Developmental coordination disorder in Swedish 7-year-old children. *Journal of the American Academy of Child and Adolescent Psychiatry, 38,* 820–828.

Kadesjo, B., & Gillberg, C. (2001). The comorbidity of ADHD in the general population of Swedish school-age children. *Journal of Child Psychology and Psychiatry, 42,* 487–492.

Kaplan, B. J., McNichol, J., Conte, R. A., & Moghadam, H. K. (1987). Sleep disturbance in preschool-aged hyperactive and nonhyperactive children. *Pediatrics, 80,* 839–844.

Karatekin, C. (2004). A test of the integrity of the components of Baddeley's model of working memory in attention-deficit/hyperactivity disorder (ADHD). *Journal of Child Psychology and Psychiatry, 45,* 912–926.

Karatekin, C., & Asarnow, R. F. (1998). Working memory in childhood-onset schizophrenia and attention-deficit/hyperactivity disorder (ADHD). *Psychiatry Research, 80,* 165–176.

Kaufman, A. S., & Kaufman, N. L. (1983). *Kaufman Assessment Battery for Children.* Circle Pines, MN: American Guidance Service.

Keith, R. W., & Engineer, P. (1991). Effects of methylphenidate on the auditory processing abilities of children with attention deficit-hyperactivity disorder. *Journal of Learning Disabilities, 24,* 630–636.

Keltner, D., Moffitt, T. E., & Stouthamer-Loeber, M. (1995). Facial expressions of emotion and psychopathology in adolescent boys. *Journal of Abnormal Psychology, 104,* 644–652.

Kendall, P., & Braswell, L. (1985). *Cognitive-behavioral therapy for impulsive children.* New York: Guilford Press.

Kesner, R. P., Hopkins, R. O., & Fineman, B. (1994). Item and order dissociation in humans with prefrontal cortex damage. *Neuropsychologia, 32,* 881–891.

Kitchens, S. A., Rosen, L. A., & Braaten, E. B. (1999). Differences in anger, aggression, depression, and anxiety between ADHD and non-ADHD children. *Journal of Attention Disorders, 3,* 77–83.

Klorman, R. (1992). Cognitive event-related potentials in attention deficit disorder. In S. E. Shaywitz & B. A. Shaywitz (1992). *Attention deficit disorder comes of age: Toward the twenty-first century* (pp. 221–244). Austin, TX: PRO-ED.

Klorman, R., Brumaghim, J. T., Coons, H. W., Peloquin, L., Strauss, J., Lewine, J. D., et al. (1988). The contributions of event-related potentials to understanding effects of stimulants on information processing in attention deficit disorder. In L. M. Bloomingdale & J. A. Sergeant (Eds.), *Attention deficit disorder: Criteria, cognition, intervention* (pp. 199–218). London: Pergamon Press.

Klorman, R., Hazel-Fernandez, L. A., Shaywitz, S. E., Fletcher, J. M., Marchione, K. E., Holahan, J. M., et al. (1999). Executive functioning deficits in attention-deficit are independent of oppositional defiant or reading disorder. *Journal of the American Academy of Child and Adolescent Psychiatry, 38,* 1148–1155.

Knouse, L. E., Bagwell, C. L., Barkley, R. A., & Murphy, K. R. (in press). Accuracy of self-evaluation in adults with attention-deficit hyperactivity disorder. *Journal of Attention Disorders.*

Kohlberg, L., Yaeger, J., & Hjertholm, E. (1968). Private speech: Four studies and a review of theories. *Child Development, 39,* 691–736.

Kohn, A. (1989, November). Suffer the restless children. *Atlantic Monthly,* pp. 90–100.

Krouse, J. P., & Kaufman, J. M. (1982). Minor physical anomalies in exceptional children: A review and critique of research. *Journal of Abnormal Child Psychology, 10,* 247–264.

Kuntsi, J., Oosterlaan, J., & Stevenson, J. (2001). Psychological mechanisms in hyperactivity: I. Response inhibition deficit, working memory impairment, delay aversion, or something else? *Journal of Child Psychology and Psychiatry, 42,* 199–210.

Kupietz, S. S., Camp, J. A., & Weissman, A. D. (1976). Reaction time performance of behaviorally deviant children: Effects of prior preparatory interval and reinforcement. *Journal of Child Psychology and Psychiatry, 17,* 123–131.

Lalloo, R., Sheiham, A., & Nazroo, J. Y. (2003). Behavioural characteristics and accidents: Findings form the Health Survey for England, 1997. *Accident Analysis and Prevention, 35,* 661–667.

Lambert, N. M. (1995, June). *Analysis of driving histories of ADHD subjects.* Final report to the National Highway Traffic Safety Administration.

Lambert, N. M., & Sandoval, J. (1980). The prevalence of learning disabilities in a sample of children considered hyperactive. *Journal of Abnormal Child Psychology, 8,* 33–50.

Landau, S., Berk, L. E., & Mangione, C. (1996, March). *Private speech as a problem-solving strategy in the face of academic challenge: The failure of impulsive children to get their act together.* Paper presented at the meeting of the National Association of School Psychologists, Atlanta, GA.

Langley, J., McGee, R., Silva, P., & Williams, S. (1983). Child behavior and accidents. *Journal of Pediatric Psychology, 8,* 181–189.

LaVeck, B., Hammond, M. A., & LaVeck, G. D. (1980). Minor congenital anomalies and behavior in different home environments. *Journal of Pediatrics, 97,* 940–941.

Lecendreux, M., Konofal, E., Bouvard, M., Falissard, B., & Mouren-Simeoni, M. (2000). Sleep and alertness in children with ADHD. *Journal of Child Psychology and Psychiatry, 41,* 803–812.

Leibson, C. L., Katusic, S. K., Barbaresi, W. J., Ransom, J., & O'Brien, P. C. (2001). Use and costs of medical care for children and adolescents with and without attention-deficit/hyperactivity disorder. *Journal of the American Medical Association, 285,* 60–66.

Lerer, R. J. (1977). Do hyperactive children tend to have abnormal palmar creases?: Report of a suggestive association. *Clinical Pediatrics, 16,* 645–647.

Loeber, R. (1990). Development and risk factors of juvenile antisocial behavior and delinquency. *Clinical Psychology Review, 10,* 1–42.

Loeber, R., Burke, J. D., Lahey, B. B., Winters, A., & Zera, M. (2000). Oppositional defiant and conduct disorder: A review of the past 10 years, Part I. *Journal of the American Academy of Child and Adolescent Psychiatry, 39,* 1–17.

Loge, D. V., Staton, D., & Beatty, W. W. (1990). Performance of children with ADHD on tests sensitive to frontal lobe dysfunction. *Journal of the American Academy of Child and Adolescent Psychiatry, 29,* 540–545.

Loo, S. K., & Barkley, R. A. (in press). Clinical utility of EEG in attention deficit hyperactivity disorder. *Applied Developmental Neuropsychology.*

Lorch, E. P., Milich, R., Sanchez, R. P., van den Broek, P., Baer, S., Hooks, K., et al. (2000). Comprehension of televised stories in boys with attention deficit/hyperactivity disorder and nonreferred boys. *Journal of Abnormal Psychology, 109,* 321–330.

Lorch, E. P., O'Neill, K., Berthiaume, K. S., Milich, R., Eastham, D., & Brooks, T. (2004). Story comprehension and the impact of studying on recall in children with attention deficit hyperactivity disorder. *Journal of Clinical Child and Adolescent Psychology, 33,* 506–515.

Lorch, E. P., Sanchez, R. P., van den Broek, P., Milich, R., Murphy, E. L., Lorch, R. F., Jr., et al. (1999). The relation of story structure properties to recall of television stories in young children with attention-deficit hyperactivity disorder and nonreferred peers. *Journal of Abnormal Child Psychology, 27,* 293–309.

Lou, H. C., Henriksen, L., & Bruhn, P. (1984). Focal cerebral hypoperfusion in children with dysphasia and/or attention deficit disorder. *Archives of Neurology, 41,* 825–829.

Lou, H. C., Henriksen, L., Bruhn, P., Borner, H., & Nielsen, J. B. (1989). Striatal dysfunction in attention deficit and hyperkinetic disorder. *Archives of Neurology, 46,* 48–52.

Lucker, J. R., Geffner, D., & Koch, W. (1996). Perception of loudness in children with ADD and without ADD. *Child Psychiatry and Human Development, 26,* 181–190.

Ludlow, C., Rapoport, J., Brown, G., & Mikkelson, E. (1979). The differential effects of dextroamphetamine on the language and communication skills of hyperactive and normal children. In R. Knights & D. Bakker (Eds.), *Rehabilitation, treatment, and management of learning disorders.* Baltimore: University Park Press.

Lufi, D., Cohen, A., & Parish-Plass, J. (1990). Identifying ADHD with the WISC-R and the Stroop Color and Word Test. *Psychology in the Schools, 27,* 28–34.

Luk, S. (1985). Direct observations studies of hyperactive behaviors. *Journal of the American Academy of Child and Adolescent Psychiatry, 24,* 338–344.

Luman, M., Oosterlaan, J., & Sergeant, J. A. (2005). The impact of reinforcement contingencies on AD/HD: A review and theoretical appraisal. *Clinical Psychology Review, 25,* 183–213.

Lynam, D., Moffitt, T., & Stouthamer-Loeber, M. (1993). Explaining the relation between IQ and delinquency: Class, race, test motivation, school failure, or self-control? *Journal of Abnormal Psychology, 102,* 187–196.

MacLeod, D., & Prior, M. (1996). Attention deficits in adolescents with ADHD and other clinical groups. *Child Neuropsychology, 2,* 1–10.

Mangels, J. A., Ivry, R. B., & Shimizu, N. (1998). Dissociable contributions of the prefrontal and neocerebellar cortex to time perception. *Cognitive Brain Research, 7,* 15–39.

Mangus, R. S., Bergman, D., Zieger, M., & Coleman, J. J. (2004). Burn injuries in children with attention-deficit/hyperactivity disorder. *Burns, 30,* 148–150.

Manheimer, D. I., & Mellinger, G. D. (1967). Personality characteristics of the child accident repeater. *Child Development, 38,* 491–513.

Marcotte, A. C., & Stern, C. (1997). Qualitative analysis of graphomotor output in children with attentional disorders. *Child Neuropsychology, 3,* 147–153.

Marcotte, A. C., Thacher, P. V., Butters, M., Bortz, J., Acebo, C., & Carskadon, M. A. (1998). Parental report of sleep problems in children with attentional and learning disorders. *Journal of Developmental and Behavioral Pediatrics, 19,* 178–186.

Mariani, M., & Barkley, R. A. (1997). Neuropsychological and academic functioning in preschool children with attention deficit hyperactivity disorder. *Developmental Neuropsychology, 13,* 111–129.

McGee, R., & Share, D. L. (1988). Attention deficit disorder—hyperactivity and academic failure: Which comes first and what should be treated? *Journal of the American Academy of Child and Adolescent Psychiatry, 27,* 318–327.

McGee, R., Stanton, W. R., & Sears, M. R. (1993). Allergic disorders and attention deficit disorder in children. *Journal of Abnormal Child Psychology, 21,* 79–88.

McGee, R., Williams, S., & Feehan, M. (1992). Attention deficit disorder and age of onset of problem behaviors. *Journal of Abnormal Child Psychology, 20,* 487–502.

McGee, R., Williams, S., Moffitt, T., & Anderson, J. (1989). A comparison of 13–year old boys with attention deficit and/or reading disorder on neuropsychological measures. *Journal of Abnormal Child Psychology, 17,* 37–53.

McGee, R., Williams, S., & Silva, P. A. (1984). Behavioral and developmental characteristics of aggressive, hyperactive, and aggressive–hyperactive boys. *Journal of the American Academy of Child Psychiatry, 23,* 270–279.

McGinnis, J. (1997, September). Attention deficit disaster. *The Wall Street Journal.*

McInnes, A., Humphries, T., Hogg-Johnson, S., & Tannock, R. (2003). Listening comprehension and working memory are impaired in attention-deficit hyperactivity disorder irrespective of language impairment. *Journal of Abnormal Child Psychology, 31,* 427–443.

McMahon, S. A., & Greenberg, L. M. (1977). Serial neurologic examination of hyperactive children. *Pediatrics, 59,* 584–587.

Meaux, J. B., & Chelonis, J. J. (2003). Time perception differences in children with and without ADHD. *Journal of Pediatric Health Care, 17,* 64–71.

Melnick, S. M., & Hinshaw, S. P. (2000). Emotion regulation and parenting in AD/HD and comparison boys: Linkages with social behaviors and peer preference. *Journal of Abnormal Child Psychology, 28,* 73–86.

Methany, A. P., Jr., & Fisher, J. E. (1984). Behavioral perspectives on children's accidents. In M. Wolraich & D. K. Routh (Eds.), *Advances in behavioral pediatrics* (Vol. 5, pp. 221–263). Greenwich, CT: JAI Press.

Michon, J. A., & Jackson, J. L. (1984). Attentional effort and cognitive strategies in the processing of temporal information. *Annals of the New York Academy of Sciences, 423,* 298–321.

Milberger, S., Biederman, J., Faraone, S. V., Chen, L., & Jones, J. (1996). ADHD is associated with early initiation of cigarette smoking in children and adolescents. *Journal of the American Academy of Child and Adolescent Psychiatry, 36,* 37–44.

Milich, R. (in press). The response of children with ADHD to failure: If at first you don't succeed, do you try, try again? *School Psychology Review.*

Milich, R., Hartung, C. M., Martin, C. A., & Haigler, E. D. (1994). Behavioral disinhibition and underlying processes in adolescents with disruptive behavioral disorders. In D. K. Routh (Ed.), *Disruptive behavior disorders in childhood* (pp. 109–138). New York: Plenum Press.

Milich, R., & Kramer, J. (1985). Reflections on impulsivity: An empirical investigation of impulsivity as a construct. In K. Gadow & I. Bialer (Eds.), *Advances in learning and behavioral disabilities* (Vol. 3, pp. 57–94). Greenwich, CT: JAI Press.

Milich, R., & Loney, J. (1979). The factor composition of the WISC for hyperkinetic/MBD males. *Journal of Learning Disabilities, 12,* 67–70.

Mimura, M., Kinsbourne, M., & O'Connor, M. (2000). Time estimation by patients with frontal lesions and by Korsakoff amnesics. *Journal of the International Neuropsychological Society, 6,* 517–528.

Mischel, W., Shoda, Y., & Peake, P. K. (1988). The nature of adolescent competencies predicted by preschool delay of gratification. *Journal of Personality and Social Psychology, 54,* 687–696.

Mitchell, E. A., Aman, M. G., Turbott, S. H., & Manku, M. (1987). Clinical characteristics and serum essential fatty acid levels in hyperactive children. *Clinical Pediatrics, 26,* 406–411.

Moffitt, T. E. (1990). Juvenile delinquency and attention deficit disorder: Boys' developmental trajectories from age 3 to 15. *Child Development, 61,* 893–910.

Moffitt, T. E., & Silva, P. A. (1988). Self-reported delinquency, neuropsychological deficit, and history of attention deficit disorder. *Journal of Abnormal Child Psychology, 16,* 553–569.

Monastra, V. J., Lubar, J. F., & Linden, M. (2001). The development of a quantitative electroencephalographic scanning process for attention deficit-hyperactivity disorder: Reliability and validity studies. *Neuropsychology, 15*(1), 136–144.

Monastra, V. J., Lubar, J. F., Linden, M., VanDeusen, P., Green, G., Wing, W., Phillips, A., & Fenger, T. N. (1999). Assessing attention deficit hyperactivity disorder via quantitative electroencephalography: An initial validation study. *Neuropsychology, 13,* 424–433.

Mori, L., & Peterson, L. (1995). Knowledge of safety of high and low active–impulsive boys: Implications for child injury prevention. *Journal of Clinical Child Psychology, 24,* 370–376.

Moss, W. L., & Sheiffe, W. A. (1994). Can we differentially diagnose an attention deficit disorder without hyperactivity from a central auditory processing problem? *Child Psychiatry and Human Development, 25,* 85–96.

Munir, K., Biederman, J., & Knee, D. (1987). Psychiatric comorbidity in patients with attention deficit disorder: A controlled study. *Journal of the American Academy of Child and Adolescent Psychiatry, 26,* 844–848.

Murphy, K. R., & Barkley, R. A. (1996). Prevalence of DSM-IV symptoms of ADHD in adult licensed drivers: Implications for clinical diagnosis. *Journal of Attention Disorders, 1,* 147–161.

Murphy, K. R., Barkley, R. A., & Bush, T. (2001). Executive functions in young adults with attention deficit hyperactivity disorder, *Neuropsychology, 15,* 211–220.

Nada-Raja, S., Langley, J. D., McGee, R., Williams, S. M., Begg, D. J., & Reeder, A. I. (1997). Inattentive and hyperactive behaviors and driving offenses in adolescence. *Journal of the American Academy of Child and Adolescent Psychiatry, 36,* 515–522.

Neef, N. A., Bicard, D. F., & Endo, S. (2001). Assessment of impulsivity and the development of self-control by students with attention deficit hyperactivity disorder. *Journal of Applied Behavioral Analysis, 34,* 397–408.

Newman, J. P., Patterson, C. M., & Kosson, D. S. (1987). Response perseveration in psychopaths. *Journal of Abnormal Psychology, 96,* 145–148.

Newman, J. P., & Wallace, J. F. (1993). Diverse pathways to deficient self-regulation: Implications for disinhibitory psychopathology in children. *Clinical Psychology Review, 13,* 699–720.

Nigg, J. T. (2001). Is ADHD an inhibitory disorder? *Psychological Bulletin, 125,* 571–596.

Nigg, J. T., Hinshaw, S. P., Carte, E. T., & Treuting, J. J. (1998). Neuropsychological correlates of childhood attention-deficit/hyperactivity disorder: Explainable by comorbid disruptive behavior or reading problems? *Journal of Abnormal Psychology, 107,* 468–480.

Ohan, J. L., & Johnston, C. (2002). Are the performance overestimates given by boys with ADHD self-protective? *Journal of Clinical Child Psychology, 31,* 230–241.

Oosterlaan, J., & Sergeant, J. A. (1995). Response choice and inhibition in ADHD, anxious, and aggressive children: The relationship between S-R compatibility and stop signal task. In J. A. Sergeant (Ed.), *Eunethydis: European approaches to hyperkinetic disorder* (pp. 225–240). Amsterdam: University of Amsterdam.

Ott, D. A., & Lyman, R. D. (1993). Automatic and effortful memory in children exhibiting attention deficit hyperactivity disorder. *Journal of Clinical Child Psychology, 22,* 420–427.

Owens, J. S., & Hoza, B. (2003). The role of inattention and hyperactivity/impulsivity in the positive illusory bias. *Journal of Consulting and Clinical Psychology, 71,* 680–691.

Ownby, R. L., & Matthews, C. G. (1985). On the meaning of the WISC-R third factor: Relations to selected neuropsychological measures. *Journal of Consulting and Clinical Psychology, 53,* 531–534.

Parry, P. A., & Douglas, V. I. (1983). Effects of reinforcement on concept identification in hyperactive children. *Journal of Abnormal Child Psychology, 11,* 327–340.

Pastor, M. A., Artieda, J., Jahanshahi, M., & Obeso, J. A. (1992). Performance of repetitive wrist movements in Parkinson's disease. *Brain, 115,* 875–891.

Pelham, W. E., Bender, M. E., Caddell, J., Booth, S., & Moorer, S. H. (1985). Methylphenidate and children with attention deficit disorder. *Archives of General Psychiatry, 42,* 948–952.

Pelham, W. E., Milich, R., & Walker, J. L. (1986). Effects of continuous and partial reinforcement and methylphenidate on learning in children with attention deficit disorder. *Journal of Abnormal Psychology, 95,* 319–325.

Pennington, B. F., Grossier, D., & Welsh, M. C. (1993). Contrasting cognitive deficits in attention deficit disorder versus reading disability. *Developmental Psychology, 29,* 511–523.

Pless, I. B., Taylor, H. G., & Arsenault, L. (1995). The relationship between vigilance deficits and traffic injuries involving children. *Pediatrics, 95,* 219–224.

Porrino, L. J., Rapoport, J. L., Behar, D., Sceery, W., Ismond, D. R., & Bunney, W. E., Jr. (1983). A naturalistic assessment of the motor activity of hyperactive boys. *Archives of General Psychiatry, 40,* 681–687.

Prior, M., Leonard, A., & Wood, G. (1983). A comparison study of preschool children diagnosed as hyperactive. *Journal of Pediatric Psychology, 8,* 191–207.

Purvis, K. L., & Tannock, R. (1997). Language abilities in children with attention deficit hyperactivity disorder, reading disabilities, and normal controls. *Journal of Abnormal Child Psychology, 25,* 133–144.

Quay, H. C. (1988). Attention deficit disorder and the behavioral inhibition system: The relevance of the neuropsychological theory of Jeffrey A. Gray. In L. M. Bloomingdale & J. Sergeant (Eds.), *Attention deficit disorder: Criteria, cognition, intervention* (pp. 117–125). Oxford, UK: Pergamon Press.

Quay, H. C. (1997). Inhibition and attention deficit hyperactivity disorder. *Journal of Abnormal Child Psychology, 25,* 7–13.

Quinn, P. O., & Rapoport, J. L. (1974). Minor physical anomalies and neurological status in hyperactive boys. *Pediatrics, 53,* 742–747.

Quinn, P. O., Renfield, M., Burg, C., & Rapoport, J. L. (1977). Minor physical anomalies: A newborn screening and 1-year follow-up. *Journal of the American Academy of Child Psychiatry, 16,* 662–669.

Rabiner, D., Coie, J. D., & the Conduct Problems Prevention Research Group. (2000). Early attention problems and children's reading achievement: A longitudinal investigation. *Journal of the American Academy of Child and Adolescent Psychiatry, 39,* 859–867.

Radonovich, K. J., & Mostofsky, S. H. (2003). *Duration judgments in children with ADHD suggest deficient utilization of temporal information rather than general impairment in timing.* Unpublished manuscript, Johns Hopkins School of Medicine (Kennedy Krieger Institute).

Rao, S. M., Harrington, D. L., Haaland, K. Y., Bobholz, J. A., Cox, R. W., & Binder, J. R. (1997). Distributed neuronal systems underlying the timing of movements. *Journal of Neuroscience, 17,* 5528–5535.

Rapoport, J. L., Pandoni, C., Renfield, M., Lake, C. R., & Ziegler, M. G. (1977). Newborn dopamine beta hydroxylase, minor physical anomalies, and infant temperament. *American Journal of Psychiatry, 134,* 676–679.

Rapport, M. D., DuPaul, G. J., Stoner, G., & Jones, J. T. (1986). Comparing classroom and clinic measures of attention deficit disorder: Differential, idiosyncratic, and dose–response effects of methylphenidate. *Journal of Consulting and Clinical Psychology, 54,* 334–341.

Rapport, M. D., Scanlan, S. W., & Denney, C. B. (1999). Attention-deficit/hyperactivity disorder and scholastic achievement: A model of dual developmental pathways. *Journal of Child Psychology and Psychiatry, 40,* 1169–1183.

Rapport, M. D., Tucker, S. B., DuPaul, G. J., Merlo, M., & Stoner, G. (1986). Hyperactivity and frustration: The influence of control over and size of rewards in delaying gratification. *Journal of Abnormal Child Psychology, 14,* 181–204.

Reader, M. J., Harris, E. L., Schuerholz, L. J., & Denckla, M. B. (1994). Attention deficit hyperactivity disorder and executive dysfunction. *Developmental Neuropsychology, 10,* 493–512.

Reebye, P. N. (1997, October). *Diagnosis and treatment of ADHD in preschoolers.* Paper presented at the annual meeting of the American Academy of Child and Adolescent Psychiatry, Toronto.

Reynolds, C. (1984). Clinical measurement issues on learning disabilities. *Journal of Special Education, 17,* 560–567.

Riccio, C. A., Hynd, G. W. Cohen, M. J., Hall, J., & Molt, L. (1994). Comorbidity of central auditory processing disorder and attention-deficit hyperactivity disorder. *Journal of the American Academy of Child Psychiatry, 33,* 849–857.

Riccio, C. A., Wolfe, M. E., Romine, C., Davis, B., & Sullivan, J. R. (2004). The Tower of London and neuropsychological assessment of ADHD in adults. *Archives of Clinical Neuropsychology, 19,* 661–671.

Roizen, N. J., Blondis, T. A., Irwin, M., & Stein, M. (1994). Adaptive functioning in children with attention-deficit hyperactivity disorder. *Archives of Pediatric and Adolescent Medicine, 148,* 1137–1142.

Rosen, B. N., & Peterson, L. (1990). Gender differences in children's outdoor play injuries: A review and an integration. *Clinical Psychology Review, 10,* 187–205.

Rosenbaum, M., & Baker, E. (1984). Self-control behavior in hyperactive and nonhyperactive children. *Journal of Abnormal Child Psychology, 12,* 303–318.

Rosenthal, R. H., & Allen, T. W. (1978). An examination of attention, arousal, and learning dysfunctions of hyperkinetic children. *Psychological Bulletin, 85,* 689–715.

Roth, N., Beyreiss, J., Schlenzka, K., & Beyer, H. (1991). Coincidence of attention deficit disorder and atopic disorders in children: Empirical findings and hypothetical background. *Journal of Abnormal Child Psychology, 19,* 1–13.

Rothenberger, A. (1995). Electrical brain activity in children with hyperkinetic syndrome: Evidence of a frontal cortical dysfunction. In J. A. Sergeant (Ed.), *Eunethydis: European approaches to hyperkinetic disorder* (pp. 255–270). Amsterdam: University of Amsterdam.

Rowe, R., Maughan, B., & Goodman, R. (2004). Childhood psychiatric disorder and unintentional injury: Findings from a national cohort study. *Journal of Pediatric Psychology, 29,* 119–130.

Rubia, K., Noorloos, J., Smith, A., Gunning, B., & Sergeant, J. (2003). Motor timing deficits in community and clinical boys with hyperactive behavior: The effect of methylphenidate on motor timing. *Journal of Abnormal Child Psychology, 31,* 301–313.

Rucklidge, J. J., & Tannock, R. (2002). Neuropsychological profiles of adolescents with ADHD: Effects of reading difficulties and gender. *Journal of Child Psychology and Psychiatry, 43,* 988–1003.

Sadeh, A., Gruber, R., & Raviv, A. (2003). The effects of sleep restriction and extension on school-age children: What a difference an hour makes. *Child Development, 74,* 444–455.

Sadeh, M., Ariel, R., & Inbar, D. (1996). Rey-Osterrieth and Taylor Complex Figures: Equivalent measures of visual organization and visual memory in ADHD and normal children. *Child Neuropsychology, 2,* 63–71.

Safer, D., & Allen, R. (1976). *Hyperactive children.* New York: Wiley.

Sagvolden, T., Wultz, B., Moser, E. I., Moser, M., & Morkrid, L. (1989). Results from a comparative neuropsychological research program indicate altered reinforcement mechanisms in children with ADD. In T. Sagvolden & T. Archer (Eds.), *Attention deficit dis-*

order: *Clinical and basic research* (pp. 261–286). Hillsdale, NJ: Erlbaum.

Sanchez, R. P., Lorch, E. P., Milich, R., & Welsh, R. (1999). Comprehension of televised stories by preschool children with ADHD. *Journal of Clinical Child Psychology, 28,* 376–385.

Satterfield, J. H., Hoppe, C. M., & Schell, A. M. (1982). A prospective study of delinquency in 110 adolescent boys with attention deficit disorder and 88 normal adolescent boys. *American Journal of Psychiatry, 139,* 795–798.

Schachar, R. J., Tannock, R., & Logan, G. (1993). Inhibitory control, impulsiveness, and attention deficit hyperactivity disorder. *Clinical Psychology Review, 13,* 721–740.

Schwebel, D. C., Brezausek, C. M., Ramey, S. L., & Ramey, C. T. (2004). Interactions between child behavior patterns and parenting: Implications for children's unintentional injury risk. *Journal of Pediatric Psychology, 29,* 93–104.

Schweitzer, J. B., & Sulzer-Azaroff, B. (1995). Self-control in boys with attention-deficit hyperactivity disorder: Effects of added stimulation and time. *Journal of Child Psychology and Psychiatry, 36,* 671–686.

Seguin, J. R., Arseneault, L., Boulerice, B., Harden, P. W., & Tremblay, R. E. (2002). Response perseveration in adolescent boys with stable and unstable histories of physical aggression: The role of underlying processes. *Journal of Child Psychology and Psychiatry, 43,* 481–494.

Seidman, L. J., Benedict, K. B., Biederman, J., Bernstein, J. H., Seiverd, K., Milberger, S., et al. (1995). Performance of children with ADHD on the Rey–Osterrieth Complex Figure: A pilot neuropsychological study. *Journal of Child Psychology and Psychiatry, 36,* 1459–1473.

Seidman, L. J., Biederman, J., Faraone, S. V., Milberger, S., Norman, D., Seiverd, K., et al. (1995). Effects of family history and comorbidity on the neuropsychological performance of children with ADHD: Preliminary findings. *Journal of the American Academy of Child and Adolescent Psychiatry, 34,* 1015–1024.

Seidman, L. J., Biederman, J., Faraone, S. V., Weber, W., & Ouellette, C. (1997). Toward defining a neuropsychology of attention deficit–hyperactivity disorder: Performance of children and adolescence from a large clinically referred sample. *Journal of Consulting and Clinical Psychology, 65,* 150–160.

Seidman, L. J., Biederman, J., Monuteaux, M. C., Doyle, A. E., & Faraone, S. V. (2001). Learning disabilities and executive dysfunction in boys with attention-deficit/hyperactivity disorder. *Neuropsychology, 15,* 544–556.

Semrud-Clikeman, M., Biederman, J., Sprich-Buckminster, S., Lehman, B. K., Faraone, S. V., & Norman, D. (1992). Comorbidity between ADDH and learning disability: A review and report in a clinically referred sample. *Journal of the American Academy of Child and Adolescent Psychiatry, 31,* 439–448.

Semrud-Clikeman, M., Guy, K., Griffin, J. D., & Hynd,

G. W. (2000). Rapid naming deficits in children and adolescents with reading disabilities and attention deficit hyperactivity disorder. *Brain and Language, 74,* 70–83.

Senior, N., Towne, D., & Huessy, D. (1979). Time estimation and hyperactivity: A replication. *Perceptual and Motor Skills, 49,* 289–290.

Sergeant, J., & van der Meere, J. (1988). What happens when the hyperactive child commits an error? *Psychiatry Research, 24,* 157–164.

Sergeant, J., & van der Meere, J. J. (1990). Convergence of approaches in localizing the hyperactivity deficit. In B. B. Lahey & A. E. Kazdin (Eds.), *Advances in clinical child psychology* (Vol. 13, pp. 207–245). New York: Plenum Press.

Shallice, T., Marzocchi, G. M., Coser, S., Del Savio, M., Meuter, R. F., & Rumiati, R. I. (2002). Executive function profile of children with attention deficit hyperactivity disorder. *Developmental Neuropsychology, 21,* 43–71.

Shapiro, E. G., Hughes, S. J., August, G. J., & Bloomquist, M. L. (1993). Processing emotional information in children with attention deficit hyperactivity disorder. *Developmental Neuropsychology, 9,* 207–224.

Shapiro, S. K., Quay, H. C., Hogan, A. E., & Schwartz, K. P. (1988). Response perseveration and delayed responding in undersocialized aggressive conduct disorder. *Journal of Abnormal Psychology, 97,* 371–373.

Shaw, G. A., & Brown, G. (1990). Laterality and creativity concomitants of attention problems. *Developmental Neuropsychology, 6,* 39–57.

Shaw, G. A., & Brown, G. (1999). Arousal, time estimation, and time use in attention-disordered children. *Developmental Neuropsychology, 16,* 227–242.

Shaywitz, S. E., & Shaywitz, B. A. (1984). Diagnosis and management of attention deficit disorder: A pediatric perspective. *Pediatric Clinics of North America, 31,* 429–457.

Sieg, K. G., Gaffney, G. R., Preston, D. F., & Hellings, J. A. (1995). SPECT brain imaging abnormalities in attention deficit hyperactivity disorder. *Clinical Nuclear Medicine, 20,* 55–60.

Siegel, R. A. (1978). Probability of punishment and suppression of behavior in psychopathic and non-psychopathic offenders. *Journal of Abnormal Psychology, 87,* 514–522.

Siklos, S., & Kerns, K. A. (2004). Assessing multitasking in children with ADHD using a modified Six Elements Test. *Archives of Clinical Neuropsychology, 19,* 347–361.

Silberg, J., Rutter, M., Meyer, J., Maes, H., Hewitt, J., Simonoff, E., et al. (1996). Genetic and environmental influences on the covariation between hyperactivity and conduct disturbance in juvenile twins. *Journal of Child Psychology and Psychiatry, 37,* 803–816.

Skinner, B. F. (1953). *Science and human behavior.* New York: Macmillan.

Skinner, B. F. (1969). *Contingencies of reinforcement: A*

theoretical analysis. New York: Appleton-Century-Crofts.

Sleator, E. K., & Pelham, W. E. (1986). *Attention deficit disorder.* Norwalk, CT: Appleton-Century-Crofts.

Slusarek, M., Velling, S., Bunk, D., & Eggers, C. (2001). Motivational effects on inhibitory control in children with ADHD. *Journal of the American Academy of Child and Adolescent Psychiatry, 40,* 355–363.

Smith, A., Taylor, E., Rogers, J. W., Newman, S., & Rubia, K. (2002). Evidence for a pure time perception deficit in children with ADHD. *Journal of Child Psychology and Psychiatry, 43,* 529–542.

Solanto, M. V. (1990). The effects of reinforcement and response-cost on a delayed response task in children with attention deficit hyperactivity disorder: A research note. *Journal of Child Psychology and Psychiatry, 31,* 803–808.

Solanto, M. V., Wender, E. H., & Bartell, S. S. (1997). Effects of methylphenidate and behavioral contingencies on sustained attention in attention-deficit hyperactivity disorder: A test of the reward dysfunction hypothesis. *Journal of Child and Adolescent Psychopharmacology, 7,* 123–136.

Sonuga-Barke, E. J. S., Dalen, L., Daley, D., & Remington, B. (2002). Are planning, working memory, and inhibition associated with individual differences in preschool ADHD symptoms? *Developmental Neuropsychology, 21,* 255–272.

Sonuga-Barke, E. J. S., Lamparelli, M., Stevenson, J., Thompson, M., & Henry, A. (1994). Behaviour problems and pre-school intellectual attainment: The associations of hyperactivity and conduct problems. *Journal of Child Psychology and Psychiatry, 35,* 949–960.

Sonuga-Barke, E. J. S., Taylor, E., & Hepinstall, E. (1992). Hyperactivity and delay aversion: II. The effect of self versus externally imposed stimulus presentation periods on memory. *Journal of Child Psychology and Psychiatry, 33,* 399–409.

Sonuga-Barke, E. J. S., Taylor, E., Sembi, S., & Smith, J. (1992). Hyperactivity and delay aversion: I. The effect of delay on choice. *Journal of Child Psychology and Psychiatry, 33,* 387–398.

Sparrow, S. S., Balla, D. A., & Cicchetti, D. V. (1984). *Vineland Adaptive Behavior Scales.* Circle Pines, MN: American Guidance Service.

Spencer, T. J., Biederman, J., Harding, M., O'Donnell, D., Faraone, S. V., & Wilens, T. E. (1996). Growth deficits in ADHD children revisited: Evidence for disorder-associated growth delays? *Journal of the American Academy of Child and Adolescent Psychiatry, 35,* 1460–1469.

Stein, D., Pat-Horenczyk, R., Blank, S., Dagan, Y., Barak, Y., & Gumpel, T. P. (2002). Sleep disturbances in adolescents with symptoms of attention-deficit/hyperactivity disorder. *Journal of Learning Disabilities, 35,* 268–275.

Stein, M. A. (1999). Unravelling sleep problems in treated and untreated children with ADHD. *Journal of Child and Adolescent Psychopharmacology, 9,* 157–168.

Stein, M. A., Mendelsohn, J., Obermeyer, W. H., Amromin, J., & Benca, R. (2001). Sleep and behavior problems in school-aged children. *Pediatrics, 107*(4), 1–9.

Stein, M. A., Szumowski, E., Blondis, T. A., & Roizen, N. J. (1995). Adaptive skills dysfunction in ADD and ADHD children. *Journal of Child Psychology and Psychiatry, 36,* 663–670.

Sternberg, R. J., & Lubart, T. I. (1996). Investing in creativity. *American Psychologist, 51,* 677–688.

Stevens, J., Quittner, A. L., Zuckerman, J. B., & Moore, S. (2002). Behavioral inhibition, self-regulation of motivation, and working memory in children with attention deficit hyperactivity disorder. *Developmental Neuropsychology, 21,* 117–139.

Stewart, M. A., Pitts, F. N., Craig, A. G., & Dieruf, W. (1966). The hyperactive child syndrome. *American Journal of Orthopsychiatry, 36,* 861–867.

Stewart, M. A., Thach, B. T., & Friedin, M. R. (1970). Accidental poisoning and the hyperactive child syndrome. *Diseases of the Nervous System, 31,* 403–407.

Still, G. F. (1902). Some abnormal psychical conditions in children. *Lancet, i,* 1008–1012, 1077–1082, 1163–1168.

Swensen, A. R., Allen, A. J., Kruesi, M. P., Buesching, D. P., & Goldberg, G. (2004). *Risk of premature death from misadventure in patients with attention-deficit/hyperactivity disorder.* Unpublished manuscript, Eli Lilly Co., Indianapolis, IN.

Swensen, A. R., Birnbaum, H. G., Hamadi, R. B., Greenberg, P., Cremieux, P., & Secnik, K. (2004). Incidence and costs of accidents among attention-deficit/hyperactivity disorder patients. *Journal of Adolescent Health, 35,* 346e1–346e9.

Swensen, A. R., Birnbaum, H. G., Secnik, K., Marynchenko, M., Greenberg, P., & Claxton, A. (2003). Attention-deficit/hyperactivity disorder: Increased costs for patients and their families. *Journal of the American Academy of Child and Adolescent Psychiatry, 42,* 1415–1423.

Szatmari, P., Offord, D. R., & Boyle, M. H. (1989). Correlates, associated impairments, and patterns of service utilization of children with attention deficit disorders: Findings from the Ontario Child Health Study. *Journal of Child Psychology and Psychiatry, 30,* 205–217.

Tannock, R. (1996, January). *Discourse deficits in ADHD: Executive dysfunction as an underlying mechanism?* Paper presented at the annual meeting of the International Society for Research in Child and Adolescent Psychopathology, Santa Monica, CA.

Tannock, R., Purvis, K. L., & Schachar, R. J. (1992). Narrative abilities in children with attention deficit hyperactivity disorder and normal peers. *Journal of Abnormal Child Psychology, 21,* 103–117.

Tannock, R., & Schachar, R. (1996). Executive dysfunction as an underlying mechanism of behaviour and language problems in attention deficit hyperactivity disorders. In J. H. Beitchman, N. J. Cohen, M.

M. Konstantareas, & R. Tannock (Eds.), *Language learning and behavior disorders: Developmental, biological, and clinical perspective* (pp. 128–155). New York: Cambridge University Press.

Tant, J. L., & Douglas, V. I. (1982). Problem-solving in hyperactive, normal, and reading-disabled boys. *Journal of Abnormal Child Psychology, 10,* 285–306.

Tarver-Behring, S., Barkley, R. A., & Karlsson, J. (1985). The mother–child interactions of hyperactive boys and their normal siblings. *American Journal of Orthopsychiatry, 55,* 202–209.

Taylor, E., Sandberg, S., Thorley, G., & Giles, S. (1991). *The epidemiology of childhood hyperactivity.* London: Oxford University Press.

Tripp, G., & Alsop, B. (1999). Sensitivity to reward frequency in boys with attention deficit hyperactivity disorder. *Journal of Clinical Child Psychology, 28,* 366–375.

Tripp, G., & Alsop, B. (2001). Sensitivity to reward delay in children with attention deficit hyperactivity disorder (ADHD). *Journal of Child Psychology and Psychiatry, 42,* 691–698.

Trites, R. L., Tryphonas, H., & Ferguson, H. B. (1980). Diet treatment for hyperactive children with food allergies. In R. M. Knight & D. Bakker (Eds.), *Treatment of hyperactive and learning disordered children* (pp. 151–166). Baltimore: University Park Press.

Trommer, B. L., Hoeppner, J. B., Rosenberg, R. S., Armstrong, K. J., & Rothstein, J. A. (1988). Sleep disturbances in children with attention deficit disorder. *Annals of Neurology, 24,* 325–332.

Ullman, D. G., Barkley, R. A., & Brown, H. W. (1978). The behavioral symptoms of hyperkinetic children who successfully responded to stimulant drug treatment. *American Journal of Orthopsychiatry, 48,* 425–437.

van der Meere, J., Gunning, W. B., & Stemerdink, N. (1996). Changing response set in normal development and in ADHD children with and without tics. *Journal of Abnormal Child Psychology, 24,* 767–786.

van der Meere, J., Hughes, K. A., Borger, N., & Sallee, F. R. (1995). The effect of reward on sustained attention in ADHD children with and without CD. In J. A. Sergeant (Ed.), *Eunethydis: European approaches to hyperkinetic disorder* (pp. 241–253). Amsterdam: University of Amsterdam.

van der Meere, J., & Sergeant, J. (1988a). Focused attention in pervasively hyperactive children. *Journal of Abnormal Child Psychology, 16,* 627–640.

van der Meere, J., & Sergeant, J. (1988b). Controlled processing and vigilance in hyperactivity: Time will tell. *Journal of Abnormal Child Psychology, 16,* 641–656.

van der Meere, J., Shalev, R., Borger, N., & Gross-Tsur, V. (1995). Sustained attention, activation and MPH in ADHD: A research note. *Journal of Child Psychology and Psychiatry, 36,* 697–703.

van der Meere, J., Vreeling, H. J., & Sergeant, J. (1992).

A motor presetting study in hyperactive, learning disabled and control children. *Journal of Child Psychology and Psychiatry, 33,* 1347–1354.

Velting, O. N., & Whitehurst, G. J. (1997). Inattention-hyperactivity and reading achievement in children from low-income families: A longitudinal model. *Journal of Abnormal Child Psychology, 25,* 321–331.

Vitulli, W. F., & Nemeth, Y. (2001). Perception of time: Variations in verbal content and delay of estimation. *Perceptual and Motor Skills, 92,* 316–318.

Vitulli, W. F., & Shepherd, H. (1996). Time estimation: Effects of cognitive task, presentation rate, and delay. *Perceptual and Motor Skills, 83,* 1387–1394.

Voelker, S. L., Carter, R. A., Sprague, D. J., Gdowski, C. L., & Lachar, D. (1989). Developmental trends in memory and metamemory in children with attention deficit disorder. *Journal of Pediatric Psychology, 14,* 75–88.

Vygotsky, L. S. (1978). *Mind in society.* Cambridge, MA: Harvard University Press.

Vygotsky, L. S. (1987). Thinking and speech. In *The collected works of L. S. Vygotsky: Vol. 1. Problems in general psychology* (N. Minick, Trans.). New York: Plenum Press.

Wakefield, J. C. (1992). The concept of mental disorder: On the boundary between biological facts and social values. *American Psychologist, 47,* 373–388.

Wakefield, J. C. (1997). Normal inability versus pathological disability: Why Ossorio's definition of mental disorder is not sufficient. *Clinical Psychology: Science and Practice, 4,* 249–258.

Walcott, C. M., & Landau, S. (2004). The relation between disinhibition and emotion regulation in boys with attention deficit hyperactivity disorder. *Journal of Clinical Child and Adolescent Psychology, 33,* 772–782.

Waldrop, M. F., Bell, R. Q., & Goering, J. D. (1976). Minor physical anomalies and inhibited behavior in elementary school girls. *Journal of Child Psychology and Psychiatry, 17,* 113–122.

Waldrop, M. F., Bell, R. Q., McLaughlin, B., & Halverson, C. F., Jr. (1978). Newborn minor physical anomalies predict short attention span, peer aggression, and impulsivity at age 3. *Science, 199,* 563–564.

Walker, N. W. (1982). Comparison of cognitive tempo and time estimation by young boys. *Perceptual and Motor Skills, 54,* 715–722.

Weiss, G., & Hechtman, L. (1993). *Hyperactive children grown up* (2nd ed.). New York: Guilford Press.

Weiss, G., Hechtman, L., Perlman, T., Hopkins, J., & Wener, A. (1979). Hyperactives as young adults: A controlled prospective tenyear followup of 75 children. *Archives of General Psychiatry, 36,* 675–681.

Welner, Z., Welner, A., Stewart, M., Palkes, H., & Wish, E. (1977). A controlled study of siblings of hyperactive children. *Journal of Nervous and Mental Disease, 165,* 110–117.

Werry, J. S., Elkind, G. S., & Reeves, J. S. (1987). Attention deficit, conduct, oppositional, and anxiety disorders in children: III. Laboratory differences. *Journal of Abnormal Child Psychology, 15,* 409–428.

Werry, J. S., Minde, K., Guzman, A., Weiss, G., Dogan, K., & Hoy, E. (1972). Studies on the hyperactive child: VII. Neurological status compared with neurotic and normal children. *American Journal of Orthopsychiatry, 42,* 441–451.

Weyandt, L. L., & Willis, W. G. (1994). Executive functions in school-aged children: Potential efficacy of tasks in discriminating clinical groups. *Developmental Neuropsychology, 19,* 27–38.

Whalen, C. K., Henker, B., Collins, B. E., McAuliffe, S., & Vaux, A. (1979). Peer interaction in structured communication task: Comparisons of normal and hyperactive boys and of methylphenidate (Ritalin) and placebo effects. *Child Development, 50,* 388–401.

Wigal, T., Swanson, J. M., Douglas, V. I., Wigal, S. B., Stoiber, C. M., & Fulbright, K. K. (1993). *Reinforcement effects on frustration and persistence in children with attention-deficit hyperactivity disorder.* Unpublished manuscript, University of California Medical School–Irvine, Irvine, CA.

Wilens, T. E., Biederman, J., & Spencer, T. (1994). Clonidine for sleep disturbances associated with attention-deficit hyperactivity disorder. *Journal of the American Academy of Child and Adolescent Psychiatry, 33,* 424–426.

Wilkison, P. C., Kircher, J. C., McMahon, W. M., & Sloane, H. N. (1995). Effects of methylphenidate on reward strength in boys with attention-deficit hyperactivity disorder. *Journal of the American Academy of Child and Adolescent Psychiatry, 34,* 877–885.

Willcutt, E. G., Pennington, B. F., Boada, R., Ogline, J. S., Tunick, R. A., Chhabildas, N. A., et al. (2001). A comparison of the cognitive deficits in reading disability and attention-deficit/hyperactivity disorder. *Journal of Abnormal Psychology, 110,* 157–172.

Winsler, A. (1998). Parent–child interaction and private speech in boys with ADHD. *Applied Developmental Science, 2,* 17–39.

Winsler, A., Diaz, R. M., Atencio, D. J., McCarthy, E. M., & Chabay, L. A. (2000). Verbal self-regulation over time in preschool children at risk for attention and behavior problems. *Journal of Child Psychology and Psychiatry, 41,* 875–886.

Woodward, L. J., Fergusson, D. M., & Horwood, L. J. (2000). Driving outcomes of young people with attentional difficulties in adolescence. *Journal of the American Academy of Child and Adolescent Psychiatry, 39,* 627–634

Wu, K. K., Anderson, V., & Castiello, U. (2002). Neuropsychological evaluation of deficits in executive functioning for ADHD children with or without learning disabilities. *Developmental Neuropsychology, 22,* 501–531.

Zahn, T. P., Krusei, M. J. P., & Rapoport, J. L. (1991). Reaction time indices of attention deficits in boys with disruptive behavior disorders. *Journal of Abnormal Child Psychology, 19,* 233–252.

Zakay, D. (1990). The evasive art of subjective time measurement: Some methodological dilemmas. In R. A. Block (Ed.), *Cognitive models of psychological time* (pp. 59–84). Hillsdale, NJ: Erlbaum.

Zakay, D. (1992). The role of attention in children's time perception. *Journal of Experimental Child Psychology, 54,* 355–371.

Zakay, D., & Block, M. (1997). Temporal cognition. *Current Directions in Psychological Science, 6,* 12–16.

Zametkin, A. J., Liebenauer, L. L., Fitzgerald, G. A., King, A. C., Minkunas, D. V., Herscovitch, P., et al. (1993). Brain metabolism in teenagers with attention-deficit hyperactivity disorder. *Archives of General Psychiatry, 50,* 333–340.

Zametkin, A. J., Nordahl, T. E., Gross, M., King, A. C., Semple, W. E., Rumsey, J., et al. (1990). Cerebral glucose metabolism in adults with hyperactivity of childhood onset. *New England Journal of Medicine, 323,* 1361–1366.

Zentall, S. S. (1985). A context for hyperactivity. In K. D. Gadow & I. Bialer (Eds.), *Advances in learning and behavioral disabilities* (Vol. 4, pp. 273–343). Greenwich, CT: JAI Press.

Zentall, S. S. (1988). Production deficiencies in elicited language but not in the spontaneous verbalizations of hyperactive children. *Journal of Abnormal Child Psychology, 16,* 657–673.

Zentall, S. S., & Smith, Y. N. (1993). Mathematical performance and behaviour of children with hyperactivity with and without coexisting aggression. *Behaviour Research and Therapy, 31,* 701–710.

Zentall, S. S., Smith, Y. N., Lee, Y. B., & Wieczorek, C. (1994). Mathematical outcomes of attention-deficit hyperactivity disorder. *Journal of Learning Disabilities, 27,* 510–519.

Comorbid Disorders, Social and Family Adjustment, and Subtyping

RUSSELL A. BARKLEY

This chapter discusses the psychiatric disorders that are often coexisting (comorbid) with Attention-Deficit/Hyperactivity Disorder (ADHD). In addition, it reviews what is known about the social relations between children with ADHD and their parents and peers. Along the way, parental adjustment and psychiatric disorders are also discussed, as they have a clear bearing both on the etiology of a child's disorders and on the implementation of treatments via the family. Finally, this chapter explores the critical issue of subtypes of ADHD, which may be clinically useful in subdividing the quite heterogeneous population of those diagnosed with the disorder into more homogeneous and clinically meaningful subgroups.

COEXISTING PSYCHIATRIC DISORDERS

The reasons why disorders may coexist with each other have been nicely reviewed by Angold, Costello, and Erkanli (1999). Common underlying etiologies may lead to both disorders (genetics, family environment, etc.), or two disorders may be correlated with a third that accounts for their relationship. But apparent comorbidity can also be an artifact of methodological problems in research, such as referral bias, ascertainment bias, overlap in symptoms on diagnostic symptom lists, and other factors. Angold et al. (1999) have computed odds ratios reflecting the likelihood that two disorders will coexist with each other, based on their meta-analysis of community samples; the results of their computations are cited below under the headings for each type of disorder that may coexist with ADHD. Use of community samples was important, because clinic-referred samples can demonstrate an overlap of disorders that is based mainly if not entirely on referral biases in how those samples were referred to and obtained from those particular clinics.

There is no doubt that a diagnosis of ADHD conveys a significant risk for other coexisting psychiatric disorders. Such findings refute not only the naive claims that ADHD is a myth, but also the claims that ADHD is otherwise a benign condition about which one need not be concerned or seek treatment. In one study using a large community sample, up to 44% of children with ADHD had at least one other psychiatric disorder, 32% had two others, and 11% had at least three other disorders (Szatmari, Offord, & Boyle, 1989). These figures are often higher among clinic-referred samples of children with ADHD, given that children with multiple disorders are more likely to be referred for treatment, as well as that the greater severity of a disorder often increases the odds that it will be associated with other disorders. For instance, in their study of both preschool and school-age samples of clinically referred children diagnosed with ADHD, Wilens et al. (2002) found that 75% of their preschool children and 80% of their school-age sample had at least one other disorder besides ADHD, with an average of 1.4 additional disorders. Another study of 111 children with ADHD found much the same result (Pfiffner et al., 1999).

As a group, children with ADHD are rated as having more symptoms of disruptive behavior (oppositional and conduct problems), anxiety, depression or dysthymia, and low self-esteem than either nondisabled children or children with learning disabilities (LDs) who do not have ADHD (Brown, 2000a; Biederman, Faraone, Mick, Moore, & Lelon, 1996; Bohline, 1985; Breen & Barkley, 1983, 1984; Jensen, Burke, & Garfinkel, 1988; Jensen, Shervette, Xenakis, & Richters, 1993; Margalit & Arieli, 1984; Weiss, Hechtman, & Perlman, 1978). I consider each of these forms of comorbidity (as well as some others) separately, though they too may coexist with each other in the presence of ADHD.

Anxiety Disorders

Earlier studies at Massachusetts General Hospital suggested that 27–30% of children with ADHD met criteria for an anxiety disorder, such as Overanxious Disorder (Biederman, Newcorn, & Sprich, 1991; Munir, Biederman, & Knee, 1987). Szatmari, Offord, and Boyle (1989), in their large epidemiological survey, found that 17% of girls and 21% of boys with ADHD between 4 and 11 years of age had at least one anxiety or mood disorder, while these figures rose to 24% for boys and 50% for girls during the adolescent years. Jensen et al. (1993) found that nearly 49% of their sample of children with ADHD had an anxiety disorder, depression, or both, while Pfiffner et al. (1999) reported that 43% of clinic-referred boys had an anxiety disorder alone and another 23% had both anxiety and depression. Other studies have also found that between 13% and 30% of children with ADHD have a

comorbid anxiety or mood disorder (Anderson, Williams, McGee, & Silva, 1987; Bird et al., 1988; Jensen et al., 1988; Cohen, Velez, Brook, & Smith, 1989). In their study of both preschool and school-age samples of clinically referred children with ADHD, Wilens et al. (2002) found that 28% of preschoolers and 33% of school-age children had at least two or more anxiety disorders (one of which was typically a phobia), with the age at onset of the anxiety disorders being 2.6 to 3.0 years. The large Multimodal Treatment Study of ADHD (MTA) also found that 33–39% of its clinic-referred sample ($n = 498$) having ADHD, Combined Type (ADHD-C), also had an anxiety disorder (March et al., 2000; Newcorn et al., 2001).

These individual studies, along with reviews of the literature on the overlap of ADHD with anxiety disorders, reported a range of 10–50% and suggested that about 25–35% of children with ADHD, on average, were likely to have such a disorder (Biederman et al., 1991; Tannock, 2000). Conversely, about 15–30% of children diagnosed clinically with anxiety disorders were likely to have ADHD (Tannock, 2000). Peterson, Pine, Cohen, and Brook (2001) consistently noted a relationship between ADHD and anxiety disorders across four follow-up periods in their longitudinal study of 976 children, suggesting that this is a real comorbidity rather than a coincidence or referral bias.

Angold et al. (1999) found that the odds of ADHD and anxiety disorders' being comorbid within a community sample ranged from 2.1 to 4.3, with a median of 3.0. This relationship remained significant even after the investigators controlled for the presence of other disorders, such as depression, Conduct Disorder (CD), or Oppositional Defiant Disorder (ODD). An odds ratio of 1.0 indicates no significant association between two disorders, while a ratio significantly different from 1.0 implies an affiliation between the disorders. It is clear from the Angold et al. meta-analysis that ADHD and anxiety disorders are significantly comorbid, such that the presence of one results in a three-fold increase in the odds of the second disorder. For instance, in one study of 9- to 13-year-olds ($n = 1,015$), the prevalence of ADHD by *Diagnostic and Statistical Manual of Mental Disorders*, third edition, revised (DSM-III-R) criteria was 1.9%, while that for an anxiety disorder was 5.5%. Approximately 4.3% of children with anxiety disorders had ADHD, while 12.8% of children with ADHD had an anxiety disorder, resulting in an odds ratio of 2.6 concerning the association of these two types of disorders (see Table 3 in Angold et al., 1999). In short, the affiliation between these two types of disorders is significantly greater than expected by chance alone. Yet the vast majority of children with one disorder do not have the other. And surprisingly, follow-up studies to date of children with ADHD into young adulthood have not reported elevated rates of anxiety disorders at that age (Fischer, Barkley, Smallish, & Fletcher, 2002; Mannuzza, Gittelman-Klein, Bessler, Malloy, & LaPadula, 1993; Mannuzza, Klein, Bessler, Malloy, & LaPadula, 1998; Weiss & Hechtman, 1993).

The nature of anxiety symptoms among children with the comorbid conditions does not appear to differ from those seen in children who have only an anxiety disorder (Tannock, 2000), though few studies actually exist on this issue. The MTA seems to suggest that anxiety in ADHD-C may be more closely related to ODD and generally disruptive behavior than to fearfulness (March et al., 2000). But the presence of anxiety with ADHD in some studies does seem to alter the expression of ADHD. Anxiety was associated with a significantly reduced level of impulsivity below that seen in children with ADHD but without anxiety in some studies, though the latter remained more impulsive than nondisabled children (Epstein, Goldberg, Conners, & March, 1997; Gordon, Mettelman, & Irwin, 1990; Pliszka, 1989, 1992; Tannock, 2000). But others have not found this to be the case or have even found the opposite (Tannock, 2000). Consistent with the notion that anxiety decreases impulsivity, however, were the findings of the large MTA (see Chapter 20). This project studied 498 clinic referred children with ADHD-C and found that those with associated anxiety disorders demonstrated significantly greater levels of inattention than impulsivity relative to those children not having an anxiety disorder. Girls with comorbid ADHD and anxiety disorders made significantly fewer impulsive errors on a continuous-performance test (CPT) than did girls having only ADHD. Yet the presence of anxiety may also increase problems in performing cognitively complex tasks, such as those involving working memory (Tannock, 2000). Surprisingly, Tannock (2000) also cited otherwise unpublished data that the comorbid group

may actually have a higher risk of aggressive symptoms than do children with only ADHD; this is unexpected, given that impulsivity and aggression are often highly correlated. Low self-esteem has also been associated with comorbid internalizing disorders (including anxiety disorders), whereas it is often in the average range in children having ADHD alone (Bussing, Zima, & Perwein, 2000; see also Chapter 3), but it is not clear whether this is due to the large overlap between anxiety and depression. As will be noted below, low self-esteem is typically problematic mainly in samples with ADHD and comorbid depression. Though not always consistent, research does seem to suggest that the presence of anxiety alters the clinical presentation of ADHD to some degree—perhaps in the direction of greater inattention and poorer working memory but less impulsive behavior, and possibly more so in girls.

The developmental and family life histories of children with the comorbid conditions may also differ from those having ADHD alone. Tannock (2000) suggests that children with comorbid anxiety and ADHD may have a higher risk for perinatal complications (problems with pregnancy, delivery, or the early neonatal period) than do children with ADHD and no anxiety disorders. The former may also experience greater stressful life events, and may report lower levels of self-esteem, than do children only having ADHD (Jensen, Martin, & Cantwell, 1997; Tannock, 2000). As I discuss in a later section of this chapter and in Chapter 5, the family members of children with ADHD have a markedly higher risk for having ADHD themselves. But where children present with ADHD and anxiety disorders, there also appears to be a threefold increase in risk that relatives will also have anxiety disorders (Tannock, 2000); this indicates a strong familial occurrence of anxiety disorders, not just to ADHD. Research does suggest, however, that the anxiety disorders in families of children with ADHD are transmitted independently within these families, with the higher rate of anxiety disorders representing an artifact of referral bias to mental health clinics (Biederman, Faraone, & Lapey, 1992; Biederman & Faraone, 1997). Finally, at the time of the preceding edition (Barkley, 1998), research suggested that the presence of anxiety with ADHD might reduce the likelihood of a positive response to stimulant medications (Jensen et al.,

1997; Tannock, 2000). But the subsequent MTA has contradicted this notion in finding no impact of comorbid anxiety on stimulant responding (March et al., 2000). So this issue is far from settled. As for psychosocial treatment response, Antshel and Remer (2003) found that children having ADHD and elevated anxiety were more likely to respond to a social skills training program than were children with ADHD alone. Consistent with this finding was that from the MTA, where a comorbid anxiety disorder increased the likelihood of a positive response to the combined medication and psychosocial treatment package (March et al., 2000). With such a limited pool of research to draw on, it is safe to say at this time that the manner in which the coexistence of anxiety disorders with ADHD may affect the clinical presentation, course, and response to treatment is clearly in need of more research before confident conclusions can be drawn.

It should be noted here that although Posttraumatic Stress Disorder (PTSD) and Obsessive–Compulsive Disorder (OCD) are both classified in DSM-IV(-TR) as anxiety disorders, each of them differs from the other anxiety disorders in important respects, and so they are discussed separately in later sections of this chapter. Also the research above often did not include them, warranting their separate review later in the chapter.

Mood Disorders

Depressive Disorders

Symptoms of depression are often elevated among clinical samples of children with ADHD (Jensen et al., 1988, 1997; Treuting & Hinshaw, 2001), with the highest levels occurring among those children having comorbid aggression (or ODD/CD). Symptoms reflecting low self-esteem, however, are chiefly associated with aggression and particularly depression in samples with ADHD, and are otherwise not especially problematic when ADHD is found alone (Bussing et al., 2000; see Chapter 3).

A review of the literature on the comorbidity of Major Depressive Disorder (MDD) or Dysthymic Disorder ADHD cases found a range between 15% and 75% (Spencer, Wilens, Biederman, Wozniak, & Harding-Crawford, 2000). However, most studies reported rates of 9–32% of children with ADHD having MDD (Biederman et al., 1991). Up to 20% of chil-

dren with ADHD seen in a pediatric clinic and up to 38% of those seen in a psychiatric clinic may have comorbid MDD (Spencer et al., 2000). Pffiffner et al. (1999) studied 111 clinic-referred boys with ADHD and 66 control boys referred to the same outpatient clinic but not diagnosed as having ADHD. They found that while just 5% had depression alone (vs. 11% of boys without ADHD), another 21% had depression with an anxiety disorder (vs. 15% of the psychiatric control group). All of this suggests a clear comorbidity of ADHD with depression, with an average risk of 25–30%.

A large portion of this research on comorbidity has been conducted by researchers at the Child Psychopharmacology Unit of the Massachusetts General Hospital, headed by Joseph Biederman. Wilens et al. (2002), in their study of preschool and school-age clinical groups with ADHD, reported that Dysthymia Disorder occurred in 5% of both age groups, while MDD was diagnosed in nearly half of their samples (42% and 47%, respectively). Biederman, Mick, and Faraone (1998) have argued that this association reflects an overlap of two clinical disorders, and that the depression evident in ADHD is not just a reflection of demoralization over failures in major life activities. Yet, surprisingly, early longitudinal studies of children with ADHD followed to adulthood did not report significantly elevated rates of mood disorders (Mannuzza et al., 1993, 1998; Spencer et al., 2000; Weiss & Hechtman, 1993). A more recent follow-up study (Fischer et al., 2002), in contrast, found that 27% of these children had MDD by young adulthood, but that it was primarily predicted by presence of lifetime CD. Similarly, Peterson et al. (2001) found that ADHD was consistently related to depression across four follow-up periods from childhood to young adulthood in their study of 976 children.

The inverse relationship is less clear, but the weight of evidence suggests some elevated risk of ADHD among youth diagnosed with depression (Spencer et al., 2000). One early study of depressed boys, for instance, found that rates of ADHD were not significantly elevated but that levels of other disruptive behavior, such as oppositional and conduct problems, were so (Jensen et al., 1988). In contrast, a study by Brumback et al. (1977) found that 63% of children with depression had hyperactivity. A study of adults with MDD also found that 16% self-reported symptoms from childhood sufficient to warrant a retrospective diagnosis of ADHD, while 12% reported persistence of these symptoms into adulthood (Alpert et al., 1996). Both figures for ADHD are greater than population prevalence estimates for either children or adults (see Chapter 2).

Large studies of community samples can shed further light on the existence and nature of this comorbid relationship. In their meta-analysis of such studies, Angold et al. (1999) reported a median odds ratio of 5.5 for the comorbidity of ADHD and MDD, with a range from 3.5 to 8.4; this was significantly greater than that seen between ADHD and anxiety disorders, noted above. Undoubtedly, then, ADHD and MDD show a greater level of association than expected by chance alone. But depression is also strongly associated with ODD/CD and with anxiety, raising the possibility that the presence of one of these latter disorders is what mediates the relationship between ADHD and MDD. This was suggested in the Fischer et al. (2002) follow-up study, where lifetime CD predicted occurrence of MDD. This was also evident in evidence provided by Angold et al. (1999), where the association of ADHD with depression was greatly reduced when the investigators controlled for comorbidity of ADHD with ODD/CD and with anxiety. In other words, the relationship of ADHD and depression may be an epiphenomenon (Angold et al., 1999) that arises only because of the association of ADHD with ODD/CD and ADHD with anxiety. In the absence of these other two types of disorders, ADHD may not have an association with depression.

The comorbidity of depression with ADHD is often associated with a poorer outcome than either disorder alone (Spencer et al., 2000). This comorbidity is also a marker for a history of greater family and personal stress, and greater parental symptoms of depression and other mood disorders (see Jensen et al., 1997, and Spencer et al., 2000; for reviews). Though this finding is not well established, this group of comorbid children may respond better to antidepressants than do those children with ADHD but without comorbidity for internalizing symptoms (Biederman, Baldessarini, Wright, Keenan, & Faraone, 1993; Jensen et al., 1997). Unlike anxiety disorders, MDD does demonstrate a familial linkage with ADHD, such that risk for one disorder in children predisposes to risk for the other disorder not only in these children, but also among family members of the comorbid children (Biederman, Faraone, & Lapey, 1992; Biederman & Faraone, 1997). Thus ADHD and MDD may share underlying familial etiological factors (Spencer et al., 2000). As noted above, though, ODD and CD are also elevated among these comorbid children and among their family members, and could in part explain the link of ADHD with MDD. Obviously the jury is not in yet on the reason why ADHD and depression share such an elevated comorbidity, but the overlap of both with ODD/CD provides one tantalizing explanation.

Bipolar I Disorder

Bipolar I Disorder (BPD) occurs in approximately 1% of children (Lewinsohn, Klein, & Seeley, 1995), and fewer than 0.4% of adults with BPD may have had the onset of the disorder in childhood (Spencer et al., 2000). BPD is a serious, severe, and potentially life-threatening mental disorder (Carlson, 1990; Geller & Luby, 1997). The relationship of ADHD to BPD, or manic–depression, remains controversial at this writing (see the debate of Biederman with Klein, Pine, & Klein in the *Journal of the American Academy of Child and Adolescent Psychiatry, 1998, 37*, pp. 1091–1099; see also Carlson, 1998), and has received considerable attention since the preceding edition of this text was published. Part of the controversy concerns the definition of and diagnostic criteria for BPD as these are applied to children in the DSM-IV(-TR). For children, episodes of mania are not required for a diagnosis of BPD; severely irritable mood can be substituted. Also, rather than the typical episodic expression of manic–depression as it often occurs in adults, BPD in children may be chronic (Carlson, 1998). These changes to the diagnostic criteria when applied to children create an obvious overlap between the diagnosis of BPD and that of severe ODD when it coexists with ADHD, in which irritability often exists as part of the symptom complex for ODD.

Moreover, the fact that many features of ADHD also appear on the symptom list for mania creates even further diagnostic confusion and possible overlap that is merely an artifact of symptoms lists. For instance, the symptoms of mania can include inflated self-esteem, decreased need for sleep, more talkativeness than usual, distractibility, psychomotor agitation, and excessive involvement in pleasurable activities that have a high potential for painful consequences. All of these, to some degree, are found to a greater-than-usual extent in children with ADHD (see Chapter 3). Children with ADHD demonstrate a positive illusory bias in their self-evaluations, show significantly more insomnia, are certainly more talkative than normal, are obviously distractible (by definition), demonstrate psychomotor agitation (hyperactivity), and often engage in risk-taking and highly impulsive behavior that may have painful consequences—particularly if ADHD co-occurs with CD. Such symptom overlap creates a substantial dilemma for clinicians attempting to conduct a differential diagnosis of BPD from ADHD. Yet the irritability seen in BPD may be markedly more severe than in ODD, in that it is characterized by "affective storms" involving prolonged and highly aggressive and destructive behavior (Spencer et al., 2000), whereas that of ODD is often milder, episodic, and likely to be provoked by parental commands (see Chapter 10). The thinking disorder seen in BPD may also be more than just excessive speech and illogical thought, which also characterize ADHD (see Chapter 3); those with BPD show evidence of thought disorder that may be more bizarre or psychotic-like (Nieman & Delong, 1987; Spencer et al., 2000). Geller et al. (1998) compared 60 older children and adolescents with BPD to 60 youth with ADHD. They found that those with BPD demonstrated symptoms of elevated mood and grandiosity (as would be expected if mania were present), as well as hypersexuality, decreased need for sleep, racing thoughts, risk-taking behavior, talkativeness and pressured speech, and inflated self-esteem more often than those with ADHD. These findings suggest that frequency/severity of these symptoms is, in part, a helpful distinguishing feature between these two disorders. However, the groups did not differ in hyperactivity (hyperenergy) or distractibility, suggesting that these symptoms are not helpful to differential diagnosis.

With these unresolved controversies in mind, we can consider the findings on comorbidity, mostly derived from the Massachusetts General Hospital research team. Milberger, Biederman, Faraone, Murphy, and Tsuang (1995) found that 11% of their children with ADHD had BPD; the figure was 10% among girls with ADHD (Biederman, 1997). In a separate study, Biederman et al. (1992) found BPD

in 13% of children with ADHD seen at a child psychiatry clinic and 10% of children seen in a health maintenance organization. In a 4-year follow-up involving many of these children, 12% of the adolescents with ADHD now met criteria for BPD (Biederman, Faraone, Mick, Wozniak, et al., 1996). Another study reported that 20–27% of children with ADHD also had BPD (Spencer et al., 2000; Wozniak et al., 1995). The subjects with BPD were considerably more impaired in their functioning than were those with ADHD alone, experiencing a greater risk for hospitalization and for additional forms of psychopathology (Biederman, Faraone, Mick, Wozniak, et al., 1996; Biederman et al., 1995; Wozniak et al., 1995). More recently, Wilens et al. (2002) reported rates of comorbidity in their clinic-referred samples; they found that 26% of preschool children with ADHD and 18% of school-age children qualified for a diagnosis of BPD. Children with both BPD and ADHD also appeared to experience an earlier onset to their BPD than did those without ADHD (Faraone, Biederman, Wozniak, et al., 1997), with the average age of onset for BPD being between 2.6 and 3.0 years of age when it coexisted with ADHD (Wilens et al., 2002). In a small study of adults with BPD, Sachs, Baldassano, Truman, and Guille (2000) also found that BPD had an earlier age of onset when it was comorbid with ADHD (12 years vs. 20 years). Those with this comorbidity often have a greater likelihood of comorbidity with other disorders (depression, psychosis, ODD/CD) than do those with ADHD alone (Spencer et al., 2000), and may show a poorer response to acute lithium therapy than those with mania alone (Strober et al., 1998).

Faraone, Biederman, Wozniak, et al. (1997) suggest that ADHD with BPD constitutes a distinct familial subtype of ADHD (see also Spencer et al., 2000). When children with ADHD are subdivided into those who do or do not have BPD, both groups demonstrate a higher rate of ADHD among their relatives. Only that subgroup of children with both ADHD and BPD have a higher rate of BPD (36% vs. 6%) among their relatives (Faraone, Biederman, & Monuteaux, 2001; Spencer et al., 2000). This research group has also suggested that those who have both ADHD and BPD may overlap genetically with that subgroup of individuals who have both ADHD and CD (Faraone & Biederman, 1997). Thus children with ADHD appear to have a small but significant risk for BPD (6–27%), whereas children with childhood-onset BPD have a very high probability of having ADHD (91–98%) (Spencer et al., 2000; Wozniak et al., 1995). Yet adolescents with BPD have a substantially lower rate of ADHD (11%) (Lewinsohn et al., 1995).

To address the possibility that the comorbidity of ADHD with BPD might be purely an artifact of the overlap of symptom lists (see above), Milberger et al. (1995) used a subtraction method to remove the symptom overlap and found that 47% of the children with both ADHD and BPD retained the latter diagnosis. This suggests that about 6–10% of children with ADHD may have a legitimate comorbidity for BPD that is not an artifact of merely having more severe ADHD symptoms. Nor does ascertainment source necessarily account for this overlap, given that Biederman, Russell, Soriano, Wozniak, and Faraone (1998) found that children recruited for a study of ADHD compared to those recruited for a study of mania both had two obvious disorders when their comorbidity was observed to exist in either recruitment source. Muddying this conclusion, however, is the fact that follow-up studies to date of children with ADHD into adulthood have not identified BPD as occurring significantly more often than in control groups (Fischer et al., 2002).

Oppositional Defiant and Conduct Disorders

It is widely accepted by scientists studying children with ADHD that they display a greater degree of difficulties with oppositional and defiant behavior, aggressiveness and conduct problems, and even antisocial behavior than typical children do. Over 65% of clinic-referred samples may show significant problems with stubbornness, defiance or refusal to obey, temper tantrums, and verbal hostility toward others (Loney & Milich, 1982; Stewart, Pitts, Craig, & Dieruf, 1966). Studies suggest that from 45% to 84% of children and adolescents with ADHD will meet full diagnostic criteria for ODD either alone or with CD (Barkley, DuPaul, & McMurray, 1990; Barkley & Biederman, 1997; Biederman et al., 1992; Faraone & Biederman, 1997; Fischer, Barkley, Edelbrock, & Smallish, 1990; Cohen et al., 1989; Pfiffner et al., 1999; Wilens et al., 2002), with an average across studies of at least 55% (Biederman et al., 1991). For instance, Wilens

et al. (2002) reported that 62% of their preschool-age children with ADHD and 59% of their school-age sample also had ODD. These same studies also indicate that as many as 15–56% of children with ADHD and 44–50% of adolescents will be diagnosed as having the more serious problem of CD (see also Szatmari, Boyle, & Offord, 1989; Wilens et al., 2002). Whereas ODD may occur by itself in the absence of CD, CD rarely occurs alone in children with ADHD, almost always being seen in the context of ODD. For instance, Pfiffner et al. (1999) found that just 1% of their 111 boys with ADHD and 3% of their psychiatric control group without ADHD were diagnosed with CD alone. Another 43% of the group with ADHD and 26% of the control group had CD with ODD, while the figures for ODD alone were 41% and 35%, respectively. Similarly, Bird, Gould, and Staghezza (1993) found that 93% of their Puerto Rican children having ADHD also had either ODD or CD.

The most common types of conduct problems found in these studies are lying, stealing, truancy, and (to a lesser degree), physical aggression. Peterson et al. (2001) observed in their longitudinal study of 976 children followed to young adulthood that ADHD showed a consistent relationship to ODD/CD across all four follow-up time periods. Again, all this implies a true comorbidity between these disorders and not just referral bias, chance, or an artifact of ascertainment of disorders.

The meta-analysis by Angold et al. (1999) of 21 different community studies reported a median odds ratio of 10.7 (range 7.7 to 14.8) between ADHD and CD/ODD, making it the most likely comorbidity between ADHD and any other set of disorders. And this relationship does not appear to be an artifact of the coexistence of a third type of disorder with these two, such as depression or anxiety.

Children with comorbid ADHD and CD/ODD appear to have higher levels of impulsivity than children with only ADHD or with ADHD and an anxiety disorder (Lynam, 1998). They also have more impulsive behavior than hyperactive behavior, and committed more impulsive errors on a CPT than children with ADHD and an anxiety disorder in one study (Newcorn et al., 2001). This implies that the presence of comorbid ODD/CD in ADHD augurs for a more severe form of ADHD.

Some earlier investigators expressed the belief that ADHD and conduct problems were the same or quite similar disorders (Shapiro & Garfinkel, 1986; Stewart, deBlois, & Cummings, 1981). Obviously this notion could have arisen from their striking comorbidity, as noted above. But research now indicates that relatively pure cases of both can be found, and that these disorders are likely to have different correlates and outcomes (for reviews, see Hinshaw, 1987; Jensen et al., 1997; Newcorn & Halperin, 2000; Werry, 1988). Children with CD usually come from backgrounds with greater social adversity and have a higher prevalence of psychiatric disorders (particularly Antisocial Personality Disorder, substance dependence and abuse, MDD, and CD) among their parents and relatives than children with ADHD but without significant conduct problems (Faraone, Biederman, Jetton, & Tsuang, 1997; Jensen et al., 1997; Loeber, Burke, Lahey, Winters, & Zera, 2000; McGee, Williams, & Silva, 1984b; Newcorn & Halperin, 2000; Reeves, Werry, Elkind, & Zametkin, 1987; Schachar & Tannock, 1995; Szatmari, Boyle, & Offord, 1989). In contrast, children with ADHD are more likely to have developmental delays and cognitive deficits than are those with CD (Hinshaw, 1987; McGee, Williams, & Silva, 1984a; Newcorn & Halperin, 2000; Schachar & Tannock, 1995; Szatmari, Boyle, & Offord, 1989). Neurobiological differences between the two disorders may also be emerging; though findings are still tentative, they support a role of the serotonergic system in aggression but not in ADHD, while dopaminergic mechanisms seem more likely in ADHD than in aggression (for reviews, see Newcorn & Halperin, 2000). When children have both disorders, they often display the mixture of cognitive and attention/inhibitory deficits typical of ADHD, as well as a greater likelihood of factors associated with social adversity, family psychiatric problems, and family conflict (Barkley, Fischer, Edelbrock, & Smallish, et al., 1991; Jensen et al., 1997; Newcorn & Halperin, 2000; Schachar & Tannock, 1995). They are also more likely to have an earlier onset of their antisocial activities, greater persistence of those activities, more school disciplinary consequences, greater substance use and abuse, more traffic offenses and vehicular crashes, and generally a worse overall outcome than are those children with ADHD but without CD (Barkley, Fischer, Edelbrock, & Smallish, 1990; Barkley et al., 1991; Jensen et al., 1997; Moffitt, 1990). All of this supports

the distinctiveness of ADHD and CD, despite their high degree of comorbidity. Where both disorders occur, the correlates, risks, and outcomes for each disorder are also likely to be present in combination (additive) if not actually worse (synergistic).

Several possibilities exist for explaining this striking comorbidity of ADHD with ODD/CD. One is that ADHD is a developmental precursor to ODD/CD. Evidence available, however, suggests that ODD and CD should be distinguished from each other in addressing this issue. Symptoms of hyperactive–impulsive behavior (but not inattention) do predict later ODD symptoms (Burns & Walsh, 2002), and the combination of the two increases the stability of ODD from the preschool to the school-age period (Lavigne et al., 2001; Speltz, McClellan, DeKlyen, & Jones, 1999). Hence ADHD may even cause or at least contribute to risk for ODD alone. But studies suggest that ODD by itself in samples with ADHD is not a precursor to later CD and may not be especially stable over later development (August, Realmuto, Joyce, & Hektner, 1999). In fact, ODD alone declines significantly with age, while CD increases with age. It is only the combination of ODD with CD that is likely to explain the persistence of ODD into adolescence (Maughan, Rowe, Messer, Goodman, & Meltzer, 2004). Though ADHD and ODD are distinct disorders, when they coexist, the features are largely additive rather than unique to the comorbid group (Gadow & Nolan, 2002).

Therefore, the early onset and persistence of CD symptoms, which often co-occur with ODD symptoms, are the hallmark of the unique group with comorbid ADHD + ODD/ CD. The available evidence suggests that ADHD is not so much a precursor to CD as a comorbidity with an early-onset and rather severe form of CD (Maughan et al., 2004; Newcorn & Halperin, 2000). ADHD + CD is a more severe subtype of ADHD in which the outcomes are often worse than is seen in ADHD alone (Barkley, Fischer, Smallish, & Fletcher, 2004). Unless signs of early aggressiveness or other CD features are present, children with ADHD do not seem to be more prone to developing CD or to greater antisocial activities in later life, even if they have ODD (Barkley et al., 2004; Lynam, 1998). Thus children with ADHD + CD (regardless of ODD status) are those who constitute a possibly unique group, not those with ADHD + ODD alone.

As just noted, another possibility is that the ADHD + CD combination represents a unique disorder or subtype of ADHD. That is, the disorders do not just coexist additively, but represent a unique combination or even unique disorder from ADHD alone. The family histories of the comorbid group suggest this possibility, given that they show elevated rates of both disorders (as well as depression and substance use disorders). But as noted above for depression, the link between ADHD and depression may be partly or wholly mediated by the link of ADHD with ODD/CD (Angold et al., 1999). The genetic findings concerning the two disorders also suggest this. Whereas a common genetic factor was shown to contribute to the comorbidity of ADHD with ODD/CD, other genetic factors were also found to be contributing to ODD/CD (Nadder, Rutter, Silberg, Maes, & Eaves, 2002). A recent meta-analysis of studies on the issue concluded, albeit tentatively, that the results do not support merely a synergistic combination of two otherwise distinct disorders when they are found to coexist. Instead, the combination may represent a unique condition (Waschbusch, 2002). Supporting this view were the following findings:

- The prevalence for the combination of disorders is higher than would be expected from simply the overlap of two separate disorders, and they co-occur more highly than would be expected by chance.
- The group with ADHD + CD demonstrates more severe symptoms (at least on parent and teacher ratings, but not lab measures) both of ADHD and of CD than are seen in either disorder alone.
- Aggressive behavior (particularly of the hostile, as opposed to instrumental, form) in the group with ADHD + CD may be more evident and more persistent when provoked than is evident in either group alone.
- Those with the combination show a wider range of antisocial activities than do those with either disorder alone.
- Those with ADHD + CD are likely to have a lower Verbal IQ than those with either disorder alone.
- Those with the combination have more severe problems with social functioning—especially in peer relations, social cognition, and social rejection—than are evident in either group alone.

- Those with ADHD + CD are more likely to show early psychopathic traits, such as callousness and lack of empathy or emotion toward others (see also Lynam, 1998).
- Those with the combination may have an earlier onset of problems, especially conduct problems, than those with either disorder alone.
- Those with ADHD + CD may be more likely to demonstrate adult Antisocial Personality Disorder and antisocial offending than those with either disorder alone (see also Lynam, 1998).
- Those with the combination are more likely to have both ADHD and CD at adult outcome than are those with either disorder alone.

All of these findings suggest that the ADHD + CD combination is probably a unique disorder in its own right and is more severe than either disorder alone. The combination shows an earlier emergence and more severe and stable symptoms than are found for either disorder alone, as well as a unique developmental pathway (Lynam, 1998; Waschbusch, 2002). Patterson, Degarmo, and Knutson (2000) have provided data to show that this pathway is characterized by an earlier onset of ADHD symptoms, early antisocial conduct in the child, the presence of disrupted parenting, and the presence of antisocial parents. In fact, disrupted parenting may be even more a correlate of CD than of ODD (Rowe, Maughan, Pickles, Costello, & Angold, 2002); it may also reflect antisocial characteristics of the parents in their own right, and not just a social environmental cause (Patterson et al., 2000). This is consistent with evidence that some cases of CD have a markedly high genetic contribution that may be influenced by within-family environment, but that there is also a cross-situational form of CD that is entirely genetically influenced with no family environment contribution (Scourfield, Van den Bree, Martin, & McGuffin, 2004). Other research suggests that early-onset noncompliance and covert antisocial behavior may also typify this group (Lee & Hinshaw, 2004).

Note that CD is highly associated with later substance use disorders. Rather than treat the latter as separate comorbidities, I will deal with them instead in Chapter 6 as developmental risks and adverse outcomes for ADHD (especially ADHD + CD).

Posttraumatic Stress Disorder

PTSD is a relatively new disorder, first introduced with the publication of DSM-III. Since the preceding edition of this book, a few papers and a review of the literature have been published on the possible comorbidity of ADHD with PTSD. The literature remains small and is not especially definitive in its conclusions, but some broad interpretations can be ventured at this time. Wozniak et al. (1999) used data from a longitudinal study of 260 children and adolescents with and without ADHD, and systematically and comprehensively evaluated them for trauma exposure and PTSD. They found no meaningful differences between the group with ADHD and the control group in trauma exposure or PTSD. Approximately 12% of the group with ADHD had been exposed to some type of traumatic event, compared to 7% of the control group, but the difference was not statistically significant. Trauma exposure was associated with the development of new-onset MDD in both groups since the baseline evaluation. But among those with ADHD, the presence of BPD at baseline was associated with a significantly greater risk for trauma exposure. Of those children with ADHD exposed to trauma during follow-up, just 2 (1%) developed PTSD. Overall, approximately 9% of the trauma-exposed children across the entire study sample developed PTSD, suggesting that most children do not develop PTSD after exposure to traumatic events. Those children with both ADHD and trauma had somewhat lower Global Assessment of Functioning scores at follow-up. The authors concluded that there was no meaningful association of ADHD with trauma or PTSD, but that childhood BPD was an important antecedent for later trauma.

Similarly, Ford et al. examined a large sample (*n* = 165) of children seen in an outpatient psychiatric clinic for trauma exposure (both victimization and nonvictimization). Although they found an initial association of both ADHD and ODD with having been exposed to victimization trauma, they found no relationship between ADHD and trauma exposure after appropriately controlling for various child and family factors that could potentially confound this relationship. However, ODD remained significantly associated with likelihood of victimization trauma, regardless of whether it coexisted with ADHD or not. This makes some sense, given the frequent association of

ODD with disrupted parenting, family social adversities, and parental psychopathology (see the discussion of ODD/CD, above). Indeed, Ford et al. found that family psychopathology was a significant predictor of victimization in the study samples. Victimization trauma was found to contribute uniquely to a child's risk for ODD but not for ADHD. The percentages of children exposed to any traumatic events were 63% for those with ADHD, 62% for those with ODD, 91% for those with ADHD + ODD, and 48% for those with adjustment disorders; only the group with comorbid ADHD + ODD was significantly different from the control group. This difference was entirely accounted for by experiences of victimization trauma rather than by nonvictimization events, such as accidents, injuries, or illness exposure.

In further analyses of these samples, the authors found that 6% of children with ADHD were likely to have PTSD, while 24% of children with ODD and 22% of children with both ADHD and ODD qualified for the PTSD diagnosis (Ford et al., 2000). Only the two groups with ODD were significantly different from the control group of children diagnosed with adjustment disorders (0% occurrence of PTSD) and showed significantly elevated PTSD-specific symptoms (hyperarousal, sleep disturbance, generalized arousal, and startle response). Since ODD may have a substantial overlap in clinical presentation with BPD, it is not clear from this study whether it is actually childhood BPD within the ODD group that accounts for this relationship. Even so, ODD is the more common disorder among outpatient referrals and, for now at least, should be taken as a significant risk factor for victimization trauma.

The converse relationship between these disorders may be somewhat different. Children with PTSD appear to have a higher-than-expected comorbidity with ADHD, ranging from 14% to 46% (Weinstein, Steffelbach, & Biaggio, 2000). However, Wozniak et al. (1999) did not find a significantly elevated level of ADHD among their subsets of children with trauma exposure or PTSD. It is likely that these studies of children with PTSD have not controlled for confounding variables, which may account for elevated levels of ADHD in some studies. The weight of the evidence to date suggests that although children with PTSD may have elevated levels of ADHD in some cases, there exists no causal or meaningful relationship between the two disorders. It also is not clear from these studies of children with PTSD whether the authors subdivided the children with both ADHD and PTSD by the presence of any additional comorbid disorders shown above to be related to trauma exposure and PTSD, these being BPD and ODD. It may well be the comorbidity of these latter two disorders with ADHD that accounts for the elevated rate of ADHD found in some studies among children with PTSD.

Tic Disorders
and Obsessive–Compulsive Disorder

Tics are a common occurrence in childhood, occurring in between 4% and 18% of children and adolescents, and having a high probability of remission by adolescence (Peterson et al., 2001). Tourette syndrome (TS) is a far rarer and more severe tic disorder, occurring at rates of 1–5 cases in 1,000 individuals. OCD is often found in 1.8–5.5% of adolescents and approximately 3.3% of young adults (see Peterson et al., 2001). The relationship of ADHD to these two types of disorders (tic disorders and OCD) has received scant attention in the scientific literature. As will become apparent below, I group tic disorders and OCD together in this section becomes of their clear relationship to each other—made most apparent in TS, where both motor and vocal tics commonly coexist with obsessive and compulsive behavior or with frank OCD (American Psychiatric Association, 2000; Spencer et al., 1998).

In the largest study to date on this issue, Peterson et al. (2001) followed 976 children prospectively into early adulthood and examined the relationship among ADHD, tic disorders, and OCD. The authors found no impressive relationship between ADHD and tic disorders. Both tics and ADHD declined significantly across the follow-up periods, whereas OCD declined initially by adolescence and then increased in early adulthood (3.3%). Tics and OCD were significantly related to each other at adolescence and again at young adulthood, while OCD was associated with ADHD at both time points. The authors examined the extent to which a diagnosis of one disorder earlier in time predicted risk for the other diagnoses at later time points. The presence of tics at both childhood and early adolescence predicted the presence of OCD by young adulthood. Al-

though early ADHD predicted tics and OCD at later time points, the relationship to tics was exceptionally modest. The Peterson et al. (2001) study suggests some relationship between childhood ADHD and adult OCD, but clearly most of their children with ADHD did not develop OCD or tic disorders, and vice versa. Moreover, this relationship of ADHD to later OCD has not been borne out by longitudinal studies of large samples of children with ADHD followed to adulthood (Fischer et al., 2002; Mannuzza et al., 1993, 1998; Weiss & Hechtman, 1993), where no significant elevation in OCD among children with ADHD has been evident in comparison to community control groups. Hence, the risk of having OCD among children with ADHD is not a clear one, and at most may be 3–5%. The inverse relationship may be different. Studies suggest that 6–33% of children with OCD may have ADHD (Brown, 2000b), and that when these disorders are found together, they represent true comorbidity rather than the OCD symptoms' merely being a phenotypic equivalent of ADHD (Geller et al., 2002).

Spencer et al. (1999) evaluated 128 children with ADHD and 110 control children and found a significantly elevated rate of tic disorders (other than TS) in the group with ADHD (34% vs. 6%). When these children were followed up 4 years later, 65% of the cases of tic disorders had remitted, versus just 20% of the cases of ADHD. As in the Peterson et al. (2001) study, the presence of ADHD at baseline predicted a slightly increased risk for tic disorders at the 4-year follow-up (20% occurrence). In a separate study, Spencer et al. (2001) found a modestly elevated rate of lifetime tic disorders among clinically referred adults diagnosed with ADHD (12%), compared to their control group (4%); the tic disorders also showed a high probability of remission. In both studies, the presence of a tic disorder did not appear to alter the clinical presentation or course of ADHD, in terms of the ADHD's severity or effects on global functioning. The few available studies appear to suggest a slightly elevated risk of tic disorders (other than TS) among children with ADHD, but such disorders have a high rate of remission and little impact on ADHD course, impairment, or general global functioning.

No evidence appears to point to a higher-than-normal frequency of TS among children with ADHD (Peterson et al., 2001). But as the severity of tic disorders increases, the likelihood of these disorders' being comorbid with ADHD also increases, such that between 25% and 85% of those with TS have comorbid ADHD (Comings, 2000). In his own study of 361 individuals with TS, Comings (2000) reported a prevalence of 61.5% having ADHD. And so it appears that a one-way comorbidity may exist between ADHD and TS, in which children with ADHD appear to have little if any elevated risk for TS, while patients with TS have a strikingly high risk for having comorbid ADHD.

Autistic Spectrum Disorders

The overlap of ADHD with autistic spectrum disorders has probably received the least attention of all in the literature on comorbidity in ADHD. This is due, in part, to the common practice of ruling out children with autism, Asperger syndrome, or other pervasive developmental disorders (PDDDs) from even entering studies of ADHD. This practice was based on the belief that children with PDDs display a high likelihood of ADHD-like symptoms as a consequence of their often severe and pervasive disorder. Autistic spectrum disorders therefore may create a phenocopy of "faux ADHD," whereas those with ADHD cannot have autism or other PDDs, if only by definition. As a consequence, the prevalence of PDDs among children with ADHD has not been identified, to my knowledge.

Recently, investigators have argued that although the two types of disorders are distinct from each other, cases of comorbidity may well exist, at least if autistic spectrum disorders are the starting point for case ascertainment. For instance, Goldstein and Schwebach (2004) recently reported a retrospective chart review of 57 clinic-referred cases involving either PDD Not Otherwise Specified (NOS), autism, or ADHD. They found that 26% of the children with PDD NOS or autism met criteria for a diagnosis of ADHD-C and 33% met criteria for ADHD, Predominantly Inattentive Type (ADHD-PI), suggesting that the majority (59%) of those with PDD NOS or autism had comorbid ADHD. So, while the likelihood that children with ADHD may have comorbid autistic spectrum disorders is unknown (and probably quite low, given the rare incidence of the latter disorders), the likelihood that children with autistic spectrum disorders may also

have ADHD seems high—perhaps again, as in the case of TS, illustrating a one-way comorbidity.

SOCIAL RELATIONSHIPS

This section examines the difficulties that children with ADHD often have in their family and peer relationships.

Parent–Child Interactions

Research finds that ADHD affects the interactions of children with their parents, and hence the manner in which parents may respond to these children. In general, these families are characterized as manifesting greater intrafamily conflict, especially between the parents and the children with ADHD, than is evident in control families (Danforth, Barkley, & Stokes, 1991; Johnston & Mash, 2001; Smith, Brown, Bunke, Blount, & Christophersen, 2002). Children with ADHD are more talkative, negative, and defiant; less compliant and cooperative; more demanding of assistance from others; and less able to play and work independently of their mothers (Barkley, 1985; Danforth et al., 1991; DuPaul, McGoey, Eckert, & VanBrakle, 2001; Gomez & Sanson, 1994; Johnston & Mash, 2001; Mash & Johnston, 1982). Their mothers appear to be less responsive to their questions, more negative and directive, and less rewarding of their behavior (Danforth et al., 1991; DuPaul et al., 2001).

More generally, the parental reactions of parents of children with ADHD appear to be characterized by a more lax yet overreactive disciplinary style, more maladaptive coping styles, coercive (negative/ineffective) management tactics, greater expressed emotion, and more negative parental perceptions of their relationships with their children than are evident in families of nondisabled children (DuPaul et al., 2001; Gerdes, Hoza, & Pelham, 2003; Harvey, Danforth, Ulaszek, & Eberhardt, 2001; Hoza et al., 2000; McKee, Harvey, Danforth, Ulaszek, & Friedman, 2004; O'Leary, Slep, & Reid, 1999; Peris & Hinshaw, 2003). The views of fathers and mothers of children with ADHD may differ, however. Singh (2003) compared the perspectives of both parents (39 mothers and 22 fathers), using in-depth interviews. In regard to fathers' perspectives on their children's ADHD and its treatment, he characterized the fathers as either "reluctant believers" or "tolerant nonbelievers." These fathers were more likely to be resistant to a medical framework for understanding their sons' behavior, identified themselves more often in their sons' behavior, and were more resistant to drug treatment than were mothers. Singh concluded that these findings may help to explain the frequent absence of fathers from clinical evaluations of their children and from participation in research on children with ADHD. In the MTA, Hoza et al. (2000) reported that mothers of children with ADHD-C were more likely than fathers to have an external locus of control; the mothers also had lower self-esteem, lower parenting efficacy, and a greater tendency to attribute noncompliance to their children's bad mood.

Interestingly, children with ADHD may not perceive their relations with their parents as being any more negative than children in control groups perceive theirs to be (Gerdes et al., 2003). This is certainly in keeping with the positive illusory bias often found in the judgments of children with ADHD about their competence and performance (see Chapter 3).

Some gender differences between parents are also evident in parents' interactions with their offspring who have ADHD. Mothers of children with ADHD have been shown to give both more commands and more rewards to sons with ADHD than to daughters with ADHD (Barkley, 1989; Befera & Barkley, 1984), but also to be more emotional and acrimonious in their interactions with their sons (Buhrmester, Camparo, Christensen, Gonzalez, & Hinshaw, 1992; Taylor, Sandberg, Thorley, & Giles, 1991). Children with ADHD seem to be somewhat less problematic for their fathers than for their mothers (Buhrmester et al., 1992; Tallmadge & Barkley, 1983), but even the latter interactions are different from those of typical father–child dyads. Research demonstrates that mother–child conflicts may result in increased father–child conflicts when mothers and fathers interact jointly (triadically) with their hyperactive children, especially hyperactive boys (Buhrmester et al., 1992). Such increased maternal negativity and acrimony toward sons in these interactions have been shown to predict greater noncompliance in classroom and play settings and greater covert stealing away from home, even when the levels of the children's own negativity and of parental psychopathology are statistically controlled for in the analyses (Anderson, Hinshaw, & Simmel, 1994).

These negative parent–child interaction patterns occur in the preschool-age group (Cohen, Sullivan, Minde, Novak, & Keens, 1983; Cunningham & Boyle, 2002; DuPaul et al., 2001; Keown & Woodward, 2002) and may be at their most negative and stressful (to the parents) in this age range (Mash & Johnston, 1982, 1990). With increasing child age, the degree of conflict in these interactions lessens, but it remains higher than in typical families into later childhood (Barkley, Karlsson, & Pollard, 1985; Mash & Johnston, 1982) and adolescence (Barkley, Anastopoulos, Guevremont, & Fletcher, 1992; Barkley et al., 1991; Edwards, Barkley, Laneri, Fletcher, & Metevia, 2001; Peris & Hinshaw, 2003). Negative parent–child interactions in childhood have been observed to be significantly predictive of continuing parent–child conflicts 8–10 years later, when the children with ADHD are adolescents (Barkley et al., 1991).

Important in this line of family research has been the discovery that *the presence of comorbid ODD and especially CD is associated with most of the conflicts* noted in the interactions of mothers with children and adolescents having ADHD (Barkley, Anastopoulos, et al., 1992; Barkley et al., 1991). In a large study of children with ADHD, Johnston, Murray, Hinshaw, Pelham, and Hoza (2002) were able to show that the reduced maternal responsiveness, warmth, sensitivity, and acceptance to child behavior described earlier were chiefly associated with conduct problems or ODD-like symptoms, not with ADHD symptoms. Maternal responsiveness was also associated with maternal depressive symptoms in this study, perhaps suggesting one pathway in which parental psychological adjustment may affect parent–child relations—a subject that is only beginning to be explored (Johnston & Mash, 2001). Another mechanism may be child care workload, in that mothers of children with ADHD who spent more time in employment with a lighter child care workload had a greater sense of parenting well-being and fewer conduct problems in their children, whereas father employment had the opposite effect (greater child care workload was associated with lower maternal parenting well-being and greater conduct problems) (Harvey, 1998).

In a sequential analysis of parent–teen interaction sequences, investigators have noted that it is the immediate or first lag in the sequence that is most important in determining the behavior of the other member of the dyad (Fletcher, Fischer, Barkley, & Smallish, 1996). That is, the behavior of each member is determined mainly by the immediately preceding behavior of the other member, and not by earlier behaviors of either member in the chain of interactions. The interactions in families of teens with comorbid ADHD and ODD reflect a strategy best characterized as "tit for tat," in that the type of behavior (positive, neutral, or negative) of each member is most influenced by the same type of behavior emitted immediately preceding it. Mothers of teens with ADHD only or of nondisabled teens are more likely to utilize positive and neutral behaviors, regardless of the immediately preceding behavior of their teens; this has been characterized as a "be nice and forgive" strategy, which is thought to be more mature and more socially successful for both parties in the long run (Fletcher et al., 1996). Even so, those families having children with ADHD alone are still found to be deviant from typical families in these interaction patterns and in expressed emotion, even after comorbid conduct problems are controlled for (Fletcher et al., 1996; Keown & Woodward, 2002; Peris & Hinshaw, 2003; Woodward, Taylor, & Dowdney, 1998).

Parents of children with ADHD, more than parents of nondisabled children, appear to sense that the disruptive behavior of their children is internally rather than externally caused, less controllable by the children, and more stable over development (Johnston & Freeman, 1997). In contrast, they evaluate the prosocial behavior of their children with ADHD as less internal and less stable than control parents see that of their children.

The interaction conflicts in families of children with ADHD are not limited to parent–child interactions. Increased conflicts have been observed between children with ADHD and their siblings, relative to typical child–sibling dyads (Mash & Johnston, 1983; Taylor et al., 1991). Few differences have been noted between mothers' interactions with their children who have ADHD and their interactions with the siblings of these children (Tarver-Behring, Barkley, & Karlsson, 1985) but research on that issue is sorely limited.

Research on the larger domain of family functioning has also shown that parents of children with ADHD experience more parenting stress, more role dissatisfaction, and a decreased sense of parenting competence and self-esteem (Anastopoulos, Guevremont, Shelton, & DuPaul, 1992; Breen & Barkley, 1988; DuPaul et al., 2001; Fischer, 1990; Johnston, 1996; Mash & Johnston, 1990; Podolski & Nigg, 2001). Of interest is that one study comparing subtypes of children with ADHD found no differences in levels of distress between the families of children with ADHD-C and with ADHD-PI (Podolski & Nigg, 2001). In that study, mothers' reports of role distress were related more to child inattention and oppositional/conduct problems; fathers' role distress was most associated with the latter domain of behavioral problems, but not with severity of ADHD symptoms. Harrison and Sofronoff (2002) further studied maternal reports of distress and depression in managing their children with ADHD, and found that it was best predicted by severity of the children's behavioral disturbance and the mothers' perceived level of control over the children's behavior. Likewise, Bussing et al. (2003) found that level of caregiver strain among parents in a large community sample of 200 high-risk children was increased among mothers as a function of male gender of the children, level of inattention, and degree of ODD symptoms.

Increased alcohol consumption in parents of children with ADHD has also been documented (Cunningham, Benness, & Siegel, 1988; Pelham & Lang, 1993), along with decreased extended family contacts (Cunningham et al., 1988), and increased marital conflict, separations, and divorce, as well as maternal depression (Befera & Barkley, 1984; Cunningham & Boyle, 2002; Cunningham et al., 1988; Barkley, Fischer, et al., 1990; Lahey, Piacentini, et al., 1988; Taylor et al., 1991). Again, the comorbid association of ADHD with ODD, and especially CD, is linked to even greater degrees of parenting stress, parental psychopathology, marital discord, and divorce than is ADHD only (Barkley, Anastopoulos, et al., 1992; Barkley, Fischer, et al., 1990; Barkley et al., 1991; Johnston, 1996; Lahey, Piacentini, et al., 1988; Taylor et al., 1991). Interestingly, Pelham and Lang (1993) have shown that the increased alcohol consumption in these parents is, in part, a direct function of their stressful interactions with their children who have ADHD.

Research has demonstrated that the primary direction of effects within these interactions is from child to parent (Fischer, 1990; Mash & Johnston, 1990), rather than the reverse. That is, much of the disturbance in the interaction seems to stem from the effects of a child's excessive, impulsive, unruly, noncompliant, and emotional behavior on a parent, rather than from the effects of the parent's behavior on the child. This finding was documented primarily through studies evaluating the effects of stimulant medication on the behavior of children with ADHD and their interaction patterns with their mothers. Such research found that medication improves the compliance of these children and reduces their negative, talkative, and generally excessive behavior, so that their parents reduce their levels of directive and negative behavior as well (Barkley & Cunningham, 1979; Barkley, Cunningham, & Karlsson, 1983; Danforth et al., 1991; Humphries, Kinsbourne, & Swanson, 1978). These medication effects are noted even in the preschool-age group of children with ADHD (Barkley, 1988), as well as in older children (Barkley, Karlsson, Pollard, & Murphy, 1985) and in children of both sexes (Barkley, 1989). Besides a general reduction in the negative, disruptive, and conflict-ridden interaction patterns of these children with their parents when the children are treated with stimulant medication, general family functioning also seems to improve (Schachar, Taylor, Weiselberg, Thorley, & Rutter, 1987).

These patterns of disruptive, intrusive, excessive, negative, and emotional social interactions have also been found to occur in the interactions between children with ADHD and their teachers (DuPaul et al., 2001; Whalen, Henker, & Dotemoto, 1980). Like the interactions of such children with their parents, their interactions with their teachers have also been shown to be significantly improved by administration of stimulant medication (Whalen et al., 1980).

One can therefore conclude that the parent–child relations in families of children with ADHD are likely to be characterized by greater conflict, coercion, and stress; more lax and overreactive discipline; and less adaptive parental coping more generally than those in typical families. Much of this conflict seems to arise from the children's ADHD and its impact on family functioning. Yet parenting behavior, parental characteristics (depression and general psychopathology), and possibly even parental

employment patterns may be associated with— if not contributory to—these interaction problems. Such conflict, negative emotion, stress, and limited parental adaptive coping and responsiveness are likely to be at their highest among families whose children have ADHD comorbid with ODD/CD than in families of children with ADHD alone. As we will see below, these are also the families having the greatest degrees of parental psychopathology and social adversity as well.

Peer Relations

Pelham and Bender (1982) once estimated that more than 50% of children with ADHD have significant problems in social relationships with other children. Mothers (Campbell & Paulauskas, 1979), teachers (Barkley, DuPaul, & McMurray, 1990), and peers (Johnston, Pelham, & Murphy, 1985; Pope, Bierman, & Mumma, 1989) find hyperactive children to be significantly more aggressive, disruptive, domineering, intrusive, noisy, and socially rejected in their social relations than typical children, especially if they are male, and particularly if they are aggressive (DuPaul et al., 2001; Hinshaw & Melnick, 1995; Milich, Landau, Kilby, & Whitten, 1982; Pelham & Bender, 1982). Evidence of such social impairments extends to adolescents with ADHD as well (Bagwell, Molina, Pelham, & Hoza, 2001). Girls with ADHD are also likely to exhibit more aggression (both direct and relational aggression) than typical girls, have greater difficulty sustaining relationships over time, and as a result are more likely to be rejected by other girls (Blachman & Hinshaw, 2002; Mikami & Hinshaw, 2003).

Studies that have directly observed these peer interactions suggest that the inattentive, disruptive, off-task, immature, provocative, aggressive, and noncompliant behaviors of children with ADHD quickly elicit a pattern of controlling and directive behavior from their peers when they must work together (Clark, Cheyne, Cunningham, & Siegel, 1988; Cunningham & Siegel, 1987; Hinshaw, 1992; Hinshaw & Melnick, 1995; Stroes, Alberts, & van der Meere, 2003; Whalen, Henker, Collins, Finck, & Dotemoto, 1979; Whalen, Henker, Collins, McAuliffe, & Vaux, 1979). A recent study observed children with ADHD interacting with an unfamiliar child and found them to be less involved with the peer, to talk more to themselves, and to direct their attention less to the peer than did control children (Stroes et al., 2003). There also seems to be a tendency for children with ADHD to accept other such children as playmates more readily than do nondisabled children (Hinshaw & Melnick, 1995). In regard to their communication patterns, children with ADHD in these studies have been found to talk more, but to be less efficient in organizing and communicating information to peers with whom they are asked to work. Moreover, despite talking more, these children are less likely to respond to the questions or verbal interactions of their peers. Hence, there is clearly less reciprocity in the social exchanges between these children and their peers (Cunningham & Siegel, 1987; Landau & Milich, 1988; Stroes et al., 2003). Children with ADHD have also been shown to have less knowledge about social skills and appropriate behavior with others (Grenell, Glass, & Katz, 1987). Among these children, those who are the most sensation-seeking, emotionally reactive, aggressive, and noncompliant receive the greatest disapproval from their peers, whether they are girls or boys (Bagwell et al., 2001; DuPaul et al., 2001; Hinshaw & Melnick, 1995; Mikami & Hinshaw, 2003). But for girls with ADHD, anxious/depressed behavior is also associated with greater peer rejection (Mikami & Hinshaw, 2003).

One large study examined the relationship between ADHD and bullying/victimization, using a sample of 1,315 middle school students (Unnever & Cornell, 2003). It found that children with ADHD were both more likely to engage in bullying (13% vs. 8%) and to be victimized in bullying episodes (34% vs. 22%) than were control students. The study found that ADHD was related to bullying of others as a consequence of the degree of low self-control manifested by these children. But their likelihood of being victimized by other bullies was independent of their level of self-control; it had more to do with other ADHD symptoms and with being overweight.

Some research suggests that children with ADHD tend to have a more external locus of control than do nondisabled children (Linn & Hodge, 1982). That is, they are more likely to view the events that happen to them as outside their personal control or due to "fate." (See also the discussion of positive illusory bias in Chapter 3). They also tend to have more inflated perceptions of themselves, their likeli-

hood of success in tasks, and the extent to which others like them than do nondisabled children (Diener & Milich, 1997; Milich & Greenwell, 1991; Milich & Okazaki, 1991; O'Neill & Douglas, 1991; again, see also Chapter 3). Although this finding may indicate an immaturity in the development of self-awareness and perceptions, given that younger children tend to overestimate their own abilities, substantial research suggests that this inflated self-assessment may in part be a form of self-protection (Diener & Milich, 1997; Milich, 1994); that is, it is an effort to present themselves in the best possible light, to protect their self-esteem and mask their self-perceived incompetence. But as noted in Chapter 3, this is not the entire story, because self-protection does not appear to explain their overestimated competence in other areas in which they are deficient, such as academics. ADHD may therefore interfere with self-awareness apart from this conscious effort to protect self-esteem. Some evidence suggests that children with ADHD also encode social cues less well, express less optimism about future events, and generate fewer responses to problematic social situations than do nondisabled children (Matthys, Cuperus, & van Engeland, 1999; Zentall, Cassady, & Javorsky, 2001).

Those children with ADHD who are also aggressive or have ODD/CD may display this same problem with encoding cues, but also manifest an additional tendency to overinterpret the actions of others toward them as actually having hostile intentions, and are therefore more likely to respond with aggressive counterattacks to minimal if any provocation (Matthys, Cuperus, & van Engeland, 1999; Milich & Dodge, 1984). Waschbusch et al. (2002) have found that children with comorbid ADHD + ODD/CD are more easily provoked to become aggressive at lower levels of provocation and may carry a grudge longer than do either children with ADHD alone or control children may. Such communication problems, skills deficits, attribution biases, and interaction conflicts could easily lead children with ADHD, especially those who are aggressive, to be rejected as playmates by their classmates and neighborhood peers in very short order. Many have noted that it takes few social exchanges over a period of only 20–30 minutes between children with ADHD and nondisabled children for the latter children to find the former disruptive, unpredictable, and aggressive, and hence to react to them with aversion, criticism, rejection, and sometimes even counter-aggression. Certainly the nondisabled children are likely to withdraw from the children with ADHD when opportunities to do so arise (Milich et al., 1982; Pelham & Bender, 1982; Pelham & Milich, 1984).

PARENTAL PSYCHIATRIC DISORDERS

ADHD in Parents (and Other Relatives)

More than 30 years ago, reports were appearing that biological parents and other relatives of hyperactive children were more likely to have had hyperactivity themselves in childhood (Morrison & Stewart, 1973), with 5% of mothers and 15% of fathers reporting this problem (vs. 2% in the control group). More recent studies have corroborated these earlier and less methodologically sophisticated studies. They indicate that the risk to biological parents of children with ADHD is probably greater than these initial studies indicated. For instance, the large MTA reported that parents of children with ADHD-C had significantly higher symptoms of ADHD than did control parents, both by self-report and by the reports of others (Epstein et al., 2000). In general, it seems that 12–20% of the mothers and 9–54% of the fathers of children with ADHD may also have ADHD themselves (Alberts-Corush, Firestone, & Goodman, 1986; Chronis et al., 2003; Deutsch et al., 1982; Singer, Stewart, & Pulaski, 1981). For instance, Faraone and Biederman (1997) reported that 13% of fathers of girls with ADHD and 21% of the girls' mothers had ADHD. Nigg and Hinshaw (1998) found that 20% of the mothers and 54% of the fathers of 80 boys with ADHD also had ADHD, while these figures were just 4% and 0%, respectively, for the mothers and fathers in their community control group (*n* = 62). This greater risk of ADHD is also seen among the biological siblings of children with ADHD; approximately 17–37% may have the disorder (Faraone & Biederman, 1997; Welner, Welner, Stewart, Palkes, & Wish, 1977). In general, the average risk of ADHD among the first-degree biological relatives of children with ADHD is between 25% and 37% (Biederman, Gastfriend, & Jellinek, 1986; Biederman, Baldessarini, Wright, Knee, & Harmatz, 1989; Biederman, Munir, & Knee, 1987), or five to seven times the risk in the general population.

In a small study of mothers having ADHD, Weinstein, Apfel, and Weinstein (1998) found that these women had higher levels of neuroticism, lower levels of conscientiousness, and a greater incidence of psychiatric disorders among their relatives. They also had a greater likelihood of having been sexually abused, greater alcohol abuse in their own families of origin, and more difficulties in their own daily living than women without ADHD.

Other Disorders in Parents

Parents of children with ADHD are also more likely to experience a variety of other psychiatric disorders. Early studies reported that the most common of these appeared to be conduct problems and antisocial behavior (25–28%), alcoholism (14–25%), hysteria or affective disorder (10–28%), and LDs (Cantwell, 1972; Faraone & Biederman, 1997; Morrison & Stewart, 1973; Singer et al., 1981). In their study, Nigg and Hinshaw (1998) found that 25–39% of mothers of their group with ADHD had MDD (vs. 18% for their control group). The rate for fathers was not different between the groups (ADHD = 11–15%, controls = 9%). Fathers of the group with ADHD, in contrast, reported higher rates of Generalized Anxiety Disorder (4–11%) than control fathers did (0%); the same was true for mothers (ADHD = 11–18%, controls = 2–6%). Biederman and colleagues (Biederman, 1997; Biederman et al., 1987, 1989; Faraone & Biederman, 1997) also reported a higher prevalence of mood disorders, particularly MDD, among the parents and siblings of children with ADHD (27–32%) than among the relatives of control children (6%). Similar results were obtained in the study by Chronis et al. (2003), where 37–43% of mothers reported a mood disorder and 23–27% reported an anxiety disorder at some time in their lives. In that same study, 15–17% of mothers and 13–31% of fathers of the group with ADHD reported a childhood history of ODD/CD, compared to 7% of the mothers and 15% of the fathers in the control group.

Less attention has been paid to substance use disorders among the parents of children with ADHD. Nigg and Hinshaw (1998) found only a higher rate of cocaine abuse/dependence among the fathers of the group with ADHD + ODD than among those of children with ADHD only, but not in comparison to their control group (17%). Chronis et al.

(2003) found a higher rate of cocaine abuse/dependence only for the mothers of their group with ADHD, as well as a higher rate of stimulant abuse. Alcohol abuse/dependence did not differ between the groups in either of these studies. Even if they are not abusing alcohol, however, parents of children with ADHD consume more alcohol than do those of nondisabled children (Cunningham et al., 1988). Pfiffner et al. (1999) found that the risks for disorders seen in children with ADHD were consistent with the risks for disorders seen in the parents. That is, parents' risk for externalizing disorders was linked only to children's risk for such disorders (ODD, CD), whereas parents' risk for internalizing disorders (anxiety, depression) was linked only to the children's risk for those same disorders.

The presence of depression in mothers of children with ADHD appears to result in some distortion in their reports of both behavior problems and depressive symptoms in their children, relative to the reports of nondepressed mothers with children having ADHD (Chi & Hinshaw, 2002; Mick, Santangelo, Wypij, & Biederman, 2000). Even after such distortions are accounted for, however, the behavior problems and depression of their children are still significantly greater than those seen in control groups, suggesting that maternal perceptual distortions do not account entirely for the elevated rates of these problems among their children with ADHD.

Family Psychiatric Disturbance and Child CD

In 1983, August and Stewart suggested that the greater incidence of antisocial behavior and alcoholism among these first-degree relatives of children with ADHD was primarily found among relatives of children with ADHD who also had conduct problems and antisocial behavior. Children free of these comorbid problems often had only a greater history of ADHD and LDs among their relatives. The greater family histories of alcoholism and of antisocial behavior, therefore, were associated mainly with antisocial behavior in children, rather than with ADHD per se (Stewart et al., 1980). These findings have been replicated in subsequent studies (Biederman et al., 1987; Faraone & Biederman, 1997), in which up to 46% of the first-degree relatives of children with ADHD and comorbid ODD/CD also had

ODD, CD, or Antisocial Personality Disorder, as compared to only 5–13% of the relatives of children with pure ADHD. A study by Lahey, Piacentini, et al. (1988) likewise demonstrated this clear relationship between familial antisocial behavior and affective disorders in relatives on the one hand, and antisocial behavior in children with ADHD on the other. As noted above, Pfiffner et al. (1999) similarly observed that ODD/CD among parents was significantly linked to risk for ODD/CD among the children with ADHD. More recently, Chronis et al. (2003) found only an elevated risk of ADHD among both mothers and fathers of children with ADHD alone. Among children with the ADHD + ODD/CD combination, they observed greater maternal mood disorders, anxiety disorders, and cocaine/stimulant dependence, as well as greater paternal ODD/CD (in childhood). Sex of the child with ADHD did not appear to result in any differences in this risk to family members if the child had comorbid CD (Faraone & Biederman, 1997). Taken together, this body of evidence clearly indicates a relationship between the severity of aggressive and oppositional behavior in children with ADHD, and the degree of antisocial behavior, substance misuse, and mood/anxiety disorders among their parents and extended relatives. In other words, children with ADHD but with little or no aggressive behavior are likely to have considerably fewer of these psychiatric disorders among their parents than are children with ADHD and ODD. However, children in the latter group are likely to have fewer of these problems in their parents than do children with ADHD and mixed ODD/CD, who have the highest rates of these disorders among all the subgroups with ADHD.

Nigg and Hinshaw (1998) have also found that only children with ADHD + ODD/CD have parents with personality traits that are significantly different from control children. For instance, fathers of children with these comorbid disorders showed lower levels of agreeableness, higher neuroticism, and more Generalized Anxiety Disorder. Mothers with higher neuroticism, lower conscientiousness, and greater depression also had children with ADHD more likely to engage in overt antisocial activities during a summer camp, while higher rates of child covert antisocial behavior were associated only with paternal history of substance abuse (greater) and paternal openness (higher).

SUBTYPING OF ADHD

As can be seen from the foregoing review, children with ADHD are a heterogeneous group who are believed to have in common the characteristics of developmentally inappropriate levels of inattention, and in most cases hyperactivity–impulsivity. Despite these apparent commonalities, children so diagnosed are acknowledged to present with a diversity of related psychiatric symptoms/disorders, family backgrounds, developmental courses, and responses to treatments. Given this diversity, increasing scientific attention has been paid to developing approaches to identifying more homogeneous, clinically meaningful subtypes of ADHD. Such subtyping approaches are clinically useful if they provide important information about differing comorbidities, etiologies, developmental courses, outcomes, or responses to therapies between the subtypes. In short, they must show some value beyond the differences that would be expected on the measures on which the subtyping occurred or those measures known to be related to them. Many ways of subtyping ADHD have been employed—some without much clinical merit, such as sorting children with ADHD on the presence or absence of reading disorders (Halperin, Gittelman, Klein, & Rudel, 1984). Three approaches to subtyping, however, have proven promising or have established themselves as clinically useful.

Subtyping on Presence or Absence of Hyperactivity–Impulsivity

One subtyping approach introduced in DSM-III (American Psychiatric Association, 1980) and resurrected later in DSM-IV (American Psychiatric Association, 1994) is based on the presence or absence of significant degrees of overactivity. In DSM-III, children diagnosed with Attention Deficit Disorder (ADD) were subtyped as having ADD with Hyperactivity (ADD + H) or ADD without Hyperactivity (ADD – H). This method of creating subtypes was later removed in the DSM-III-R (American Psychiatric Association, 1987), given the lack of research at that time on the utility of this approach. But it returned in DSM-IV (see Chapter 2) with the label ADHD, Predominantly Inattentive Type (ADHD-PI), and with the use now of hyperactivity–impulsivity as the feature that is either ruled in or out to create the sub-

types. More thorough reviews of this literature can be found elsewhere (Barkley, Grodzinsky, & DuPaul, 1992; Lahey & Carlson, 1992; Goodyear & Hynd, 1992); see particularly the excellent review by Milich, Ballentine, and Lynam (2001), along with commentaries by other leading experts. Indeed, Milich et al. have gone so far as to argue that individuals diagnosed with ADHD-PI may in fact have a distinct disorder, or at least that significant subset of them with characteristics reflecting sluggish cognitive tempo (SCT)—a conclusion with which I agree.

In what follows, children previously diagnosed with ADD + H are now referred to as having ADHD, Combined Type (ADHD-C), while those having ADD – H are described as having ADHD-PI, in keeping with current diagnostic terminology. Several of the early studies on this issue found few if any important differences between these types (Maurer & Stewart, 1980; Rubinstein & Brown, 1984). Later ones, however, indicated that children with ADHD-C were more likely to be male, to be oppositional and aggressive, to be more rejected by peers, to have lower self-esteem, to be more depressed, and in some cases to be more impaired in cognitive and motor test performance than children with ADHD-PI (Barkley, DuPaul, & McMurray, 1990; Berry, Shaywitz, & Shaywitz, 1985; Cantwell & Baker, 1992; Carlson, Lahey, Frame, Walker, & Hynd, 1987; Gadow et al., 2004; Hern & Hynd, 1992; Hynd et al., 1991; Johnson, Altmaier, & Richman, 1999; Lahey, Schaughency, Hynd, Carlson, & Nieves, 1987; King & Young, 1982; Maedgen & Carlson, 2000; Morgan, Hynd, Riccio, & Hall, 1996; Wheeler & Carlson, 1994; Willcutt, Pennington, Chhabildas, Friedman, & Alexander, 1999; see Milich et al., 2001, for a more thorough review). In contrast, children with ADHD-PI are more likely to have math disorders; possibly to have more internalizing symptoms; to have relatives with more internalizing problems; to be shy, passive, and withdrawn in their peer relations (rather than rejected outright); to have more deficits in social knowledge; and possibly to be less responsive to stimulant medication (Hodgens, Cole, & Boldizar, 2000; Maedgen & Carlson, 2000; Milich et al., 2001). Children with ADHD-C are consistently found to be more impaired and to have a more severe disorder than children with ADHD-PI, overall, though both types are more impaired than control groups (Faraone, Biederman, Weber, & Russell, 1998; Graetz, Sawyer, Hazell, Arney, & Baghurst, 2001; Milich et al., 2001).

Our own study of these subtypes found that more than twice as many children with ADHD-C as with ADHD-PI are diagnosed with ODD (41% vs. 19%), using DSM-III-R criteria, and more than three times as many are diagnosed with CD (21% vs. 6%) (Barkley, DuPaul, & McMurray, 1990). This is not surprising, since research suggests that hyperactive–impulsive behavior is more closely associated with oppositional and conduct problems than is inattentive behavior (Crystal, Ostrander, Chen, & August, 2001; Willcutt et al., 1999). The children with ADHD-C may also be more likely to have speech and language problems, greater marital discord between their parents, and more maternal psychiatric disorders (Cantwell & Baker, 1992), although the evidence base here is quite slim. In contrast, children with ADHD-PI have been characterized as more anxious, daydreamy, lethargic, and sluggish than children with ADHD-PI when teacher ratings of classroom adjustment are used (Edelbrock, Costello, & Kessler, 1984; Lahey, Shaughency, Strauss, & Frame, 1984; Lahey et al., 1987). These and other items (staring, slow-moving, easily confused) have come to be known as the SCT subset of items (Milich et al., 2001), which may be more useful in subtyping children with ADHD than just the inattention symptoms in DSM-IV(-TR) (see Chapter 2). That is, the subset of children with ADHD-PI who exhibit SCT may be most distinctive from those with ADHD-C (Carlson & Mann, 2002; McBurnett, Pfiffner, & Frick, 2001). The characteristics of SCT form a distinct factorial dimension from the inattention symptoms listed in DSM-IV(-TR) (Milich et al., 2001; Todd, Rasmussen, Wood, Levy, & Hay, 2004), arguing for their use in creating more homogeneous subtypes of ADHD in future studies of this issue.

Our own study also found children with both subtypes to have been retained in grade (32% in each group) and placed in special education considerably more often than our nondisabled control children (45% vs. 53%). However, we found that children with ADHD-C were more likely to have been placed in special classes for children with behavior disorders (emotional disturbances) than the children with ADHD-PI (12% vs. 0%), whereas the latter children were more likely to be in classes

for children with LDs (53%) than children with ADHD-C (34%). Both groups of children had equivalent rates of LDs, but the additional problems with conduct and antisocial behavior are likely to result in the assignment of children with ADHD-C to the programs for behavioral disturbances rather than for LDs.

Unfortunately, few studies have directly addressed whether ADHD-C and ADHD-PI are subtypes of the same type of disorder or whether they represent qualitatively different disorders, despite the similar levels of deviance on teacher rating scales of inattention. Such an examination would require a more comprehensive and objective assessment of different components of attention in both groups. In the one study that used four different types of reaction time tasks to study cognitive processing, few meaningful differences between the subtypes were obtained (Hynd et al., 1989). However, these reaction time tasks do not necessarily evaluate the different components of attention as viewed from neuropsychological models (Mirsky, 1996; Posner, 1987); thus the question of whether these subtypes involve the same type of attention disturbance remains unanswered. The results of our own study of these subtypes imply that the attention disturbances are not identical. We (Barkley, DuPaul, & McMurray, 1990) found that the children with ADHD-PI performed considerably worse on the Coding subtest of the Wechsler Intelligence Scale for Children—Revised and on a measure of consistent retrieval of verbal information from memory. The children with ADHD-C did not differ from nondisabled subjects on either of these measures. These findings intimate that children with ADHD-PI may have more of a problem with memory, perceptual–motor speed, or even more central cognitive processing speed, whereas children with ADHD-C manifest more problems with behavioral disinhibition and poor attention to tasks, in addition to their overactivity. Consistent with this notion of different neurological mechanisms underlying these disorders were the preliminary findings of Garcia-Zanchez, Estevez-Gonzalez, Suarez-Romero, and Junque (1997), who observed greater evidence for right-hemisphere dysfunction on neuropsychological tests in children with ADHD-PI than in those with ADHD-C. Others have not found distinctive neuropsychological differences between the subtypes, however (Chhabildas, Pennington, & Willcutt, 2001; Nigg, Blaskey, Huang-Pollack,

& Rappley, 2002), or have found adolescents with ADHD-PI to be more impulsive on the Stroop test and more impaired on a digit span task (Schmidtz et al., 2002)—differences often associated more with the ADHD-C in other studies. Problematic in these studies is that none of them used the specific SCT symptoms to subdivide their ADHD-PI cases, and so the merits of the SCT subclassification approach for neuropsychological findings remain untested.

Such differences in the types of attention affected in these groups of children would be expected to have different neuroanatomical loci (Mirsky, 1996; Posner, 1987). ADHD-C may be a problem in the functional level of prefrontal–limbic pathways, particularly the striatum (Lou, Henriksen, & Bruhn, 1984; Lou, Henriksen, Bruhn, Borner, & Nielsen, 1989), whereas ADHD-PI may involve more posterior associative cortical areas and/or cortical–subcortical feedback loops, perhaps including the hippocampal system (Heilman, Voeller, & Nadeau, 1991; Hynd et al., 1991; Posner, 1987). Shaywitz et al. (1986) observed that small samples of children with ADHD-C showed a different response than children with ADHD-PI did in growth hormone and prolactin levels in blood plasma when placed on methylphenidate. The authors imply that ADHD-C may involve a problem with dopamine, whereas ADHD-PI may selectively involve norepinephrine. One study of epinephrine excretion in urine found elevated levels only in children with ADHD-PI, and a significant correlation between such excretion and severity of inattention (Anderson et al., 2000). Such excretions could reflect problems peripherally in the adrenomedullary functioning of these children, or more centrally in dysregulation of norepinphrine systems in the brain. These neuropsychological and neurochemical hypotheses regarding ADHD-PI are quite conjectural at present. Nevertheless, they hint at the possibility of eventually identifying two distinctive attention disorders in children, and they corroborate distinctions already being made in the study of normal attention processes in the basic neurosciences (Mirsky, 1996; Posner, 1987).

In general, these results suggest that children with ADHD-C have considerably different patterns of psychiatric comorbidity from those of children with ADHD-PI: They are at significantly greater risk for other disruptive behavior disorders, academic placement in programs for behavioral disturbances, school suspensions, and psychotherapeutic interventions than are children with ADHD-PI. These patterns of comorbidity, along with the findings of different family psychiatric histories, suggest that these are actually dissimilar psychiatric disorders rather than subtypes of a shared disturbance in attention processes.

An early survey (Szatmari et al., 1989a) indicated that the prevalence of these two disorders within the study population was quite different, especially in the childhood years (6–11 years of age). ADHD-PI was considerably less prevalent than ADHD-C in this epidemiological study: Only 1.4% of boys and 1.3% of girls had ADHD-PI, whereas 9.4% of boys and 2.8% of girls had ADHD-C. These figures changed considerably in the adolescent age groups, in which 1.4% of males and 1% of females had ADHD-PI, and 2.9% of males and 1.4% of females had ADHD-C. In other words, the rates of ADHD-PI remained relatively stable across these developmental age groupings, whereas ADHD-C, especially in males, showed a considerable decline in prevalence with age. Among all children with either type of ADHD, about 78% of boys and 63% of girls would have ADHD-C.

However, later studies have contradicted this survey in finding ADHD-PI to be considerably more prevalent than Szatmari et al. (1989a) originally indicated. Baumgaertel, Wolraich, and Dietrich (1995) found that 3.2% had ADHD-PI, whereas 6.4% had ADHD-C. When the more recent DSM-IV criteria for subtyping were employed, 9% of the children met criteria for ADHD-PI whereas 8.8% had the Predominantly Hyperactive–Impulsive Type (ADHD-PHI) and ADHD-C. Using DSM-IV, Graetz et al. (2001) found that 3.7% of Australian children had ADHD-PI, 1.9% had ADHD-C, and 1.9% had ADHD-PHI. Hudziak et al. (1998) used latent class and factor analyses to form these subtypes and found a prevalence of 4% for ADHD-PI, 3.7% for ADHD-C, and 2.2% for ADHD-PHI. The differences in these studies probably arise from the fact that the Szatmari et al. (1989a) study did not use DSM symptom lists, but subtypes based on ratings of items related to inattention and to hyperactive–impulsive behavior, whereas the other studies employed symptom lists from the DSM.

It remains to be seen just how stable ADHD-PI is over development. No longitudinal studies have employed sufficiently large samples with ADHD-PI to make any conclusions about their outcomes. Unfortunately, at present little is known about which types of treatment may be more effective with ADHD-PI, whereas much is known about the treatment of ADHD-C (see Part III of this volume). A few studies exist on the response of these two types to different doses of stimulant medication and hint at possible differences (ADHD-PI is less responsive) (Barkley, DuPaul, & McMurray, 1990; Famularo & Fenton, 1987; Milich et al., 2001; Saul & Ashby, 1986; Sebrechts et al., 1986; Ullmann & Sleator, 1985). Antshel and Remer (2003) found that ADHD-PI may be more responsive to social skills training than ADHD-C, while the MTA (see Chapter 20) suggested that ADHD-PI may be more responsive to psychosocial treatment packages more generally when combined with medications. More research is to be encouraged on the response of these different subtypes (or disorders) to other types of behavioral, educational, and pharmacological interventions.

Subtyping on Presence or Absence of Aggression

Another, more widely accepted subtyping approach that has already demonstrated considerable clinical significance is based on aggression (Loney, Kramer, & Milich, 1981; Loney & Milich, 1982) or the presence of comorbid ODD/CD. As noted earlier in this chapter, much evidence has accumulated that shows important differences between children having ADHD alone and those having ADHD + ODD/CD.

In general, children with both ADHD and ODD/CD display significantly greater levels of physical aggression, lying, and stealing, as well as more rejection by peers, than either children with pure ADHD or those with pure aggression do (Loney, Langhorne, & Paternite, 1978; Milich et al., 1982; Waschbusch et al., 2002; Walker, Lahey, Hynd, & Frame, 1987; see also the earlier discussion of comorbid ODD/CD, parent–child relations, and parental psychiatric disorders). These children also display different patterns of social attribution (Milich & Dodge, 1984), often viewing others' actions as intentionally aggressive against them. They are typically rated as more severely maladjusted (McGee et al., 1984b; Moffitt, 1990), and have a poorer adolescent and young adult outcome

(Barkley, Fischer, et al., 1990; Milich & Loney, 1979; Weiss & Hechtman, 1993), than do children having ADHD alone. Finally, children who have both ADHD and ODD/CD have greater levels of parental and family psychopathology (particularly antisocial conduct, MDD, and substance use disorders), as well as greater social adversity, than do children with either disorder alone. Indeed, some have argued that ADHD with CD may represent a distinct familial subtype of ADHD (Waschbusch et al., 2002; see above). Clearly, the use of ODD/CD for subtyping of children with ADHD has been of great scientific and clinical utility.

Subtyping on Presence or Absence of Internalizing Symptoms

A third approach to subtyping ADHD, considerably less studied than the two discussed previously, is based on the presence and degree of anxiety and depression (often referred to as "internalizing symptoms") in children with ADHD (see the earlier discussions of anxiety and mood disorders; see also Jensen et al., 1997, and Tannock, 2000, for reviews). This subtyping model is based on studies showing that children who had relatively high ratings of internalizing symptoms were more likely to have poor or adverse responses to stimulant medication (DuPaul, Barkley, & McMurray, 1994; Pliszka, 1989; Taylor, 1983; Voelker, Lachar, & Gdowski, 1983), though this has recently been questioned (March et al., 2002; Tannock, 2000). Children with ADHD and anxiety may be more appropriate for antidepressant medications (Biederman et al., 1993; Pliszka, 1989). Results of other studies suggest the possibility that within the broader population of individuals having ADHD, those with greater internalizing symptoms as children may have less impulsivity, more impaired working memory, and a greater likelihood of mood and anxiety disorders in adolescence (Tannock, 2000). Research shows that some anxiety disorders and depressive symptoms in childhood may evolve into other types of anxiety or mood disorders or even MDD in later childhood or adolescence (Cantwell & Baker, 1989). However, no studies have specifically examined the stability and differential course of ADHD with and without significant internalizing symptoms; thus the actual clinical predictive value of this subtyping approach remains unstudied.

SUMMARY

This chapter indicates that beyond the myriad cognitive, academic, developmental, and medical risks that exist in children with ADHD (and have been described in Chapter 3), a high probability of having comorbid psychiatric disorders also exists. Up to 75% or more of children diagnosed with ADHD are destined to have at least one of these additional disorders. The co-occurrence of mood and anxiety disorders with ADHD is only somewhat less than that for ODD and CD, with at least 25–50% or more of children with ADHD experiencing these internalizing forms of psychopathology. Although BPD co-occurs with ADHD considerably less often than do the anxiety and the other mood disorders, its occurrence is still 6–10 times greater than would be expected in a population without ADHD, and BPD is probably one of the most serious and impairing of the comorbidities that may exist with ADHD. PTSD, OCD, TS, and autistic spectrum disorders may not be overrepresented among children with ADHD, but children diagnosed with those disorders may show elevated rates of ADHD.

Besides these comorbid disorders, children with ADHD are significantly more likely to experience problems in their relationships with family members, peers, and teachers, particularly if they fall into the subgroup with significant levels of aggression or ODD/CD. The family members of children with ADHD are also more likely to experience ADHD, among other disorders; once again, these risks to family members are highest in the group with comorbid ODD/CD.

Finally, this chapter has examined various approaches to the subtyping of ADHD. Results suggest that subtyping on the basis of presence or absence of hyperactive–impulsive behavior, as in DSM-IV(-TR), may actually be distinguishing two separate disorders rather than two subtypes having the same attentional disturbance and risks for comorbid conditions. Certainly ADHD-PI appears to be more benign, and possibly less developmentally stable, than ADHD-C. Subtyping children with ADHD on the basis of comorbid ODD/CD distinguishes a group having considerably greater family problems, social adversity, and parental psychopathology, as well as a greater risk for later academic maladjustment, social rejection, early substance experimentation and abuse,

and more persistent antisocial/criminal activities. This approach to subtyping ADHD may be exceptionally useful for identifying those children with among the highest risks for long-term maladjustment—perhaps second only to the risks of children with ADHD and comorbid BPD. Children with ADHD and comorbid internalizing symptoms form a somewhat less risk-prone subtype, but one that may still be clinically useful for identifying children who are somewhat less impulsive than their counterparts without such symptoms; they also may respond less well to stimulant medications, but possibly better to antidepressants. In recent years, then, there has been a considerable advance in our understanding of ADHD and how it may best be subgrouped to yield clinically valuable information.

KEY CLINICAL POINTS

✓ Anxiety disorders may occur in 10–50% of clinic-referred children with ADHD (average 25–35%; odds ratio of 3.0), and ADHD may occur in 15–30% of children with anxiety disorders. Although anxiety disorders may be associated with less severe impulsivity, they may be associated with more severe inattention and, arguably, a poorer response to stimulant medication.

✓ Major Depressive Disorder (MDD) can occur in 15–75% of clinic-referred youth with ADHD (average 25–30%; odds ratio of 5.5), and 16–63% of those with MDD may experience ADHD. When comorbid with ADHD, MDD may signal a greater likelihood of ODD/CD, a poorer outcome, and greater parental psychological maladjustment (including MDD and/or ADHD).

✓ Bipolar I Disorder (BPD) in children remains controversial due to unresolved conceptual and diagnostic issues. It may occur in 6–27% of clinic-referred children with ADHD (average 6–10% after subtraction of overlapping symptoms), but follow-up studies to date find no greater incidence of BPD in such children by adulthood. However, ADHD is highly likely (90%+) in cases of childhood-onset BPD. When present in cases of ADHD, BPD signals a greater likelihood of BPD in the family history and a significantly poorer course and outcome.

✓ Up to 84% of clinic-referred children with ADHD will have comorbid Oppositional Defiant Disorder (ODD) (average 45–55%; odds ratio for ODD/CD of 10.7). When present without CD, ODD may not signal a worse course or outcome, but when mixed with CD, it signals a much poorer course (see below).

✓ Conduct Disorder (CD) can be found in 15–56% of clinical cases of ADHD (average 35–45%; odds ratio for ODD/CD of 10.7). When CD is present in cases of ADHD, it is nearly always associated with ODD as well and has a much earlier onset than when CD develops in the absence of ADHD. The presence of CD signals a more severe form of ADHD, and the comorbidity probably constitutes a unique subtype, with highly persistent antisocial activities, a higher level of impulsivity, greater emotional expression, distorted attributional biases about the intentions of others, more easily provoked aggression, more sustained social grudges, a greater likelihood of MDD and of substance use disorders, a greater likelihood of adult Antisocial Personality Disorder, and a more significantly impaired family of origin.

✓ PTSD does cause ADHD, or vice versa. PTSD does not appear to be elevated in or significantly related to clinically diagnosed ADHD alone (1–6%). However, when ODD and especially BPD are comorbid conditions with ADHD, the risk for exposure to trauma (especially victimization forms of trauma) and PTSD is significantly higher (22–24% for PTSD in mixed ADHD + ODD or ADHD + BPD). Approximately 14–46% of children with PTSD may have ADHD, but this elevated incidence may be due to the comorbidity of ADHD with ODD and BPD, as shown above.

✓ Tourette syndrome (TS) or other tic disorders are not more common among children with ADHD in community samples, but non-TS tic disorders may be mildly elevated in clinic-referred samples with ADHD (12–34%). In clinically diagnosed cases of TS, ADHD may be a common comorbidity (25–85%). When present in cases of ADHD, tic disorders (other than TS) have a high probability of remission and appear to have little or no influence on clinical status or course.

✓ No data exist on the prevalence of autistic spectrum disorders in children with ADHD, but ADHD may occur in 26% of children with autistic spectrum disorders.

✓ Clinic-referred children with ADHD often manifest poor peer relationships (50–70%) and greater social rejection. Such social problems are highest in the group with comorbid ADHD + ODD/CD, where (as noted above) greater social aggression, higher expressed emotion, lower thresholds for provoked aggression, and more persistent aggression may be found, along with biased misattribution of intentions of others.

✓ ADHD is associated with significant conflict in parent–child relationships, characterized by less child compliance to parental requests, poor sustained compliance, and greater requests for assistance, along with more parental commands, reprimands, and punishment. Parent–child conflict and poor parental disciplinary style are highest in the families of children with comorbid ADHD + ODD/CD. The same appears to be true for teacher–child interactions.

✓ Parents of children with ADHD manifest greater parenting stress, lowered sense of parenting competence, more lax and overreactive discipline, greater use of coercive tactics, and more negative perceptions of their relations with their children. Again, these characteristics are more severe in families of children with comorbid ADHD + ODD/CD.

✓ Parents of children with ADHD are more likely to have ADHD themselves. When the children have comorbid ODD/CD, parents are more likely to show MDD, ODD/CD, Antisocial Personality Disorder, and arguably substance use disorders, as well as greater marital problems and social disadvantage.

✓ ADHD can be usefully subtyped by the presence or absence of hyperactivity–impulsivity, as in DSM-IV(-TR)'s subtypes of ADHD, Combined Type (ADHD-C) and ADHD, Predominantly Inattentive Type (ADHD-PI). Among those with ADHD-PI, the subset having symptoms of sluggish cognitive tempo (SCT) may actually have a qualitatively distinct disorder of attention. Individuals with SCT are likely to be more passive, withdrawn, sluggish, lethargic, spacey, or daydreamy; are less likely to have ODD or CD; and may be more likely to manifest internalizing symptoms or disorders.

✓ As noted above, the comorbidity of ADHD with CD/ODD may constitute a unique subtype of ADHD, with more severe symptoms, more domains of impairment, an earlier onset of both disorders, more persistent antisocial behavior, a greater risk for substance dependence/abuse, a greater risk for antisocial behavior or Antisocial Personality Disorder in adulthood, and a greater family history of these same disorders, as well as greater social disadvantage/adversity.

✓ ADHD with internalizing symptoms may arguably constitute another subtype, given that such cases appear to have reduced impulsivity, a greater family history of anxiety and mood disorders, and possibly a poorer response to stimulant medication.

REFERENCES

Alberts-Corush, J., Firestone, P., & Goodman, J. T. (1986). Attention and impulsivity characteristics of the biological and adoptive parents of hyperactive and normal children. *American Journal of Orthopsychiatry, 56,* 413–423.

Alpert, J. E., Maddocks, A., Nierenberg, A. A., O'Sullivan, R., Pava, J. A., Worthington, J. J., et al. (1996). Attention deficit hyperactivity disorder in childhood among adults with major depression. *Psychiatry Research, 62,* 213–219.

American Psychiatric Association. (1980). *Diagnostic and statistical manual of mental disorders* (3rd ed.). Washington, DC: Author.

American Psychiatric Association. (1987). *Diagnostic and statistical manual of mental disorders* (3rd ed., rev.). Washington, DC: Author.

American Psychiatric Association. (1994). *Diagnostic and statistical manual of mental disorders* (4th ed.). Washington, DC: Author.

American Psychiatric Association. (2000). *Diagnostic and statistical manual of mental disorders* (4th ed., text rev.). Washington, DC: Author.

Anastopoulos, A. D., Guevremont, D. C., Shelton, T. L., & DuPaul, G. J. (1992). Parenting stress among families of children with attention deficit hyperactivity disorder. *Journal of Abnormal Child Psychology, 20,* 503–520.

Anderson, C. A., Hinshaw, S. P., & Simmel, C. (1994). Mother–child interactions in ADHD and comparison boys: Relationships with overt and covert externalizing behavior. *Journal of Abnormal Child Psychology, 22,* 247–265.

Anderson, G., Dover, M. A., Yang, B. P., Holahan, J.

M., Shaywitz, S. A., Marchione, K. E., et al. (2000). Adrenomedullary function during cognitive testing in attention-deficit/hyperactivity disorder. *Journal of the American Academy of Child and Adolescent Psychiatry, 39,* 635–643.

Anderson, J. C., Williams, S., McGee, R., & Silva, P. A. (1987). DSM-III disorders in preadolescent children. *Archives of General Psychiatry, 44,* 69–76.

Angold, A., Costello, E. J., & Erkanli, A. (1999). Comorbidity. *Journal of Child Psychology and Psychiatry, 40,* 57–88.

Antshel, K. M., & Remer, R. (2003). Social skills training in children with attention deficit hyperactivity disorder: A randomized–controlled clinical trial. *Journal of Clinical Child and Adolescent Psychology, 32,* 153–165

August, G. J., Realmuto, G. M., Joyce, T., & Hektner, J. M. (1999). Persistence and desistance of oppositional defiant disorder in a community sample of children with ADHD. *Journal of the American Academy of Child and Adolescent Psychiatry, 38,* 1262–1270.

August, G. J., & Stewart, M. A. (1983). Family subtypes of childhood hyperactivity. *Journal of Nervous and Mental Disease, 171,* 362–368.

Bagwell, C. L., Molina, B., Pelham, W. E., & Hoza, B. (2001). Attention-deficit hyperactivity disorder and problems in peer relations: Predictions from childhood to adolescence. *Journal of the American Academy of Child and Adolescent Psychiatry, 40,* 1285–1292.

Barkley, R. A. (1985). The social interactions of hyperactive children: Developmental changes, drug effects, and situational variation. In R. McMahon & R. Peters (Eds.), *Childhood disorders: Behavioral–developmental approaches* (pp. 218–243). New York: Brunner/Mazel.

Barkley, R. A. (1988). The effects of methylphenidate on the interactions of preschool ADHD children with their mothers. *Journal of the American Academy of Child and Adolescent Psychiatry, 27,* 336–341.

Barkley, R. A. (1989). Hyperactive girls and boys: Stimulant drug effects on mother–child interactions. *Journal of Child Psychology and Psychiatry, 30,* 379–390.

Barkley, R. A. (1998). *Attention-deficit hyperactivity disorder: A handbook for diagnosis and treatment* (2nd ed.). New York: Guilford Press.

Barkley, R. A., Anastopoulos, A. D., Guevremont, D. G., & Fletcher, K. F. (1992). Adolescents with attention deficit hyperactivity disorder: Mother–adolescent interactions, family beliefs and conflicts, and maternal psychopathology. *Journal of Abnormal Child Psychology, 20,* 263–288.

Barkley, R. A., & Biederman, J. (1997). Towards a broader definition of the age of onset criterion for attention deficit hyperactivity disorder. *Journal of the American Academy of Child and Adolescent Psychiatry, 36,* 1204–1210.

Barkley, R. A., & Cunningham, C. E. (1979). The effects of methylphenidate on the mother–child interactions of hyperactive children. *Archives of General Psychiatry, 36,* 201–208.

Barkley, R. A., Cunningham, C., & Karlsson, J. (1983). The speech of hyperactive children and their mothers: Comparisons with normal children and stimulant drug effects. *Journal of Learning Disabilities, 16,* 105–110.

Barkley, R. A., DuPaul, G. J., & McMurray, M. B. (1990). A comprehensive evaluation of attention deficit disorder with and without hyperactivity. *Journal of Consulting and Clinical Psychology, 58,* 775–789.

Barkley, R. A., Fischer, M., Edelbrock, C. S., & Smallish, L. (1990). The adolescent outcome of hyperactive children diagnosed by research criteria: I. An 8-year prospective follow-up study. *Journal of the American Academy of Child and Adolescent Psychiatry, 29,* 546–557.

Barkley, R. A., Fischer, M., Edelbrock, C. S., & Smallish, L. (1991). The adolescent outcome of hyperactive children diagnosed by research criteria: III. Mother–child interactions, family conflicts, and maternal psychopathology. *Journal of Child Psychology and Psychiatry, 32,* 233–256.

Barkley, R. A., Fischer, M., Smallish, L., & Fletcher, K. (2004). Young adult follow-up of hyperactive children: Antisocial activities and drug use. *Journal of Child Psychology and Psychiatry, 45,* 195–211.

Barkley, R. A., Grodzinsky, G., & DuPaul, G. (1992). Frontal lobe functions in attention deficit disorder with and without hyperactivity: A review and research report. *Journal of Abnormal Child Psychology, 20,* 163–188.

Barkley, R. A., Karlsson, J., & Pollard, S. (1985). Effects of age on the mother–child interactions of hyperactive children. *Journal of Abnormal Child Psychology, 13,* 631–638.

Barkley, R. A., Karlsson, J., Pollard, S., & Murphy, J. V. (1985). Developmental changes in the mother–child interactions of hyperactive boys: Effects of two dose levels of Ritalin. *Journal of Child Psychology and Psychiatry, 26,* 705–715.

Baumgaertel, A., Wolraich, M. L., & Dietrich, M. (1995). Comparison of diagnostic criteria for attention deficit disorders in a German elementary school sample. *Journal of the American Academy of Child and Adolescent Psychiatry, 34,* 629–638.

Befera, M., & Barkley, R. A. (1984). Hyperactive and normal girls and boys: Mother–child interactions, parent psychiatric status, and child psychopathology. *Journal of Child Psychology and Psychiatry, 26,* 439–452.

Berry, C. A., Shaywitz, S. E., & Shaywitz, B. A. (1985). Girls with attention deficit disorder: A silent majority? A report on behavioral and cognitive characteristics. *Pediatrics, 75,* 801–809.

Biederman, J. (1997, October). *Returns of comorbidity in girls with ADHD.* Paper presented at the annual meeting of the American Academy of Child and Adolescent Psychiatry, Toronto.

Biederman, J., Baldessarini, R. J., Wright, V., Keenan, K., & Faraone, S. V. (1993). A double-blind placebo controlled study of desipramine in the treatment of ADD: III. Lack of impact of comorbidity and family history factors on clinical response. *Journal of the American Academy of Child and Adolescent Psychiatry, 32,* 199–204.

Biederman, J., Baldessarini, R. J., Wright, V., Knee, D., & Harmatz, J. S. (1989). A double-blind placebo controlled study of desipramine in the treatment of ADD: I. Efficacy. *Journal of the American Academy of Child and Adolescent Psychiatry, 28,* 777–784.

Biederman, J., & Faraone, S. V. (1997, October). *Patterns of comorbidity in girls with ADHD.* Paper presented at the annual meeting of the American Academy of Child and Adolescent Psychiatry, Toronto.

Biederman, J., Faraone, S. V., & Lapey, K. (1992). Comorbidity of diagnosis in attention-deficit hyperactivity disorder. *Child and Adolescent Psychiatry Clinics of North America, 1,* 335–360.

Biederman, J., Faraone, S., Mick, E., Moore, P., & Lelon, E. (1996). Child Behavior Checklist findings further support comorbidity between ADHD and major depression in a referred sample. *Journal of the American Academy of Child and Adolescent Psychiatry, 35,* 734–742.

Biederman, J., Faraone, S., Mick, E., Wozniak, J., Chen, L., Ouellette, C., et al. (1996). Attention-deficit hyperactivity disorder and juvenile mania: An overlooked comorbidity? *Journal of the American Academy of Child and Adolescent Psychiatry, 35,* 997–1008.

Biederman, J., Gastfriend, D. R., & Jellinek, M. S. (1986). Desipramine in the treatment of children with attention deficit disorder. *Journal of Clinical Psychopharmacology, 6,* 359–363.

Biederman, J., Mick, E., & Faraone, S. V. (1998). Depression in attention deficit hyperactivity disorder (ADHD) children: "True depression" or demoralization? *Journal of Affective Disorders, 47,* 113–122.

Biederman, J., Munir, K., & Knee, D. (1987). Conduct and oppositional disorder in clinically referred children with attention deficit disorder: A controlled family study. *Journal of the American Academy of Child and Adolescent Psychiatry, 26,* 724–727.

Biederman, J., Newcorn, J., & Sprich, S. (1991). Comorbidity of attention deficit hyperactivity disorder with conduct, depressive, anxiety, and other disorders. *American Journal of Psychiatry, 148,* 564–577.

Biederman, J., Russell, R., Soriano, J., Wozniak, J., & Faraone, S. V. (1998). Clinical features of children with both ADHD and mania: Does ascertainment source make a difference? *Journal of Affective Disorders, 51,* 101–112.

Biederman, J., Wozniak, J., Kiely, K., Ablon, S., Faraone, S., Mick, E., et al. (1995). CBCL clinical scales discriminate prepubertal children with structured-interview-derived diagnosis of mania from those with ADHD. *Journal of the American Academy of Child and Adolescent Psychiatry, 34,* 464–471.

Bird, H. R., Canino, G., Rubio-Stipec, M., Gould, M. S., Ribera, I., Sesman, M., et al. (1988). Estimates of the prevalence of childhood maladjustment in a community survey in Puerto Rico. *Archives of General Psychiatry, 45,* 1120–1126.

Bird, H. R., Gould, M. S., & Staghezza, B. M. (1993). Patterns of diagnostic comorbidity in a community sample of children aged 9 through 16 years. *Journal of the American Academy of Child and Adolescent Psychiatry, 32,* 361–368.

Blachman, D. R., & Hinshaw, S. P. (2002). Patterns of friendship among girls with and without attention-deficit/hyperactivity disorder. *Journal of Abnormal Child Psychology, 30,* 625–640.

Bohline, D. S. (1985). Intellectual and effective characteristics of attention deficit disordered children. *Journal of Learning Disabilities, 18,* 604–608.

Breen, M., & Barkley, R. A. (1983). The Personality Inventory for Children (PIC): Its clinical utility with hyperactive children. *Journal of Pediatric Psychology,* 359–366.

Breen, M., & Barkley, R. A. (1984). Psychological adjustment in learning disabled, hyperactive, and hyperactive/learning disabled children using the Personality Inventory for Children. *Journal of Clinical Child Psychology, 13,* 232–236.

Breen, M., & Barkley, R. A. (1988). Parenting stress with ADDH girls and boys. *Journal of Pediatric Psychology, 13,* 265–280.

Brown, T. E. (Eds.). (2000a). *Attention-deficit disorders and comorbidities in children, adolescents and adults.* Washington, DC: American Psychiatric Press.

Brown, T. E. (2000b). Attention-deficit disorders with obsessive–compulsive disorder. In T. E. Brown (Ed.), *Attention-deficit disorders and comorbidities in children, adolescents, and adults* (pp. 209–230). Washington, DC: American Psychiatric Press.

Buhrmeister, D., Camparo, L., Christensen, A., Gonzalez, L. S., & Hinshaw, S. P. (1992). Mothers and fathers interacting in dyads and triads with normal and hyperactive sons. *Developmental Psychology, 28,* 500–509.

Burns, G. L., & Walsh, J. A. (2002). The influence of ADHD-hyperactivity/impulsivity symptoms on the development of oppositional defiant disorder symptoms in a 2-year longitudinal study. *Journal of Abnormal Child Psychology, 30,* 245–256.

Bussing, R., Gary, F., Mason, D. M., Leon, C. E., Sinha, K., & Garvan, C. W. (2003). Child temperament, ADHD, and caregiver strain: Exploring relationships in an epidemiological sample. *Journal of the American Academy of Child and Adolescent Psychiatry, 42,* 184–192.

Bussing, R., Zima, B. T., & Perwein, A. R. (2000). Self-esteem in special education children with ADHD: Relationship to disorder characteristics and medication use. *Journal of the American Academy of Child and Adolescent Psychiatry, 39,* 1260–1269.

Campbell, S. B., & Paulauskas, S. (1979). Peer relations in hyperactive children. *Journal of Child Psychology and Psychiatry, 20,* 233–246.

Cantwell, D. P. (1972). Psychiatric illness in the families of hyperactive children. *Archives of General Psychiatry, 27,* 414–427.

Cantwell, D. P., & Baker, L. (1989). Stability and natural history of DSM-III childhood diagnoses. *Journal of the American Academy of Child and Adolescent Psychiatry, 28,* 691–700.

Cantwell, D. P., & Baker, L. (1992). Association between attention deficit-hyperactivity disorder and learning disorders. In S. E. Shaywitz & B. A. Shaywitz (Eds.), *Attention deficit disorder comes of age: Toward the twenty-first century* (pp. 145–164). Austin, TX: PRO-ED.

Carlson, C. L., Lahey, B. B., Frame, C. L., Walker, J., & Hynd, G. W. (1987). Sociometric status of clinic-referred children with attention deficit disorders with and without hyperactivity. *Journal of Abnormal Child Psychology, 15,* 537–547.

Carlson, C. L., & Mann, M. (2002). Sluggish cognitive tempo predicts a different pattern of impairment in the attention deficit hyperactivity disorder, predominantly inattentive type. *Journal of Clinical Child and Adolescent Psychology, 31,* 123–129.

Carlson, G. A. (1990). Child and adolescent mania: Diagnostic considerations. *Journal of Child Psychology and Psychiatry, 31,* 331–342.

Carlson, G. A. (1998). Mania and ADHD: Comorbidity or confusion? *Journal of Affective Disorders, 51,* 177–187.

Chhabildas, N., Pennington, B. F., & Willcutt, E. G. (2001). A comparison of the neuropsychological profiles of the DSM-IV subtypes of ADHD. *Journal of Abnormal Child Psychology, 29,* 529–540.

Chi, T. C., & Hinshaw, S. P. (2002). Mother–child relationships of children with ADHD: The role of maternal depressive symptoms and depression-related distortions. *Journal of Abnormal Child Psychology, 30,* 387–400.

Chronis, A. M., Lahey, B. B., Pelham, W. E., Jr., Kipp, H. I., Baumann, B. L., & Lee, S. S. (2003). Psychopathology and substance abuse in parents of young children with attention-deficit/hyperactivity disorder. *Journal of the American Academy of Child and Adolescent Psychiatry, 42,* 1424–1432.

Clark, M. L., Cheyne, J. A., Cunningham, C. E., & Siegel, L. S. (1988). Dyadic peer interaction and task orientation in attention-deficit-disordered children. *Journal of Abnormal Child Psychology, 16,* 1–15.

Cohen, N. J., Sullivan, J., Minde, K., Novak, C., & Keens, S. (1983). Mother–child interaction in hyperactive and normal kindergarten-aged children and the effect of treatment. *Child Psychiatry and Human Development, 13,* 213–224.

Cohen, P., Velez, C. N., Brook, J., & Smith, J. (1989). Mechanisms of the relation between perinatal problems, early childhood illness, and psychopathology in late childhood and adolescence. *Child Development, 60,* 701–709.

Comings, D. E. (2000). Attention-deficit/hyperactivity disorder with Tourette syndrome. In T. E. Brown (Ed.), *Attention-deficit disorders and comorbidities in children, adolescents, and adults* (pp. 363–392). Washington, DC: American Psychiatric Press.

Crystal, D. S., Ostrander, R., Chen, R. S., & August, G. J. (2001). Multimethod assessment of psychopathology among DSM-IV subtypes of children with attention-deficit/hyperactivity disorder: self-, parent, and teacher reports. *Journal of Abnormal Child Psychology, 29,* 189–205.

Cunningham, C. E., Benness, B. B., & Siegel, L. S. (1988). Family functioning, time allocation, and parental depression in the families of normal and ADDH children. *Journal of Clinical Child Psychology, 17,* 169–177.

Cunningham, C. E., & Boyle, M. H. (2002). Preschoolers at risk for attention-deficit hyperactivity disorder and oppositional defiant disorder: Family, parenting, and behavioral correlates. *Journal of Abnormal Child Psychology, 30,* 555–569.

Cunningham, C. E., & Siegel, L. S. (1987). Peer interactions of normal and attention-deficit disordered boys during free-play, cooperative task, and simulated classroom situations. *Journal of Abnormal Child Psychology, 15,* 247–268.

Danforth, J. S., Barkley, R. A., & Stokes, T. F. (1991). Observations of parent–child interactions with hyperactive children: Research and clinical implications. *Clinical Psychology Review, 11,* 703–727.

Deutsch, C. K., Swanson, J. M., Bruell, J. H., Cantwell, D. P., Weinberg, F., & Baren, M. (1982). Over-representation of adoptees in children with the attention deficit disorder. *Behavioral Genetics, 12,* 231–238.

Diener, M. B., & Milich, R. (1997). Effects of positive feedback on the social interactions of boys with attention deficit hyperactivity disorder: A test of the self-protective hypothesis. *Journal of Clinical Child Psychology, 26,* 256–265.

DuPaul, G. J., Barkley, R. A., & McMurray, M. B. (1994). Response of children with ADHD to methylphenidate: Interaction with internalizing symptoms. *Journal of the American Academy of Child and Adolescent Psychiatry, 33,* 894–903.

DuPaul, G. J., McGoey, K. E., Eckert, T., & VanBrakle, J. (2001). Preschool children with attention-deficit/hyperactivity disorder: Impairments in behavioral, social, and school functioning. *Journal of the American Academy of Child and Adolescent Psychiatry, 40,* 508–515.

Edelbrock, C. S., Costello, A., & Kessler, M. D. (1984). Empirical corroboration of attention deficit disorder. *Journal of the American Academy of Child and Adolescent Psychiatry, 23,* 285–290.

Edwards, F., Barkley, R., Laneri, M., Fletcher, K., & Metevia, L. (2001). Parent–adolescent conflicts and parent and teen psychological adjustment in teenagers with ADHD and ODD: The role of maternal depression. *Journal of Abnormal Child Psychology, 29,* 557–572.

Epstein, J. N., Conners, C. K., Erhardt, D., Arnold, L. E., Hechtman, L., Hinshaw, S. P., et al. (2000). Familial aggregation of ADHD characteristics. *Journal of Abnormal Child Psychology, 28,* 585–600.

Epstein, J. N., Goldberg, N. A., Conners, C. K., & March, J. S. (1997). The effects of anxiety on continuous performance test functioning in an ADHD clinic sample. *Journal of Attention Disorders, 2,* 45–52.

Famularo, R., & Fenton, T. (1987). The effect of methylphenidate on school grades in children with attention deficit disorder without hyperactivity: A preliminary report. *Journal of Clinical Psychiatry, 48,* 112–114.

Faraone, S. V., & Biederman, J. (1997, October). *Familial transmission of attention-deficit/hyperactivity disorder and comorbid disorders.* Paper presented at the annual meeting of the American Academy of Child and Adolescent Psychiatry, Toronto.

Faraone, S. V., Biederman, J., Jetton, J. G., & Tsuang, M. T. (1997). Attention deficit disorder and conduct disorder: Longitudinal evidence for a familial subtype. *Psychological Medicine, 27,* 291–300.

Faraone, S. V., Biederman, J., & Monuteaux, M. C. (2001). Attention deficit hyperactivity disorder with bipolar disorder in girls: Further evidence for a familial subtype. *Journal of Affective Disorders, 64,* 19–26.

Faraone, S. V., Biederman, J., Weber, W., & Russell, R. L. (1998). Psychiatric, neuropsychological, and psychosocial features of DSM-IV subtypes of attention-deficit/hyperactivity disorder: Results from a clinically referred sample. *Journal of the American Academy of Child and Adolescent Psychiatry, 37,* 185–193.

Faraone, S. V., Biederman, J., Wozniak, J., Mundy, E., Mennin, D., & O'Donnell, D. (1997). Is comorbidity with ADHD a marker for juvenile-onset mania? *Journal of the American Academy of Child and Adolescent Psychiatry, 36,* 1046–1055.

Fischer, M. (1990). Parenting stress and the child with attention deficit hyperactivity disorder. *Journal of Clinical Child Psychology, 19,* 337–346.

Fischer, M., Barkley, R. A., Edelbrock, C. S., & Smallish, L. (1990). The adolescent outcome of hyperactive children diagnosed by research criteria: II. Academic, attentional, and neuropsychological status. *Journal of Consulting and Clinical Psychology, 58,* 580–588.

Fischer, M., Barkley, R. A., Smallish, L., & Fletcher, K. (2002). Young adult follow-up of hyperactive children: Self-reported psychiatric disorders, comorbidity, and the role of childhood conduct problems. *Journal of Abnormal Child Psychology. 30,* 463–475.

Fletcher, K., Fischer, M., Barkley, R. A., & Smallish, L. (1996). A sequential analysis of the mother–adolescent interactions of ADHD, ADHD/ODD, and normal teenagers during neutral and conflict discussions. *Journal of Abnormal Child Psychology, 24,* 271–297.

Ford, J. D., Racusin, R., Daviss, W. B., Ellis, C. G., Thomas, J., Rogers, K., et al. (1999). Trauma exposure among children with oppositional defiant disorder and attention deficit-hyperactivity disorder. *Journal of Consulting and Clinical Psychology, 67,* 786–789.

Ford, J. D., Racusin, R., Ellis, C. G., Daviss, W. B., Reiser, J., Fleischer, A., et al. (2000). Child maltreatment, other trauma exposure, and posttraumatic symptomatology among children with oppositional defiant and attention deficit hyperactivity disorders. *Child Maltreatment, 5,* 205–217.

Gadow, K. D., Drabick, D. A. G., Loney, J., Sprafkin, J., Salisbury, H., Azizian, A., et al. (2004). Comparison of ADHD symptom subtypes as source-specific syndromes. *Journal of Child Psychology and Psychiatry, 45,* 1135–1149.

Gadow, K. D., & Nolan, E. E. (2002). Differences between preschool children with ODD, ADHD, and ODD + ADHD symptoms. *Journal of Child Psychology and Psychiatry, 43,* 191–201.

Garcia-Sanchez, C., Estevez-Gonzalez, A., Suarez-Romero, E., & Junque, C. (1997). Right hemisphere dysfunction in subjects with attention-deficit disorder with and without hyperactivity. *Journal of Child Neurology, 12,* 107–115.

Geller, B., & Luby, J. (1997). Child and adolescent bipolar disorder: A review of the past 10 years. *Journal of the American Academy of Child and Adolescent Psychiatry, 36,* 1168–1176.

Geller, B., Williams, M., Zimerman, B., Frazier, J., Beringer, L., & Warner, K. L. (1998). Prepubertal and early adolescent bipolarity differentiate from ADHD by manic symptoms, grandiose delusions, ultra-rapid or ultradian cycling. *Journal of Affective Disorders, 51,* 81–91.

Geller, D. A., Biederman J., Faraone, S. V., Cradock, K., Hagermoser, L., Zaman, N., et al. (2002). Attention-deficit/hyperactivity disorder in children and adolescents with obsessive–compulsive disorder: Factor or artifact? *Journal of the American Academy of Child and Adolescent Psychiatry, 41,* 52–58.

Gerdes, A. C., Hoza, B., & Pelham, W. E. (2003). Attention-deficit/hyperactivity disordered boys' relationships with their mothers and fathers: Child, mother, and father perceptions. *Development and Psychopathology, 15,* 363–382.

Goldstein, S., & Schwebach, A. J. (2004). The comorbidity of pervasive developmental disorder and attention deficit hyperactivity disorder: Results of a retrospective chart review. *Journal of Autism and Developmental Disorders, 34,* 329–339.

Gomez, R., & Sanson, A. V. (1994). Mother–child interactions and noncompliance in hyperactive boys with and without conduct problems. *Journal of Child Psychology and Psychiatry, 35,* 477–490.

Goodyear, P., & Hynd, G. (1992). Attention deficit disorder with (ADDH) and without (ADDWO) hyperactivity: Behavioral and neuropsychological differentiation. *Journal of Clinical Child Psychology, 21,* 273–304.

Gordon, M., Mettelman, B. B., & Irwin, M. (1990, August). *The impact of comorbidity on ADHD laboratory measures.* Paper presented at the annual meeting of the American Psychological Association, Boston.

Graetz, B. W., Sawyer, M. G., Hazell, P. L., Arney, F., & Baghurst, P. (2001). Validity of DSM-IV ADHD subtypes in a nationally representative sample of Australian children and adolescents. *Journal of the American Academy of Child and Adolescent Psychiatry, 40,* 1410–1417.

Grenell, M. M., Glass, C. R., & Katz, K. S. (1987). Hyperactive children and peer interaction: Knowledge and performance of social skills. *Journal of Abnormal Child Psychology, 15,* 1–13.

Halperin, J. M., Gittelman, R., Klein, D. F., & Rudel, R. G. (1984). Reading-disabled hyperactive children: A distinct subgroup of attention deficit disorder with hyperactivity? *Journal of Abnormal Child Psychology, 12,* 1–14.

Harrison, C., & Sofronoff, K. (2002). ADHD and parental psychological distress: Role of demographics, child behavioral characteristics, and parental cognitions. *Journal of the American Academy of Child and Adolescent Psychiatry, 41,* 703–711.

Harvey, E. (1998). Parental employment and conduct problems among children with attention-deficit/hyperactivity disorder: An examination of child care workload and parenting well-being as mediating variables. *Journal of Social and Clinical Psychology, 17,* 476–490.

Harvey, E., Danforth, J. S., Ulaszek, W. R., & Eberhardt, T. L. (2001). Validity of the Parenting Scale for parents of children with attention-deficit hyperactivity disorder. *Behaviour Research and Therapy, 39,* 731–743.

Heilman, K. M., Voeller, K. K. S., & Nadeau, S. E. (1991). A possible pathophysiological substrate of attention deficit hyperactivity disorder. *Journal of Child Neurology, 6,* 74–79.

Hern, K. L., & Hynd, G. W. (1992). Clinical differentiation of the attention deficit disorder subtypes: Do sensorimotor deficits characterize children with ADDWO? *Archives of Clinical Neuropsychology, 7,* 77–83.

Hinshaw, S. P. (1987). On the distinction between attentional deficits/hyperactivity and conduct problems/aggression in child psychopathology. *Psychological Bulletin, 101,* 443–447.

Hinshaw, S. P. (1992). Externalizing behavior problems and academic underachievement in childhood and adolescence: Causal relationships and underlying mechanisms. *Psychological Bulletin, 111,* 127–155.

Hinshaw, S. P., & Melnick, S. M. (1995). Peer relationship in boys with attention deficit hyperactivity disorder with and without comorbid aggression. *Developmental Psychopathology, 7,* 627–647.

Hodgens, J. B., Cole, J., & Boldizar, J. (2000). Peer-based differences among boys with ADHD. *Journal of Clinical Child Psychology, 29,* 443–452.

Hoza, B., Owens, J. S., Pelham, W. E., Swanson, J, M., Conners, C. K., Hinshaw, S. P., et al. (2000). Parent cognitions as predictors of child treatment response in attention-deficit/hyperactivity disorder. *Journal of Abnormal Child Psychology, 28,* 569–584.

Hudziak, J. J., Heath, A. C., Madden, P. F., Reich, W., Bucholz, K. K., Slutske, W., et al. (1998). Latent class and factor analysis of DSM-IV ADHD: A twin study of female adolescents. *Journal of the American Academy of Child and Adolescent Psychiatry, 37,* 848–857.

Humphries, T., Kinsbourne, M., & Swanson, J. (1978). Stimulant effects on cooperation and social interaction between hyperactive children and their mothers. *Journal of Child Psychology and Psychiatry, 19,* 13–22.

Hynd, G. W., Lorys, A. R., Semrud-Clikeman, M., Nieves, N., Huettner, M. I. S., & Lahey, B. B. (1991). Attention deficit disorder without hyperactivity: A distinct behavioral and neurocognitive syndrome. *Journal of Child Neurology, 6,* S37–S43.

Hynd, G. W., Nieves, N., Conner, R., Stone, P., Town, P., Becker, M. G., et al. (1989). Speed of neurocognitive processing in children with attention deficit disorder with and without hyperactivity. *Journal of Learning Disabilities, 22,* 573–580.

Jensen, J. B., Burke, N., & Garfinkel, B. D. (1988). Depression and symptoms of attention deficit disorder with hyperactivity. *Journal of the American Academy of Child and Adolescent Psychiatry, 27,* 742–747.

Jensen, P. S., Martin, D., & Cantwell, D. P. (1997). Comorbidity in ADHD: Implications for research, practice, and DSM-V. *Journal of the American Academy of Child and Adolescent Psychiatry, 36,* 1065–1079.

Jensen, P. S., Shervette, R. E., III, Xenakis, S. N., & Richters, J. (1993). Anxiety and depressive disorders in attention deficit disorder with hyperactivity: New findings. *American Journal of Psychiatry, 150,* 1203–1209.

Johnson, B. D., Altmaier, E. M., & Richman, L. C. (1999). Attention deficits and reading disabilities: Are immediate memory defects additive? *Developmental Neuropsychology, 15,* 213–226.

Johnston, C. (1996). Parent characteristics and parent–child interactions in families of nonproblem children and ADHD children with higher and lower levels of oppositional-defiant disorder. *Journal of Abnormal Child Psychology, 24,* 85–104.

Johnston, C., & Freeman, W. (1997). Attributions of child behavior in parents of children with behavior disorders and children with attention deficit–hyperactivity disorder. *Journal of Consulting and Clinical Psychology, 65,* 636–645.

Johnston, C., & Mash, E. J. (2001). Families of children with attention-deficit/hyperactivity disorder: Review and recommendations for future research. *Clinical Child and Family Psychology Review, 4,* 183–207.

Johnston, C., Murray, C., Hinshaw, S. P., Pelham, W. E., Jr., & Hoza, B. (2002). Responsiveness of interactions of mothers and sons with ADHD: Relations to maternal and child characteristics. *Journal of Abnormal Child Psychology, 30,* 77–88.

Johnston, C., Pelham, W. E., & Murphy, H. A. (1985). Peer relationships in ADDH and normal children: A developmental analysis of peer and teacher ratings. *Journal of Abnormal Child Psychology, 13,* 89–100.

Keown, L. J., & Woodward, L. J. (2002). Early parent–child relations and family functioning of preschool boys with pervasive hyperactivity. *Journal of Abnormal Child Psychology, 30,* 541–553.

King, C., & Young, R. (1982). Attentional deficits with and without hyperactivity: Teacher and peer perceptions. *Journal of Abnormal Child Psychology, 10,* 483–496.

Lahey, B. B., & Carlson, C. L. (1992). Validity of the diagnostic category of attention deficit disorder without hyperactivity: A review of the literature. In S. E. Shaywitz & B. A. Shaywitz (Eds.), *Attention deficit disorder comes of age: Toward the twenty-first century* (pp. 119–144). Austin, TX: PRO-ED.

Lahey, B. B., Piacentini, J. C., McBurnett, K., Stone, P., Hartdagen, S., & Hynd, G. (1988). Psychopathology in the parents of children with conduct disorder and hyperactivity. *Journal of the American Academy of Child and Adolescent Psychiatry, 27,* 163–170.

Lahey, B. B., Schaughency, E., Hynd, G., Carlson, C., & Nieves, N. (1987). Attention deficit disorder with and without hyperactivity: Comparison of behavioral characteristics of clinic-referred children. *Journal of the American Academy of Child Psychiatry, 26,* 718–723.

Lahey, B. B., Schaughency, E., Strauss, C., & Frame, C. (1984). Are attention deficit disorders with and without hyperactivity similar or dissimilar disorders? *Journal of the American Academy of Child Psychiatry, 23,* 302–309.

Landau, S., & Milich, R. (1988). Social communication patterns of attention deficit-disordered boys. *Journal of Abnormal Child Psychology, 16,* 69–81.

Lavigne, J. V., Cicchetti, C., Gibbons, R. D., Binns, H. J., Larsen, L., & DeVito, C. (2001). Oppositional defiant disorder with onset in preschool years: Longitudinal stability and pathways to other disorders. *Journal of the American Academy of Child and Adolescent Psychiatry, 40,* 1393–1400.

Lee, S. S., & Hinshaw, S. P. (2004). Severity of adolescent delinquency among boys with and without attention deficit hyperactivity disorder: Predictions from early antisocial behavior and peer status. *Journal of Clinical Child and Adolescent Psychology, 33,* 705–716.

Lewinsohn, P. M., Klein, D. N., & Seeley, J. R. (1995). Bipolar disorders in a community sample of older adolescents: Prevalence, phenomenology, comorbidity, and course. *Journal of the American Academy of Child and Adolescent Psychiatry, 34*, 454–463.

Linn, R. T., & Hodge, G. K. (1982). Locus of control in childhood hyperactivity. *Journal of Consulting and Clinical Psychology, 50*, 592–593.

Loeber, R. (1990). Development and risk factors of juvenile antisocial behavior and delinquency. *Clinical Psychology Review, 10*, 1–42.

Loeber, R., Burke, J. D., Lahey, B. B., Winters, A., & Zera, M. (2000). Oppositional defiant and conduct disorder: A review of the past 10 years, Part I. *Journal of the American Academy of Child and Adolescent Psychiatry, 39*, 1–17.

Loney, J., Kramer, J., & Milich, R. (1981). The hyperkinetic child grows up: Predictors of symptoms, delinquency, and achievement at follow-up. In K. Gadow & J. Loney (Eds.), *Psychosocial aspects of drug treatment for hyperactivity*. Boulder, CO: Westview Press.

Loney, J., Langhorne, J., & Paternite, C. (1978). An empirical basis for subgrouping the hyperkinetic/minimal brain dysfunction syndrome. *Journal of Abnormal Psychology, 87*, 431–444.

Loney, J., & Milich, R. (1982). Hyperactivity, inattention, and aggression in clinical practice. In D. Routh & M. Wolraich (Eds.), *Advances in developmental and behavioral pediatrics* (Vol. 3, pp. 113–147). Greenwich, CT: JAI Press.

Lou, H. C., Henriksen, L., & Bruhn, P. (1984). Focal cerebral hypoperfusion in children with dysphasia and/or attention deficit disorder. *Archives of Neurology, 41*, 825–829.

Lou, H. C., Henriksen, L., Bruhn, P., Borner, H., & Nielsen, J. B. (1989). Striatal dysfunction in attention deficit and hyperkinetic disorder. *Archives of Neurology, 46*, 48–52.

Lynam, D. R. (1998). Early identification of the fledgling psychopath: Locating the psychopathic child in the current nomenclature. *Journal of Abnormal Psychology, 107*, 566–575.

Maedgen, J. W., & Carlson, C. L. (2000). Social functioning and emotional regulation in the attention deficit hyperactivity disorder subtypes. *Journal of Clinical Child Psychology, 29*, 30–42.

Mannuzza, S., Gittelman-Klein, R., Bessler, A., Malloy, P., & LaPadula, M. (1993). Adult outcome of hyperactive boys: Educational achievement, occupational rank, and psychiatric status. *Archives of General Psychiatry, 50*, 565–576.

Mannuzza, S., Klein, R., Bessler, A., Malloy, P., & LaPadula, M. (1998). Adult psychiatric status of hyperactive boys grown up. *American Journal of Psychiatry, 155*, 493–498.

March, J. S., Swanson, J. M., Arnold, L. E., Hoza, B., Conners, C. K., Hinshaw, S. P., et al. (2000). Anxiety as a predictor and outcome variable in the Multimodal Treatment Study of Children with ADHD (MTA). *Journal of Abnormal Child Psychology, 28*, 527–542.

Margalit, M., & Arieli, N. (1984). Emotional and behavioral aspects of hyperactivity. *Journal of Learning Disabilities, 17*, 374–376.

Mash, E. J., & Johnston, C. (1982). A comparison of mother–child interactions of younger and older hyperactive and normal children. *Child Development, 53*, 1371–1381.

Mash, E. J., & Johnston, C. (1983). Sibling interactions of hyperactive and normal children and their relationship to reports of maternal stress and self-esteem. *Journal of Clinical Child Psychology, 12*, 91–99.

Mash, E. J., & Johnston, C. (1990). Determinants of parenting stress: Illustrations from families of hyperactive children and families of physically abused children. *Journal of Clinical Child Psychology, 19*, 313–328.

Matthys, W., Cuperus, J. M., & van Engeland, H. (1999). Deficient social problem-solving in boys with ODD/CD, with ADHD, and with both disorders. *Journal of the American Academy of Child and Adolescent Psychiatry, 38*, 311–321.

Maughan, B., Rowe, R., Messer, J., Goodman, R., & Meltzer, H. (2004). Conduct disorder and oppositional defiant disorder in a national sample: developmental epidemiology. *Journal of Child Psychology and Psychiatry, 45*, 609–621.

Maurer, R. G., & Stewart, M. (1980) Attention deficit disorder without hyperactivity in a child psychiatric clinic. *Journal of Clinical Psychiatry, 41*, 232–233.

McBurnett, K., Pfiffner, L. J., & Frick, P. J. (2001). Symptom properties as a function of ADHD type: An argument for continued study of sluggish cognitive tempo. *Journal of Abnormal Child Psychology, 29*, 207–213.

McGee, R., Williams, S., & Silva, P. A. (1984a). Behavioral and developmental characteristics of aggressive, hyperactive, and aggressive–hyperactive boys. *Journal of the American Academy of Child Psychiatry, 23*, 270–279.

McGee, R., Williams, S., & Silva, P. A. (1984b). Background characteristics of aggressive, hyperactive, and aggressive–hyperactive boys. *Journal of the American Academy of Child and Adolescent Psychiatry, 23*, 280–284.

McKee, T. E., Harvey, E., Danforth, J. S., Ulaszek, W. R., & Friedman, J. L. (2004). The relation between parental coping styles and parent–child interactions before and after treatment for children with ADHD and oppositional disorder. *Journal of Clinical Child and Adolescent Psychology, 33*, 158–168.

Mick, E., Santangelo, S. L., Wypij, D., & Biederman, J. (2000). Impact of maternal depression on ratings of comorbid depression in adolescents with attention-deficit/hyperactivity disorder. *Journal of the American Academy of Child and Adolescent Psychiatry, 39*, 314–319.

Mikami, A. Y., & Hinshaw, S. P. (2003). Buffers of peer rejection among girls with and without ADHD: The role of popularity with adults and goal-directed solitary play. *Journal of Abnormal Child Psychology, 31,* 381–397.

Milberger, S., Biederman, J., Faraone, S. V., Murphy, J., & Tsuang, M. T. (1995). Attention deficit hyperactivity disorder and comorbid disorders: Issues of overlapping symptoms. *American Journal of Psychiatry, 152,* 1783–1800.

Milich, R. (1994). The response of children with ADHD to failure: If at first you don't succeed, do you try, try again? *School Psychology Review, 23,* 11–18.

Milich, R., Ballentine, A. C., & Lynam, D. R. (2001). ADHD/combined type and ADHD predominantly inattentive type are distinct and unrelated disorders. *Clinical Psychology: Science and Practice, 8,* 463–488.

Milich, R., & Dodge, K. A. (1984). Social information processing in child psychiatric populations. *Journal of Abnormal Child Psychology, 12,* 471–490.

Milich, R., & Greenwell, L. (1991, December). *An examination of learned helplessness among attention-deficit hyperactivity disordered boys.* Paper presented at the annual meeting of the Association for Advancement of Behavior Therapy, New York.

Milich, R., Landau, S., Kilby, G., & Whitten, P. (1982). Preschool peer perceptions of the behavior of hyperactive and aggressive children. *Journal of Abnormal Child Psychology, 10,* 497–510.

Milich, R., & Loney, J. (1979). The role of hyperactive and aggressive symptomatology in predicting adolescent outcome among hyperactive children. *Journal of Pediatric Psychology, 4,* 93–112.

Milich, R., & Okazaki, M. (1991). An examination of learned helplessness among attention-deficit hyperactivity disordered boys. *Journal of Abnormal Child Psychology, 19,* 607–623.

Mirsky, A. F. (1996). Disorders of attention: A neuropsychological perspective. In R. G. Lyon & N. A. Krasnegor (Eds.), *Attention, memory, and executive function* (pp. 71–96). Baltimore: Brookes.

Moffitt, T. E. (1990). Juvenile delinquency and attention deficit disorder: Boys' developmental trajectories from age 3 to 15. *Child Development, 61,* 893–910.

Morgan, A. E., Hynd, G. W., Riccio, C. A., & Hall, J. (1996). Validity of DSM-IV ADHD predominantly inattentive and combined types: Relationship to previous DSM diagnoses/subtype differences. *Journal of the American Academy of Child and Adolescent Psychiatry, 35,* 325–333.

Morrison, J., & Stewart, M. (1973). The psychiatric status of the legal families of adopted hyperactive children. *Archives of General Psychiatry, 28,* 888–891.

Munir, K., Biederman, J., & Knee, D. (1987). Psychiatric comorbidity in patients with attention deficit disorder: A controlled study. *Journal of the American Academy of Child and Adolescent Psychiatry, 26,* 844–848.

Nadder, T. S., Rutter, M., Silberg, J. L., Maes, H. H., & Eaves, L. J. (2002). Genetic effects on the variation and covariation of attention-deficit hyperactivity disorder (ADHD) and oppositional-defiant disorder/conduct disorder (ODD/CD) symptomatologies across informant and occasion of measurement. *Psychological Medicine, 32,* 39–53.

Newcorn, J. H., & Halperin, J. M. (2000). Attention-deficit disorders with oppositionality and aggression. In T. E. Brown (Ed.), *Attention-deficit disorders and comorbidities in children, adolescents, and adults* (pp. 171–208). Washington, DC: American Psychiatric Press.

Newcorn, J. H., Halperin, J. M., Jensen, P. S., Abikoff, H. B., Arnold, L. E., Cantwell, D. P., et al. (2001). Symptom profiles in children with ADHD: Effects of comorbidity and gender. *Journal of the American Academy of Child and Adolescent Psychiatry, 40,* 137–146.

Nieman, G. W., & Delong, R. (1987). Use of the Personality Inventory for Children as an aid in differentiating children with mania from children with attention deficit disorder with hyperactivity. *Journal of the American Academy of Child and Adolescent Psychiatry, 26,* 381–388.

Nigg, J. T., Blaskey, L. G., Huang-Pollock, C. L., & Rappley, M. D. (2002). Neuropsychological executive functions in DSM-IV ADHD subtypes. *Journal of the American Academy of Child and Adolescent Psychiatry, 41,* 59–66.

Nigg, J. T., & Hinshaw, S. P. (1998). Parent personality traits and psychopathology associated with antisocial behaviors in childhood attention-deficit hyperactivity disorder. *Journal of Child Psychology and Psychiatry, 39,* 145–159.

O'Leary, S. G., Slep, A. M. S., & Reid, M. J. (1999). A longitudinal study of mothers' overreactive discipline and toddlers externalizing behavior. *Journal of Abnormal Child Psychology, 27,* 331–341.

O'Neill, M. E., & Douglas, V. I. (1991). Study strategies and story recall in attention-deficit hyperactivity disorder and reading disability. *Journal of Abnormal Child Psychology, 19,* 671–692.

Patterson, G. R., Degarmo, D. S., & Knutson, N. (2000). Hyperactive and antisocial behaviors: Comorbid or two points in the same process? *Development and Psychopathology, 12,* 91–106.

Pelham, W. E., & Bender, M. E. (1982). Peer relationships in hyperactive children: Description and treatment. In K. D. Gadow & I. Bialer (Eds.), *Advances in learning and behavioral disabilities* (Vol. 1, pp. 365–436). Greenwich, CT: JAI Press.

Pelham, W. E., & Lang, A. R. (1993). Parental alcohol consumption and deviant child behavior: Laboratory studies of reciprocal effects. *Clinical Psychology Review, 13,* 763–784.

Pelham, W. E., & Milich, R. (1984). Peer relationships in children with hyperactivity/attention deficit disorder. *Journal of Learning Disabilities, 17,* 560–567.

Peris, T. S., & Hinshaw, S. P. (2003). Family dynamics and preadolescent girls with ADHD: The relationship between expressed emotion, ADHD symptomatology, and comorbid disruptive behavior. *Journal of Child Psychology and Psychiatry, 44,* 1177–1190.

Peterson, B. S., Pine, D. S., Cohen, P., & Brook, J. S. (2001). Prospective, longitudinal study of tic, obsessive–compulsive, and attention-deficit/hyperactivity disorders in an epidemiological sample. *Journal of the American Academy of Child and Adolescent Psychiatry, 40,* 685–695.

Pfiffner, L. J., McBurnett, K., Lahey, B. B., Loeber, R., Green, S., Frick, P. J., et al. (1999). Association of parental psychopathology to the comorbid disorders of boys with attention-deficit hyperactivity disorder. *Journal of Consulting and Clinical Psychology, 67,* 881–893.

Pliszka, S. R. (1989). Effect of anxiety on cognition, behavior, and stimulant responding in ADHD. *Journal of the American Academy of Child and Adolescent Psychiatry, 28,* 882–887.

Pliszka, S. R. (1992). Comorbidity of attention-deficit hyperactivity disorder and overanxious disorder. *Journal of the American Academy of Child and Adolescent Psychiatry, 31,* 197–203.

Podolski, C., & Nigg, J. T. (2001). Parent stress and coping in relation to child ADHD severity and associated child disruptive behavior problems. *Journal of Clinical Child Psychology, 30,* 503–513.

Pope, A. W., Bierman, K. L., & Mumma, G. H. (1989). Relations between hyperactive and aggressive behavior and peer relations at three elementary grade levels. *Journal of Abnormal Child Psychology, 17,* 253–267.

Posner, M. (1987). *Structures and functions of selection attention.* Washington, DC: American Psychological Association.

Reeves, J. C., Werry, J., Elkind, G. S., & Zametkin, A. (1987). Attention deficit, conduct, oppositional, and anxiety disorders in children: II. Clinical characteristics. *Journal of the American Academy of Child and Adolescent Psychiatry, 26,* 133–143.

Rowe, R., Maughan, B., Pickles, A., Costello, E. J., & Angold, A. (2002). The relationship between DSM-IV oppositional defiant disorder and conduct disorder: Findings from the Great Smoky Mountains Study. *Journal of Child Psychology and Psychiatry, 43,* 365–373.

Rubinstein, R. S., & Brown, R. T. (1984). An evaluation of the validity of the diagnostic category of attention deficit disorder. *American Journal of Orthopsychiatry, 54,* 398–414.

Sachs, G. S., Baldassano, C. F., Truman, C. J., & Guille, C. (2000). Comorbidity of attention deficit hyperactivity disorder with early- and late-onset bipolar disorder. *American Journal of Psychiatry, 157,* 466–468.

Saul, R. C., & Ashby, C. D. (1986). Measurement of whole blood serotonin as a guide for prescribing psychostimulant medication for children with attention deficits. *Clinical Neuropharmacology, 9,* 189–195.

Schachar, R., & Tannock, R. (1995). Test of four hypotheses for the comorbidity of attention-deficit hyperactivity disorder and conduct disorder. *Journal of the American Academy of Child and Adolescent Psychiatry, 34,* 639–648.

Schachar, R., Taylor, E., Weiselberg, M., Thorley, G., & Rutter, M. (1987). Changes in family function and relationships in children who respond to methylphenidate. *Journal of the American Academy of Child and Adolescent Psychiatry, 26,* 728–732.

Schmidtz, M., Cadore, L., Paczko, M., Kipper, L., Chaves, M., Rohde, L. A., et al. (2002). Neuropsychological performance in DSM-IV ADHD subtypes: An exploratory study with untreated adolescents. *Canadian Journal of Psychiatry, 47,* 863–869.

Scourfield, J., Van den Bree, M., Martin, N., & McGuffin, P. (2004). Conduct problems in children and adolescents: A twin study. *Archives of General Psychiatry, 61,* 489–496.

Sebrechts, M. M., Shaywitz, S. E., Shaywitz, B. A., Jatlow, P., Anderson, G. M., & Cohen, D. J. (1986). Components of attention, methylphenidate dosage, and blood levels in children with attention deficit disorder. *Pediatrics, 77,* 222–228.

Shapiro, S., & Garfinkel, B. (1986). The occurrence of behavior disorders in children: The interdependence of attention deficit disorder and conduct disorder. *Journal of the American Academy of Child Psychiatry, 25,* 809–919.

Shaywitz, S. E., Shaywitz, B. A., Jatlow, P. R., Sebrechts, M., Anderson, G. M., & Cohen, D. T. (1986). Biological differentiation of attention deficit disorder with and without hyperactivity: A preliminary report. *Annals of Neurology, 21,* 363.

Singer, S. M., Stewart, M. A., & Pulaski, L. (1981). Minimal brain dysfunction: Differences in cognitive organization in two groups of index cases and their relatives. *Journal of Learning Disabilities, 14,* 470–473.

Singh, I. (2003). Boys will be boys: Fathers' perspectives on ADHD symptoms, diagnosis, and drug treatment. *Harvard Review of Psychiatry, 11,* 308–316.

Smith, A. J., Brown, R. T., Bunke, V., Blount, R. L., & Christophersen, E. (2002). Psychological adjustment and peer competence of siblings of children with attention-deficit/hyperactivity disorder. *Journal of Attention Disorders, 5,* 165–176.

Speltz, M. L., McCllelan, J., DeKlyen, M., & Jones, K. (1999). Preschool boys with oppositional defiant disorder: Clinical presentation and diagnostic change. *Journal of the American Academy of Child and Adolescent Psychiatry, 38,* 838–845.

Spencer, T., Biederman, J., Coffey, B., Geller, D., Wilens, T., & Faraone, S. (1999). The 4-year course of tic disorders in boys with attention-deficit/hyperactivity disorder. *Archives of General Psychiatry, 56,* 842–847.

Spencer, T., Biederman, J., Faraone, S., Mick, E., Coffey, B., Geller, D., et al. (2001). Impact of tic disorders on

ADHD outcome across the life cycle: Findings from a large group of adults with and without ADHD. *American Journal of Psychiatry, 158*, 611–617.

Spencer, T., Biederman, J., Harding, M., O'Donnell, D., Wilens, T., Faraone, S., et al. (1998). Disentangling the overlap between Tourette's disorder and ADHD. *Journal of Child Psychology and Psychiatry, 39*, 1037–1044.

Spencer, T., Wilens, T., Biederman, J., Wozniak, J., & Harding-Crawford, M. (2000). Attention-deficit/hyperactivity disorder with mood disorders. In T. E. Brown (Ed.), *Attention-deficit disorders and comorbidities in children, adolescents, and adults* (pp. 79–124). Washington, DC: American Psychiatric Press.

Stewart, M. A., deBlois, S., & Cummings, C. (1980). Psychiatric disorder in the parents of hyperactive boys and those with conduct disorder. *Journal of Child Psychology and Psychiatry, 21*, 283–292.

Stewart, M. A., Pitts, F. N., Craig, A. G., & Dieruf, W. (1966). The hyperactive child syndrome. *American Journal of Orthopsychiatry, 36*, 861–867.

Strober, M., DeAntonio, M., Schmidt-Lackner, L., Freeman R., Lampert, C., & Diamond, J. (1998). Early childhood attention deficit hyperactivity disorder predicts poorer response to acute lithium therapy in adolescent mania. *Journal of Affective Disorders, 51*, 145–151.

Stroes, A., Alberts, E., & van der Meere, J. J. (2003). Boys with ADHD in social interaction with a nonfamiliar adult: An observational study. *Journal of the American Academy of Child and Adolescent Psychiatry, 42*, 295–302.

Szatmari, P., Boyle, M., & Offord, D. R. (1989). ADDH and conduct disorder: Degree of diagnostic overlap and differences among correlates. *Journal of the American Academy of Child and Adolescent Psychiatry, 28*, 865–872.

Szatmari, P., Offord, D. R., & Boyle, M. H. (1989). Ontario Child Health Study: Prevalence of attention deficit disorder with hyperactivity. *Journal of Child Psychology and Psychiatry, 30*, 219–230.

Tallmadge, J., & Barkley, R. A. (1983). The interactions of hyperactive and normal boys with their mothers and fathers. *Journal of Abnormal Child Psychology, 11*, 565–579.

Tannock, R. (2000). Attention-deficit/hyperactivity disorder with anxiety disorders. In T. E. Brown (Ed.), *Attention-deficit disorders and comorbidities in children, adolescents, and adults* (pp. 125–170). Washington, DC: American Psychiatric Press.

Tarver-Behring, S., Barkley, R. A., & Karlsson, J. (1985). The mother–child interactions of hyperactive boys and their normal siblings. *American Journal of Orthopsychiatry, 55*, 202–209.

Taylor, E. A. (1983). Drug response and diagnostic validation. In M. Rutter (Ed.), *Developmental neuropsychiatry* (pp. 348–368). New York: Guilford Press.

Taylor, E. A., Sandberg, S., Thorley, G., & Giles, S. (1991). *The epidemiology of childhood hyperactivity.* London: Oxford University Press.

Todd, R. D., Rasmussen, E. R., Wood, C., Levy, F., & Hay, D. A. (2004). Should sluggish cognitive tempo symptoms be included in the diagnosis of attention-deficit/hyperactivity disorder? *Journal of the American Academy of Child and Adolescent Psychiatry, 43*, 588–597.

Treuting, J. J., & Hinshaw, S. P. (2001). Depression and self-esteem in boys with attention-deficit/hyperactivity disorder: Associations with comorbid aggression and explanatory attributional mechanisms. *Journal of Abnormal Child Psychology, 29*, 23–39.

Ullmann, R. K., & Sleator, E. K. (1985). Attention deficit disorder children with and without hyperactivity: Which behaviors are helped by stimulants? *Clinical Pediatrics, 24*, 547–551.

Unnever, J. D., & Cornell, D. G. (2003). Bullying, self-control, and ADHD. *Journal of Interpersonal Violence, 18*, 129–147.

Voelker, S. L., Lachar, D., & Gdowski, C. L. (1983). The Personality Inventory for Children and response to methylphenidate: Preliminary evidence for predictive validity. *Journal of Pediatric Psychology, 8*, 161–169.

Waschbusch, D. A. (2002). A meta-analytic examination of comorbid hyperactive–impulsive–attention problems and conduct problems. *Psychological Bulletin, 128*, 118–150.

Waschbusch, D. A., Pelham, W. E., Jennings, J. R., Greiner, A. R., Tarter, R. E., & Moss, H. B. (2002). Reactive aggression in boys with disruptive behavior disorders: Behavior, physiology, and affect. *Journal of Abnormal Child Psychology, 30*, 641–656.

Walker, J. L., Lahey, B. B., Hynd, G. W., & Frame, C. (1987). Comparison of specific patterns of antisocial behavior in children with conduct disorder with and without coexisting hyperactivity. *Journal of Consulting and Clinical Psychology, 55*, 910–913.

Weinstein, C. S., Apfel, R. J., & Weinstein, S. R. (1998). Description of mothers with ADHD with children with ADHD. *Psychiatry, 61*, 12–19.

Weinstein, D., Steffelbach, D., & Biaggio, M. (2000). Attention-deficit hyperactivity disorder and posttraumatic stress disorder: Differential diagnosis in childhood sexual abuse. *Clinical Psychology Review, 20*, 359–378.

Weiss, G., & Hechtman, L. (1993). *Hyperactive children grown up* (2nd ed.). New York: Guilford Press.

Weiss, G., Hechtman, L., & Perlman, T. (1978). Psychiatric status of hyperactives as adults: School, employer, and self-rating scales obtained during ten-year follow-up evaluation. *American Journal of Orthopsychiatry, 48*, 438–445.

Welner, Z., Welner, A., Stewart, M., Palkes, H., & Wish, E. (1977). A controlled study of siblings of hyperactive children. *Journal of Nervous and Mental Disease, 165*, 110–117.

Werry, J. S. (1988). Differential diagnosis of attention deficits and conduct disorders. In L. Bloomingdale & J. Sergeant (Eds.), *Attention deficit disorder: Criteria, cognition, intervention* (pp. 83–96). New York: Pergamon Press.

Whalen, C. K., Henker, B., Collins, B. E., Finck, D., & Dotemoto, S. (1979). A social ecology of hyperactive boys: Medication effects in systematically structured classroom environments. *Journal of Applied Behavior Analysis, 12,* 65–81.

Whalen, C. K., Henker, B., Collins, B. E., McAuliffe, S., & Vaux, A. (1979). Peer interaction in structured communication task: Comparisons of normal and hyperactive boys and of methylphenidate (Ritalin) and placebo effects. *Child Development, 50,* 388–401.

Whalen, C. K., Henker, B., & Dotemoto, S. (1980). Methylphenidate and hyperactivity: Effects on teacher behaviors. *Science, 208,* 1280–1282.

Wheeler, J., & Carlson, C. L. (1994). The social functioning of children with ADD with hyperactivity and ADD without hyperactivity: A comparison of their peer relations and social deficits. *Journal of Emotional and Behavioral Disorders, 2,* 2–12.

Wilens, T. E., Biederman, J., Brown, S., Tanguay, S., Monuteaux, M. C., Blake, C., et al. (2002). Psychiatric comorbidity and functioning in clinically-referred preschool children and school-age youth with ADHD. *Journal of the American Academy of Child and Adolescent Psychiatry, 41,* 262–268.

Willcutt, E. G., Pennington, B. F., Chhabildas, N. A., Friedman, M. C., & Alexander, J. (1999). Psychiatric comorbidity associated with DSM-IV ADHD in a nonreferred sample of twins. *Journal of the American Academy of Child and Adolescent Psychiatry, 38,* 1355–1362.

Woodward, L., Taylor, E., & Dowdney, L. (1998). The parenting and family functioning of children with hyperactivity. *Journal of Child Psychology and Psychiatry, 39,* 161–169.

Wozniak, J., Biederman, J., Kiely, K., Ablon, S., Faraone, S. V., Mundy, E., et al. (1995). Mania-like symptoms suggestive of childhood-onset bipolar disorder in clinically referred children. *Journal of the American Academy of Child and Adolescent Psychiatry, 34,* 867–876.

Wozniak, J., Harding-Crawford, M., Biederman, J., Faraone, S. V., Spencer, T. J., Taylor, A., et al. (1999). Antecedents and complications of trauma in boys with ADHD: Findings from a longitudinal study. *Journal of the American Academy of Child and Adolescent Psychiatry, 38,* 48–55.

Zentall, S. S., Cassady, J. C., & Javorsky, J. (2001). Social comprehension of children with hyperactivity. *Journal of Attention Disorders, 5,* 11–24.

Etiologies

RUSSELL A. BARKLEY

Considerable research has accumulated on various etiologies for Attention-Deficit/Hyperactivity Disorder (ADHD) since the preceding edition of this text. Despite some inconsistencies across studies, labs, samples, and measures, broad conclusions are now possible about the causes of ADHD. There is even less doubt now among senior investigators in this field than there was at the time of the preceding edition that although multiple etiologies may lead to ADHD, evidence points to neurological and genetic factors as the greatest contributors to this disorder. Our knowledge of the final common neurological pathway through which these factors produce their effects on behavior has been further increased by converging lines of evidence from cerebral blood flow studies; studies of brain electrical activity using computer-averaging techniques; studies using neuropsychological tests sensitive to frontal lobe dysfunction (see Chapter 3); and neuroimaging studies using positron emission tomography (PET), magnetic resonance imaging (MRI), and functional MRI (fMRI). Neurochemical abnormalities that may underlie ADHD have still proven extremely difficult to document with any certainty, though some inferences about them are possible from some research results and from the medications that appear to be of

most benefit for the disorder (dopamine and norepinephrine reuptake inhibitors and agonists; see Chapters 17–19, 22). Even so, evidence is converging on a probable neurological network for ADHD. As much or more research has also occurred on the genetics of ADHD, and the two disciplines are beginning to converge in studies that combine their methods to examine the effects of particular genes (allele polymorphisms) on particular brain structures and their functioning.

Just as important is the fact that in the past decade, no credible social-environmental theory or even hypothesis concerning causation in ADHD has been developed that either is consistent with the known scientific findings on the disorder, or has any explanatory or predictive value for understanding the disorder and driving further scientific research in testing it (i.e., falsifiability). And given what is now known, nor could there be, because studies of twins and families have made it abundantly clear that the majority of variation in the behavioral traits constituting ADHD is the result of genetic factors. What little variation remains is best explained by unique events that befall the individual child, often prenatally, and are not shared by other family members. Those events include biological (nongenetic) hazards that cause neurological injury, such as alcohol and tobacco exposure during pregnancy, premature delivery (especially with minor brain hemorrhaging), early lead poisoning, stroke, and frank brain trauma, to name just a few. We are very near to reaching the time when we can conclude unequivocally that ADHD cannot and does not arise from purely social factors, such as child rearing, family conflict, marital/couple difficulties, insecure infant attachment, television or video games, the pace of modern life, or interactions with peers. This is not to say that such social factors may not have some influence on these children, and particularly on the extent and diversity of impairments the children may experience or their risk for developing comorbid disorders, such as Major Depressive Disorder (MDD), anxiety disorders, Oppositional Defiant Disorder (ODD) and Conduct Disorder (CD). Evidence suggests some role for the social environment in the onset, course, and severity of those comorbid conditions. But the prevailing evidence makes it clear that those social factors do not create ADHD or contribute through some social mechanism to causing this disorder.

NEUROLOGICAL FACTORS

Various etiologies have been proposed for ADHD. Brain damage was initially proposed as a chief cause of ADHD symptoms (see Chapter 1); such damage was thought to result from known brain infections, trauma, or other injuries or complications occurring during pregnancy or at the time of delivery. Several studies show that brain damage, particularly hypoxic/anoxic types of insults, is indeed associated with greater attention deficits and hyperactivity (Cruickshank, Eliason, & Merrifield, 1988; O'Dougherty, Nuechterlein, & Drew, 1984). ADHD symptoms also occur more often in children with seizure disorders (Hesdorffer et al., 2004; Holdsworth & Whitmore, 1974) and with focal stroke to the putamen (Max et al., 2002). However, most children with ADHD have no history of significant brain injuries, and such injuries are unlikely to account for the majority of children with this condition (Rutter, 1977, 1983).

Throughout the 20th century, investigators repeatedly noted the similarities between symptoms of ADHD and those produced by lesions or injuries to the frontal lobes more generally

and the prefrontal cortex specifically (Benton, 1991; Heilman, Voeller, & Nadeau, 1991; Levin, 1938; Mattes, 1980; see Chapter 1). Both children and adults suffering injuries to the prefrontal region demonstrate deficits in sustained attention, inhibition, regulation of emotion and motivation, and the capacity to organize behavior across time (Fuster, 1997; Grattan & Eslinger, 1991; Stuss & Benson, 1986). Evidence continues to mount that ADHD is associated, at least in part, with structural and/or functional differences from normal in the frontal lobes, basal ganglia, and cerebellum, and possibly the anterior cingulate.

Neuropsychological Studies

Much of the neuropsychological evidence pertaining to ADHD has been reviewed in Chapters 2 and 3. A large number of studies have used neuropsychological tests of frontal lobe functions; indeed, this number has nearly doubled since the preceding edition of this text. These studies, as noted earlier, have often found deficits on tests believed to assess executive functioning and, by inference, the structures contributing to it (frontal lobes, basal ganglia, and cerebellum) (Barkley, 1997; Bradley & Golden, 2001; Frazier, Demaree, & Youngstrom, 2004; Hendren, De Backer, & Pandina, 2000; Hervey, Epstein, & Curry, 2004; Tannock, 1998). When consistent, the results of these tests suggest that disinhibition of behavioral responses is evident, in addition to difficulties with working memory, planning, verbal fluency, behavioral timing, motor coordination and sequencing, and other frontal–striatal–cerebellar functions. Adults with ADHD display similar deficits on neuropsychological tests of executive functions (Hervey et al., 2004; Seidman, 1997). Moreover, research shows that not only do the siblings of children with ADHD who also have ADHD show similar executive function deficits, but even those siblings who do not actually manifest ADHD appear to have milder yet significant impairments in these same executive functions (Seidman, 1997; Seidman, Biederman, Faraone, Weber, & Ouellette, 1997). Such findings imply a possible genetically linked risk for executive function deficits in families that have ADHD in their children, even if symptoms of ADHD are not fully manifested in some family members. Evidence does suggest that the executive deficits in ADHD arise from the same substantial shared genetic liability as do the ADHD symptoms themselves (Coolidge, Thede, & Young, 2000).

Neurological Studies

It is only within the past two decades that more direct research findings pertaining to neurological integrity in ADHD have increasingly supported the view of a neurodevelopmental origin for the disorder. Studies using *psychophysiological measures* of nervous system (central and autonomic) electrical activity, variously measured (electroencephalograms [EEGs], galvanic skin responses, heart rate deceleration, etc.), have been inconsistent in demonstrating group differences between children with ADHD and control children. But when differences from controls are found, they are consistently in the direction of diminished arousal or reactive arousal in those with ADHD (for reviews, see Ferguson & Pappas, 1979; Hastings & Barkley, 1978; Rosenthal & Allen, 1978; Ross & Ross, 1982). Such findings have been evident in more recent research as well (Borger & van der Meere, 2000; Beauchaine et al., 2001; Herpertz et al., 2001) and may point to impaired right prefrontal mechanisms underlying response inhibition (Pliszka, Liotti, & Woldorff, 2000).

Far more consistent are the results of quantitative EEG (QEEG) and evoked response potential (ERP) measures, often taken in conjunction with performance on vigilance tests (El-Sayed, Larsson, Persson, & Rydelius, 2002; Frank, Lazar, & Seiden, 1992; Johnstone, Barry, & Anderson, 2001; Klorman et al., 1988; Monastra, Lubar et al., 1999; see Loo & Barkley, in press, for a recent review). Subtype differences in ERPs may also exist, but this issue requires more extensive research (Johnstone et al., 2001). Although results have varied substantially across these studies (see Tannock, 1998, for a review), the most consistent pattern for QEEG research is increased slow-wave or theta activity, particularly in the frontal lobe, and decreased beta activity (Baving, Laucht, & Schmidt, 1999; Chabot & Serfontein, 1996; Kuperman, Johnson, Arndt, Lindgren, & Wolraich, 1996; Loo & Barkley, in press; Mann, Lubar, Zimmerman, Miller, & Muenchen, 1992; Matsuura et al., 1993; Monastra, Lubar, & Linden, 2001). Children with ADHD have been found to have smaller amplitudes in the late positive components of

their ERPs. These late components are believed to be a function of the prefrontal regions of the brain, are related to poorer performances on vigilance tests, and are corrected by stimulant medication (Johnstone et al., 2001; Klorman et al., 1988; Kuperman et al., 1996; Pliszka et al., 2000). The EEG improvements from stimulant medication have been recently shown to be partly a function of the DAT1 gene allele, particularly in its 10-repeat form (Loo et al., 2003), which some studies suggest may be overrepresented in some forms of ADHD (Levy & Hay, 2001). Thus, although the evidence is far from conclusive, evoked response patterns related to sustained attention and inhibition suggest that children with ADHD have an underresponsiveness to stimulation that can be corrected by stimulant medication.

Several studies have examined cerebral blood flow using single-photon emission computed tomography (SPECT) in children with ADHD and nondisabled children (see Hendren et al., 2000, for a review). These studies have consistently shown decreased blood flow to the prefrontal regions (particularly in the right frontal area) and pathways connecting these regions to the limbic system via the striatum—specifically, its anterior region known as the caudate—and to the cerebellum (Lou, Henriksen, & Bruhn, 1984, 1990; Lou, Henriksen, Bruhn, Borner, & Nielsen, 1989; Sieg, Gaffney, Preston, & Hellings, 1995). Degree of blood flow in the right frontal region has been correlated with behavioral severity of the disorder and with reduced EEG activity, while that in more posterior regions and the cerebellum seems related to degree of motor impairment (Gustafsson, Thernlund, Ryding, Rosen, & Cederblad, 2000). Blood flow in these regions appears to be affected by methylphenidate, a stimulant often used to treat ADHD (Langleben et al., 2002).

Studies using PET to assess cerebral glucose metabolism have found diminished metabolism in adults with ADHD, particularly in the frontal region (Schweitzer et al., 2000; Zametkin et al., 1990) but have been far less consistent with teens and children (for reviews, see Ernst, 1996, and Tannock, 1998; see also Ernst, Cohen, Liebenauer, Jons, & Zametkin, 1997; Ernst et al., 1994; Zametkin et al., 1993). Using a radioactive tracer that indicates dopamine activity, Ernst et al. (1999) were able to show abnormal dopamine activity in the right midbrain region of children with ADHD; the severity of symptoms was correlated with the degree of this abnormality. Ernst et al. (2003) later studied adults with ADHD during a decision-making task, and found them to be less likely to activate the hippocampal and insular regions and more likely to use the right anterior cingulate than healthy controls. These demonstrations of an association between the metabolic activity of certain brain regions on the one hand, and symptoms of ADHD and associated executive deficits on the other, are critical to proving a connection between the findings pertaining to brain activation and the behaviors constituting ADHD.

Very early studies of the gross structure of the brain as portrayed by computed tomography (CT) did not show differences between children with ADHD and nondisabled children (B. A. Shaywitz, Shaywitz, Byrne, Cohen, & Rothman, 1983), but greater brain atrophy was found in adults with ADHD who had a history of substance abuse (Nasrallah et al., 1986). The substance abuse, however, seems more likely to account for the latter results than does the ADHD.

Studies using MRI and its greater resolution of brain structure than CT often find differences in the structure (mainly size) of selected brain regions in those with ADHD relative to control groups (Tannock, 1998). Initial studies by Hynd and colleagues examined the region of the left and right temporal lobes associated with auditory detection and analysis (planum temporale) in children with ADHD, learning disabilities (LDs, in reading), or no disability. For some time, researchers studying reading disorders have focused on these brain regions, given their connection to the analysis of speech sounds. Both the children with ADHD and those with LDs were found to have smaller right-hemisphere plana temporale than the control group, whereas only those with LDs had smaller left plana temporale (Hynd, Semrud-Clikeman, Lorys, Novey, & Eliopulos, 1990). In the next study, the corpus callosum was examined in those with ADHD. This structure assists with the interhemispheric transfer of information. Those with ADHD were found to have a smaller callosum, particularly in the area of the genu and splenium and that region just anterior to the splenium (Hynd et al., 1991). An attempt to replicate this finding, however, failed to show any differences between children with ADHD and control children in the size or shape of the entire corpus

callosum, with the exception of the region of the splenium (posterior portion), which again was significantly smaller in the subjects with ADHD (Semrud-Clikeman et al., 1994).

Later studies have indicated significantly smaller anterior right frontal regions, smaller size of the caudate nucleus, possibly reversed asymmetry in the size of the head of the striatum (caudate), and smaller globus pallidus regions in children with ADHD compared to control subjects (Aylward et al., 1996; Castellanos et al., 1994, 2002; Filipek et al., 1997; Hendren et al., 2000; Hynd et al., 1993; Singer et al., 1993). The putamen, however, has not been found to be smaller in children with ADHD (Aylward et al., 1996; Castellanos et al., 1996; Singer et al., 1993). Besides reduced size, there is some evidence of reduced neurometabolite activity in the right frontal region (Yeo et al., 2003), with the degree of this activity being associated with degree of attention problems on a continuous-performance test. The size of the basal ganglia and right frontal lobe has been shown in other studies as well to correlate with the degree of impairment in inhibition and attention in children having ADHD (Casey et al., 1997; Semrud-Clikeman et al., 2000). The study by Filipek et al. (1997) did find smaller posterior volumes of white matter in both hemispheres in the regions of the parietal and occipital lobes, which might be consistent with the earlier studies showing smaller volumes of the corpus callosum in this same area. Castellanos et al. (1996) suggest that such differences in corpus callosal volume, particularly in the posterior regions, may be more closely related to LDs (which are often found in a large minority of children with ADHD) than to ADHD itself.

Numerous studies (Castellanos et al., 1996, 2001, 2002; Durston et al., 2004) have also found smaller cerebellar volume in those with ADHD, especially in a central region known as the vermis. This would be consistent with the view that the cerebellum plays a major role in executive functioning and the motor-presetting aspects of sensory perception that derive from planning and other executive actions (Akshoomoff & Courchesne, 1992; Diamond, 2000; Houk & Wise, 1995), and that these functions may be deficient in children with ADHD.

The results for the smaller size of the caudate nucleus are quite consistent across studies, but are inconsistent in indicating which side of the caudate may be smaller. The work by Hynd et al. (1993), discussed earlier, found the left caudate to be smaller than normal in subjects with ADHD. The study by Filipek et al. (1997) found the same result. However, Castellanos et al. (1996) also reported a smaller caudate, but found this to be on the right side. The typical human brain is believed to demonstrate a relatively consistent asymmetry in volume, in favor of the right frontal cortical region's being larger than the left (Giedd et al., 1996). This led Castellanos et al. (1996) to conclude that a lack of frontal asymmetry (a smaller-than-normal right frontal region) probably mediates the expression of ADHD. However, whether this asymmetry of the caudate (right side > left side) is actually true of nondisabled individuals is debatable, as other studies found the opposite pattern in their nondisabled control subjects (Filipek et al., 1997; Hynd et al., 1993). As Filipek and colleagues noted, many of these differences in the findings of studies regarding which side of the caudate is more affected in subjects with ADHD could readily be explained by subject and procedural differences, as well as by differences in defining the boundaries of the caudate. More consistent across these studies are the findings of smaller right prefrontal cortical regions and smaller caudate volume, regardless of whether it is more on the right than the left side.

Studies using fMRI find children with ADHD and nondisabled children to have differing patterns of activation during attention and inhibition tasks, particularly in the right prefrontal region, the basal ganglia (striatum, globus pallidus, and putamen), and the cerebellum (Rubia et al., 1999; Teicher et al., 2000; Vaidya et al., 1998; Yeo et al., 2003). Again, the demonstrated linkage of brain structure and function with psychological measures of ADHD symptoms and executive deficits is exceptionally important in such research, to permit causal inferences to be made about the role of these brain abnormalities in the cognitive and behavioral deficits constituting ADHD. A recent study (Durston et al., 2004) suggests that the reduced size of the brain (by about 3–5%), particularly in the right frontal area, found in children with ADHD may be evident as well in their siblings without ADHD; perhaps this is consistent with the increased familial risk for the disorder and a spectrum of the phenotype for ADHD within these families. But the reduced volume of the cerebellum was also found to be specific only to the children with ADHD and was not evident in the unaffected siblings, implying that this region may be directly related to the pathophysiology of the disorder itself.

Others reviewing this literature over the last two decades have reached similar conclusions—namely, that abnormalities in the development of the frontal–striatal–cerebellar regions probably underlie the development of ADHD (Arnsten, Steere, & Hunt, 1996; Benton, 1991; Gualtieri & Hicks, 1985; Hendren et al., 2000; Mattes, 1980; Mercugliano, 1995; Pontius, 1973; Tannock, 1998). These regions are shown in Figure 5.1.

Neurotransmitter Deficiencies

Possible neurotransmitter dysfunction or imbalances have been proposed, resting chiefly on the responses of children with ADHD to dopamine and norepinephrine reuptake inhibitors and agonists (see Pliszka, McCracken, & Maas, 1996, for a review). Given the findings that nondisabled children show a positive, albeit lesser, response to stimulants (Rapoport et al., 1978), evidence from drug responding by itself cannot be used to support a neurochemical abnormality in ADHD. However, some direct evidence from studies of cerebral spinal fluid indicates decreased brain dopamine in children with ADHD compared to nondisabled children (Halperin et al., 1997; Raskin, Shaywitz, Shaywitz, Anderson, & Cohen, 1984). Evidence from other studies using blood and urinary metabolites of brain neurotransmitters have proven conflicting in their results (S. E. Shaywitz, Shaywitz, Cohen, & Young, 1983; S. E. Shaywitz et al., 1986; Zametkin & Rapoport, 1986). What limited evidence there is seems to point to a selective deficiency in the availability of both dopamine and norepinephrine, but this evidence cannot be considered conclusive at this time.

Although direct evidence for neurotransmitter difficulties' being associated with ADHD in children has proven inconclusive, results from animal research and that on typical humans suggests that they may be involved in ADHD. Sagvolden, Johansen, Aase, and Russell (in press) have recently proposed a dynamic neurodevelopmental theory of ADHD (Combined and Predominantly Hyperactive–Impulsive Types) based on altered dopamine function, that can arise from hypofunctioning in

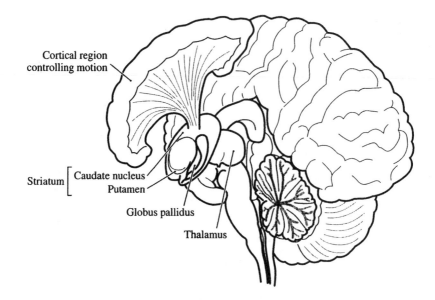

FIGURE 5.1. Diagram of the human brain showing the right hemisphere, and particularly the location of the striatum, globus pallidus, and thalamus. Most of the left hemisphere has been cut away up to the prefrontal lobes to reveal the striatum and other midbrain structures. Adapted with permission from an illustration by Carol Donner from page 53 of the article by M. B. H. Youdin & P. Riederer (1997). Understanding Parkinson's disease. *Scientific American, 276* (January), pp. 52–59. Copyright by *Scientific American*, 415 Madison Avenue, New York, NY 10017-1111.

one of three dopamine branches identified in the brain. Low functioning in a mesolimbic pathway in the brain produces an altered sensitivity to reinforcement and deficient extinction of previously reinforced behavior, which could give rise to the delay aversion, hyperactivity, impulsivity, and poor sustained attention. Low functioning in the mesocortical dopamine pathway could also give rise to deficient attention toward a target, as well as to poor planning and executive functioning. Finally, low functioning in the nigral–striatal dopamine pathway results in impaired modulation of motor behavior and deficient learning and memory, which could give rise to the motor delay, clumsiness, and poor motor inhibition seen in ADHD. Predispositions to low functioning in these dopamine pathways are hypothesized to interact with each other and with surrounding environmental factors to amplify or alter these initial predispositions. The theory provides a more comprehensive explanation of symptoms and deficits associated with ADHD (see Chapters 2 and 3), while generating some testable hypotheses concerning which of these should be associated with hypofunctioning in particular pathways. Future research is clearly in order

before this innovative attempt to account for ADHD via these neurotransmitter pathways can be properly evaluated, however.

Pregnancy and Birth Complications

Pregnancy and birth complications are of interest to researchers in ADHD because they can have a detrimental effect on brain development. Some studies have not found a greater incidence of such complications in children with ADHD than in nondisabled children (Barkley, DuPaul, & McMurray, 1990). But others clearly have. For instance, Claycomb, Ryan, Miller, and Schnakenberg-Ott (2004) found that mother's age at delivery (younger), educational level (lower), time between onset of labor and birth (longer), and presence of delivery complications accounted for 42% of the variance in ADHD. The study, however, did not control for maternal ADHD symptoms, which may have resulted in the younger age at delivery and lower educational level of the mothers. The latter maternal characteristics may simply be markers for maternal ADHD, and so may explain their being associated with the children's ADHD.

Others have found a slightly higher prevalence of unusually short or long labor, fetal distress, forceps delivery, and toxemia or eclampsia (Hartsough & Lambert, 1985; Minde, Webb, & Sykes, 1968). Nichols and Chen (1981) found that low birth weight was associated with an increased risk of hyperactivity, inattention, disruptive behavior, and poor school adjustment. These results have been subsequently replicated (Breslau et al., 1996; Schothorst & van Engeland, 1996; Sykes et al., 1997; Szatmari, Saigal, Rosenbaum, & Campbell, 1993). After controlling for other factors that might be associated with low birth weight and ADHD (maternal smoking, alcohol use, ADHD, socioeconomic status [SES], etc.), Mick, Biederman, Faraone, Sayer, and Kleinman (2002) continued to find low birth weight to be three times more common in children with ADHD than in control children, perhaps accounting for nearly 14% of all ADHD cases. It is not merely low birth weight that seems to pose the risk for symptoms of ADHD or the disorder itself (among other psychiatric disorders), but the extent of white matter abnormalities due to birth injuries, such as parenchymal lesions and/or ventricular enlargement (Whittaker et al., 1997).

In one very unusual study, Sharp et al. (2003) studied possible environmental contributions to ADHD by identifying monozygotic (MZ) twins in which only one twin was affected by ADHD. Given the striking genetic contribution to ADHD and the very high concordance rate for it in MZ twin pairs, such a study might find it difficult to find MZ twin pairs in which only one twin was affected. This was precisely the case, in that out of 297 pairs initially screened for the study, just 10 pairs were eventually found in which the twins were discordant for the disorder. Consistent with the authors' hypothesis that the affected twin would be more likely to have birth complications (a nongenetic explanation for the twins' discordance on ADHD), the study found that the affected twin was smaller at birth and more likely to have experienced a breech delivery.

Several studies suggest that mothers of children with ADHD conceive these children at a younger age than that of mothers of control children, and that such pregnancies may have a greater risk of adversity (Claycomb et al., 2004; Denson, Nanson, & McWatters, 1975; Hartsough & Lambert, 1985; Minde et al., 1968). Because pregnancy complications are more likely to occur among young mothers, mothers of children with ADHD may have a higher risk for such complications, which may act neurologically to predispose their children toward ADHD. However, the complications that have been noted to date are rather mild and hardly compelling evidence of pre- or perinatal brain damage as a cause of ADHD. Furthermore, large-scale epidemiological studies have generally not found a strong association between pre- or perinatal adversity and symptoms of ADHD once other factors are taken into account, such as maternal smoking and alcohol use (see later) as well as low SES, all of which may predispose to perinatal adversity and hyperactivity (Goodman & Stevenson, 1989; Nichols & Chen, 1981; Werner et al., 1968).

Stress during pregnancy has also been examined in a few studies, and their results have been inconclusive. They suggest a modest contribution of stress to ADHD symptoms in the offspring of these pregnancies, but this finding is hardly definitive, given the many methodological problems evident to date (for a review, see Linnet et al., 2003). For instance, Van den Bergh and Marcoen (2004) evaluated mothers and their firstborn children and found that maternal state anxiety during pregnancy explained 22% of the variance in symptoms of ADHD in the offspring of the pregnancy, with anxiety during the 12th to 22nd week being specifically implicated. Such stress may result in some programming effect on the fetal brain. Nevertheless, neither the parents nor the children had clinically diagnosed ADHD; no attempt was made to control for maternal ADHD and its genetic contribution to level of child ADHD; and no evidence of actual neural programming was evaluated in the study. Therefore, the results remain merely correlational—suggesting some association of maternal anxiety to child ADHD, but not clarifying what the direction of effect might be or whether the presence of a third variable explains (confounds) these results.

One study found that the season of a child's birth was significantly associated with risk for ADHD, at least among those subgroups that also had either LDs or no psychiatric comorbidity (Mick, Biederman, & Faraone, 1996). Birth in September was overrepresented in these subgroups of children with ADHD. The authors conjecture that the season of birth may serve as a proxy for the timing of seasonally mediated viral infections to which these mothers and their fetuses may have been exposed, and that such infections may account for approximately 10% of cases of ADHD.

GENETIC FACTORS

No evidence exists to show that ADHD is the result of abnormal chromosomal structures (as in Down syndrome), their fragility (as in fragile X or transmutations), or extra chromosomal material (as in XXY syndrome). Children with such chromosomal abnormalities may show greater problems with attention, but such abnormalities are very uncommon in children with ADHD. By far the greatest research evidence suggests that ADHD is highly hereditary in nature, making heredity one of the best-substantiated etiologies for ADHD.

Family Aggregation Studies

Multiple lines of research support such a conclusion. For years, researchers have noted the higher prevalence of psychopathology in the parents and other relatives of children with ADHD. In particular, higher rates of ADHD, conduct problems, substance abuse, and depression have been repeatedly observed in these studies (Barkley et al., 1990; Biederman et al., 1992; Pauls, 1991). Research shows that between 10% and 35% of the immediate family members of children with ADHD are also likely to have the disorder, with the risk to siblings of these children being approximately 32% (Biederman et al., 1992; Biederman, Keenan, & Faraone, 1990; Levy & Hay, 2001; Welner, Welner, Stewart, Palkes, & Wish, 1977). Higher-than-expected rates of family aggregation of the disorder have been found in African American families, similar to rates reported in families of European American children (Samuel et al., 1997). And these higher rates are as evident in the families of girls as of boys with ADHD (Faraone et al., 2000; Faraone & Doyle, 2001). Even more striking is the finding that if a parent has ADHD, the risk to the offspring is 57% (Biederman et al., 1995). Further evidence for the familial clustering of ADHD in families of affected children came from a study by Smalley et al. (2000), in which they identified families having at least two affected children with ADHD (n = 132).

They then assessed the 256 parents in these families for various psychiatric disorders and found that 55% of the families had at least one parent with a lifetime diagnosis of ADHD. Thus ADHD clusters far more than would be expected from the base rate of the disorder among biological relatives of children or adults with the disorder, strongly implying a hereditary basis to this condition.

Interestingly, research by Faraone and Biederman (1997) at Massachusetts General Hospital suggests that MDD among family members of children with ADHD may be a nonspecific expression of the same genetic contribution that is related to ADHD. This is based on their findings that family members of children with ADHD are at increased risk for MDD, whereas individuals who have MDD have first-degree relatives at increased risk for ADHD.

Some research suggests that ADHD with CD may be a distinct familial subtype of ADHD (Faraone, Biederman, Mennin, Russell, & Tsuang, 1998). Using sibling pairs in which both siblings had ADHD, Smalley et al. (2000) have also recently supported this view through findings that CD significantly clusters among the families of only those sib-pairs having CD. And another study has likewise supported this view by finding that while ADHD and ODD/CD have a shared genetic contribution, there are additional unique genetic contributions to ODD/CD (Nadder, Rutter, Silberg, Maes, & Eaves, 2002).

Some research has also suggested that females who manifest ADHD may need to have a greater genetic loading (higher family member prevalence) than do males with ADHD in order to express the disorder (Smalley et al., 2000; Faraone & Doyle, 2001). Further research using twins (described below) supports this view, in finding that females appear to have a higher threshold for expression of the disorder than do males with ADHD (Rhee, Waldman, Hay, & Levy, 1999).

Adoption Research

Another line of evidence for genetic involvement in ADHD has emerged from studies of adopted children. Cantwell (1975) and Morrison and Stewart (1973) both reported higher rates of hyperactivity in the biological parents of hyperactive children than in the adoptive parents of such children. Both studies suggest that hyperactive children are more likely to resemble their biological parents than their adoptive parents in their levels of hyperactivity. Yet both studies were retrospective, and both failed to study the biological parents of the adopted hyperactive children as a comparison group (Pauls, 1991). Cadoret and Stewart (1991) studied 283 male adoptees and found that if one of the biological parents had been judged delinquent or to have an adult criminal conviction, the adopted-away sons had a higher likelihood of having ADHD. A later study (van den Oord, Boomsma, & Verhulst, 1994), using biologically related and unrelated pairs of international adoptees, identified a strong genetic component (47% of the variance) in scores on the Attention Problems dimension of the Child Behavior Checklist—a rating scale commonly used in research in child psychopathology. This particular scale has a strong association with (but is certainly not equivalent to) a diagnosis of ADHD (Biederman, Milberger, Faraone, Guite, & Warburton, 1994), and it is often used in research to select subjects with the disorder. A more recent study by Sprich, Biederman, Crawford, Mundy, and Faraone (2000) compared the rates of ADHD in the first-degree adoptive relatives of 25 adopted children with ADHD, compared to the relatives of nonadopted children with ADHD and to those of nonadopted control children with ADHD. They found that just 6% of the relatives of the adopted children with ADHD had ADHD—a figure very close to the prevalence of ADHD in adults in the population (see Chapter 2)—suggesting that the children's ADHD did not arise from family environmental transmission. However, families of the nonadopted ADHD children had 18% of their relatives diagnosed with ADHD, compared to 3% for the control group. Thus, like the family association studies discussed earlier, these adoption studies point to a strong possibility of a significant hereditary contribution to hyperactivity or ADHD.

Twin Studies

Studies of twins provide a third avenue of evidence for a genetic contribution to ADHD. The evidence is both substantial in scope and striking in the magnitude of the genetic role in this disorder. Early studies demonstrated a greater agreement (concordance) for symptoms of hyperactivity and inattention between MZ twins than between dizygotic (DZ) twins (Goodman & Stevenson, 1989; O'Connor, Foch, Sherry, & Plomin, 1980; Willerman, 1973). Studies of very small samples of twins (Heffron, Martin, & Welsh, 1984; Lopez, 1965) found complete (100%) concordance for MZ twins for hyperactivity, and far less agreement for DZ twins. Other large-scale twin studies are also quite consistent with these findings (Edelbrock, Rende, Plomin, & Thompson, 1995; Gillis, Gilger, Pennington, & DeFries, 1992; Levy & Hay, 1992, 2001; Thapar, Holmes, Poulton, & Harrington, 1999). For instance, Gilger, Pennington, and DeFries (1992) found that if one twin was diagnosed as having ADHD, the concordance for the disorder was 81% in MZ twins and 29% in DZ twins. Sherman, McGue, and Iacono (1997) found that the concordance for MZ twins having ADHD (mother-identified) was 67%, versus 0% for DZ twins. Stevenson (1994) summarized the status of twin studies on symptoms of ADHD up to that time by stating that the average heritability is .80 for symptoms of this disorder (range .50–.98).

Numerous large-scale twin studies subsequently conducted have been remarkably consistent with this conclusion, demonstrating that the majority of variance (70–95%) in the traits of ADHD is a result of genetic factors (averaging approximately 80%+), and that such a genetic contribution may increase as the scores along this trait become more extreme, although this latter point is debatable (Coolidge et al., 2000; Faraone, 1996; Gjone, Stevenson, & Sundet, 1996; Gjone, Stevenson, Sundet, & Eilertsen, 1996; Hudziak, 1997; Kuntsi & Stevenson, 2000; Levy, Hay, McStephen, Wood, & Waldman, 1997; Nadder et al., 2002; Rhee, Waldman, Hay, & Levy, 1995; Sherman, Iacono, & McGue, 1997; Sherman, McGue, & Iacono, 1997; Silberg et al., 1996; Thapar, Hervas, & McGuffin, 1995; Thapar, Harrington, Ross, & McGuffin, 2000; Todd et al., 2001; van den Oord, Verhulst, & Boomsma, 1996). This remains so even when just attention problems are rated in twin studies by parents (Reitveld, Hudziak, Bartels, van Beijsterveldt, & Boomsma, 2004) or teachers (Groot, de Sonneville, Stins, & Boomsma, 2004). Thus twin studies indicate that the average heritability of ADHD is at least .80–.90 and can be higher than this when clinical diagnostic criteria serve as the basis for determining ADHD (Rhee et al., 1999). This research adds substantially more evidence to that already found in family and adoption studies supporting a strong genetic basis to ADHD and its behavioral symptoms. As noted earlier, some research now suggests that females have a higher threshold than males for expression of the disorder in their phenotype, implying that females must receive a stronger familial genetic contribution before expressing the disorder than in males must. This may well account for the 3:1 male-to-female ratio in ADHD (Rhee et al., 1999).

But twin studies can also tell us as much about environmental contributions as they do about genetic factors affecting the expression of a trait (Faraone, 1996; Pike & Plomin, 1996; Plomin, 1995). Across the twin studies conducted to date, the results have been reasonably consistent in demonstrating that the shared environment contributes little, if any, explanation to individual differences in the traits underlying ADHD (hyperactive–impulsive–inattentive); it accounts for typically 0–13% of the variance among individuals, which is not statistically significant (Levy & Hay, 2001; Levy et al., 1997; Sherman, Iacono, & McGue, 1997; Silberg et al., 1996; Thapar et al., 1999). Similar findings have been noted for other forms of child psychopathology (Pike & Plomin, 1996). Such shared environmental factors include SES and family educational/occupational status, the general home environment, family nutrition, toxins that may be present in the home environment (especially lead), parental and child-rearing characteristics that are common or shared across children in the family, and other such nongenetic factors that are common to the twins under investigation in these studies. In their totality, such shared environmental factors seem to account for 0–6% of individual differences on average in the behavioral trait(s) related to ADHD. It is for this reason that little emphasis is placed here on purely environmental or social factors as involved in the causation of ADHD. The numerous twin studies have not been able to support such common environmental factors as contributing much of significance to individual differences in symptoms of ADHD.

The twin studies cited above have also been able to indicate the extent to which individual differences in ADHD symptoms are the result of nonshared environmental factors. Such factors include not only those typically thought of as involving the social environment, but also all

biological factors that are nongenetic in origin. Factors in the nonshared environment are those events or conditions that will have uniquely affected only one twin and not the other. Besides biological hazards or neurologically injurious events that may have befallen only one member of a twin pair, the nonshared environment also includes those differences in the manner in which parents may have treated each child. Parents do not interact with all their children in an identical fashion, and such unique parent–child interactions are believed to make more of a contribution to individual differences among siblings than factors about the home and child rearing that are common to all children in the family are thought to make. Twin studies to date have suggested that approximately 9–20% of the variance in hyperactive–impulsive–inattentive behaviors or ADHD symptoms can be attributed to such nonshared environmental (nongenetic) factors (Levy & Hay, 2001; Levy et al., 1997; Sherman, Iacono, & McGue, 1997; Silberg et al., 1996; Thapar et al., 1999). Research suggests that the nonshared environmental factors also contribute disproportionately more to individual differences in other forms of child psychopathology than do factors in the shared environment (Pike & Plomin, 1996). Thus, if researchers are interested in identifying environmental contributors to ADHD, these twin studies suggest that such research should focus on those biological, interactional, and social experiences that are specific and unique to the individual, rather than those that are part of the common environment to which other siblings have been exposed.

Molecular Genetic Research

Early quantitative genetic analyses of the large sample of families studied in Boston by Biederman and his colleagues suggested that a single gene may account for the expression of the disorder (Faraone et al., 1992). Later research suggests that more than one gene is highly likely to be involved in the expression of the disorder. Research has focused much attention on dopamine-regulating genes, given the positive response of ADHD cases to dopamine agonists and reuptake inhibitors, as well as the large role of dopamine in the striatum and frontal cortex (two regions implicated in ADHD). At least five different forms of dopamine have been identified in the brain, and five different dopamine receptors (D1–D5) have been identified, each produced by a different gene (Barr, 2001). D1 and D5 receptors are believed to generate stimulatory signals, while D2–D4 receptors are believed to transmit inhibitory signals. The sensitivity of the receptors to dopamine appears to be determined in part by the particular sequence (substitutions, deletions, or more often number of repeats) of the gene, known as a "polymorphism."

The focus of research initially was on the DRD2 gene—that is, the gene for the D2 dopamine receptor. This was based on findings of its increased association with alcoholism, Tourette syndrome, and ADHD (Blum, Cull, Braverman, & Comings, 1996; Comings et al., 1991). But later many others failed to replicate this association of ADHD with DRD2 (Gelernter et al., 1991; Kelsoe et al., 1989; Fisher et al., 2002).

Another gene related to dopamine receptor sensitivity is the gene for the D4 receptor, or DRD4, particularly in its 48-bp form and with 7 or more repeats of it. The number of repeats in humans ranges from 2 to 10 (Barr, 2001). The 7-repeat version of this polymorphism was initially found to be overrepresented in children with ADHD (LaHoste et al., 1996). Such a finding is quite interesting, because this gene was previously associated with the personality trait of high novelty-seeking behavior (though the issue remains arguable). It also affects pharmacological responsiveness, and the gene's impact on postsynaptic sensitivity is primarily found in the frontal and prefrontal cortical regions believed to be associated with executive functions and attention (Barr, 2001; Swanson et al., 1998). The finding of an overrepresentation of the 7-repeat version of the DRD4 48-bp polymorphism has now been replicated in many subsequent studies, using not only children with ADHD, but also adolescents and adults with the disorder (Grady et al., 2003; Swanson et al., 1998; Sonuhara et al., 1997; Faraone et al., 1999; see Faraone, Doyle, Mick, & Biederman, 2001, for a meta-analysis). Approximately 29% of these samples with ADHD seem to have the 7-repeat allele, which may serve as a marker for a more homogeneous phenotype within this population. This is one of the few genes identified so far that has been reliably associated with a sizable subgroup of individuals with ADHD (DiMaio, Grizenko, & Joober, 2003; Faraone et al., 2001). Grady and colleagues (2003) have recently shown that it

may be novel variation (allelic heterogeneity) in the DRD4 7-repeat alleles that contributes to risk for ADHD, rather than the risk arising from just one particular sequence of this allele. Also, this 7-repeat form of the gene has recently been related to greater impulsivity on laboratory measures, as well as higher measured activity levels, in children with ADHD who possessed this form of the gene than in those who did not (Langley et al., 2004).

Two studies suggest that the D5 dopamine receptor gene, DRD5, may have some association with ADHD (Daly, Hawi, Fitzgerald, & Gill, 1999). One of these findings came from the first entire genome-wide scan for genetic loci involved in ADHD (Fisher et al., 2002). This same scan was unable to find an association of DRD4 or DAT1 (see below) with ADHD, buts its sample size was small, thereby limiting its power to detect genes making small contributions to the disorder. It also suggested that the 13p16 region on chromosome 16 may contain a gene or genes associated with ADHD—a finding that continued to hold up when the sample size of affected sibling pairs was increased from 126 to 203 pairs (Smalley et al., 2002). A fascinating finding here is that this same region has been linked in three separate genome-wide scans to autism, implying that one or more genes on this region may create a susceptibility to both disorders (Smalley et al., 2002).

The dopamine transporter gene (DAT1) also has been implicated in a number of studies of ADHD children (Cook et al., 1995; Cook, Stein, & Leventhal, 1997; Daly et al., 1999; Gill, Daly, Heron, Hawi, & Fitzgerald, 1997; Waldman et al., 1998). One study found that a 10-repeat form of this gene may be related to poorer response to methylphenidate (Winsberg & Comings, 1999). That study also found that the DRD2 and DRD4 alleles were not related to drug response. However, here again other laboratories have not been able to replicate this association (Swanson et al., 1997). The gene is believed to be active during fetal brain development and may contribute to the density of dopamine transporters (reuptake mechanisms) on the nerve cell.

More recently, the long polymorphism of the DBH gene (Taq I) has also been implicated in our Milwaukee longitudinal study of hyperactive children followed to adulthood (Mueller et al., 2003). This gene is believed to regulate the extent of dopamine-beta-hydroxylase (a chemical known to contribute to the conversion of dopamine to norepinephrine) in the brain. Two other studies have also suggested that this gene may have a small association with the disorder, and this issue is deserving of further research (Daly et al., 1999; Wigg et al., 2002). Clearly, research into the genetic mechanisms involved in the transmission of ADHD across generations promises to be an exciting and fruitful area of research endeavor over the next decade, as the human genome is further mapped and better understood.

TOXINS

As the twin and quantitative genetic studies suggest, the environment may play some role in individual differences in symptoms of ADHD; however, these may involve biological events, not just family influences or those influences within the psychosocial realm. As noted previously, variance in the expression of ADHD that may be a result of "environmental sources" means all nongenetic sources more generally. These include pre-, peri-, and postnatal complications and malnutrition, as well as diseases, trauma, and other neurologically compromising events that may occur during the development of the nervous system before and after birth. Among these various biologically compromising events, several have been repeatedly linked to risks for inattention and hyperactive behavior.

One such event is exposure to environmental toxins, and especially lead. Elevated body lead burden has been shown to have a small but consistent and statistically significant relationship to the symptoms constituting ADHD (Baloh, Sturm, Green, & Gleser, 1975; David, 1974; de la Burde & Choate, 1972, 1974; Needleman et al., 1979; Needleman, Schell, Bellinger, Leviton, & Alfred, 1990). However, even at relatively high levels of lead, fewer than 38% of children are rated as having the behavior of hyperactivity on a teacher rating scale (Needleman et al., 1979), implying that most lead-poisoned children do not develop symptoms of ADHD. And most children with ADHD, likewise, do not have significantly elevated lead burdens, although one study indicates that their lead levels may be higher than those in control subjects (Gittelman & Eskinazi, 1983). Studies that have controlled for the presence of potentially confounding fac-

tors in this relationship have found the association between body lead (in blood or dentition) and symptoms of ADHD to be .10–.19; the more factors controlled, the more likely the relationship is to fall below .10 (Fergusson, Fergusson, Horwood, & Kinzett, 1988; Silva, Hughes, Williams, & Faed, 1988; Thomson et al., 1989). This finding suggests that no more than 4% (at best) of the variance in the expression of these symptoms in children with elevated lead is explained by their lead levels. Moreover, two serious methodological issues plague even the better-conducted studies in this area:

1. None of the studies used clinical criteria for a diagnosis of ADHD to determine precisely what percentage of lead-burdened children actually had the disorder; all simply used behavior ratings of only a small number of items for inattention or hyperactivity.
2. None of the studies assessed for the presence of ADHD in the parents and controlled its contribution to the relationship. Given the high heritability of ADHD, this factor alone could attenuate the already small correlation between lead and symptoms of ADHD by as much as a third to a half its present levels.

Other types of environmental toxins found to have some relationship to inattention and hyperactivity are prenatal exposures to alcohol and tobacco smoke (Bennett, Wolin, & Reiss, 1988; Denson et al., 1975; Mick et al., 2002; Milberger, Biederman, Faraone, Chen, & Jones, 1996; Nichols & Chen, 1981; S. E. Shaywitz, Cohen, & Shaywitz, 1980; Streissguth et al., 1984; Streissguth, Bookstein, Sampson, & Barr, 1995). The relationship between maternal smoking during pregnancy and ADHD remains significant even after symptoms of ADHD in the mother are controlled for (Mick et al., 2002; Milberger et al., 1996), and maternal smoking shows the strongest association with risk for ADHD; maternal alcohol consumption has been less reliably documented as a risk factor (see Linnet et al., 2003, for a review), but remains impressive (O'Malley & Nanson, 2002).

Recently, elevated levels of phenylalanine in mothers with phenylketonuria have been associated with higher levels of hyperactive–impulsive symptoms in their offspring, whereas when children experienced phenylketonuria it was more likely to be associated with symptoms of inattention (Antshel & Waisbren, 2003). This study implies that phenylalanine may be contributing to some degrees of ADHD in some children, and that the timing of exposure to high levels of phenylalanine affects the two symptom dimensions of ADHD differently.

STREPTOCOCCAL INFECTION

Some research had previously suggested that Obsessive–Compulsive Disorder (OCD) and Tourette syndrome may be sequelae of prior exposure to streptococcal infection (Kiessling, Marcotte, & Culpepper, 1993; Singer et al., 1998). In some individuals, such infections may result in autoimmune system antibodies that cross-react with and compromise neural proteins, particularly in the basal ganglia of the brain. Peterson et al. (2000) examined 105 individuals having OCD, chronic tic disorder, or ADHD, and 37 controls without any disorder. Levels of antistreptococcal antibody titers in blood were measured, as was the integrity of the basal ganglia (via MRI). Results indicated that ADHD was significantly related to such antibodies, even after the effects of OCD and tic disorders were controlled for, and that those antibodies were related to basal ganglia volume. Though such findings need to be replicated, they suggest that some cases of ADHD could arise from or be exacerbated by streptococcal infection. Even if this is so for only a small percentage of cases, this finding is important in further supporting a significant role of the basal ganglia in the creation of ADHD symptoms.

SIDE EFFECTS OF MEDICATIONS

Some evidence indicates that the medications used to treat seizure disorders, particularly phenobarbital and phenytoin (dilantin), are likely to result in increased problems with inattention and hyperactivity in children taking these medications (Committee on Drugs, 1985). Between 9% and 75% of children given phenobarbital are likely to develop hyperactivity or to have any preexisting ADHD symptoms worsened by this drug (Committee on Drugs, 1985; Wolf & Forsythe, 1978). However, a more recent study suggests that although such symptoms are more common in children treated with phenobarbital, few if any of these children meet full clinical criteria for ADHD (Brent, Crumrine, Varma, Allen, & Allman, 1987). Instead, more of the children treated with this medication are likely to be diagnosed as depressed or irritable. Considering that few children with ADHD are taking these medications, such drugs cannot be considered to be a major cause of ADHD in the population. It would still be advisable, however, for clinicians working with children who have both ADHD and epilepsy to be cautious about the possibility that certain types of anticonvulsants may worsen such a preexisting condition.

Some clinical anecdotal evidence suggests that methylxanthines, such as theophylline (a medication often used in treating asthma) and caffeine, may cause such side effects as inattention and hyperactivity. These effects do not reach degrees that could be considered to warrant a diagnosis of ADHD, but they may sufficiently predispose a child on these medications to be somewhat poorer at paying attention in school, or they may exacerbate the symptoms of a child who already has ADHD. A meta-analysis of the research literature (Stein, Krasowski, Leventhal, Phillips, & Bender, 1996) found no evidence of significant deleterious effects of either theophylline or caffeine on behavioral or cognitive functioning.

PSYCHOSOCIAL FACTORS

A few environmental theories of ADHD were proposed nearly 30 years ago (Block, 1977; Willis & Lovaas, 1977), but they have not shown any consistency with the subsequent scientific literature or received much direct research attention. Willis and Lovaas (1977) claimed that hyperactive behavior was the result of poor stimulus control by maternal commands, and that this poor regulation of behavior arose from poor parental management of the children. But if that were the case, ADHD would demonstrate a substantial contribution from shared or rearing environment in the numerous twin studies conducted to date (see above), and the exact opposite has been the result. There is no significant contribution of rearing or common environment to the behaviors that constitute ADHD.

Others have also conjectured that ADHD results from difficulties in parents' overstimulating approach to caring for and managing children as well as from parental psychological problems (Carlson, Jacobvitz, & Sroufe, 1995; Jacobvitz & Sroufe, 1987; Silverman & Ragusa, 1992). But these theories have not been clear in articulating just how the deficits in behavioral inhibition and other cognitive deficits commonly associated with clinically diagnosed ADHD, as described in Chapters 2 and 3 of this volume, could arise from such social factors. Moreover, many of these studies proclaiming to have evidence of parental characteristics as potentially causative of ADHD did not use clinical diagnostic criteria to identify children as having ADHD; instead, they relied merely on elevated parental ratings of hyperactivity or laboratory demonstrations of distractibility to classify the children as having ADHD (Carlson et al., 1995; Silverman & Ragusa, 1992). Nor have these theories received much support in the available literature that has studied clinically diagnosed children with ADHD (see Danforth, Barkley, & Stokes, 1991, and Johnston & Mash, 2001, concerning parent–child interactions and family issues). Again, in view of the fact that the twin studies discussed previously show no significant contributions of the common or shared environment to the expression of ADHD symptoms, theories based entirely on social explanations of the origins of ADHD are difficult to take seriously, especially when they do not explain the precise social mechanism by which this effect is supposed to occur.

Despite the large role heredity seems to play in ADHD symptoms, they remain malleable to unique environmental influences and nonshared social learning. The actual severity of the symptoms, their continuity over development, the types of secondary symptoms, and the outcome of the disorder are related in varying degrees to environmental factors (Biederman et al., 1996; Milberger, Biederman, Faraone, Guite, & Tsuang, 1997; van den Oord & Rowe, 1997; Weiss & Hechtman, 1993). Yet even here care must be taken in interpreting these findings as evidence of a pure environmental contribution to ADHD, because many measures of family functioning and adversity also show that there is a strong heritable contribution to them, largely owing to the presence of symptoms and disorders in the parents similar to those evident in the children (Pike & Plomin, 1996; Plomin, 1995). Thus there is a genetic contribution to the family environment—a fact that often goes overlooked in studies of family and social factors involved in ADHD.

Moreover, as noted in Chapter 4, several investigators attempted to evaluate the direction of effects within parent–child interactions. They did so by investigating the effects of stimulant medication and placebo on these mother–child interactions. The studies consistently found that the medications resulted in significant improvements in children's hyperactivity and compliance. There was a corresponding reduction in mothers' use of commands, direction, and negative behavior when the children were on medication, indicating that much of the negative behavior of the mothers appeared to be in response to the difficult behavior of these children (Barkley & Cunningham, 1979; Barkley, Karlsson, Strzelecki, & Murphy, 1984; Barkley, Karlsson, Pollard, & Murphy, 1985; Cunningham & Barkley, 1979; Humphries, Kinsbourne, & Swanson, 1978).

Taken together, these findings suggest that the overly critical, commanding, and negative behavior of mothers of hyperactive children is most likely a reaction to the difficult, disruptive, and noncompliant behavior of these children rather than a cause of it. And such disrupted parenting is likely to not only be a reaction to the children's behavioral control problems, but may also arise from the parents' own ADHD and the higher likelihood that the parents may experience other psychological disorders, such as depression, anxiety, antisocial behaviors or Antisocial Personality Disorder, and substance dependence or abuse. This is not to say that the manner in which parents attempt to manage their children's ADHD behavior cannot exacerbate it or maintain higher levels of conflict between parent and children over time. Studies have shown that the continuation of hyperactive behavior over development, and especially the maintenance of oppositional behavior in these children, are related in part to parents' use of commands, criticism, and an overcontrolling and intrusive style of management (Barkley, Fischer, Edelbrock, & Smallish, 1991; Campbell, 1987, 1989; Campbell & Ewing, 1990). But all this tells us is that comorbid ODD/CD when seen in ADHD may in part be a function of parental management practices; it does not mean that a child's ADHD is a result of those practices. Indeed, recent twin studies suggest that the high association of ADHD with ODD/CD is likely to be the result of a shared genetic liability for these two disorders, with ODD/CD also being influenced by additional genetic factors (Nadder et al., 2002). Theories of the causation of ADHD can no longer be based solely or even primarily on social factors, such as parental characteristics, caregiving abilities, child management, or other family environmental factors.

As discussed in Chapter 1, Block (1977) proposed that an increase in "cultural tempo" in modern Western civilization may account for the prevalence of hyperactivity in these countries. Precisely what was meant by "cultural tempo" was not operationally defined; nor was evidence presented to suggest that either less developed cultures or Eastern cultures have less hyperactivity than do more developed or Western cultures. This theory and its modification by Ross and Ross (1982) remain speculative and would seem to be almost scientifically untestable. Moreover, such theories once again conflict with a wealth of information on the genetics and heritability of this behavior pattern and disorder, and on the nonsignificant role of the common environment (this tempo would be considered an aspect of that environment)—all of which would argue against those theories as explanations for the occurrence of most ADHD in children.

One psychosocial factor that has received recent attention in the popular media is the degree of children's exposure to television. In the week of April 14, 2004, on the Cable News Network's (CNN's) *Anderson Cooper 360°* show, Sanja Gupta, MD, CNN's medical advisor, and Anderson Cooper committed an elementary fallacy so common that it is taught in virtually every "Introduction to Statistics" course taught at college—the misinterpretation of correlation as causation. Gupta and Cooper were discussing a paper just published that month in the journal *Pediatrics*. The paper suggested that early television exposure is associated with later increased attention problems in childhood. Gupta and Cooper took this paper to imply that ADHD, or at least its attention symptoms, could arise from watching too much television in early childhood. And they admonished viewers to warn parents about this detrimental effect and (if viewers were parents themselves) to reduce TV viewing so as to reduce the risk of their children's having ADHD. These media personalities were not the only ones to misconstrue a correlation as a cause. Other media outlets and many critics of ADHD

seemed to do likewise, judging by the number of calls and e-mails I received that month about this paper. This is not the first time that a belief that television contributes to inattention or ADHD has been proffered. A syndicated columnist and family therapist, John Rosemond, has made this claim in several of his columns. The *Pediatrics* article therefore deserves more careful scrutiny here.

Christakis, Zimmerman, DiGiuseppe, and McCarty (2004) used data from the National Longitudinal Survey of Youth to examine the relationship between hours of television viewed at ages 1 and 3 years with attention problems at age 7 years, as measured by 5 items from the Hyperactivity subscale of the Behavior Problems Index. They defined children as having an attention problem if they were 1.2 standard deviations above the mean on this set of 5 items. Using this very generous definition of attention problems, they classified 10% of their sample as having such problems at age 7 years. The authors then used logistic regression analyses to evaluate the association between early TV exposure with later attention problems. They found that hours of television exposure at ages 1 and 3 years was significantly associated with being classified as having attention problems at age 7 years (odds ratio of 1.09 for both analyses). The analyses statistically controlled for a number of other variables as covariates, including gestational age, maternal tobacco and alcohol exposure during this pregnancy, number of children at home, single-parent versus two-parent household, emotional support, cognitive stimulation, maternal depression and self-esteem, and others.

These authors hypothesized that early TV viewing shortens children's attention spans because of the unrealistic pace with which TV events unfold in relation to real life. The mechanism for this causal influence was suggested to be exposure to TV during critical periods of synaptic development in brain neurons. Somehow, though the mechanism was left unspecified, TV portrayals of events were proposed to alter synaptic connections in neuronal networks related to attention, so that these shorten the children's attention span. The authors claimed that their findings supported their hypothesis. However, to their credit, they did note that their study design permitted no causal inferences from these associations. Despite this acknowledged limitation of the study, the authors went on anyway to conclude that "we added inattention to the previously studied deleterious consequences of excessive television viewing, including violent behavior and obesity" (Christakis et al., 2004, p. 711). They further stated that "our findings suggest that preventive action can be taken with respect to attention problems in children" (p. 711) by limiting their exposure to TV during formative years of brain development and that this "may reduce children's subsequent risk of developing ADHD" (p. 711). In short, while acknowledging that the study could say nothing about causation, they nevertheless drew causal conclusions and made treatment recommendations based on such conclusions.

Several things are remarkable about this study and its mistaken conclusions, apart from the popular media attention it received:

• As the authors rightly noted, this study can say absolutely nothing about early TV exposure *causing* attention problems in children. And it surely cannot speak to whether early TV viewing affects synaptic connections in the brain in the hypothesized manner, given that no such neuronal connections were studied. All it has demonstrated is an association, and a weak one at that. A correlation, no matter how strong, cannot prove a causal connection between the related variables. The causal arrow in this case could just as easily point the other way: Attention problems may cause children to watch more TV (as opposed to doing other things that require more sustained attention). This makes just as much sense as the causal direction the authors wished to imply—that TV exposure causes attention problems.

• The authors appeared to be exceptionally biased toward environmental (especially social) causes of attention problems. Although they acknowledged that their analyses did not adjust for other possible variables (most notably, genetic factors) that may mediate the relationship they found between TV and attention problems, they then went on to blame parental homemaking as another potential cause of attention problems: "For example, parents who were distracted, neglectful, or otherwise preoccupied might have allowed their children to watch excessive amounts of television *in addition to having created a household environment that promoted the development of attention problems*" (p. 712; emphasis added). Missing here is the very real possibility that genetics may actually mediate this relationship.

Nowhere did these authors even acknowledge that each parent shares half of his or her genes with offspring. Why should that matter? Because attention problems like those found in ADHD have a strikingly high genetic influence (average heritability of .80 across studies, and higher among studies using DSM symptom lists; Thapar et al., 1999; Levy & Hay, 2001). That means that 80% or more of the variation in attention problems in children is the result of genetic effects. Moreover, twin studies to date have found no compelling evidence that the shared or rearing environment makes any contribution to these symptoms, despite incorrect assertions by these authors that twin studies are flawed, as they do not measure the environment. All environmental variance found in twin studies is accounted for by unique events—things twins and siblings do *not* have in common as they grow up together. TV viewing within families is often a shared event among children in the family, not a unique event specific to just one of them. Twin studies therefore tell us that the causal direction offered by Christakis et al. (2004) for TV's causing attention problems is not likely to be the case. Their correlation probably results from some other, unstudied variable, and the chief candidate is shared family genetics for attention problems. Thus it is just as plausible (if not more so) that children with attention problems have parents with attention problems, and that such people with shorter attention spans are likely to watch more television and to leave their children in rooms with TVs on as babysitters. The TV viewing habits are simply a "red herring" or marker for those who already have attention problems—not necessarily a cause of them.

• Let's examine the results of another study published in 2004 that can shed light on this issue. It measured attention in a similar fashion to the Christakis et al. (2004) study—via parent ratings of attention, activity, and impulsivity problems, using items from the Child Behavior Checklist. As it just so happens, the study (Reitveld et al., 2004) assessed children's attention problems at age 3, and then later at age 7—the same time frame as the Christakis et al. study. (It also assessed them again at ages 10 and 12 years). The beauty of the Reitveld et al. study is that it was a longitudinal study of 11,938 twins, and so tells us a great deal about genetic and environmental factors that can explain the variation in attention problems.

Christakis et al. assessed only TV viewing at age 3 (and 1), but not attention problems, which they evaluated only later at age 7. The Reitveld et al. study can therefore tell us not only about the genetic contribution to attention problems at age 3 years, but also about its stability over a time period comparable to that of the Christakis et al. study. Reitveld et al. found that average heritability across ages for attention problems ranged from .70 to .74. All residual variation in this trait was due entirely to unique environmental effects (events not shared among twins or siblings). *None was accounted for by shared events.* The authors concluded as well that the stability of attention problems in these twins was accounted for by genetic factors. What does this mean for interpreting the Christakis et al. results? It suggests that the children with attention problems at age 7 were highly likely to have already had attention problems at age 3 (and probably 1), and that the presence of those problems at both ages and their persistence over development are largely explained by genetic factors, along with a more modest contribution of the unique events befalling these children. They are not due to any shared event, such as TV viewing within the family.

• In our Milwaukee follow-up study, Mariellen Fischer and I just recently found the same association as Christakis et al. did between ADHD and TV viewing. Yet we did not trumpet this association to the world as yet another detrimental effect of television. Indeed, we have yet to publish it, largely because it is not very interesting. We examined hyperactive children we have followed for over 13 years and who are now in their early 20s, and we asked them how they spent their leisure time. (As an aside, as many as 46–66% of these children still have ADHD in adulthood.) We found that these young adults watched significantly more TV, read significantly less, and spent more time talking on the phone with friends than did the young adults in the control group we have followed over the same period of time. Now if we were to interpret our results in the same causal direction as Christakis et al. interpreted theirs, we could assert, "Not only does TV viewing cause ADHD even in your 20s, but so do not reading very much and talking excessively with your friends on the phone." Following the logic of Christakis et al., we could then go so far as to caution the public not only not to watch so much TV, but also to read more

and to talk less on the phone, so as to reduce their subsequent risk of developing ADHD. In contrast to Christakis et al., however, we saw our findings in just the opposite light: People who have long-standing problems with attention read less, watch TV more, and talk more on the phone. Why would we flip the causal arrow here in the opposite direction from Christakis et al.'s arrow? Because of the far too numerous twin studies finding that environmental events such as these make no contribution to attention problems.

• It also deserves note that the size of the relationship Christakis et al. found (the odds ratio) is clinically trivial, despite being statistically significant. Using large samples, as these authors did, can make very small associations between variables become statistically significant, which seems to be what happened here. That does not mean we should craft public policy or even draw causal connections on the basis of them. An odds ratio of 1.00, for instance, means that there is no association between the two variables above that expected by chance alone. A ratio of greater than 1.00 (say, 2.00) means that an increase in TV viewing of an hour per day may double the chances of having an attention problem at age 7 over the base rate for the sample being studied (10%). This study found a ratio of 1.09, which means that an increase in early TV viewing increased the chances of having attention problems at age 7 by about 9%. This is not a big deal, and certainly not one on which to base admonitions to parents and professionals to start limiting children's television exposure so as to reduce their later risks for ADHD. As a contrast, consider this: The gene known as DRD4 in its long allele form (7 or more repeats) has been shown in a meta-analysis of several separate genetic studies to increase the likelihood of having ADHD by 50% (average odds ratio of 1.50) (Faraone et al., 2001). This microscopic piece of DNA has an association with attention problems (ADHD symptoms) more than five times greater than the TV viewing studied by Christakis et al. Even more impressive is the odds ratio of a child's having ADHD if a parent has the disorder—it's a whopping 8.00 (Levy & Hay, 2001). This means that children with attention problems are very likely to have parents with similar traits.

• Also worth mentioning is the fact (Christalos et al., noted in their discussion) that they really did not measure or clinically diagnose ADHD in this sample, which means that their results have only a very modest bearing on the issue of what causes ADHD. The authors used just 5 items that are only broadly similar to some of the 18 symptoms in the diagnostic criteria for ADHD in the *Diagnostic and Statistical Manual of Mental Disorders*. And they defined children as having an attention problem if they were a mere 1.2 standard deviations about the mean—a threshold resulting in 10% of their sample being so classified. Yet they then went on to imply that early TV viewing may increase the risk for later ADHD, and that limiting such early exposure may reduce this risk. It is a big conceptual stretch from a rating scale using 5 dichotomously scored items of behavioral problems to the clinical diagnosis of ADHD.

• Further examination of the study shows that Christakis et al. (2004) had no way of assessing whether the children were actually watching the television that was on in the same room as they may have been occupying. As such, the methods of this study tell us only about children's being in a room with a TV on, not their TV viewing. The study could be telling us as much about parental caretaking behavior as about child television viewing, if not more. It may tell us that parents who give less attention to their children and instead use TV to babysit their children for longer-than-normal periods of time have children with attention problems. As noted above, this does not necessarily imply that the parental behavior is the cause of the attention problems in their children. It is just as possible that inattentive parents have inattentive children by virtue of shared genetics and the personality traits they influence.

• Christakis et al. also confessed that they had no way of assessing the content of the programs the children may have been watching. Given that children in the 1- to 3-year-old range may well have been viewing educational programs, such as those on public television (PBS) (e.g., *Mr. Rogers' Neighborhood* or *Sesame Street*), does this mean that exposure to such programs contributes to later ADHD? In other words, does it matter what the content of the programs were, or is it merely quantity of exposure that is so harmful? Interestingly, the authors were reluctant to go there. In yet another revelation of their interpretive biases, they confided that educational programs might well have had a *beneficial* effect and moderated

their results, thereby making those results a conservative estimate of TV's potential harm to children's attention spans. This seems to be a case of having their cake and eating it too: "TV is bad for your children's attention," they want to say, but they are quick to dismiss educational TV from this indictment. Yet the study found that it was the amount of exposure that was associated with attention problems and not the content of programming, which was not measured at all.

To conclude, the Christakis et al. (2004) study is a classic example of how investigator bias and the mass media propensity for sound bites and glibness, both coupled with a deeply held societal desire to blame parents for the problems of their children can all lead to the public's being fed an exceptionally mistaken impression—that TV viewing causes ADHD. In fact, this particular study found only a very weak association between early TV *exposure* and later attention and activity problems. It does not mean anything about TV *viewing's causing* later attention problems, much less later ADHD. It could just as easily mean that attention problems lead to watching more TV, or (more likely) that both attention problems and TV viewing are mediated by some unmeasured variable (family ADHD genetics).

SUMMARY

It should be evident from the research reviewed here that neurological and genetic factors make a substantial contribution both to symptoms of ADHD and to the occurrence of the disorder per se. Various genetic and neurological etiologies (e.g., pregnancy and birth complications, acquired brain damage, toxins, infections, and genetic effects) can give rise to the disorder, probably through some disturbance in a final common pathway in the nervous system. That final common pathway appears to date to be the integrity of the prefrontal cortical–striatal–cerebellar network. It now appears that hereditary factors play the largest role in the occurrence of ADHD symptoms in children. The condition can also be caused or exacerbated by pregnancy complications, exposure to toxins, or neurological disease. Social factors alone cannot be supported as causal of this disorder, but such factors may contribute to the forms of comorbid disorders associated with ADHD. Cases of ADHD can also arise without a genetic predisposition to the disorder, provided that the children are exposed to significant disruption or neurological injury to this final common neurological pathway, but this would seem to account for only a small minority of such cases. In general, then, research conducted since the preceding edition of this text has further strengthened the evidence for genetic and developmental neurological factors as the probable primary causes of ADHD, while greatly reducing the support for purely social factors as having a role in the causation of this disorder.

KEY CLINICAL POINTS

✓ There is no currently available credible scientific theory of ADHD that can account for its existence by purely social means.

✓ The totality of evidence indicates that neurological and genetic factors play a substantial role in the origins and expression of this disorder.

✓ Neuropsychological research finds substantial evidence for deficits in behavioral inhibition, sustained attention (task persistence), resistance to distraction, and executive functioning (the internalization of speech, verbal working memory, temporal–sequential working memory, motor coordination and the timing of fine motor movements, emotional and motivational self-regulation, verbal fluency, and planning) (see Chapter 3). The executive functions are known to be mediated by the prefrontal cortex and its networks with the basal ganglia and cerebellum, suggesting that these regions may play a prime role in ADHD.

✓ Psychophysiological research demonstrates reduced arousal to stimulation (particularly on averaged evoked responses); diminished sensitivity to reinforcement; and increased slow-wave or theta activity (associated with drowsiness and poor focus of attention) and decreased beta or fast-wave activity (associated with decreased concentration and persistence) on EEG.

✓ Studies of cerebral blood flow indicate reduced flow to the frontal lobes, striatum, and cerebellum, consistent with underactivity in these regions.

✓ PET scan studies are inconsistent, but suggest some reduced activation in the insular and hippocampal regions and greater activation in the right anterior cingulate during decision-making tasks.

✓ MRI studies indicate smaller total brain size, with greatest reductions in brain volumes of the anterior frontal lobes (mainly on the right), the basal ganglia, and the cerebellar vermis (mainly on the right). Some evidence also suggests a possible involvement of the anterior cingulate. Reduced right frontal volume has also been found in siblings of children with ADHD who do not have ADHD themselves, suggesting a potential endophenotype for the disorder.

✓ Studies using fMRI indicate differences from typical brain activity in the frontal region, basal ganglia, and cerebellum.

✓ Deficits in specific neurotransmitters have not been definitively established, but a clear role for dopamine and norepinephrine is suggested by the positive response of those with ADHD to stimulants (dopamine reuptake inhibitors and agonists) and atomoxetine (norepinephrine reuptake inhibitors), and by the distribution of these two neurotransmitters in the brain regions implicated in ADHD.

✓ Pregnancy complications are associated with risk for ADHD, especially maternal smoking, maternal alcohol consumption, low birth weight and associated minor brain hemorrhaging, possibly maternal phenylalanine levels, and arguably stress/anxiety during pregnancy.

✓ Family studies show a markedly elevated risk of ADHD among the biological relatives of children with ADHD (10–35%) rising to a risk of 55% to at least one parent in families with two affected children. Parental ADHD coveys a risk to offspring of up to 57%. Adoption studies indicate no increased risk of ADHD among adoptive parents of adopted children with ADHD, further supporting a genetic contribution to ADHD.

✓ Numerous studies of large samples of twins in many countries find a genetic contribution accounting for 50–95% of the variation in the traits constituting ADHD, averaging 80% or higher. No significant contribution of shared or common environmental factors (rearing environment) has been evident, whereas nonshared or unique environmental factors make a small but significant contribution to variation in these traits. The strong genetic contribution to ADHD is now a "fact in the bag," and the consistent absence of a rearing environmental contribution rules out within-family factors as contributing to the expression of the disorder, but suggests some role for unique events in the lives of children (pregnancy complications, biohazards, developmental risks, and possibly unique social effects).

✓ Molecular genetic studies find that the greatest reliable gene polymorphism associated with ADHD is the DRD4 (48-bp) 7+-repeat polymorphism, with the next strongest body of evidence supporting a role for the DAT1 480-bp (long) polymorphism. Several studies have recently suggested a possible involvement of the DBH Taq I allele and the DRD5 allele.

✓ Several toxins have been associated with risk for ADHD, two of which are maternal smoking and alcohol consumption (as noted above). A third appears to be elevated body lead burden during the first 2–3 years of child development.

✓ One study suggests a potential contribution of streptococcal infection to some cases of ADHD, wherein the infection triggers an immune response of antibodies that destroy cells of the basal ganglia.

✓ Some older anticonvulsant medications (phenobarbital and phenytoin [Dilantin]) may create or exacerbate symptoms of ADHD.

✓ Evidence for a contribution of psychosocial factors to ADHD is weak. The recent suggestion that television viewing during early childhood may play a contributing role in ADHD was overstated and has not been replicated.

REFERENCES

Akshoomoff, N. A., & Courchesne, E. (1992). A new role for the cerebellum in cognitive operations. *Behavioral Neurosciences, 106,* 731–738.

Antshel, K. M., & Waisbren, S. E. (2003). Developmental timing of exposure to elevated levels of phenylalanine is associated with ADHD symptom expression. *Journal of Abnormal Child Psychology, 31,* 565–574.

Arnsten, A. F. T., Steere, J. C., & Hunt, R. D. (1996). The contribution of alpha2 noradrenergic mechanism to prefrontal cortical cognitive function. *Archives of General Psychiatry, 53,* 448–455.

Aylward, E. H., Reiss, A. L., Reader, M. J., Singer, H. S., Brown, J. E., & Denckla, M. B. (1996). Basal ganglia volumes in children with attention-deficit hyperactivity disorder. *Journal of Child Neurology, 11,* 112–115.

Baloh, R., Sturm, R., Green, B., & Gleser, G. (1975). Neuropsychological effects of chronic asymptomatic increased lead absorption. *Archives of Neurology, 32,* 326–330.

Barkley, R. A. (1997). *ADHD and the nature of self-control.* New York: Guilford Press.

Barkley, R. A., & Cunningham, C. E. (1979). The effects of methylphenidate on the mother–child interactions of hyperactive children. *Archives of General Psychiatry, 36,* 201–208.

Barkley, R. A., DuPaul, G. J., & McMurray, M. B. (1990). A comprehensive evaluation of attention deficit disorder with and without hyperactivity. *Journal of Consulting and Clinical Psychology, 58,* 775–789.

Barkley, R. A., Fischer, M., Edelbrock, C. S., & Smallish, L. (1991). The adolescent outcome of hyperactive children diagnosed by research criteria: III. Mother–child interactions, family conflicts, and maternal psychopathology. *Journal of Child Psychology and Psychiatry, 32,* 233–256.

Barkley, R. A., Karlsson, J., Pollard, S., & Murphy, J. V. (1985). Developmental changes in the mother–child interactions of hyperactive boys: Effects of two dose levels of Ritalin. *Journal of Child Psychology and Psychiatry, 26,* 705–715.

Barkley, R. A., Karlsson, J., Strzelecki, E., & Murphy, J. (1984). The effects of age and Ritalin dosage on the mother–child interactions of hyperactive children. *Journal of Consulting and Clinical Psychology, 52,* 750–758.

Barr, C. L. (2001). Genetics of childhood disorders: XXII. ADHD, Part 6: The dopamine D4 receptor gene. *Journal of the American Academy of Child and Adolescent Psychiatry, 40,* 118–121.

Baving, L., Laucht, M., & Schmidt, M. H. (1999). Atypical frontal activation in ADHD: Preschool and elementary school boys and girls. *Journal of the American Academy of Child and Adolescent Psychiatry, 38,* 1363–1371.

Beauchaine, T. P., Katkin, E. S., Strassberg, Z., & Snarr, J. (2001). Disinhibitory psychopathology in male adolescents: Discriminating conduct disorder from attention-deficit/hyperactivity disorder through concurrent assessment of multiple autonomic states. *Journal of Abnormal Psychology, 110,* 610–624.

Bennett, L. A., Wolin, S. J., & Reiss, D. (1988). Cognitive, behavioral, and emotional problems among school-age children of alcoholic parents. *American Journal of Psychiatry, 145,* 185–190.

Benton, A. (1991). Prefrontal injury and behavior in

children. *Developmental Neuropsychology, 7,* 275–282.

Biederman, J., Faraone, S. V., Keenan, K., Benjamin, J., Krifcher, B., Moore, C., et al. (1992). Further evidence for family-genetic risk factors in attention deficit hyperactivity disorder: Patterns of comorbidity in probands and relatives in psychiatrically and pediatrically referred samples. *Archives of General Psychiatry, 49,* 728–738.

Biederman, J., Faraone, S. V., Mick, E., Spencer, T., Wilens, T., Kiely, K., et al. (1995). High risk for attention deficit hyperactivity disorder among children of parents with childhood onset of the disorder: A pilot study. *American Journal of Psychiatry, 152,* 431–435.

Biederman, J., Faraone, S., Milberger, S., Curtis, S., Chen, L., Marrs, A., et al. (1996). Predictors of persistence and remission of ADHD into adolescence: Results from a four-year prospective follow-up study. *Journal of the American Academy of Child and Adolescent Psychiatry, 35,* 343–351.

Biederman, J., Keenan, K., & Faraone, S. V. (1990). Parent-based diagnosis of attention deficit disorder predicts a diagnosis based on teacher report. *Journal of the American Academy of Child and Adolescent Psychiatry, 29,* 698–701.

Biederman, J., Milberger, S., Faraone, S. V., Guite, J., & Warburton, R. (1994). Associations between childhood asthma and ADHD: Issues of psychiatric comorbidity and familiality. *Journal of the American Academy of Child and Adolescent Psychiatry, 33,* 842–848.

Block, G. H. (1977). Hyperactivity: A cultural perspective. *Journal of Learning Disabilities, 110,* 236–240.

Blum, K., Cull, J. G., Braverman, E. R., & Comings, D. E. (1996). Reward deficiency syndrome. *American Scientist, 84,* 132–145.

Borger, N., & van der Meere, J. (2000). Visual behaviour of ADHD children during an attention test: An almost forgotten variable. *Journal of Child Psychology and Psychiatry, 41,* 525–532.

Bradley, J. D. D., & Golden, C. J. (2001). Biological contributions to the presentation and understanding of attention-deficit/hyperactivity disorder: A review. *Clinical Psychology Review, 21,* 907–929.

Brent, D. A., Crumrine, P. K., Varma, R. R., Allan, M., & Allman, C. (1987). Phenobarbital treatment and major depressive disorder in children with epilepsy. *Pediatrics, 80,* 909–917.

Breslau, N., Brown, G. G., DelDotto, J. E., Kumar, S., Exhuthachan, S., Andreski, P., et al. (1996). Psychiatric sequelae of low birth weight at 6 years of age. *Journal of Abnormal Child Psychology, 24,* 385–400.

Cadoret, R. J., & Stewart, M. A. (1991). An adoption study of attention deficit/hyperactivity/aggression and their relationship to adult antisocial personality. *Comprehensive Psychiatry, 32,* 73–82.

Campbell, S. B. (1987). Parent-referred problem three-year-olds: Developmental changes in symptoms. *Journal of Child Psychology and Psychiatry, 28,* 835–846.

Campbell, S. B. (1990). *Behavior problems in preschool children.* New York: Guilford Press.

Campbell, S. B., & Ewing, L. J. (1990). Follow-up of hard-to-manage preschoolers: Adjustment at age nine years and predictors of continuing symptoms. *Journal of Child Psychology and Psychiatry, 31,* 891–910.

Cantwell, D. (1975). *The hyperactive child.* New York: Spectrum.

Carlson, E. A., Jacobvitz, D., & Sroufe, L. A. (1995). A developmental investigation of inattentiveness and hyperactivity. *Child Development, 66,* 37–54.

Casey, B. J., Castellanos, F. X., Giedd, J. N., Marsh, W. L., Hamburger, S. D., Schubert, A. B., et al. (1997). Implication of right frontostriatal circuitry in response inhibition and attention-deficit/hyperactivity disorder. *Journal of the American Academy of Child and Adolescent Psychiatry, 36,* 374–383.

Castellanos, F. X., Giedd, J. N., Berquin, P. C., Walter, J. M., Sharp, W., Tran, T., et al. (2001). Quantitative brain magnetic resonance imaging in girls with attention-deficit/hyperactivity disorder. *Archives of General Psychiatry, 58,* 289–295.

Castellanos, F. X., Giedd, J. N., Eckburg, P., Marsh, W. L., Vaituzis, C., Kaysen, D., et al. (1994). Quantitative morphology of the caudate nucleus in attention deficit hyperactivity disorder. *American Journal of Psychiatry, 151,* 1791–1796.

Castellanos, F. X., Giedd, J. N., Marsh, W. L., Hamburger, S. D., Vaituzis, A. C., Dickstein, D. P., et al. (1996). Quantitative brain magnetic resonance imaging in attention-deficit hyperactivity disorder. *Archives of General Psychiatry, 53,* 607–616.

Castellanos, F. X., Lee, P. P., Sharp, W., Jeffries, N. O., Greenstein, D. K., Clasen, L. S., et al. (2002). Developmental trajectories of brain volume abnormalities in children and adolescents with attention-deficit/hyperactivity disorder. *Journal of the American Medical Association, 288,* 1740–1748.

Chabot, R. J., & Serfontein, G. (1996). Quantitative electroencephalographic profiles of children with attention deficit disorder. *Biological Psychiatry, 40,* 951–963.

Christakis, D. A., Zimmerman, F. J., DiGiuseppe, D. L., & McCarty, C. A. (2004). Early television exposure and subsequent attentional problems in children. *Pediatrics, 113,* 708–713.

Claycomb, C. D., Ryan, J. J., Miller, L. J., & Schnakenberg-Ott, S. D. (2004). Relationships among attention deficit hyperactivity disorder, induced labor, and selected physiological and demographic variables. *Journal of Clinical Psychology, 60,* 689–693.

Comings, D. E., Comings, B. G., Muhleman, D., Dietz, G., Shahbahrami, B., Tast, D., et al. (1991). The dopamine D2 receptor locus as a modifying gene in neuropsychiatric disorders. *Journal of the American Medical Association, 266,* 1793–1800.

Committee on Drugs, American Academy of Pediatrics. (1985). Behavioral and cognitive effects of anti-convulsant therapy. *Pediatrics, 76,* 644–647.

Cook, E. H., Stein, M. A., Krasowski, M. D., Cox, N. J., Olkon, D. M., Kieffer, J. E., et al. (1995). Association of attention deficit disorder and the dopamine transporter gene. *American Journal of Human Genetics, 56,* 993–998.

Cook, E. H., Stein, M. A., & Leventhal, D. L. (1997). Family-based association of attention-deficit/hyperactivity disorder and the dopamine transporter. In K. Blum & E. P. Noble (Eds.), *Handbook of psychiatric genetics* (pp. 297–310). Boca Raton, FL: CRC Press.

Coolidge, F. L., Thede, L. L., & Young, S. E. (2000). Heritability and the comorbidity of attention deficit hyperactivity disorder with behavioral disorders and executive function deficits: A preliminary investigation. *Developmental Neuropsychology, 17,* 273–287.

Cruickshank, B. M., Eliason, M., & Merrifield, B. (1988). Long-term sequelae of water near-drowning. *Journal of Pediatric Psychology, 13,* 379–388.

Cunningham, C. E., & Barkley, R. A. (1979). The inter-actions of hyperactive and normal children with their mothers during free play and structured task. *Child Development, 50,* 217–224.

Daly, G., Hawi, Z., Fitzgerald, M., & Gill, M. (1999). Mapping susceptibility loci in attention deficit hyperactivity disorder: Preferential transmission of parental alleles at DAT1, DBH, and DRD5 to affected children. *Molecular Psychiatry, 4,* 192–196.

Danforth, J. S., Barkley, R. A., & Stokes, T. F. (1991). Observations of parent–child interactions with hyperactive children: Research and clinical implications. *Clinical Psychology Review, 11,* 703–727.

David, O. J. (1974). Association between lower level lead concentrations and hyperactivity. *Environmental Health Perspective, 7,* 17–25.

de la Burde, B., & Choate, M. (1972). Does asymptomatic lead exposure in children have latent sequelae? *Journal of Pediatrics, 81,* 1088–1091.

de la Burde, B., & Choate, M. (1974). Early asymptomatic lead exposure and development at school age. *Journal of Pediatrics, 87,* 638–642.

Denson, R., Nanson, J. L., & McWatters, M. A. (1975). Hyperkinesis and maternal smoking. *Canadian Psychiatric Association Journal, 20,* 183–187.

Diamond, A. (2000). Close interrelation of motor development and cognitive development and of the cerebellum and prefrontal cortex. *Developmental Psychology, 71,* 44–56.

DiMaio, S., Grizenko, N., & Joober, R. (2003). Dopamine genes in attention-deficit hyperactivity disorder: A review. *Journal of Psychiatric Neuroscience, 28,* 27–38.

Durston, S., Hulshoff, H. E., Schnack, H. G., Buitelaar, J. K., Steenhuis, M. P., Minderaa, R. B., et al. (2004). Magnetic resonance imaging of boys with attention-deficit/hyperactivity disorder and their unaffected siblings. *Journal of the American Academy of Child and Adolescent Psychiatry, 43,* 332–240.

Edelbrock, C. S., Rende, R., Plomin, R., & Thompson, L. (1995). A twin study of competence and problem behavior in childhood and early adolescence. *Journal of Child Psychology and Psychiatry, 36,* 775–786.

El-Sayed, E., Larsson, J. O., Persson, H. E., & Rydelius, P. (2002). Altered cortical activity in children with attention-deficit/hyperactivity disorder during attentional load task. *Journal of the American Academy of Child and Adolescent Psychiatry, 41,* 811–819.

Ernst, M. (1996). Neuroimaging in attention-deficit/hyperactivity disorder. In G. R. Lyon & J. Rumsey (Eds.), *Neuroimaging: A window to the neurological foundations of learning and behavior in children* (pp. 95–118). Baltimore: Brookes.

Ernst, M., Cohen, R. M., Liebenauer, L. L., Jons, P. H., & Zametkin, A. J. (1997). Cerebral glucose metabolism in adolescent girls with attention-deficit/hyperactivity disorder. *Journal of the American Academy of Child and Adolescent Psychiatry, 36,* 1399–1406.

Ernst, M., Kimes, A. S., London, E. D., Matochik, J. A., Eldreth, D., Tata, S., et al. (2003). Neural substrates of decision making in adults with attention deficit hyperactivity disorder. *American Journal of Psychiatry, 160,* 1061–1070.

Ernst, M., Liebenauer, L. L., King, A. C., Fitzgerald, G. A., Cohen, R. M., & Zametkin, A. J. (1994). Reduced brain metabolism in hyperactive girls. *Journal of the American Academy of Child and Adolescent Psychiatry, 33,* 858–868.

Ernst, M., Zametkin, A. J., Matochik, J. A., Pascualvaca, D., Jons, P. H., & Cohen, R. M. (1999). High midbrain [^{18}F]DOPA accumulation in children with attention deficit hyperactivity disorder. *American Journal of Psychiatry, 156,* 1209–1215.

Faraone, S. V. (1996). Discussion of "Genetic influence on parent-reported attention-related problems in a Norwegian general population twin sample." *Journal of the American Academy of Child and Adolescent Psychiatry, 35,* 596–598.

Faraone, S. V., & Biederman, J. (1997). Do attention deficit hyperactivity disorder and major depression share familial risk factors? *Journal of Nervous and Mental Disease, 185,* 533–541.

Faraone, S. V., Biederman, J., Chen, W. J., Krifcher, B., Keenan, K., Moore, C., et al. (1992). Segregation analysis of attention deficit hyperactivity disorder. *Psychiatric Genetics, 2,* 257–275.

Faraone, S. V., Biederman, J., Mennin, D., Russell, R., & Tsuang, M. T. (1998). Familial subtypes of attention deficit hyperactivity disorder: A 4-year follow-up study of children from antisocial–ADHD families. *Journal of Child Psychology and Psychiatry, 39,* 1045–1053.

Faraone, S. V., Biederman, J., Mick, E., Williamson, S., Wilens, T., Spencer, T., et al. (2000). Family study of girls with attention deficit hyperactivity disorder. *American Journal of Psychiatry, 157,* 1077–1083.

Faraone, S. V., Biederman, J., Weiffenbach, B., Keith, T., Chu, M. P., Weaver, A., et al. (1999). Dopamine D4 gene 7-repeat allele and attention deficit hyperactivity disorder. *American Journal of Psychiatry, 156,* 768–770.

Faraone, S. V., & Doyle, A. E. (2001). The nature and heritability of attention-deficit/hyperactivity disorder. *Child and Adolescent Psychiatric Clinics of North America, 10,* 299–316.

Faraone, S. V., Doyle, A. E., Mick, E., & Biederman, J. (2001). Meta-analysis of the association between the 7-repeat allele of the dopamine D4 receptor gene and attention deficit hyperactivity disorder. *American Journal of Psychiatry, 158,* 1052–1057.

Ferguson, H. B., & Pappas, B. A. (1979). Evaluation of psychophysiological, neurochemical, and animal models of hyperactivity. In R. L. Trites (Eds.), *Hyperactivity in children.* Baltimore: University Park Press.

Fergusson, D. M., Fergusson, I. E., Horwood, L. J., & Kinzett, N. G. (1988). A longitudinal study of dentine lead levels, intelligence, school performance, and behaviour. *Journal of Child Psychology and Psychiatry, 29,* 811–824.

Filipek, P. A., Semrud-Clikeman, M., Steingard, R. J., Renshaw, P. F., Kennedy, D. N., & Biederman, J. (1997). Volumetric MRI analysis comparing subjects having attention-deficit hyperactivity disorder with normal controls. *Neurology, 48,* 589–601.

Fisher, S. E., Francks, C., McCracken, J. T., McGough, J. J., Marlow, A. J., MacPhie, L., et al. (2002). A genomewide scan for locu involved in attention-deficit/hyperactivity disorder. *American Journal of Human Genetics, 70,* 1183–1196.

Frank, Y., Lazar, J. W., & Seiden, J. A. (1992). Cognitive event-related potentials in learning-disabled children with or without attention-deficit hyperactivity disorder [Abstract]. *Annals of Neurology, 32,* 478.

Frazier, T. W., Demaree, H. A., & Youngstrom, E. A. (2004). Meta-analysis of intellectual and neuropsychological test performance in attention-deficit/hyperactivity disorder. *Neuropsychology, 18,* 543–555.

Fuster, J. M. (1997). *The prefrontal cortex* (3rd ed.). New York: Raven Press.

Gelernter, J. O., O'Malley, S., Risch, N., Kranzler, H. R., Krystal, J., Merikangas, K., et al. (1991). No association between an allele at the D2 dopamine receptor gene (DRD2) and alcoholism. *Journal of the American Medical Association, 266,* 1801–1807.

Giedd, J. N., Snell, J. W., Lange, N., Rajapakse, J. C., Casey, B. J., Kozuch, P. L., et al. (1996). Quantitative magnetic resonance imaging of human brain development: Ages 4–18. *Cerebral Cortex, 6,* 551–560.

Gilger, J. W., Pennington, B. F., & DeFries, J. C. (1992). A twin study of the etiology of comorbidity: Attention-deficit hyperactivity disorder and dyslexia. *Journal of the American Academy of Child and Adolescent Psychiatry, 31,* 343–348.

Gill, M., Daly, G., Heron, S., Hawi, Z., & Fitzgerald, M. (1997). Confirmation of association between attention deficit hyperactivity disorder and a dopamine transporter polymorphism. *Molecular Psychiatry, 2,* 311–313.

Gillis, J. J., Gilger, J. W., Pennington, B. F., & DeFries, J.

C. (1992). Attention deficit disorder in reading-disabled twins: Evidence for a genetic etiology. *Journal of Abnormal Child Psychology, 20,* 303–315.

Gittelman, R., & Eskinazi, B. (1983). Lead and hyperactivity revisited. *Archives of General Psychiatry, 40,* 827–833.

Gjone, H., Stevenson, J., & Sundet, J. M. (1996). Genetic influence on parent-reported attention-related problems in a Norwegian general population twin sample. *Journal of the American Academy of Child and Adolescent Psychiatry, 35,* 588–596.

Gjone, H., Stevenson, J., Sundet, J. M., & Eilertsen, D. E. (1996). Changes in heritability across increasing levels of behavior problems in young twins. *Behavior Genetics, 26,* 419–426.

Goodman, R., & Stevenson, J. (1989). A twin study of hyperactivity: II. The aetiological role of genes, family relationships, and perinatal adversity. *Journal of Child Psychology and Psychiatry, 30,* 691–709.

Grady, D. L., Chi, H.-C., Ding, Y.-C., Smith, M., Wang, E., Schuck, S., et al. (2003). High prevalence of rare dopamine receptor D4 alleles in children diagnosed with attention-deficit hyperactivity disorder. *Molecular Psychiatry, 8,* 536–545.

Grattan, L. M., & Eslinger, P. J. (1991). Frontal lobe damage in children and adults: A comparative review. *Developmental Neuropsychology, 7,* 283–326.

Groot, A. S., de Sonneville, L. M. J., Stins, J. F., & Boomsma, D. I. (2004). Familial influences on sustained attention and inhibition in preschoolers. *Journal of Child Psychology and Psychiatry, 45,* 306–314.

Gualtieri, C. T., & Hicks, R. E. (1985). Neuropharmacology of methylphenidate and a neural substrate for childhood hyperactivity. *Psychiatric Clinics of North America, 8,* 875–892.

Gustafsson, P., Thernlund, G., Ryding, E., Rosen, I., & Cederblad, M. (2000). Associations between cerebral blood-flow measured by single photon emission computer tomography (SPECT), electroencephalogram (EEG), behaviour symptoms, cognition and neurological soft signs in children with attention-deficit hyperactivity disorder (ADHD). *Acta Paediatrica, 89,* 830–835.

Halperin, J. M., Newcorn, J. H., Koda, V. H., Pick, L., McKay, K. E., & Knott, P. (1997). Noradrenergic mechanisms in ADHD children with and without reading disabilities: A replication and extension. *Journal of the American Academy of Child and Adolescent Psychiatry, 36,* 1688–1697.

Hartsough, C. S., & Lambert, N. M. (1985). Medical factors in hyperactive and normal children: Prenatal, developmental, and health history findings. *American Journal of Orthopsychiatry, 55,* 190–210.

Hastings, J., & Barkley, R. A. (1978). A review of psychophysiological research with hyperactive children. *Journal of Abnormal Child Psychology, 7,* 413–437.

Heffron, W. A., Martin, C. A., & Welsh, R. J. (1984). Attention deficit disorder in three pairs of monozygotic twins: A case report. *Journal of the American Academy of Child Psychiatry, 23,* 299–301.

Heilman, K. M., Voeller, K. K. S., & Nadeau, S. E. (1991). A possible pathophysiological substrate of attention deficit hyperactivity disorder. *Journal of Child Neurology, 6,* 74–79.

Hendren, R. L., De Backer, I., & Pandina, G. J. (2000). Review of neuroimaging studies of child and adolescent psychiatric disorders from the past 10 years. *Journal of the American Academy of Child and Adolescent Psychiatry, 39,* 815–828.

Herpertz, S. C., Wenning, B., Mueller, B., Qunaibi, M., Sass, H., & Herpetz-Dahlmann, B. (2001). Psychological responses in ADHD boys with and without conduct disorder: Implications for adult antisocial behavior. *Journal of the American Academy of Child and Adolescent Psychiatry, 40,* 1222–1230.

Hervey, A. S., Epstein, J. N., & Curry, J. F. (2004). Neuropsychology of adults with attention-deficit/hyperactivity disorder: A meta-analytic review. *Neuropsychology, 18,* 485–503.

Hesdorffer, D. C., Ludvigsson, P., Olafsson, E., Gudmundsson, G., Kjartansson, O., & Hauser, W. A. (2004). ADHD as a risk factor for incident unprovoked seizures and epilepsy in children. *Archives of General Psychiatry, 61,* 731–736.

Holdsworth, L., & Whitmore, K. (1974). A study of children with epilepsy attending ordinary schools: I. Their seizure patterns, progress, and behaviour in school. *Developmental Medicine and Child Neurology, 16,* 746–758.

Houk, J. C., & Wise, S. P. (1995). Distributed modular architectures linking basal ganglia, cerebellum, and cerebral cortex: Their role in planning and controlling action. *Cerebral Cortex, 2,* 95–110.

Hudziak, J. (1997, October). *The genetics of attention deficit hyperactivity disorder.* Paper presented at the annual meeting of the American Academy of Child and Adolescent Psychiatry, Toronto.

Humphries, T., Kinsbourne, M., & Swanson, J. (1978). Stimulant effects on cooperation and social interaction between hyperactive children and their mothers. *Journal of Child Psychology and Psychiatry, 19,* 13–22.

Hynd, G. W., Hern, K. L., Novey, E. S., Eliopulos, D., Marshall, R., Gonzalez, J. J., et al. (1993). Attention-deficit hyperactivity disorder and asymmetry of the caudate nucleus. *Journal of Child Neurology, 8,* 339–347.

Hynd, G. W., Semrud-Clikeman, M., Lorys, A. R., Novey, E. S., & Eliopulos, D. (1990). Brain morphology in developmental dyslexia and attention deficit disorder/hyperactivity. *Archives of Neurology, 47,* 919–926.

Hynd, G. W., Semrud-Clikeman, M., Lorys, A. R., Novey, E. S., Eliopulos, D., & Lyytinen, H. (1991). Corpus callosum morphology in attention deficit-hyperactivity disorder: Morphometric analysis of MRI. *Journal of Learning Disabilities, 24,* 141–146.

Jacobvitz, D., & Sroufe, L. A. (1987). The early caregiver–child relationship and attention-deficit disorder with hyperactivity in kindergarten: A prospective study. *Child Development, 58,* 1488–1495.

Johnston, C., & Mash, E. J. (2001). Families of children with attention-deficit/hyperactivity disorder: Review and recommendations for future research. *Clinical Child and Family Psychology Review, 4,* 183–207.

Johnstone, S. J., Barry, R. J., & Anderson, J. W. (2001). Topographic distribution and developmental time-course of auditory event-related potentials in two subtypes of attention-deficit hyperactivity disorder. *International Journal of Psychophysiology, 42,* 73–94.

Kelsoe, J. R., Ginns, E. I., Egeland, J. A., Gerhard, D. S., Goldstein, A. M., Bale, S. J., et al. (1989). Reevaluation of the linkage relationship between chromosome 11p loci and the gene for bipolar affective disorder in the Old Order Amish. *Nature, 342,* 238–243.

Kiessling, L. S., Marcotte, A. C., & Culpepper, L. (1993). Antineuronal antibodies in movement disorders. *Pediatrics, 92,* 39–43.

Klorman, R., Brumaghim, J. T., Coons, H. W., Peloquin, L., Strauss, J., Lewine, J. D., et al. (1988). The contributions of event-related potentials to understanding effects of stimulants on information processing in attention deficit disorder. In L. M. Bloomingdale & J. A. Sergeant (Eds.), *Attention deficit disorder: Criteria, cognition, intervention* (pp. 199–218). London: Pergamon Press.

Kuntsi, J., & Stevenson, J. (2000). Hyperactivity in children: A focus on genetic research and psychological theories. *Clinical Child and Family Psychology Review, 3,* 1–23.

Kuperman, S., Johnson, B., Arndt, S., Lindgren, S., & Wolraich, M. (1996). Quantitative EEG differences in a nonclinical sample of children with ADHD and undifferentiated ADD. *Journal of the American Academy of Child and Adolescent Psychiatry, 35,* 1009–1017.

LaHoste, G. J., Swanson, J. M., Wigal, S. B., Glabe, C., Wigal, T., King, N., et al. (1996). Dopamine D4 receptor gene polymorphism is associated with attention deficit hyperactivity disorder. *Molecular Psychiatry, 1,* 121–124.

Langleben, D. D., Acton, P. D., Austin, G., Elman, I., Krikorian, G., Monterosso, J. R., et al. (2002). Effects of methylphenidate discontinuation on cerebral blood flow in prepubescent boys with attention deficit hyperactivity disorder. *Journal of Nuclear Medicine, 43,* 1624–1629.

Langley, K., Marshall, L., van den Bree, M., Thomas, H., Owen, M., O'Donovan, M., et al. (2004). Association of the dopamine D4 receptor gene 7-repeat allele with neuropsychological test performance of children with ADHD. *American Journal of Psychiatry, 161,* 133–138.

Levin, P. M. (1938). Restlessness in children. *Archives of Neurology and Psychiatry, 39,* 764–770.

Levy, F., & Hay, D. (1992, February). *ADHD in twins and their siblings*. Paper presented at the meeting of the International Society for Research in Child and Adolescent Psychopathology, Sarasota, FL.

Levy, F., & Hay, D. A. (2001). *Attention, genes, and attention-deficit hyperactivity disorder*. Philadelphia: Psychology Press.

Levy, F., Hay, D. A., McStephen, M., Wood, C., & Waldman, I. (1997). Attention-deficit hyperactivity disorder: A category or a continuum? Genetic analysis of a large-scale twin study. *Journal of the American Academy of Child and Adolescent Psychiatry, 36*, 737–744.

Linnet, K. M., Dalsgaard, S., Obel, C., Wisborg, K., Henriksen, T. B., Rodriquez, A., et al. (2003). Maternal lifestyle factors in pregnancy risk of attention deficit hyperactivity disorder and associated behaviors: Review of the current literature. *American Journal of Psychiatry, 160*, 1028–1040.

Loo, S. K., & Barkley, R. A. (in press). Clinical utility of EEG in attention deficit hyperactivity disorder. *Applied Developmental Neuropsychology*.

Loo, S. K., Specter, E., Smolen, A., Hopfer, C., Teale, P. D., & Reite, M. L. (2003). Functional effects of the DAT1 polymorphism on EEG measures in ADHD. *Journal of the American Academy of Child and Adolescent Psychiatry, 42*, 986–993.

Lopez, R. (1965). Hyperactivity in twins. *Canadian Psychiatric Association Journal, 10*, 421–425.

Lou, H. C., Henriksen, L., & Bruhn, P. (1984). Focal cerebral hypoperfusion in children with dysphasia and/or attention deficit disorder. *Archives of Neurology, 41*, 825–829.

Lou, H. C., Henriksen, L., & Bruhn, P. (1990). Focal cerebral dysfunction in developmental learning disabilities. *Lancet, 335*, 8–11.

Lou, H. C., Henriksen, L., Bruhn, P., Borner, H., & Nielsen, J. B. (1989). Striatal dysfunction in attention deficit and hyperkinetic disorder. *Archives of Neurology, 46*, 48–52.

Mann, C., Lubar, J. F., Zimmerman, A. W., Miller, C. A., & Muenchen, R. A. (1992). Quantitative analysis of EEG in boys with attention-deficit hyperactivity disorder: Controlled study with clinical implications. *Pediatric Neurology, 8*, 30–36.

Matsuura, M., Okuba, Y., Toru, M., Kojima, T., He, Y., Hou, Y., et al. (1993). A cross-national EEG study of children with emotional and behavioral problems: A WHO collaborative study in the Western Pacific region. *Biological Psychiatry, 34*, 59–65.

Mattes, J. A. (1980). The role of frontal lobe dysfunction in childhood hyperkinesis. *Comprehensive Psychiatry, 21*, 358–369.

Max, J. E., Fox, P. T., Lancaster, J. L., Kochunov, P., Mathews, K., Manes, F. F., et al. (2002). Putamen lesions and the development of attention-deficit/hyperactivity symptomatology. *Journal of the American Academy of Child and Adolescent Psychiatry, 41*, 563–571.

Mercugliano, M. (1995). Neurotransmitter alterations in attention-deficit/hyperactivity disorder. *Mental Retardation and Developmental Disabilities Research Reviews, 1*, 220–226.

Mick, E., Biederman, J., & Faraone, S. V. (1996). Is season of birth a risk factor for attention-deficit hyperactivity disorder? *Journal of the American Academy of Child and Adolescent Psychiatry, 35*, 1470–1476.

Mick, E., Biederman, J., Faraone, S. V., Sayer, J., & Kleinman, S. (2002). Case–control study of attention-deficit hyperactivity disorder and maternal smoking, alcohol use, and drug use during pregnancy. *Journal of the American Academy of Child and Adolescent Psychiatry, 41*, 378–385.

Milberger, S., Biederman, J., Faraone, S. V., Chen, L., & Jones, J. (1996). Is maternal smoking during pregnancy a risk factor for attention deficit hyperactivity disorder in children? *American Journal of Psychiatry, 153*, 1138–1142.

Milberger, S., Biederman, J., Faraone, S. V., Guite, J., & Tsuang, M. T. (1997). Pregnancy, delivery, and infancy complications and attention deficit disorder: Issues of gene–environment interaction. *Biological Psychiatry, 41*, 65–75.

Minde, K., Webb, G., & Sykes, D. (1968). Studies on the hyperactive child: VI. Prenatal and perinatal factors associated with hyperactivity. *Developmental Medicine and Child Neurology, 10*, 355–363.

Monastra, V. J., Lubar, J. F., & Linden, M. (2001). The development of a quantitative electroencephalographic scanning process for attention deficit-hyperactivity disorder: Reliability and validity studies. *Neuropsychology, 15*, 136–144.

Monastra, V. J., Lubar, J. F., Linden, M., VanDeusen, P., Green, G., Wing, W., et al. (1999). Assessing attention deficit hyperactivity disorder via quantitative electroencephalography: An initial validation study. *Neuropsychology, 13*, 424–433.

Morrison, J., & Stewart, M. (1973). The psychiatric status of the legal families of adopted hyperactive children. *Archives of General Psychiatry, 28*, 888–891.

Mueller, K., Daly, M., Fischer, M., Yiannoutsos, C. T., Bauer, L., Barkley, R. A., et al. (2003). Association of the dopamine beta hydroxylase gene with attention deficit hyperactivity disorder: Genetic analysis of the Milwaukee longitudinal study. *American Journal of Medical Genetics, 119B*, 77–85.

Nadder, T. S., Rutter, M., Silberg, J. L., Maes, H. H., & Eaves, L. J. (2002). Genetic effects on the variation and covariation of attention-deficit hyperactivity disorder (ADHD) and oppositional-defiant disorder/conduct disorder (ODD/CD) symptomatologies across informant and occasion of measurement. *Psychological Medicine, 32*, 39–53.

Nasrallah, H. A., Loney, J., Olson, S. C., McCalley-Whitters, M., Kramer, J., & Jacoby, C. G. (1986). Cortical atrophy in young adults with a history of hyperactivity in childhood. *Psychiatry Research, 17*, 241–246.

Needleman, H. L., Gunnoe, C., Leviton, A., Reed, R., Peresie, H., Maher, C., et al. (1979). Deficits in psychologic and classroom performance of children with elevated dentine lead levels. *New England Journal of Medicine, 300,* 689–695.

Needleman, H. L., Schell, A., Bellinger, D. C., Leviton, L., & Alfred, E. D. (1990). The long-term effects of exposure to low doses of lead in childhood: An 11-year follow-up report. *New England Journal of Medicine, 322,* 83–88.

Nichols, P. L., & Chen, T. C. (1981). *Minimal brain dysfunction: A prospective study.* Hillsdale, NJ: Erlbaum.

O'Connor, M., Foch, T., Sherry, T., & Plomin, R. (1980). A twin study of specific behavioral problems of socialization as viewed by parents. *Journal of Abnormal Child Psychology, 8,* 189–199.

O'Dougherty, M., Nuechterlein, K. H., & Drew, B. (1984). Hyperactive and hypoxic children: Signal detection, sustained attention, and behavior. *Journal of Abnormal Psychology, 93,* 178–191.

O'Malley, K. D., & Nanson, J. (2002). Clinical implications of a link between fetal alcohol spectrum disorder and attention-deficit hyperactivity disorder. *Canadian Journal of Psychiatry, 47,* 349–354.

Pauls, D. L. (1991). Genetic factors in the expression of attention-deficit hyperactivity disorder. *Journal of Child and Adolescent Psychopharmacology, 1,* 353–360.

Peterson, B. S., Leckman, J. F., Tucker, D., Scahill, L., Staib, L., Zhang, H., et al. (2000). Preliminary findings of antistreptococcal antibody titers and basal ganglia volumes in tic, obsessive–compulsive, and attention-deficit/hyperactivity disorders. *Archives of General Psychiatry, 57,* 364–372.

Pike, A., & Plomin, R. (1996). Importance of nonshared environmental factors for childhood and adolescent psychopathology. *Journal of the American Academy of Child and Adolescent Psychiatry, 35,* 560–570.

Pliszka, S. R., Liotti, M., & Woldorff, M. G. (2000). Inhibitory control in children with attention-deficit/hyperactivity disorder: Event-related potentials identify the processing component and timing of an impaired right-frontal response-inhibition mechanism. *Biological Psychiatry, 48,* 238–246.

Pliszka, S. R., McCracken, J. T., & Maas, J. W. (1996). Catecholamines in attention deficit/hyperactivity disorder: Current perspectives. *Journal of the American Academy of Child and Adolescent Psychiatry, 35,* 264–272.

Plomin, R. (1995). Genetics and children's experiences in the family. *Journal of Child Psychology and Psychiatry, 36,* 33–68.

Pontius, A. A. (1973). Dysfunction patterns analogous to frontal lobe system and caudate nucleus syndromes in some groups of minimal brain dysfunction. *Journal of the American Medical Women's Association, 26,* 285–292.

Rapoport, J. L., Buchsbaum, M. S., Zahn, T. P., Weingarten, H., Ludlow, C., & Mikkelsen, E. J. (1978). Dextroamphetamine: Cognitive and behav-

ioral effects in normal prepubertal boys. *Science, 199,* 560–563.

Raskin, L. A., Shaywitz, S. E., Shaywitz, B. A., Anderson, G. M., & Cohen, D. J. (1984). Neurochemical correlates of attention deficit disorder. *Pediatric Clinics of North America, 31,* 387–396.

Reitveld, M. J. H., Hudziak, J. J., Bartels, M., van Beijsterveldt, C. E. M., & Boomsma, D. I. (2004). Heritability of attention problems in children: Longitudinal results from a study of twins, age 3 to 12. *Journal of Child Psychology and Psychiatry, 45,* 577–588.

Rhee, S. H., Waldman, I. D., Hay, D. A., & Levy, F. (1995). Sex differences in genetic and environmental influences on DSM-III-R attention-deficit hyperactivity disorder (ADHD). *Behavior Genetics, 25,* 285–293.

Rhee, S. H., Waldman, I. D., Hay, D. A., & Levy, F. (1999). Sex differences in genetic and environmental influences on DSM-III-R attention-deficit hyperactivity disorder. *Journal of Abnormal Psychology, 108,* 24–41.

Rosenthal, R. H., & Allen, T. W. (1978). An examination of attention, arousal, and learning dysfunctions of hyperkinetic children. *Psychological Bulletin, 85,* 689–715.

Ross, D. M., & Ross, S. A. (1982). *Hyperactivity: Research, theory and action.* New York: Wiley.

Rubia, K., Overmeyer, S., Taylor, E., Brammer, M., Williams, S. C. R., Simmons, A., et al. (1999). Hypofrontality in attention deficit hyperactivity disorder during higher-order motor control: A study with functional MRI. *American Journal of Psychiatry, 156,* 891–896.

Rutter, M. (1977). Brain damage syndromes in childhood: Concepts and findings. *Journal of Child Psychology and Psychiatry, 18,* 1–21.

Rutter, M. (1983). Introduction: Concepts of brain dysfunction syndromes. In M. Rutter (Ed.), *Developmental neuropsychiatry* (pp. 1–14). New York: Guilford Press.

Sagvolden, T., Johansen, E. B., Aase, H., & Russell, V. A. (in press). A dynamic developmental theory of attention-deficit/hyperactivity disorder (ADHD) predominantly hyperactive/impulsive and combined subtypes. *Behavioral and Brain Sciences.*

Samuel, V., George, P., Thornell, A., Curtis, S., Taylor, A., Brome, D., et al. (1997, October). *A pilot controlled family study of ADHD in African-American children.* Paper presented at the annual meeting of the American Academy of Child and Adolescent Psychiatry, Toronto.

Schothorst, P. F., & van Engeland, H. (1996). Long-term behavioral sequelae of prematurity. *Journal of the American Academy of Child and Adolescent Psychiatry, 35,* 175–183.

Schweitzer, J. B., Faber, T. L., Grafton, S. T., Tune, L. E., Hoffman, J. M., & Kilts, C. D. (2000). Alterations in the functional anatomy of working memory in adult attention deficit/hyperactivity disorder. *American Journal of Psychiatry, 157,* 278–280.

Seidman, L. J. (1997, October). *Neuropsychological findings in ADHD children: Findings from a sample of high-risk siblings.* Paper presented at the annual meeting of the American Academy of Child and Adolescent Psychiatry, Toronto.

Seidman, L. J., Biederman, J., Faraone, S. V., Weber, W., & Ouellette, C. (1997). Toward defining a neuropsychology of attention deficit-hyperactivity disorder: Performance of children and adolescence from a large clinically referred sample. *Journal of Consulting and Clinical Psychology, 65,* 150–160.

Semrud-Clikeman, M., Filipek, P. A., Biederman, J., Steingard, R., Kennedy, D., Renshaw, P., et al. (1994). Attention-deficit hyperactivity disorder: Magnetic resonance imaging morphometric analysis of the corpus callosum. *Journal of the American Academy of Child and Adolescent Psychiatry, 33,* 875–881.

Semrud-Clikeman, M., Steingard, R. J., Filipek, P., Biederman, J., Bekken, K., & Renshaw, P. F. (2000). Using MRI to examine brain–behavior relationships in males with attention deficit disorder with hyperactivity. *Journal of the American Academy of Child and Adolescent Psychiatry, 39,* 477–484.

Sharp, W. S., Gottesman, R. F., Greenstein, D. K., Ebens, C. L., Rapoport, J. L., & Castellanos, F. X. (2003). Monozygotic twins discordant for attention-deficit/hyperactivity disorder: Ascertainment and clinical characteristics. *Journal of the American Academy of Child and Adolescent Psychiatry, 42,* 93–97.

Shaywitz, B. A., Shaywitz, S. E., Byrne, T., Cohen, D. J., & Rothman, S. (1983). Attention deficit disorder: Quantitative analysis of CT. *Neurology, 33,* 1500–1503.

Shaywitz, S. E., Cohen, D. J., & Shaywitz, B. E. (1980). Behavior and learning difficulties in children of normal intelligence born to alcoholic mothers. *Journal of Pediatrics, 96,* 978–982.

Shaywitz, S. E., Shaywitz, B. A., Cohen, D. J., & Young, J. G. (1983). Monoaminergic mechanisms in hyperactivity. In M. Rutter (Ed.), *Developmental neuropsychiatry* (pp. 330–347). New York: Guilford Press.

Shaywitz, S. E., Shaywitz, B. A., Jatlow, P. R., Sebrechts, M., Anderson, G. M., & Cohen, D. J. (1986). Biological differentiation of attention deficit disorder with and without hyperactivity: A preliminary report. *Annals of Neurology, 21,* 363.

Sherman, D. K., Iacono, W. G., & McGue, M. K. (1997). Attention-deficit hyperactivity disorder dimensions: A twin study of inattention and impulsivity–hyperactivity. *Journal of the American Academy of Child and Adolescent Psychiatry, 36,* 745–753.

Sherman, D. K., McGue, M. K., & Iacono, W. G. (1997). Twin concordance for attention deficit hyperactivity disorder: A comparison of teachers' and mothers' reports. *American Journal of Psychiatry, 154,* 532–535.

Sieg, K. G., Gaffney, G. R., Preston, D. F., & Hellings, J. A. (1995). SPECT brain imaging abnormalities in attention deficit hyperactivity disorder. *Clinical Nuclear Medicine, 20,* 55–60.

Silberg, J., Rutter, M., Meyer, J., Maes, H., Hewitt, J., Simonoff, E., et al. (1996). Genetic and environmental influences on the covariation between hyperactivity and conduct disturbance in juvenile twins. *Journal of Child Psychology and Psychiatry, 37,* 803–816.

Silva, P. A., Hughes, P., Williams, S., & Faed, J. M. (1988). Blood lead, intelligence, reading attainment, and behaviour in eleven year old children in Dunedin, New Zealand. *Journal of Child Psychology and Psychiatry, 29,* 43–52.

Silverman, I. W., & Ragusa, D. M. (1992). A short-term longitudinal study of the early development of self-regulation. *Journal of Abnormal Child Psychology, 20,* 415–435.

Singer, H. S., Giuliano, J. D., Hansen, B. H., Hallett, J. J., Laurino, J. P., Benson, M., et al. (1998). Antibodies against human putamen in children with Tourette syndrome. *Neurology, 50,* 1618–1624.

Singer, H. S., Reiss, A. L., Brown, J. E., Aylward, E. H., Shih, B., Chee, E., et al. (1993). Volumetric MRI changes in basal ganglia of children with Tourette's syndrome. *Neurology, 43,* 950–956.

Smalley, S. L., Kustanovich, V., Minassian, S. L., Stone, J. L., Ogdie, M. N., McGough, J. J., et al. (2002). Genetic linkage of attention-deficit/hyperactivity disorder on chromosome 16p13, in a region implicated in autism. *American Journal of Human Genetics, 71,* 959–963.

Smalley, S. L., McGough, J. J., Del'Homme, M., NewDelman, J., Gordon, E., Kim, T., et al. (2000). Familial clustering of symptoms and disruptive behaviors in multiplex families with attention-deficit/hyperactivity disorder. *Journal of the American Academy of Child and Adolescent Psychiatry, 39,* 1135–1143.

Sonuhara, G. A., Barr, C., Schachar, R. J., Tannock, R., Roberts, W., Malone, M. A., et al. (1997, October). *Association study of the dopamine D4 receptor gene in children and adolescents with ADHD.* Paper presented at the annual meeting of the American Academy of Child and Adolescent Psychiatry, Toronto.

Sprich, S., Biederman, J., Crawford, M. H., Mundy, E., & Faraone, S. V. (2000). Adoptive and biological families of children and adolescents with ADHD. *Journal of the American Academy of Child and Adolescent Psychiatry, 39,* 1432–1437.

Stein, M. A., Krasowski, M., Leventhal, B. L., Phillips, W., & Bender, B. G. (1996). Behavioral and cognitive effects of methylxanthines: A meta-analysis of theophylline and caffeine. *Archives of Pediatric and Adolescent Medicine, 150,* 284–288.

Stevenson, J. (1994, June). *Genetics of ADHD.* Paper

presented at the meeting of the Professional Group for ADD and Related Disorders, London.

Streissguth, A. P., Bookstein, F. L., Sampson, P. D., & Barr, H. M. (1995). Attention: Prenatal alcohol and continuities of vigilance and attentional problems from 4 through 14 years. *Development and Psychopathology, 7,* 419–446.

Streissguth, A. P., Martin, D. C., Barr, H. M., Sandman, B. M., Kirchner, G. L., & Darby, B. L. (1984). Intrauterine alcohol and nicotine exposure: Attention and reaction time in 4-year-old children. *Developmental Psychology, 20,* 533–541.

Stuss, D. T., & Benson, D. F. (1986). *The frontal lobes.* New York: Raven Press.

Swanson, J. M., Sunohara, G. A., Kennedy, J. L., Regino, R., Fineberg, E., Wigal, E., et al. (1998). Association of the dopamine receptor D4 (DRD4) gene with a refined phenotype of attention deficit hyperactivity disorder (ADHD): A family-based approach. *Molecular Psychiatry, 3,* 38–42.

Sykes, D. H., Hoy, E. A., Bill, J. M., McClure, B. G., Halloiday, H. L., & Reid, M. M. (1997). Behavioral adjustment in school of very low birthweight children. *Journal of Child Psychology and Psychiatry, 38,* 315–325.

Szatmari, P., Saigal, S., Rosenbaum, P., & Campbell, D. (1993). Psychopathology and adaptive functioning among extremely low birthweight children at eight years of age. *Development and Psychopathology, 5,* 345–357.

Tannock, R. (1998). Attention deficit hyperactivity disorder: Advances in cognitive, neurobiological, and genetic research. *Journal of Child Psychology and Psychiatry, 39,* 65–100.

Teicher, M. H., Anderson, C. M., Polcari, A., Glod, C. A., Maas, L. C., & Renshaw, P. F. (2000). Functional deficits in basal ganglia of children with attention-deficit/hyperactivity disorder shown with functional magnetic resonance imaging relaxometry. *Nature Medicine, 6,* 470–473.

Thapar, A., Harrington, R., Ross, K., & McGuffin, P. (2000). Does the definition of ADHD affect heritability? *Journal of the American Academy of Child and Adolescent Psychiatry, 39,* 1528–1536.

Thapar, A., Hervas, A., & McGuffin, P. (1995). Childhood hyperactivity scores are highly heritable and show sibling competition effects: Twin study evidence. *Behavior Genetics, 25,* 537–544.

Thapar, A., Holmes, J., Poulton, K., & Harrington, R. (1999). Genetic basis of attention deficit and hyperactivity. *British Journal of Psychiatry, 174,* 105–111.

Thomson, G. O. B., Raab, G. M., Hepburn, W. S., Hunter, R., Fulton, M., & Laxen, D. P. H., (1989). Blood-lead levels and children's behaviour: Results from the Edinburgh lead study. *Journal of Child Psychology and Psychiatry, 30,* 515–528.

Todd, R. D., Rasmussen, E. R., Neuman, R. J., Reich, W., Hudziak, J. J., Bucholz, K. F., et al. (2001). Familiality and heritability of subtypes of attention deficit hyperactivity disorder in a population sample of adolescent female twins. *American Journal of Psychiatry, 158,* 1891–1898.

Vaidya, C. J., Austin, G., Kirkorian, G., Ridlehuber, H. W., Desmond, J. E., Glover, G. H., et al. (1998). Selective effects of methylphenidate in attention deficit hyperactivity disorder: A functional magnetic resonance study. *Proceedings of the National Academy of Sciences USA, 95,* 14494–14499.

Van Den Bergh, B. R. H., & Marcoen, A. (2004). High antenatal maternal anxiety is related to ADHD symptoms, externalizing problems, and anxiety in 8- and 9-year-olds. *Child Development, 75,* 1085–1097.

van den Oord, E. J. C., Boomsma, D. I., & Verhulst, F. C. (1994). A study of problem behaviors in 10- to 15-year-old biolo lgically related and unrelated international adoptees. *Behavior Genetics, 24,* 193–205.

van den Oord, E. J. C., & Rowe, D. C. (1997). Continuity and change in children's social maladjustment: A developmental behavior genetic study. *Developmental Psychology, 33,* 319–332.

van den Oord, E. J. C., Verhulst, F. C., & Boomsma, D. I. (1996). A genetic study of maternal and paternal ratings of problem behaviors in 3-year-old twins. *Journal of Abnormal Psychology, 105,* 349–357.

Waldman, I. D., Rowe, D. C., Abramowitz, A., Kozel, S. T., Mohr, J. H., Sherman, S. L., et al. (1998). Association and linkage of the dopamine transporter gene and attention-deficit hyperactivity disorder in children: Heterogeneity owing to diagnostic subtype and severity. *American Journal of Human Genetics, 63,* 1767–1776.

Weiss, G., & Hechtman, L. (1993). *Hyperactive children grown up* (2nd ed.). New York: Guilford Press.

Welner, Z., Welner, A., Stewart, M., Palkes, H., & Wish, E. (1977). A controlled study of siblings of hyperactive children. *Journal of Nervous and Mental Disease, 165,* 110–117.

Werner, E. E., Bierman, J. M., French, F. W., Simonian, K., Connor, A., Smith, R. S., et al. (1968). Reproductive and environmental casualties: A report on the 10-year follow-up of the children of the Kauai pregnancy study. *Pediatrics, 42,* 112–127.

Whittaker, A. H., Van Rossem, R., Feldman, J. F., Schonfeld, I. S., Pinto-Martin, J. A., Torre, C., et al. (1997). Psychiatric outcomes in low-birth-weight children at age 6 years: Relation to neonatal cranial ultrasound abnormalities. *Archives of General Psychiatry, 54,* 847–856.

Wigg, K., Zai, G., Schachar, R., Tannock, R., Roberts, W., Malone, M., et al. (2002). Attention deficit hyperactivity disorder and the gene for dopamine beta-hydroxylase. *American Journal of Psychiatry, 159,* 1046–1048.

Willerman, L. (1973). Activity level and hyperactivity in twins. *Child Development, 44,* 288–293.

Willis, T. J., & Lovaas, I. (1977). A behavioral approach to treating hyperactive children: The parent's role. In

J. B. Millichap (Ed.), *Learning disabilities and related disorders* (pp. 119–140). Chicago: Year Book Medical.

Winsberg, B. G., & Comings, D. E. (1999). Association of the dopamine transporter gene (DAT1) with poor methylphenidate response. *Journal of the American Academy of Child and Adolescent Psychiatry, 38,* 1474–1477.

Wolf, S. M., & Forsythe, A. (1978). Behavior disturbance, phenobarbital, and febrile seizures. *Pediatrics, 61,* 728–731.

Yeo, R. A., Hill, D. E., Campbell, R. A., Vigil, J., Petropoulos, H., Hart, B., et al. (2003). Proton magnetic resonance spectroscopy investigation of the right frontal lobe in children with attention-deficit/hyperactivity disorder. *Journal of the American Academy of Child and Adolescent Psychiatry, 42,* 303–310.

Youdin, M. B. H., & Riederer, P. (1997). Understanding Parkinson's disease. *Scientific American, 276,* 52–59.

Zametkin, A. J., Liebenauer, L. L., Fitzgerald, G. A., King, A. C., Minkunas, D. V., Herscovitch, P., et al. (1993). Brain metabolism in teenagers with attention-deficit hyperactivity disorder. *Archives of General Psychiatry, 50,* 333–340.

Zametkin, A. J., Nordahl, T. E., Gross, M., King, A. C., Semple, W. E., Rumsey, J., et al. (1990). Cerebral glucose metabolism in adults with hyperactivity of childhood onset. *New England Journal of Medicine, 323,* 1361–1366.

Zametkin, A. J., & Rapoport, J. L. (1986). The pathophysiology of attention deficit disorder with hyperactivity: A review. In B. B. Lahey & A. E. Kazdin (Eds.), *Advances in clinical child psychology* (Vol. 9, pp. 177–216). New York: Plenum Press.

CHAPTER 6

ADHD in Adults

Developmental Course and Outcome of Children
with ADHD, and ADHD in Clinic-Referred Adults

RUSSELL A. BARKLEY

The symptoms of Attention-Deficit/Hyperactivity Disorder (ADHD) appear to arise relatively early in childhood, with the mean age of onset being between 3 and 5 years (see Chapter 2), and ranging between infancy and as late as 12 years (Applegate et al., 1997; Barkley & Biederman, 1997). Although most cases may develop before age 7 years, in a sizable minority of cases the children may have had their ADHD characteristics for quite some time, but these traits did not interfere with their academic or social functioning until later childhood. Thus the onset of impairment may succeed the onset of symptoms by several years or more. This seems to occur with regard to academic impairment in very bright or gifted children with ADHD, whose superior intellect allows them to pass through the early grades of school without difficulty, because they do not need to apply much effort to be successful. As the workload at home and school increases in length and complexity, and greater demands for responsibility and self-control are made, such children become impaired by their deficits. This interface between environmental demands and child capabilities seems important in determining the degree to which a child's ADHD will prove disabling throughout his or her development.

This chapter first discusses the developmental course and adult outcome of children with ADHD, as revealed by many different follow-up studies, including my own research in this area with Mariellen Fischer at the Medical College of Wisconsin. It then discusses the much smaller literature on the nature of ADHD among clinic-referred adults seeking services for their disorder. The two populations are not the same. As will become evident below, among children with ADHD followed to adulthood, some no longer qualify fully for the diagnosis of the disorder. This is not the case among clinic-referred adults diagnosed with the disorder, all of whom so qualify. When individuals with childhood ADHD are followed into adulthood, very few such individuals are seeking clinical assistance for themselves (at least not in their 20s and early 30s), whereas nearly all clinic-referred adults are so motivated. These and other differences that will become apparent later make it necessary to keep these two literatures on ADHD in adults separate.

FACTORS ASSOCIATED WITH RISK FOR DEVELOPING ADHD

Certain parental characteristics have been noted to be associated with risk for ADHD in children of those parents, as described previously (see Chapters 4 and 5). Chief among these is parental ADHD, which can increase the odds of a child of that parents' having ADHD by eight times, or approximately 30–54% (Biederman et al., 1995; Milberger, Biederman, Faraone, Guite, & Tsuang, 1997). Although early studies in this area implied that parents with depression, alcoholism, Conduct Disorder (CD), and Antisocial Personality Disorder may be more likely to have children with ADHD (Cantwell, 1975; Morrison & Stewart, 1973), these disorders are actually comorbid with ADHD in most cases. It is the adult ADHD in such cases that is the likely risk factor, and not alcoholism or CD alone. However, as noted in Chapters 4 and 5, depression and ADHD seem to share an underlying genetic vulnerability to each other, as do ADHD and CD. In this case, it is not the comorbid disorders per se that increase the risk, but their shared genetic basis, which could easily be predisposing toward all of them in combination in the parent (and hence in the offspring of that parent). As for alcoholism, the risk may arise through the additional mechanism of maternal drinking during pregnancy which, as noted in Chapter 5, is a risk factor for ADHD in the offspring of that pregnancy (odds ratio of about 2.5). And since mothers who drink during pregnancy often smoke as well, the contribution of maternal smoking could increase this risk by another 2.5 times, as also noted in Chapter 5 (see also Linnet et al., 2003; Milberger, Biederman, Faraone, Guite, et al., 1997). The mechanism by which the risk to offspring can arise in these circumstances is therefore complex; it is likely to be a combination of shared genetic liability between parent and child with the teratogenic effects of maternal smoking and drinking, which may directly affect the child's developing brain *in utero*.

Having a hyperactive sibling may also be a predictor of higher risk of hyperactivity among other children in the family, because of the high genetic risk it conveys to biologically related siblings (again, see Chapter 5). Goodman and Stevenson (1989) estimated this risk to be approximately 13–17% for female siblings and 27–30% for male siblings, regardless of whether the hyperactive proband is male or female. Earlier, Welner, Welner, Stewart, Palkes, and Wish (1977) found a 35% risk of hyperactivity in siblings of children diagnosed with hyperactivity. In general, the risk to immediate family members if a child in the family has ADHD is between 12% and 29%, and this risk is elevated whether the child is a male or female or whether European American or African American samples are used (Faraone et al., 2000; Samuel et al., 1999). In short, families with an existing history of ADHD among their relatives, especially the immediate parents and siblings, are more likely to have hyperactivity or ADHD in their children than are those families without such familial disorders. Other family risk factors associated with the early emergence and persistence of ADHD symptoms are low maternal education and socioeconomic status (SES) and single parenthood or father desertion (Nichols & Chen, 1981; Palfrey, Levine, Walker, & Sullivan, 1985); however, these may not remain significant once parental ADHD is controlled (Milberger, Biederman, Faraone, Guite, et al., 1997).

Several studies cited in Chapter 5 showed that pregnancy complications and problems at time of delivery are more likely for children with ADHD than for nondisabled children. In their large epidemiological study, Nichols and Chen (1981) found that the following pregnancy factors, in decreasing order of importance, were predictive of later hyperactivity in children: number of cigarettes smoked per day, maternal convulsions, maternal hospitalizations, fetal distress, and placental weight. And as Chapter 5 has also noted, younger-than-usual motherhood may be another risk factor for offspring ADHD (Claycomb, Ryan, Miller, & Schnakenberg-Ott, 2004), possibly due to a greater likelihood of such mothers' actually having ADHD themselves (see the discussion of young adults' pregnancy risks below), and also due to the increased antenatal risks such pregnancies are likely to suffer.

Certain neonatal and infancy variables have been studied for their association with ADHD. Nichols and Chen (1981) found delayed motor development, smaller head circumference at birth and at 12 months of age, meconium staining, neonatal nerve damage, primary apnea, and low birth weight, among others, to be predictive of later hyperactivity to a low but significant degree (regression weights below .19). Prematurity of delivery has also been noted in

Chapter 5 to be repeatedly associated with a greater risk for later ADHD in childhood, particularly in children with evidence of parenchymal injuries or ventricular enlargement (Bradley & Golden, 2001; Whittaker et al., 1997). Moreover, greater health problems and delayed motor development were found by others to be associated with a higher risk for early and persistent ADHD symptoms (Hartsough & Lambert, 1985; Palfrey et al., 1985).

"Temperament" refers to early and relatively persistent personality characteristics of children, such as activity level, intensity or degree of energy in a response, persistence or attention span, demandingness of others, quality of mood (e.g., irritability or quickness to anger or display emotion), adaptability or capacity to adjust to change, and rhythmicity (i.e., the regularity of sleep–waking periods, eating, and elimination). The early emergence of excessive activity level, short durations of responding to objects, low persistence of pursuing objects with which to play, strong intensity of response, and parent-reported negativity or demandingness in infancy are more often found in children with ADHD than in nondisabled or clinical control groups of young children (Barkley, DuPaul, & McMurray, 1990; Nigg, Goldsmith, & Sachek, 2004). Some of these factors, such as high activity level, short attention span, and difficult temperament in general, also predict the persistence of these behavioral problems into the preschool years (Campbell, 1990; Carlson, Jacobvitz, & Sroufe, 1995; Deater-Deckard, Dodge, Bates, & Petit, 1998; Jacobvitz & Sroufe, 1987; Keenan, Shaw, Delliquadri, Giovannelli, & Walsh, 1998; McInerny & Chamberlin, 1978; Palfrey et al., 1985; Prior, Leonard, & Wood, 1983) and thus may provide some linkage between research on temperamental traits and the disorder of ADHD (Nigg et al., 2004).

One aspect of a difficult temperament is negativity (high fear, greater distress at parental limit setting, or generally greater emotional expression). But infant negativity specifically may not be associated with externalizing problems later on when it is measured objectively, apart from parent reports of such. For instance, Belsky, Hsieh, and Crnic (1998) followed 125 children through infancy to early childhood and found that directly observed infant negativity was not a risk factor for later externalizing problems or impulsivity, but more neg-

ative mothering was so associated, whereas more positive fathering was associated with better inhibition. Campbell (1990) also found that the existence of a negative, critical, and commanding style of child management by mothers of children with preschool hyperactivity was associated with the persistence of hyperactivity by ages 4, 6, and 9 years. Others (Cameron, 1978; Earls & Jung, 1987) also found that prediction of behavioral problems in childhood was greatly enhanced by considering parent psychiatric distress, hostility, and marital discord, in addition to preschool temperament. Such developmental risks are likely to be transactional, in that child features such as noncompliance, lack of persistence, and very early onset of externalizing behavior interact with parental responsiveness and rejection as well as peer relations to predict later elevated externalizing behavior (Deater-Deckard et al., 1998; Shaw et al., 1998). And so, while negativity per se may not be a risk factor for later externalizing problems, other features of the child's temperament (activity, attention) and family (disrupted parenting) clearly are so.

The problem with these studies for our purposes, however, is twofold. First, they did not separate out child ADHD specifically from the broader class of externalizing problems, which includes symptoms of Oppositional Defiant Disorder (ODD) and CD. As Chapters 4 and 5 have noted, ADHD may not arise from parental behavior, but ODD and CD are certainly associated in part with quality of parenting. This makes it likely that these findings on early childhood predictors of externalizing problems may have arisen more from the inclusion of ODD and CD in the measures of such problems than from the inclusion of ADHD. Second, the studies did not evaluate the parents for ADHD, nor did they control for genetic similarities in traits between parents and children. Thus, although rejecting and negative parents may have disruptive and aggressive children, the relationship is mediated by their shared genetic predispositions toward hostility and is not necessarily a direct effect of parenting on child behavior.

The appearance of early and persistent problems with activity, inhibition, and persistence of attention, however, is clearly associated with ADHD in the preschool years (ages 2–5) (Carlson et al., 1995; Jacobvitz & Sroufe, 1987; Palfrey et al., 1985; Prior et al., 1983). For instance, we (Shelton et al., 1998) screened a large sample of children entering kindergarten for high levels of hyperactive–impulsive–inattentive and aggressive behaviors, and found that the majority (80%) qualified for a diagnosis of ADHD upon more careful clinical evaluation. These traits also predicted a continuation of both ADHD symptoms and aggression or conduct problems on entry into formal schooling (Barkley, Shelton, et al., 2002; see also Buss, Block, & Block, 1980; Campbell, 1990; Earls & Jung, 1987; Fagot, 1984; Fischer, Rolf, Hasazi, & Cummings, 1984; Garrison, Earls, & Kindlon, 1984; Halverson & Waldrop, 1976; Palfrey et al., 1985). Such traits also predict greater reading and academic achievement delays, poorer social skills and relations, greater use of special educational services (22–46%), and greater likelihood of being on medication (14–29%) by second grade (Barkley, Shelton, et al., 2002; Mariani & Barkley, 1997; Palfrey et al., 1985). In addition, adaptive disability (i.e., levels of adaptive functioning below a standard score of 80) in combination with high levels of ADHD symptoms predicted an even greater level of academic and social impairment, as well as risk for later ODD (46–60%) and CD (9–30%) (Barkley, Shelton, et al., 2002). Children whose inattentive–hyperactive symptoms are sufficiently severe to warrant a diagnosis of ADHD in childhood are quite likely to continue to receive this diagnosis 3 years later in elementary school (72%) (Barkley, Shelton, et al., 2002); 8–10 years later, in adolescence (70–80%) (Barkley, Fischer, Edelbrock, & Smallish, 1990; Beitchman, Wekerle, & Hood, 1987; Lerner, Inui, Trupin, & Douglas, 1985; Weiss & Hechtman, 1993); and even later, in young adulthood (46–66%) (Barkley, Fischer, Smallish, & Fletcher, 2002).

Taken together, these findings suggest that it is possible to identify children at risk for developing an early and persistent pattern of ADHD symptoms prior to their entrance into kindergarten, and perhaps even as early as 2–3 years of age. A combination of both child and parental variables seems the most useful. The following factors would appear to be useful as potential predictors of the early emergence and persistence of ADHD in children: (1) family, especially parental, history of ADHD; (2) maternal smoking and alcohol consumption, and poor maternal health during pregnancy; (3) prematurity and/or significantly low birth weight; (4) poor infant health and developmental motor delays; (5) the early emergence of high activity level, impersistence, and (parent-reported) demandingness in infancy; (6) preschool adaptive disability; and (7) critical/directive/rejecting parental behavior in early childhood. The last factor seems to be associated more with comorbidity for ODD/CD than for ADHD. Some studies have examined factors that may be protective against the development of ADHD or its persistence from early childhood to school age. They, of course, tend to be the opposite of those risk factors noted above, and are (1) higher parental education, (2) better infant health, (3) higher cognitive ability, (4) absence of adaptive disability, (5) better language skills, and (6) greater family stability (see Campbell, 1987, 1990; Palfrey et al., 1985; Weithorn & Kagan, 1978).

PRESCHOOL CHILDREN WITH ADHD

The appearance of significantly inattentive and overactive behavior by age 3 years, in itself, is not indicative of a persistent pattern of ADHD into later childhood in at least 50–90% of those children so characterized. Palfrey et al. (1985) noted that approximately 5% of their total sample of children, or about 10% of those with concerns about inattention, eventually developed a pattern of persistent inattention that was predictive of behavior problems, low academic achievement, and need for special educational services by second grade. Campbell (1990) also showed that among difficult-to-manage 3-year-olds, those whose problems still existed by age 4 years were much more likely to be considered clinically hyperactive and to have difficulties with their hyperactivity, as well as conduct problems, by ages 6 and 9 years. Therefore, both the degree of ADHD symptoms *and* their duration determine which children are likely to show a chronic course of their ADHD symptoms throughout later development. All this means is that concerns about ADHD-like symptoms at an early age do not a diagnosis make. But once such symptoms reach the point where a clinical diagnosis of ADHD is warranted in a preschooler, the chances of a persistent disorder become markedly higher, with over 70% continuing to so qualify 3 years later (Barkley, Shelton, et al., 2002). Those who no longer qualify for the diagnosis are not necessarily within the nondisabled range; many remaining simply continue to have subthreshold cases of the disorder.

Parents of children with this durable pattern of ADHD in this age group describe them as restless, always up and on the go, acting as if driven by a motor, and frequently climbing on and getting into things. They are more likely to encounter accidental injuries as a result of their overactive, inattentive, impulsive, and often fearless pattern of behavior. "Childproofing" the home at this age becomes essential to reduce the risk of injury or poisoning. Persistent in their wants, demanding of parental attention, and often insatiable in their curiosity about their environment, preschoolers with ADHD pose a definite challenge to the child-rearing skills of their parents. Such children require far more frequent and closer monitoring of their ongoing conduct than do typical preschoolers; at times they have to be tethered to allow parents to complete necessary household functions requiring their undivided attention. Noncompliance is common, and at least 30–60% are actively defiant or oppositional, especially if they are boys. Although temper tantrums may be common instances even for typical preschoolers, their frequency and intensity are often exacerbated in children with ADHD. Mothers of these children are likely to find themselves giving far more commands, directions, criticism, supervision, and punishment than do mothers of typical preschoolers (Barkley, 1988; Battle & Lacey, 1972; Campbell, 1990; Cohen & Minde, 1981; Danforth, Barkley, & Stokes, 1991). Although the mothers of preschoolers with ADHD are likely to report feeling competent in their sense of knowing how to manage children, this finding will progressively decline as these children grow older and parents find that the techniques used to manage typical children are less effective with children with ADHD (Mash & Johnston, 1983; Johnston & Mash, 2001). The coexistence of additional difficulties, such as sleep problems, toilet-training difficulties, and/or motor and speech delays, in a small to moderate percentage of children with ADHD is likely to further tax the patience and competence of many of their parents. No wonder, then, that mothers of preschoolers with ADHD report their lives to be much more stressful in their parental roles than do either mothers of typical preschoolers or mothers of older children with ADHD (Fischer, 1990; Mash & Johnston, 1982, 1983; Johnston & Mash, 2001).

Should such a child happen to have a mother whose own mental health is compromised by psychiatric problems, such as depression, anxiety, or hysteria, or whose marriage or couple relationship is in trouble, the combination of negative child temperament with a psychologically distressed caregiver could be potentially explosive and increase the risk of physical abuse to the child, particularly if the child's irritability is a function of childhood Bipolar I Disorder (see Chapter 4). This same situation may also arise when the father of this child has alcoholism, exhibits antisocial behavior, or is highly aggressive within the family. Research indicates that this combination of parent and child characteristics is a strong predictor of children's going on to develop significant aggressive behavior or ODD; it is an especially strong predictor of CD (again, see Chapter 4).

Placement of these children in day care or preschool is likely to bring additional distress as personnel begin to complain about the children's disruptive behavior, aggression toward others in many cases, and difficulties in being managed. Such children are often noted to be out of their seats, wandering the room inappropriately, disrupting the play activities of other children, excessively demanding during peer interactions, and especially vocally noisy and talkative (Barkley, Shelton, et al., 2002; Campbell, Endman, & Bernfield, 1977; Campbell, Schleifer, & Weiss, 1978; Schleifer et al., 1975; Shelton et al., 1998). It is not uncommon for the more active and aggressive of these children with ADHD actually to be "kicked out" of preschool; so begins the course of school adjustment problems afflicting many of these children throughout their compulsory educational careers. Other children with ADHD—especially those who are not oppositional or aggressive, who have a milder level of ADHD, or who are intellectually brighter—may have few or no difficulties with the demands of a typical day care or preschool program. This is especially true if the program lasts only half a day for a few days each week, and if it is conducted in the morning hours when the children are better behaved.

Difficulties in obtaining babysitters for their children, especially the ones more severe ADHD and oppositional symptoms, is reported by mothers of children with ADHD at this age during clinical interviews. This difficulty may result in a greater restriction of both socializing with other adults and the ability to carry out the typical and necessary errands within the community needed to care for a household. For single parents of children with ADHD, these limitations may prove more frequent and distressing, as there is no other adult with whom to share the burden of raising such children.

As preschool children with ADHD approach entry into formal schooling, research suggests that they are already at high risk for academic failure. Not only does their symptom picture predispose them to be less ready to learn in school, but they are also more likely to be behind in basic academic readiness skills (e.g., prereading abilities, simple math concepts, and fine motor skills) (Barkley, Shelton, et al., 2002; Mariani & Barkley, 1997; Shelton et al., 1998). And, as noted in Chapter 3, they may be somewhat less intelligent than their peers and significantly delayed in their adaptive functioning.

CHILDREN WITH ADHD IN MIDDLE CHILDHOOD

Most of the research reviewed so far in this volume was done on children of elementary school age, making earlier chapters a good description of the problems of this age group. Once children with ADHD enter school, a major social burden is placed on them that will last at least the next 12 years of their lives; this burden is formal, compulsory education in a relatively homogenized environment that is unlikely to cater to their unorthodox behavior. Studies suggest that school is the area of greatest impact on these children's ADHD (Barkley, Fischer, et al., 1990; Biederman, 1997) and will create the greatest source of distress for many of them and their parents. The abilities to sit still, attend, listen, obey, inhibit impulsive behavior, cooperate, organize actions, and follow through on instructions, as well as to share, play well, keep promises, and interact pleasantly with other children, are essential to negotiating a successful academic career—beyond those cognitive and achievement skills needed to master the curriculum itself. It is not surprising that the vast majority of children with ADHD will have been identified as deviant in their behavior by entry into formal schooling, particularly first grade. Parents not

only have to contend with the ongoing behavioral problems at home noted in the discussion of the preschool years, but now have the additional burden of helping their children adjust to the academic and social demands of school. Regrettably, these parents must also tolerate the complaints of some teachers who see the children's problems at school as stemming entirely from home problems or poor child-rearing abilities in the parents.

Often at this age, parents must confront decisions about whether to retain the children in kindergarten because of "immature" behavior and/or slow academic achievement. Although the impact of retention at kindergarten is uncertain, the effects of retaining a child once formal schooling has begun are not likely to contribute to a positive outcome. Indeed, retention now actually appears to create several adverse consequences, including increased aggression, loss of motivation to learn, peer problems, and increased likelihood of quitting school (Pagani, Tremblay, Vitaro, Boulerice, & McDuff, 2001). The fact that many schools now assign homework, even to first-graders, places an additional demand on both a parent and a child to accomplish these tasks together. It is not surprising to see that homework time becomes another area in which conflict now arises in the family. For those 20–35% of children with ADHD who are likely to have a reading disorder, this disorder will be soon noted as the child tries to master the early reading tasks at school. Such children are doubly impaired in their academic performance by the combinations of these disabilities. Among those who will develop math and writing disorders, these problems often go undetected until several years into elementary school. Even in the absence of comorbid learning disabilities, almost all children with ADHD are haunted by their highly erratic educational performance over time: On some days they perform at or near normal levels of ability and accomplish all assignments, while on other days they fail quizzes and tests and do not complete assigned work. Disorganized desks, lockers, coat closet spaces, and even notebooks are highly characteristic of these children, forcing others to step in periodically and reorganize their materials to try to facilitate better academic performance.

At home, parents often complain that their children with ADHD do not accept household chores and responsibilities as well as do other children their age. Greater supervision of and assistance with these daily chores and self-help activities (dressing, bathing, etc.) are common and lead to the perception that these children are quite immature. Although temper tantrums are likely to decline, as they do in typical children, children with ADHD are still more likely to emit such behavior when frustrated than typical children. Relations with siblings may become tense as the siblings grow tired and exasperated at trying to understand and live with so disruptive a force as a brother or sister with ADHD. Some siblings develop resentment over the greater burden of work they often carry compared to their hyperactive siblings. Certainly, siblings are often jealous of the greater amount of time children with ADHD receive from their parents, especially those siblings who are younger than the affected children. (And some siblings, given the high heritability of ADHD, may also have ADHD themselves, further adding to the family turmoil.) At an age when other children are entering extracurricular community and social activities, such as clubs, music lessons, sports, and Scouts, children with ADHD are likely to find themselves barely tolerated in these group activities or outright ejected from them in some cases. Parents frequently find that they must intervene in these activities on behalf of their children to explain and apologize for their behavior and transgressions to others, to try to aid the children in coping better with the social demands, or to defend their children against sanctions that may be applied for their unacceptable conduct.

An emerging pattern of social rejection will have appeared by now, if not earlier, in over half of all children with ADHD because of their poor social skills (as described in Chapter 3). Even when a child with ADHD displays appropriate or prosocial behavior toward others, it may be at such a high rate or intensity that it elicits rejection by and avoidance of the child in subsequent situations, or even punitive responses from his or her peers (again, see Chapter 3). This rejection can present a confusing picture to the child attempting to learn appropriate social skills. This high rate of behavior, vocal noisiness, and tendency to touch and manipulate objects more than is typical for age combine to make the child with ADHD overwhelming, intrusive, and even aversive to others.

By later childhood and preadolescence, these patterns of academic, familial, and social conflicts have become well established for many children with ADHD. At least 40–85% have developed ODD (see Chapter 4), and as many as 25–50% are likely to develop symptoms of antisocial behavior or CD between 7 and 10 years of age. The most common among these symptoms are lying, petty thievery, and resistance to the authority of others. At least 25% or more may have problems with fighting with other children. For the socially aggressive subgroup, bragging or boasting about fictitious accomplishments, cheating others at games or in schoolwork, and in some cases truancy from school may also be seen. Only a minority of children with ADHD who have not developed some comorbid psychiatric (ODD/CD), academic (learning disability and underachievement), or social disorder by this time. Those with pure ADHD whose attention problems are most prominent are likely to have the best adolescent outcomes, experiencing problems primarily with academic performance and eventual attainment (Fergusson, Lynskey, & Horwood, 1997; Weiss & Hechtman, 1993). For others, an increasing pattern of familial conflict and antisocial behavior in the community may begin to appear or to worsen where it already exists. Such family conflicts often prove particularly recalcitrant to treatment (Barkley, Guevremont, Anastopoulos, & Fletcher, 1992; see also Chapter 14). The majority of children with ADHD (60–80%) by this time have been placed on a trial of stimulant medication, and over half have participated in some type of individual and family therapy (Barkley, DuPaul, & McMurray, 1990; Barkley, Fischer, et al., 1990; Faraone et al., 1993; Munir, Biederman, & Knee, 1987; Semrud-Clikeman et al., 1992). Approximately 30–45% will also be receiving formal special educational assistance for their academic difficulties by the time they enter adolescence.

ADOLESCENT OUTCOME

At the outset, it needs to be noted that no follow-up studies have focused on the Predominantly Inattentive Type of ADHD or that subset with sluggish cognitive tempo (see Chapter 2). All of what follows applies only to the Combined or Predominantly Hyperactive–Impulsive Types of the disorder. Despite a decline in their levels of hyperactivity and an improvement in their attention span and impulse control (Fischer, Barkley, Smallish, & Fletcher, 2005; Hart, Lahey, Loeber, Applegate, & Frick, 1995; Schmidt & Moll, 1995), 70–80% of children with ADHD are likely to continue to display these symptoms into adolescence to an extent inappropriate for their age group (Barkley, Fischer, et al., 1990; Barkley, Anastopoulos, Guevremont, & Fletcher, 1991). As Ross and Ross (1976) indicated nearly 30 years ago, the adolescent years of individuals with ADHD may be some of the most difficult because of the increasing demands for independent, responsible conduct, as well as the emerging social and physical changes inherent in puberty. Issues of identity, peer group acceptance, dating and courtship, and physical development and appearance erupt as a second source of demands and distress with which these adolescents must now cope. Sadness, Major Depressive Disorder (MDD) in as many as 25–30% of cases, poor self-confidence, diminished hopes of future success, and concerns about school completion may develop.

Follow-up studies published during the past 20+ years have done much to dispel the notion that ADHD is typically outgrown by the adolescent years. These studies have consistently demonstrated that up to 80% of children diagnosed as hyperactive in childhood continue to display their symptoms to a significant degree in adolescence and young adulthood (August, Stewart, & Holmes, 1983; Barkley, Fischer, et al., 1990; Biederman, Faraone, Milberger, Curtis, et al., 1996; Brown & Borden, 1986; Cantwell & Baker, 1989; Claude & Firestone, 1995; Gittelman, Mannuzza, Shenker, & Bonagura, 1985; Lambert, Hartsough, Sassone, & Sandoval, 1987; Schmidt & Moll, 1995; Thorley, 1984; Weiss & Hechtman, 1993). In general, these studies indicate that between 30% and 80% of these children continue to be impaired by their symptoms in adolescence or to meet current diagnostic criteria for ADHD. More recent studies using more contemporary and rigorous diagnostic criteria consistently find higher rates of ADHD symptom persistence than earlier, less methodologically rigorous studies have found. As many as 25–55% of adolescents display oppositional or antisocial behavior or outright CD (Biederman, Faraone, Milberger, Curtis et al., 1996; Biederman, Faraone, et al., 1997; see Chapter 4), and 30–58% have failed at least one grade in school (Barkley et al., 1991; Barkley, Fischer et

al., 1990; Brown & Borden, 1986). Other studies clearly show these children to be significantly behind matched control groups in academic performance at follow-up (Fischer, Barkley, Edelbrock, & Smallish, 1990; Lambert et al., 1987; Weiss & Hechtman, 1993). Research has been less consistent in documenting whether hyperactive children are at greater risk for substance abuse than typical children upon reaching adolescence, with some finding a greater occurrence of alcohol or drug use (Blouin, Bornstein, & Trites, 1978; Hoy, Weiss, Minde, & Cohen, 1978; Loney, Kramer, & Milich, 1981), and others finding it only for drug use (Gittelman et al., 1985; Minde et al., 1971; Weiss & Hechtman, 1993). Most of these studies followed groups of clinically diagnosed hyperactive children. When epidemiologically derived samples were used, rates of antisocial behavior, academic failure, and continuation of ADHD symptoms remained higher than in matched control samples, but less than half that reported in the clinical samples (Lambert et al., 1987).

A significant limitation of many of these studies, particularly those initiated in the early 1970s, was the lack of consensus criteria for the diagnosis of hyperactivity or ADHD. Many of these early studies relied exclusively on the referral of children based on parental or teacher complaints of hyperactivity and clinical diagnosis as the primary inclusion criteria. None of these studies used standardized child behavior rating scales to establish a cutoff score for their subjects' degree of deviance in terms of ADHD symptoms. Considering that many children termed "normal" may also have parent or teacher complaints of inattentiveness, hyperactivity, or impulsivity, it is likely that previous studies have been overly inclusive, permitting many children with borderline or marginal ADHD characteristics to be included in their samples. The result could be a considerably more positive outcome of the hyperactive sample and a sample with much higher remission rates than if more rigorous research selection criteria were employed, as is now customary in more recent studies. All these studies were begun, and many were completed, prior to the publication of consensus diagnostic criteria for ADHD in the third edition of the *Diagnostic and Statistical Manual of Mental Disorders* (DSM-III; American Psychiatric Association, 1980) or DSM-III-R (American Psychiatric Association, 1987), leading to tremendous variation across studies in their selection criteria.

A more detailed picture of the adolescent outcome of children with ADHD has emerged in several outcome studies that did use DSM criteria at follow-up, if not at study entry (Barkley, Fischer, et al., 1990; Biederman, Faraone, Milberger, Curtis, et al. 1996; Fischer et al., 1990). The following results are from our Milwaukee study (Barkley, Fischer, et al., 1990) of a large sample of children with ADHD and nondisabled children followed prospectively 8–10 years after their initial evaluation. Unlike past studies, the clinic-referred children diagnosed with hyperactivity in the present study fulfilled a set of rigorous research criteria designed to select a sample of children who were truly developmentally deviant in their symptoms relative to same-age typical children.

The initial sample consisted of 158 children designated as "hyperactive" and 81 designated as "normal," all between 4 and 12 years of age. A total of 123 hyperactive children and 66 normal children were located for the adolescent follow-up, and agreed to be interviewed and complete our questionnaires either in person or by telephone (interview) and mail (rating scales). This number represents a total of 78% of the original sample for the hyperactive group and 81% for the normal group. These recruitment rates compare favorably to the prospective follow-up studies by Lambert et al. (1987) and Gittelman et al. (1985), in which the average recruitment rate was between 72% and 85%, and are considerably higher than those in most of the earlier follow-up studies (Weiss & Hechtman, 1993). In the hyperactive group, 12 of the subjects (9.7%) were female and 111 were male; in the normal group, 4 of the subjects (6.1%) were female and 62 were male.

Comorbidity for Other Disruptive Behavior Disorders

We examined the rates of the occurrence of disruptive behavior disorder diagnoses in both groups of children. We also calculated the number of symptoms within each disorder that represented 2 standard deviations above the mean (97th percentile) for the normal adolescents. We did so because the DSM-III-R cutoff scores for these disorders were based on field trials of primarily elementary-age children, in whom

one would expect a greater occurrence of the ADHD characteristics and a lesser degree of CD symptoms within the typical population at that age range. Because these symptoms are known to vary considerably with age, it is likely that the cutoff scores may have been overinclusive for some age groups and underinclusive for others.

We found that the vast majority of our hyperactive subjects (71.5%) met the DSM-III-R criteria for ADHD, with a mean number of 9 symptoms versus only 1.5 in the control group. Furthermore, when the cutoff of 2 standard deviations above the mean for the normal group was used to make the diagnosis for ADHD, the cutoff score had to be adjusted downward to 6 rather than 8 of 14 symptoms. Using this norm-referenced cutoff score resulted in a larger percentage of the hyperactive group (83.3%) being eligible for a diagnosis of ADHD in adolescence. The mean age of onset for the subjects' ADHD symptoms was 3.7 years. More than 59% of the hyperactive group met DSM-III-R criteria for a diagnosis of ODD, compared to 11% of the control group, and this rate did not change appreciably when the cutoff score of 2 standard deviations from the normal mean was substituted as the diagnostic cutoff point (5 or more symptoms). Approximately 43% of the hyperactive group qualified for a DSM-III-R diagnosis of CD, as compared to only 1.6% of the control group. Again, readjusting the symptom cutoff score based on the 2-standard-deviations mark for the normal control group results in a lowering of the cutoff score from 3 symptoms to 2 and led to a much larger percentage of the hyperactive group being diagnosed with CD (60%). The mean age of onset for ODD was 6.7 and for CD was 6 years.

Table 6.1 reports the relative rates of occurrence for each of the DSM symptoms within each of the three disruptive behavior disorders. Among the ADHD symptoms, it seems that difficulties with attention and instruction following were the most problematic for this group at adolescent outcome. Among the ODD symptoms, arguing and irritable or touchy manner were the most frequent. As one might expect, the occurrence for each symptom of CD was considerably less than for these other two disorders, but for the majority of these symptoms the rate in the hyperactive group was still significantly greater than that seen in the normal adolescents.

TABLE 6.1. Prevalence of Disruptive Behavior Disorders and Symptoms at Outcome

Diagnosis/symptom	Hyperactives (%)	Normals (%)	p
Attention-Deficit/Hyperactivity Disorder			
Fidgets	73.2	10.6	<.01
Difficulty remaining seated	60.2	3.0	<.01
Easily distracted	82.1	15.2	<.01
Difficulty waiting turn	48.0	4.5	<.01
Blurts out answers	65.0	10.6	<.01
Difficulty following instructions	83.7	12.1	<.01
Difficulty sustaining attention	79.7	16.7	<.01
Shifts from one uncompleted task to another	77.2	16.7	<.01
Difficulty playing quietly	39.8	7.6	NS
Talks excessively	43.9	6.1	<.01
Interrupts others	65.9	10.6	<.01
Doesn't seem to listen	80.5	15.2	<.01
Loses things needed for tasks	62.6	12.1	<.01
Engages in physically dangerous behavior	37.4	3.0	<.01
Oppositional Defiant Disorder			
Argues with adults	72.4	21.1	<.01
Defies adult requests	55.3	9.1	<.01
Deliberately annoys others	51.2	13.6	<.01
Blames others for own mistakes	65.9	16.7	<.01
Acts touchy or easily annoyed by others	70.7	19.7	<.01
Angry or resentful	50.4	10.6	<.01
Spiteful or vindictive	21.1	0.0	NS
Swears	40.7	6.1	<.01
Conduct Disorder			
Stolen without confrontation	49.6	7.6	<.01
Runs away from home overnight (2+ times)	4.9	3.0	NS
Lies	48.8	4.5	<.01
Deliberately engaged in fire setting	27.6	0.0	<.01
Truant	21.1	3.0	<.01
Broken in home, building, or car	9.8	1.5	NS
Deliberately destroyed others' property	21.1	4.5	<.01
Physically cruel to animals	15.4	0.0	<.01
Forced someone into sexual activity	5.7	0.0	NS
Used a weapon in a fight	7.3	0.0	NS
Physically fights	13.8	0.0	NS
Stolen with confrontation	0.8	0.0	NS
Physically cruel to people	14.6	0.0	<.01

Note. p values listed in last column are for chi-square or *t*-test results, as appropriate. NS means the statistical test was not significantly different between the groups. Age of onset for each disorder is not reported for the normal subjects, given that the vast majority of these subjects did not have these disorders at outcome. From Barkley, Fischer, Edelbrock, and Smallish (1990). Copyright 1990 by Lippincott Williams & Wilkins. Reprinted by permission.

Auto Accidents

Prior research (Weiss & Hechtman, 1993) suggested that hyperactive adolescents have a higher incidence of automobile accidents than do nondisabled adolescents. Our study of a sample of teens with ADHD followed prospectively for 3–5 years found that they were significantly more likely to have had an auto crash, to have had more such crashes, to have more bodily injuries associated with such accidents, and to be at fault more often for such accidents. They were also more likely to receive traffic citations, particularly for speeding (Barkley, Guevremont, Anastopolous, DuPaul, & Shelton, 1993). As Chapter 3 has indicated, these initial findings have now been substantially replicated in later studies, such that the risk of driving problems for those with ADHD is now documented to a far greater extent than at the time of the preceding edition of this text (see Barkley, 2004).

Substance Use and Abuse

Previous research has been equivocal concerning whether the rates of substance use and abuse among hyperactive adolescents differ from those of typical adolescents. Table 6.2 presents the rates of occurrence for 10 specific categories of substance use in our study (Barkley, Fischer, et al., 1990). Cigarette use was the only category of substance use that sig-

nificantly differentiated our hyperactive and nondisabled teenagers, according to the teens' self-reports. A previous follow-up study by Gittelman et al. (1985) found that the differences between clinically diagnosed hyperactive children and the control group in substance use at adolescent outcome were primarily accounted for by those hyperactive teens who received a diagnosis of CD. In agreement, a more recent study using an epidemiologically derived sample reported by Lynskey and Fergusson (1995) found that rates of adolescent substance use and abuse were elevated only in children with ADHD who had comorbid conduct problems as children. We separated our hyperactive subjects into those who were purely hyperactive and those who also had CD. In agreement with the studies above, we found that the purely hyperactive subjects had no greater use of cigarettes, alcohol, or marijuana than did normal subjects. However, the hyperactive sub-

TABLE 6.2. Illicit Substance Use at Outcome as Reported by Mother and Adolescent for Hyperactive and Normal Groups, and for Hyperactive Subjects Subgrouped as to the Presence or Absence of Conduct Disorder

Substance	Entire sample (%)			Hyperactives (%)		
	Hyperactives	Normals	p	w/CD	w/o CD	p
	By mother's report					
Cigarettes	48.8	30.3	NS	65.2	32.2	<.01
Alcohol	41.5	22.7	NS	54.3	29.0	NS
Marijuana	15.4	7.6	NS	28.3	4.8	<.01
Hashish	0.0	1.5	NS	0.0	0.0	NS
Cocaine	0.8	0.0	NS	2.2	0.0	NS
Stimulants	1.6	0.0	NS	4.3	0.0	NS
Sedatives	0.8	0.0	NS	2.2	0.0	NS
Tranquilizers	1.6	0.0	NS	2.2	1.6	NS
Heroin	0.0	0.0	NS	0.0	0.0	NS
Hallucinogens	0.0	0.0	NS	0.0	0.0	NS
	By adolescent's report					
Cigarettes	48.0	26.7	.02	63.6	35.7	<.01
Alcohol	40.0	21.7	NS	57.7	33.9	NS
Marijuana	17.0	5.0	NS	27.3	8.9	NS
Hashish	7.0	1.7	NS	11.4	3.6	NS
Cocaine	4.0	0.0	NS	9.1	0.0	NS
Stimulants	6.0	0.0	NS	4.5	7.1	NS
Sedatives	2.0	0.0	NS	4.5	0.0	NS
Tranquilizers	1.0	0.0	NS	2.3	0.0	NS
Heroin	0.0	0.0	NS	0.0	0.0	NS
Hallucinogens	2.0	1.7	NS	4.5	0.0	NS

Note. p values are the probability levels for the results of the chi-square analyses between the groups. NS means that the statistical test results were not significant. w/CD means with Conduct Disorder as diagnosed by DSM-III-R criteria, while w/o CD means without Conduct Disorder. From Barkley, Fischer, et al. (1990). Copyright 1990 by Lippincott Williams & Wilkins. Reprinted by permission.

jects with CD displayed rates of use of these substances two to five times higher than those of the other two groups. Biederman, Faraone, et al. (1997) also found that a higher percentage (40%) of their adolescents with ADHD qualified for a diagnosis of substance dependence or abuse compared to a control group, although 33% of their control group met such criteria as well.

Academic Outcome

The academic outcome of the hyperactive adolescents was considerably poorer in our Milwaukee study than that of the normal adolescents, with at least three times as many hyperactive children having failed a grade (29.3% vs. 10%), been suspended (46.3% vs. 15.2%), or been expelled (10.6% vs. 1.5%). Among another sample of clinic-referred teenagers with ADHD, we found a similar risk for school retention and suspension (Barkley et al., 1991). Almost 10% of the Milwaukee hyperactive sample followed into adolescence had quit school at this follow-up point, compared to none of the normal sample (Barkley, Fischer, et al., 1990). The mean number of grade retentions (0.33 vs. 0.11), suspensions (3.69 vs. 0.35), and expulsions (0.14 vs. 0.02) was also significantly greater within the hyperactive than within the normal group. We also found that the levels of academic achievement on standard tests were significantly below average on tests of math, reading, and spelling, falling toward the lower end of the normal range (standard scores between 90 and 95).

We again examined whether the presence of CD at follow-up within the hyperactive group accounted for these greater-than-normal rates of academic failure. The results indicated that although hyperactivity alone increased the risk of suspension (30.6% of the purely hyperactive group vs. 15.2% of controls) and dropping out of school (4.8% of the purely hyperactivegroup vs. 0% of controls), the additional diagnosis of CD greatly increased these risks (67.4% were suspended and 13% dropped out). Moreover, the presence of CD accounted almost entirely for the increased risk of expulsion within the hyperactive group, in that the purely hyperactive group did not differ from the normal group in expulsion rate (1.6 vs. 1.5%), whereas 21.7% of the hyperactive group with CD had been expelled from school. In contrast, the increased risk of grade retention in the hyperac-

tive group was entirely accounted for by hyperactivity, with no further risk accounted for by comorbid CD.

Treatment Received

Table 6.3 shows the extent of various interventions received in the ensuing 8–10 years since initial evaluation and their durations for both groups. Not surprisingly, more of the hyperactive children had received medication and individual and group therapy, as well as special educational services, than had the normal children. Similar results were found in our later study of clinic-referred adolescents having ADHD (Barkley et al., 1991). In terms of their duration of treatment among those receiving it, the hyperactive children had received a substantial period of stimulant medication treatment (mean of 36 months) and individual and family therapy (16 and 7 months, respectively), as well as special educational assistance for learning, behavioral, and speech disorders (65, 59, and 40 months, respectively), during the past 8 years (Barkley, Fischer, et al., 1990; Fischer et al., 1990). This pattern is similar to that found in our study of clinic-referred teens with ADHD (Barkley et al., 1991) and by Lambert et al. (1987) in their follow-up of 58 hyperactive and control teens.

Conclusions and Integration with Past Research

The results of the Milwaukee follow-up study are consistent with those of many other adolescent outcome studies in finding children with hyperactivity/ADHD to be at substantially higher risk for negative outcomes in the domains of psychiatric, social, legal, academic, and family functioning than a control group of normal children followed concurrently (August et al., 1983; Biederman, Faraone, Milberger, Curtis, et al., 1996; Biederman, Faraone, Milberger, Guite, et al., 1996; Brown & Borden, 1986; Thorley, 1984; Weiss & Hechtman, 1993). In contrast to early studies that followed hyperactive children into adolescence, however, our research found a substantially greater number of hyperactive children with negative outcomes in many of these domains of functioning than was previously demonstrated in studies using less rigorous entry criteria. Our rates for continuing ADHD were very similar to the rate of 68% having ADHD

TABLE 6.3. Treatment History of the Hyperactive and Normal Groups at Teen Outcome

Type of treatment	Hyperactives	Normals	p
Medication			
Methylphenidate	80.5%	0.0	<.01
Duration	36.1 mo	0.0	<.01
D-Amphetamine	3.3%	0.0	NS
Duration	1.1 mo	0.0	NS
Pemoline	19.5%	0.0	<.01
Duration	2.6 mo	0.0	NS
Tranquilizers	1.6%	0.0	NS
Duration	0.1 mo	0.0	NS
Other psychotropic drugs	14.6%	3.0%	NS
Duration	0.4 mo	3.0 mo	NS
Individual psychotherapy	63.4%	13.6%	<.01
Duration	16.3 mo	2.0 mo	<.01
Group psychotherapy	17.9%	4.5%	<.02
Duration	1.8 mo	0.1 mo	NS
Family therapy	49.6%	24.2%	<.01
Duration	7.2 mo	1.4 mo	<.01
Inpatient psychiatric treatment	9.8%	1.5%	NS
Duration	0.3 mo	0.03 mo	NS
Residential psychiatric treatment	8.9%	0.0	NS
Duration	1.9 mo	0.0	NS
Foster care	4.9%	0.0	NS
Duration	1.7 mo	0.0	NS
Special educational services			
Learning disability classes	32.5%	3.0%	<.01
Duration	65.5 mo	48.0 mo	NS
Behavior disorder classes	35.8%	6.1%	<.01
Duration	59.1 mo	37.5 mo	NS
Speech therapy	16.3%	1.5%	<.01
Duration	40.2 mo	6.0 mo	<.01
Other			
Biological mother in therapy	46.3%	28.8%	NS
Biological father in therapy	21.1%	13.6%	NS
Biological mother and father received marital therapy	30.9%	19.7%	NS

Note. p values are the probability levels for the results of the chi-square analyses between the groups. NS means that the statistical test results were not significant. From Barkley, Fischer, et al. (1990). Copyright 1990 by Lippincott Williams & Wilkins. Reprinted by permission.

at some time since age 13 years found in the Gittelman et al. (1985) adult outcome study, and considerably higher than the 43% continuing to exhibit hyperactivity in the Lambert et al. (1987) study. Nevertheless, the rates are equal to those found by August et al. (1983), as well as those found by Claude and Firestone (1995), Biederman, Faraone, Milberger, Curtis, et al. (1996), and Cantwell and Baker (1989). In any case, our findings make it clear that when rigorous criteria are used to diagnose children with hyperactivity or ADHD (Barkley, 1981, 1982), these criteria select a group of children whose symptom deviance remains highly stable over time (8–10 years), with the vast majority of them (70–80+%) continuing to have this disorder into adolescence.

Yet the research of Weiss and Hechtman (1993) suggests that although present, these primary ADHD symptoms are not the major concerns of either parents or adolescents at outcome. Instead, poor schoolwork, social difficulties with peers, problems related to authority (especially at school), and low self-esteem are major concerns at this developmental stage. Our results, discussed later, lend considerable credence to these concerns, as did my later study with Gwenyth Edwards on clinic-referred teens (Edwards, Barkley, Laneri, Fletcher, & Metevia, 2001). A review of the concerns of parents of children with ADHD, however, would probably indicate that the first three of these concerns are the primary reasons they also seek clinical services for their children. Social conflict within the family would probably be listed as the fourth concern of these childhood years. This finding suggests to me that at any stage in the course of development, the concerns expressed by parents of children with ADHD will stem primarily from the impact of the children's deficits on their functioning in the school, in the family, and within the peer group, and not from the ADHD symptoms per se. Only later in development is one likely to see the impact of the ADHD symptoms on personal satisfaction and self-acceptance, and thus problems such as low self-esteem may then emerge as significant concerns of the adolescent or young adult with ADHD. Once again it appears that when ADHD symptoms are not disabling to individual children or adolescents, they are of considerably less concern to the caregivers of these individuals than when they are proving especially disabling to

these youth in meeting environmental expectations.

The rates of antisocial behavior and CD in our study were also higher than those seen in most early follow-up studies, but are consistent with those found in more recent studies, such as those by Biederman and colleagues (Biederman, Faraone, Milberger, Guite, et al., 1996; Biederman, Faraone, et al., 1997). Most early studies of adolescent outcome found between 22% and 30% of their hyperactives subjects engaging in antisocial acts (see Brown & Borden, 1986, for a review; see also Mendelson, Johnson, & Stewart, 1971; Zambelli, Stam, Maintinsky, & Loiselle, 1977). Gittelman et al. (1985) reported that 45% of their sample met DSM-III criteria for CD at some time since age 13 years of age. Biederman, Faraone, et al. (1997) found that 42% of their adolescents had CD. Our results are similar to these two studies in finding that 43% of our hyperactive subjects could be diagnosed with CD according to the more recent DSM-III-R criteria. The most common antisocial acts were stealing, thefts outside the home, and fire setting. This subgroup of hyperactive teens would be at substantial risk for later criminal activities in adulthood. Antisocial activities in adolescence seem to be highest among those children with hyperactivity or ADHD who have had comorbid conduct problems or CD earlier in childhood (August et al., 1983; Biederman, Faraone, Milberger, Curtis, et al., 1996; Claude & Firestone, 1995; Fischer et al., 1990; Satterfield, Swanson, Schell, & Lee, 1994; Weiss & Hechtman, 1993). This does not mean that children with ADHD but without comorbid CD carry no higher risk for later antisocial activities as adolescence, for they do seem to show such an elevated risk over nondisabled children (Satterfield et al., 1994; Taylor, Chadwick, Hepinstall, & Danckaerts, 1996). It only means that the risk is considerably increased, should conduct problems or CD also exist during childhood.

Like many of the other follow-up studies discussed earlier (see also Wilson & Marcotte, 1996), our study found a significantly higher rate of academic performance problems in the hyperactive than in the control group. Our hyperactive teens were three times more likely to have failed a grade or been suspended, and over eight times more likely to have been expelled or dropped out of school, than the normal controls at adolescent outcome (Fischer, Barkley, Smallish, & Fletcher, 2002). Our rates for truancy were comparable to those (17%) reported in other follow-up studies (Mendelson et al., 1971). The level of grade repetition was 20–49% in our studies of teenagers, falling somewhat below that found in previous follow-up studies (56–70%; Ackerman, Dykman, & Peters, 1977; Mendelson et al., 1971; Minde et al., 1971; Stewart, Mendelson, & Johnson, 1973; Weiss, Minde, Werry, Douglas, & Nemeth, 1971). Perhaps the availability of special educational services in the later 1970s had something to do with this diminution in rates of grade retention in later follow-up studies such as our own. In general, it appears that academic performance difficulties in adolescence are associated with having persistent ADHD since childhood, whereas school disciplinary actions such as suspensions and expulsions are more closely linked to comorbid conduct problems or CD than to ADHD alone (Barkley, Fischer, et al., 1990; Wilson & Marcotte, 1996). The children with ADHD who have the lowest levels of adaptive functioning in childhood are also the most likely to have comorbid psychiatric disorders and academic impairments in adolescence (Barkley, Fischer, et al., 2002; Greene, Biederman, Faraone, Sienna, & Garcia-Jetton, 1997; Wilson & Marcotte, 1996).

Our findings for substance use are consistent with those of many other studies (see Tercyak, Peshkin, Walker, & Stein, 2002, for a review). We found that a greater number of our hyperactive teens had smoked cigarettes or marijuana, whereas Hartsough and Lambert (1985) found only cigarette use to be greater in hyperactive than in normal adolescents. Borland and Heckman (1976) also found more of their hyperactive subjects to be smoking cigarettes than their brothers at follow-up. All of these results certainly point to a higher-than-normal risk for cigarette use among hyperactive adolescents. Follow-up studies conducted after our own have done much to refine our understanding of this risk. For instance, Milberger, Biederman, Faraone, Chen, and Jones (1997) followed 6- to 17-year-olds with and without ADHD for 4 years and found that ADHD was specifically associated with a higher risk for initiating cigarette smoking even after they controlled for SES, psychiatric comorbidity, and intelligence. Molina, Smith, and Pelham (1999) reported in a study of 202 adolescents that ADHD was as-

sociated with increased use of all substances, including nicotine, only when it was associated with comorbid CD. Yet they also found that the impulsive–hyperactive dimension of ADHD within this comorbid group was most closely associated with this elevated risk of substance use. In partial agreement with these results, Burke, Loeber, and Lahey (2001) followed 177 clinic-referred boys with ADHD to age 15 years and likewise found that 51% of these teens reported tobacco use, but that this risk was only elevated in the comorbid group of CD with ADHD. Unlike the Molina et al. (1999), these authors found that the inattention dimension was specifically associated with a 2.2 times greater risk for tobacco use by adolescence, even after they controlled for other factors known to be associated with such use (CD, poor parental communication, ethnicity, etc.). Tercyak, Lerman, and Audrain (2002) also confirmed this linkage of not only ADHD but specifically its inattention symptoms with the risk for cigarette use by adolescence. Even mild levels of ADHD symptoms appear to elevate this risk for smoking (Whalen, Jamner, Henker, Delfino, & Lozano, 2002). Given the stimulant-like action of nicotine on the dopamine transporter in the striatum of the brain and its similarity to the effects of methylphenidate on that site (Krause et al., 2002), these findings suggest that greater nicotine use among those with ADHD could be a form of self-medication.

Concerning alcohol use, Blouin et al. (1978), in a retrospective study, were among the first to report that children with hyperactivity may be more at risk than control children for adolescent alcohol use (57% of their hyperactive subjects vs. 20% of the controls). Weiss and Hechtman (1993) also found somewhat more of their hyperactive subjects, as teenagers, to have used nonmedical substances, particularly alcohol, than did their control subjects. Biederman, Wilens, et al. (1997) found that 40% of their teens with ADHD had some form of substance dependence or abuse. With the exception of the study by Hartsough and Lambert (1985), there is some consistency across studies in finding hyperactive adolescents to be at somewhat higher risk for alcohol use than nondisabled adolescents. These and other studies have also documented a greater frequency of substance use among adolescents with ADHD (Chilcoat & Breslau, 1999). Most of these studies have concurred with our own in finding that the elevated risk for alcohol and substance use and abuse in adolescence is to be found primarily among children with hyperactivity or ADHD who also had conduct problems or frank CD in childhood (August et al., 1983; Barkley, Fischer, et al., 1990; Biederman, Wilens, et al., 1997; Claude & Firestone, 1995; Gittelman et al., 1985; Lynskey & Fergusson, 1995; Wilson & Marcotte, 1996). Likewise, youth diagnosed with alcohol dependence have a markedly higher incidence of ADHD and CD, with the developmental sequence being a progression from initial alcohol or tobacco use to marijuana and then to other street drugs (Kuperman et al., 2001). Such findings are quite consistent with studies of community samples in showing that CD, but not ADHD, is associated with greater risk for substance use, dependence, and abuse (Armstrong & Costello, 2002). Once again, the attention symptoms and associated executive functioning deficits seen in ADHD may be most predictive of later substance use problems (Tapert, Baratta, Abrantes, & Brown, 2002). This greater use of drugs among youth with combined ADHD and CD may contribute to further problems with learning, memory retention, and attention problems (Tapert, Granholm, Leedy, & Brown, 2002).

Predictors of Adolescent Outcome

Several follow-up studies of hyperactive children have examined the degree to which certain childhood and family characteristics at study entry predict the adolescent outcomes of such children (August et al., 1983; Biederman, Faraone, Milberger, Guite, et al., 1996; Fergusson, Lynskey, & Horwood, 1996; Fischer, Barkley, Fletcher, & Smallish, 1993b; Lambert et al., 1987; Paternite & Loney, 1980; Taylor et al., 1996; Weiss & Hechtman, 1993). No single predictor, by itself, seems especially useful in prophesizing the adolescent outcome of children with ADHD. The combination of several factors is important in such an exercise, but even then the predictor power remains low. The following predictors appear to be useful:

• First, the SES of the family and general level of intelligence of the child are positively related to outcome, especially to academic outcome, eventual educational attainment, and level of employment. Family SES is also related to the severity of ADHD symptoms at out-

come, with children from lower-SES families having significantly higher degrees of ADHD.
• Second, the degree to which children experience peer relationship problems predicts the degree to which they will experience interpersonal problems in adolescence and adulthood.
• Third, the degree of aggressiveness and conduct problems in childhood predicts a poorer outcome in many different domains of adjustment, including poorer educational adjustment and attainment, poorer social relationships, and increased risk for substance abuse. As expected, childhood aggression is also related to adolescent delinquency and antisocial offenses.
• Fourth, the degree to which parental psychopathology, particularly a family history of ADHD, is present in the families of children with ADHD is associated with an increased risk of psychiatric and emotional problems in the children themselves by late adolescence. Families whose members have not only ADHD but comorbid conduct problems, antisocial behavior, and substance dependence and abuse are particularly likely to have children with ADHD who experience greater difficulties in adolescence.
• Fifth, the degree of conflict and hostility in the interactions between parents and their children with ADHD is significantly associated with the degree to which parent–child conflicts as well as generally aggressive behavior are present in adolescence.
• And sixth, the degree of ADHD in childhood is related only to the degree of academic attainment in adolescence.

To date, research has not found the type or extent of childhood intervention to have much impact on the adolescent or young adult outcome of children with ADHD. Indeed, it seems to correlate negatively with outcome in naturalistic follow-up studies where random assignment to treatments has not been employed; that is, the more services the children have received across their development, the worse their prognosis in some particular domain of outcome seems to be (Fischer, Barkley, Fletcher, & Smallish, 1993a). This finding, however, can be seen to be an artifact of the severity of disorder: More severely affected children receive more treatment and are also likely to have worse outcomes, thus making duration or range of treatment a marker for the severity of disorder. Some hope for the success of interventions with ADHD is held out by the results of multimodal treatment studies (see Chapter 20). These have found that a combination of medication, special education, parent counseling, and training in child management, classroom consultation, and individual counseling of the children may, if maintained over several years into early adolescence, alter the prognosis for ADHD children so long as treatment is sustained.

ADULT OUTCOME

Only a few studies have followed samples of hyperactive children into adulthood. Most of this research is nicely summarized in the excellent text by Weiss and Hechtman (1993) and in a review by Klein and Mannuzza (1991). When appropriate, the results from the more recent follow-up study of Mannuzza, Gittelman-Klein, Bessler, Malloy, and LaPadula (1993) and from my own follow-up study in Milwaukee with Mariellen Fischer and Kenneth Fletcher (Barkley, Fischer, et al., 2002; Barkley, Fischer, Smallish, & Fletcher, in press) are noted.

Persistence of ADHD in Adulthood

Adult outcome studies of large samples of clinic-referred children with hyperactivity, or what is now diagnosed as ADHD, are few in number. Only four follow-up studies have retained at least 50% or more of their original samples into adulthood. These are the Montréal study by Weiss, Hechtman, and their colleagues (see Weiss & Hechtman, 1993); the New York City study by Mannuzza, Klein, and colleagues (see Mannuzza, Klein, Bessler, Malloy, & LaPadula, 1998); the Swedish study by Rasmussen and Gillberg (2001); and our Milwaukee study. The results regarding the persistence of disorder into young adulthood (middle 20s) are mixed. The Montréal study (n = 103) found that two-thirds of its original sample (n = 64; mean age of 25 years) claimed to be troubled as adults by at least one or more disabling core symptoms of their original disorder (restlessness, impulsivity, or inattention), and that 34% had at least moderate to severe levels of hyperactive, impulsive, and inattentive symptoms (Weiss & Hechtman, 1993, p. 73). In Sweden (n = 50), Rasmussen and Gillberg

(2001) obtained similar results: 49% of probands reported marked symptoms of ADHD at age 22 years, compared to 9% of controls. Formal diagnostic criteria for ADHD, as in DSM-III or later editions, were not employed at any of the outcome points in either study, however. A follow-up study in China (Wenwei, 1996) found that nearly 70% of 197 children diagnosed 15 years earlier as having minimal brain dysfunction persisted in having symptoms of ADHD into young adulthood (ages 20–33 years; mean 25.5 years).

In contrast, the New York study has followed two separate cohorts of hyperactive children and has used DSM criteria to assess the persistence of the disorder. This study found that 31% of their initial cohort (n = 101) and 43% of their second cohort (n = 94) met DSM-III criteria by ages 16–23 (mean age 18.5 years) (Gittelman et al., 1985; Mannuzza, Klein, Bonagura, et al., 1991). Eight years later (mean age 26 years), however, these figures fell to 8% and 4%, respectively (when DSM-III-R criteria were used) (Mannuzza et al., 1993, 1998). Those results might imply that the vast majority of hyperactive children no longer qualify for the diagnosis of ADHD by adulthood.

The disparity in persistence to age 25 years between the New York study and the other two studies might have resulted in part from differences in their selection criteria. All three studies were begun before systematic DSM criteria existed. The Montréal study accepted children who had received a clinical diagnosis of hyperactivity based on significant levels of restlessness and poor concentration that were longstanding symptoms and caused problems at both home and school. Nevertheless, explicit criteria for level of deviance in these symptoms, age of onset, pervasiveness, or other more exact criteria were not applied. The Swedish study selected children initially for having minimal brain dysfunction, and a subset of these children also had elevated teacher ratings of ADHD symptoms. Subsequently, 85% received a DSM-IV diagnosis of ADHD (American Psychiatric Association, 1994).

In contrast, the New York study required a clinical diagnosis of DSM-II Hyperkinetic Reaction of Childhood (American Psychiatric Association, 1968); significantly elevated ratings of hyperactivity from parents, teachers, or clinical staff on the Conners rating scales; an IQ of 85 or higher; and absence of gross neurological disorders or psychosis. Children with high levels of aggressive behavior or conduct problems were excluded from this study, however—a procedure not used in the Montréal or Swedish studies. This probably ruled out many children with CD from participation (Mannuzza et al., 1993), and thus may have limited the severity of ADHD within the New York cohorts. More severe levels of ADHD are often associated with more severe levels of aggression and CD (Achenbach, 1991; Hinshaw, 1987). For these reasons, it is possible that while the New York study followed a more rigorously selected group of hyperactive children, their sample may also have been less severely disabled than those in the other studies. By contrast, the Milwaukee project followed a large sample of rigorously selected hyperactive children to adulthood, and conduct problems were not used to screen children out of the study.

The interpretation of the relatively low rate of persistence of ADHD into adulthood, particularly for the New York study, is clouded by at least two issues apart from differences in selection criteria. One is that the source of information about the disorder changed in all of these studies from that used at the childhood and adolescent evaluations to that used at the adult outcome. At study entry and at adolescence, all studies used the reports of others (parents and typically teachers). By midadolescence, all found that the majority of hyperactive participants (70%+) continued to manifest significant levels of the disorder (Klein & Mannuzza, 1991)—findings consistent with other adolescent follow-up studies using DSM-III and III-R (70–86%; American Psychiatric Association, 1980, 1987) and parental reports (August et al., 1983; Barkley, Fischer, et al., 1990; Claude & Firestone, 1995). In young adulthood (approximately age 26 years), however, both the New York and Montréal studies switched to self-reports of disorder.

The rather marked decline in persistence of ADHD from adolescence to adulthood in these studies could have stemmed from this change in source of information. Indeed, the New York study found this to be likely when, at late adolescence (mean age of 18–19 years), they interviewed both the teenagers and their parents about the teens' psychiatric status (Mannuzza & Gittelman, 1986). There was a marked disparity between the reports of parents and teens concerning the presence of ADHD (11% vs. 27%; agreement 74%, kappa = .19). Other research also suggests that the correlation be-

tween older children's (age 11) self-reports of externalizing symptoms, such as those involved in ADHD, and those of parents and teachers is quite low ($r = .16–.32$; Henry, Moffitt, Caspi, Langley, & Silva, 1994). Thus the changing sources of reporting in longitudinal studies on behavioral disorders could be expected to lead to marked differences in estimates of persistence of these disorders.

The question obviously arises as to whose assessment of the probands is more accurate. This would depend on the purpose of the assessment, but the prediction of impairment in major life activities would seem to be an important one in research on psychiatric disorders. After all, the very definition of "disorder" may hinge on the demonstration of harm or impairment to the individual (Wakefield, 1999). The Milwaukee study examined this issue by interviewing both the participants and their parents about ADHD symptoms at the young adult follow-up. It then examined the relationship of each source's reports to significant outcomes in major life activities (education, occupation, social, etc.) after controlling for the contribution made by the other source.

A second limitation in establishing persistence of ADHD into adulthood is the contradiction inherent between the current conceptualization of it and the criteria actually used to diagnose it. ADHD has long been conceptualized as a developmental disability. This implies that it is a disorder because its symptoms occur to a degree that is *developmentally inappropriate* and thereby cause impairment in major life activities. All developmental disorders are diagnosed on the basis of developmental relativity—age-inappropriateness in comparison to peers. That is because they reflect delays in the rate of development of a typical psychological attribute, and not static pathological states or absolute deficits in or losses of formerly typical functioning.

From this perspective, the presence of ADHD at any stage in life must be partly determined by using age-relative thresholds for diagnostic symptom lists. However, such thresholds are not provided in the DSM. Despite requiring developmental inappropriateness, a fixed symptom threshold is imposed across all ages. Given that the frequency of ADHD symptoms declines substantially in normal populations with age (DuPaul, Power, Anastopoulos, & Reid, 1998; Hart et al., 1995), this application of a fixed threshold across a developmentally declining frequency curve means that the fixed threshold is becoming stricter or statistically rarer with age. Two predictable outcomes will flow from this circumstance. First, the diagnostic criteria will become less valid (sensitive to the disorder) with age—a situation noted in both the DSM-III-R and DSM-IV field trials (Applegate et al., 1997; Spitzer, Davies, & Barkley, 1990). And second, many of those having the disorder as children will appear to have outgrown the disorder by adulthood, when in fact they have only outgrown the criteria—as noted in Chapter 2 of the present book.

To examine this issue, ADHD was determined in the Milwaukee study (Barkley, Fischer, et al., 2002) not only according to the DSM-III-R threshold, but also by a developmentally referenced cutoff. The 98th percentile, or +2 standard deviations above the normal mean, was chosen for several reasons. It was the threshold used to select the probands for the study in childhood. It is also the one most commonly recommended in clinical practice for the interpretation of rating scale elevations as being significant (Achenbach, 1991; DuPaul et al., 1998). And it is used as the demarcation on intelligence and adaptive behavior inventories for the diagnosis of another developmental disorder, that being mental retardation.

We found that only 3–5% of our hyperactive subjects qualified for a DSM-III-R diagnosis of ADHD when the decision was based on their self-report at young adult follow-up (mean age approximately 20 years) (Barkley, Fischer, et al., 2002). However, when we subsequently interviewed their parents about the presence of disorder, using DSM-IV criteria, the rate rose to 42%. And if an empirical criterion for presence of disorder was employed with these same parent reports (e.g., 2+ standard deviations above the mean for the normal control group on the DSM-IV symptoms), 66% of the hyperactive subjects exceeded this cutoff score and could be said to have retained the disorder. Thus the persistence of ADHD into adulthood is very much a matter of the source of information and the diagnostic criteria being employed, with parent reports not only yielding a far higher rate of persistence, but also being more predictive of various impairments in major life activities (Barkley, Fischer, et al., 2002). If DSM criteria were applied to the subject's own self-reports, low rates of persistence of ADHD were found in this study. But if parent reports of the subjects continued to be used, as they were in the prior follow-up assessments (and in other studies of ADHD into adolescence), persistence of disorder was 14 times greater. And if an empirical criterion was established for the disorder, rates were nearly 23 times greater. This helps to explain the low rate of persistence of ADHD predicted by Hill and Schoener (1996). They relied heavily on these results to conjecture that, given a continuation of such trends, the disorder should occur in fewer than 2 in 1,000 adults by age 30 years or later. That review suffered from numerous other methodological and conceptual flaws that undermined their conclusions (see Barkley, 1998, pp. 202–206). This and other information (see Chapter 2, this volume) suggest that the DSM criteria become increasingly insensitive to the disorder with age. This information also implies that subjects with ADHD may be prone to seriously underreporting their symptoms of the disorder, relative to what others may say about them—a problem we noted at the adolescent follow-up point as well (Fischer et al., 1993b).

Other Psychiatric Diagnoses and Impairments

Three of the aforementioned follow-up studies examined the extent to which the clinic-referred hyperactive children were at risk for other adult psychiatric disorders, apart from ongoing hyperactivity or ADHD. No study documented an excess degree of mood or anxiety disorders (Klein & Mannuzza, 1991; Rasmussen & Gillberg, 2001; Weiss & Hechtman, 1993). All three studies reported a significantly elevated occurrence of Antisocial Personality Disorder in their hyperactive (vs. control) samples (Montréal = 23% vs. 2.4% of controls; New York = 27% vs. 8% in late adolescence, and 12–18% vs. 2–3% in adulthood; Sweden = 18% vs. 2.1%) (Mannuzza et al., 1993, 1998; Mannuzza, Klein, & Addalli, 1991; Rasmussen & Gillberg, 2001; Weiss, Hechtman, Milroy, & Perlman, 1985). Except for alcohol use, substance use disorders were also somewhat more common in the hyperactive children at adulthood in the New York study, being 16% (vs. 3%) by age 18 years and 12–16% by age 26 years (Gittelman et al., 1985; Mannuzza et al., 1993, 1998). The opposite was true in the smaller Swedish study, where only alcohol use disorders occurred significantly more often than in controls (24% vs. 4%) (Rasmussen & Gillberg, 2001). The Milwaukee study sought to replicate the results of these earlier investigations by examining presence of DSM-III-R psychiatric disorders at young adult follow-up. We hypothesized an elevated risk for Antisocial Personality Disorder and drug use disorders among the hyperactive group, in view of our earlier results.

The three previous longitudinal studies of hyperactive children discussed above did not find an elevated prevalence of mood disorders in young adulthood (Klein & Mannuzza, 1991; Weiss & Hechtman, 1993, pp. 74–77). This is surprising given that MDD is often overrepresented in samples of clinic-referred children (24%) and adults (17-31%) with ADHD (see Chapter 4), and that epidemiological studies of children show a significant comorbid association of ADHD to MDD (Angold, Costello, & Erkanli, 1999). One reason for this disparity between the rates in follow-up studies and those of clinic-referred children, at least in the New York study, may have been the latter study's exclusion of children with significant conduct problems as their primary concern. MDD may be more prevalent among children with ADHD who also have ODD and CD. Indeed, a meta-analysis of epidemiological studies of comorbidity found that the link between ADHD and MDD was mediated by the link between both of these disorders and ODD/CD (Chapter 4). In the absence of that link, ADHD may not predispose to MDD.

The Milwaukee follow-up study (Fischer et al., 2002) found that the hyperactive group had a significantly higher risk for any non-drug-related psychiatric disorders than the community control group (59% vs. 36%) at the young adult follow-up. More of the hyperactive group met criteria for Major Depressive Disorder (26%), and for Histrionic (12%), Antisocial (21%), Passive–Aggressive (18%), and Borderline (14%) Personality Disorders at follow-up than the control group. Severity of childhood conduct problems contributed to the risk for Passive–Aggressive, Borderline, and Antisocial Personality Disorders. But it only affected risk for Antisocial Personality Disorder after we controlled for severity of teen CD, which also contributed to the risk for these same three disorders. Examination for comorbidity among these disorders indicated that presence of either Borderline or Antisocial Personality Disorder significantly increased the risk for MDD and the other significant personality disorders.

Anxiety disorders and mania were not overrepresented in our hyperactive sample at follow-up, in keeping with the results of all prior follow-up studies. Yet these disorders exist with significant frequency in samples of clinic-referred children, where anxiety disorders may occur in as many 25% and mania in up to 17–19% (Chapter 4). The reasons for this disparity between longitudinal studies of hyperactive children and studies of clinic-referred ADHD children are unclear. Further research is clearly in order to clarify the actual level of risk for these comorbid mood and anxiety disorders in children with hyperactivity/ADHD.

As was the case at the midadolescent follow-up (Barkley, Fischer, et al., 1990), the hyperactive group in the present study continued to be more likely than the control group to use mental health services throughout their high school years. The hyperactive probands were more likely to have received stimulant medication treatment as well. The picture after high school, once individuals became more independent of their parents, is quite different. By early adulthood, fewer members of the hyperactive group had received treatment in the ensuing years since leaving high school, though this level was still significantly greater than in the control group.

Antisocial Activities and Drug Use

Although the association of childhood ADHD and conduct problems with adolescent CD and substance use have become increasingly well established (Loeber, Burke, Lahey, Winters, & Zera, 2000; see also discussion above), the risks for antisocial activities and substance use in young adulthood are less certain. Only a handful of studies of children clinically diagnosed with ADHD or hyperactivity have followed them into adulthood to evaluate their ongoing risks for antisocial activities and substance use at this developmental stage. Just four follow-up studies (other than our own) seem to exist that used large clinic-referred samples, had control groups, retained at least 50% of their original samples into adulthood, and examined for antisocial behavior and drug use by young adulthood. These consist of the Montréal follow-up study (clinical *n* = 103) conducted by Weiss, Hechtman, and their colleagues (see Weiss & Hechtman, 1993); the

New York City longitudinal study of two separate cohorts (n's = 101, 94) conducted by Mannuzza, Klein, and colleagues (see Mannuzza et al., 1993, 1998; Mannuzza, Gittelman, Konig, & Giampino, 1989); the Los Angeles study (n = 89) conducted by Satterfield and colleagues (Satterfield & Schell, 1997); and the Swedish follow-up study (n = 50) conducted by Rasmussen and Gillberg (2001).

In the Montréal, New York, and Swedish studies, antisocial activity occurred in a significant minority of probands by adulthood, as evident in the higher proportion of Antisocial Personality Disorder in the hyperactive (vs. control) samples by young adulthood (see "Other Psychiatric Diagnoses and Impairments," above). Criminal arrests have also been shown to be higher among hyperactive children followed to adulthood (Babinski, Hartsough, & Lambert, 1999; Rasmussen & Gillberg, 2001; Satterfield & Schell, 1997). Except for alcohol use, drug use disorders were also found to be somewhat more common in the hyperactive children at adulthood in the New York study (again, see "Other Psychiatric Diagnoses ... "), although in the smaller

Swedish study only alcohol use disorders occurred significantly more often than in controls. These results show that at least some children with ADHD are at risk for adult arrests, antisocial behaviors or disorders, and substance use disorders. Although documenting arrest rates and clinical disorders by adulthood is certainly informative, more precise information on the specific forms of antisocial activities and drug use by the probands would help to further clarify the nature and risks for maladjustment in the adult outcome of ADHD.

To turn to our Milwaukee young adult follow-up (Barkley, Fischer, Smallish, & Fletcher, 2004), we found that more of the hyperactive group committed a variety of antisocial acts and had been arrested for doing so (corroborated through official arrest records) than did the community control group. These are shown in Table 6.4. The hyperactive group also committed a higher frequency of property theft, disorderly conduct, assault with fists, carrying a concealed weapon, and illegal drug possession, as well as more arrests (see Table 6.5). Our study extends the results of prior follow-up studies in several important respects:

TABLE 6.4. Proportion of Hyperactive and Control Groups That Ever Committed Various Antisocial Activities by Young Adulthood or Were Arrested (Self-Reported and Official Records)

Activity	Hyperactive %	(#)	Control %	(#)	χ^2	p	Eta
Stolen property	85	(125)	64	(47)	12.19	<.001	.235
Stolen money	50	(73)	36	(26)	3.89	.049	.133
Broken into a home	20	(29)	8	(6)	4.83	.028	.148
Disorderly conduct	69	(101)	53	(39)	4.92	.026	.150
Assault with fists	74	(109)	52	(38)	10.74	.001	.221
Assault with a weapon	22	(32)	7	(5)	7.76	.005	.188
Robbery or mugging	4	(6)	0	(0)	3.06	NS	.118
Set serious fires	15	(22)	5	(4)	4.21	.04	.138
Carried concealed weapon	38	(56)	11	(8)	17.41	<.001	.281
Forced someone into sex	1	(1)	0	(0)	0.50	NS	.048
Had sex with prostitute	2	(3)	0	(0)	1.51	NS	.083
Took money to have sex	2	(3)	0	(0)	1.51	NS	.083
Ran away from home	31	(45)	16	(12)	5.10	.024	.152
Illegal drug possession	52	(76)	42	(31)	1.66	NS	.087
Illegal drug sales	24	(35)	20	(15)	0.29	NS	.037
Ever arrested (self-reported)	54	(79)	37	(27)	5.48	.019	.158
Arrested 2+ times	39	(58)	12	(9)	16.95	<.001	.278
Arrested 3+ times	27	(40)	11	(8)	7.55	.006	.185
Misdemeanor arrest (official)	24	(35)	11	(8)	5.02	.025	.151
Felony arrest (official)	27	(40)	11	(8)	7.42	.006	.183

Note. %, percent of group; (#), number committing this act; χ^2, chi-square; p, probability associated with the chi-square statistic; Eta, effect size; Official, derived from the official state crime records. Sample sizes are 147 for the hyperactive and 73 for the control groups. From Barkley, Fischer, Smallish, and Fletcher (2004). Copyright 2004 by the Association of Child Psychology and Psychiatry. Reprinted by permission.

TABLE 6.5. Comparison of Hyperactive and Control Groups on Frequency of Antisocial Activities at Young Adult Outcome

Activity	Hyperactive		Control		F	p	Eta^2
	M	SD	M	SD			
Stolen property	15.2	25.1	4.7	10.6	11.53	.001	.050
Stolen money	4.4	10.6	2.3	6.8	2.52	NS	.011
Broken into a home	1.8	8.4	0.5	2.7	1.66	NS	.008
Disorderly conduct	16.3	28.4	7.6	17.6	5.78	.017	.026
Assault with fists	12.7	22.8	3.8	10.8	10.02	.002	.044
Assault with a weapon	2.0	8.1	0.3	1.8	3.25	NS	.015
Robbery or mugging	0.1	0.4	0.0	0.0	2.55	NS	.012
Set serious fires	0.4	2.6	0.1	0.7	1.06	NS	.005
Carried concealed weapon	10.3	21.3	3.3	12.7	6.65	.011	.030
Forced someone into sex[a]	0.1	0.4	0.0	0.0	0.00	NS	.000
Had sex with prostitute	0.1	0.3	0.0	0.0	1.14	NS	.005
Took money to have sex	0.1	0.2	0.0	0.0	1.34	NS	.006
Ran away from home	2.1	6.0	1.1	5.0	1.53	NS	.007
Illegal drug possession	183.5	295.3	105.0	232.1	3.94	.048	.018
Illegal drug sales[b]	7.9	17.6	3.8	11.4	3.21	NS	.006
Arrested (self-reported)	3.5	8.4	0.7	1.5	7.52	.007	.033
Total arrests[c]	1.1	2.1	0.2	0.6	0.77	NS	.004

Note. M, percent of group; *SD*, standard deviation; Eta^2, effect size for the *F* test. Sample sizes are 147 for the hyperactive and 73 for the control groups. From Barkley et al. (2004). Copyright 2004 by the Association of Child Psychology and Psychiatry. Reprinted by permission.
[a]Age served as a covariate in this analysis.
[b]Duration of follow-up served as a separate factor in this analysis (*F* test is for main effect of group).
[c]Age and IQ score served as covariates in this analysis, while duration of follow-up also served as a separate factor (*F* test is for the main effect of group). Scores for total arrests were derived from the official state crime records.

• We identified a wider range of offenses among the hyperactive group than had been previously reported.

• We unearthed two relatively robust underlying dimensions to these antisocial activities, which we called Predatory–Overt and Drug-Related, and each of which accounted for more than 20% of the variance in antisocial activities. Additional factors were discovered pertaining to sexual deviance–theft, fire setting, and sexual assault. But each accounted for less than 10% of the variance, each consisted mainly of just one or two antisocial actions each, and those actions occurred relatively infrequently, leading us to view those factors as not particularly reliable or stable.

• We found that the hyperactive group differed primarily from the control group only on the Drug-Related antisocial dimension, not on the Predatory–Overt dimension. Such a distinction in the nature of antisocial activities toward which hyperactive children may be predisposed has not been previously reported.

• We found that this group difference in Drug-Related antisocial activities was related to severity of ADHD in childhood, adolescence, and adulthood, after we controlled for the contribution of both ADHD and severity of conduct problems at the earlier developmental period. Only severity of childhood conduct problems made an additional significant contribution to predicting this form of young adult antisocial behavior beyond severity of childhood ADHD. Severity of teen CD and adult CD made no significant additional contributions to this dimension of adult antisocial behavior, once we controlled for severity of childhood conduct problems. All this implies that severity of ADHD may be the principal risk factor for determining the frequency of Drug-Related antisocial behavior committed by young adulthood.

• Other longitudinal studies have found that severity of childhood ADHD symptoms is specifically associated with risk for later drug use, apart from the better-established association of childhood conduct problems with later drug use (Babinski et al., 1999; Kaplow, Curran, Dodge, & the Conduct Problems Prevention Research Group, 2002). To our knowledge, however, this is the first time that ADHD has been linked to drug-related antisocial activities, and that such a contribution has been established apart from any made by severity of childhood, teen, or adult CD.

• Finally, we were able to extend prior follow-up research on hyperactive children by evaluating the degree to which severity of teen CD and teen drug use contributed independently of each other to antisocial activity by adulthood. Such an examination was initiated primarily to explore previous suggestions (Brook, Whiteman, Finch, & Cohen, 1996) that teen drug use may contribute additional risk to antisocial activities by young adulthood, apart from its well-known affiliation with severity of teen CD. Our results supported this hypothesis, but only for certain types of young adult antisocial activities. Drug use did not contribute independently to the Predatory–Overt dimension of antisocial activities by young adulthood, apart from severity of teen CD. Teen CD, however, was significantly predictive of this dimension of antisocial behavior by young adulthood, in keeping with numerous prior longitudinal studies finding such a linkage (Brook et al., 1996; Satterfield & Schell, 1997; Loeber et al., 2000). In contrast, teen substance use was significantly predictive of the Drug-Related dimension of antisocial behavior by young adulthood, apart from any contribution of teen CD to this dimension. In fact, teen drug use seemed to mediate the link of teen CD to this form of young adult criminal behavior. These results are quite consistent with the findings of Brook et al. (1996) that teen drug use contributes additional risk for later young adult delinquency, apart from teen delinquency. Our results also are in keeping with those of Ridenour et al. (2002), showing that adolescent drug use before 18 years of age significantly increased the risk of adult antisocial behavior. Our findings go further in showing that at least among our groups, teen drug use contributed chiefly to the dimension of Drug-Related antisocial activities rather than that of Predatory–Overt antisocial behavior.

• In a related study, the hyperactive group was found to have an increased expected criminal cost of $37,830 per person (in dollar values for the year 2000), compared to the control group and with all else held equal (Swensen et al., 2004).

Given the well-known association of CD with risk of drug use, we subdivided our hyperactive subjects into those who did and did not have lifetime CD by young adulthood (self-reported), and compared them to the control group for their frequency of use of various drugs. These results are shown in Table 6.6. Our results found significant group differences for 9 of the 11 drug use activities we surveyed.

TABLE 6.6. Comparison of Hyperactive Only, Hyperactive with Conduct Disorder (Lifetime), and Control Groups on Self-Reported Frequency of Substance Use at Young Adulthood

Substance	(1) H only		(2) H + CD		(3) Control		F	p	Contrasts
	M	SD	M	SD	M	SD			
Average # of drinks per week	6.8	10.6	15.4	21.5	8.0	10.1	6.82	.001	1,3 < 2
# times drunk in past 3 mo	3.4	6.2	1.9	21.3	6.6	9.1	8.26	.001	1,3 < 2
# times passed out in past 3 mo	3.3	4.3	16.2	32.2	5.4	9.0	4.98	.009	1,3 < 2
Marijuana	89.4	199.4	510.1	308.1	153.2	275.2	46.09	<.001	1,3 < 2
Cocaine	5.8	53.7	40.5	150.7	1.9	8.2	4.00	.02	1,3 < 2
Hallucinogens	2.4	7.1	9.5	13.0	3.8	8.7	9.63	<.001	1,3 < 2
Amphetamines[a]	3.3	14.2	9.8	21.1	0.2	1.0	9.63	.001	1,3 < 2
Narcotics	<0.1	0.1	0.8	4.3	0.4	2.6	1.87	NS	—
Sedatives[a]	0.8	5.4	5.0	13.2	0.8	6.0	4.95	.008	1,3 < 2
Other drugs	0.8	4.7	4.3	12.0	2.2	9.4	2.82	NS	—
# times used drugs in past 3 mo	3.0	11.8	25.0	36.0	5.5	14.7	20.05	<.001	1,3 < 2

Note. Sample sizes are 101 for the hyperactive only, 46 for the hyperactive with Conduct Disorder, and 73 for the control groups, except for the conditional measure of "# of times passed out in past 3 months," where sample sizes were 44, 24, and 36, respectively. Inquiring about that question was conditional on the participant's having answered yes to having gotten drunk in the past 3 months. H only, hyperactive only; H + CD, hyperactive with Conduct Disorder. From Barkley et al. (2004). Copyright 2004 by the Association of Child Psychology and Psychiatry. Reprinted by permission.
[a]This measure was analyzed by a 2 × 2 ANOVA (group × follow-up duration).

In all cases, it was the hyperactive group having CD that accounted for these differences, with there being no significant differences between the purely hyperactive and control groups in any form of drug use. As with many other studies, these results again demonstrate that the joint occurrence of CD with ADHD is the major risk factor for drug use by young adulthood, rather than hyperactivity/ADHD alone (Chilcoat & Breslau, 1999; Flory, Lynam, Milich, Leukefeld, & Clayton, 2001; Kuperman et al., 2001; Mannuzza et al., 1993; Molina et al., 1999).

Having reaffirmed this general association once more, the present study went further to show that drug use among our participants could be reduced to approximately three underlying dimensions, which we labeled Hard Drug Use, Grass/LSD Use, and Alcohol Use. As above, we found that the subgroup of hyperactive children having CD by young adulthood accounted for the significant group differences along all three of these dimensions. However, for Alcohol Use this group did not differ from the purely hyperactive group but did from the control group, implying that the purely hyperactive group may also be prone to greater use of this particular substance.

In studying predictors of these dimensions of drug use, we found that it was principally severity of both teen ADHD and especially teen CD (after we controlled for teen ADHD) that contributed significantly to the Hard Drug Use dimension, not childhood severity of either set of symptoms or severity of ADHD in young adulthood. Only severity of teen CD contributed significantly to the prediction of drug use along the other two dimensions (Grass/LSD Use, Alcohol Use). Our results are generally in keeping with those of other studies, particularly that of White, Xie, Thompson, Loeber, & Stouthamer-Loeber (2001), in showing the major contribution of teen CD to later drug use; however, they differ from White et al.'s in that severity of teen ADHD did not contribute to level of marijuana use. This difference may be due to differences in samples and methods, given that White et al. (2001) employed an epidemiologically derived sample and examined frequencies of specific drug use, as opposed to employing underlying principal components of drug use as we did.

Our study also sought to determine the degree to which teen CD independently contributed to risk for drug use by young adulthood,

apart from the contribution made by teen drug use. Neither teen CD nor drug use made a significant contribution to Grass/LSD Use by young adulthood. Teen drug use contributed to adult Hard Drug Use and seemed to mediate the relationship of teen CD to this dimension of adult drug use. For Alcohol Use, again, teen drug use made a greater contribution than did teen CD, though controlling for teen CD weakened the contribution of teen drug use.

At first glance, it seems paradoxical that drug-related antisocial activities should be increased in hyperactive children and should be largely related to severity of ADHD symptoms at each developmental stage, whereas it is mainly severity of lifetime CD in conjunction with hyperactivity that increases the frequency of drug use. Why this discrepancy between predictors of drug use and those of drug-related antisocial activities should have been found is unclear. We can only conjecture that while lifetime CD is primarily the risk factor for greater drug use, severity of ADHD creates a greater predisposition toward engaging in antisocial activities that are related to drug possession and sale, perhaps because of the increased impulsivity ADHD conveys. Or it may be that drug use has a disproportionate impact on those with ADHD, predisposing them toward greater antisocial activities than might be the case in the absence of ADHD. Further research is certainly needed to clarify the issue.

Cognitive Functioning

Follow-up studies of children with hyperactivity/ADHD into adulthood have not focused on the extent to which the deficits in executive functioning or other cognitive deficits so well documented in child ADHD (see Chapters 2 and 3) may be present at adulthood. Only one previous follow-up study has examined executive functioning in children with hyperactivity or ADHD at young adult outcome (Hopkins, Perlman, Hechtman, & Weiss, 1979). This study found that the hyperactive group manifested significant deficits in executive functioning including attention, impulse control, and resistance to distraction, relative to the control group. These differences remained despite measurable improvement in these abilities since the adolescent follow-up evaluation. At least a third or more of hyperactive children may no longer qualify for the diagnosis of ADHD by young adulthood (Barkley, Fischer, et al.,

2002). Thus it is not clear in the Hopkins et al. study whether the executive functioning deficits found in the hyperactive group were primarily characteristic of those meeting the diagnostic criteria for ADHD by adulthood, or whether they typified even those hyperactive children no longer qualifying for that disorder.

Given the dearth of longitudinal studies objectively evaluating the presence of ADHD symptoms and executive functioning deficits at young adult follow-up in their samples with hyperactivity or ADHD, the Milwaukee study (Fischer et al., 2005) incorporated commonly used tests of several executive functions (including inattention and inhibition) at the young adult follow-up, as well as direct behavioral observations of ADHD-related behavior. We also examined the degree to which any deficits in these domains were a function of current ADHD at follow-up. Several measures used here were also collected at the adolescent follow-up, permitting examination of possible developmental changes on them as well. The results suggested that those hyperactive children who had a diagnosis of ADHD in young adulthood were primarily the ones who were significantly impaired in attention and inhibition compared to the control group. These young adults were also observed to display significantly greater symptoms of ADHD during performance of a continuous-performance test (CPT) and a letter cancellation task than did the control group (and, in the latter instance, than did the hyperactive subjects who did not have ADHD by adulthood). Only on a measure of reaction time were those hyperactive participants who did not receive a diagnosis of ADHD in adulthood different from the control group in their functioning. These findings are quite consistent with those found at the earlier adolescent follow-up, where the hyperactive group performed more poorly than the control group on this identical measure of attention and inhibition and on direct observations of their ADHD symptoms during a math task (Fischer et al., 1990).

In the only other follow-up study to objectively document executive functioning in these domains, Hopkins et al. (1979) also found their hyperactive group to demonstrate greater errors on a measure of cognitive impulsiveness (Matching Familiar Figures Test) than did their control group. They also noted slower scanning time, fewer correct responses, and more errors on a test of attention (Embedded Figures Test) among the hyperactive group, as well as slower performance and a tendency for more errors on a task assessing response inhibition (interference control; the Stroop Color–Word Test). Our study went further than that of Hopkins et al. in demonstrating that the subset of hyperactive children who met diagnostic criteria for ADHD in adulthood were chiefly the ones who differed from control participants in executive functioning (attention, inhibition, and ADHD-related behavior during task performances). Taken together, these findings suggest that cognitive deficits characteristic of hyperactive children are present at the young adult stage of this disorder, but that this may be largely determined by the presence of current ADHD. Like Hopkins et al. (1979), we also showed that both the hyperactive and control groups improved in their attention and inhibition from adolescence to adulthood, while remaining significantly different from each other across this period of development.

Academic Attainment

The trends toward lower academic achievement and ability, and more grade retentions, suspensions, and expulsions, that are evident in the adolescent years increase; by adulthood, the percentages of children with ADHD having difficulties in these areas are even greater than those percentages noted in adolescence and, of course, greater than those of control subjects. Hyperactive groups in previous follow-up studies into adulthood had less education, achieved lower academic grades, failed more of their courses, were more often retained in grade, failed to graduate from high school, and did not attend college than control groups (Lambert, 1988; Mannuzza et al., 1993, 1998; Weiss & Hechtman, 1993).

The Milwaukee study (Barkley et al., in press) found that more than three times as many hyperactive subjects as community controls had been retained in grade at least once (42% vs. 13%) during their schooling or had been suspended from high school at least once (60% vs. 18%). The hyperactive group members had also completed fewer years of education, and had a lower grade point average (1.69 vs. 2.56 out of a possible 4.0) and class ranking in their last year of schooling (69th percentile vs. 49th percentile), than those in the control group. In addition, more of the hyperactive group had received special educational services while in high school. Of significant social and economic impact, however, was the finding that 32% of the hyperactive group had failed to complete high school, compared to none of the members of the control group. Substantially fewer hyperactive than control children had ever enrolled in college (21% vs 78%) or were currently attending at this follow-up point (15% vs. 66%). In the Montréal follow-up study, approximately 20% attempted a college program but only 5% completed a university degree program, compared to over 41% of control children (Weiss & Hechtman, 1993). These findings demonstrate that the educational domain is a major one for impaired functioning and reduced attainment for children growing up with ADHD.

Unique to this follow-up study was our examination of grade retention in school as a possible risk factor for failing to complete high school in the hyperactive group, over and above other possible factors that might mediate this relationship. Although special education in high school and lifetime severity of CD symptoms were both significantly predictive of this outcome, retention in grade made am additional significant contribution to failing to complete high school, consistent with the results of Pagani et al. (2001). Pagani et al. (2001) were able to show that grade retention results in a significant loss of motivation to learn in school, reduced academic performance, and significant peer relationship problems, as well as greater persistence (and a potential worsening) of anxious, inattentive, and disruptive behavior following retention. Their results were independent of the characteristics the children brought to the situation prior to or at the time of retention, as well as of their subsequent developmental trajectories predicted by such characteristics. Both studies suggest that grade retention is not a satisfactory solution to the problems of disruptive youth.

Employment Functioning

Results from past studies suggest that adolescents with ADHD are no different in their job functioning from nondisabled adolescents (Weiss & Hechtman, 1993). However, these findings need to be qualified by the fact that most jobs taken by adolescents are unskilled or only semiskilled and are usually part-time. As children with ADHD enter adulthood and take on full-time jobs that require skilled labor,

independence of supervision, acceptance of responsibility, and periodic training in new knowledge or skills, their deficits in attention, impulse control, regulation of activity, and organizational skills could begin to handicap them on the job. The findings from the few outcome studies that have examined job functioning suggest that this may be the case. Two prior studies examined occupational status by adulthood and reported their hyperactive groups to rank significantly lower than control groups (Mannuzza et al., 1993; Weiss & Hechtman, 1993). In the Montréal study, employer ratings revealed significantly worse job performance in the hyperactive than in the control group (Weiss & Hechtman, 1993), and more of the hyperactive group had also reported having been fired or laid off from employment than had members of the control group. The Milwaukee follow-up study (Barkley et al., in press) obtained employer ratings of work performance at the young adult assessment and found that hyperactive subjects were rated as performing significantly more poorly at work than control subjects were.

Adults with ADHD were likely to have lower SES than their brothers or control subjects in these studies, and to move and change jobs more often, but also to have more part-time jobs outside their full-time employment. Employers have been found to rate children with ADHD in adulthood as less adequate in fulfilling work demands, less likely to be working independently and to complete tasks, and less likely to be getting along well with supervisors. In the Montréal study, they also did more poorly on job interviews than control individuals did (Weiss & Hechtman, 1993). And these adults reported that they were more likely to find certain tasks at work too difficult for them. Finally, those adults with ADHD were more likely to have been fired from jobs, as well as to have been laid off from work, than were control subjects. In general, adults with ADHD appear to have a poorer work record and lower job status than nondisabled adults (Weiss & Hechtman, 1993). These findings were recently corroborated in our Milwaukee follow-up study as well.

Social Relations

Weiss and Hechtman (1993) are the only previous investigators to have specifically studied the social skills of hyperactive children followed into adulthood. Their findings indicate greater social skills and interaction problems for these adults, particularly in the areas of heterosocial skills (male–female interactions) and assertion. Like this earlier follow-up study, the Milwaukee study (Barkley et al., in press) found greater social impairment in the hyperactive than in the control children by young adulthood. The hyperactive participants reported having significantly fewer social acquaintances and close friends at follow-up, and reported more problems with keeping friends, than did control group members. As for dating, the proportion of both groups currently dating someone did not differ (60%+ for both groups), but the hyperactive group reported having had more dating partners since high school than the control group reported. These results cannot speak to the reasons for this greater turnover in dating partners in the hyperactive group. But a longitudinal study of a large community sample conducted by Woodward, Fergusson, and Horwood (2002) found that children with childhood-onset antisocial behavior had significantly higher rates of partnership difficulties, including greater partnership violence perpetration and victimization, interpartner conflict, and ambivalence about their relationships. Given that a greater proportion of our hyperactive than of our control children had childhood conduct problems and lifetime CD symptoms, such partner difficulties might be expected to occur more often in the hyperactive children by adulthood.

Sexual Activity

In the Montréal follow-up study (Weiss & Hechtman, 1993), sexual adjustment problems were described by as many as 20% of the hyperactive group in adulthood—a figure far greater than that of the control group (i.e., 2.4%). For this reason, we chose to examine sexual activity in the Milwaukee follow-up study (Barkley et al., in press). We questioned subjects about their sexual activities as part of the evaluation at the young adult follow-up point. We found that while the frequency of sexual intercourse within the past year did not differ between the groups, the hyperactive group started having sexual intercourse significantly earlier (15 vs. 16 years of age), and reported having twice as many total sex partners by follow-up and more within the past year, than the control group reported. We found no

group differences in risk for any sexual dysfunctions. Nor were there any differences in sexual orientation (hetero- vs. homosexuality) by follow-up. But more than nine times as many hyperactive group members had been involved in a pregnancy as a biological parent than control group members (38% vs 4%) by this follow-up. For females, this risk was even greater (68% vs. 16%), although the small number of females per group reduced the power of this comparison and its likely reliability. By follow-up (mean age 20 years), 37 children had been born to the hyperactive group members, compared to just 1 for the control group. Four times more hyperactive than control group members had also contracted a sexually transmitted disease (17% vs 4%), and more than twice as many had been tested for HIV (54% vs 21%), though fortunately none reported a positive test result. All of this suggests that children with hyperactivity may lead a higher-risk sexual lifestyle upon reaching sexual maturity, since they have a greater likelihood of being early parents by young adulthood and of contracting sexually transmitted diseases.

Our examination of potential predictors of several of these risks within the hyperactive group showed that greater lifetime CD symptoms and lower IQ were associated with earlier initiation of sexual intercourse. The risk of involvement in an early pregnancy was also predicted by lifetime CD symptoms only, at least for males in this group (the pool of females was too low to provide adequate power, and no predictors reached significance for it). Although our findings are novel to the field of follow-up studies of hyperactive children, they are consistent with the Dunedin longitudinal study of a large community sample of children, in which 19% of participants had become fathers by age 26 years (Jaffee, Caspi, Moffitt, Taylor, & Dickson, 2001). These researchers found that a history of conduct problems, among other variables, significantly increased the risk for early fatherhood among the 499 males they followed to adulthood.

Driving

As noted in Chapter 3, the study by Weiss and Hechtman (1993) found that significantly more of their hyperactive subjects as adults had been involved in motor vehicle crashes and had received speeding tickets, compared to their control group. We found similar results in adolescents with ADHD followed over the first 3–5 years of their initial driving careers (see "Adolescent Outcome," above). Greater driving performance problems and adverse outcomes have since been well documented in the adolescent and adult outcomes of children with ADHD (Barkley, 2004). At the young adult assessment in the Milwaukee outcome study (Fischer, Barkley, Smallish, & Fletcher, in press), more of the hyperactive group reported having been ticketed for reckless driving and driving without a license, having hit-and-run crashes, and having their licenses suspended or revoked. Official driving records also revealed that a greater proportion of this group had received traffic citations and a greater frequency of license suspensions. The cost of damage in their initial crashes was significantly greater in the hyperactive than in the control group as well. Both self-report and other ratings of actual driving behavior revealed less safe driving practices being used by the hyperactive group, while observations by driving instructors during a behind-the-wheel road test indicated significantly more impulsive errors in driving. Driving performance on a simulator further revealed slower and more variable reaction times, greater impulsive errors (false alarms, poor rule following), more steering variability, and more scrapes and crashes of the simulated vehicle against road boundaries than in the control group. These findings corroborate prior research on clinic-referred teens and adults with ADHD (Barkley, 2004), and they add to a growing literature on the significant driving risks associated with hyperactivity/ADHD at all levels of driving performance.

Predictors of Adult Outcome

Weiss and Hechtman (1993) reported on potential predictors of adult outcome in their prospectively followed group of hyperactive children. Their results suggest that the previously discussed predictors of adolescent outcome may be useful in predicting adult outcome as well. The emotional adjustment of their hyperactive subjects as adults was related to the emotional climate of their homes (particularly the mental health of family members) in childhood, and to the emotional stability and intelligence of the subjects themselves. It is important to note here that emotional stability as measured in this study was highly related to child-

hood aggression, making these results consistent with those for predictors of adolescent outcome, when childhood aggression was highly related to many aspects of adolescent adjustment. Friendships in these adults were also related to the early emotional climate of the home. Academic attainment (grades completed) was best predicted by a combination of factors: childhood intelligence, hyperactivity, poor child-rearing practices, parental SES, and the emotional climate of the home. The employment functioning of these adults was significantly related to their childhood intelligence estimates and their relationships with adults.

Weiss and Hechtman (1993) also found that earlier antisocial behavior was significantly associated with being fired from a greater number of jobs and (in combination with earlier hyperactivity and relationships with adults) with general work record as rated by current employers. The likelihood of committing criminal offenses in adulthood was most closely associated with childhood emotional instability (aggression), and to a lesser degree with intelligence, hyperactivity, SES, mental health of family members, emotional climate in the home, and parental overprotectiveness in child rearing. Not surprisingly, these same factors were associated with the likelihood of later nonmedical drug use.

Despite the discovery of these significant predictors of outcome, the amount of variance accounted for by any one predictor in the outcomes under study has been exceptionally small. In general, no single childhood factor is likely to be of much use in predicting the adult adjustment of individuals with ADHD. As Weiss and Hechtman (1993) argued, the combination of child cognitive ability (intelligence) and emotional stability (aggression, low frustration tolerance, greater emotionality) with family environment (mental health of family members, SES, emotional climate of home) and child-rearing practices provides a considerably more successful prediction of adult outcome.

In contrast, Loney et al. (1981) found that only IQ and the number of siblings in the family was predictive of outcome—in this case, a diagnosis of Antisocial Personality Disorder—whereas only IQ was related to later alcoholism. No other childhood predictors were found to predict various outcomes in adulthood in this study. The New York follow-up study, however, was not able to identify any significant predictors of outcome after controlling for chance associations among the large number of statistical tests often conducted in such research (Klein & Mannuzza, 1991). As noted earlier, the best predictor in the Milwaukee outcome study has been the presence of CD by adolescence or young adulthood, which is predictive of greater antisocial activity, arrest rates, drug use, dropping out of school, and teen pregnancy.

One study (Lambert & Hartsough, 1998) suggested that childhood treatment with stimulants appeared to predict a greater use of substances, particularly nicotine and cocaine, by adolescence and adulthood. However, 13 other studies as well as the Milwaukee study have not replicated this finding, which appears to have been the result of not controlling for lifetime CD (Barkley, Fischer, Smallish, & Fletcher, 2003; Wilens, Faraone, Biederman, & Gunawardene, 2003).

CLINIC-REFERRED ADULTS DIAGNOSED WITH ADHD

Over the past 20 years, a still small but increasing body of scientific literature has begun to emerge on the nature of ADHD as it is likely to appear in adults who are self-referred to clinics specializing in the treatment of adults with ADHD (see Goldstein & Ellison, 2002; Spencer, 2004). As noted in the introduction to this chapter, there is reason to suspect that these individuals will not manifest identical problems to those children followed to adulthood who were diagnosed with ADHD as children. Although it is clear that both groups experience the same disorder (O'Donnell, McCann, & Pluth, 2001; Wilens, Faraone, & Biederman, 2004), comorbidity and other associated conditions and risks may differ significantly, warranting this separate section of this chapter dedicated to research on clinic-referred adults.

Popular books on the subject of adults with ADHD abound (Gordon & McClure, 1996; Hallowell & Ratey, 1994; Kelly & Ramundo, 1992; Murphy & LeVert, 1994; Solden, 1995; Weiss, 1992), and a few clinical textbooks for professionals have also appeared (Goldstein & Ellison, 2002; Nadeau, 1995; Wender, 1995; Weiss, Hechtman, & Weiss, 1999). But, for all their good intentions, many of the assertions made in popular books about the nature of clinic-referred adults diagnosed with ADHD

have not been put to the empirical test of controlled scientific research. For instance, some claim that adults with ADHD are more intelligent, more creative, more "lateral" in their thinking, more optimistic, and better able to handle crises than those without the disorder. To my knowledge, none of these claims has any scientific support at this time. The information obtained from such clinical cases is also fraught with various confounding variables, not the least of which are referral bias and comorbid psychiatric disorders. Useful as they may initially be when a vacuum exists in scientific information about a disorder, such case reports still remain purely anecdotal wisdom, for better or worse. Studies of relatively large samples of clinic-referred adults with ADHD have been published in the past 15 years, however. Their results speak to both the legitimacy and the specificity of this diagnosis in adults (Wilens et al., 2004), if the follow-up studies of children with ADHD reviewed earlier were not sufficient evidence of such.

Even without the suggested modifications to the DSM-IV(-TR) diagnostic criteria for ADHD set forth in Chapter 2 of this volume, these criteria as published can be used successfully in the clinical diagnosis of adult self-referrals. Doing so, however, is likely to identify only those with more serious or severe cases of the disorder, given that the frequency with which typical adults endorse 6 or more of the DSM symptoms in either the inattention or the hyperactivity–impulsivity symptom categories declines significantly with age (see Murphy & Barkley, 1996b). The male-to-female ratio found in adults diagnosed with ADHD ranges from 1.8:1 to 2.6:1 (Barkley, Murphy, & Kwasnik, 1996b; Biederman et al., 1993; Murphy & Barkley, 1996b; Roy-Byrne et al., 1997). This ratio is similar to or only slightly lower than those reported in community prevalence studies of ADHD in children using DSM criteria (see Chapter 2), but is well below the ratio of males to females often seen in clinic-referred samples of children with ADHD. This last ratio, of course, is likely to be driven by a referral bias, given that boys are more aggressive than girls with ADHD and thus are more likely to be referred for evaluation and treatment. In any case, the DSM diagnostic criteria for ADHD do appear to identify a group of individuals who are impaired in their daily adaptive functioning and show patterns of deficits in both clinical interviews and psychological testing comparable to those patterns found in children diagnosed with ADHD (Mick, Faraone, & Biederman, 2004).

Presenting Symptoms

Adults with ADHD who had a prior diagnosis of ADHD as children are highly likely to endorse many of the individual symptoms in the DSM-IV(-TR) symptom list to a greater degree than control groups do (O'Donnell et al., 2001). Two studies reported together by Span, Earleywine, and Strybel (2002) suggest that the two-factor or two-dimensional nature of the DSM symptom groupings may actually better separate into three factors by adulthood (inattention, impulsivity, and hyperactivity). Kevin Murphy and I (1996b) also found three factors when we factor-analyzed the results of a survey of more than 700 general-population adults, in which we found that the verbal impulsive items seemed to form a weaker third factor apart from inattention and hyperactivity–impulsivity. This might imply that verbal impulsivity becomes a distinct problem for adults apart from hyperactivity and behavioral (motor) impulsivity with which it is associated in children.

In a review of the charts of more than 170 adults with ADHD who presented to our adult ADHD clinic during its first few years of operation, Kevin Murphy and I (Murphy & Barkley, 1996) identified a number of symptoms beyond those in the DSM about which these adults were complaining. Table 6.7 summarizes these complaints. As this table suggests, the types of symptoms reported by adults with ADHD are similar to the difficulties reported for children and adolescents with ADHD by their parents and teachers, especially as these pertain to school functioning. It is as if the very same difficulties that teens with ADHD experience in school have been translated to the adult employment setting and now become the difficulties that adults with ADHD and their employers are likely to notice. And such difficulties are quite close to those described in the theoretical model of ADHD developed in Chapter 7.

In general, the chief presenting complaints in adults with ADHD who refer themselves to clinics are quite consistent with conceptualizations of this disorder as involving impairments in attention, inhibition, activity regulation, and especially self-regulation.

Comorbid Psychiatric Disorders

Just as do children and adolescents diagnosed with ADHD, adults given a clinical diagnosis of ADHD have considerably higher amounts of comorbid ODD and CD than do either clinical control groups without a diagnosis of ADHD or typical, nonreferred adults. Approximately 24–35% of clinic-referred adults diagnosed with ADHD have ODD and 17–25% manifest CD, either currently or over the course of their earlier development (Barkley, Murphy, & Kwasnik, 1996a; Biederman et al., 1993; Murphy & Barkley, 1996b; Spencer, 1997). These figures are below those reported in studies of children with ADHD, particularly studies of hyperactive children followed to adulthood, where levels of ODD and CD may be double these reported for adults diagnosed with ADHD (Barkley, Fischer, et al., 1990; Fischer et al., 2002; Weiss & Hechtman, 1993; see also the "Adolescent Outcome" section). Among adult relatives of children having ADHD who also meet criteria for ADHD, 53% have had ODD and 33% have had CD at some time in their lives (Biederman et al., 1993)—figures closer to those seen in follow-up studies of children with hyperactivity or ADHD. Antisocial Personality Disorder is often an associated adult outcome in a large minority of those adolescents who have CD; thus it is not surprising to find that 7–18% of adults diagnosed with ADHD qualify for a diagnosis of this personality disorder (Biederman et al., 1993; Shekim, Asarnow, Hess, Zaucha, & Wheeler, 1990). Even among those who do not qualify for this diagnosis, many receive higher-than-normal ratings on the personality traits associated with it (Tzelepis, Schubiner, & Warbasse, 1995).

One of our studies (Murphy, Barkley, & Bush, 2002) corroborates these earlier reports. We compared 60 adults with the Combined Type of ADHD to 36 adults with the Predominantly Inattentive Type and 64 community control adults (ages 17–27). Our results appear in Tables 6.8 and 6.9. Both groups with ADHD also presented with a greater likelihood of Dysthymic Disorder, alcohol dependence/abuse, cannabis dependence/abuse, and learning disorders than control adults. And both reported greater psychological distress on all scales of the Symptom Checklist 90—R than the control group. The two groups with ADHD differed in only a few respects: Those with the Combined Type were more likely to have

TABLE 6.7. Frequent Presenting Complaints of Adults with ADHD Self-Referred to Clinics

Poor school/work performance related to . . .

Deficient sustained attention to reading, paperwork, lectures, etc.
Poor reading comprehension
Easily bored by tedious material or tasks
Poor organization, planning, and preparation
Procrastination until deadlines are imminent
Subjectively restless; objectively fidgety
Less able to initiate and sustain effort to uninteresting tasks
Highly distractible when context demands concentration
Trouble staying in a confined space or context, such as dull meetings (not a phobia)
Impulsive decision making
Cannot work well independently of supervision
Does not listen carefully to directions
Less able to follow through on instructions or assignments
Frequent impulsive job changes; more often fired from employment
Poor academic grades for ability
Often late for work/appointments
Frequently misplacing things
Forgetful of things that must be done
Poor sense of time; deficient time management
Trouble thinking clearly and using sound judgment, especially under stressful conditions
Generally poor self-discipline
Less able to pursue goals as well as others

Poor interpersonal skills

Difficulties making friendships; fewer friends than others
Significant marital problems; more likely to divorce
Impulsive comments to others
Quick to anger or frustration
Verbally abusive to others when angered
Poor follow-through on commitments
Perceived by others as self-centered and immature
Often failing to see others' needs or activities as important
Poor listening skills
Trouble sustaining friendships or intimate relations

Emotional problems

Low self-esteem
Dysthymic
Quick-tempered
Proneness to emotional upset or hysteria
Demoralized over chronic failures, often since childhood
Generalized Anxiety Disorder
Poor regulation of emotions

Antisocial behavior

Full Antisocial Personality Disorder (10–15+%)
Substance dependence/abuse (10–20%)
More frequent lying and stealing
History of physical aggression toward others
Greater likelihood of criminal activities and arrests

(continued)

TABLE 6.7. *(continued)*

Adaptive behavior problems

Chronic employment difficulties
Generally less educated than others of their cognitive ability
Poor financial management; failure to pay bills on time, frequent impulse purchases, and excess debt
Poor driving habits; frequent traffic accidents, violations, and license suspensions
Perceiving themselves as less adequate in child care/management if they have children
Trouble organizing/maintaining home; poor housekeeping
More chaotic personal and family routines
Less health-conscious than others (poor exercise, diet, weight control, management of cholesterol; increased likelihood of smoking and alcohol consumption; riskier sexual lifestyle, less likely to employ birth control or disease protection during sex, more sexual partners than typical, and greater likelihood of having children at an early age)

ODD, to experience interpersonal hostility and paranoia, to have attempted suicide, and to have been arrested (40%) than those with the Predominantly Inattentive Type (19%; 12% for controls). Both groups with ADHD had significantly less education (13 vs. 14.3 years for controls), were less likely to have graduated from college (6–7% vs. 24% for controls), and were more likely to have received special edu-cational placement in high school (17-25% vs. 3% for controls). And both groups were more likely to have previously received psychiatric medication and other mental health services than control adults. Yet only 36–50% of these adults with ADHD had ever been previously diagnosed with that disorder.

Given the relationship of adult ADHD to adult Antisocial Personality Disorder, one

TABLE 6.8. Comorbidity of Clinical Psychiatric Diagnoses (DSM-IV) in Clinic-Referred Adults with ADHD and Community Control Adults

Clinical disorders	ADHD-C[a] (%) (n = 60)	ADHD-PI[b] (%) (n = 36)	Control (%) (n = 64)	χ^2	$p =$	Cont.[c]
Axis I disorders						
Oppositional Defiant Disorder	45.0	19.4	0.0	38.05	.001	1 > 2,3
Conduct Disorder	5.0	2.8	0.0	3.19	NS	—
Major Depressive Disorder	13.3	8.3	3.1	4.43	NS	—
Dysthymic Disorder	25.0	16.7	1.5	14.91	.001	1,2 > 3
Any anxiety disorder	8.3	5.6	1.5	3.08	NS	—
Personality and substance use disorders						
Antisocial Personality Disorder	6.7	0.0	0.0	6.90	NS	—
Alcohol dependence/abuse	36.7	27.8	6.2	17.52	.001	1,2 > 3
Cannabis dependence/abuse	20.0	19.4	1.5	11.88	.001	1,2 > 3
Other drug dependence/abuse	6.7	0.0	0.0	6.90	NS	—
Other disorders						
Any eating disorder	6.7	8.3	0.0	5.10	NS	—
Learning disorders	38.3	41.7	0.0	33.82	.001	1,2 > 3

Note. Adapted from Murphy, Barkley, and Bush (2002). Copyright 2002 by Lippincott Williams & Wilkins. Adapted by permission.
[a]ADHD-C, ADHD, Combined Type.
[b]ADHD-PI, ADHD Predominantly Inattentive Type.
[c]Results for the pairwise contrasts among the groups if significant.

TABLE 6.9. Psychological Maladjustment (Symptom Checklist 90—Revised *T* Scores)

Measure	ADHD-C[a]		ADHD-PI[b]		Control		F^2	$p <$	Cont.[c]
	M	SD	M	SD	M	SD			
Somatization	58.9	12.3	58.9	12.1	45.3	7.8	31.12	.001	1,2 > 3
Obsessive–Compulsive	71.8	9.4	70.4	11.3	49.2	9.3	96.81	.001	1,2 > 3
Interpersonal Sensitivity	69.7	11.3	68.3	10.5	51.2	9.3	57.49	.001	1,2 > 3
Depression	67.5	12.2	68.5	9.3	48.3	9.2	66.87	.001	1,2 > 3
Hostility	69.7	11.2	64.0	9.6	48.0	7.7	83.65	.001	1 > 2 > 3
Anxiety	61.7	12.4	60.8	10.2	48.1	5.1	37.06	.001	1,2 > 3
Paranoid Ideation	66.0	10.9	61.5	12.8	48.9	9.1	41.85	.001	1 > 2 > 3
Psychoticism	65.9	12.7	65.8	10.0	47.9	6.9	60.30	.001	1,2 > 3

Note. Group *n*'s as in Table 6.8. Adapted from Murphy, Barkley, and Bush (2002). Copyright 2002 by Lippincott Williams & Wilkins. Adapted by permission.
[a]ADHD-C, ADHD, Combined Type.
[b]ADHD-PI, ADHD Predominantly Inattentive Type.
[c]Results for the pairwise contrasts among the groups if significant.

would not be surprised to find ADHD over-represented in adult prison populations. I am aware of just two published studies on the issue, however (Eyestone & Howell, 1994; Rasmussen, Almvik, & Levander, 2001). In the first study, a random sampling of 102 inmates in the Utah State Prison was employed (Eyestone & Howell, 1994). Results indicated that 25.5% of those inmates evaluated qualified for a diagnosis of adult ADHD. This diagnosis required the subjects to have self-reported significant symptoms of the disorder since childhood and to meet DSM-III-R criteria for ADHD. Of interest in the study was its finding of a strong association between adult ADHD and MDD in this population, where the prevalence of MDD was also 25.5%. The overlap of the two disorders was 47%, with evidence that increasing severity of ADHD symptoms was associated with increasing risk for MDD. Eyestone and Howell also cited an unpublished master's thesis by Favarino that was reported to have found a similar prevalence rate for adult ADHD in a prison population. The more recent study, by Rasmussen et al. (2001), was conducted in a representative Norwegian prison population (*n* = 82) and used the Wender Utah Rating Scale for determining childhood retrospective reports of ADHD. These researchers found that 46% met the recommended cutoff score for probable ADHD, while another 18% surpassed the threshold suggestive of further screening for the disorder. For current ADHD, the researchers used the Brown scales for adult ADHD and found that 30% met the recommended threshold for the

disorder and another 16% had sufficiently high symptoms to warrant further evaluation. Given the problems with self-reports cited earlier, these figures are probably underestimates.

Substance dependence and abuse are known to occur to a more frequent degree among children with hyperactivity or ADHD who develop CD by adolescence or Antisocial Personality Disorder by adulthood. Adults clinically diagnosed with ADHD seem to be no exception to this rule. Studies have found lifetime rates of alcohol dependence or abuse ranging between 21% and 53% of adults diagnosed with ADHD, whereas 8–32% may manifest some other form of substance dependence or abuse (Barkley et al., 1996b; Biederman et al., 1993; Murphy & Barkley, 1996b; Minde et al., 2003; Murphy et al., 2002; Roy-Byrne et al., 1997; Shekim et al., 1990; Wilens, 2004). Tzelepis et al. (1995) reported that 36% of their 114 adults with ADHD had experienced misuse of alcohol, 21% of cannabis, 11% of cocaine or other stimulants, and 5% of multiple substances. Moreover, at the point of their initial evaluation, 13% met criteria for alcohol dependence or abuse within the past month. The highest risks for substance use disorders appear to be among those adults with ADHD who may also have comorbid CD, Antisocial Personality Disorder, or Bipolar I Disorder (Wilens, 2004).

Approximately 25% of children with ADHD have an anxiety disorder (see Chapter 4). Most studies of ADHD in adults likewise find an overrepresentation of these disorders. The corresponding figures among adults are 24–43%

for Generalized Anxiety Disorder and 52% for a history of Overanxious Disorder (Barkley et al., 1996a; Biederman et al., 1993; Minde et al., 2003; Murphy & Barkley, 1996b; Shekim et al., 1990). But not all studies of ADHD in adults have found this to be the case. We (Murphy et al., 2002) did not find anxiety or depression to be overrepresented in a clinical sample with ADHD, though these findings were based on clinical diagnoses and not formal structured interviews. Neither did the Murphy and Barkley (1996b) and Roy-Byrne et al. (1997) studies. The prevalence of anxiety disorders among adults with ADHD who are relatives of children with clinically diagnosed ADHD, however, is 20%; again, this suggests some comorbidity with ADHD (Biederman et al., 1993). Yet, using structured clinical interviews, we have not found a higher occurrence of anxiety disorders in our hyperactive children followed to adulthood in Milwaukee than in our control group of nonreferred children (see the earlier discussion of the Milwaukee study).

As discussed in Chapter 4, MDD does seem to have some inherent affinity with ADHD. Approximately 16–31% of adults meeting ADHD diagnostic criteria also have MDD (Barkley et al., 1996b; Biederman et al., 1993; Murphy & Barkley, 1996b; Roy-Byrne et al., 1997; Tzelepis et al., 1995). Dysthymic Disorder, a milder form of depression, has been reported to occur in 19–37% of clinic-referred adults diagnosed with ADHD (Murphy & Barkley, 1996b; Murphy et al., 2002; Roy-Byrne et al., 1997; Shekim et al., 1990; Tzelepsis et al., 1995). Some follow-up studies have not been able to document an increased risk for depression among hyperactive children followed to adulthood (see earlier discussions). However, our Milwaukee follow-up study of a large sample of hyperactive children has recently found a prevalence of 28% for MDD by young adulthood—a finding quite consistent with the studies on adults diagnosed with ADHD. Even so, a few studies comparing clinic-referred adults with ADHD to adults seen at the same clinic without ADHD have not found a higher incidence of depression among the adults with ADHD (Murphy & Barkley, 1996a; Roy-Byrne et al., 1997). Rucklidge and Kaplan (1997) reported one of the few studies of women with ADHD and found them to report more symptoms of depression, anxiety, stress, and low self-esteem, as well as a more external locus of control, than did women in the control group.

Obsessive–Compulsive Disorder (OCD) was initially reported to occur in 14% of clinically diagnosed adults with ADHD (Shekim et al., 1990). However, Tzelepis et al. (1995) were unable to replicate this finding and reported that only 4% of their adults met diagnostic criteria for OCD. Roy-Byrne et al. (1997) similarly reported a 4.3–6.5% prevalence rate, which was not significantly different from their clinical control group. Spencer (1997) reported that OCD was more common (12%) only among those adults with a comorbid tic disorder, whereas the figure for those adults with ADHD but without tics was approximately 2%. Thus OCD does not appear to be significantly associated with ADHD in clinic-referred adults unless Tourette syndrome or other tic disorders are also present.

Intelligence and Academic Functioning

Studies of ADHD in children often find their IQ to be significantly below those of control groups; the difference averages about 7–10 points (see Chapter 3). This does not seem to be the case for clinic-referred adults with ADHD, whose IQ scores generally fall in the average range and are comparable to those for control groups of clinic-referred adults (Barkley et al., 1996b; Murphy & Barkley, 1996b; Murphy et al., 2002). Although Biederman et al. (1993) found that their adults diagnosed with ADHD had IQ scores significantly below those of their control groups, the IQ scores for the adults with ADHD were 107–110, nearly identical to the results of our own studies of such adults. The adults with ADHD in the Biederman et al. (1993) study therefore seem to differ significantly from the control groups' only by virtue of the control groups having above-average IQs (110–113).

Adults diagnosed with ADHD seem to have a likelihood of problems in academic functioning at some time during their schooling, similar to that found in children with ADHD who have been followed over development. Between 16% and 40% of clinic-referred adults have repeated a grade, in keeping with the figures reported for ADHD in children and discussed earlier in this chapter (Barkley et al., 1996b; Biederman et al., 1993; Murphy & Barkley, 1996b). Up to 43% have also received some form of extra tutoring services in their academic histories to assist them with their schooling (Biederman et al., 1993). My colleagues and I have found that 16–28% of young adult samples with ADHD have received special educational services (Barkley et al., 1996b; Murphy et al., 2002)—a figure about half that found in hyperactive children followed to young adulthood, but still higher than usual. Consistent with these studies, Roy-Byrne et al. (1997) also found clinic-referred adults with ADHD to have a significantly greater frequency of achievement difficulties in school, grade retentions, and special educational services. A history of behavioral problems and school suspensions is also significantly more common in clinic-referred adults with ADHD than in clinical control groups (Murphy & Barkley, 1996b). Yet young adults with ADHD seen in clinics are far more likely to have graduated from high school (78–92%) and attended college (68%) than are clinic-referred children with ADHD followed to adulthood (see above), for whom the high school graduation rate is only about 64%. Some studies indicate that clinic-referred adults with ADHD may have less education than adults without ADHD seen at the same clinic (Roy-Byrne et al., 1997)—a finding consistent with adult follow-up studies of hyperactive children (Mannuzza et al., 1993). Others, in contrast, have not found this to be the case (Murphy & Barkley, 1996b; Murphy et al., 2002).

Concerning actual academic achievement skills, adults diagnosed with ADHD have been found to perform significantly more poorly on tests of math than those in control groups (Biederman et al., 1993). Only those adults with ADHD who were relatives of children with ADHD were found to be significantly lower on tests of reading in this study. Others have also found clinic-referred adults with ADHD to perform more poorly on reading achievement tests than do control groups from the same clinic (Roy-Byrne et al., 1997). Yet the mean scores on both achievement tests in these studies were still within the average range for these adults with ADHD. Still, these findings are in keeping with studies of children with ADHD, who are almost routinely found to be below average in their academic achievement skills (see Chapter 3). The prevalence of learning disabilities in adults diagnosed with ADHD is well below that found in children, ranging from 0% to

12% (Barkley et al., 1996b; Biederman et al., 1993; Matochik, Rumsey, Zametkin, Hamburger, & Cohen, 1996).

All this suggests that although clinically diagnosed adults with ADHD experience some of the same types of academic difficulties in their histories as do children with hyperactivity or ADHD followed over development, their intellectual levels are higher, and their likelihood of having academic difficulties is considerably less in most respects.

This higher level of intellectual and academic functioning in clinic-referred ADHD adults makes sense, given that they are self-referred to clinics in comparison to children with ADHD. This fact makes it much more likely that these adults have employment, health insurance, and a sufficient educational level to be so employed and insured, as well as a sufficient level of intellect and self-awareness to perceive themselves as needing assistance for their psychiatric problems and difficulties in adaptive functioning. Children with ADHD brought to clinics by their parents are less likely to have these attributes by the time they reach adulthood. They are not as well educated, are having considerable problems sustaining employment, are more likely to have a history of aggression and antisocial activities, and are not as self-aware of their symptoms as adults having ADHD who are self-referred to clinics (see earlier discussions). As already discussed, only 3–5% of the hyperactive children followed to adulthood in our Milwaukee study endorsed sufficient symptoms to receive a clinical diagnosis of ADHD, but that figure was 48% if their parents' reports were employed. This suggests that children with ADHD who are brought to clinics as children may have a more severe form of ADHD—or one that at least predisposes them to more severe impairments and a greater likelihood of comorbid oppositional, conduct, and antisocial problems or disorders—than do adults self-referred to clinics and diagnosed then as having ADHD.

Neuropsychological Findings

As in children with ADHD, research into the neuropsychology of ADHD in adults has expanded substantially since the preceding edition of this text. These studies have used similar or even the same neuropsychological tests employed with children with ADHD, and have often obtained comparable results (see Chapter

3, this volume; see also Hervey, Epstein, & Curry, 2004, for a meta-analysis on adults with ADHD). Matochik et al. (1996) compared 21 adults with ADHD against the norms provided with the neuropsychological tests. They found that performance on the Arithmetic and Digit Span subtests of on the Wechsler Adult Intelligence Scale—Revised were significantly below average, suggesting nonverbal working memory problems, as are often found in children with ADHD. Other studies (Barkley et al., 1996b; Kovner et al., 1997) also found adults with ADHD to perform more poorly on the Digit Span subtest, again indicating difficulties with verbal working memory (see Chapter 3). In contrast, tests of verbal learning, memory, and fluency have shown mixed results, with some studies finding no differences from control groups (Barkley et al., 1996b; Holdnack, Moberg, Arnold, Gur, & Gur, 1995; Kovner et al., 1997), while others have done so (Jenkins et al., 1998; Lovejoy et al., 1999), especially when larger samples are used (Johnson et al., 2001). This implies that statistical power in the earlier studies may have been limited by smaller sample sizes.

Performance on the Wisconsin Card Sort Test (WCST) has been found (Barkley et al., 1996b) to be within the average range in young adults with ADHD. Others have also not found performance on the WCST to discriminate groups of adults with ADHD from control groups (Holdnack et al., 1995; Johnson et al., 2001; Seidman, 1997; Rapport, Van Voorhis, Tzelepis, & Friedman, 2001; see Hervey et al., 2004, for a meta-analysis). Only the study by Weyandt, Rice, Linterman, Mitzlaff, and Emert (1998) found differences between their groups on this task. Studies of childhood ADHD also obtained quite inconsistent results on the WCST, with most finding no group differences (see Chapter 3; see also the meta-analysis by Frazier, Demaree, & Youngstrom, 2004). This suggests that ADHD does not have an adverse impact on whatever neuropsychological function is being tapped by the WCST (typically thought of as flexibility; Mirsky, 1996).

We (Barkley et al., 1996b) compared a small sample of young adults with ADHD ($n = 25$) to a control group ($n = 23$) on measures of creativity. No group differences were found, as was the case in later studies (Murphy, Barkley, & Bush, 2001; Rapport et al., 2001). Rapport et al., however, did find more perseverative and nonperseverative errors on their design fluency

task in their group with ADHD compared to their control group.

Adults with ADHD were also found in two studies (Barkley et al., 1996b; Murphy, Barkley, & Bush, 2001) to perform significantly worse on a nonverbal working memory task (the Simon tone–color game, in which increasing lengthy sequences of tone–color key presses must be imitated). Dowson et al. (2003) likewise found impaired spatial working memory in their group with ADHD, compared to adults with Borderline Personality Disorder and controls.

In a later study, McClean et al. (2004) found adults with ADHD ($n = 19$) to perform more poorly on a computerized cognitive battery assessing spatial working memory, planning, and set shifting, and to be slower to respond to targets in a go/no-go task, than their matched control group ($n = 19$). A much larger study by Nigg et al. (in press) evaluated 105 adults with ADHD and 90 control adults; these researchers reduced their executive function battery by factor analysis to an overall Executive factor and a separate Speed factor (response output), and found the group with ADHD to perform more poorly on both factors. The earlier study by Johnson et al. (2001) likewise found adults with ADHD to perform more poorly on tests of response speed, as have others using very small samples (Himelstein & Halperin, 2000; Kovner et al., 1997). These studies are in keeping with similar deficits noted in childhood ADHD (see Chapter 3). Symptoms of inattention in the Nigg et al. study were more closely related to the Executive factor, while both inattention and hyperactivity–impulsivity symptoms were related to the Speed factor. The study is significant for demonstrating that these results were not a function of age, IQ, comorbid disorders, gender, or educational level.

Studies of children with ADHD that employ CPTs frequently find them to perform these tasks more poorly than do control groups (see Chapter 3), whether the differences involve omission errors (reflecting inattention), commission errors (reflecting inhibition), or reaction time. Many studies of adults with ADHD have found similar deficits. We (Barkley et al., 1996a) found that our young adults with ADHD demonstrated more omission and commission errors than the control group on a CPT. So did three other studies (Epstein, Conners, Erhardt, March, & Swanson, 1997; Gansler et al., 1998; Seidman, 1997), while other studies found that only commission errors differentiated their subjects with ADHD and control participants (Ossman & Mulligan, 2003; Shaw & Giambra, 1993). Roy-Byrne et al. (1997) compared adults diagnosed with ADHD ("probable ADHD") to a group having current adult ADHD symptoms without persuasive childhood history ("possible ADHD") and to a clinical control group, using the Conners CPT. They found that those adults with possible ADHD had significantly poorer composite CPT scores than those in the control group, and that the group with probable ADHD fell between these two groups. Holdnack et al. (1995) also found poorer CPT performance in adults with ADHD, though in this instance it was on the measure of reaction time only and not omission or commission errors. Weyandt, Mitzlaff, and Thomas (2002) found more omission errors in their group with ADHD than their control group. Deficits in inhibition have also been noted on other tests besides CPTs, such as the Stroop task (Hervey et al., 2004; Lovejoy et al., 1999; Rapport et al., 2001), antisaccade tasks (Nigg, Butler, Huang-Pollack, & Henderson, 2002), and negative priming and stopping tasks (Nigg et al., 2002; Ossman & Mulligan, 2003). Such results indicate that response inhibition is significantly impaired in adults with ADHD, as it is in childhood ADHD (Chapter 3).

Two studies have examined distractibility in adults. One studied college students with a history of hyperactivity in childhood and found greater intrusive task-unrelated thoughts during performance on a CPT (Shaw & Giambra, 1993). Another study found clinically diagnosed adults with ADHD to show greater performance problems on a test when background noise occurred during the task (Corbett & Stanczak, 1999).

For the most part, neuropsychological studies of adults with ADHD have employed very small sample sizes, often well below those necessary for adequate statistical power to detect small to moderate effect sizes (group differences) in such research. As a consequence, the failure to find group differences on some measures for which differences have been found in the literature on childhood ADHD may simply be a result of low power. In an effort to address this problem, my colleagues and I compared adults with ADHD (n = 105; ages 17–28 years) to a community control group (n = 64) on 14

measures of executive functions and olfactory identification, using a 2 (groups) × 2 (gender) design (Murphy et al., 2001). Our results appear in Table 6.10. The group with ADHD performed significantly worse on 11 of these 14 measures, including the Stroop Color–Word Test, a measure of inhibition and interference control, and measures of verbal working memory (digit span) and fluency. Measures of attention and inhibition from a CPT also revealed deficits in the adults with ADHD, similar to those seen in childhood ADHD. Consistent with studies of patients having frontal lobe damage, we found adults with ADHD to make more errors on a smell identification test than did control adults. No gender differences were evident on any measures. No differences were found in the group with ADHD as a function of ADHD subtype or comorbid ODD. These results are in agreement with many studies above, particularly the large study by Nigg et al. (in press), in finding executive and response speed deficits associated with adult ADHD. We concluded that the executive function deficits found in childhood ADHD exist in young adults with ADHD and are largely not influenced by comorbidity. And just as in childhood ADHD (see Chapter 3), we found these adults with ADHD to be more impaired in time reproduction than were the control adults (Barkley, Murphy, & Bush, 2001).

One neuropsychological study examined expressed emotion and affect recognition in adults with ADHD. It found the adults with ADHD to show a greater intensity of expressed emotion and a greater deficit in affect recognition than control adults (Rapport, Friedman, Tzelepis, & Van Voorhis, 2002). In the control group, expressed emotion facilitated affect recognition; in the group with ADHD, the opposite was the case. The results are in keeping with my earlier theory of ADHD (see Chapter 7), in which affect regulation is hypothesized to be impaired in the disorder. Another study in this same lab also found adults with ADHD to use less emotion-laden words to describe scenes involving emotional interactions (Friedman et al., 2003).

Adaptive Functioning

Few studies have examined the adaptive functioning of clinic-referred adults with ADHD in comparison to those in control groups. In

TABLE 6.10. Group Means and Standard Deviations for the Executive Function and Olfaction Measures on Adults with ADHD (*n* = 105) and a Community Control Group (*n* = 64)

Measure	ADHD			Control			ANOVA	
	n	*M*	*SD*	*n*	*M*	*SD*	*F*	*p*
Interference control								
Stroop interference %	96	52.2	37.2	64	74.0	29.4	12.04	.001
Stroop number completed	96	102.9	13.5	64	110.2	5.0	11.38	.001
Stroop number of errors	96	1.1	1.6	64	0.8	1.3	0.29	NS
Inattention								
CPT variability of RT	105	13.6	11.4	64	7.5	4.9	16.21	.001
CPT omission errors	105	4.8	7.9	64	1.8	3.0	6.28	.013
WAIS-III Digit Symbol	101	56.6	12.0	63	64.2	10.9	12.73	.001
Response inhibition								
CPT hit RT	105	399.5	267.9	64	355.1	78.6	0.74	NS
CPT commission errors	105	14.0	8.1	64	10.8	6.8	8.61	.004
Verbal working memory								
WAIS-III Digit Span	104	16.5	3.9	64	18.0	3.7	5.25	.023
Nonverbal working memory								
Simon: Longest sequence	104	9.8	2.8	64	11.1	3.4	10.12	.002
Verbal/ideational fluency								
COWAT F-A-S Test	104	36.2	13.0	64	40.5	8.6	10.07	.002
Object Usage Test	105	16.9	7.2	64	17.1	5.2	.003	NS
Smell identification								
Smell test error score	96	3.2	2.4	57	2.2	1.9	5.46	.021
Smell test percentile	96	56.7	28.4	57	67.6	26.8	5.94	.016

Note. ANOVA, results for the univariate analysis of variance; *F*, results of *F* test; *p*, statistical probability for the *F* test if significant (<.05); *SD*, standard deviation; WAIS-III, Wechsler Adult Intelligence Scale—Third edition; CPT, continuous-performance test; RT, reaction time; COWAT, Controlled Oral Word Association Test. Adapted from Murphy, Barkley, and Bush (2001). Copyright 2001 by the American Psychological Association. Adapted by permission.

one such study of 172 adults with ADHD, we (Murphy & Barkley, 1996b) reported that adults with ADHD were more likely to have divorced and remarried than control adults and tended to report less marital satisfaction in their current marriages (*p* < .08). More adults with ADHD had been fired from employment (53% vs. 31%), had impulsively quit a job (48% vs. 16%), and reported chronic employment difficulties (77% vs. 57%). These adults also had changed jobs significantly more often than those in the control group (6.9 times vs. 4.6). Such findings for employment difficulties are in keeping with the outcomes of follow-up studies of hyperactive children (see above).

Friedman et al. (2003) found adults with ADHD to describe themselves as less socially competent, yet more sensitive toward violations of social norms, than their control group. A study of marital and family functioning in adults with ADHD found that these functions were more impaired in families including an adult with ADHD, regardless of parent gender, than in control families (Minde et al., 2003). In keeping with the genetic contribution recognized in the disorder (Chapter 5), 43% of the offspring of the adults with ADHD also met diagnostic criteria for the disorder.

As suggested earlier in this chapter, children with hyperactivity or ADHD followed into later adolescence are likely to have more negative driving outcomes than are control subjects followed over this same period. Several studies of adults with ADHD have inquired about their driving risks. In these studies, adults with ADHD were more likely to have received speeding tickets, to have received more of them, and to have had more motor vehicle accidents (Barkley et al., 1996a; Barkley, Murphy, DuPaul, & Bush, 2002; Murphy & Barkley, 1996b; see Barkley, 2004, for a review). Consistent across studies is the observation that more adults with ADHD have had their licenses suspended or revoked than those in the control groups (24–32% vs. 4%). In the two studies of driving risks and behavior, we (Barkley et al., 1996a; Barkley, Murphy, et al., 2002) also found that adults with ADHD were more likely to have been involved in crashes that resulted in bodily injuries, and were rated by themselves and others as demonstrating significantly less sound driving practices during driving, than were the control adults. We obtained the official driving records as well, which corroborated many of these findings. In the Barkley et al. (1996a) study, adults with ADHD had more driving violations on their official records (including speeding tickets), and were indeed more likely to have had their licenses suspended or revoked (48% vs. 9%) and to experience such suspensions more often

(mean of 1.5 vs. 0.1 episodes). The differences between groups for officially recorded crashes were marginally significant ($p < .08$), both for the percentage of subjects having crashes (80% vs. 52%) and for the total number of such crashes on their records (means of 0.8 vs. 0.3). The problems with driving in these young adults could not be attributed to poor driving knowledge, as no differences between the groups were found on an extensive assessment of such knowledge. However, these young adults, when tested on a computer-simulated driving task, displayed more erratic steering of the vehicle and had more scrapes and crashes while operating this simulated vehicle than did subjects in the control group. The results of our later study of a larger sample of adults with ADHD appear in Tables 6.11 and 6.12. Here again, there were numerous differences between the driving histories of adults with ADHD and those of control adults; these findings only further reinforce the previously established adverse impact of ADHD on driving.

Thus it appears that, like children with ADHD followed into adolescence and young adulthood, adults with ADHD who refer themselves to clinics are likely to have significantly poorer driving habits and a greater risk of various negative driving outcomes than are nondisabled or clinical control groups of adults.

TABLE 6.11. Group Means and Standard Deviations for the Frequency Scores from the Driving History Interview and Official Driving Record

| Measure | ADHD | | | Control | | | | |
	n	M	SD	n	M	SD	t	p <
Self-reported history								
Total tickets for traffic violations	88	11.7	20.6	44	4.8	3.2	3.07	.001
License suspensions or revocations	105	0.5	1.26	64	0.1	.21	3.57	.001
Vehicular crashes as driver	105	1.9	2.4	64	1.2	1.1	2.55	.006
If so, at faults in vehicular crashes	75	1.3	1.2	43	0.9	0.8	2.43	.008
Damage caused in first crash ($)	76	4,221.2	8,051.8	43	1,665.6	2,229.6	2.60	.005
Speeding ticket	88	3.9	5.2	44	2.4	1.5	2.55	.006
Official DMV records								
Tickets for traffic violations	105	5.1	8.4	63	2.1	2.4	3.45	.001
License suspensions or revocations	105	1.1	2.2	63	0.3	0.7	3.34	.001
Vehicular crashes as driver	105	0.6	0.9	63	0.4	0.8	1.33	—
Speeding ticket	105	1.6	2.0	63	1.0	1.2	2.46	.007

Note. All results reported are for *t* tests except for five measures, the analyses of which employed analysis of covariance. *t*, results for the *t* test; *p*, one-tailed statistical probability for the *t* test (where Levene's test for equality of variances was statistically significant at .05 level, the *t* test for unequal variances is reported); *SD*, standard deviation; DMV, Department of Motor Vehicles. Adapted from Barkley, Murphy, DuPaul, and Bush (2002). Copyright 2002 by the International Neuropsychological Society. Adapted by permission.

TABLE 6.12. Negative Driving Outcomes (Categorical Answers) from the Driving History Interview and the Official Driving Record

Measure	ADHD		Control		χ^2	p
	n	% Yes	n	% Yes		
Self-reported history						
Drove illegally before licensed to do so	105	63.8	64	40.6	8.64	.003
12 or more traffic citations	105	20.0	64	3.1	9.63	.001
5 or more speeding citations	105	20.0	64	3.1	9.63	.001
License suspended or revoked	105	21.9	64	4.7	9.05	.002
3 or more vehicular crashes	105	25.7	64	9.4	6.76	.007
3 or more at-fault vehicular crashes	105	7.6	64	3.1	1.44	—
$6,000 or more damage in first crash	76	19.7	43	7.0	3.48	—
Official DMV record						
Ever ticketed for traffic violations	105	80.0	64	59.4	8.45	.003
7 or more traffic tickets	105	20.0	64	6.3	5.96	—
4 or more speeding tickets	105	11.4	64	3.1	3.61	—
License suspended or revoked	105	35.2	64	20.3	4.25	—
2 or more vehicular crashes	105	17.1	64	12.5	0.66	—

Note. n, total sample size per group used in the analysis; % Yes, percentage of each group responding affirmatively; χ^2, results for the chi-square test; *p*, probability for the chi-square test (one-sided Fisher's exact test), if significant; DMV, Department of Motor Vehicles. Adapted from Barkley, Murphy, DuPaul, and Bush (2002). Copyright 2002 by the International Neuropsychological Society. Adapted by permission.

KEY CLINICAL POINTS

✔ Early predictors of risk for ADHD in early childhood are family history of ADHD, the emergence of difficult temperament in the preschool years, high activity levels combined with inattentive and impulsive behavior, and motor coordination difficulties in the preschool period.

✔ Throughout their development, children with ADHD are at greatest risk for academic problems (both in skill development and in behavioral adjustment). There is a higher risk for grade retention, suspensions and expulsions, and special educational services at school, as well as a high risk for failure to complete formal schooling.

✔ Their second greatest risk is for oppositional behavior and antisocial conduct; such conduct itself becomes a strong predictor of adolescent substance use and abuse, as well as later adult Antisocial Personality Disorder and criminality.

✔ The third domain of impairment is social, with a greater risk for peer rejection.

✔ By adolescence, high-risk sexual activities lead to a markedly higher risk for teen pregnancy (30–40%) and a fourfold increase in risk for sexually transmitted diseases.

✔ In adolescence and adulthood, a greater number of driving problems have been documented, including more accidents, traffic citations (especially for speeding), and license suspensions.

✔ As adults, children with ADHD are likely to be less educated, to be underachieving in their occupational settings, and to be having problems with working independently of supervision.

✔ Research on clinic-referred adults with ADHD indicates that they have somewhat lower educational and social risks (but a similar pattern to those risks) than children with ADHD followed into adulthood. These risks include greater comorbid psychiatric diagnoses (conduct problems, Antisocial Personality Disorder, depression, and probably anxiety).

✔ Adults with ADHD also have adaptive functioning impairments (social, occupational, educational), as do children with hyperactivity or ADHD followed into adulthood.

✔ These self-referred adults with ADHD are also likely to have problems in the same areas of neuropsychological functioning as children with ADHD do, particularly on measures of inhibition, working memory, and other executive functions.

✓Differences between self-referred adults with ADHD and children with ADHD followed to adulthood are chiefly in their levels of oppositional, conduct, or antisocial problems or disorders (these are somewhat lower in self-referred adults), and in intellectual and academic functioning (self-referred adults may be more intelligent, have better achievement skills, and be better educated).

✓ADHD among clinic-referred adults is a valid adult psychiatric disorder.

REFERENCES

Achenbach, T. M. (1991). *Manual for the Child Behavior Checklist/4–18 and 1991 Profile*. Burlington, VT: Author.

Ackerman, P., Dykman, R., & Peters, J. E. (1977). Teenage status of hyperactive and nonhyperactive learning disabled boys. *American Journal of Orthopsychiatry, 47*, 577–596.

American Psychiatric Association. (1968). *Diagnostic and statistical manual of mental disorders* (2nd ed.). Washington, DC: Author.

American Psychiatric Association. (1980). *Diagnostic and statistical manual of mental disorders* (3rd ed.). Washington, DC: Author.

American Psychiatric Association. (1987). *Diagnostic and statistical manual of mental disorders* (3rd ed., rev.). Washington, DC: Author.

American Psychiatric Association. (1994). *Diagnostic and statistical manual of mental disorders* (4th ed.). Washington, DC: Author.

Angold, A., Costello, E. J., & Erkanli, A. (1999). Comorbidity. *Journal of Child Psychology and Psychiatry, 40*, 57–88.

Applegate, B., Lahey, B. B., Hart, E. L., Waldman, I., Biederman, J., Hynd, G. W., et al. (1997). Validity of the age of onset criterion for ADHD: A report from the DSM-IV field trials. *Journal of the American Academy of Child and Adolescent Psychiatry, 36*, 1211–1221.

Armstrong, T. D., & Costello, E. J. (2002). Community studies on adolescent substance use, abuse, or dependence and psychiatric comorbidity. *Journal of Consulting and Clinical Psychology, 70*, 1224–1239.

August, G. J., Stewart, M. A., & Holmes, C. S. (1983). A four-year follow-up of hyperactive boys with and without conduct disorder. *British Journal of Psychiatry, 143*, 192–198.

Babinski, L. M., Hartsough, C. S., & Lambert, N. M. (1999). Childhood conduct problems, hyperactivity–impulsivity, and inattention as predictors of adult criminal activity. *Journal of Child Psychology and Psychiatry, 40*, 347–355.

Barkley, R. A. (1981). *Hyperactive children: A handbook for diagnosis and treatment*. New York: Guilford Press.

Barkley, R. A. (1982). Specific guidelines for defining hyperactivity in children (attention deficit disorder with hyperactivity). In B. Lahey & A. Kazdin (Eds.), *Advances in clinical child psychology* (Vol. 5, pp. 137–180). New York: Plenum Press.

Barkley, R. A. (1988). The effects of methylphenidate on the interactions of preschool ADHD children with their mothers. *Journal of the American Academy of Child and Adolescent Psychiatry, 27*, 336–341.

Barkley, R. A. (1998). *Attention-deficit hyperactivity disorder: A handbook for diagnosis and treatment* (2nd ed.). New York: Guilford Press.

Barkley, R. A. (2004). Driving impairments in teens and young adults with attention-deficit/hyperactivity disorder. *Psychiatric Clinics of North America, 27*(2), 233–260.

Barkley, R. A., Anastopoulos, A. D., Guevremont, D. G., & Fletcher, K. F. (1991). Adolescents with attention deficit hyperactivity disorder: Patterns of behavioral adjustment, academic functioning, and treatment utilization. *Journal of the American Academy of Child and Adolescent Psychiatry, 30*, 752–761.

Barkley, R. A., & Biederman, J. (1997). Towards a broader definition of the age of onset criterion for attention deficit hyperactivity disorder. *Journal of the American Academy of Child and Adolescent Psychiatry, 36*, 1204–1210.

Barkley, R. A., DuPaul, G. J., & McMurray, M. B. (1990). A comprehensive evaluation of attention deficit disorder with and without hyperactivity. *Journal of Consulting and Clinical Psychology, 58*, 775–789.

Barkley, R. A., Fischer, M., Edelbrock, C. S., & Smallish, L. (1990). The adolescent outcome of hyperactive children diagnosed by research criteria: I. An 8-year prospective follow-up study. *Journal of the American Academy of Child and Adolescent Psychiatry, 29*, 546–557.

Barkley, R. A., Fischer, M., Smallish, L., & Fletcher, K. (2002). The persistence of attention-deficit/hyperactivity disorder into young adulthood as a function of reporting source and definition of disorder. *Journal of Abnormal Psychology, 111*, 279–289.

Barkley, R. A., Fischer, M., Smallish, L., & Fletcher, K. (2003). Does the treatment of ADHD with stimulant medication contribute to illicit drug use and abuse in adulthood?: Results from a 15-year prospective study. *Pediatrics, 111*, 109–121.

Barkley, R. A., Fischer, M., Smallish, L., & Fletcher, K. (2004). Young adult follow-up of hyperactive children: Antisocial activities and drug use. *Journal of Child Psychology and Psychiatry, 45*, 195–211.

Barkley, R. A., Fischer, M., Smallish, L., & Fletcher, K.

(in press). Young adult outcome of hyperactive children: Educational, occupational, social, sexual, and financial functioning. *Journal of the American Academy of Child and Adolescent Psychiatry.*

Barkley, R. A., Guevremont, D. G., Anastopoulos, A. D., DuPaul, G. J., & Shelton, T. L. (1993). Driving-related risks and outcomes of attention deficit hyperactivity disorder in adolescents and young adults: A 3–5-year follow-up survey. *Pediatrics, 92,* 212–218.

Barkley, R. A., Guevremont, D. G., Anastopoulos, A. D., & Fletcher, K. (1992). A comparison of three family therapy programs for treating family conflicts in adolescents with attention-deficit hyperactivity disorder. *Journal of Consulting and Clinical Psychology, 60,* 450–462.

Barkley, R. A., Murphy, K. R., & Bush, T. (2001). Time estimation and reproduction in young adults with attention deficit hyperactivity disorder (ADHD). *Neuropsychology, 15,* 351–360.

Barkley, R. A., Murphy, K. R., DuPaul, G. J., & Bush, T. (2002). Driving in young adults with attention deficit hyperactivity disorder: Knowledge, performance, adverse outcomes, and the role of executive functioning. *Journal of the International Neuropsychological Society, 8,* 655–672.

Barkley, R. A., Murphy, K. R., & Kwasnik, D. (1996a). Psychological adjustment and adaptive impairments in young adults with ADHD. *Journal of Attention Disorders, 1,* 41–54.

Barkley, R. A., Murphy, K. R., & Kwasnik, D. (1996b). Motor vehicle driving competencies and risks in teens and young adults with ADHD. *Pediatrics, 98,* 1089–1095.

Barkley, R. A., Shelton, T. L., Crosswait, C., Moorehouse, M., Fletcher, K., Barrett, S., et al. (2002). Preschool children with disruptive behavior: Three-year outcome as a function of adaptive disability. *Development and Psychopathology, 14,* 45–67.

Battle, E. S., & Lacey, B. (1972). A context for hyperactivity in children, over time. *Child Development, 43,* 757–773.

Beitchman, J. H., Wekerle, C., & Hood, J. (1987). Diagnostic continuity from preschool to middle childhood. *Journal of the American Academy of Child and Adolescent Psychiatry, 26,* 694–699.

Belsky, J., Hsieh, K., & Crnic, K. (1998). Mothering, fathering, and infant negativity as antecedents of boys' externalizing problems and inhibition at age 3 years: Differential susceptibility to rearing experience? *Development and Psychopathology, 10,* 301–309.

Biederman, J. (1997, October). *Returns of comorbidity in girls with ADHD.* Paper presented at the annual meeting of the American Academy of Child and Adolescent Psychiatry, Toronto.

Biederman, J., Faraone, S. V., Mick, E., Spencer, T., Wilens, T., Kiely, K., et al. (1995). High risk for attention deficit hyperactivity disorder among children of parents with childhood onset of the disorder: A pilot study. *American Journal of Psychiatry, 152,* 431–435.

Biederman, J., Faraone, S. V., Milberger, S., Curtis, S., Chen, L., Marrs, A., et al. (1996). Predictors of persistence and remission of ADHD into adolescence: Results from a four-year prospective follow-up study. *Journal of the American Academy of Child and Adolescent Psychiatry, 35,* 343–351.

Biederman, J., Faraone, S., Milberger, S., Guite, J., Mick, E., Chen, L., et al. (1996). A prospective 4-year follow-up study of attention-deficit hyperactivity and related disorders. *Archives of General Psychiatry, 53,* 437–446.

Biederman, J., Faraone, S., Spencer, T., Wilens, T., Norman, D., Lapey, K. A., et al. (1993). Patterns of psychiatric comorbidity, cognition, and psychosocial functioning in adults with attention deficit hyperactivity disorder. *American Journal of Psychiatry, 150,* 1792–1798.

Biederman, J., Faraone, S. V., Taylor, A., Sienna, M., Williamson, S., & Fine, C. (1997, October). *Diagnostic continuity between child and adolescent ADHD: Findings from a longitudinal clinical sample.* Paper presented at the annual meeting of the American Academy of Child and Adolescent Psychiatry, Toronto.

Biederman, J., Wilens, T., Mick, E., Faraone, S. V., Weber, W., Curtis, S., et al. (1997). Is ADHD a risk factor for psychoactive substance use disorders?: Findings from a four-year prospective follow-up study. *Journal of the American Academy of Child and Adolescent Psychiatry, 36,* 21–29.

Blouin, A. G., Bornstein, M. A., & Trites, R. L. (1978). Teenage alcohol abuse among hyperactive children: A five year follow-up study. *Journal of Pediatric Psychology, 3,* 188–194.

Borland, H. L., & Heckman, H. K. (1976). Hyperactive boys and their brothers: A 25-year follow-up study. *Archives of General Psychiatry, 33,* 669–675.

Bradley, J. D. D., & Golden, C. J. (2001). Biological contributions to the presentation and understanding of attention-deficit/hyperactivity disorder: A review. *Clinical Psychology Review, 21,* 907–929.

Brook, J. S., Whiteman, M., Finch, S. J., & Cohen, P. (1996). Young adult drug use and delinquency: Childhood antecedents and adolescent mediators. *Journal of the American Academy of Child and Adolescent Psychiatry, 35,* 1584–1592.

Brown, R. T., & Borden, K. A. (1986). Hyperactivity in adolescence: Some misconceptions and new directions. *Journal of Clinical Child Psychology, 15,* 194–209.

Burke, J. D., Loeber, R., & Lahey, B. B. (2001). Which aspects of ADHD are associated with tobacco use in early adolescence? *Journal of Child Psychology and Psychiatry, 42,* 493–502.

Buss, D. M., Block, J. H., & Block, J. (1980). Preschool activity level: Personality correlates and developmental implications. *Child Development, 51,* 401–408.

Cameron, J. R. (1978). Parental treatment, children's temperament, and the risk of childhood behavioral problems: II. Initial temperament, parental attitudes, and the incidence and form of behavioral problems. *American Journal of Orthopsychiatry, 48*, 140–147.

Campbell, S. B. (1987). Parent-referred problem three-year-olds: Developmental changes in symptoms. *Journal of Child Psychology and Psychiatry, 28*, 835–846.

Campbell, S. B. (1990). *Behavior problems in preschool children*. New York: Guilford Press.

Campbell, S. B., Endman, M., & Bernfield, G. (1977). A three-year follow-up of hyperactive preschoolers into elementary school. *Journal of Child Psychology and Psychiatry, 18*, 239–249.

Campbell, S. B., Schleifer, M., & Weiss, G. (1978). Continuities in maternal reports and child behaviors over time in hyperactive and comparison groups. *Journal of Abnormal Child Psychology, 6*, 33–45.

Cantwell, D. P. (1975). *The hyperactive child*. New York: Spectrum.

Cantwell, D. P., & Baker, L. (1989). Stability and natural history of DSM-III childhood diagnoses. *Journal of the American Academy of Child and Adolescent Psychiatry, 28*, 691–700.

Carlson, E. A., Jacobvitz, D., & Sroufe, L. A. (1995). A developmental investigation of inattentiveness and hyperactivity. *Child Development, 66*, 37–54.

Chilcoat, H. D., & Breslau, N. (1999). Pathways from ADHD to early drug use. *Journal of the American Academy of Child and Adolescent Psychiatry, 38*, 1347–1354.

Claude, D., & Firestone, P. (1995). The development of ADHD boys: A 12-year follow-up. *Canadian Journal of Behavioural Science, 27*, 226–249.

Claycomb, C. D., Ryan, J. J., Miller, L. J., & Schnakenberg-Ott, S. D. (2004). Relationships among attention deficit hyperactivity disorder, induced labor, and selected physiological and demographic variables. *Journal of Clinical Psychology, 60*, 689–693.

Cohen, N. J., & Minde, K. (1981). The "hyperactive syndrome" in kindergarten children: Comparison of children with pervasive and situational symptoms. *Journal of Child Psychology and Psychiatry, 24*, 443–455.

Corbett, B., & Stanczak, D. E. (1999). Neuropsychological performance of adults evidencing attention-deficit hyperactivity disorder. *Archives of Clinical Neuropsychology, 14*, 373–387.

Danforth, J. S., Barkley, R. A., & Stokes, T. F. (1991). Observations of parent–child interactions with hyperactive children: Research and clinical implications. *Clinical Psychology Review, 11*, 703–727.

Deater-Deckard, K., Dodge K. A., Bates, J. E., & Petit, G. S. (1998). Multiple risk factors in the development of externalizing behavior problems: Group and individual differences. *Development and Psychopathology, 10*, 469–493.

Dowson, J. H., McClean, A., Bazanis, E., Toone, B., Young, S., Robbins, T. W., & Sahakian, B. (2003). Impaired spatial working memory in adults with attention-deficit/hyperactivity disorder: Comparisons with performance in adults with borderline personality disorder and in controls. *Acta Psychiatrica Scandinavica, 110*, 45–54.

DuPaul, G. J., Power, T. J., Anastopoulos, A. D., & Reid, R. (1998). *The ADHD Rating Scale–IV: Checklists, norms, and clinical interpretation*. New York: Guilford Press.

Earls, F., & Jung, K. G. (1987). Temperament and home environment characteristics as causal factors in the early development of childhood psychopathology. *Journal of the American Academy of Child and Adolescent Psychiatry, 26*, 491–498.

Edwards, F., Barkley, R., Laneri, M., Fletcher, K., & Metevia, L. (2001). Parent–adolescent conflicts and parent and teen psychological adjustment in teenagers with ADHD and ODD: The role of maternal depression. *Journal of Abnormal Child Psychology, 29*, 557–572.

Epstein, J. N., Conners, C. K., Erhardt, D., March, J. S., & Swanson, J. M. (1997). Asymmetrical hemispheric control of visual–spatial attention in adults with attention deficit hyperactivity disorder. *Neuropsychology, 11*, 467–473.

Eyestone, L. L., & Howell, R. J. (1994). An epidemiological study of attention-deficit hyperactivity disorders and major depression in a male prison population. *Bulletin of the American Academy of Psychiatry and Law, 22*, 181–193.

Fagot, B. (1984). The consequences of problem behavior in toddler children. *Journal of Abnormal Child Psychology, 12*, 385–396.

Faraone, S. V., Biederman, J., Mick, E., Williamson, S., Wilens, T., Spencer, T., et al. (2000). Family study of girls with attention deficit hyperactivity disorder. *American Journal of Psychiatry, 157*, 1077–1083.

Fergusson, D. M., Lynskey, M. T., & Horwood, L. J. (1996). Factors associated with continuity and changes in disruptive behavior patterns between childhood and adolescence. *Journal of Abnormal Child Psychology, 24*, 533–553.

Fergusson, D. M., Lynskey, M. T., & Horwood, L. J. (1997). Attention difficulties in middle childhood and psychosocial outcomes in young adulthood. *Journal of Child Psychology and Psychiatry, 38*, 633–644.

Fischer, M. (1990). Parenting stress and the child with attention deficit hyperactivity disorder. *Journal of Clinical Child Psychology, 19*, 337–346.

Fischer, M., Barkley, R. A., Edelbrock, C. S., & Smallish, L. (1990). The adolescent outcome of hyperactive children diagnosed by research criteria, II: Academic, attentional, and neuropsychological status. *Journal of Consulting and Clinical Psychology, 58*, 580–588.

Fischer, M., Barkley, R. A., Fletcher, K., & Smallish, L.

(1993a). The stability of dimensions of behavior in ADHD and normal children over an 8 year period. *Journal of Abnormal Child Psychology, 21,* 315–337.

Fischer, M., Barkley, R. A., Fletcher, K., & Smallish, L. (1993b). The adolescent outcome of hyperactive children diagnosed by research criteria: V. Predictors of outcome. *Journal of the American Academy of Child and Adolescent Psychiatry, 32,* 324–332.

Fischer, M., Barkley, R. A., Smallish, L., & Fletcher, K. (2002). Young adult follow-up of hyperactive children: Self-reported psychiatric disorders, comorbidity, and the role of childhood conduct problems. *Journal of Abnormal Child Psychology. 30,* 463–475.

Fischer, M., Barkley, R. A., Smallish, L., & Fletcher, K. (2005). Executive functioning in hyperactive children as young adults: Attention, inhibition, and response perseveration and the impact of comorbidity. *Developmental Neuropsychology, 27,* 107–133.

Fischer, M., Barkley, R. A., Smallish, L., & Fletcher, K. (in press). Hyperactive children as young adults: Driving ability, safe driving behavior, and adverse driving outcomes. *Accident Analysis and Prevention.*

Fischer, M., Rolf, J. E., Hasazi, J. E., & Cummings, L. (1984). Follow-up of a preschool epidemiological sample: Cross-age continuities and predictions of later adjustment with internalizing and externalizing dimensions of behavior. *Child Development, 55,* 1317–1350.

Flory, K., Lynam, D., Milich, R., Leukefeld, C., & Clayton, R. (2001, August). *Attention deficit hyperactivity disorder as a moderator of the relation between conduct disorder and drug abuse.* Poster presented at the annual meeting of the American Psychological Association, San Francisco.

Frazier, T. W., Demaree, H. A., & Youngstrom, E. A. (2004). Meta-analysis of intellectual and neuropsychological test performance in attention-deficit/hyperactivity disorder. *Neuropsychology, 18,* 543–555.

Friedman, S. R., Rapport, L. J., Lumley, M., Tzelepis, A., Van Voorhis, A., Stettner, L., et al. (2003). Aspects of social and emotional competence in adult attention-deficit/hyperactivity disorder. *Neuropsychology, 17,* 50–58.

Gansler, D. A., Fucetola, R., Krengel, M., Stetson, S., Zimering, R., & Makary, C. (1998). Are there cognitive subtypes in adult attention deficit/hyperactivity disorder? *Journal of Nervous and Mental Disease, 186,* 776–781.

Garrison, W., Earls, F., & Kindlon, D. (1984). Temperament characteristics in the third year of life and behavioral adjustment at school entry. *Journal of Clinical Child Psychology, 13,* 298–303.

Gittelman, R., Mannuzza, S., Shenker, R., & Bonagura, N. (1985). Hyperactive boys almost grown up: I. Psychiatric status. *Archives of General Psychiatry, 42,* 937–947.

Goldstein, S., & Ellison, A. T. (2002). *Clinicians' guide to adult ADHD: Assessment and intervention.* San Diego, CA: Academic Press.

Goodman, J. R., & Stevenson, J. (1989). A twin study of hyperactivity: II. The aetiological role of genes, family relationships, and perinatal adversity. *Journal of Child Psychology and Psychiatry, 30,* 691–709.

Gordon, M., & McClure, F. D. (1996). *The down and dirty guide to adult ADD.* DeWitt, NY: GSI.

Greene, R. W., Biederman, J., Faraone, S. V., Sienna, M., & Garcia-Jetton, J. (1997). Adolescent outcome of boys with attention-deficit/hyperactivity disorder and social disability: Results from a 4-year longitudinal follow-up study. *Journal of Consulting and Clinical Psychology, 65,* 758–767.

Hallowell, E. M., & Ratey, J. J. (1994). *Driven to distraction.* New York: Pantheon.

Halverson, C. F., & Waldrop, M. F. (1976). Relations between preschool activity and aspects of intellectual and social behavior at age 7.5 years. *Developmental Psychology, 12,* 107–112.

Hart, E. L., Lahey, B. B., Loeber, R., Applegate, B., & Frick, P. J. (1995). Developmental changes in attention-deficit hyperactivity disorder in boys: A four-year longitudinal study. *Journal of Abnormal Child Psychology, 23,* 729–750.

Hartsough, C. S., & Lambert, N. M. (1985). Medical factors in hyperactive and normal children: Prenatal, developmental, and health history findings. *American Journal of Orthopsychiatry, 55,* 190–210.

Henry, B., Moffitt, T. E., Caspi, A., Langley, J., & Silva, P. A. (1994). On the "remembrance of things past": A longitudinal evaluation of the retrospective method. *Psychological Assessment, 6,* 92–101.

Hervey, A. S., Epstein, J. N., & Curry, J. F. (2004). Neuropsychology of adults with attention-deficit/hyperactivity disorder: A meta-analytic review. *Neuropsychology, 18,* 495–503.

Hill, J. C., & Schoener, E. P. (1996). Age-dependent decline of attention deficit hyperactivity disorder. *American Journal of Psychiatry, 153,* 1143–1146.

Himelstein, J., & Halperin, J. M. (2000). Neurocognitive functioning in adults with attention-deficit/hyperactivity disorder. *CNS Spectrums, 5,* 58–64.

Hinshaw, S. P. (1987). On the distinction between attentional deficits/hyperactivity and conduct problems/aggression in child psychopathology. *Psychological Bulletin, 101,* 443–447.

Holdnack, J. A., Moberg, P. J., Arnold, S. E., Gur, R. C., & Gur, R. E. (1995). Speed of processing and verbal learning deficits in adults diagnosed with attention deficit disorder. *Neuropsychiatry, Neuropsychology, and Behavioral Neurology, 8,* 282–292.

Hopkins, J., Perlman, T., Hechtman, L., & Weiss, G. (1979). Cognitive style in adults originally diagnosed as hyperactives. *Journal of Child Psychology and Psychiatry, 20,* 209–216.

Hoy, E., Weiss, G., Minde, K., & Cohen, N. (1978). The hyperactive child at adolescence: Cognitive, emotional, and social functioning. *Journal of Abnormal Child Psychology, 6*, 311–324.

Jacobvitz, D., & Sroufe, L. A. (1987). The early caregiver–child relationship and attention-deficit disorder with hyperactivity in kindergarten: A prospective study. *Child Development, 58*, 1488–1495.

Jaffee, S., Caspi, A., Moffitt, T., Taylor, A., & Dickson, N. (2001). Predicting early fatherhood and whether young fathers live with their children: Prospective findings and policy reconsiderations. *Journal of Child Psychology and Psychiatry, 42*, 803–815.

Jenkins, M., Cohen, R., Malloy, P., Salloway, S., Johnson, E. G., Penn, J., et al. (1998). Neuropsychological measures which discriminate among adults with residual symptoms of attention deficit disorder and other attentional complaints. *The Clinical Neuropsychologist, 12*, 74–83.

Johnson, D. E., Epstein, J. N., Waid, L. R., Latham, P. K., Voronin, K. E., & Anton, R. F. (2001). Neuropsychological performance deficits in adults with attention deficit/hyperactivity disorder. *Archives of Clinical Neuropsychology, 16*, 587–604.

Johnston, C., & Mash, E. J. (2001). Families of children with attention-deficit/hyperactivity disorder: Review and recommendations for future research. *Clinical Child and Family Psychology Review, 4*, 183–207.

Kaplow, J. B., Curran, P. J., Dodge, K. A., & the Conduct Problems Prevention Research Group. (2002). Child, parent, and peer predictors of early onset substance use: A multisite longitudinal study. *Journal of Abnormal Child Psychology, 30*, 199–216.

Keenan, K., Shaw, D., Delliquadri, E., Giovannelli, J., & Walsh, B. (1998). Evidence for the continuity of early problem behaviors: Application of a developmental model. *Journal of Abnormal Child Psychology, 26*, 441–454.

Kelly, K., & Ramundo, P. (1992). *You mean I'm not lazy, stupid, or crazy?* Cincinnati, OH: Tyrell & Jerem.

Klein, R. G., & Mannuzza, S. (1991). Long-term outcome of hyperactive children: A review. *Journal of the American Academy of Child and Adolescent Psychiatry, 30*, 383–387.

Kovner, R., Budman, C., Frank, Y., Sison, C., Lesser, M., & Halperin, J. M. (1997). *Neuropsychological testing in adult attention deficit hyperactivity disorder: A pilot study.* Unpublished manuscript, North Shore University Hospital, Manhasset, NY.

Krause, K. H., Dresel, S. H., Krause, J., Kung, H. F., Tatsch, K., & Ackenheil, M. (2002). Stimulant-like action of nicotine on striatal dopamine transporter in the brain of adults with attention deficit hyperactivity disorder. *International Journal of Neuropsychopharmacology, 5*, 111–113.

Kuperman, S., Schlosser, S. S., Kramer, J. R., Bucholz, K., Hesselbrock, V., Reich, T., et al. (2001). Developmental sequence from disruptive behavior diagnosis to adolescent alcohol dependence. *American Journal of Psychiatry, 158*, 2022–2026.

Lambert, N. M. (1988). Adolescent outcomes for hyperactive children. *American Psychologist, 43*, 786–799.

Lambert, N. M., & Hartsough, C. S. (1998). Prospective study of tobacco smoking and substance dependencies among samples of ADHD and non-ADHD participants. *Journal of Learning Disabilities, 31*, 533–544.

Lambert, N. M., Hartsough, C. S., Sassone, S., & Sandoval, J. (1987). Persistence of hyperactive symptoms from childhood to adolescence and associated outcomes. *American Journal of Orthopsychiatry, 57*, 22–32.

Lerner, J. A., Inui, T. S., Trupin, E. W., & Douglas, E. (1985). Preschool behavior can predict future psychiatric disorders. *Journal of the American Academy of Child Psychiatry, 24*, 42–48.

Linnet, K. M., Dalsgaard, S., Obel, C., Wisborg, K., Henriksen, T. B., Rodriguez, A., et al. (2003). Maternal lifestyle factors in pregnancy risk of attention deficit hyperactivity disorder and associated behaviors: Review of the current literature. *American Journal of Psychiatry, 160*, 1028–1040.

Loeber, R., Burke, J. D., Lahey, B. B., Winters, A., & Zera, M. (2000). Oppositional defiant and conduct disorder: A review of the past 10 years, Part I. *Journal of the American Academy of Child and Adolescent Psychiatry, 39*, 1468–1484.

Loney, J., Kramer, J., & Milich, R. (1981). The hyperkinetic child grows up: Predictors of symptoms, delinquency, and achievement at follow-up. In K. Gadow & J. Loney (Eds.), *Psychosocial aspects of drug treatment for hyperactivity.* Boulder, CO: Westview Press.

Lovejoy, D. W., Ball, J. D., Keats, M., Stutts, M. L., Spain, E. H., Janda, L., et al. (1999). Neuropsychological performance of adults with attention deficit hyperactivity disorder (ADHD): Diagnostic classification estimates for measures of frontal lobe/executive functioning. *Journal of the International Neuropsychological Society, 5*, 222–233.

Lynskey, M. T., & Fergusson, D. M. (1995). Childhood conduct problems, attention deficit behaviors, and adolescent alcohol, tobacco, and illicit drug use. *Journal of Abnormal Child Psychology, 23*, 281–302.

Mannuzza, S., & Gittelman, R. (1986). Informant variance in the diagnostic assessment of hyperactive children as young adults. In J. E. Barrett & R. M. Rose (Eds.), *Mental disorders in the community* (pp. 243–254). New York: Guilford Press.

Mannuzza, S., Gittelman, R., Konig, P. H., & Giampino, T. L. (1989). Hyperactive boys almost grown up: VI. Criminality and its relationship to psychiatric status. *Archives of General Psychiatry, 46*, 1073–1079.

Mannuzza, S., Gittelman-Klein, R., Bessler, A., Malloy, P., & LaPadula, M. (1993). Adult outcome of hyperactive boys: Educational achievement, occupational rank, and psychiatric status. *Archives of General Psychiatry, 50*, 565–576.

Mannuzza, S., Klein, R. G., & Addalli, K. A. (1991). Young adult mental status of hyperactive boys and their brothers: A prospective follow-up study. *Journal of the American Academy of Child and Adolescent Psychiatry, 30,* 743–751.

Mannuzza, S., Klein, R., Bessler, A., Malloy, P., & LaPadula, M. (1998). Adult psychiatric status of hyperactive boys grown up. *American Journal of Psychiatry, 155,* 493–498.

Mannuzza, S., Klein, R. G., Bonagura, N., Malloy, P., Giampino, H., & Addalli, K. A. (1991). Hyperactive boys almost grown up: Replication of psychiatric status. *Archives of General Psychiatry, 48,* 77–83.

Mariani, M., & Barkley, R. A. (1997). Neuropsychological and academic functioning in preschool children with attention deficit hyperactivity disorder. *Developmental Neuropsychology, 13,* 111–129.

Mash, E. J., & Johnston, C. (1982). A comparison of mother–child interactions of younger and older hyperactive and normal children. *Child Development, 53,* 1371–1381.

Mash, E. J., & Johnston, C. (1983). Sibling interactions of hyperactive and normal children and their relationship to reports of maternal stress and self-esteem. *Journal of Clinical Child Psychology, 12,* 91–99.

Matochik, J. A., Rumsey, J. M., Zametkin, A. J., Hamburger, S. D., & Cohen, R. M. (1996). Neuropsychological correlates of familial attention-deficit hyperactivity disorder in adults. *Neuropsychiatry, Neuropsychology, and Behavioral Neurology, 9,* 186–191.

McClean, A., Dowson, J., Toone, B., Young, S., Bazanis, E., Robbins, T. W., et al. (2004). Characteristic neurocognitive profile associated with adult attention-deficit/hyperactivity disorder. *Psychological Medicine, 34,* 681–692.

McInerny, T., & Chamberlin, R. W. (1978). Is it feasible to identify infants who are at risk for later behavioral problems?: The Carey Temperament Questionnaire as a prognostic tool. *Clinical Pediatrics, 17,* 233–238.

Mendelson, W., Johnson, N., & Stewart, M. A. (1971). Hyperactive children as teenagers: A follow-up study. *Journal of Nervous and Mental Disease, 153,* 273–279.

Mick, E., Faraone, S. V., & Biederman, J. (2004). Age-dependent expression of attention-deficit/hyperactivity disorder symptoms. *Psychiatric Clinics of North America, 27*(2), 215–224.

Milberger, S., Biederman, J., Faraone, S. V., Chen, L., & Jones, J. (1997). ADHD is associated with early initiation of cigarette smoking in children and adolescents. *Journal of the American Academy of Child and Adolescent Psychiatry, 36,* 37–44.

Milberger, S., Biederman, J., Faraone, S. V., Guite, J., & Tsuang, M. T. (1997). Pregnancy, delivery, and infancy complications and attention deficit disorder: Issues of gene–environment interaction. *Biological Psychiatry, 41,* 65–75.

Minde, K., Eakin, L., Hechtman, L., Ochs, L., Bouffard, R., Greenfield, B., et al. (2003). The psychosocial functioning of children and spouses of adults with ADHD. *Journal of Child Psychology and Psychiatry, 44,* 637–646.

Minde, K., Lewin, D., Weiss, G., Lavigueur, H., Douglas, V., & Sykes, E. (1971). The hyperactive child in elementary school: A 5-year, controlled follow-up. *Exceptional Children, 38,* 215–221.

Mirsky, A. F. (1996). Disorders of attention: A neuropsychological perspective. In R. G. Lyon & N. A. Krasnegor (Eds.), *Attention, memory, and executive function* (pp. 71–96). Baltimore: Brookes.

Molina, B. S. G., Smith, B. H., & Pelham, W. E. (1999). Interactive effects of attention deficit hyperactivity disorder and conduct disorder on early adolescent substance use. *Psychology of Addictive Behaviors, 13,* 348–358.

Morrison, J., & Stewart, M. (1973). The psychiatric status of the legal families of adopted hyperactive children. *Archives of General Psychiatry, 28,* 888–891.

Munir, K., Biederman, J., & Knee, D. (1987). Psychiatric comorbidity in patients with attention deficit disorder: A controlled study. *Journal of the American Academy of Child and Adolescent Psychiatry, 26,* 844–848.

Murphy, K., & Barkley, R. A. (1996a). Attention deficit hyperactivity disorder in adults. *Comprehensive Psychiatry, 37,* 393–401.

Murphy, K., & Barkley, R. A. (1996b). Prevalence of DSM-IV symptoms of ADHD in adult licensed drivers: Implications for clinical diagnosis. *Journal of Attention Disorders, 1,* 147–161.

Murphy, K. R., Barkley, R. A., & Bush, T. (2001). Executive functions in young adults with attention deficit hyperactivity disorder, *Neuropsychology, 15,* 211–220.

Murphy, K. R., Barkley, R. A., & Bush, T. (2002). Young adults with ADHD: Subtype differences in comorbidity, educational, and clinical history. *Journal of Nervous and Mental Disease, 190,* 147–157.

Murphy, K. R., & LeVert, S. (1994). *Out of the fog.* New York: Hyperion.

Nadeau, K. G. (Ed.). (1995). *A comprehensive guide to attention deficit disorder in adults: Research, diagnosis, and treatment.* New York: Brunner/Mazel.

Nichols, P. L., & Chen, T. C. (1981). *Minimal brain dysfunction: A prospective study.* Hillsdale, NJ: Erlbaum.

Nigg, J. T., Butler, K. M., Huang-Pollock, C. L., & Henderson, J. M. (2002). Inhibitory processes in adults with persistent childhood onset ADHD. *Journal of Consulting and Clinical Psychology, 70,* 153–157.

Nigg, J. T., Goldsmith, H. H., & Sacheck, J. (2004). Temperament and attention deficit hyperactivity disorder: The development of a multiple pathway model. *Journal of Clinical Child and Adolescent Psychology, 33,* 42–53.

Nigg, J. T., Stavro, G., Ettenhofer, M., Hambrick, D., Miller, T., & Henderson, J. M. (in press). Executive functions and ADHD in adults: Evidence for selective effects on ADHD symptom domains. *Journal of Abnormal Psychology.*

O'Donnell, J. P., McCann, K. K., & Pluth, S. (2001). Assessing adult ADHD using a self-report symptom checklist. *Psychological Reports, 88,* 871–881.

Ossman, J. M., & Mulligan, N. W. (2003). Inhibition and attention deficit hyperactivity disorder in adults. *American Journal of Psychology, 116,* 35–50.

Palfrey, J. S., Levine, M. D., Walker, D. K., & Sullivan, M. (1985). The emergence of attention deficits in early childhood: A prospective study. *Journal of Developmental and Behavioral Pediatrics, 6,* 339–348.

Pagani, L., Tremblay, R., Vitaro, F., Boulerice, B., & McDuff, P. (2001). Effects of grade retention on academic performance and behavioral development. *Development and Psychopathology, 13,* 297–315.

Paternite, C., & Loney, J. (1980). Childhood hyperkinesis: Relationships between symptomatology and home environment. In C. K. Whalen & B. Henker (Eds.), *Hyperactive children: The social ecology of identification and treatment* (pp. 105–141). New York: Academic Press.

Prior, M., Leonard, A., & Wood, G. (1983). A comparison study of preschool children diagnosed as hyperactive. *Journal of Pediatric Psychology, 8,* 191–207.

Rapport, L. J., Friedman, S. L., Tzelepis, A., & Van Voorhis, A. (2002). Experienced emotion and affect recognition in adult attention-deficit hyperactivity disorder. *Neuropsychology, 16,* 102–110.

Rapport, L. J., Van Voorhis, A., Tzelepis, A., & Friedman, S. R. (2001). Executive functioning in adult attention-deficit hyperactivity disorder. *The Clinical Neuropsychologist, 15,* 479–491.

Rasmussen, K., Almvik, R., & Levander, S. (2001). Attention deficit hyperactivity disorder, reading disability, and personality disorders in a prison population. *Journal of the American Academy of Psychiatry and the Law, 29,* 186–193.

Rasmussen, P., & Gillberg, C. (2001). Natural outcome of ADHD with developmental coordination disorder at age 22 years: A controlled, longitudinal, community-based study. *Journal of the American Academy of Child and Adolescent Psychiatry, 39,* 1424–1431.

Ridenour, T. A., Cottler, L. B., Robins, L. N., Compton, W. M., Spitznagel, E. L., & Cunningham-Williams, R. M. (2002). Test of the plausibility of adolescent substance use playing a causal role in developing adulthood antisocial behavior. *Journal of Abnormal Psychology, 111,* 144–155.

Ross, D. M., & Ross, S. A. (1976). *Hyperactivity: Research, theory, and action.* New York: Wiley.

Roy-Byrne, P., Scheele, L., Brinkley, J., Ward, N., Wiatrak, C., Russo, J., et al. (1997). Adult attention-deficit hyperactivity disorder: Assessment guidelines based on clinical presentation to a specialty clinic. *Comprehensive Psychiatry, 38,* 133–140.

Rucklidge, J. J., & Kaplan, B. J. (1997). Psychological functioning of women identified in adulthood with attention-deficit/hyperactivity disorder. *Journal of Attention Disorders, 2,* 167–176.

Samuel, V. J., George, P., Thornell, A., Curtis, S., Taylor, A., Brome, D., et al. (1999). A pilot controlled family study of DSM-III-R and DSM-IV ADHD in African-American children. *Journal of the American Academy of Child and Adolescent Psychiatry, 38,* 34–39.

Satterfield, J. H., & Schell, A. (1997). A prospective study of hyperactive boys with conduct problems and normal boys: Adolescent and adult criminality. *Journal of the American Academy of Child and Adolescent Psychiatry, 36,* 1726–1735.

Satterfield, J. H., Swanson, J. M., Schell, A., & Lee, F. (1994). Prediction of antisocial behavior in attention-deficit hyperactivity disorder boys from aggression/defiance scores. *Journal of the American Academy of Child and Adolescent Psychiatry, 33,* 185–190.

Schleifer, M., Weiss, G., Cohen, N. J., Elman, M., Cvejic, H., & Kruger, E. (1975). Hyperactivity in preschoolers and the effect of methylphenidate. *American Journal of Orthopsychiatry, 45,* 38–50.

Schmidt, M. H., & Moll, G. H. (1995). The course of hyperkinetic disorders and symptoms: A ten-year prospective longitudinal field study. In J. Sergeant (Ed.), *Eunethydis: European approaches to hyperkinetic disorder* (pp. 191–207). Amsterdam: University of Amsterdam.

Seidman, L. J. (1997, October). *Neuropsychological findings in ADHD children: Findings from a sample of high-risk siblings.* Paper presented at the annual meeting of the American Academy of Child and Adolescent Psychiatry, Toronto.

Semrud-Clikeman, M., Biederman, J., Sprich-Buckminster, S., Lehman, B. K., Faraone, S. V., & Norman, D. (1992). Comorbidity between ADDH and learning disability: A review and report in a clinically referred sample. *Journal of the American Academy of Child and Adolescent Psychiatry, 31,* 439–448.

Shaw, D. S., Winslow, E. B., Owens, E. B., Vondra, J. I., Cohen, J. E., & Bell, R. Q. (1998). The development of early externalizing problems among children from low-income families: A transformational perspective. *Journal of Abnormal Child Psychology, 26,* 95–107.

Shaw, G. A., & Giambra, L. (1993). Task-unrelated thoughts of college students diagnosed as hyperactive in childhood. *Developmental Neuropsychology, 9,* 17–30.

Shekim, W., Asarnow, R. F., Hess, E., Zaucha, K., & Wheeler, N. (1990). An evaluation of attention deficit disorder—residual type. *Comprehensive Psychiatry, 31(5),* 416–425.

Shelton, T. L., Barkley, R. A., Crosswait, C., Moorehouse, M., Fletcher, K., Barrett, S., et al. (1998). Psychiatric and psychological morbidity as a function of adaptive disability in preschool children with aggressive and hyperactive–impulsive–inattentive behavior. *Journal of Abnormal Child Psychology, 26,* 475–494.

Solden, S. (1995). *Women with attention deficit disorder*. Grass Valley, CA: Underwood.

Span, S. A., Earleywine, M., & Strybel, T. Z. (2002). Confirming the factor structure of attention deficit hyperactivity disorder symptoms in adult, nonclinical samples. *Journal of Psychopathology and Behavioral Assessment, 24*, 129–136.

Spencer, T. (1997, October). *Chronic tics in adults with ADHD*. Paper presented at the annual meeting of the American Academy of Child and Adolescent Psychiatry, Toronto.

Spencer, T. (Ed.). (2004). Adult attention-deficit/hyperactivity disorder [Special issue]. *Psychiatric Clinics of North America, 27*(2).

Spitzer, R. L., Davies, M, & Barkley, R. A. (1990). The DSM-III-R field trial of disruptive behavior disorders. *Journal of the American Academy of Child and Adolescent Psychiatry, 2*, 690–697.

Stewart, M. A., Mendelson, W. B., & Johnson, N. E. (1973). Hyperactive children as adolescents: How they describe themselves. *Child Psychiatry and Human Development, 4*, 3–11.

Swensen, A. R., Secnik, K., Buesching, D. P., Barkley, R. A., Fischer, M., & Fletcher, K. E. (2004). *Young adult outcome of hyperactive/ADHD children: Cost of criminal behavior*. Unpublished manuscript, Eli Lilly Co., Indianapolis, IN.

Tapert, S. F., Baratta, M. V., Abrantes, A. M., & Brown, S. A. (2002). Attention dysfunction predicts substance involvement in community youths. *Journal of the American Academy of Child and Adolescent Psychiatry, 41*, 680–686.

Tapert, S. F., Granholm, E., Leedy, N. G., & Brown, S. A. (2002). Substance use and withdrawal: Neuropsychological functioning over 8 years in youth. *Journal of the International Neuropyschological Society, 8*, 873–883.

Taylor, E., Chadwick, O., Hepinstall, E., & Danckaerts, M. (1996). Hyperactivity and conduct problems as risk factors for adolescent development. *Journal of the American Academy of Child and Adolescent Psychiatry, 35*, 1213–1226.

Tercyak, K. P., Lerman, C., & Audrain, J. (2002). Association of attention-deficit/hyperactivity disorder symptoms with levels of cigarette smoking in a community sample of adolescents. *Journal of the American Academy of Child and Adolescent Psychiatry, 41*, 799–805.

Tercyak, K. P., Peshkin, B. N., Walker, L. R., & Stein, M. A. (2002). Cigarette smoking among youth with attention-deficit/hyperactivity disorder: Clinical phenomenology, comorbidity, and genetics. *Journal of Clinical Psychology in Medical Settings, 9*, 35–50.

Thorley, G. (1984). Review of follow-up and followback studies of childhood hyperactivity. *Psychological Bulletin, 96*, 116–132.

Tzelepis, A., Schubiner, H., & Warbasse, L. H., III. (1995). Differential diagnosis and psychiatric comorbidity patterns in adult attention deficit disorder. In K. Nadeau (Ed.), *A comprehensive guide to attention deficit disorder in adults: Research, diagnosis, and treatment* (pp. 35–57). New York: Brunner/Mazel.

Wakefield, J. C. (1999). Evolutionary versus prototype analyses of the concept of disorder. *Journal of Abnormal Psychology, 108*, 374–399.

Weiss, G., & Hechtman, L. (1993). *Hyperactive children grown up* (2nd ed.). New York: Guilford Press.

Weiss, G., Hechtman, L., Milroy, T., & Perlman, T. (1985). Psychiatric status of hyperactives as adults: A controlled prospective 15-year follow-up of 63 hyperactive children. *Journal of the American Academy of Child Psychiatry, 23*, 211–220.

Weiss, G., Minde, K., Werry, J., Douglas, V., & Nemeth, E. (1971). Studies on the hyperactive child: VIII. Five year follow-up. *Archives of General Psychiatry, 24*, 409–414.

Weiss, L. (1992). *ADD in adults*. Dallas, TX: Taylor.

Weiss, M., Hechtman, L. T., & Weiss, G. (1999). *ADHD in adulthood: A guide to current theory, diagnosis, and treatment*. Baltimore: Johns Hopkins University Press.

Weithorn, C. J., & Kagan, E. (1978). Interaction of language development and activity level on performance of first graders. *American Journal of Orthopsychiatry, 48*, 148–159.

Welner, Z., Welner, A., Stewart, M., Palkes, H., & Wish, E. (1977). A controlled study of siblings of hyperactive children. *Journal of Nervous and Mental Disease, 165*, 110–117.

Wender, P. (1995). *Attention-deficit hyperactivity disorder in adults*. New York: Oxford University Press.

Wenwei, Y. (1996). An investigation of adult outcome of hyperactive children in Shanghai. *Chinese Medical Journal, 109*, 877–880.

Weyandt, L. L., Mitzlaff, L., & Thomas, L. (2002). The relationship between intelligence and performance on the Test of Variables of Attention (TOVA). *Journal of Learning Disabilities, 35*, 114–120.

Weyandt, L. L., Rice, J. A., Linterman, I., Mitzlaff, L., & Emert, E. (1998). Neuropsychological performance of a sample of adults with ADHD, developmental reading disorder, and controls. *Developmental Neuropsychology, 16*, 643–656.

Whalen, C. K., Jamner, L. D., Henker, B., Delfino, R. J., & Lozano, J. M. (2002). The ADHD spectrum and everyday life: Experience sampling of adolescent moods, activities, smoking, and drinking. *Child Development, 73*, 209–227.

White, H. R., Xie, M., Thompson, W., Loeber, R., & Stouthamer-Loeber, M. (2001). Psychopathology as a predictor of adolescent drug use trajectories. *Psychology of Addictive Behaviors, 15*, 210–218.

Whittaker, A. H., Van Rossem, R., Feldman, J. F., Schonfeld, I. S., Pinto-Martin, J. A., Torre, C., et al. (1997). Psychiatric outcomes in low-birth-weight children at age 6 years: Relation to neonatal cranial ultrasound abnormalities. *Archives of General Psychiatry, 54*, 847–856.

Wilens, T. E. (2004). Attention-deficit/hyperactivity disorder and the substance use disorders: The nature of the relationship, subtypes at risk, and treatment issues. *Psychiatric Clinics of North America, 27*(2), 283–302.

Wilens, T. E., Faraone, S. V., & Biederman, J. (2004). Attention-deficit/hyperactivity disorder in adults. *Journal of the American Medical Association, 292,* 619–623.

Wilens, T. E., Faraone, S. V., Biederman, J., & Gunawardene, S. (2003). Does stimulant therapy of attention deficit/hyperactivity disorder beget later substance abuse?: A meta-analytic review of the literature. *Pediatrics, 11,* 179–185.

Wilson, J. M., & Marcotte, A. C. (1996). Psychosocial adjustment and educational outcome in adolescents with a childhood diagnosis of attention deficit disorder. *Journal of the American Academy of Child and Adolescent Psychiatry, 35,* 579–587.

Woodward, L. J., Fergusson, D. M., & Horwood, L. J. (2002). Romantic relationships of young people with childhood and adolescent onset antisocial behavior problems. *Journal of Abnormal Child Psychology, 30,* 231–243.

Zambelli, A. J., Stam, J. S., Maintinsky, S., & Loiselle, D. L. (1977). Auditory evoked potential and selective attention in formerly hyperactive boys. *American Journal of Psychiatry, 134,* 742–747.

CHAPTER 7

A Theory of ADHD

RUSSELL A. BARKLEY

It is the intent of this chapter to provide an update to the theory of Attention-Deficit/Hyperactivity Disorder (ADHD) presented in the preceding edition of this text. This theory is based on a model of the development of self-regulation that should help explain many of the myriad cognitive deficits associated with the disorder (see Chapter 3, this volume). The scientific basis for this hybrid model of self-regulation and of the executive functions that provide for self-regulation has been presented in detail elsewhere (Barkley, 1997a, 1997b, 2001), along with the scientific evidence for the model's applicability to ADHD. Those bodies of evidence are not repeated here. Suffice it to say that a growing body of evidence supports much, though by no means all, of this model and its appropriateness for understanding ADHD. The fact that not all of the model is currently supported by data matters relatively little. Theories of ADHD are time-limited tools that for the moment strive to offer a richer conceptualization of the nature of the disorder, by providing a number of new, untested hypotheses about the nature of additional cognitive deficits likely to be seen in ADHD that have received little or no previous research attention. Theories, moreover, should not only be insightful, innovative, and testable (falsifiable), but should also serve to guide efforts at designing interventions. It is fair to say that the theory set forth here achieves these goals better than any existing or previous theory of this disorder, in my immodest opinion, although it is far from perfect. Again, no theory ever is so. One does not ask for perfection in a theory, particularly in its debut, but utility in advancing the field of inquiry. And this theory has certainly been one major impetus (though by no means the only one) to the explosion of neuropsychological research on ADHD since the preceding edition. This body of research has more than doubled in size in that period of time, and many of the new studies are efforts to test some of this theory's predicted conditional relationships among the various components of executive functioning and how they may be affected by ADHD.

THE NEED FOR A BETTER THEORY OF ADHD

As I have stated elsewhere (Barkley, 1997a, 1997b), a new paradigm for understanding the nature of ADHD is needed for a number of reasons. To begin with, research on ADHD up through the mid-1990s was nearly atheoretical, at least regarding the basic nature of the disorder. Much of the research into that nature had been mainly exploratory and descriptive, with four exceptions. One exception was Herbert Quay's use of Jeffrey Gray's neuropsychological model of anxiety to explain the origin of the poor inhibition seen in ADHD (Quay, 1988a, 1988b, 1997). The Quay–Gray model, described in Chapter 1 of this volume, states that the impulsivity characterizing ADHD arises from diminished activity in the brain's behavioral inhibition system (BIS). That system is said to be sensitive to signals of conditioned punishment that, when detected, result in increased activity in the BIS and a resulting inhibitory effect on behavior. This theory predicts that those with ADHD should prove less sensitive to such signals, particularly in passive avoidance paradigms (Quay, 1988a; Milich, Hartung, Martin, & Haigler, 1994). For a more recent discussion of the use of this model for ADHD and Conduct Disorder (CD), and the mixed results of research into it, see the article by Beauchaine, Katkin, Strassberg, and Snarr (2001). With the exception of predictions about the response of children with ADHD to various contingencies of reward and punishment, this model provides no explanation for the emerging evidence for executive deficits associated with ADHD.

The second exception to the mainly descriptive nature of research into the essence of ADHD has been the work of Sergeant and van der Meere (1988; Sergeant, 1995a, 1995b, 1996; van der Meere, van Baal, & Sergeant, 1989) on their cognitive energetic model of ADHD. These researchers have been successfully employing information-processing theory and its associated energetic model (arousal, activation, and effort) in the isolation of the central deficits in ADHD as they might be delineated within that paradigm (Sergeant, 1995b). But this approach actually does not set forth a theory of ADHD; it mainly predicts that the inattention and impulsivity involved in the disorder arise from relatively low levels of arousal and a capacity to activate cognitive energetic resources toward tasks. Like Quay's model, this one also makes no attempt to broaden its explanatory power to include executive functioning and self-regulation.

The third exception is the work of Schachar, Tannock, and Logan (1993) on the inhibitory deficits associated with ADHD. This approach draws on the "race" model of Logan, in which environmental stimuli are seen as initiating signals for both activation and inhibition of responding. These signals race against each other

to determine whether behavior toward the stimulus event will be initiated or inhibited. The first signal to reach the motor control system, in essence, wins the race and determines the nature of the eventual response (approach/responding or withdrawal/inhibition of responding). Using the stop signal paradigm discussed in Chapter 2 (this volume), these investigators and others (Oosterlaan & Sergeant, 1995, 1996; Luman, Oosterlaan, & Sergeant, 2005), showed that the principal deficits in ADHD appear to be both a slower initiation of response inhibition and an inability to disengage or shift responding when signaled to do so within this task. Once more, no discussion of other cognitive deficits (e.g., verbal fluency, time reproduction, delayed internalized language, planning, etc.) now known to be associated with ADHD, or of how they may arise out of the disorder, has been ventured.

Finally, there is the hypothesis of Edward Sonuga-Barke (Sonuga-Barke, 2002; Sonuga-Barke, Taylor, & Hepinstall, 1992), who essentially claims that the impulsivity seen in ADHD arises from the disorder's producing an aversion to delay or waiting, so that children with ADHD act to terminate delay intervals more quickly than do nondisabled children. Research on this hypothesis has produced some interesting yet mixed results (Luman et al., 2005). Again, however, the larger sphere of executive deficits is not addressed in this hypothesis.

Like the Quay–Gray hypothesis of ADHD, these research paradigms have generally reached the conclusion that ADHD involves a central deficiency in response inhibition or delay aversion (albeit qualified by some additional deficits, depending on the paradigm). As noted in Chapter 2, I and others (Nigg, 2001) have also reached the same conclusion, based on the substantial body of research supporting it. All these research programs are concerned with the origin of this inhibitory deficit within their respective paradigms. They are to some extent complementary rather than contradictory approaches to understanding ADHD. Sergeant and van der Meere go further than Quay, Schachar et al. or Sonuga-Barke in also concluding that the inhibitory deficit in ADHD is associated with additional deficiencies in motor presetting (response selection) and in effort or arousal. But all these researchers make no effort at large-scale theory construction to provide a unifying account of the various cognitive deficits associated with ADHD. I began my theory construction where these other paradigms have left off: with the premise that ADHD does indeed represent a developmental delay in processes related to response inhibition. I then went on to show how behavioral inhibition is essential to the internalization or privatization of public behavior and the effective execution of four executive functions (privatized acts of self-regulation) that control the motor system in the initiation and performance of goal-directed, future-oriented behavior (Barkley, 1997b). The theory is not concerned so much with the origin of the inhibitory deficits in ADHD—whether they arise from a deficient energetic pool of arousal, from diminished sensitivity to signals of punishment, from a delay aversion, or from a lop-sided race between excitatory and inhibitory stimuli to control a motor response. Instead, this theory goes on to explain that, regardless of its origin, a deficit in the inhibition of behavior will produce an adverse impact on executive functioning, self-regulation, and the cross-temporal organization of behavior toward the future.

This theory provides a needed definition of self-regulation, articulates the cognitive components (executive functions) that contribute to it, specifies the primacy of behavioral inhibition within the theory and the evidence for such a conclusion, and sets forth a motor control component that is poorly regulated by the executive system in ADHD. Most important, the model generates many more new, testable predictions about additional cognitive and behavioral deficits in ADHD deserving of further study than do these other paradigms of ADHD. The present paradigm, then, does not contradict these earlier attempts at a theory of the nature of ADHD; instead, it complements them, builds on them, and broadens our understanding of ADHD to include the concepts of self-control and executive functioning.

A second reason why a theory of ADHD is sorely needed is that the current clinical view of ADHD (i.e., that of the Diagnostic and Statistical Manual of Mental Disorders [DSM-IV]; American Psychiatric Association 1994, 2000) is purely descriptive, detailing as it does two broad categories of behavioral deficits (inattention and hyperactivity–impulsivity) that are believed to constitute the disorder. This descriptive approach to ADHD, helpful as it has been for the purpose of clinical diagnosis, cannot readily account for the many other cognitive

and behavioral deficits that have emerged in studies of ADHD (see Chapter 3).

In particular, a theory must explain the nature of the inattention that plagues those with this disorder, given that attention is a multidimensional construct (Mirsky, 1996). It must also explain the link that exists between poor behavioral inhibition (hyperactivity–impulsivity) and the sister impairment of inattention, or whatever this latter symptom turns out to be. These two dimensions are correlated to a moderate but significant degree ($r = .49-.56$; Achenbach & Edelbrock, 1983; Hudziak, 1997). What does this dimension labeled "inattention" represent if not a deficit in attention? Why is it associated to only a moderate degree with problems of behavioral inhibition in this disorder? Why do the apparent problems with "inattention" seem to arise later in the development of this disorder than do the problems with hyperactive–impulsive behavior, as noted in Chapter 2 of this text? Again, the current clinical consensus view of ADHD makes no attempt to address such questions.

Any credible theory of ADHD also must link these two dimensions of hyperactive–impulsive behavior and inattention with the concept of executive or metacognitive functions, because most if not all of the additional cognitive deficits associated with ADHD (noted in Chapter 3) seem to fall within the realm of self-regulation or executive functions (Barkley, 1995, 1997a, 1997b; Denckla, 1994, 1996; Douglas, 1983, 1988; Douglas, Barr, Desilets, & Sherman, 1995; Grodzinsky & Diamond, 1992; Pennington & Ozonoff, 1996; Seidman et al., 1995; Torgesen, 1994; Welsh, Pennington, & Grossier, 1991; Weyandt & Willis, 1994). Why and how are the hyperactive–impulsive and inattentive symptoms of ADHD linked to problems with executive functions and self-control? What are those executive functions, exactly? Once more, the present clinical view of ADHD as mainly an attention deficit fails miserably in answering such important questions in psychological research on the disorder.

For a theory of ADHD to be persuasive, moreover, it must ultimately bridge the literature on ADHD with the larger literatures of developmental psychology and developmental neuropsychology as they pertain to self-regulation and the executive functions. In most instances, past studies of ADHD have not been based on studies of typical developmental processes, nor have efforts been made to interpret their findings in the light of extant findings in the developmental-psychological literature. Likewise, researchers in developmental psychology and developmental neuropsychology have typically failed to draw on the findings accruing in their respective literatures on self-regulation and executive functions, respectively, to enlighten each other's understanding of these processes (as Welsh & Pennington, 1988, previously noted). And rarely have researchers in these two disciplines drawn on the substantial scientific knowledge accumulated on ADHD to illuminate the study of these typical processes. But if it is to be argued that ADHD arises from a deviation from or a disruption in typical developmental processes, then these typical processes must be specified in explaining ADHD. And bridges must be built from the findings on ADHD to the findings on these typical processes. The current view of ADHD makes no such attempt to link the understanding of the disorder with an understanding of typical child development in the areas of behavioral inhibition, self-control, and executive functions. The present theory does so (see Barkley, 1997b).

Furthermore, any theory of ADHD must prove to be useful as a scientific tool. Not only must it better explain what is already known about ADHD, but it must make explicit predictions about new phenomena that were not previously considered in the literature on ADHD, or that may have received only cursory research attention. New theories often predict new constructs and relationships among constructs or elements that existing theories or descriptions did not predict. Those new predictions can serve as hypotheses that drive research initiatives. And such hypothesis testing can also provide a means for falsifying the theory. The present description of ADHD in the DSM provides no such utility as a scientific tool. This fact does not detract from the utility of the DSM view of ADHD as a clinical diagnostic tool (as noted in Chapter 2), for diagnosis is a different enterprise from the one being discussed here. But as an instrument to advance the scientific understanding of ADHD, the current consensus view of the disorder is grossly inadequate.

A final reason for a new model of ADHD is that the current DSM view treats the subtypes of ADHD as sharing qualitatively identical deficits in attention, while differing only in the presence or absence of hyperactive–impulsive

symptoms. As noted in Chapter 4, it is doubtful that the problems with inattention associated with hyperactive–impulsive behavior actually lie in the realm of attention. It is more likely, as will be argued here, that this inattention actually reflects defective executive functioning. By contrast, those problems seen in ADHD, Predominantly Inattentive Type—and especially in that subset having sluggish cognitive tempo (SCT; see Chapter 2)—may represent a qualitatively distinct attention or cognitive deficit from that evident in ADHD, Combined Type (Milich, Ballentine, & Lynam, 2001). The present theory does not try to explain the nature of SCT symptoms.

CONSTRUCTING THE THEORY OF SELF-REGULATION AND ADHD

Elsewhere (Barkley, 1997a, 1997b), I have reviewed several previous models of the executive or prefrontal lobe functions developed by others in neuropsychology, noted their points of overlap and distinction, argued for their combination into a hybrid model, and discussed evidence from both neuropsychology and developmental psychology for the existence of behavioral inhibition and four separable executive functions. Research consistently shows these functions to be mediated by the prefrontal regions of the brain, and to be disrupted by damage or injury to these various regions. The hybrid model presented in this chapter is therefore a theory of prefrontal lobe functions (and related networks in the basal ganglia and cerebellum), particularly the executive function system. It is also a developmental-neuropsychological model of human self-regulation. This theory specifies that behavioral inhibition is the first component in the model and the foundation for the others; specifically, it is critical to the development, privatization, and proficient performance of the four executive functions. It permits them, creates their internalization, supports their occurrence, and protects them from interference, just as it does for the generation and execution of the cross-temporal goal-directed behavioral structures developed from these executive functions. The four executive functions are nonverbal working memory; internalization of speech (verbal working memory); the self-regulation of affect/motivation/arousal; and reconstitution (planning and generativity). These executive functions can shift behavior from control by the immediate environment to control by internally represented forms of information through their influence over the last component of the model, motor control. Before I describe each component, it is first necessary to define the terms "behavioral inhibition," "self-regulation," and "executive functions" as I use them here.

Behavioral Inhibition

"Behavioral inhibition," like "attention," is multidimensional. In the present discussion, it refers to three interrelated processes that, though distinguishable from each other, are treated here for simplicity of explication as a single construct: (1) inhibiting the initial prepotent response to an event; (2) stopping an ongoing response or response pattern, thereby permitting a delay in the decision to respond or to continue responding; and (3) protecting this period of delay and the self-directed responses that occur within it from disruption by competing events and responses (interference control). Not only the delay in responding that results from response inhibition, or the self-directed actions within it, are protected, but also the eventual execution of the goal-directed responses generated from those self-directed actions (Fuster, 1997).

The "prepotent response" is defined as that response for which immediate reinforcement (positive or negative) is available or has been previously associated with that response. Both forms of reinforcement need to be considered prepotent. Some prepotent responses do not function to gain an immediate positive reinforcer as much as to escape or avoid immediate aversive, punitive, or otherwise undesirable consequences (negative reinforcement). It is hypothesized that both forms of prepotent responses are difficult for those with ADHD to inhibit. This may help us to understand the delay aversion conjectured by Sonuga-Barke to be involved in ADHD. Almost by definition, delay or waiting is unreinforcing or boring if not outright aversive, and so individuals with ADHD may act to terminate or escape from such aversiveness. But this problem, in the present theory, is believed to be part of a larger inhibitory deficit.

The initiation of self-regulation must begin with inhibiting the prepotent response from occurring or with interrupting an ongoing response pattern that is proving ineffective. This inhibition or interruption creates a delay in responding during which the executive functions can occur. Thus the executive functions are dependent on inhibition for their effective execution and for their regulation over the motor programming and execution component of the model (motor control). Figure 7.1 shows this component of the model, where it exerts a direct influence over the behavioral programming and motor control system of the brain, as indicated by the downward arrow between these two functions.

Behavioral inhibition does not directly cause the four executive functions (the intermediate boxes in Figure 7.2; see below) to occur, but merely sets the occasion for their performance and protects that performance from interference. To visibly represent this crucial point, the lines I eventually use in Figure 7.2 to connect

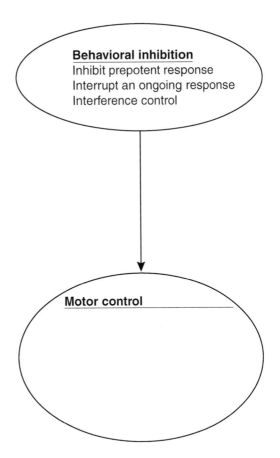

FIGURE 7.1. Diagram showing the influence of the behavioral inhibition system on the motor control system. From Barkley (1997b). Copyright 1997 by The Guilford Press. Reprinted by permission.

the component of behavioral inhibition to those other four executive functions are blunted. But because these executive functions themselves produce direct and causal effects on the motor programming and execution system, lines with arrowheads are placed between each of these executive functions and aimed at the motor control system to convey that direct, controlling influence.

Preventing a prepotent response from occurring is critical to self-control. The individual cannot engage in self-control to maximize later outcomes related to a particular event if he or she has already acted to maximize the immediate ones related to that event or context. This is particularly evident when there is a conflict between the valences of the immediate and later outcomes (immediately rewarding outcomes that lead to later and larger punitive ones, or immediately aversive ones that lead to later and larger rewarding ones). Such situations create a conflict for the individual between sources of behavioral control (typically external and temporally immediate information vs. internal, temporally distant information), and so impose a demand on the individual to utilize self-directed, private forms of behavior and information to manage this conflict situation successfully. In essence, this situation reflects a battle between the external now and the internally represented hypothetical future. That future stands no chance of affecting current behavior if the individual cannot inhibit responding to the moment to give the sense of time and the future a chance to influence that behavior.

The capacity to interrupt an ongoing sequence of behavior is likewise critical to self-regulation. If the individual is currently engaged in a pattern or series of responses, and feedback for those responses is signaling their apparent ineffectiveness, this sequence of behavior must be interrupted—the sooner the better. Such flexibility in ongoing behavior must exist that allows behavior to be altered quickly as the exigencies of the situation change and the individual detects those changes. This presupposes a degree of self-monitoring and awareness of immediately past responses and their outcomes. That monitoring permits the individual to read the signs in the trail of past behavior for information that may signal the need to shift response patterns. This self-monitoring function is probably contributed by the nonverbal working memory com-

ponent of the model. Thus the capacity to interrupt ongoing response patterns probably reflects an interaction of inhibition with working memory to achieve this end, creating both a sensitivity to errors and the appearance of flexibility in the individual's ongoing performance in a task or situation. Once interrupted, the delay in responding is again used for further self-directed action by the executive functions, which will give rise to a new and ideally more effective pattern of responding toward the task or situation. The detection of the errors in the past and in the ongoing behavioral performance, as well as the new pattern of behavior that will eventually be generated from analysis of feedback, are both believed to arise from the working memory components of this theory. However, the behavioral inhibition component must still become engaged to halt the current stream of responses to permit such analysis, synthesis, and midcourse correction to occur, thereby redirecting the motor programming and execution system onto this new tack of responding.

The third inhibitory process in this component of the model is interference control. Interference control is as important to self-regulation as are the other inhibitory processes, especially during the delay in responding when the other executive functions are at work. As Fuster (1997) noted, this is a time that is particularly vulnerable to both external and internal sources of interference. The world does not stop changing around or within an individual just because his or her responses to it have temporarily ceased and covert forms of self-directed behavior are engaged. New events playing out around the individual may be disruptive to those executive functions taking place during the delay; the more similar those events are to the information being generated by these executive functions (private behaviors), the more difficult it is to protect those functions from disruption, distortion, or perversion. For instance, imagine you are trying to rehearse a long distance phone number to call while the person next to you is reciting a string of digits. This thought experiment easily demonstrates the need for interference control. Likewise, sources of internal interference may arise, such as other ideas that occur in association with the ones that are the focus of the executive actions but are not relevant to the goal. And the immediate past contents of working memory must be cleansed or suppressed, so that they are not carried forward into the formulation of the new goal-directed behavioral structure and thereby disrupt its construction and performance. All this requires inhibition that protects the self-regulatory actions of the individual from interference. Figure 7.2 shows this aspect of the model. The schematic diagram of the model now shows the inhibition system having not only a direct influence over the motor control system, but also a supportive and protective role in regard to the other four executive functions (the boxes for which have been left blank for the moment).

The inhibitory process involved in the third form of behavioral inhibition (interference control) can be thought of as freedom from distractibility. It may be separable from that involved in delaying a prepotent response or ceasing an ongoing response. Indeed, as others have argued (see Goldman-Rakic, 1995; Roberts & Pennington, 1996), it may be an inherent part of the executive function of working or representational memory. As noted previously, the second form of inhibition (ceasing ongoing responses) may arise as an interaction of the working memory function (which retains information about outcomes of immediately past performance that feed forward to planning the next response) with the ability to inhibit prepotent responses (Fuster, 1997), thereby creating a sensitivity to errors. If so, this second form of inhibition also may be distinguishable from these other forms. Nevertheless, some of the previous neuropsychological models on which the present one was developed clustered them as forms of inhibition. That fact, along with research (reviewed in Chapter 2) suggesting that all three inhibitory activities are impaired in ADHD, led to their treatment here as a single global construct for the time being. But since the preceding edition of this text, it is becoming increasingly evident that the inhibition of prepotent responses, termed "executive inhibition" by Nigg (2001), may be the most impaired in ADHD.

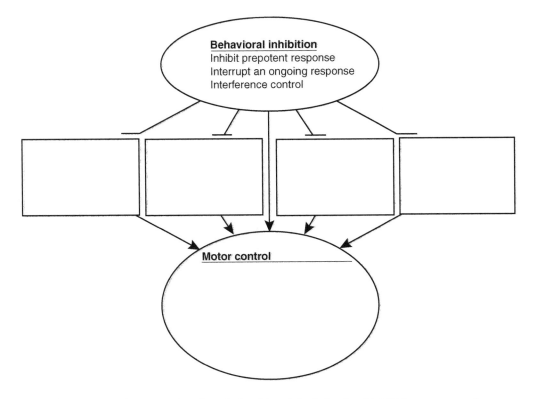

FIGURE 7.2. Diagram demonstrating the relationship of the behavioral inhibition system to four executive functions (boxes) and their relationship to the motor control system. From Barkley (1997b). Copyright 1997 by The Guilford Press. Reprinted by permission.

Self-Regulation

I have argued that inhibition is crucial to creating a delay between an event and our response to it. This results in a decoupling of the normal stimulus–response arrangement, building in a pause or waiting period. Self-control (or self-regulation) is not possible without such a delay and decoupling, because it will be in this delay that the self-directed actions that constitute self-control can occur. "Self-control" is defined as any response or chain of responses by the individual that changes his or her own behavior so as to alter the probability of a later consequence. Six key ingredients implicit in this definition deserve notice (Barkley, 1997b):

1. "Self-regulation" means behavior by an individual that is directed at the individual, rather than at the environmental event that may have initiated the self-regulation. It is self-directed action.

2. Such self-regulatory actions are designed to alter the probability of a subsequent response by the individual. That is, these actions are designed to change subsequent behavior.

3. Behaviors that are classified as self-regulatory serve to change the likelihood of a later rather than an immediate outcome. They are future-directed. This process achieves a net maximization of beneficial consequences across both short- and long-term outcomes of a response for the individual, particularly when there is a discrepancy between the valences of the short- and long-term outcomes. The individual is striving to create a net maximization of the immediate and the delayed consequences.

4. For self-control to occur or even to be desired by individuals, they must have developed a preference for the often larger long-term over the usually smaller short-term outcomes of behavior. There is an increasing preference for larger delayed rewards over smaller immediate ones across development until approximately the early 30s (Green, Fry, & Meyerson, 1994). In short, if individuals do not conceive of the future or value later consequences, then there is no point to self-control. They may as well act impulsively and maximize the momentary consequences.

5. Self-regulatory actions by an individual have as an inherent property the bridging of time delays among the elements comprising behavioral contingencies. As long as there is lit-

tle or no time between events and the individual's responses, and between these responses and their outcomes, there is little or even no need for self-regulation. This is simply Skinnerian learning. However, when time delays are introduced between these elements, self-directed actions must be undertaken to bridge them successfully—that is, to bind them together into a contingency, despite the delays in time—so as to maximize the longer-term outcomes. Thus a capacity for the cross-temporal organization of behavioral contingencies is implicit in the definition of self-regulation.

6. For self-control to occur, some neuropsychological or mental faculty must exist that permits this capacity to bind the parts of the contingency together, despite large gaps in time between them. It requires a sense of time, the ability to conjecture the future, and the ability to put both of these to use in the organization and execution of behavior. To conjecture the future, the past must be capable of recall and analysis to detect patterns among chains of events and their behavioral contingencies. It is from the recall of the past that such hypothetical futures can be constructed. This mental faculty is, I believe, working memory (see below).

The Executive Functions

This leads to the next construct in the model—that of the "executive functions." What are they? Neuropsychology seems to have been grappling with their definition, but has offered no satisfying account or operational definition to date (Barkley, 2001). As noted previously, behavioral inhibition delays the decision to respond to an event. This gives self-control time to act. The self-directed actions occurring during the delay in the response constitute, I believe, the executive functions. They are often not publicly observable, although it is likely that in early development many of them are so. Over development, they may become progressively more private or covert in form. The development of internalized, self-directed speech (see Chapter 3) seems to exemplify this process. Although eventually "internalized" (or, better yet, "privatized,") these self-directed actions remain essentially self-directed forms of behavior, despite the fact that they have become less observable or even unobservable. Therefore, the term "executive functions" refers here to a specific class of self-directed actions by the individual that are being used for self-regulation toward the future.

There are four such classes of self-directed actions, I believe, meaning that there are four types of executive functions. Despite having distinct labels, they are believed to share a common purpose: to internalize or privatize behavior so as to anticipate change and to guide behavior toward that anticipated future. All this is done, as already noted, to maximize the long-term outcomes or benefits for the individual. I believe that these four executive functions share a common characteristic: All represent private, covert forms of behavior that at one time in early child development and in human evolution were entirely public behavior and directed at managing others and the environment. They have become turned back on the self (self-directed) as a means to control one's own behavior, and have become increasingly covert, privatized, or "internalized" in form over human evolution and over a child's maturation. The four are often called by neuropsychologists "nonverbal working memory," "verbal working memory," "emotion regulation," and "planning" or "generativity." Such terms obscure the public behavioral origins of each function, however. Nonverbal working memory is, I believe, the privatization of sensory–motor activities (resensing to or behaving toward the self). Verbal working memory is self-directed, private speech—the internalization of speech, as Vygotsky (1978, 1987) conceived it. The third executive function (emotion regulation) is the self-regulation of affect, motivation, and arousal. It occurs in large part, I believe, as a consequence of the first two executive functions (self-directed behavior and speech), as well as the privatization of emotional behavior and its associated motivational features. Finally, planning, generativity, or what Bronowski (1977) called "reconstitution" represents the internalization of play.

If, as I believe, the executive functions represent the privatization or internalization of self-directed behavior to anticipate change in the environment (the future), this change represents essentially the concept of time. Thus what the internalization of behavior achieves is the internalization of a conscious sense of time, which is then applied to the organization of behavior in anticipation of the changes in the environment—events that probably lie ahead in time. Such behavior is therefore future-oriented, and the individual who employs it can be said to be goal-directed, purposive, and intentional in his or her actions. I believe that, like language and its internalization during child development, this developmental process of privatizing behavior and a sense of time is universal and instinctive to humans; it is not merely a product of cultural training. Indeed, as I have explained elsewhere, culture would be impossible without this process. It makes some sense, then, that behavioral inhibition should be so instrumentally related to this process, for it is probably behavioral inhibition that assists with the suppression of those initially observable self-directed actions that make up each type of executive function (internalized behavior).

Although I believe that each of these executive functions is capable of being dissociated from the others, they are interactive and interreliant in their naturally occurring state. We do not experience them as separate, but as coexistent and interactive, like the parts of a symphony played simultaneously by different sections of the orchestra. This is a critical point. It is the action of these functions in concert that permits and produces human self-regulation. Deficits in any particular executive function will produce a relatively distinct impairment in self-regulation, different from the impairment in self-control produced by deficits in the other functions. And this is also a crucial point: There is not one form of self-regulation, but four types of self-control, each of which can be separately impaired.

Undoubtedly, these executive functions and the future-directed behavior they permit do not all arise suddenly or simultaneously in human development. Instead, they develop in stages and probably evolved as such in earlier hominids and humans. I believe that they are probably staggered in their sequence during maturation; that is, in early childhood only one form exists, while at later ages two, then three, then finally all four forms of self-control (executive abilities) exist. I have conjectured that behavioral inhibition arises first, quite likely in parallel with the nonverbal working memory function. This is followed by the internalization of speech, then the internalization of affect and motivation, and then lastly by the internalization of play, or the reconstitution component of the model. Though these stages in the development of self-control are speculative, they constitute a testable feature of this model, as is the larger generic process of internalizing or privatizing of behavior. The sequence of stages here may not be correct, though there is certainly evidence that inhibition and nonverbal working memory are the first to arise in child development (Barkley, 1997b). Nor is it clear that the internalization of speech necessarily precedes that of affect/motivation. It seems to me that the internalized affect/motivation component actually depends on and is in large part a result of the internalization of both sensory–motor activities (nonverbal working memory) and speech. Far more research is surely needed on the development of these executive functions and their sequential staging, but I have placed my bets, which is what a good theory needs to do to be falsifiable. I only wish to emphasize here the prospect of stage-related sequencing in their development.

Behavioral inhibition and the four executive functions it supports influence the motor system, wresting it from complete control by the immediate environment to bring behavior under the possible control of internal information, the concept of time (change) it represents, and the probable future, and thus to make behavior goal-directed. I have labeled the motor component of the model "motor control/fluency/syntax." This label emphasizes not only the features of control or management of the motor system that these executive functions afford, but also the synthetic capacity for generating a diversity of novel, complex, publicly observable motor responses and their sequences in a goal-directed manner. Such complex behavior requires an ideational syntax that is placed for now within the reconstitution component of the model, yet which must be translated into actual motor responding. Thus, although the generation of ideational syntax is placed under the reconstitution component, its translation into the actual execution of motor sequences is placed within the motor control component.

As in constructing a model from Tinkertoys, I build the hybrid model one piece at a time. Although I represent the components of the model as geometric shapes (see Figures 7.1 to 7.7), I do not intend to represent them as stages in an information-processing model, as if they were some cognitive schematic diagram. I prefer instead to think of the rectangular boxes as representing simply different forms of private, self-directed, and often covert behavior. Nor is the particular configuration of these boxes in-tended to be a critical element of the model. The functions that these boxes represent are what I wish to emphasize here, as well as their sequential staging and hierarchical configuration, which are difficult to represent on the two-dimensional page. The executive functions depend on behavioral inhibition. The motor control component depends on both inhibition and those executive functions if behavior is to be internally guided (self-regulated) in the service of a goal (the future). Beyond intending to convey this set of conditional relations, the exact arrangement of the boxes in the model is open to debate, though I think its arrangement here has some merit.

As these executive functions develop in a child, one should witness a gradual shift in those things that are guiding and controlling the child's behavior. Others may exist, but at least four such progressive shifts seem evident to me:

- A change from being controlled by purely external events to being guided by increasingly internal forms of information, many of which deal with the future (images, speech, motivation, etc.)—that is, a change from external to internal control.
- A shift from having to be entirely controlled and managed by others to increasingly controlling him- or herself—in short, a shift from control by others to self-control.
- A change from being aware of and entirely responsive to events in the moment or temporal now to increasingly being aware of and directed toward later, future events—briefly, a change from focusing on the now to focusing on the future.
- Finally, a shift toward increasingly valuing larger, delayed consequences over smaller, immediate ones—in other words, the development of deferred gratification.

By adulthood (specifically, ones 30's) the pinnacle of self-regulation (social maturity) is achieved: The adult of our species is primarily guided by internal information as much as or more than by external events, is typically controlling him- or herself rather than requiring control by others, is largely demonstrating goal-directed behavior toward future events, and is concerned with maximizing the future consequences of his or her actions more than the immediate ones.

Nonverbal Working Memory:
Covert Sensory–Motor Action toward the Self

"Nonverbal working memory" is defined as the capacity to maintain internally represented information in mind or online that will be used to control a subsequent response. It represents covert sensing toward oneself. But sensing is also behaving, and so one should think of this component as representing sensory–motor action toward oneself. What is being re-sensed by this process is not just some past event or its sensory representations, but the entire behavioral contingency related to the event (event,

response, and outcome). Figure 7.3 illustrates this component of the model. And although it includes all forms of sensory–motor behavior of which humans are capable (sight, hearing, smell, taste, and touch), two of these are particularly important to human self-regulation: covert visual imagery (re-seeing to oneself) and covert audition (re-hearing to oneself). These two internalized, covert sensory–motor activities, along with the other types of sensory behavior, generate an internal stream of information that is then used to guide behavior across time toward a goal. One envisions a possible future and works toward that future, us-

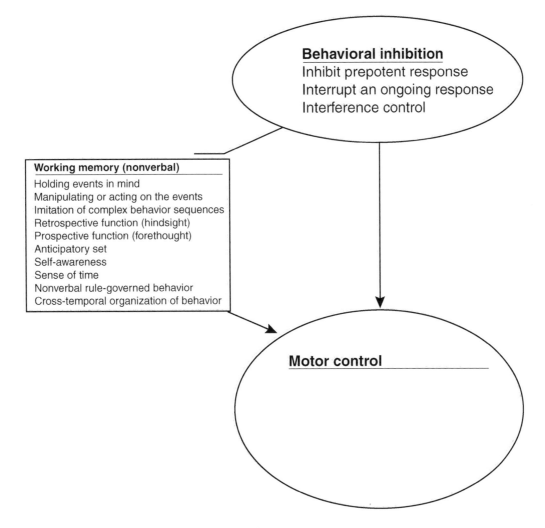

FIGURE 7.3. Diagram illustrating the functions of the nonverbal working memory system and its relationship to the behavioral inhibition and motor control systems. From Barkley (1997b). Copyright 1997 by The Guilford Press. Reprinted by permission.

ing the imagery as a guide. Even though I use the neuropsychological term "nonverbal working memory" in this discussion to represent these self-directed forms of sensory–motor behavior, it is important to keep in mind the forms of private behavior the term represents— private re-sensing to the self.

The reactivations of prior sensory representations are the means by which past events that may be relevant to the moment are *held in mind*. When we see to ourselves, we are covertly reactivating the images of the past, just as when we hear, taste, or smell to ourselves, we are reactivating and maintaining prior sensory representations within these modalities. The numbers and types of such past events that can be reactivated and held online at any one time, as well as the length or complexity of their temporal sequence, probably increase with development. Eventually, we develop the capability not only to hold such events or series of events in mind, but also to *manipulate or act on the events* as task demands may necessitate. As I note later, this ability to manipulate, analyze, and synthesize such sensory–motor representations is likely to represent a later, more highly developed ability of the working memory systems that is discussed further under the planning or reconstitution component of the model.

I have elsewhere speculated that this executive ability probably underlies the power of individuals to *imitate complex sequences of behavior* demonstrated by others (Barkley, 1997b, 2001). This could explain one basis for its evolution in humans and related species that demonstrate a power to imitate. Imitation is a powerful tool by which we humans learn new behavior. The power to imitate requires the capacity to retain a mental representation of the behavior of another person that is to be imitated. We do not so much copy the actions of another as copy our images of those actions. In many cases, this representation will be through visual imagery or covert audition. The more lengthy and complex are the sequences of new behavior that we are expected to imitate, the greater will be the demand of such tasks on working memory systems. This permits a child to progress from immediate imitation to delayed imitation and then to vicarious learning (doing the opposite of what is witnessed, should it prove ineffective or punitive).

The ability to reactivate the images and sounds of the past and to prolong their exis-

tence in mind during a delay in responding is the basis for *hindsight*. Through this function, an individual's pertinent history is able to come forward into the moment to help him or her select the optimal response to an event and to aid in guiding that eventual response. A delay in responding is critical to engaging in hindsight. Adults admonish young children to "stop and think before they act," a capacity that Virginia Douglas (1972) believed to be impaired in those with ADHD. Over development, the individual builds up a progressively larger archive of such past sensory representations that can be reactivated during delay periods as they appear pertinent to the formulation of a response in the present situation. Important in such recall of the past is the ability to keep the temporal sequence of these past events in a correct order, to guide the correct sequence of responses that will be based on them. Therefore, a syntax must exist for recall and ongoing representation of events within working memory (Butters, Kaszniak, Glisky, Eslinger, & Schachter, 1994; Fuster, 1997; Godbout & Doyon, 1995; Grafman, 1995; McAndrews & Milner, 1991; Milner, 1995; Sirigu et al., 1995).

A corollary or temporally symmetrical function arises out of hindsight, and that is *foresight* or *forethought*. That is, the reactivation of prior sensory representations appears to be carried forward in time to prepare to activate the motor response patterns associated with those prior events. The individual demonstrates a preparation to act. The reactivation and prolongation of past sensory events across time lead to a priming of the motor responses associated with those events. In this way, hindsight creates forethought and a preparation to act.

The recall of the past permits the anticipation of a hypothetical future, which acts to prepare or prime a set of motor responses directed toward that future, known as the *anticipatory set*. Hindsight represents the more sensory aspects of this process (the reactivation of past sensory experiences), whereas the forethought linked with it represents the more motor aspects of this process, or the presetting and priming of motor response patterns associated with those sensory events in anticipation of the future. For an individual eventually to initiate these primed or preset motor responses, an ongoing comparison of the sequence of events playing out in the external world with the sequence of sensory events being represented in working memory must be operating. That is, the person is tracking internal information against external events. Such a comparative process will instruct the timing of the release of the primed responses. Negative feedback, or information about one's errors during task performance, should be a particularly important source of self-regulating information. This feedback indicates a discrepancy between the actual current state (external situation) and the internally represented desired state of affairs (the goal), and the inadequacy of the current plans for achieving that outcome. The negative feedback must be temporarily held in mind to assist with correcting and refining the internally represented plans, which then feed forward to result in changes in behavior that may better achieve the desired state. Thus a sensitivity to errors and a flexibility of behavioral responding should be consequences of effective self-regulation.

The referencing of the past to inform and regulate present behavior and direct it toward the future most likely contributes to *self-awareness*. Past events and behaviors involving oneself are being reactivated and prolonged (held in mind) to prepare for a future for oneself, out of which probably arises an awareness of oneself.

The retention of a sequence of events in working memory appears to provide the basis for the human *sense of time,* or, more properly, the human capacity to manage behavior relative to time—what laypeople refer to as "time management." When one holds such sequences in mind and makes comparisons among the events in the sequence, a sense of both time and temporal durations appears to arise (Brown, 1990; Michon & Jackson, 1984). The processing of events in a sequence, or what is essentially temporal information, is not automatic but requires effort. This effort reflects a form of "attention," and that temporally focused attention is likely to be afforded through the working memory system. The judgment of temporal durations requires that attention to internal and external sources of temporal information (change) be increased and that attention to purely spatial information be decreased; this suggests that the sense of time, as a result of its dependence on working memory, requires the protection from interference that is provided by inhibition. It also may help to explain why behavioral inhibition appears to be related to

the capacity to accurately estimate and especially to reproduce temporal durations (see Chapter 3).

Working memory and the hindsight, forethought, and time management it permits may contribute to or even underlie the development of an increasing preference for delayed over immediate rewards, as discussed previously. Such a preference would seem to be a prerequisite for the development of self-control, given that the ultimate function of self-control is the maximization of future over immediate consequences.

In a way, the development of hindsight and forethought creates a window on time (past, present, future) of which the individual is aware. The opening of that temporal window probably increases across development—at least up to age 30, if the development of a preference for delayed over immediate rewards is any indication. Across child and adolescent development, the individual develops the capacity to organize and direct behavior toward events that lie increasingly distant in the future. By adulthood (ages 20–30), behavior is typically being organized to deal with events of the near future (8–12 weeks ahead). This time horizon can be extended to events even further into the future if the consequences associated with those events are particularly salient (Fingerman & Perlmutter, 1994). This sequence then may represent, as Fuster (1997) suggested, the overarching function of the prefrontal cortex: *the cross-temporal organization of behavior.* Wheeler, Stuss, and Tulving (1997) referred to this same capacity as "autonoetic awareness," a function they believe is localized more to the right than to the left prefrontal region. The temporal period over which such cross-temporal behavior can be organized is expected to be considerably shorter in young children and to increase across development as this cortex matures. One means, then, of judging the maturity of a person's time horizon at differing ages is to examine the average period prior to an event that typically results in the initiation of preparatory behaviors.

Once an individual begins to think about, anticipate, and prepare for future exigencies and to value delayed over merely immediate consequences, this should be accompanied by a willingness to share, cooperate, and reciprocate the sharing of others; that is, reciprocal altruism should arise. After all, if you have no sense of the future, sharing what you have with others makes no sense, because all you can appreciate at the moment is the loss of your own hard-earned assets. But if you can sense the future, you come to realize that sharing and social cooperation are a form of social insurance policy against the vagaries of future resources, so that giving up some excess resources to another person now can be reciprocated by him or her in the future, when the other person may have more resources than you. Humans have been repeatedly described as selfish altruists or cooperators, and this executive function may underlie the capacity for doing so.

If the mental representation of past events in working memory ultimately initiates and guides the motor responses associated with those events, then such mental representations take on the power of rules in governing behavior. Rule-governed behavior and its characteristics have been discussed in Chapter 3 of this volume. Working memory, therefore, seems to afford the individual a capacity for *nonverbal rule-governed behavior*. All of the foregoing are reasonably testable predictions of this theory.

To reiterate, sensory–motor action to the self (nonverbal working memory) probably gives rise to mental imagery, hindsight, forethought, a preparation to act, time management, imitation and vicarious learning, and social reciprocity. It is my guess (Barkley, 2001) that social reciprocity may have come first, absolutely crucial as it has been to human group survival in environments having wide swings in resources over time. This may have led the evolution of this system toward imitation, vicarious learning, and finally foresight and time management.

Internalization of Speech (Verbal Working Memory)

Developmental psychologists (Berk & Potts, 1991; Kopp, 1982) and developmental neuropsychologists (Vygotsky, 1978, 1987) have emphasized the importance of the internalization of speech for the development of self-control. Yet this process seems to have gone relatively unnoticed or been underemphasized in modern considerations of brain functions. Luria (1961) and Vygotsky (1967), and later Diaz and Berk (1992), argued that the influence of private speech on self-control certainly may be reciprocal: Inhibitory control contributes to the internalization of speech, which contributes to even greater self-restraint and self-guidance. Despite

this reciprocity, initial primacy within this bi-directional process is given here to behavioral (motor) inhibition.

Figure 7.4 demonstrates this component of the hybrid model. Although it is discussed here as representing the internalization of speech, it is believed to comprise what some neuropsychologists have considered "verbal working memory" or the "articulatory (phonological) loop" (Baddeley & Hitch, 1994). The capacity to converse with oneself in a quasi-dialogue brings about a number of important features for self-regulation. Self-directed speech is believed to provide a means for *reflection and description*, by which the individual covertly labels, describes, and verbally contemplates the nature of an event or situation prior to responding to that event. Private speech also provides a means for *self-questioning* through language, creating an important means for self-interrogation of the past and thereby a source of *problem-solving ability*, as well as a means of formulating rules and plans. Eventually, rules about rules *(meta-rules)* can be generated into a hierarchically arranged system that resembles the concept of "metacognition" in developmental psychology (Flavell, Miller, & Miller, 1993). The interaction of self-speech (verbal working memory) with self-sensing (nonverbal working memory) may contribute to three other mental abilities: the ability to comply at a later time with a rule given in the moment (see "Deficient Rule-Governed Behavior," Chapter 3, and also Hayes, Gifford, & Ruckstuhl, 1996), *reading comprehension* (holding in mind what we have silently read to ourselves), and *moral reasoning* (internalizing the rules of the culture).

Self-Regulation of Affect/Motivation/Arousal

We humans have the capacity not only to privately sense and behave to ourselves, but also to emote to or motivate ourselves as an integral part of this process of private, self-directed actions. And this capacity is what provides the drive, in the absence of external rewards, that fuels our persistence in goal-directed action. This is how the delay to future outcomes is bridged (Fuster, 1997). Figure 7.5 shows this component of the hybrid model.

Everyone recognizes that external events elicit emotional reactions of varying degrees, along with the motor responses to those events. But, as Damasio (1994, 1995) and others

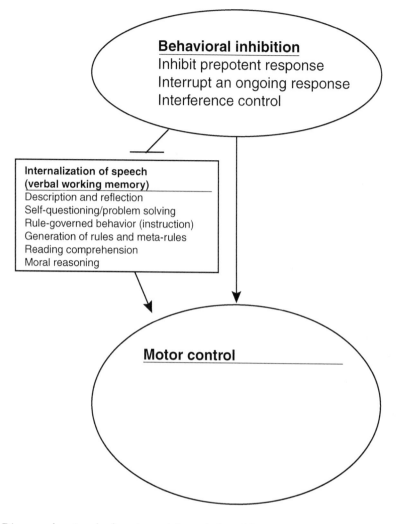

FIGURE 7.4. Diagram showing the functions of the verbal working memory system and its relationship to the behavioral inhibition and motor control systems. From Barkley (1997b). Copyright 1997 by The Guilford Press. Reprinted by permission.

(Fuster, 1997) have noted, the internally generated events arising from visual imagery, audition, and self-speech are also paired with affective and motivational tones, or somatic markers. Covert visual imagery and covert self-speech, among other forms of covert self-directed behavior, produce not only private images and verbalizations, but also the private emotional charges associated with them.

The power to inhibit and delay prepotent responses to events brings with it this power to delay the expression of those emotional reactions that would have been elicited by the event and whose expression would have been a part of the performance of those prepotent re-

sponses. Just as the delaying of a prepotent response permits a period for self-regulation through the use of internally generated and self-directed behavior (e.g., imagery and private speech), so the delaying of the affective response to the emotional charge of that event permits it likewise to undergo a change as a function of self-directed, private action. We can modify, moderate, and otherwise alter our own emotional reactions to events. The covert deliberations concerning the decision to respond not only result in a modification of the eventual response to the event, but also affect the eventual emotional charge (if any) that is emitted in conjunction with that response. This modification

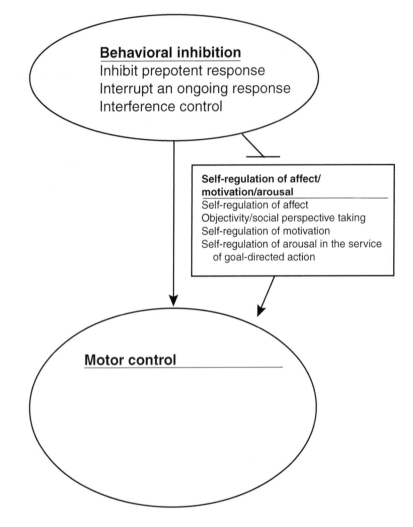

FIGURE 7.5. Diagram showing the functions of the self-regulation of affect/motivation/arousal system to the behavioral inhibition and motor control systems. From Barkley (1997b). Copyright 1997 by The Guilford Press. Reprinted by permission.

of the initial emotional response prior to its public display could be achieved through private imagery, in which images that have a different emotional charge are used to offset the ones that may have been initially associated with the event. For instance, an external event that is especially frustrating and anger-provoking may lead us to delay our emotional response, giving us time to talk to ourselves privately, calm ourselves down, use images and words that are soothing and positive, and thereby quell or greatly reduce the eventual emotional display. Such use of private action to countermand or counterbalance the initial emotional charge of external events contributes

to the development of *emotional self-control* (Kopp, 1982).

Self-directed emotions may become progressively more private or covert in form over development, eventually being internalized and having little or no publicly observable manifestations, except perhaps for their associated reactions in the autonomic nervous system (heart rate, skin conductance, respiration rate, flushed skin, etc.). Among the variety of human emotions, the negative array of emotions may be most in need of such self-control, given that we live in social groups with others on whom we must depend and can ill afford to offend (Kopp, 1982). This is because negative affect may prove more socially unacceptable, thereby producing more salient, long-term negative social consequences than such positive emotions as laughter or affection. For this reason, negative prepotent emotions are more likely to be in need of inhibition and self-regulation than are positive emotional reactions to events.

Such a process permits the original affective charge of an event to be separated and modified during the period of delayed responding. Thus not only is the eventual response made more deliberate, conscious, and reasoned, but so is the eventual emotional tone that is associated with it. Impulsive prepotent responses are often charged with far more raw emotion than those responses that are emitted after a delay and a period of self-regulation. That is, internally guided behavior, such as that governed by rules, is often associated with significantly less emotion than behavior that is impulsive and contingency-shaped (Skinner, 1969). The delay in the emotional response and the self-regulation of that response would seem to permit individuals the capacity for *objectivity* (Bronowski, 1977), and even the ability to *consider the perspective of another* in determining the eventual response to an event.

Also included in this component is the *self-regulation of drive or motivational and arousal states* that support the execution of goal-directed actions and persistence toward the goal. Motivation and arousal are included here for the simple reason that they constitute the very definition of an emotion—a motivational state. Lang (1995) has cogently argued that the array of human emotions can be reduced to a two-dimensional grid, of which one dimension is motivation (reinforcement and punishment) and the other is level of arousal. Other researchers in the field of emotion likewise associate it with motivational properties (see Ekman & Davidson, 1994, for reviews). Emotions are the results of a continual appraisal that takes place as an individual moves about and interacts with the external world, informing the individual about the significance of events for his or her own concerns (self-interest). The emotions have motivational or reinforcing significance; they motivate action in response to an event that elicits them and may induce adjustments to energy resources or level of activation as a consequence (Frijda, 1994). This would argue that the ability to self-regulate and even induce emotional states as needed in the service of goal-directed behavior also brings with it the

ability to regulate and even induce motivation, drive, and arousal states in support of such behavior. This, I argue, is the mental module from which intrinsic motivation (drive, willpower, persistence, determination, "stick-to-it-tiveness," etc.) springs and is used to sustain goal-directed behavior in the absence of external consequences for doing so.

Planning or Reconstitution

Figure 7.6 illustrates the planning or reconstitution component of the hybrid model. It represents, first, two important interrelated activities: *analysis and synthesis* (Bronowski, 1977). "Analysis" means the ability to take the units of behavioral sequences apart, as can be seen in the capacity to dismember a sentence into its component elements (words), to dismember words into their syllables, or even to break syllables into their phonological units. Units of behavior are built into sequences, and these behavioral structures can be combined into more complex sequences, which can be hierarchically organized into more complex sequences having subroutines of sequences within them, and so on. This is what gives human behavior its complex and hierarchically organized nature. The subhierarchies of which such complex hierarchies are composed, as well as their own behavioral units and subunits, can be taken apart in this process of analysis. These behavioral units can then be recombined to create novel behaviors and sequences of behaviors out of previously learned responses, in a process Bronowski called "synthesis."

The analytical and synthetic functions are evident not just in human speech, but in nonverbal forms of fine and gross motor behavior. For instance, consider the human capacity to play the piano. The rapid assembling of such fine motor gestures by an accomplished pianist into such extraordinarily complex sequences of the movements of digits on both hands simultaneously when playing a concerto is a marvel of human ability unduplicated in any other animal species. And although this nicely demonstrates the synthetic function of behavior of which I speak here, the capacity to break down these same gestures into their component parts and even to their individual keystrokes illustrates the analytical function just as nicely. The recombination of these dismembered units (synthesis) once again results in a novel sequence of fine motor actions, not to mention a

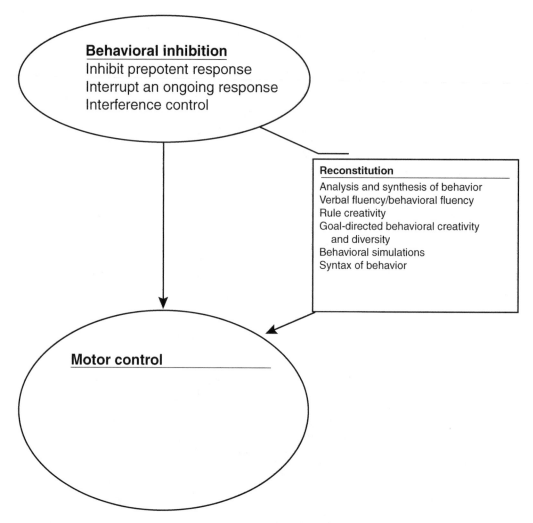

FIGURE 7.6. Diagram demonstrating the functions of the reconstitution system and its relationship to the behavioral inhibition and motor control systems. From Barkley (1997b). Copyright 1997 by The Guilford Press. Reprinted by permission.

new melody from the sounds those gestures create on the keyboard. Many examples of other forms of complex human motor responses and their reconstitution to provide new behavioral structures could be used to illustrate this process (ballet, modern dance, gymnastics, drawing, handwriting, etc.), but the point here should be evident. Humans have a tremendous capacity to analyze (dismember) their past behavioral repertoire and then to synthesize (recombine) its components into novel chains and hierarchies of responses. This capacity confers a substantial inventive or generative power on their behavior.

It is likely that this module can be subdivided into a verbal and a nonverbal subcomponent, as working memory can. I deal with them in combination here for simplicity's sake. *Verbal fluency* is one manifestation of this reconstitutive function. It is evident through the person's capacity to rapidly and effectively assemble the units of language to create a diversity of verbal responses. But it is also evident in *nonverbal* or *behavioral fluency.* Thus fine or gross motor fluency, written fluency, musical or vocal fluency, and even design fluency are also manifestations of this process of reconstitution. Whenever a goal must be accomplished, regardless of the form of behavior that may be required to attain it, the reconstitutive function will be available to act on the archive of previously acquired structures of those forms of behavior to assist with generating a range of novel, complex structures that may be of value in the attainment of that goal. Reconstitution, then, is the source or generator of behavioral diversity and novelty—not only in language and the rules that language can be used to formulate (*rule creativity*), but in nonverbal behavior as well. In a sense, then, the reconstitutive function contributes to *goal-directed behavioral flexibility and creativity*: the power to assemble multiple potential responses for the resolution of a problem or the attainment of a future goal. Such new response assemblies are, in a way, *simulations of behaviors* that can be covertly constructed and tested before one is eventually selected for performance. And that is a good definition of "planning."

A problem arises, however, when such analytical and synthetic functions are operative. The combination of units of behavior must be based on a syntax or set of rules governing the sequencing of such units and especially their contingent "if–then" relations. Just as many recombinations of genes or their sequences are harmful or even deadly, so too may be many potential recombinations of behavior, proving themselves to be utterly useless or even life-threatening (e.g., squeezing the trigger *before* aiming the gun). A syntax for assembling units of behavior into proper and potentially useful sequences undoubtedly exists, just as one exists for the composition of words into sentences (grammar). Thus the *syntax of behavior* is placed within this component, little understood as it seems to be at the moment. Such a syntax probably has much to do with aspects of causality or event contingencies in the external world as the individual has previously encountered them.

The metaprocess at work (reconstitution) on each of these domains of verbal and nonverbal mental information may turn out to be rather similar to the other, or even the same process. It may operate as a relatively random process with some constraints in its parsing and reconstituting of units of behavioral information, much as meiosis may parse and then recombine sequences of DNA. This process of trial and error—testing, recombining, testing again, and recombining—is akin to that of natural selection itself. And so, as Campbell (1960) has noted, new original ideas arise as a consequence of a form of cognitive natural selection, or "ideational Darwinism."

Motor Control/Fluency/Syntax

The internal, covert forms of self-directed behavior that comprise the executive functions and the information they generate come increasingly to control the actions of the behavioral programming and execution systems across child development. This gives behavior not only an increasingly deliberate, reasoned, and dispassionate nature, but also a more purposive, intentional, and future-oriented one as well. These executive functions produce observable effects on behavioral responding and motor control. Many of these effects have been either directly mentioned or implied earlier in the discussion of each executive function. I reiterate those effects on motor control here to complete the model; Figure 7.7 shows this completed model.

As a result of this internal regulation of behavior, both sensory input and motor behavior that are unrelated to the goal and its internally represented behavioral structures become *minimized or even suppressed* during task- or goal-directed performances. This protective suppression of prepotent responding (impulsivity) occurs not only during the operation of these executive functions, but also during the *execution of the goal-directed responses* they generate. Once goal-directed actions are formulated and prepared for transfer to the motor execution system, in the form of *novel/complex motor sequences*, the motivation or drive necessary to maintain these sequences of goal-directed behavioral structures must be recruited or self-induced. This induction may happen automatically as a result of the affective and motivational states that are associated with the internally represented information held in working memory and used to formulate the goal-directed behavior. Regardless of precisely how it arises, such a recruitment of motivation in the service of goal-directed behavior, when combined with working memory and interference control, drives that behavior toward its intended destination. The total process creates *goal-directed persistence*—a persistence that is characterized by willpower, self-discipline, determination, single-mindedness of purpose, and a driven or intentional quality.

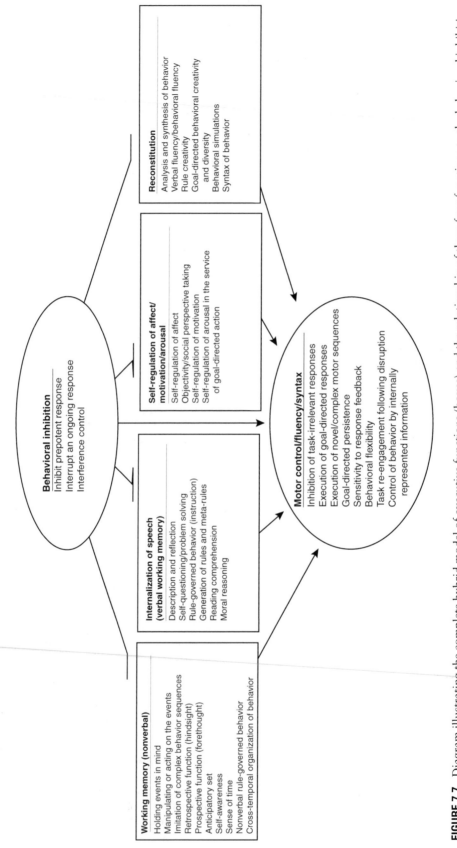

FIGURE 7.7. Diagram illustrating the complete hybrid model of executive functions (boxes) and the relationship of these four functions to the behavioral inhibition and motor control systems. From Barkley (1997b). Copyright 1997 by The Guilford Press. Reprinted by permission.

Throughout the execution of goal-directed behavior, the self-awareness features of working memory permit the feedback from the last response(s) to be held in mind (retrospective function), in order to feed forward (prospective function) in modifying subsequent responding, thereby creating *a sensitivity to errors*. Just as important, when interruptions in this chain of goal-directed behaviors occur (e.g., by distraction), the individual is able to *disengage, respond to the interruption, and then reengage the original goal-directed sequence* because the plan for that goal-directed activity has been held in mind despite interruption. Thus inhibition sets the occasion for the engagement of the four executive functions, which then provide considerably greater *control over behavior by the internally represented information* they generate. This in turn provides for the cross-temporal organization of behavior—the organization of behavior relative to time and the future.

THE PLACE OF SUSTAINED ATTENTION IN THE MODEL

If the current model of self-control and executive functions is to be at all applicable to ADHD, it must identify not only the nature of the inhibitory deficiencies known to be associated with this disorder (which I have done), but also the difficulties with inattention, particularly poor sustained attention, involved in this disorder. This relationship can now be readily understood as resulting from the interaction of the inhibitory module with those executive functions that provide for the control of behavior by internally represented information (especially covert imagery, rules, and self-motivation). Interference control seems particularly critical to the persistence of goal-directed behavior, which I believe represents a special form of sustained attention. It is self-sustained attention (persistence) rather than externally reinforced persistence. When responses that are under the control and guidance of internally represented information must be sustained over long periods, the individual must resist responding to distractions that may arise both internally and externally during task performance or pursuit of a goal. This resistance is provided by the interference control functions of the inhibitory module. The individual must also formulate and hold in mind the goal of the

task and the plan for attaining that goal, so that it serves as a template for constructing the necessary behavioral structures to that end. Thus the working memory functions may be involved in goal-directed persistence as well. But, most important, the individual must also kindle, sustain, and renew internally represented sources of drive and motivation that continuously support behavior toward the goal, in the absence of external sources of reinforcement or motivation for doing so.

These covert, self-controlling functions are not necessary in situations or tasks in which the individual's pattern of responding is simply being maintained by the prevailing schedule of immediate reinforcement. That form of sustained responding is not being internally guided, but is a function of the motivational factors in the immediate task and context; it is, in a sense, externally maintained attention or sustained responding.

The type of sustained attention that is internally guided is better termed "goal-directed persistence," and its origin lies in self-regulation and the interaction of the executive functions, especially self-regulation of motivation and effort. The other type of sustained attention is better termed "contingency-shaped or context-dependent responding," and its origins lie in the nature of those immediate contingencies operating within the task or setting and the individual's contact with them. Both these forms of sustained attention appear as sustained responding to the casual observer. Their differences in origins and in the sources maintaining them, however, can be readily detected by removing any source of immediate reinforcement that may be provided by the task or external context. This removal should have little or no effect on goal-directed persistence that is being internally (covertly) mediated or guided, while resulting in a significant decline in or extinction of sustained responding that is contingency-shaped and maintained by the external consequences prevailing in the task. It is the former (goal-directed, internally guided) type of persistence, and not the latter (contingency-shaped, externally regulated) form of sustained attention, that is predicted here to be disrupted in ADHD. This, it would seem, is why children with ADHD can sustain their attention to video games or other activities they enjoy for extended periods of time, but cannot pay attention to their homework for more than a few minutes of sustained persistence. The former is externally reinforced behavior, while the latter must be internally guided and motivated.

Most measures of sustained attention in psychological and neuropsychological research on this construct are actually assessing goal-directed persistence rather than contingency-shaped sustained attention. Subjects are given an instruction as to how to perform the task, and this instruction becomes both a rule and a goal. Quite often, such a task involves little if any reinforcement within the task; this is what one sees in continuous-performance tests, which require that subjects sustain their responding toward the rule or goal in the absence of external reinforcement. Consequently, such tasks do not assess sustained attention of the contingency-shaped sort, but goal-directed persistence of the internally guided form. Neuroimaging and other neuropsychological studies have found that the right prefrontal region is more likely to be involved in the performance of tasks involving the type of behavioral or motor persistence I describe here (Goldberg & Podell, 1995; Kertesz, Nicholson, Cancelliere, Kassa, & Black, 1985; Knight, Grabowecky, & Scabini, 1995; Pardo, Fox, & Raichle, 1991; Rueckert & Grafman, 1996). Other neuroimaging research shows that this region seems to be smaller in those with ADHD (Castellanos et al., 1996; Filipek et al., 1997; see Chapter 5), perhaps explaining why those with ADHD may have difficulties on such tasks.

The involvement of the prefrontal cortex is probably not necessary for the contingency-shaped type of sustained attention. The goal-directed form, however, is dependent on the prefrontal cortex and the executive functions that cortex and its networks permit.

EXTENDING THE THEORY TO ADHD

Increasing evidence (see Chapter 5) suggests that ADHD may arise from deficiencies in the development, structure, and function of the prefrontal cortex and its networks with other brain regions, especially with the striatum and cerebellum. Therefore, any model of prefrontal executive functions, such as that developed here, should also offer great promise as a model for understanding ADHD. Increasing evidence also indicates that ADHD is a disorder of self-regulation. Once more, then, theories of self-regulation should have much to offer us in understanding ADHD. The present

theory achieves both—offering a model of how self-regulation may develop, showing how it is linked to behavioral inhibition, and explaining how executive functioning is related to both of these constructs. In short, inhibition creates a delay in responding to events, thereby partially decoupling the event from our response to it. In this delay or gap will arise self-directed actions that function to change our behavior so as to maximize future over immediate consequences (self-regulation). The self-directed actions being used in this process are the executive functions. No clearer explanation of why inhibition is linked to self-regulation and both are linked to executive functioning currently exists in the neuropsychological literature, nor is there a better operational definition of executive functioning, to my mind. Just as interesting in this model is its clear explication of how the executive functions are likely to arise in development—and probably of how they arose in human evolution—through the internalization (or, more accurately, privatization) of self-directed actions.

Compelling evidence exists that ADHD comprises a deficit in the development of behavioral inhibition (see Chapter 2). The hybrid model of executive functions developed in Figure 7.7 posits that the three subcomponents of behavioral inhibition make a fundamental contribution to the creation and effective performance of four executive functions: nonverbal working memory, verbal working memory (internalized speech), the self-regulation of affect/motivation/arousal, and reconstitution. It does so because it permits the privatization or internalization of behavior that forms these executive functions. The inhibitory deficit that characterizes ADHD disrupts this formation and execution of the executive functions, and thus disrupts their control of goal-directed motor behavior by the internally represented information they generate. In short, the inhibitory deficit in ADHD delays and disrupts the internalization of behavior that forms the executive functions, and thereby has an adverse impact on the self-regulation they afford to the individual.

Although I use the terms "deficit" or "deficiency" here interchangeably, it is worth noting that what I mean is that they refer to relative delays in the development of the abilities under discussion. To some, the term "deficiency" implies that a function or ability once existed at a fully operational level and then was lost or impaired through some pathological process. This is not the meaning I wish to imply here for that term. Those with ADHD are behind in the proficiency of the executive abilities because they are behind their peers in their development of behavioral inhibition. But in using or implying the term "delay" here, I also do not wish to connote that the ability under discussion is expected eventually to catch up with that of the typical peer group—in other words, that there exists some temporary lag in a developmental process that will be made up later on. Just as mental retardation is taken to imply a chronic developmental delay in general cognitive ability that is not outgrown with time or maturation (though relative gains may be made), so do I wish to impart a similar meaning here when I state that ADHD represents a developmental delay in behavioral inhibition and the executive functions (self-regulation) dependent on it.

Given all this, those with ADHD can be said to have impairments in all of the executive functions and the subfunctions listed beneath them in Figure 7.7 as a consequence of the poor inhibition. Consequently, they can be said to manifest the difficulties evident in the motor control component of this model as well. Here, then, is a relatively comprehensive theory of ADHD that links the delay in behavioral inhibition well recognized to be involved in the disorder with problems in the executive functions, self-regulation, and self-management relative to time. This means that ADHD is not just a deficit in behavioral inhibition, but also a deficit (secondarily) in executive functioning and self-regulation as a consequence of that inhibitory impairment. This deficit results in a renegade motor control system that is not under the same degree of control by internally represented information, time, and the future as would be evident in the typical peer group of an individual with ADHD. As it emerges, then, ADHD becomes a disorder of self-management relative to time and the social future (time management).

It is quite possible that I may be wrong about some of the relationships specified above. After all, no theory in science is perfect as formulated. This does not mean that the present theory is not useful as a scientific tool that can drive programmatic research testing its predicted arrangements. Theories are but ships that we build, sail, and test, so as to build better ships. For instance, it seems likely now, given 10 years to ponder it, that both inhibition

and working memory develop simultaneously in a form of codevelopment. The first executive function requires inhibition, and inhibition needs a reason to explain its development (it is necessary for self-directed sensory–motor action). If so, then ADHD may not only be a primary deficit in inhibition, but also a primary deficit in working memory (what the DSM is calling "attention"). I am honestly not certain of this arrangement, and so for now I will leave things as they were when first proposed (Barkley, 1997a, 1997b), with working memory as a secondary consequence of ADHD stemming from its inhibitory deficit. But I fully recognize that research may show them both to be "primary" in the disorder. So be it. A theorist has to place his or her bets if theories are to be testable, and I have done so (Barkley, 1997b). Likewise, its quite conceivable that nonverbal working memory can be further subdivided into its temporal and spatial aspects, with evidence suggesting that ADHD may have a more deleterious effect on the temporal–sequential processes in working memory than on the spatial ones—perhaps because, as I have noted in Chapter 3, the former processes demand more effortful control and place a greater load on working memory. Time will tell.

TESTABLE PREDICTIONS FROM THE THEORY

For the sake of students and fellow scientists wishing to further test and falsify this theory of self-regulation and ADHD, let me here set forth some (though by no means all) of its testable predictions—some of which have been supported by research (see Chapter 3), while others await further study. Children and adults with ADHD, Combined Type should manifest the following deficits, with some depending upon the age at which they are studied; this is to say that if a process described below is not yet developed or proficient in typical children, it cannot yet be found to be deficient in children with ADHD. It is also to say that if typical children have been proficient in a capacity for many years, it is likely at a certain point that children with ADHD will eventually attain some proficiency at that task because the disorder is a *delay* in development, not a total *loss* of ability. If such a task is too easy for both groups to accomplish, no group difference would be expected in the results, even if those with

ADHD are delayed in the larger developmental domain being tested.

Behavioral Inhibition

ADHD involves deficits in three aspects of behavioral inhibition: (1) inhibiting the prepotent response (the urge to act on the moment); (2) inhibiting ongoing responses that are proving ineffective, so as to be sensitive to their errors and thereby to discover and shift to more effective responses; and (3) inhibiting responses to task-irrelevant events (distractibility), known as "interference control."

Sensing toward the Self

The deficits noted above will interfere with the development of self-directed actions (sensory–motor action), and especially the use of visual imagery and private audition (hearing to the self), as means of regulating behavior.

• This interference arises because inhibition is needed to delay the response to the temporal now and its immediate and compelling events, as well as to begin privatizing (suppressing) the publicly observable or overt aspects of those self-directed actions the individual will use to self-regulate. Why self-directed actions need to become private or internalized in form is an interesting question for evolutionary psychology, the answer to which will be conjectured below. But here the point is that if private self-directed behavior is a form of thinking—as Skinner, Vygotsky, and Bronowski earlier believed it to be—then children with ADHD are thinking out loud more than others, when they should be engaging in private action or thought like others of their age.

• The nonverbal working memory system may have arisen in evolution to permit a capacity for reciprocal altruism (selfish cooperation) and social exchange within human groups, probably so that early humans could address problems associated with wide swings in resource availability. Humans also engage in "non-zero-sum" interactions (see Wright, 2000), which involve joining together to accomplish a common goal that no single individual could achieve alone; it is the root of social cooperation. Whatever the problems were that these activities solved for early humans, the capacities for such social exchange (often delayed

across time) and for joining with others to accomplish larger goals require evolved mental mechanisms to support them. If these are functions of the working memory system, then children with ADHD will demonstrate deficits related to reciprocal altruism (social exchange), sharing, and cooperation in these activities. This may help us to understand their substantial problems with peer relationships. Sharing and cooperation depend on a capacity to wait and to sense the future implications of what a person does with others; if some individuals cannot stop and think (see the probable future) before they act, they are far less likely to share, cooperate, keep promises, exchange goods and services, and otherwise engage in social reciprocity and the non-zero-sum interactions that are the heart of human social groups. Conscious cooperation, and especially conscious altruism and its inherent delay in social exchange, require a sense of the social future. ADHD should impair that sense, thereby impairing the social behavior dependent on that sense.

• Once a capacity for holding an image (or sound) in mind is attained, many of those images will be of the behavior of others in the social group. Here, I believe, arises the capacity for imitative learning. Humans cannot copy each other's behavior, because it is rather ephemeral. They are actions that disappear from the world, once performed. Copying the behavior of another, it seems to me, requires the ability to hold an image of that behavior in mind, so as to sustain its existence mentally for a sufficient period of time to permit it to be duplicated. The image is therefore the template from which the imitative response will be constructed. No imagery, no imitation. If such images of the actions of others can then be stored in long-term memory for later recall, then a further capacity for delayed imitation can arise, so that what is witnessed at one time in a given social context can be duplicated at a later time and in another social context. Imitation is doing what others do. Vicarious learning is a broader capacity that involves imitation, as well as sometimes doing the opposite of what others do. For instance, if Peter observes Paul engaging in a behavior that leads to Paul's being punished, injured, or even killed, Peter's image of this contingency arrangement can subsequently be used to suppress that same behavior in his own repertoire. Peter can learn from

Paul's mistakes. And so develops the capacity to use the behavior and learning of others for self-change and improvement. In doing so, Peter has saved himself an exceptional amount of time and effort that is required for trial-and-error (operant) learning. I have argued above that this capacity to retain images of the actions of others to be used, now or later, for imitation or vicarious learning depends on the nonverbal working memory system. To the extent that ADHD adversely affects this system, children with ADHD should be less capable of imitating the behavior of others (particularly complex sequences that will tax working memory capacity), and they will be less capable of self-improvement through the larger capacity of vicarious learning.

• When one is capable of reactivating images of past experience, hindsight arises. And when those images that are relevant to the current context can be held in mind and studied for recurrent patterns, those patterns can be carried forward in time to serve as a best guests of the future—an expectation. Hindsight has now generated foresight, or an ability to anticipate the likely future. Such images and associated expectations can then generate a capacity for anticipatory preparations to act when the time arrives to do so. This too seems to arise from the nonverbal working memory system. And again, to the extent that ADHD disrupts that system, we should find that those with the disorder act without due regard to hindsight, foresight, and their associated anticipatory preparations for the likely impending future. In short, they are less likely to stop and think before they act, the thinking here being hindsight–foresight.

• This problem for those with ADHD should be evident as well in the content of their speech with others and their interactions with them, as well as in how they elect to spend their time and energies. They do not stop and consider (much less verbally refer to) their past experience and its associated images, so as to consider and verbally discuss the future when it is essential to do so. It is not that they cannot do so at all whenever they are asked about their past or even their future; it is that they do not do so at the crucial junctures in the stream of their ongoing activities when it would be wise to do so. This is a point that needs to be made repeatedly: The problem is not so much with knowing as with doing or using. This issue ap-

pears in regard to all of the executive functions discussed here.

• The images we are capable of holding in mind constitute our own individual history and include images of ourselves and our past behavior. By frequently referring to such images about ourselves, we develop autonoetic awareness, or a sense of ourselves across time. This is self-awareness within a temporal sense. Once again, to the degree that ADHD interferes with the capacity to review past experiences online and in mind, it also interferes with awareness of self across time. Is this the origin of the positive illusory bias so well established now in children with ADHD—their inability to appreciate how poorly they may actually perform certain activities, relative to their typical peers?

• Holding images and other information in mind from the past and projecting them forward in time to anticipate the future probably contributes to the conscious sense of time itself—and, just as important, to the capacity to use that sense of time in order to govern behavior, make it more timely, and make preparations to act on future events in a timely manner. Might not this be the origin of the time reproduction problems so consistently evident in children, teens, and adults with ADHD (see Chapter 3)? This is in its largest scope, time management, or the management of oneself relative to the sense of time. And it too should be impaired in those with ADHD. Complaints of procrastination, lack of punctuality, and a failure to give due regard for the time, timing, and timeliness of their actions should be rife about those with the disorder.

• If individuals do not consider time and the future before taking action, as I argue that those with ADHD are less likely to do, then they will not place greater value on larger, later future rewards over the more obvious, immediate, and usually smaller ones. The value of future consequences should be more steeply discounted than is the case with typical peers. Some suggestion of this differential discounting of future consequences has already been evident in studies of children and teens with ADHD (see Chapter 3), but it deserves far greater research attention than it has received to date.

• If children with ADHD do not think about and utilize their sense of time, we could easily predict that they will be less likely to talk about time in their general conversations with others, and that they will be later in doing so in their development than when typical children first begin to make verbal references to past, future, and time more generally.

Speech to the Self

As noted above, speech to the self progresses from being directed at others in early childhood, to being self-directed yet still overt by ages 3–5 years, and eventually to covert self-speech in middle to late childhood. With this progressive privatization comes a shift from description to include self-instruction, as well as an increasing power of language to guide motor behavior. We should (and do!) find that just as children with ADHD may be delayed in nonverbal working memory, particularly its temporal–sequential aspects, so too are they delayed in their privatization of self-speech (see Chapter 3). Although such a delay in a fascinating developmental progression is interesting in its own right, it also suggests a delay in the power of self-regulation that self-directed speech probably evolved to provide.

- Children with ADHD will be deficient in the capacity of language generally and self-directed speech particularly to guide motor behavior. Rule-governed behavior should prove problematic for these individuals.
- Children with ADHD will engage in greater public speech (excessive talking) and less private speech, given that they are thinking out loud, as noted earlier, when others are thinking covertly.
- Self-speech also provides a source of problem solving, because it permits typical individuals to interrogate or question themselves so as to better elicit useful information from their memory and experiences. Self-questioning in problem solving should be less proficient in those with ADHD.
- One somewhat unexpected prediction about this delay in self-directed speech (verbal working memory) in those with ADHD is that it should also be associated with a progressive deficit in reading, viewing, and listening comprehension. Take reading, for instance. Silent reading to oneself requires self-directed covert speech, but it also requires that what is said (read) to the self be held in mind or online so as to extract its meaning. Words as arbitrary utterances derive their meanings, directly or indi-

rectly, from the images and actions that they symbolically represent. What is read must be held in mind, so as to more fully appreciate the nonverbal semantic content it was intended to convey. Because ADHD interferes with working memory (both verbal and nonverbal), those with the disorder should have greater difficulty holding in mind the content of what is read, and therefore should be less proficient in understanding what is read. As many clinical patients with ADHD will describe, when reading they often forget what was read at the top portion of the page by the time they have reached the middle or lower portion of the page, and therefore must return to the top to read it once again. We should also find that they retain only the most obvious and concrete aspects of the story, while being less proficient at understanding and retaining the more complex and subtle features of plot and sequence. Given that this is a working memory problem, it should affect not just reading, but listening to story narratives and even viewing televised content. Although there is growing evidence that this is indeed the case (see Chapter 3), what this theory provides is the reason it would be expected to be found in the first place in those with the disorder—another testable prediction.

- Also unexpected (at first) is the prediction that such a disorder of internalized speech and verbal working memory should lead to a delay in moral development and the capacity to be socialized into the rules of the group or larger culture. If speech is not being internalized well, then the rules that it conveys will likewise not be internalized well. Part of moral development springs from the sense of the social future described above and the social consciousness it affords—"Do unto others as you would have them do unto you." But part of moral development is also internalizing codified rules of conduct that instruct right from wrong. The difficulties with internalizing speech and using rules to guide behavior predicted to be associated with ADHD should also be expected to create some adverse impact on moral conduct in those with the disorder.
- Consider also that if those with ADHD are less able to consider the future consequences of their actions before they act, and are less capable of remembering and of following through on rules, instructions, and advice more generally, should they not also then be less able to follow through on promises and commit-

ments made to others, even if these were sincerely made at the outset?

Self-Regulation of Emotion/Motivation

Given the foregoing discussion of how emotional self-regulation may arise, and with it motivational self-regulation, one can predict that children with ADHD will have difficulties in moderating and self-regulating emotional states, thereby displaying raw and impulsive emotions more than typical children do.

• They will also have difficulties in creating and sustaining self-motivation. Self-motivation provides the drive, determination, stick-to-it-tiveness, persistence, and willpower to "stay the course" and continue persisting toward tasks and future goals in the absence of externally provided reinforcement or punishment. Those with ADHD will not be as capable of these actions, and so will not be as capable of sustaining effortful behavior toward goals in the absence of external consequences for doing so.

• The corollary of this prediction is that those with ADHD are more dependent than others on such externally provided consequences for their drive states and persistence toward tasks and goals than are typical children or adults. In part, then, ADHD is "MDD"—motivation deficit disorder. I believe this predicts and explains why those with ADHD can sustain their attention and activity toward tasks (e.g., video games) that provide frequent external consequences or that the individuals find enjoyable to do, yet cannot sustain their attention and activity toward tasks, such as homework or chores, which provide no such frequent schedule of consequences.

• But emotion equals more than just a motivational state; it also comprises a dimension of arousal. If those with ADHD cannot regulate emotional states, then almost by definition they cannot self-regulate states of arousal as well as others of their age. Self-arousal and self-activation toward goals and tasks will be less successful in those with ADHD.

Self-Directed Play (Planning and Generativity)

I believe that the fourth executive function represents the internalization of play, or analysis and synthesis. The capacity to take things apart and recombine them into novel sequences and structures applies not just to objects, but, more importantly, to our own behavioral sequences and hierarchical structures. We don't just play with objects (or words); we play with the behaviors that so affect and create them. Typical children will progress from overt physical or manual as well as verbal play to covert forms of these self-directed actions. They will come to be able to manipulate the nonverbal and verbal contents of working memory, taking apart and recombining them into novel recombinations. Many of these products will be useless or nonsensical, but a few will be exceptionally creative, innovative, and useful new ideas that can be put into play for problem solving, goal attainment, and their associated social effectiveness.

• Those with ADHD should show a delay in the progressive privatizing of overt manual and verbal play to their covert forms. They will have a greater need than typical children to manipulate material manually or play with language publicly in their task performance and problem solving.

• And when mental problem solving, planning, or fluency (defined as generating a diversity of responses on demand), those with ADHD will be less proficient at doing so than are their peers. One can easily see the probable adverse impacts of this on mental arithmetic, digit span backward, verbal and design fluency, and planning tasks, all of which require manipulating the content of working memory for successful performance.

• This unit of the executive system provides for effective problem solving, particularly when obstacles are encountered in pursuit of goals. It affords one the ability to rapidly construct and mentally test out various behavioral options for resolving the problem (planning) before selecting that which seems to address the problem most effectively. Those with ADHD should be less proficient at such problem solving than typical individuals.

• When typical individuals are recombining the parts of the world or their own behavioral units into new sequences, a syntax will prove essential to doing so effectively; order and timing are crucial in many aspects of their actions. This theory predicts that those with ADHD will have greater problems with such a syntax, showing greater errors in these recombinatorial activities having to do with sequence and timing, and hence the utility of these new ideas. Here then may arise the organizational difficulties so apparent in the drawing, writing, speech, actions, general task performance, and social functioning of those with ADHD.

• This executive unit is not just for planning and goal-directed behavioral innovation. It is also likely to be the source of critical thinking—the mechanism by which competing forms of information, response options, and their consequences are weighed for their likely long-term benefits (or, more technically, risk–benefit tradeoffs). Such critical thinking is not merely an activity of science or the academic life, but an essential part of daily social life for all of us. It is a means of social self-defense in which we can respond to and defend against the efforts of others to influence us socially for their own self-interests. Without such a means of critically considering the proposals, advice, instructions, sales pitches, or other means of social persuasion (or even coercion) to which we are subjected on a daily basis, we would be inherently gullible—easy prey for the salespeople, charlatans, shysters, cranks, and other social predators we encounter. This should mean that those with ADHD are less capable of such social self-defense; less capable of critically weighing the substantial efforts of social influence by others to which they are exposed daily; and hence more suggestible, gullible, and socially manipulable for others' self-interests and social ends. And they should be least capable of defending themselves in this way when it is most useful to do so.

Here then are some of the many testable predictions that such a model provides for understanding the development of self-regulation and of ADHD. Others, as they pertain to the clinical understanding and management of the disorder, will be evident below. It is fair to say (all arrogance and conceit aside) that such a model truly does make more testable predictions about both ADHD and related features of typical development than any previous theory of the disorder has done. No other contemporary theory or hypothesis about the nature of ADHD even comes close to affording such an extensive blueprint for programmatic research, such a deeper insight into the likely nature of this disorder, and (as I show below) such utility in proposing interventions for the management

of the disorder. Imperfect as this theory undoubtedly is, its utility in comparison to its competitors cannot be faulted. And that is really all one can ask of a theory in its often all-too-brief conceptual shelf life.

IMPLICATIONS FOR UNDERSTANDING ADHD

Let's "cut to the chase": What does this theory mean for understanding and managing ADHD? What is its utility or practical cash value for doing so, apart from the numerous testable predictions elaborated above? Elsewhere I have gone into great detail regarding the implications of this theoretical model for understanding, diagnosing, assessing, and treating ADHD (Barkley, 1997b). Some of these points are sufficiently important to be reiterated here for their clinical utility.

ADHD as a Disorder of Performance, Not of Skill

The totality of the deficits associated with ADHD serve to cleave thought from action, knowledge from performance, past and future from the moment, and the sense of time from the rest of behavior more generally. This definition means that ADHD is not a disorder of knowing what to do, but of doing what one knows. It produces a disorder of applied intelligence by partially dissociating the crystallized intelligence of prior knowledge from its application in the day-to-day stream of adaptive social functioning. ADHD, then, is a disorder of performance more than a disorder of skill—a disability in the "when" and "where" rather than in the "how" or "what" of behavior. Those with ADHD often know what they should do or should have done before, but knowing provides little consolation to them, little influence over their behavior, and often much irritation to others. Such knowledge seems to matter little when they are actually behaving at particular moments. The executive system is where the "rubber" of past experience and knowledge meets the "road" of ongoing social performance and effectiveness, and ADHD partially decouples them. What is known is not likely to be done when doing it matters most.

Events predicted to lie in the distant future will elicit planning and anticipatory behaviors in others at a far greater future time horizon than is likely to be seen in those with ADHD. Those with ADHD may not begin to make preparations, if at all, until the event is far closer in time, imminent, or already upon them. They have literally a myopia (nearsightedness) to the future. This pattern is a recipe for a life of chaos and crisis, in which a person with ADHD tries to prepare for future events only at the last minute, if at all. Individuals with ADHD squander their energies dealing with the emergencies or urgencies of the more temporal now, when a few moments of earlier forethought and planning could have eased the burden and likely avoided the crisis. ADHD greatly constricts the temporal window or time horizon over which those with the disorder consider the consequences of their actions, keeping them from coping with the probable future as well as others do. As this theory shows, this is not a choice; it is through no fault of their own that they find themselves in this predicament. The neuropsychological mechanisms (executive functions) for doing so are not operating as effectively for them as for typical individuals.

ADHD and Personal Responsibility

I fully appreciate the conundrum that such conclusions about ADHD pose for the notion of personal accountability and responsibility within society. The argument here could be used by some to seek a legal finding of "diminished capacity" in the mental status of those with ADHD. As that capacity was originally conceived in common law, it was the power to consider one's actions in light of past experience and future consequences as best as one can know them—to deliberate the outcomes of one's acts in relation to time. In a way, those seeking to make such a case would be correct in this analysis: ADHD does create a diminished capacity to deliberate on the outcomes of one's actions, at least in the heat of the moment.

It is clear that ADHD disrupts the cross-temporal organization of behavior, loosens the binding of past and future consequences to the deliberations on current behavior, and lessens the capacity to bridge delays among the elements of a behavioral contingency (events, responses, and outcomes). Given this circumstance, I submit that the required response of others to the poor self-control shown by those with ADHD is *not* to eliminate the outcomes of their actions and to excuse them from personal accountability. It is to temporally tighten up those consequences, emphasizing more immediate accountability. Consequences must be made more immediate, increased in their frequency, made more "external" and salient, and provided more consistently than is likely to be the case for the natural consequences associated with human conduct. Providing more feedback more often is the resulting conclusion; more accountability and holding to responsibility, not less, are the watchwords in helping those with ADHD. Their problem is not so much being held accountable for the outcomes of their actions, but *the delays in that accountability* that are often inherent in those natural outcomes. The most salient natural outcomes of our behavior are often those that are delayed in time, such as eventually being retained in grade after several years of poor school performance, being suspended from school after years of repeated misconduct in that environment, and being arrested and jailed for years of impulsive criminal conduct. The provision of more proximal consequences more often should preclude or minimize the likelihood of these more harmful, socially damaging, yet temporally distant natural outcomes of the conduct of those with ADHD.

Therefore, ADHD is not an excuse but an explanation—not a reason to dismiss outright the ultimate consequences of actions, but a reason to increase accountability by making it more temporally contiguous with those actions. Time, not consequences, is the problem in life's behavioral contingencies for those with ADHD. Therefore, altering time factors, not removing outcomes, is the solution to their problem of "diminished capacity." Time and the future are the nemeses of those with ADHD, not outcomes and personal responsibility. Thus society should not absolve those with ADHD of accountability or responsibility for their actions, but it should absolve them of the moral indignation of others that often accompanies this issue, and it should strive to provide environmental accommodations that make accountability more immediate and frequent.

IMPLICATIONS FOR TREATMENT OF ADHD

Numerous implications for the clinical treatment or management of ADHD stem from the model of executive functions and self-regulation developed here and extrapolated to ADHD (see Barkley, 1997b). Space here permits a brief discussion of only the more important ones.

Blindness to Time as the Ultimate Disability

This text takes as its premise that *a blindness to time is the ultimate yet nearly invisible disability afflicting those with ADHD*. If the ultimate function of the prefrontal lobes is the mental binding of events across time so as to aim behavior more effectively at the probable future (Fuster, 1997) and ADHD is a prefrontal lobe disorder, then those with ADHD should obviously be less capable of doing so. If one cannot see spatial distances very well, the solution is corrective lenses. If one neglects events at spatial distances as a consequence of brain injury, the prescription is cognitive rehabilitation. But what are the solutions for those with a myopia or blindness to time and a neglect of events that lie at great distances ahead in time? And how can those individuals be expected to benefit from any corrective or rehabilitative treatments when the very cognitive mechanisms that subserve the use of these treatments (generalization and maintenance)—the self-regulatory or executive functions—are precisely where the damage caused by ADHD lies?

Teaching time management to a person who cannot *perform* time management, no matter how much he or she may *know* about it, is not going to prove especially fruitful. Given the information in this chapter, we should not be surprised to find that the person with ADHD often may not even show up for the appointments for such rehabilitation, or may nor show up on time, given his or her disability in performing within time. Understanding time and how one comes to organize behavior within it and toward it, then, is a major key to the mystery of understanding ADHD—a key not offered by any other theory of this disorder.

Treating at the Point of Performance

An important implication of this model is that *the most useful treatments are those in place in natural settings at the point of performance, where the desired behavior is to occur.* Ingersoll and Goldstein (1993) say that this "point of performance" seems to be a key concept in the management of those with ADHD. The further away in space and time an intervention is lo-

cated from this point of performance, the less effective it should prove to be for those having ADHD. This implication immediately suggests that clinic-delivered treatments, such as play therapy, counseling of the child, neurofeedback, cognitive therapy, or other such therapies, are not as likely to produce clinically significant improvement in ADHD (if they do so at all) as are treatments undertaken by caregivers in natural settings at the places and times the desired behavior is to be performed. Examples of the latter treatments would include behavior modification, curriculum adjustments, environmental reconfigurations, and other interventions that undertake to restructure the natural setting and its contingencies to achieve a change in the desired behavior *and to maintain that desired behavior over time*. The goal of such environmental reengineering is to help those with ADHD show what they know when it is most essential to be doing so.

Purely Symptomatic Treatment

This perspective suggests an additional implication of the model for treating those with ADHD: Any such treatment will be purely symptomatic. That is, treatments that alter the natural environment to increase desired behavior at critical points of performance will result in changes in that behavior and its maintenance over time only insofar as the treatments are maintained in those places over time. Behavioral treatments or any other environmental reengineering efforts applied at the point of performance will not alter the underlying neuropsychological and largely genetic deficits in behavioral inhibition and executive functioning. They will only provide immediate relief from these deficits by reducing or restructuring those environmental factors that appear to handicap the performance of the individual with ADHD in that setting. If the behavioral treatments and environmental structure created to sustain the behavior are eliminated, the treatment effects should largely or completely disappear.

Behavior modification treatments may be highly successful in altering behavior in the contexts in which they are applied, and in sustaining those treatment gains as long as they are applied. But the removal of the contingencies often heralds the death knell for further maintenance of these treatment gains. Nor should we expect to find that such treatments, even when in place, produce generalization of treatment effects to other settings where no such treatments are in place. Thus treatment of the individual with ADHD should not be considered a "cure" that eliminates the underlying cause of the disorder. Instead, it is a means of providing temporary improvement in the symptoms of the disorder, and even then only in those settings in which such treatments are applied. The larger goal of symptomatic treatment is the reduction of secondary harms that can befall the individual if symptoms and related impairments were left unmanaged. Treatment may be initiated to reduce those future risks that are secondary consequences of having unmanaged ADHD, but as yet, little or no evidence suggests that such benefits accrue from these short-term treatments unless they are sustained over the long term. Nevertheless, the management of behavior in the immediate environments in which it is problematic for those with ADHD is a laudable goal in and of itself, even if it is not shown to produce additional benefits for such individuals in later years. After all, the reduction of immediate distress and improvement in immediate success are legitimate treatment outcomes in their own right if they improve the immediate quality of life for these individuals.

Inhibition and Medication

This theory suggests another implication for the management of ADHD. Only a treatment that can result in improvement of the underlying neuropsychological (neurogenetic) deficit in behavioral inhibition is likely to result in an improvement of the executive functions dependent on such inhibition. The only treatments to date that have any hope of achieving this end are stimulant medications or other psychopharmacological agents that alter the probable neural substrates of ADHD in the prefrontal regions and related networks. Evidence to date suggests that this improvement in inhibition and some of the executive functions may occur as a temporary consequence of active treatment with stimulant medications, but only during the time such a medication remains within the brain (see Chapter 17, this volume). Research on stimulant treatment shows that clinical improvement in behavior occurs in as many as 75–92% of those with the Combined or Predominantly Hyperactive–Impulsive Type of

ADHD, and that such behavior comes to resemble that of typical peers in approximately 50–60% of these cases. The model of ADHD developed here, then, implies that stimulant medication is not only useful for the management of ADHD but the predominant treatment approach among those treatments currently available, because it is the only treatment known to date to produce such improvement rates, albeit temporarily.

Society may view medication treatment of children with ADHD as anathema, largely as a result of a misunderstanding of both the nature of ADHD specifically and the nature of self-control more generally. In both instances, many in society wrongly believe the causes of both ADHD and poor self-control to be chiefly social in nature. Poor child upbringing and management by the parents of the poorly self-controlled children are seen as the most likely culprits. The present model and this book more generally state that not only is this view of ADHD incorrect, but so is this view of self-regulation. ADHD is a disorder of largely genetic and neurological origins, not of child rearing (see Chapter 5). That fact and this model both imply that using medication to temporarily improve or alleviate the underlying neuropsychological dysfunction is a commendable, ethical, and professionally responsible, and humane way of proceeding with treatment for those with ADHD. This does not mean that every person with ADHD requires medication, or that medication is all that is required to manage the disorder. Depending on severity, as well as on comorbidity and the associated adaptive impairments likely to be factors in each clinical case, multiple treatments are likely to be required to address them. But it does mean that there is absolutely nothing wrong or reprehensible about the use of medication to manage a disorder having such a strong biological basis.

Externalizing Information to Manage Behavior

To turn to other specific implications of this model of ADHD for treatment, it can be reasoned that if ADHD results in an undercontrol of behavior by internally represented forms of information, then such information should be "externalized" as much as possible and whenever feasible. That is, it should be made physical and moved outside of the individual once again, as it has to have been in earlier development. The internal forms of information generated by the executive system, if they have been generated at all, appear to be extraordinarily weak in their ability to control and sustain the behavior of those with ADHD toward the future. Self-directed visual imagery, audition, and the other covert re-sensing activities that form nonverbal working memory, as well as covert self-speech, are not yielding up information of sufficient power to control behavior in this disorder (if they are functional at all at certain times and contexts). Behavior is remaining largely under the control of the salient aspects of the immediate context. The solution to this problem is not simply to nag those with ADHD to try harder or to remember what they are supposed to be working on or toward. It is instead to take charge of that immediate context and fill it with various physical cues to supplement their internal counterparts that are proving so ineffective. In a sense, clinicians treating those with ADHD must beat the environment at its own game. Sources of high-appealing distracters that may serve to subvert, pervert, or disrupt task-directed behavior should be minimized whenever possible. In their place should be cues, prompts, and other forms of information that are just as salient and appealing, yet are directly associated with or are an inherent part of the task to be accomplished. Such externalized information serves to cue these individuals to do what they know.

If the rules that are understood to be operative during classroom individual deskwork, for instance, do not seem to be controlling the behavior of a child with ADHD, they should be externalized. The rules can be externalized by posting signs around the classroom that are related to these rules, by creating a poster displayed at the front of the class, or by taping a card listing the rules to the child's desk and having the child frequently refer to this card. Verbally self-stating these rules aloud before and during these individual work performances may also be helpful for older youth with ADHD, once internal language has gained some traction with the motor system. One can also tape-record these reminders on a cassette tape that a child or youth listens to through an earphone while working. It is not the intention of this chapter to articulate the details of the many treatments that can be designed on the basis of this model. That is done in later chapters of this text. All I wish to do here is simply

to show the principle that underlies them—that is, to put external information around children with ADHD and within their sensory fields that may serve to guide their behavior into more appropriate activities. With the knowledge this model provides and a little ingenuity, many of these forms of internally represented information can be externalized for better management of the child or adult with ADHD.

An alternative to externalizing internally represented forms of information, may be removing them entirely from tasks. This is particularly true of information related to time. As I have stated earlier, time and the future are the enemies of people with ADHD when it comes to task accomplishment or performance toward a goal. An obvious solution, then, is to reduce or eliminate these problematic elements of a task when feasible. For instance, rather than assign a behavioral contingency that has large temporal gaps among its elements to someone with ADHD, those temporal gaps should be reduced whenever possible. In other words, the elements should be made more contiguous.

For example, let us consider a book report assigned to a student with ADHD. The assignment stipulates that the report is due in 2 weeks, after which it will be at least 1 week or more before the graded report is returned to the student. There is a 2-week gap between the event (assignment) and response (report) in this contingency, as well as a 1-week gap between the response and its consequence (the grade). Moreover, the grade is a rather weak source of motivation for someone with ADHD, as it is symbolic and secondary. This additional implication of the model—dealing with the requirement for more external sources of behavioral motivation to undergird task or goal-directed performances for those with ADHD—is discussed later. The important point here is that large gaps exist within this temporal contingency, and that these gaps are detrimental to the successful performance of this contingency by those with ADHD. This model suggests, instead, that instructions for the task be presented to a child with ADHD as follows: "(1) Read 1–2 pages right now from your book, then (2) write two to three sentences based on what you read, after which (3) I will give you five tokens [or some other immediate privilege] that you have earned for following this rule." Although the example may seem simplistic, the concepts underlying it are not; these concepts are critical to developing effective management programs for those with ADHD, according to this model. Gaps in time within behavioral contingencies must be reduced or eliminated whenever possible.

When they cannot be eliminated, the sense of time itself, or its passage, needs to be externalized in some way. If the individual's internal cognitive clock is not working well in guiding him or her, an external clock in the immediate context should become part of the task's performance. For instance, instead of telling a child with ADHD that he or she has 30 minutes to get some classwork, homework, or a chore done, caregivers should consider other, more helpful options. Not only does the rule of the assignment need to be more externalized— for example, by using printed rules on chore, homework, or classwork cards, as discussed previously—but the time interval itself should be as well. Caregivers can accomplish this goal by writing that number on the card to signify the time limit, and also by setting a spring-loaded kitchen cooking timer to 30 minutes and placing it before the child while he or she performs the task. Then there is little need for the child to fall back on an internal sense of this temporal duration, as I have shown that this is likely to be inaccurate in its control of behavior (see Chapter 3). Time can be externalized within tasks or settings in many ways that might prove beneficial to those with ADHD. It simply requires some cleverness to devise these. Likewise, other ways of "bridging" temporal delays—limited only by the creativity of the clinician or caregiver—may help those with ADHD. The point once again is not the issue of the particular method to be used, but the concept behind that method: Externalize time and the bridges we use across it!

Externalizing Sources of Motivation and Drive

Yet there is a major caveat to all these implications for externalizing forms of internally represented information. This caveat stems from the component of the model that deals with self-regulation of emotion, motivation, and arousal: No matter how much clinicians, educators, and caregivers externalize prompts, cues, and other signals of the internalized forms of information by which they desire the person with ADHD to be guided (stimuli, events, rules, images, sounds, etc.), doing so is likely to prove only partially and only tempo-

rarily successful. Internal sources of motivation must be augmented with more powerful external forms as well. Not only the internally represented information, but the internally generated sources of motivation associated with this information, are weak in those with ADHD. Those sources of motivation are critical to driving goal-directed behavior toward tasks, the future, and the intended outcome in the absence of external motivation in the immediate context. Addressing one form of internalized information without addressing the other is a sure recipe for ineffectual treatment. Anyone wishing to treat those with ADHD has to understand that sources of motivation must also be externalized in those contexts in which tasks are to be performed, rules followed, and goals accomplished. Complaining to these individuals about their lack of motivation (laziness), drive, willpower, or self-discipline will not suffice to correct the problem. Pulling back from assisting them to let the natural consequences occur, as if this will teach them a lesson that will correct their behavior, is likewise a recipe for disaster. Instead, artificial means of creating external sources of motivation must be arranged *at the point of performance*, in the context in which the work or behavior is desired.

For example, token systems in the form of artificial reward programs for children 5 years of age and older are among the best means to enhance the weak internal sources of motivation in ADHD. Plastic poker chips can be given throughout and at the end of the work performance, as suggested earlier in the book report example. These chips can be exchanged for access to other more salient privileges, rewards, treats, and so on that the children with ADHD may desire. The point here is not as much the technique as the concept. Rewards—in most cases, artificial or socially arranged ones—must be instituted more immediately and more often throughout a task for those with ADHD, and must be tied to more salient reinforcers that are available. Those consequences must be accessible within relatively short periods of time if the behavior of those with ADHD is to be improved. This point applies as much to mild punishments for inappropriate behavior or poor work performance as it does to rewards. And, as I have noted earlier, such artificial sources of motivation must be maintained over long periods, or the gains in performance they initially induce will not be sustained.

The methods of behavior modification are particularly well suited to achieving these ends. Many techniques exist within this form of treatment that can be applied to those with ADHD (see later chapters for such methods). What first needs to be recognized, as this model of ADHD stipulates, is that (1) internalized, self-generated forms of motivation are weak at initiating and sustaining goal-directed behavior; (2) externalized sources of motivation, often artificial, must be arranged within the context at the point of performance; and (3) these compensatory, prosthetic forms of motivation must be sustained for long periods.

Concerning the latter recommendation, it is certainly likely that with neurological maturation, those with ADHD improve their ability to self-generate motivation, as is implied in the concept of a developmental delay. They merely lag behind their normal peers in this capacity at each age at which we examine them. Thus, as for typical children, we can diminish their reliance on external sources of motivation and the intensity and frequency with which they are arranged as they mature and develop the capacity for self-motivation. This means that behavior modification programs using artificial rewards can be "thinned" or reduced in their frequency and immediacy over time as the maturation of children with ADHD results in an increase in their self-motivation ability. But this model also argues that at any age at which we work with an individual with ADHD, such external sources of motivation must still be relied on more than is usual for the individual's age, even though with less rigor, immediacy, frequency, and consistency than at earlier ages.

Addressing Deficits in Reconstitution

Thus far, I have tried to address the treatment implications for the first three executive function deficits in the model of ADHD created here: nonverbal working memory, internalized speech, and self-regulated motivation. How to deal with the problem of reconstitution predicted to be deficient in those with ADHD seems to me to be more difficult to address. If more were known about the process of analysis–synthesis and the behavioral creativity to which it gives rise, ways of externalizing this process might be more evident and useful to those with ADHD. Perhaps taking the problem assigned to an individual with ADHD and

placing its parts on some externally represented material would help, along with prompting and guidance as to how to take apart and move about these forms of information to recombine them into more useful forms. Adults seem to do this when struggling with a difficult problem; they make their previous internal forms of problem-solving behavior external. For instance, we see this when people talk to themselves out loud while solving a difficult puzzle or acquisition of a complex procedure; when they begin to doodle on a pad, playing with certain designs or relationships among pieces of critical information; when they free-associate publicly to the topic of the problem under discussion; or even when they reduce a number of words to slips of paper or pieces of magnets and then randomly reshuffle them to create new arrangements. Regardless, the point of this discussion is the same as for the other executive functions: By externalizing what should otherwise be internally represented information, and even externalizing the process by which that information is being generated and recombined, caregivers may be able to assist those with ADHD in compensating for their weak executive functions. Again, such structuring of tasks and contexts must be sustained over long periods if the gains it initially achieves are to be sustained as well.

Managing ADHD as a Chronic Disability

The foregoing discussion leads to a much more general implication of this model of ADHD: The approach taken to its management must be the same as that taken in the management of other chronic medical or psychiatric disabilities. I frequently use diabetes as an analogous condition to ADHD in trying to assist parents and other professionals in grasping this point. At the time of diagnosis, all involved realize that no cure exists as yet for the condition. Still, multiple means can provide symptomatic relief from the deleterious effects of the condition, including taking daily doses of medication and changing settings, tasks, and lifestyles. Immediately following diagnosis, the clinician designs and implements a treatment package on the condition. This package must be maintained over long periods to maintain the symptomatic relief that the treatments initially achieve. Ideally, the treatment package, so maintained, will reduce or eliminate the secondary consequences of leaving the condition unmanaged. However, each patient is different, and so is each instance of the chronic condition being treated. As a result, symptom breakthroughs and crises are likely to occur periodically over the course of treatment; these may demand reintervention, or the design and implementation of modified or entirely new treatment packages. Throughout all this management, the goal of the clinician, the family members, and the patient him- or herself is to try to achieve an improvement in the quality of life and success for the individual, though it may never be totally "normal."

KEY CLINICAL POINTS

✓ This chapter has constructed a hybrid model of the nature of executive functions (see especially Figure 7.7).

✓ The first component is behavioral inhibition, which is the foundation on which the four executive functions depend.

✓ These four functions are nonverbal working memory, verbal working memory, the self-regulation of affect/motivation/arousal, and reconstitution. All are hypothesized to be covert, self-directed forms of behavior that yield internally represented information and that exert a controlling influence over the sixth component of the model: the motor control and execution system.

✓ Redefined in terms of their behavioral equivalents, the executive functions are (1) covert, self-directed sensing (nonverbal working memory); (2) covert, self-directed speech (verbal working memory); (3) covert, self-directed affect/motivation/arousal or emoting to oneself; and (4) covert, self-directed behavioral manipulation, experimentation, and play (reconstitution). Each is believed to derive from its more public, observable counterparts in human behavior, which have become turned on the self and made progressively more private, covert, or unobservable (internalized) in form.

✓ These executive functions permit outer behavior to be guided by forms of inner action that effectively bridge delays in cross-temporal contingencies and direct behavior toward hypothetical future events (outcomes, goals, etc.).

✓ They also give rise to a new form of sustained responding (attention), apart from that form controlled by the immediate prevailing contingencies; this new sustained responding arises out of such internally guided forms of behavior directed toward a goal.

✓ Time, timing, and timeliness, then, become important concepts in understanding such goal-directed behavior and in determining it—making time and the social future, in a way, the "central executive." The ultimate purpose of these executive actions and the self-regulation relative to time they provide is the net maximization of long-term consequences for the benefit of the individual's self-interests.

✓ ADHD is a disorder of inhibiting behavior; as such, it disrupts the development and effective performance of the executive functions and the self-regulation they permit.

✓ Those with ADHD are left with a form of temporal nearsightedness or time blindness. This temporal myopia produces substantial social, educational, and occupational devastation via its disruption of day-to-day adaptive functioning relative to time and the future.

✓ A number of treatment implications flow from this model for the management of ADHD. Among them is a justification for the use of medications as a temporary corrective treatment for the underlying neuropsychological deficits in behavioral inhibition and self-control.

✓ Medications need to be accompanied by the externalization of sources of information aimed at controlling the individual's behavior.

✓ Behavioral motivation must be made external as well, by arranging artificial consequences at key places in the environment or task where they do not usually occur.

✓ Such modifications must be sustained over long periods if they are to continue to benefit the individual with ADHD.

✓ A chronic disability perspective seems more appropriate to the management of ADHD, as it is for diabetes, than would be a short-term curative model (e.g., the treatment of infection with antibiotics).

REFERENCES

Achenbach, T. M., & Edelbrock, C. S. (1983). *Manual for the Child Behavior Profile and Child Behavior Checklist.* Burlington, VT: Author.

American Psychiatric Association. (1994). *Diagnostic and statistical manual of mental disorders* (4th ed.). Washington, DC: Author.

American Psychiatric Association. (2000). *Diagnostic and statistical manual of mental disorders* (4th ed., text rev.). Washington, DC: Author.

Baddeley, A. D., & Hitch, G. J. (1994). Developments in the concept of working memory. *Neuropsychology, 8,* 1485–1493.

Barkley, R. A. (1995). Linkages between attention and executive functions. In G. R. Lyon & N. A. Krasnegor (Eds.), *Attention, memory, and executive function* (pp. 307–326). Baltimore: Brookes.

Barkley, R. A. (1997a). Behavioral inhibition, sustained attention, and executive functions: Constructing a unifying theory of ADHD. *Psychological Bulletin, 121,* 65–94.

Barkley, R. A. (1997b). *ADHD and the nature of self-control.* New York: Guilford Press.

Barkley, R. A. (2001). The executive functions and self-regulation: An evolutionary neuropsychological perspective. *Neuropsychology Review, 11,* 1–29.

Beauchaine, T. P., Katkin, E. S., Strassberg, Z., & Snarr, J. (2001). Disinhibitory psychopathology in male adolescents: Discriminating conduct disorder from attention-deficit/hyperactivity disorder through concurrent assessment of multiple autonomic states. *Journal of Abnormal Psychology, 110,* 610–624.

Berk, L. E., & Potts, M. K. (1991). Development and functional significance of private speech among attention-deficit hyperactivity disorder and normal boys. *Journal of Abnormal Child Psychology, 19,* 357–377.

Bronowski, J. (1977). Human and animal languages. In P. E. Ariotti (Ed.), *A sense of the future* (pp. 104–131). Cambridge, MA: MIT Press.

Brown, J. W. (1990). Psychology of time awareness. *Brain and Cognition, 14,* 144–164.

Butters, M. A., Kaszniak, A. W., Glisky, E. L., Eslinger, P. J., & Schacter, D. L. (1994). Recency discrimination deficits in frontal lobe patients. *Neuropsychology, 8,* 343–353.

Campbell, D. T. (1960). Blind variation and selective retention in creative thought as in other knowledge processes. *Psychological Review, 67,* 380–400.

Castellanos, F. X., Giedd, J. N., Marsh, W. L., Hamburger, S. D., Vaituzis, A. C., Dickstein, D. P., et al. (1996). Quantitative brain magnetic resonance imaging in attention-deficit hyperactivity disorder. *Archives of General Psychiatry, 53,* 607–616.

Damasio, A. R. (1994). *Descartes' error: Emotion, reason, and the human brain.* New York: Putnam.

Damasio, A. R. (1995). On some functions of the human prefrontal cortex. *Annals of the New York Academy of Sciences, 769,* 241–251.

Denckla, M. B. (1994). Measurement of executive function. In G. R. Lyon (Ed.), *Frames of reference for the assessment of learning disabilities: New views on measurement issues* (pp. 117–142). Baltimore: Brookes.

Denckla, M. B. (1996). A theory and model of executive function: A neuropsychological perspective. In G. R. Lyon & N. A. Krasnegor (Eds.), *Attention, memory, and executive function* (pp. 263–277). Baltimore: Brookes.

Diaz, R. M., & Berk, L. E. (1992). *Private speech: From social interaction to self-regulation.* Mahwah, NJ: Erlbaum.

Douglas, V. I. (1972). Stop, look, and listen: The problem of sustained attention and impulse control in hyperactive and normal children. *Canadian Journal of Behavioural Science, 4,* 259–282.

Douglas, V. I. (1983). Attention and cognitive problems. In M. Rutter (Ed.), *Developmental neuropsychiatry* (pp. 280–329). New York: Guilford Press.

Douglas, V. I. (1988). Cognitive deficits in children with attention deficit disorder with hyperactivity. In L. M. Bloomingdale & J. A. Sergeant (Eds.), *Attention deficit disorder: Criteria, cognition, intervention* (pp. 65–82). London: Pergamon Press.

Douglas, V. I., Barr, R. G., Desilets, J., & Sherman, E. (1995). Do high doses of stimulants impair flexible thinking in attention-deficit hyperactivity disorder? *Journal of the American Academy of Child and Adolescent Psychiatry, 34,* 877–885.

Ekman, P., & Davidson, R. J. (Eds.). (1994). *The nature of emotion: Fundamental questions.* New York: Oxford University Press.

Filipek, P. A., Semrud-Clikeman, M., Steingard, R. J., Renshaw, P. F., Kennedy, D. N., & Biederman, J. (1997). Volumetric MRI analysis comparing subjects having attention-deficit hyperactivity disorder with normal controls. *Neurology, 48,* 589–601.

Fingerman, K. L., & Perlmutter, M. (1994). Future time perspective and life events across adulthood. *Journal of General Psychology, 122,* 95–111.

Flavell, J. H., Miller, P. H., & Miller, S. A. (1993). *Cognitive development.* Englewood Cliffs, NJ: Prentice-Hall.

Frijda, N. H. (1994). Emotions are functional, most of the time. In P. Ekman & R. J. Davidson (Eds.), *The nature of emotion: Fundamental questions* (pp. 112–122). New York: Oxford University Press.

Fuster, J. M. (1997). *The prefrontal cortex* (3rd ed.). New York: Raven Press.

Godbout, L., & Doyon, J. (1995). Mental representation of knowledge following frontal-lobe or postrolandic lesions. *Neuropsychologia, 33,* 1671–1696.

Goldberg, E., & Podell, K. (1995). Lateralization in the frontal lobes. In H. H. Jasper, S. Riggio, & P. S. Goldman-Rakic (Eds.), *Epilepsy and the functional anatomy of the frontal lobe* (pp. 85–96). New York: Raven Press.

Goldman-Rakic, P. S. (1995). Architecture of the prefrontal cortex and the central executive. *Annals of the New York Academy of Sciences, 769,* 71–83.

Grafman, J. (1995). Similarities and distinctions among current models of prefrontal cortical functions. *Annals of the New York Academy of Sciences, 769,* 337–368.

Green, L., Fry, A. F., & Meyerson, J. (1994). Discounting of delayed rewards: A life-span comparison. *Psychological Science, 5,* 33–36.

Grodzinsky, G. M., & Diamond, R. (1992). Frontal lobe functioning in boys with attention-deficit hyperactivity disorder. *Developmental Neuropsychology, 8,* 427–445.

Hayes, S. C., Gifford, E. V., & Ruckstuhl, L. E., Jr. (1996). Relational frame theory and executive function: A behavioral analysis. In G. R. Lyon & N. A. Krasnegor (Eds.), *Attention, memory, and executive function* (pp. 279–306). Baltimore: Brookes.

Hudziak, J. (1997, October). *The genetics of attention deficit hyperactivity disorder.* Paper presented at the annual meeting of the American Academy of Child and Adolescent Psychiatry, Toronto.

Ingersoll, B., & Goldstein, S. (1993). *Attention deficit disorder and learning disabilities: Realities, myths, and controversial treatments.* New York: Doubleday.

Kertesz, A., Nicholson, I., Cancelliere, A., Kassa, K., & Black, S. E. (1985). Motor impersistence: A right hemisphere syndrome. *Neurology, 35,* 662–666.

Knight, R. T., Grabowecky, M. F., & Scabini, D. (1995). Role of human prefrontal cortex in attention control. In H. H. Jasper, S. Riggio, & P. S. Goldman-Rakic (Eds.), *Epilepsy and the functional anatomy of the frontal lobe* (pp. 21–34). New York: Raven Press.

Kopp, C. B. (1982). Antecedents of self-regulation: A developmental perspective. *Developmental Psychology, 18,* 199–214.

Lang, P. J. (1995). The emotion probe: Studies of motivation and attention. *American Psychologist, 50,* 372–385.

Luman, M., Oosterlaan, J., & Sergeant, J. A. (2005). The impact of reinforcement contingencies on AD/HD: A review and theoretical appraisal. *Clinical Psychology Review, 25,* 183–213.

Luria, A. R. (1961). *The role of speech in the regulation of normal and abnormal behavior* (J. Tizard, Ed.). New York: Liveright.

McAndrews, M. P., & Milner, B. (1991). The frontal cortex and memory for temporal order. *Neuropsychologia, 29,* 849–859.

Michon, J. A., & Jackson, J. L. (1984). Attentional effort and cognitive strategies in the processing of temporal information. *Annals of the New York Academy of Sciences, 423,* 298–321.

Milich, R., Ballentine, A. C., & Lynam, D. R. (2001). ADHD/combined type and ADHD/predominantly inattentive type are distinct and unrelated disorders. *Clinical Psychology: Science and Practice, 8,* 463–488.

Milich, R., Hartung, C. M., Matrin, C. A., & Haigler, E. D. (1994). Behavioral disinhibition and underlying processes in adolescents with disruptive behavior disorders. In D. K. Routh (Ed.), *Disruptive behavior disorders in childhood* (pp. 109–138). New York: Plenum Press.

Milner, B. (1995). Aspects of human frontal lobe function. In H. H. Jasper, S. Riggio, & P. S. Goldman-Rakic (Eds.), *Epilepsy and the functional anatomy of the frontal lobe* (pp. 67–81). New York: Raven Press.

Mirsky, A. F. (1996). Disorders of attention: A neuropsychological perspective. In R. G. Lyon & N. A. Krasnegor (Eds.), *Attention, memory, and executive function* (pp. 71–96). Baltimore: Brookes.

Nigg, J. T. (2001). Is ADHD an inhibitory disorder? *Psychological Bulletin, 125,* 571–596.

Oosterlaan, J., & Sergeant, J. A. (1995). Response choice and inhibition in ADHD, anxious, and aggressive children: The relationship between S-R compatibility and stop signal task. In J. A. Sergeant (Ed.), *Eunethydis: European approaches to hyperkinetic disorder* (pp. 225–240). Amsterdam: University of Amsterdam.

Oosterlaan, J., & Sergeant, J. A. (1996). Inhibition in ADHD, anxious, and aggressive children: A biologically based model of child psychology. *Journal of Abnormal Child Psychology, 24,* 19–36.

Pardo, J. V., Fox, P. T., & Raichle, M. E. (1991). Localization of a human system for sustained attention by positron emission tomography. *Nature, 349,* 61–64.

Pennington, B. F., & Ozonoff, S. (1996). Executive functions and developmental psychopathology. *Journal of Child Psychology and Psychiatry, 37,* 51–87.

Quay, H. C. (1988a). The behavioral reward and inhibition systems in childhood behavior disorder. In L. M. Bloomingdale (Ed.), *Attention deficit disorder: Vol. 3. New research in treatment, psychopharmacology, and attention* (pp. 176–186). New York: Pergamon Press.

Quay, H. C. (1988b). Attention deficit disorder and the behavioral inhibition system: The relevance of the neuropsychological theory of Jeffrey A. Gray. In L. M. Bloomingdale & J. Sergeant (Eds.), *Attention deficit disorder: Criteria, cognition, intervention* (pp. 117–126). New York: Pergamon Press.

Quay, H. F. (1997). Inhibition and attention deficit hyperactivity disorder. *Journal of Abnormal Child Psychology, 25,* 7–14.

Roberts, R. J., & Pennington, B. F. (1996). An integrative framework for examining prefrontal cognitive processes. *Developmental Neuropsychology, 12,* 105–126.

Rueckert, L., & Grafman, J. (1996). Sustained attention deficits in patients with right frontal lesions. *Neuropsychologia, 34,* 953–963.

Schachar, R. J., Tannock, R., & Logan, G. (1993). Inhibitory control, impulsiveness, and attention deficit hyperactivity disorder. *Clinical Psychology Review, 13,* 721–739.

Seidman, L. J., Biederman, J., Faraone, S. V., Milberger, S., Norman, D., Seiverd, K., et al. (1995). Effects of family history and comorbidity on the neuropsychological performance of children with ADHD: Preliminary findings. *Journal of the American Academy of Child and Adolescent Psychiatry, 34,* 1015–1024.

Sergeant, J. A. (1995a). Hyperkinetic disorder revisited. In J. A. Sergeant (Ed.), *Eunethydis: European approaches to hyperkinetic disorder* (pp. 7–17). Amsterdam: University of Amsterdam.

Sergeant, J. A. (1995b). A theory of attention: An information processing perspective. In G. R. Lyon & N. A. Krasnegor (Eds.), *Attention, memory, and executive function* (pp. 57–69). Baltimore: Brookes.

Sergeant, J. A. (1996, January). *The cognitive–energetic model of ADHD.* Paper presented at the annual meeting of the International Society for Research in Child and Adolescent Psychopathology, Los Angeles.

Sergeant, J. A., & van der Meere, J. (1988). What happens when the hyperactive child commits an error? *Psychiatry Research, 24,* 157–164.

Sirigu, A., Zalla, T., Pillon, B., Grafman, J., Bubois, B., & Agid, Y. (1995). *Annals of the New York Academy of Sciences, 769,* 277–288.

Skinner, B. F. (1969). *Contingencies of reinforcement: A theoretical analysis.* New York: Appleton-Century-Crofts.

Sonuga-Barke, E. J. S. (2002). Interval length and time-use by children with AD/HD: A comparison of four models. *Journal of Abnormal Child Psychology, 30,* 257–264.

Sonuga-Barke, E. J. S., Taylor, E., & Hepinstall, E. (1992). Hyperactivity and delay aversion: II. The effect of self versus externally imposed stimulus presentation periods on memory. *Journal of Child Psychology and Psychiatry, 33,* 399–409.

Torgesen, J. K. (1994). Issues in the assessment of executive function: An information-processing perspective. In G. R. Lyon (Ed.), *Frames of reference for the assessment of learning disabilities: New views on measurement issues* (pp. 143–162). Baltimore: Brookes.

van der Meere, J., van Baal, M., & Sergeant, J. (1989). The additive factor method: A differential diagnostic tool in hyperactivity and learning disability. *Journal of Abnormal Child Psychology, 17,* 409–422.

Vygotsky, L. S. (1978). *Mind in society.* Cambridge, MA: Harvard University Press.

Vygotsky, L. S. (1987). Thinking and speech. In R. W. Rieber & A. S. Carton (Eds.), *The collected works of L. S. Vygotsky: Vol. 1. Problems in general psychology* (N. Minick, Trans.). New York: Plenum Press.

Welsh, M. C., & Pennington, B. F. (1988). Assessing frontal lobe functioning in children: Views from developmental psychology. *Developmental Neuropsychology, 4,* 199–230.

Welsh, M. C., Pennington, B. F., & Grossier, D. B. (1991). A normative–developmental study of executive function: A window on prefrontal function in children. *Developmental Neuropsychology, 7,* 131–149.

Weyandt, L. L., & Willis, W. G. (1994). Executive functions in school-aged children: Potential efficacy of tasks in discriminating clinical groups. *Developmental Neuropsychology, 19,* 27–38.

Wheeler, M. A., Stuss, D. T., & Tulving, E. (1997). Toward a theory of episodic memory: The frontal lobes and autonoetic consciousness. *Psychological Bulletin, 121,* 331–354.

Wright, R. (2000). *Nonzero: The logic of human destiny.* New York: Pantheon.

PART II

ASSESSMENT

CHAPTER 8

Diagnostic Interview, Behavior Rating Scales, and the Medical Examination

RUSSELL A. BARKLEY
GWENYTH EDWARDS

The evaluation of a child (or an adult, for that matter) with Attention-Deficit/Hyperactivity Disorder (ADHD) is driven by the issues involved in each case, and not by the methods that clinicians just happen to know and prefer. For that reason, the evaluation will vary, sometimes considerably, from case to case as the issues vary, rather than consisting of the same methods for each and every case. But a core set of issues often exists across cases and can be used as a starting framework for understanding the necessary components of an appropriate assessment protocol. For example, Table 8.1 lists issues common across many cases, together with the method(s) that could be used to address each issue. The table is intended only to provide an example. The point here is for the clinician to select the best reasonable method currently available to address each issue.

As Table 8.1 indicates, the most important component in a comprehensive evaluation of a child suspected of having ADHD is the clinical interview—in this case, with the parents and, later, teachers. (The interview is of equal importance for adults presenting for evaluation of their own ADHD symptoms, as Chapter 11 of this volume describes.) In this chapter, we describe the details of conducting clinical interviews with parents, teachers, and children/adolescents when a child or adolescent is presenting for evaluation of ADHD. We also briefly discuss the essential features of the medical examination of such a child or adolescent, and the issues this examination needs to address. This discussion is followed by an overview of some of the most useful behavior rating scales to incorporate in the clinical evaluation. When it is feasible, clinicians may wish to supplement these components of the evaluation with objective assessments of the ADHD symptoms, such as psychological tests of attention or direct behavioral observations. These tests are not essential to reaching a diagnosis or to treatment planning, but they may yield further information about the presence and severity of cognitive impairments that could be associated with some cases of ADHD. These methods of assessment are discussed in Chapter 9 of this volume. Ten case examples of child/adolescent evaluations can be found in Chapter 10. Readers wishing to have many of the clinical tools referenced here can find them in a convenient format, with limited permission granted by the publisher for photocopying, in the clin-

TABLE 8.1. Common Issues in Assessment

Issue	Method
• Current concerns about the child • History of those concerns (onset, course, periodicity, etc.) • Differentiation among other disorders	• Unstructured interview • Semistructured interview • Structured interview based on the *Diagnostic and Statistical Manual of Mental Disorders* (DSM) • Well-normed behavior rating scales • Semistructured interview of developmental domains (e.g., motor, language, social, educational, etc.)
• Developmental inappropriateness of symptoms or concerns • Comorbidity • Impairments • Psychological adjustment of parents	• DSM diagnostic thresholds • Well-normed behavior rating scales • Psychological testing (see Chapter 9) • Structured, DSM-based interview • Screen of intelligence (testing) • Screen of achievement skills (testing) • Interviews with parents, teachers, etc. • Review of prior school and medical records • Adaptive functioning interviews/scales • Symptom Checklist 90—Revised • Marital/couple functioning screen • Parenting stress screen • Parental screen for ADHD (or other disorders as appropriate)
• Child and parent strengths • Community resources	• Semistructured interview • Semistructured interview and search of available professional services

ical workbook accompanying this textbook (Barkley & Murphy, 2006).

ASSESSMENT GOALS

As indicated above, clinicians should bear in mind several common goals when evaluating children for ADHD. A major goal of such an assessment is the determination of the presence or absence of ADHD, as well as the differential diagnosis of ADHD from other childhood psychiatric disorders. This differential diagnosis requires extensive clinical knowledge of these other psychiatric disorders, and readers are referred to a text on child psychopathology for a review of the major childhood disorders (see Mash & Barkley, 2003). In any child evaluation, it may be necessary to draw on measures that have norms for the individual's ethnic background (if such instruments are available), to preclude the overdiagnosis of minority children when diagnostic criteria developed on white American children are extrapolated to other ethnic groups. But diagnosis is merely a means to an end, not an end in itself.

A second purpose of the evaluation is the actual reason to diagnose: It is to begin delineating the types of interventions needed to address the psychiatric disorders and psychological, academic, and social impairments identified in the course of assessment. As noted later, these may include individual counseling, parent training in behavior management, family therapy, classroom behavior modification, psychiatric medications, and formal special educational services, to name just a few. For a more thorough discussion of treatments for childhood disorders, readers are referred to a recent text on this subject (Mash & Barkley, 2006).

Another important purpose of the evaluation is to determine conditions that often coexist with ADHD and the manner in which these conditions may affect prognosis or treatment decision making. For instance, the presence of high levels of physically assaultive behavior by a child with ADHD may indicate that a parent training program (see, e.g., the one recommended in Chapter 12 of this text) is contraindicated, at least for the time being, because such training in limit setting and behavior modification could temporarily increase child violence toward parents when limits on non-compliance with parental commands are established. Or consider the presence of high levels of anxiety specifically and internalizing symptoms more generally in children with ADHD. Research suggests that such symptoms may be a predictor of poorer responses to stimulant medication (see Chapter 17). Similarly, the presence of high levels of irritable mood, severely hostile and defiant behavior, and periodic episodes of serious physical aggression and destructive behavior may be early markers for later Bipolar I Disorder (manic–depression) in children. Oppositional behavior is almost universal in juvenile-onset Bipolar I Disorder (Wozniak et al., 1995). Such a disorder is likely to require the use of psychiatric medication in conjunction with a parent training program.

A further objective of the evaluation is to identify the pattern of the child's psychological strengths and weaknesses and to consider how these strengths and weaknesses, may be useful in treatment planning. This identification may also include gaining some impression of the parents' own abilities to carry out the treatment program, as well as the family's social and economic circumstances and the treatment resources that may (or may not) be available within their community and cultural group. Some determination also must be made of the child's eligibility for special educational services within his or her school district, if eligible disorders (such as developmental delay, learning disabilities, or speech and language problems) are present.

As the foregoing discussion illustrates, the evaluation of a child for the presence of diagnosable ADHD is but one of many purposes of the clinical evaluation. A brief discussion now follows regarding the different assessment methods that may be used in the evaluation of children with ADHD.

INFORMATION OBTAINED AT THE TIME OF REFERRAL

Surprisingly enough, the initial phase of a diagnostic interview may not be conducted by the clinician, but by a support staff member. The initial phone intake provides invaluable information when conducted by a well-trained individual; otherwise, it is a lost opportunity. When a parent calls to request an evaluation, it is useful to collect the following information:

- What is the reason for the parent's request? Is it an open-ended question, such as "What's wrong with my child?", or a specific one, such as "Does my child have ADHD?"
- Who referred the family? Is the family self-referred because members recently read a newspaper article or saw a television program which raised their concerns? Is the family referred by the child's school because of school-related rather than parental concerns? Or is the family referred by a pediatrician or another health or mental health professional who questions ADHD but wants diagnostic confirmation?
- Has the child been previously evaluated or tested by someone else? Is the family looking for a second opinion, or for a reevaluation of ADHD that was diagnosed when the child was younger?
- Does the child have any other diagnosed conditions, such as mood disorders, substance abuse, or other developmental delays? Has the child been tested and diagnosed by the school system as having learning disabilities or cognitive delays?
- Is the child already on medication? Are the parents seeking an evaluation of their child's response to medication, rather than a diagnostic evaluation? If the child is on stimulant medication, would the parents consent to withhold the medication on the day of the evaluation?

The content of the diagnostic interview is influenced by all these factors, and important information can be collected and reviewed ahead of time when the reason for the referral is clear. Thus, once the child is referred for services, the clinician (or support staff member) must glean some important details from the telephone interview. This information also allows the clinician to set in motion some initial procedures. In particular, it is important at this point to do the following: (1) obtain any necessary releases of information, to permit reports of previous professional evaluations to be sought; (2) contact the child's treating physician for further information on health status and medication treatment, if any; (3) obtain the results of the most recent evaluation from the child's school, or have the parent initiate one immediately, if school performance concerns are part of the referral complaints; (4) mail out the packet of parent and teacher behavior rating forms to be completed and returned before the initial appointment, being sure to include the written release-of-information permission form with the school forms; and (5) obtain any information from social service agencies that may be involved in providing services to this child.

INFORMATION OBTAINED IN ADVANCE OF THE INTERVIEW

A clinician may want to send out a packet of questionnaires to parents and teachers following the parents' call to the clinic but in advance of the scheduled appointment. In these days of increasing cost consciousness concerning mental health evaluations (particularly in managed care environments), efficiency of the evaluation is paramount, and time spent directly with the family is often limited and at a premium. Besides a form cover letter from the professional asking the parents to complete the packet of information, the packet may also contain the General Instruction Sheet, the Child and Family Information Form, and the Developmental and Medical History Form, all of which can be obtained for limited photocopying purposes in the clinical manual accompanying this textbook (Barkley & Murphy, 2006). This packet should also include a reasonably comprehensive child behavior rating scale that covers the major dimensions of child psychopathology, such as the Child Behavior Checklist (CBCL; Achenbach, 2001) or the Behavior Assessment System for Children (BASC-2; Reynolds & Kamphaus, 2004), to begin to screen for areas of potential psychopathology even before the appointment. Also in this packet should be a copy of a rating scale that specifically assesses ADHD symptoms. Such a form can also be found in the clinical manual by Barkley and Murphy (2006). That scale permits the clinician to obtain information ahead of the appointment concerning the presence of symptoms of Oppositional Defiant Disorder (ODD) and Conduct Disorder (CD), as well as ADHD symptoms and their severity. ODD and CD are quite common among children referred for ADHD, and it is useful to know of their presence in advance of the appointment. Or clinicians might consider using the ADHD Rating Scale–IV by DuPaul, Power, Anastopoulos, and

Reid (1998). Clinicians who wish to assess adaptive behavior via the use of a questionnaire might consider including the Normative Adaptive Behavior Checklist (NABC; Adams, 1984) in this packet. Finally, the Home Situations Questionnaire (HSQ) is included so that the clinician can gain a quick appreciation for the pervasiveness and severity of the child's disruptive behavior across a variety of home and public situations (see Barkley & Murphy, 2006, for this form and its norms). Such information is of clinical interest not only for indications of pervasiveness and severity of behavior problems, but also for focusing discussions around these situations during the evaluation and subsequent parent training program. These rating scales are discussed later.

It is useful to collect and review previous records before the interview. These might include any one or combination of the following: school report cards, standardized testing results, medical records (including neurology, audiology, optometry, speech, and occupational therapy), school individual educational plans, psychoeducational testing, psychological testing, and psychotherapy summaries.

A packet of rating scales should also be sent to the teachers of this child, with parental written permission obtained beforehand, of course. This packet could contain the teacher version of the CBCL or BASC, the School Situations Questionnaire (SSQ), and the same rating scale for assessing ADHD symptoms (see Barkley & Murphy, 2006, for the latter two scales and their norms). The Social Skills Rating System (Gresham & Elliott, 1990) might also be included if the clinician desires information about the child's social problems in school, as well as his or her academic competence. (However, too large a packet of scales may overwhelm teachers, who generally have limited time available for such requests, and thus may not return the scales if there are too many.) From these scales, the clinician can quickly see, for example, whether a teacher feels the child is functioning at grade level in various subject areas, how the child has performed on group-administered achievement or aptitude tests, or how the teacher perceives the child's general mood and behavioral functioning. If possible, it is quite useful to contact the child's teachers for a brief telephone interview prior to meeting with the family. Otherwise, a meeting can take place following the family's appointment.

Alternatively, and more traditionally, the clinician may conduct an intake interview with the parents first. Then any rating scales deemed necessary may be completed by parents and teachers. During a second session, the clinician can conduct the child interview and any testing. The feedback session with parents may be conducted during a third session. The disadvantage here, however, is that the clinician does not have the information from these scales, which could have been used to guide the interview more intelligently.

On the day of the appointment, the following still remains to be done: (1) parental and child interview; (2) completion of self-report rating scales by the parents; and (3) any psychological testing that may be indicated by the nature of the referral (intelligence and achievement testing, etc.).

PARENT INTERVIEW

The parent (often maternal) interview, although often criticized for its unreliability and subjectivity (Angold, Erkalni, Costello, & Rutter, 1996), is an indispensable part of the evaluation for any child or adolescent with possible ADHD, particularly regarding behavior at home and in community settings. No other adult is more likely than the parents to have the wealth of knowledge about, history of interactions with, or sheer time spent with a child. As stated in the practice parameters for the assessment and treatment of ADHD (American Academy of Child and Adolescent Psychiatry, 1997), the parental interview is the core of the assessment process.

Whether wholly accurate or not, parent reports provide the most ecologically valid and important source of information concerning the child's difficulties. It is the parents' complaints that often lead to the referral of the child, will affect the parents' perceptions of and reactions to the child, and will influence the parents' adherence to the treatment recommendations to be made. Moreover, the reliability and accuracy of the parental interview have much to do with the manner in which it is conducted and the specificity of the questions offered by the examiner. An interview with highly specific questions about symptoms of psychopathology, history, course, and periodicity that have been empirically demonstrated to have a high degree of association with particular disorders greatly enhances diagnostic reliability. For instance, although parents' recall may be imperfect with regard to precise times or ages of symptom onset (Angold et al., 1996), they remain quite reliable and accurate with regard to symptom presence and whether or not a diagnosis is rendered (Faraone, Biederman, & Milberger, 1995; Kentgen, Klein, Mannuzza, & Davies, 1997).

We do not typically have the child in the same room when we conduct the parental interview. Other clinicians may choose to do so; the presence of the child during the parental interview, however, raises thorny issues for the evaluation, to which an examiner must be sensitive. Some parents are less forthcoming about their concerns and the details of the child's specific problems when the child is present, because they do not wish to sensitize or embarrass the child unnecessarily or to create another reason for arguments at home about the nature of the child's problems. Others are heedless of the potential problems posed for their child by this procedure, making it even more imperative that the examiner review these issues with them before beginning the evaluation. Still other parents may use the child's presence to further publicly humiliate the child about his or her deficiencies or the distress the child has created for the family by behaving the way he or she does. Suffice it to say here that before starting the interview, the examiner must discuss and review with each family whether the advantages of having the child present are outweighed by these potential negative effects.

A structured interview, such as the Diagnostic Interview Schedule for Children (Shaffer, Fischer, Lucas, Dulcan, & Schwab-Stone, 2000) or the Diagnostic Interview for Children and Adolescents (Reich, 1997), provides the most reliable method for gathering information about existing symptoms of psychopathology in both externalizing and internalizing domains. The semistructured portion of the interview must also, however, focus on the specific complaints about the child's psychological adjustment and any functional parameters (eliciting and consequating events) associated with those problems if psychosocial and educational treatment planning is to be based on the evaluation.

Purposes

The parental interview often serves several purposes:

1. It establishes a necessary rapport between the parents and the examiner, which will prove invaluable in enlisting parental cooperation with later aspects of assessment and treatment.

2. The interview is an obvious source of highly descriptive information about the child and family, revealing the parents' particular views of the child's apparent problems and narrowing the focus of later stages and components of the evaluation. If the child is present during this interview, the examiner must be cautious not to overinterpret any informal observations of the child's behavior during this clinic visit. The office behavior of children with ADHD is often far better than that observed at home (Sleator & Ullmann, 1981). Such observations merely raise hypotheses about potential parent–child interaction problems, which can be explored in more detail with parents toward the end of this interview, as well as during later direct behavioral observations of parents and child during play and task performance together. At the end of this portion of the interview, the examiner should inquire how representative the child's immediate behavior is of that seen at home when the parent speaks with other adults in the child's presence.

3. It can readily reveal the degree of distress the child's problems are presenting to the family (especially the parent being interviewed, if only one is present), as well as the overall psychological integrity of the parent(s). Hypotheses as to the presence of parental personality or psychiatric problems (depression, hostility, marital/couple discord, etc.) may arise; if so, these will require further evaluation in subsequent components of the evaluation and consideration in formulating treatment recommendations.

4. The initial parent interview can help to focus the parents' perceptions of the child's problems on more important and more specific controlling events within the family. Parents often tend to emphasize historical or developmental causes of a global nature in discussing their child's problems, such as what they did or failed to do with the child earlier in development that has led to this problem (e.g., placing the child in infant daycare, an earlier divorce, the child's diet in earlier years, etc.). The interaction interview discussed later can serve to shift the parents' attention to more immediate antecedents and consequences surrounding child behaviors, thereby preparing the parents

for the initial stages of parent training in child management skills.

5. The interview is designed to formulate a diagnosis and to develop treatment recommendations. Although diagnosis is not always considered necessary for treatment planning (a statement of the child's developmental and behavioral deficits is often adequate), the diagnosis of ADHD does provide some utility in terms of predicting developmental course and prognosis for the child, determining eligibility for some special educational placements, and predicting potential response to a trial on stimulant medication. Many child behavior problems are believed to remit over short periods in as many as 75% of cases. However, ADHD is a relatively chronic condition, warranting much more cautious conclusions about eventual prognosis and careful preparation of the family for coping with these later problems.

6. A parental interview may serve as sheer catharsis, especially if this is the first professional evaluation of the child or if previous evaluations have proven highly conflicting in their results and recommendations. Ample time should be permitted to allow parents to ventilate any distress, hostility, or frustration. It may be helpful to note at this point that many parents of children with ADHD have reported similarly distressing, confusing, or outright hostile previous encounters with professionals and educators about their child, in addition to well-intentioned but overly enmeshed or misinformed relatives. Compassion and empathy for the plight of the parents at this point can often result in a substantial degree of rapport with and gratitude toward the examiner, and a greater motivation to follow subsequent treatment recommendations. At the very least, parents are likely to feel that they have finally found someone who truly understands the nature of their child's problems and the distress they have experienced in trying to assist the child. They may also experience relief that someone has recommendations to do something about the problems.

The suggestions that follow for interviewing parents of children with ADHD are not intended to be rigid guidelines, only areas that clinicians should consider. Each interview clearly differs according to individual child and family circumstances. Generally, those areas of importance to an evaluation include demographic information; child-related information;

school-related information; and details about the parents, other family members, and community resources that may be available to the family.

Demographic Information

If not obtained in advance, the routine demographic data concerning the child and family (e.g., ages of child and family members; child's date of birth; parents' names, addresses, employers, and occupations; and the child's school, teachers, and physician) should be obtained at the outset of the appointment. We also use this initial introductory period to review with the family any legal constraints on the confidentiality of information obtained during the interview, such as the clinician's legal duty (as required by state law) to report to state authorities instances of suspected child abuse, threats the child (or parents) may make to cause physical harm to other specific individuals (the duty to inform), and threats the child (or parents) may make about self-harm (e.g., suicide threats).

Major Parental Concerns

The interview then proceeds to the major referral concerns of the parents (and of the professional referring the child, when appropriate). A parental interview form designed by Barkley and colleagues is available in the clinical manual accompanying this text (Barkley & Murphy, 2006). It can be very helpful in collecting the information discussed later. This form contains not only major sections for the important information discussed here, but also the diagnostic criteria for ADHD as well as the other childhood disorders most likely to be seen in conjunction with ADHD (ODD, CD, anxiety disorders, mood disorders). Such a form allows clinicians to collect the essential information likely to be of greatest value to them, in a convenient and standardized format across their child client populations.

General descriptions of concerns by parents must be followed with specific questions by the examiner to elucidate the details of the problems and any apparent precipitants. Such an interview probes for the specific nature, frequency, age of onset, and chronicity of the problematic behaviors. It can also obtain information, as needed, on the situational and temporal variation in the behaviors and their con-

sequences. If the problems are chronic (which they often are), determining what prompted the referral at this time reveals much about parental perceptions of the children's problems, current family circumstances related to the problems' severity, and parental motivation for treatment.

Review of Major Developmental Domains

Following this part of the interview, the examiner should review with the parents potential problems that might exist in the developmental domains of motor, language, intellectual, academic, emotional, and social functioning. Such information greatly aids in the differential diagnosis of the child's problems. To achieve this differential diagnosis requires that the examiner have an adequate knowledge of the diagnostic features of other childhood disorders, some of which may present as similar to ADHD. For instance, many children with Asperger syndrome, other pervasive developmental disorders, or early Bipolar I Disorder may be viewed by their parents as having ADHD, since the parents are more likely to have heard about the latter disorder than the former ones and will recognize some of the qualities in their children. Questioning about inappropriate thinking, affect, social relations, and motor peculiarities may reveal a more seriously and pervasively disturbed child. Inquiry also must be made as to the presence or history of Tourette syndrome or other tic disorders in the child or the immediate biological family members. When noted, a tic disorder may result in a recommendation for the cautious use of stimulant drugs in the treatment of ADHD, or perhaps for lower doses of such medicine than typical, while monitoring any exacerbation of the child's tics (see Chapter 17).

School, Family, and Treatment Histories

The examiner should also obtain information on the school and family histories. The family history must include a discussion of potential psychiatric difficulties in the parents and siblings; marital/couple difficulties; and any family problems centered around chronic medical conditions, employment problems, or other potential stress events within the family. Of course, the examiner will want to obtain some information about prior treatments received by the child and his or her family for these presenting problems. When the history suggests potentially treatable medical or neurological conditions (allergies, seizures, Tourette syndrome, etc.), a referral to a physician is essential. Without evidence of such problems, however, referral to a physician for examination usually fails to reveal any further useful treatment information. But when the use of psychiatric medications is contemplated, a referral to a physician is clearly indicated. Of course, if the child has not had a relatively recent physical examination, then referral to a physician is essential to rule in or out other potentially treatable maladies that may pertain to the current concerns of the parents as voiced in the interview.

Information about the child's family is essential for two reasons. First, ADHD is not caused by family stress or dysfunction. Therefore, the family history can help to clarify whether the child's attention or behavioral problems are developmental in nature or are actually reactions to stressful events that have taken place. Second, a history of certain psychiatric disorders in the extended family might influence diagnostic impressions or treatment recommendations. For example, because ADHD is hereditary, a strong family history of ADHD in biological relatives lends weight to the ADHD diagnosis, especially when other diagnostic factors are questionable. A family history of Bipolar I Disorder in a child with severe behavioral problems might suggest the child to be at risk for a similar disorder, or might indicate particular medication choices that otherwise might not be considered.

The interviewer can organize this section by first asking about the child's siblings (whether there is anything significant about sibling relationships, whether siblings have any health or developmental problems). Then questions about the parents may include how long they have been married or cohabiting, the overall stability of their marriage or relationship, whether each parent is in good physical health, whether either parent has ever been given a psychiatric diagnosis, and whether either parent has had a learning disability. The clinician should always be cautious about inquiring too much into the parents' personal concerns, however. The purpose is to rule out family stress or other parental factors as a cause for or contributor to the child's difficulties and to determine what treatment recommendations may be appropriate.

In asking about extended family history, the interviewer should include maternal and paternal relatives (see clinical workbook by Barkley & Murphy, 2006).

Although it may seem tedious, it is *extremely* useful to go through the child's school history year by year, starting with preschool. The examiner should ask parents open-ended questions: "What did his teachers have to say about him?", "How did she do academically?", or "How did he get along socially?" The examiner should avoid pointed, leading questions (e.g., "Did the teacher think she had ADHD?"). Examiners should allow parents to tell them their child's story and listen for the red flags (e.g., "The teacher thought he was immature," "She had trouble with work completion," "His organizational skills were terrible," "She could not keep her hands to herself," or "He would not do homework").

Gathering a reliable school history gives the clinician two crucial pieces of the diagnostic puzzle. First, is there evidence of symptoms or characteristics of ADHD in the early school years? Second, is there evidence of impairment in the child's academic functioning as a result of these characteristics at any stage in the child's educational career? Establishing impairment is essential to distinguishing merely a high level of symptoms from valid disorders, and the school domain is often among the most likely to be impaired by ADHD.

The examiner should ask parents what strategies teachers may have attempted to help the child in class. He or she should also inquire about tutoring services, school counselors, study skills classes, or peer helpers. The examiner should find out whether, when, and why teachers referred the child for psychoeducational testing. If the child is not doing well in school, the examiner should ask whether school personnel have ever offered an explanation. As always, the examiner should listen for clues about possible problems with behavioral regulation, impulse control, or sustained attention. If the child has a diagnosed learning disability, are there problems in school that cannot be explained by the learning disability alone?

Review of Childhood Psychiatric Disorders

As part of the general parent interview, the examiner must cover the symptoms of the major child psychiatric disorders likely to be seen in children with ADHD. A review of the major childhood disorders in the fourth edition, text revision, of the *Diagnostic and Statistical Manual of Mental Disorders* (DSM-IV-TR; American Psychiatric Association, 2000) in some semistructured or structured way is imperative if any semblance of a reliable and differential approach to diagnosis and the documentation of comorbid disorders is to occur (see interview in Barkley & Murphy, 2006). As noted earlier in regard to rating scales, the examiner must exercise care in the evaluation of minority children to avoid overdiagnosing psychiatric disorders simply by virtue of ignoring differing cultural standards for child behavior. Chapter 2 (this volume) discusses ensuring that the behaviors of children are statistically deviant as well as associated with evidence of impairment in adaptive functioning or some other "harmful dysfunction." Should a parent indicate that a symptom is present, one means of precluding overidentification of psychopathology in a minority child is to ask the following question: "Do you consider this to be a problem for your child, compared to other children of the same ethnic or minority group?" Only if the parent answers "yes" is the symptom to be considered present for purposes of psychiatric diagnosis.

It may be useful to query about ODD and CD first. Many parents arrive at the diagnostic evaluation overwhelmed by emotional stress, frustrations with home behaviors, or endless criticisms about the child from the school; thus they may be inclined to say "yes" to anything. Starting with questions about ODD and CD allows these parents to get some of this frustration out of their system. Thus, when they are asked questions about ADHD, the answers are potentially more reliable and accurate.

In addition, unfortunately, some parents actually "shop" for the ADHD diagnosis. They may have an agenda that involves obtaining a diagnosis for their child that is not entirely objective. Beginning the clinical interview with the reason for referral and then the ODD questions may assist the clinician in gaining important clinical impressions about the parents' agenda. This is also why it can be extremely useful for a clinician to avoid the initial use of the word "attention" during the beginning of the interview, when he or she is inquiring about current concerns of the parents, until progressing to the DSM inattention symptom list. When the clinician asks specific questions about ADHD symptoms, the questions should

be phrased in such a way that they are concrete and descriptive.

Table 2.1 in Chapter 2 of this volume presents the diagnostic criteria for ADHD as set forth in the DSM-IV-TR. These require careful review with the parents during this interview. As suggested in Chapter 2, adjustments may need to be made to the DSM-IV-TR criteria for ADHD:

1. The cutoff scores on both the inattention and hyperactivity–impulsivity symptom sets (6 of 9) were primarily based on children ages 4–16 years in the DSM-IV field trial (Lahey et al., 1994), making the extrapolation of these thresholds to age ranges outside those in the field trial of uncertain validity. ADHD behaviors tend to decline in frequency within the population over development, again suggesting that a somewhat higher threshold may be needed for preschool children (ages 2–4).

2. The children used in the DSM-IV field trial were predominantly males (Lahey et al., 1994). Studies reliably demonstrate that parents and teachers report lower levels of those behaviors associated with ADHD in girls than in boys (Achenbach, 2001; DuPaul et al., 1998). It is possible, then, that the cutoff points on the DSM-IV-TR symptom lists, based as they are mainly on males, are unfairly high for females. Some latitude should be granted to females who are close to meeting the diagnostic criteria but may fall short by a single symptom.

3. The specific age of onset of 7 years is not particularly critical for identifying children with ADHD (Barkley & Biederman, 1997). Indeed, parental recall of age of onset is not especially reliable (Angold et al., 1996), and therefore insisting on a precise age for diagnosis is likely to reduce the reliability of the diagnosis. The field trial for the DSM-IV found that ADHD children with various ages of onset were essentially similar in the nature and severity of impairments, as long as their symptoms developed prior to ages 10–12 years (Applegate et al., 1997). Thus stipulating an age of onset of symptoms sometime in childhood is probably sufficient for purposes of clinical diagnosis. This does not mean that age of onset is meaningless, as it appears that children with earlier onsets (prior to or at school entry) may have more severe ADHD, may have greater cognitive deficits and reading problems, and may possibly be more at risk for developing comor-

bid disorders such as ODD (McGee, Williams, & Feehan, 1992) than are children with onsets after school entry. That having been said, it does not support the imposition of a fixed and early age of onset for all cases. Indeed, the DSM-IV field trial found that as many as 35% of children with ADHD, Predominantly Inattentive Type would not have met the onset of 7 as required for diagnosis. This may be consistent with the observations of McGee et al. (1992) that children with onset of inattentive symptoms after school entry had a less severe or pervasive form of the disorder most often associated with reading problems and far less risk of comorbidity with other disorders—findings typical of children with the Predominantly Inattentive Type.

4. The criterion that duration of symptoms be at least 6 months was not specifically studied in the DSM-IV field trial and was held over from earlier DSMs primarily out of tradition, as well as a desire to distinguish ADHD from situational reactions of childhood (Angold et al., 1996). Some research on preschool children suggests that a large number of 2- to 3-year-olds may manifest the symptoms of ADHD as part of this developmental period, and that these symptoms may remain present for periods of 3–6 months or longer (Campbell, 1990; Palfrey, Levine, Walker, & Sullivan, 1985). Children whose symptoms have persisted for at least 1 year or more, however, are likely to remain deviant in their behavior pattern into the elementary school years (Campbell & Ewing, 1990; Palfrey et al., 1985). Adjusting the duration criterion to 12 months would seem to make good clinical sense, to avoid misdiagnosing transient behavioral problems as ADHD.

5. The criterion that symptoms must be evident in at least two of three settings (home, school, work) essentially requires that children have significant symptoms of ADHD by both parent and teacher reports before they can qualify for the diagnosis. This requirement does not mean that both parent and teacher must give sufficient symptoms to surpass the diagnostic threshold (6 of 9). Such agreement is not likely to be found (Mitsis, McKay, Schulz, Newcorn, & Halperin, 2000). As a diagnostic requirement, it also bumps up against a methodological problem inherent in comparing parent and teacher reports: On average, the relationship of behavior ratings from these two sources tends to be fairly modest, averaging about .30 (Achenbach, McConaughy, & Howell, 1987), and this is especially so for symptoms of ADHD (Wolraich et al., 2004). However, if parent and teacher ratings are unlikely to agree across the various behavioral domains being rated, the number of children qualifying for the diagnosis of ADHD is unnecessarily limited, due mainly to such setting × source artifact. As some recent research shows, parents or teachers interpret symptoms relative to behavior and functioning most specific to the domain or setting in which they supervise the child (Gadow et al., 2004), and combining such information may be better than viewing one source as more accurately or truly rendering the child's actual adjustment than the other source. Fortunately, some evidence demonstrates that children who meet DSM criteria (in this case, DSM-III-R) by parent reports have a high probability of meeting the criteria by teacher reports (Biederman, Keenan, & Faraone, 1990). Even so, stipulating that parents and teachers *must* agree on the diagnostic criteria before a diagnosis can be rendered is probably unwise and unnecessarily restrictive. For now, to grant the diagnosis, clinicians are advised to seek evidence that symptoms of the disorder existed at some time in the past or present of the child in several settings rather than insisting on the agreement of the parents with a current teacher. Moreover, the developers of the DSM diagnosis used a blending approach in which the number of significant symptoms reported by the parent (or teacher) was combined with any new symptoms reported by the other party, giving a total symptom count across parent and teacher sources. Clinicians should use the same approach when dealing with these two sources of information in an effort to enhance diagnostic reliability and accuracy (Gadow et al., 2004; Piacentini, Cohen, & Cohen, 1992).

6. As discussed in earlier chapters, research has begun to identify a subset of children (30–50%) often diagnosed with the Predominantly Inattentive Type who may actually have a qualitatively distinct disorder of attention from that seen in ADHD, Combined Type. The symptoms most distinguishing of these children, unfortunately, are not in the DSM inattention list. But they should be reviewed nonetheless with parents when the presenting concerns appear to suggest their presence. Recall that these are

symptoms of sluggish cognitive tempo (SCT), such as being daydreamy, spacey, confused, in a fog, slow-moving or hypoactive, lethargic, slow to process information, and socially passive, reticent, or withdrawn. If such symptoms occur often or more frequently, it may signal that the child's difficulties may be more akin to SCT than to traditional ADHD.

The foregoing issues should be kept in mind when clinicians are applying the DSM criteria to particular clinical cases. It helps to appreciate the fact that the DSM represents guidelines for diagnosis, not rules of law or dogmatic prescriptions. Some clinical judgment is always going to be needed in the application of such guidelines to individual cases in clinical practice. For instance, if a child meets all criteria for ADHD including both parent and teacher agreement on symptoms, except that the age of onset for the symptoms and impairment is 9 years, should the diagnosis be withheld? No! Given the previous discussion concerning the lack of specificity for an age of onset of 7 years in ADHD, the wise clinician will grant the diagnosis anyway. Likewise, if an 8-year-old girl meets criteria for 5 of the 9 ADHD inattention or hyperactivity–impulsivity symptoms and all other conditions are met for ADHD, the diagnosis should probably be granted, given the previous comments about gender bias within these criteria. Some flexibility (and common sense), then, must be incorporated into the clinical application of any DSM criteria.

To assist clinicians with the differential diagnosis of the Combined or Predominantly Hyperactive–Impulsive Type of ADHD from other childhood mental disorders, we have compiled a list of differential diagnostic tips (see Table 8.2). Under each disorder, we list those features that would distinguish this disorder in its pure form from ADHD. However, many children with ADHD may have one or more of these disorders as comorbid conditions with their ADHD; thus the issue here is not which single or primary disorder the child has, but what other disorders besides ADHD are present and how they might affect treatment planning. Table 8.3 lists features that distinguish "pure" ADHD from ADHD that is comorbid with other disorders, as well as the likelihood that various other disorders or conditions will be comorbid with ADHD.

For years, some clinicians eschewed diagnosing children, viewing it as a mechanistic and dehumanizing practice that merely resulted in unnecessary labeling. Moreover, they felt that it got in the way of appreciating the clinical uniqueness of each case, unnecessarily homogenizing the heterogeneity of clinical cases. Some believed that labeling a child's condition with a diagnosis was unnecessary, because it was far more important to articulate the child's pattern of behavioral and developmental excesses and deficits in planning behavioral treatments. Although there may have been some justification for these views in the past, particularly prior to the development of more empirically based diagnostic criteria, this is no longer the case in view of the wealth of research that went into creating the DSM-IV(-TR) childhood disorders and their criteria and that has subsequently been produced. This is not to say that clinicians should not document patterns of behavioral deficits and excesses, as such documentation is important for treatment planning. Indeed, as DuPaul has noted (DuPaul & Ervin, 1996; DuPaul & Stoner, 2003), such a functional analysis of ADHD within the school setting may be the most useful feature of the evaluation in terms of making recommendations to teachers. But such documentation should not be used as an excuse not to diagnose at all. Furthermore, given that the protection of rights and access to educational and other services may actually hinge on awarding or withholding the diagnosis of ADHD, dispensing with diagnosis altogether could well be considered professional negligence. For these reasons and others, clinicians, along with the parents of each child referred to them, must review in some systematic way the symptom lists and other diagnostic criteria for various childhood mental disorders.

The parental interview may also reveal that one parent, usually the mother, has more difficulty managing a child with ADHD than the other does. Care should be taken to discuss differences in the parents' approaches to management and any marital/couple problems these differences may have spawned. Such difficulties in child management can often lead to reduced leisure and recreational time for the parents and increased conflict within the couple (and often within the extended family, should relatives live nearby). It is often helpful to inquire as to what the parents attribute the causes or

TABLE 8.2. Differential Diagnostic Tips for Distinguishing Other Mental Disorders from ADHD, Combined Type or Predominantly Hyperactive–Impulsive Type

ADHD, Predominantly Inattentive Type (with sluggish cognitive tempo)

- Lethargy, staring, spaceyness, and daydreaming more likely than in ADHD, Combined Type or Predominantly Hyperactive–Impulsive Type
- Sluggish cognitive tempo/slow information processing
- Lacks impulsive, disinhibited, or aggressive behavior often seen in other ADHD types
- Possibly greater family history of anxiety disorders and learning disabilities
- Makes significantly more errors in academic work
- Much lower risk for Oppositional Defiant Disorder or Conduct Disorder

Oppositional Defiant Disorder and Conduct Disorder

- Lacks impulsive, disinhibited behavior
- Defiance primarily directed toward mother or both parents initially
- Able to cooperate and complete tasks requested by others
- Lacks any problems with poor sustained attention (persistence) and marked restlessness
- Resists initiating demands, whereas children with ADHD may initiate but cannot stay on task
- Often associated with parental deficits in child management or family dysfunction
- Lacks neuromaturational delays in motor abilities

Learning disabilities

- Has a significant IQ–achievement discrepancy (+1 standard deviation)
- Places below the 10th percentile in an academic achievement skill
- Lacks an early childhood history of hyperactivity
- Attention problems arise in middle childhood and appear to be task- or subject-specific
- Not socially aggressive or disruptive
- Not impulsive or disinhibited

Anxiety/mood disorders

- Likely to have a focused, not sustained, attention deficit
- Not impulsive or aggressive; often overinhibited
- Has a strong family history of anxiety disorders
- Restlessness is more like fretful, worrisome, fearful, phobic, or panicky behavior, not the "driven," inquisitive, or overstimulated type
- Lacks preschool history of hyperactive, impulsive behavior
- Not socially disruptive; typically socially reticent

Thought disorders

- Oddities/atypical patterns of thinking not seen in ADHD
- Peculiar sensory reactions
- Odd fascinations and strange aversions
- Socially aloof, schizoid, uninterested
- Lacks concern for personal hygiene/dress in adolescence
- Atypical motor mannerisms, stereotypies, and postures
- Labile, capricious, unpredictable moods not tied to reality
- Poor empathy, often disturbed cause–effect perception
- Poor perception of meaningfulness of events

Juvenile-onset mania or Bipolar I Disorder

- Characterized by severe and persistent irritability
- Depressed mood more days than not
- Irritable/depressed mood typically punctuated by rage outbursts (destructive or violent)
- Mood swings often unpredictable or related to minimal events
- Severe temper outbursts and aggression with minimal provocation (thus ODD is often present and severe)
- Later onset of symptoms than ADHD (but comorbid early ADHD is commonplace)
- Press of speech and flight of ideas may be present
- Psychotic-like symptoms often present during manic episodes
- Family history of Bipolar I Disorder more common
- Expansive mood, grandiosity of ideas, inflated self-esteem, and high productivity (goal-directed activity periods) often seen in adults with Bipolar I Disorder are usually not present; children more often have the dysphoric type of disorder
- Sufficient symptoms of Bipolar I Disorder must be present after distractibility and hyperactivity (motor agitation) are excluded from Bipolar I symptom list in DSM-IV-TR before Bipolar I diagnosis can be granted to a child with symptoms of ADHD
- Suicidal ideation is more common in children (and suicide attempts more common in family history)

TABLE 8.3. Features That Are Likely to Discriminate "Pure" Cases of ADHD from ADHD That Is Comorbid with Other Disorders

Discriminating features

1. Difficulties with sustained attention, persistence, and resistance to distraction, and/or
2. Difficulties with impulse control, regulating activity level, and self-regulation

Consistent features

For Combined and Hyperactive–Impulsive Types:
1. Difficulties with concentration, forgetfulness, disorganization, procrastination
2. Excessively talkative, blurts out comments thoughtlessly
3. Can't wait for things, wait in line, or take turns; impatient
4. Busy, on the go, fidgety, restless

For Predominantly Inattentive Type:
1. Passive, sluggish, lethargic, or hypoactive
2. Daydreamy, spacey, easily confused, stares, "in a fog"

Variable features (comorbid conditions and their likelihood in clinic-referred cases)

1. Specific learning disabilities (20–70%)
2. Specific language disorders (15–60%)
3. Oppositional Defiant Disorder (45–65%)
4. Conduct Disorder (25–45%)
5. Dysthymic Disorder or Major Depressive Disorder (20–30%)
6. Anxiety disorders (10–25%)
7. Childhood Bipolar I Disorder (3–10%)
8. Poor peer relations (50–70%)
9. Developmental Coordination Disorder (50%+)
10. Poor educational performance (70–90%+), grade retention (25–50%), or suspension/expulsion (15–30%)

origins of their child's behavioral difficulties, because such exploration may unveil areas of ignorance or misinformation that will require attention during the initial counseling of the family about the child's disorder (or disorders) and its likely causes. The examiner also should briefly inquire about the nature of parental and family social activities to determine how isolated, or insular, the parents are from the usual social support networks in which many parents are involved. Research by Wahler (1980) shows that the degree of maternal insularity is significantly associated with severity of a child's disruptive behavior and with the likelihood of failure in subsequent parent training programs. When present to a significant degree, such a finding might support addressing the isolation as an initial goal of treatment, rather than progressing directly to child behavior management training with that family.

Psychosocial Functioning

The first topic in the portion of the interview devoted to psychosocial functioning involves peer relationships and recreational activities. A clinical diagnosis of ADHD requires impairment in the child's functioning in at least two important areas. This area could certainly be one of them. In addition, evidence of impaired peer relationships may lead to important treatment recommendations, such as additional in-school assistance with peer relationship training or a peer support group.

Parents are asked whether the child has trouble making or keeping friends, how the child behaves around other children, and how well the child fits in at school. Parents are also asked whether they have concerns about the friends with whom their child spends time (e.g., do the parents view these friends as "troublemakers"?). Finally, they are asked about recreational activities in which the child participates outside school and any problems that have occurred during those activities.

Compliance with parental requests and parental use of compensatory or motivational strategies can also be explored, especially if the clinician anticipates conducting parent training in child management skills with this family. These questions substantiate evidence of impairment in family functioning, as well as possible treatment recommendations for parent management training. If the interview on parent–child interactions discussed next is not to be used, parents are asked to describe how quickly their child complies with parental requests, whether there are discrepancies in the child's behavior with the mother and father, and whether the parents generally agree on how to manage their child. They are also asked to describe the types of disciplinary strategies they use and whether or not they have tried incentive systems to encourage more appropriate behavior.

At a later appointment, perhaps even during the initial session of parent training, the examiner may wish to pursue more details about the nature of the parent–child interactions surrounding the following of rules by the child. Parents should be questioned about the child's ability to accomplish commands and requests satisfactorily in various settings, to adhere to rules of conduct governing behavior in various situations, and to demonstrate self-control (rule following) appropriate to the child's age in the absence of adult supervision. We have found it useful to follow the format set forth in Table 8.4, in which parents are questioned about their interactions with their children in a variety of home and public situations. When problems are said to occur, the examiner follows up with the list of questions in Table 8.4. When time constraints are problematic, the

HSQ can be used to provide similar types of information. After parents complete the scale, they can be questioned about one or two of the problem situations, using the same follow-up questions as in Table 8.4. The HSQ is discussed later.

Such an approach yields a wealth of information on the nature of parent–child interactions across settings, the type of noncompliance shown by the child (stalling, starting the task but failing to finish it, outright opposition and defiance, etc.), the particular management style employed by parents to deal with noncompliance, and the particular types of coercive behaviors used by the child as part of the noncompliance.

The parental interview can then conclude with a discussion of the child's positive characteristics, psychological strengths, and attributes, as well as potential rewards and reinforcers desired by the child that will prove useful in later parent training on contingency management methods. Some parents of children with ADHD have had such chronic and pervasive management problems that, upon initial questioning, they may find it hard to report anything positive about their children. Getting them to begin thinking of such attributes is actually an initial step toward treatment, as the early phases of parent training will teach parents to focus on and attend to desirable child behaviors (see Chapter 12, this volume).

TABLE 8.4. Parental Interview Format for Assessing Child Behavior Problems at Home and in Public

Situation to be discussed	If a problem, follow-up questions to ask
Overall parent–child interactions Playing alone Playing with other children Mealtimes Getting dressed/undressed Washing and bathing When parent is on telephone Child is watching television When visitors are in your home When you are visiting someone else's home In public places (stores, restaurants, church, etc.) When father is in the home When child is asked to do chores When child is asked to do school homework At bedtime When child is riding in the car When child is left with a babysitter Any other problem situations	1. Is this a problem area? If so, then proceed with questions 2–9. 2. What does the child do in this situation that bothers you? 3. What is your response likely to be? 4. What will the child do in response to you? 5. If the problem continues, what will you do next? 6. What is usually the outcome of this situation? 7. How often do these problems occur in this situation? 8. How do you feel about these problems? 9. On a scale of 1 (no problem) to 9 (severe), how severe is this problem for you?

Note. From Barkley (1981). Copyright 1981 by The Guilford Press. Reprinted by permission.

CHILD INTERVIEW

Some time should always be spent interacting directly with the referred child. The length of this interview depends on the child's age, intellectual level, and language abilities. An important aspect of the interview is its function as a mental status exam—the opportunity for the clinician to observe the child's language skills, interpersonal skills, eye contact, and thought processing. For a preschool child, the interview may also serve merely as a time to become acquainted with the child, noting his or her appearance, behavior, developmental characteristics, and general demeanor. For an older child or adolescent, this time can be fruitfully spent inquiring about the child's views of the reasons for the referral and evaluation, views of the family's functioning, perceptions of any additional problems he or she may have, school performance, degree of acceptance by peers and classmates, and any changes in the family the child believes might make life happier at home. As with the parents, the child can be queried about potential rewards and reinforcers; this information will prove useful in later contingency management programs.

Although any clinician trained and experienced with working with children will have his or her own style of conducting an interview with a child, the clinician conducting a diagnostic evaluation for the purpose of determining the presence or absence of ADHD is encouraged to utilize a standard interview format. Standardization of the interview contributes to the reliability of the overall diagnostic process. The following format is one possible option.

• The clinician can begin by querying the child about the reason for the session. This will allow the clinician to correct any misperceptions the child might have about why he or she is seeing a mental health professional (e.g., "I'm crazy," "I'm retarded"), but it will also clarify to what extent the child is a willing participant who is actively seeking help for his or her difficulties.

• A discussion of school functioning may include questions about whether or not the child likes school, which subjects seem easiest and which the most difficult, whether the child thinks he or she could achieve higher grades, and what the child thinks might be impeding his or her progress. Additional questions might

reflect the phenomenology of ADHD from the perspective of the child:

• "Do you ever find that you've been sitting in class, and all of a sudden you realize your teacher has been talking and you have no idea what she's [or he's] talking about?"
• "Does it ever seem to take you longer to get your work done compared to other kids?"
• "Do you think your work is messier than other kids' work?"
• "Do you have trouble keeping track of things you need for school?"
• "Do you have trouble finishing your homework?"
• "Does your teacher ever have to speak to you because you're talking when you're not supposed to be talking, or fooling around when you're supposed to be working?"

• Questions about peer relationships should include probes about bullying in school. Parents may be unaware of the problem, and bullying can certainly be a source of anxiety and distraction for any child. Asking the child whether he or she has friends in school may also help to identify a child with a distorted view of peer relations, particularly if parents and teachers have reported that the child has peer relationship difficulties.

• Asking about recreational activities not only can establish a source of rapport for any future counseling sessions, but is also a way to identify the child's areas of strength or competence.

• Queries about family relations may be as simple as asking whether the child has the opportunity to do fun things with parents and siblings, but this might also be a time to probe further into the child's perceptions of his or her behavior problems at home, as well as parental disciplinary practices.

• Specific questions can assist the child in reporting about his or her general mood state. Questions such as "When are you happiest?", "Is there anything you worry about a lot?", or "What makes you angry?" can assist the child to talk about areas of emotional concern that are unknown to the parents.

Children below the ages of 9–12 years are not especially reliable in their reports of their own disruptive behavior. The problem is compounded by the frequently diminished self-awareness and impulse control typical of defiant children with ADHD (Hinshaw, 1994). These children with ODD/ADHD often show little reflection about the examiner's questions and may lie or distort information in a more socially pleasing direction. Some report that they have many friends, have no interaction problems at home with their parents, and are doing well at school, in direct contrast with the extensive parental and teacher complaints of inappropriate behavior by these children. Because of this tendency of children with ADHD to underreport the seriousness of their behavior, particularly in the realm of disruptive or externalizing behaviors (Barkley, Fischer, Edelbrock, & Smallish, 1991; Fischer, Barkley, Fletcher, & Smallish, 1993), a diagnosis of ODD or ADHD is never based solely on a child's reports. Nevertheless, children's reports of their internalizing symptoms, such as anxiety and depression, may be more reliable and thus should play some role in the diagnosis of comorbid anxiety or mood disorders in children with ADHD (Hinshaw, 1994).

Although notations of children's behavior, compliance, attention span, activity level, and impulse control in the clinic are useful, clinicians must guard against drawing any diagnostic conclusions when the children are not problematic in the clinic or office. Many children with ODD and/or ADHD do not misbehave in the clinician's office; thus reliance on such observations would clearly lead to false negatives in the diagnosis (Sleator & Ullmann, 1981). In some instances, a child's behavior with parents in the waiting area prior to the appointment may be a better indication of the child's management problems at home than is the child's behavior toward the clinician, particularly when the interaction between child and examiner is one to one.

This is not to say that the office behavior of a child is entirely meaningless. When it is grossly inappropriate or extreme, it may well signal the likelihood of problems in the child's natural settings, particularly school. It is the presence of relatively typical conduct by the child that may be an unreliable indicator of the child's behavior elsewhere. For instance, in a study of 205 children ages 4–6 years (Shelton, Barkley, et al., 1998), we examined the relationship of office behavior to parent and teacher ratings. Of these children, 158 were identified at kin-

dergarten registration as being 1.5 standard deviations above the mean (93rd percentile) on parent ratings of ADHD and ODD (aggressive) symptoms. These children were subsequently evaluated for nearly 4 hours in a clinic setting, after which the examiner completed a rating scale of each child's behavior in the clinic. We then classified the children as falling below or above the 93rd percentile on these clinic ratings, using data from a nondisabled control group. The children were also classified as falling above or below this threshold on parent ratings of home behavior and teacher ratings of school behavior, using the CBCL. We have found to date that no significant relationship exists between children's clinic behavior (typical or atypical) and the ratings of the children as typical by their parents. However, a significant relationship exists between atypical ratings in the clinic and atypical ratings by teachers: 70% of the children classified as atypical in their clinic behavior have also been classified as such by the teacher ratings of class behavior, particularly on the Externalizing behavior dimension of the CBCL. Typical behavior, however, is not necessarily predictive of typical behavior in either parent or teacher ratings. This finding suggests that atypical or significantly disruptive behavior during a lengthy clinical evaluation may be a marker for similar behavioral difficulties in a school setting. Nevertheless, the wise clinician will contact the child's teacher directly to learn about the child's school adjustment, rather than relying entirely on such inferences about school behavior from clinic behavior.

TEACHER INTERVIEW

At some point before or soon after the initial evaluation session with the family, contact with the child's teachers may be helpful to further clarify the nature of the child's problems. This contact is most likely to occur by telephone, unless the clinician works within the child's school system (in this case, see DuPaul & Stoner, 2003, for more on teacher interviewing within school systems). Interviews with teachers have all of the same merits as interviews with parents, providing a second ecologically valid source of indispensable information about the child's psychological adjustment—in this case, in the school setting. Like parent reports, teacher reports are also subject to bias, and the integrity of each informant (be it parent or teacher) must always be weighed.

Many children with ADHD have problems with academic performance and classroom behavior and the details of these difficulties need to be obtained. Initially, this information may be obtained by telephone; however, when time and resources permit, a visit to the classroom for direct observation and recording of a child's behavior can prove quite useful if further documentation of ADHD behaviors is necessary for planning later contingency management programs for the classroom. Although this scenario is unlikely to prove feasible for clinicians working outside school systems (particularly in the climate of managed health care plans, which severely restrict the evaluation time that will be compensated), for those professionals working within school systems, direct behavioral observations can prove very fruitful for diagnosis, and especially for treatment planning (Atkins & Pelham, 1992; DuPaul & Stoner, 2003).

A teacher should also be sent the rating scales mentioned earlier. They can be sent as a packet prior to the actual evaluation so that the results are available for discussion with the parents during the interview, as well as with the teacher during the subsequent telephone contact or school visit.

The teacher interview should focus on the specific nature of the child's problems in the school environment, again following a behavioral format. The settings, nature, frequency, consequent events, and eliciting events for the major behavioral problems also can be explored. The follow-up questions used in the parental interview on parent–child interactions (shown in Table 8.4) may prove useful here as well. Given the greater likelihood of the occurrence of learning disabilities in this population, teachers should be questioned about such potential disorders. When evidence suggests their existence, the evaluation of the child should be expanded to explore the nature and degree of such deficits as viewed by the teacher. Even when learning disabilities do not exist, children who have ADHD are more likely to have problems with sloppy handwriting, careless approaches to tasks, poor organization of their work materials, and academic underachievement relative to their tested abilities. Time should be taken with teachers to explore the possibility of these problems.

CHILD BEHAVIOR RATING SCALES

Rating Scales for Parent and Teacher Reports

Child behavior checklists and rating scales have become essential elements in the evaluation and diagnosis of children with behavior problems. The availability of several scales with excellent reliability and validity, as well as normative data across a wide age range of children, makes their incorporation into the assessment protocol quite convenient, extremely useful, and in many cases utterly essential for more accurately establishing developmental deviance relative to same-age and same-sex peers. As a result, it is useful to mail out a packet of these scales to parents prior to the initial appointment (as described earlier), with a request that they be returned on or before the day of the evaluation. Thus the examiner can review and score the scales before interviewing the parents; this will allow vague or significant answers to be clarified in the subsequent interview and will focus the interview on those problem areas highlighted in the responses to scale items.

Numerous child behavior rating scales for parents and teachers exist, only a few of which can be noted here. Readers are referred to other reviews (Barkley, 1988, 1990; American Academy of Child and Adolescent Psychiatry, 1997; Hinshaw & Nigg, 1999) for more details and for discussions of the requirements and underlying assumptions of behavior rating scales—assumptions all too easily overlooked in the clinical use of these instruments. Despite their limitations, behavior rating scales offer a means of gathering information from informants who may have spent months or years with a child. Apart from interviews, there is no other means of obtaining such a wealth of information with so little investment of time. The fact that such scales provide a means to quantify the opinions of others, often along qualitative dimensions, and to compare these scores to norms collected on large groups of children is further affirmation of their merits. Nevertheless, parents' and teachers' responses to behavior rating scales are opinions and are subject to the oversights, prejudices, and limitations on reliability and validity inherent in such opinions.

Initially, it is advisable to utilize a "broadband" rating scale that provides coverage of the major dimensions of child psychopathology known to exist, such as depression, anxiety, withdrawal, aggression, delinquent conduct, and (of course) inattentive and hyperactive–impulsive behavior. These scales should be completed by both parents and teachers. Such scales include the BASC-2 (Reynolds & Kamphaus, 2004) and the CBCL (Achenbach, 2001), both of which have versions for parents and teachers and satisfactory normative information. The Conners Rating Scales—Revised (Conners, 2001) can also be used with parents and teachers for this initial screening for psychopathology, but they do not provide quite the same breadth of coverage across these dimensions of psychopathology as do the aforementioned scales.

Narrow-band scales that focus specifically on the assessment of ADHD symptoms should also be employed in the initial screening of children. For this purpose, parent and teacher versions of a Disruptive Behavior Rating Scale can be found in the clinical workbook accompanying this text (Barkley & Murphy, 2006). Those scales obtain ratings of the DSM-IV (-TR) symptoms of ODD, ADHD, and CD (parent form only), as described earlier. DuPaul et al. (1998) have collected norms for another version of an ADHD rating scale. High scores alone on any of these scales do not automatically indicate a diagnosis of ADHD, however. The clinician must combine this information with that obtained from the parent and teacher interviews, as well as with his or her specialized knowledge in differential diagnosis, before rendering a specific diagnosis.

The clinician should also examine the pervasiveness of the child's behavior problems within the home and school settings, as such measures of situational pervasiveness appear to have as much stability over time as the aforementioned scales, if not more (Fischer et al., 1993). The HSQ (Barkley, 1988, 1990) provides a means for doing so (see Barkley & Murphy, 2006), and normative information for these scales is available (Altepeter & Breen, 1992; Barkley & Edelbrock, 1987; DuPaul & Barkley, 1992). The HSQ requires parents to rate their child's behavioral problems across 16 different home and public situations. The SSQ similarly obtains teacher reports of problems in 12 different school situations (see Barkley & Murphy, 2006).

The more specialized or narrow-band scales focusing on symptoms of ODD and ADHD, as well as the HSQ and SSQ, can be used to monitor treatment response when given prior to, throughout, and at the end of parent training (see Chapter 12, this volume). They can also be used to monitor the behavioral effects of medication on children with ADHD. In that case, use of the Side Effects Rating Scale is encouraged (see Barkley & Murphy, 2006).

One of the most common problem areas for children with ADHD is their academic productivity. The amount of work that these children typically accomplish at school is often substantially less than that done by their peers within the same period. Demonstrating such an impact on school functioning is often critical if children with ADHD are to be deemed eligible for special educational services (DuPaul & Stoner, 2003). The Academic Performance Rating Scale (see Barkley, 1990) was developed to provide a means of screening quickly for this domain of school functioning. It is a teacher rating scale of academic productivity and accuracy in major subject areas, with norms based on a sample of children from central Massachusetts (DuPaul, Rapport, & Perriello, 1991).

Self-Report Behavior Rating Scales for Children

Achenbach (2001) has developed a rating scale quite similar to the CBCL, which is completed by children ages 11–18 years (the Youth Self-Report form). Most items are similar to those on the parent and teacher forms of the CBCL, except that they are worded in the first person. The latest revision of this scale (Achenbach, 2001) now permits direct comparisons of results among the parent, teacher, and youth self-report forms of this popular rating scale. Research suggests that although such self-reports of children and teens with ADHD are more deviant than the self-reports of youth without ADHD, the self-reports of problems by the former youth—whether by interview or the Youth Self-Report form—are often less severe than the reports provided by parents and teachers (Fischer et al., 1993; Loeber, Green, Lahey, & Stouthamer-Loeber, 1991). The BASC-2, noted earlier, also has a self-report form that may serve much the same purpose as that for the CBCL.

The reports of children about internalizing symptoms, such as anxiety and depression, are more reliable and likely to be more valid than the reports of parents and teachers about these symptoms in their children (Achenbach et al., 1987; Hinshaw, Han, Erhardt, & Huber,

1992). For this reason, the self-reports of children and youth with ADHD should still be collected, as they may have more pertinence to the diagnosis of comorbid internalizing disorders in children than to the ADHD behavior itself.

Adaptive Behavior Scales and Inventories

Research shows that a major area of life functioning affected by ADHD is the realm of general adaptive behavior (Barkley, DuPaul, & McMurray, 1990; Barkley, Shelton, et al., 2002; Roizen, Blondis, Irwin, & Stein, 1994; Shelton, Barkley, et al., 1998). "Adaptive behavior" often refers to children's development of skills and abilities that will assist them in becoming more independent, responsible, and self-caring individuals. This domain of self-sufficiency often includes (1) self-help skills, such as dressing, bathing, feeding, and toileting requirements, as well as telling and using time, and understanding and using money; (2) interpersonal skills, such as sharing, cooperation, and trust; (3) motor skills, including both fine motor skills (zipping, buttoning, drawing, printing, use of scissors, etc.) and gross motor abilities (walking, hopping, negotiating stairs, bike riding, etc.); (4) communication skills; and (5) social responsibility, such as degree of freedom permitted within and outside the home, running errands, performing chores, and so on. So substantial and prevalent is impairment of adaptive behavior among children with ADHD that Roizen et al. (1994) have even argued that a significant discrepancy between IQ and adaptive behavior scores (expressed as standard scores) may be a hallmark of ADHD.

Several instruments are available for the assessment of this domain of functioning. The Vineland Adaptive Behavior Inventory–II (Sparrow, Cicchetti, & Balla, 2005) is probably the most commonly used measure for assessing adaptive functioning. It is an interview, however, and takes considerable time to administer. When time is of the essence, we use the NABC (Adams, 1984) to assess this domain because of its greater ease of administration. It can be included as part of the packet of rating scales sent to parents in advance of the child's appointment, for more efficient use of clinical time. The CBCL and the BASC-2 completed by parents also contain several short scales that provide a cursory screening of several areas of adaptive functioning (activities, social, and school) in children, but they are no substitutes

for the in-depth coverage provided by the Vineland-II or NABC scales.

Peer Relationship Measures

As noted earlier, children with ADHD often demonstrate significant difficulties in their interactions with peers, and such difficulties are associated with an increased likelihood of persistence of their disorder. Several different methods for assessing peer relations have been employed in research with behavior problem children, such as direct observation and recording of social interactions, peer- and subject-completed sociometric ratings, and parent and teacher rating scales of children's social behavior. Most of these assessment methods are very cumbersome to implement in clinical settings, and because most have no norms, they would be inappropriate for use in the clinical evaluation of children with ADHD. Reviews of the methods for obtaining peer sociometric ratings can be found elsewhere (Newcomb, Bukowski, & Pattee, 1993). For clinical purposes, rating scales may offer the most convenient and cost-effective means for evaluating this important domain of childhood functioning. The CBCL and BASC-2 rating forms described earlier contain scales that evaluate children's social behavior, but only a few items on each scale pertain to friendships and social relations, and thus they provide only a cursory evaluation of this domain. As discussed earlier, norms are available for these scales, permitting their use in clinical settings. Three other scales that focus specifically and in much more detail on social skills are the Matson Evaluation of Social Skills with Youngsters (Matson, Rotatori, & Helsel, 1983), the Taxonomy of Problem Social Situations for Children (Dodge, McClaskey, & Feldman, 1985), and the Social Skills Rating System (Gresham & Elliott, 1990). The last of these also has norms and a software scoring system, making it useful in clinical contexts. We have used it extensively in our research and clinical evaluations.

PARENT SELF-REPORT MEASURES

It has become increasingly apparent that child behavioral disorders, their level of severity, and their responses to interventions are in part functions of factors affecting parents and the family at large. As noted in Chapter 4 (this volume), several types of psychiatric disorders are likely to occur more often among family members of a child with ADHD than in matched groups of control children. Numerous studies have demonstrated the further influence of these disorders on the frequency and severity of behavioral problems in children with ADHD. As discussed earlier, the extent of social isolation in mothers of behaviorally disturbed children influences the severity of the children's behavioral disorders, as well as the outcomes of parent training. Separate and interactive contributions of parental psychopathology and marital/couple discord affect the decision to refer children for clinical assistance, the degree of conflict in parent–child interactions, and child antisocial behavior. The degree of parental resistance to training also depends on such factors. Assessing the psychological integrity of parents, therefore, is an essential part of the clinical evaluation of defiant children, the differential diagnosis of their prevailing disorders, and the planning of treatments stemming from such assessments. Thus the evaluation of children for ADHD is often a family assessment, rather than one of the child alone. Although space does not permit a thorough discussion of the clinical assessment of adults and their disorders, this section provides a brief mention of some assessment methods clinicians may find useful as a preliminary screening for certain variables of importance to treatment of children with ADHD.

The parents can complete these instruments in the waiting room, during the time their child is being interviewed. (To save time, some professionals may prefer to send these self-report scales out to parents in advance of their appointment, at the same time they send the child behavior questionnaires to the parents. If so, the clinician needs to prepare a cover letter sensitively explaining to parents the need for obtaining such information.) On the day of the interview, the clinician can indicate to parents that having a complete understanding of a child's behavior problems requires learning more about both the child and the parents. This process includes gaining more information about the parents' own psychological adjustment and how they view themselves as succeeding in their role as parents. The rating scales can then be introduced as one means of gaining such information. Few parents refuse to complete these scales after an introduction of this type.

Parental ADHD and ODD

Family studies of the aggregation of psychiatric disorders among the biological relatives of children with ADHD and ODD clearly demonstrate an increased prevalence of ADHD and ODD among the parents of these children (see Chapters 4 and 5, this volume). In general, there seems to be at least a 40–50% chance that one of the two parents of a child with ADHD will also have adult ADHD (15–20% of mothers and 25–30% of fathers). The manner in which ADHD in a parent may influence the behavior of an ADHD child specifically and the family environment more generally has not been well studied. It does seem to adversely affect that parent's benefiting from participation in a parent training program (Evans, Velano, & Pelham, 1994; Sonuga-Barke, Daley, & Thompson, 2002). Treatment of the parent's ADHD (with medication) results in greater success in subsequent retraining of the parent. Fortunately, parental ADHD does not appear to affect the veracity of the parents' reports about their own child with ADHD during a clinical interview (Faraone, Monuteaux, Biederman, Cohan, & Mick, 2003). Adults with ADHD also have been shown to be more likely to have problems with anxiety, depression, personality disorders, alcohol use and abuse, and marital/couple difficulties; to change their employment and residence more often; and to have less education and lower socioeconomic status than adults without ADHD (see Chapter 6). Greater diversity and severity of psychopathology among parents is particularly apparent among the subgroup of children with ADHD and comorbid ODD or CD. More severe ADHD seems to also be associated with younger parental age (Murphy & Barkley, 1996), suggesting that pregnancy during their own teenage or young adult years is more common among parents of children with ADHD than of children without ADHD. It is not difficult to see that these factors, as well as the primary symptoms of ADHD, could influence both the manner in which child behavior is managed within the family and the quality of home life for such children more generally. Some research in our clinic suggests that when a parent has ADHD, the probability that the child with ADHD will also have ODD increases markedly. These preliminary findings suggest the importance of determining the presence of ADHD and even ODD in the parents of children undergoing evaluation for the disorder.

The DSM-IV(-TR) symptom lists for ADHD and for ODD have been cast in the form of two behavior rating scales, one for current behavior and the other for recall of behavior during childhood. Some limited regional norms on 720 adults ages 17–84 years were collected (Murphy & Barkley, 1996). These two rating scales for adults, along with their norms, are provided in the clinical manual accompanying this text (Barkley & Murphy, 2006). Alternatively, clinicians may wish to use the Conners Adult ADHD Rating Scales (Conners, Erhardt, & Sparrow, 2000), which have norms on a much larger sample of adults from numerous geographic regions. Again, clinically significant scores on these scales do not by themselves warrant the diagnosis of ADHD or ODD in a parent, but they should raise suspicion in the clinician's mind about such a possibility. If so, consideration should be given to referral of the parent for further evaluation and possibly treatment of adult ADHD or ODD.

The use of such scales in screening parents of children with ADHD would be a helpful first step in determining whether the parents have ADHD. If a child meets diagnostic criteria for ADHD, and these screening scales for ADHD in the parents prove positive (clinically significant), referral of the parents for a more thorough evaluation and differential diagnosis may be in order. At the very least, positive findings from the screening will suggest the need to take them into account in treatment planning and parent training.

Marital/Couple Discord

Many instruments exist for evaluating marital/couple discord in parents. The one most often used in research on childhood disorders has been the Locke–Wallace Marital Adjustment Scale (Locke & Wallace, 1959), although its norms are sorely dated. If a scale is not used, clinicians should inquire about the status of the marital relationship as part of their clinical interview. As noted in Chapter 4, marital/couple discord, parental separation, and parental divorce are more common in parents of children with ADHD. Parents with such difficulties may have children with more severe defiant and aggressive behavior, and such parents may also be less successful in parent training programs. Screening parents for marital/couple problems,

therefore, provides important clinical information to therapists contemplating a parent training program for such parents. Clinicians are encouraged to incorporate some method of screening for marital/couple discord into their assessment battery for parents of children with defiant behavior.

Parental Depression and General Psychological Distress

Parents of children with ADHD, especially those with comorbid ODD or CD, are frequently more depressed than those of nondisabled children; this may affect their responsiveness to behavioral parent training programs. The Beck Depression Inventory–II (Beck, Steer, & Brown, 1996) is often used to provide a quick assessment of parental depression. Greater levels of psychopathology generally and psychiatric disorders specifically also have been found in parents of children with ADHD, many of whom also have ADHD themselves (Breen & Barkley, 1988; Lahey et al., 1988). One means of assessing this area of parental difficulties is the Symptom Checklist 90—Revised (SCL-90-R; Derogatis, 1995). This instrument not only has a scale assessing depression in adults, but also has scales measuring other dimensions of adult psychopathology and psychological distress. Although there is an adult self-report version of the CBCL, it has not yet gained wide acceptance among clinicians or researchers as a means of evaluating parent psychological difficulties. Whether clinicians use the SCL-90-R or some other scale, the assessment of parental psychological distress generally and psychiatric disorders particularly makes sense—in view of their likely presence among a large minority of parents of children having ADHD, and the impact those conditions might have on the children's course and the implementation of treatments typically delivered via the parents.

Parental Stress

Much research suggests that parents of children with behavior problems, especially those children with comorbid ODD and ADHD, report more stress in their families and their parental role than those of either nondisabled children or clinic-referred children (see Chapter 4). One measure frequently used in such research to evaluate this construct has been the

Parenting Stress Index (PSI; Abidin, 1995). The original PSI is a 150-item multiple-choice questionnaire that can yield six scores pertaining to child behavioral characteristics (distractibility, mood, etc.), eight scores pertaining to maternal characteristics (depression, sense of competence as a parent, etc.), and two scores pertaining to situational and life stress events. These scores can be summed to yield three domain or summary scores: Child Domain, Mother Domain, and Total Stress. A shorter version of this scale is also available (Abidin, 1986), and clinicians are encouraged to utilize it in evaluating parents of children with ADHD.

LEGAL AND ETHICAL ISSUES

Among the legal and ethical issues involved in the general practice of providing mental health services to children, several may be somewhat more likely to occur in the evaluation of children with ADHD. The first involves the issue of custody or guardianship of the child as it pertains to who can request the evaluation of the child who may have ADHD. Children with ODD, ADHD, or CD are more likely than average to come from families in which the parents have separated or divorced, or in which significant marital/couple discord may exist between the biological parents. As a result, the clinician must take care at the point of contact between the family and the clinic or professional to determine who has legal custody of the child, and particularly who has the right to request mental health services on behalf of the minor. It must also be determined in cases of joint custody (an increasingly common status in divorce/custody situations) whether the nonresident parent has the right to dispute the referral for the evaluation, to consent to the evaluation, to attend on the day of appointment, and/or to have access to the final report. This right to review or dispute mental health services may also extend to the provision of treatment to the child. Failing to attend to these issues before the evaluation can lead to contentiousness, frustration, and even legal action among the parties to the evaluation—all of which could have been avoided, had greater care been taken to iron out these issues beforehand. Although these issues apply to all evaluations of children, they may be more likely to arise in families seeking assistance for children with ADHD.

A second issue that also arises in all evaluations but may be more likely in cases involving ADHD is the duty of the clinician to disclose to state agencies any suspected physical or sexual abuse or neglect of the child. Clinicians should routinely forewarn parents of this duty to report when it applies in a particular state, *before* starting the formal evaluation procedures. In view of the greater stress that children with ADHD or ODD appear to pose for their parents, as well as the greater psychological distress their parents are likely to report, the risk for abuse of these children may be higher than average. The greater likelihood of parental ADHD or other psychiatric disorders may further contribute to this risk, resulting in a greater likelihood that evaluations of children with disruptive behavior disorders will involve suspicions of abuse. Understanding such legal duties as they apply in a given state or region, and taking care to exercise them properly yet with sensitivity to the larger clinical issues, are the responsibilities of any clinician involved in providing mental health services to children.

Increasingly, children with ADHD have been gaining access to government protections and entitlements; this makes it necessary for clinicians to be well informed about the legal issues if they are to advise parents and school staff properly and correctly. For instance, children with ADHD in the United States are now entitled to formal special educational services under the "Other Health Impaired" category of the Individuals with Disabilities Education Act (IDEA; Public Law 101-476), provided of course that their ADHD is sufficiently serious to interfere significantly with their school performance. In addition, such children also have legal protections and entitlements under Section 504 of the Rehabilitation Act of 1973 (Public Law 93-112) or the more recent Americans with Disabilities Act of 1990 (Public Law 101-336) as these apply to the provision of an appropriate education for children with disabilities (see DuPaul & Stoner, 2003, and Latham & Latham, 1992, for discussions of these entitlements). And should children with ADHD have a sufficiently severe disorder and reside in families of low economic means, they may also be eligible for financial assistance under the Social Security Act. Space precludes a more complete explication of these legal entitlements here. Readers are referred to the excellent text by attorneys Latham and Latham (1992) for a fuller account of these matters.

Suffice it to say here that clinicians working with children who have ADHD need to familiarize themselves with these various rights and entitlements if they are to be effective advocates for the children they serve.

A final legal issue related to children with ADHD pertains to legal accountability for their actions, in view of the argument made elsewhere (Barkley, 1997a) that their ADHD is a developmental disorder of self-control. Should children with ADHD be held legally responsible for the damage they may cause to property, the injury they may inflict on others, or the crimes they may commit? In short, is ADHD an excuse to behave irresponsibly without being held accountable for the consequences? The answer is unclear and deserves the attention of sharper legal minds than ours. It is our opinion, however, that ADHD explains why certain impulsive acts may have been committed, but it does not sufficiently disturb mental faculties to excuse legal accountability (as might occur, for example, under the insanity defense). Nor should ADHD be permitted to serve as an extenuating factor in the determination of guilt or the sentencing of an individual involved in criminal activities, particularly those involving violent crime. This opinion is predicated on the fact that the vast majority of children with ADHD, even those with comorbid ODD, do not become involved in violent crime as they grow up (see Chapter 4). Moreover, studies attempting to predict criminal conduct within samples of children with ADHD followed to adulthood either have not been able to find adequate predictors of such outcomes, or have found them to be so weak as to account for a paltry amount of variance in such outcomes. Moreover, the variables that may make a significant contribution to the prediction of criminal or delinquent behavior more often involve measures of parental and family dysfunction as well as social disadvantage, and much less often (if at all) involve measures of ADHD symptoms. Until this matter receives greater legal scrutiny, it seems wise to view ADHD as one of several predisposing factors for impulsive conduct, but not as a direct, primary, or immediate cause of criminal conduct.

THE PEDIATRIC MEDICAL EXAMINATION

It is essential that children being considered for a diagnosis of ADHD have a complete pedi-atric physical examination. However, such examinations are traditionally brief, relatively superficial, and as a result often unreliable and invalid for achieving a diagnosis of ADHD or identifying other comorbid behavioral, psychiatric, and educational conditions (Costello et al., 1988; Sleator & Ullmann, 1981). This is often the result of ignoring the other two essential features of the evaluation of children with ADHD: a thorough clinical interview, reviewed earlier, and the use of behavior rating scales. To diagnose and treat these children and adolescents properly, it is imperative that adequate time be committed to the evaluation to complete these components. If this is not possible, the physician is compelled to conduct the appropriate medical examination but withhold the diagnosis until the other components can be accomplished by referral to another mental health professional.

The features of the pediatric examination and the issues that must be entertained therein are described next and are taken from previous reviews of this exam by our medical colleagues Mary McMurray at the University of Massachusetts Medical Center (McMurray & Barkley, 1997) and Michelle Macias at the Medical University of South Carolina (Barkley & Macias, 2005).

The Medical Interview

Most of the contents of an adequate medical interview are identical to those described previously for the parental interview. However, greater time will clearly be devoted to a more thorough review of the child's genetic background, pre- and perinatal events, and developmental and medical history, as well as the child's current health, nutritional status, and gross sensory–motor development. Taking the time to listen to the parents' story and the child's feelings, and to explain the nature of the disorder, is one of the most important things a physician can offer a family. In this way, the evaluation process itself can often be therapeutic.

One major purpose of the medical interview that distinguishes it from the psychological interview described previously is its focus on differential diagnosis of ADHD from other *medical* conditions, particularly those that may be treatable. In rare cases, the ADHD may have arisen secondary to a clear biologically compromising event, such as recovery from severe

Reye syndrome, a hypoxic–anoxic event such as near-drowning or severe smoke inhalation, significant head trauma, or a central nervous system infection, or a cerebrovascular disease. The physician should obtain details of any such event, as well as the child's developmental, psychiatric, and educational status prior to the event and significant changes in these domains of adjustment since the event. The physician should also document ongoing treatments related to such events. In other cases, the ADHD may be associated with significant lead or other metal or toxic poisoning, which will require treatment in its own right.

It is also necessary to determine whether the child's conduct or learning problems are related to the emergence of a seizure disorder or are secondary to the medication being used to treat the disorder. As noted earlier, children who develop seizures are 2.5 times more likely to develop ADHD, and the inverse is also true (see Chapter 3). As many as 20% of children with epilepsy may have ADHD as a comorbid condition, and up to 30% may develop ADHD or have it exacerbated by the use of phenobarbital or phenytoin (Dilantin) as an anticonvulsant (Wolf & Forsythe, 1978). In such cases, changing to a different anticonvulsant may greatly reduce or even ameliorate the attentional deficits and hyperactivity of such children.

A second purpose of the medical exam is to thoroughly evaluate any coexisting conditions that may require medical management. In this case, the child's ADHD is not seen as arising from these other conditions, but as being comorbid with it. As noted in Chapter 3 (this volume), ADHD is often associated with higher risks not only for other psychiatric or learning disorders, but also for motor incoordination, enuresis, encopresis, allergies, otitis media, and greater somatic complaints in general. A pediatric evaluation is desirable or even required for many of these comorbid conditions. For instance, a child's eligibility for physical or occupational therapy at school or in a rehabilitation center may require a physician's assessment and written recommendation of the need for such. And although most cases of enuresis and encopresis are not due to underlying physiological disorders, all cases of these elimination problems should be evaluated by a physician before nutritional and behavioral interventions are begun. Even though many of these cases are "functional" in origin, medications may be prescribed to aid in their treatment, as in the use of oxybutynin, atomoxetine, or desipramine for bedwetting. Certainly children with significant allergies or asthma require frequent medical consultation and management of these conditions, often by specialists who appreciate the behavioral side effects of medications commonly used to treat them. Theophylline, for example, is increasingly recognized as affecting children's attention span and may exacerbate a preexisting case of ADHD. For these and other reasons, the role of the physician in the evaluation of ADHD should not be underestimated, despite overwhelming evidence that a medical exam by itself is inadequate as the sole basis for a diagnosis of ADHD.

A third purpose of the medical examination is to determine whether physical conditions exist that are contraindications for treatment with medications. For instance, a history of high blood pressure or cardiac difficulties warrants careful consideration about a trial on a stimulant drug or atomoxetine, given the known pressor effects of these drugs on the cardiovascular system. Some children may have a personal or family history of Tourette syndrome or other tic disorders, which would dictate caution in prescribing stimulants because of their greater likelihood of bringing out such movement disorders or increasing the occurrence of those that already exist, as may happen in over 30% of such cases. These examples merely illustrate the myriad medical and developmental factors that need to be carefully assessed in considering whether a particular child with ADHD is an appropriate candidate for drug treatment.

Physical Examination

In the course of the physical examination, height, weight, and head circumference require measurement and comparison to standardized graphs. Hearing and vision, as well as blood pressure and heart rate, should be screened. Findings suggestive of hyper- or hypotension, hyper- or hypothyroidism, lead poisoning, anemia, or other chronic illness clearly need to be documented, and further workup should be pursued. The formal neurological examination often includes testing of cranial nerves, gross and fine motor coordination, eye movements, finger sequencing, rapid alternating movements, impersistence, synkinesia, and motor overflow, choreiform movements, and tandem gait. This exam is often used to look for signs of previous central nervous system insult or of a progressive neurological condition; abnormalities of muscle tone; or a difference in strength, tone, or deep tendon reflex response between the two sides of the body. The existence of nystagmus, ataxia, tremor, decreased visual field, or fundal abnormalities should be determined and further investigation pursued when appropriate. This evaluation should be followed by a careful neurodevelopmental exam covering the following areas: motor coordination, visual perceptual skills, language skills, and cognitive functioning. Although these tests are certainly not intended to be comprehensive or even moderately in-depth evaluations of these functions, they are invaluable as quick screening methods for relatively gross deficiencies in these neuropsychological functions. When deficits are noted, follow-up with more careful and extensive neuropsychological, speech/language, motor, and academic evaluations may be necessary to document their nature and extent more fully.

Routine physical examinations of children with ADHD frequently indicate no physical problems and are of little help in diagnosing the condition or suggesting its management. However, the physician certainly needs to rule out the rare possibility of visual or hearing deficits, which may give rise to ADHD-like symptoms. Also, on physical inspection, children with ADHD may have a greater number of minor physical anomalies in outward appearance (e.g., an unusual palmar crease, two whorls of hair on the head, increased epicanthal fold, or hyperteliorism). Studies conflict on whether such findings occur more often in ADHD, but certainly they are nonspecific to it, being found in other psychiatric and developmental disorders. Examining for these minor congenital anomalies may only be beneficial when the physician suspects maternal alcohol abuse during pregnancy, to determine the presence of fetal alcohol syndrome (Shaywitz & Shaywitz, 1984). The presence of small palpebral fissures and midfacial hypoplasia with growth deficiency supports this diagnosis.

Asking about accidental injuries is an important part of this examination, given the high likelihood that children with ADHD will experience them. It may be useful to know not only about major trauma, but also about whether a child has sustained more than his or her share of cuts, bumps, scrapes, or broken bones. The impulsiveness, lack of judgment, inattention,

hyperactivity, and poor motor coordination that characterize ADHD often earn a child preferred customer status at the local emergency room (Barkley, 2001). Accidental ingestions of poisons are also more common in children with ADHD than in control children; parents should be explicitly forewarned of this likelihood and of the need for more aggressive childproofing of the home to remove these substances, as well as dangerous objects such as power tools and firearms. And burn injuries are also more common among children with ADHD. Such risks warrant admonishing parents to restrict the child's access to matches, lighters, ranges, grills, or other flammable devices.

As noted earlier, children with ADHD may be somewhat more likely to be physically abused, by virtue of the stress they may impose on already compromised caretakers. The risk for such abuse may be even more elevated in those cases having comorbid ODD, and is particularly prominent when comorbid CD or Bipolar I Disorder exists. Given that from 10% to 40% of children exposed to physically traumatic events may manifest symptoms of or meet criteria for Posttraumatic Stress Disorder (PTSD) within 4–12 weeks after exposure (see Chapter 4), the greater risk of children with ADHD/ODD and ADHD/CD for exposure to such trauma would suggest an elevated rate of PTSD among these subgroups as well.

The routine examination for growth in height and weight is also often unexceptional, although one study reported a younger bone age in children with minimal brain dysfunction, including hyperactivity (see Chapter 3). Nevertheless, when a physician contemplates a trial of a stimulant drug, accurate baseline data on physical growth, heart rate, and blood pressure are necessary against which to compare repeat exams during the drug trial or during long-term maintenance on these medications.

Similarly, the routine neurological examination is frequently unexceptional in children with ADHD. These children may display a greater prevalence of neurological "soft signs" suggestive of immature neuromaturational development, but again these are nonspecific for ADHD and can often be found in children with learning disabilities, psychosis, autism, and mental retardation, not to mention a small minority of nondisabled children. Such findings are therefore not diagnostic of ADHD, nor does their absence rule out the condition (Reeves, Werry, Elkind, & Zametkin, 1987).

Instead, findings of choreiform movements, delayed laterality development, fine or gross motor incoordination, dysdiadochokinesis, or other "soft signs" may suggest that the child requires more thorough testing by occupational or physical therapists and may need some assistance in school with fine motor tasks or adaptive physical education.

Children with ADHD may also have a somewhat higher number of atypical findings on brief mental status examinations or screening tests of higher cortical functions, especially those related to frontal lobe functions (e.g., sequential hand movement tests, spontaneous verbal fluency tests, and go/no-go tests of impulse control). When these are found, more thorough neuropsychological testing may be useful in further delineating the nature of these deficits and providing useful information to educators for making curriculum adjustments for these children. In some cases, findings on brief mental status exams may have more to do with a coexisting learning disability in a particular case than with ADHD per se. When problems with visual–spatial–constructional skills or simple language abilities are noted, they are most likely signs of a comorbid learning disorder, as they are not typical of children with ADHD generally. It is often the case that these brief mental status examinations are unexceptional. This does not necessarily imply that all higher cortical functions are intact, as these screening exams are often relatively brief and crude methods of assessing neuropsychological functions. More sensitive and lengthier neuropsychological tests may often reveal deficits not detected during a brief neurological screening or mental status exam. Even so, the routine use of extensive neuropsychological test batteries assess children with ADHD is likely to have a low yield. It should be undertaken only when there is a question of coexisting learning or processing deficits that require further clarification, and even then tests should be selected carefully to address these specific hypotheses.

Laboratory Tests

A number of studies have used various physical, physiological, and psychophysiological measures to assess potential differences between children with ADHD and other clinical or control groups of children. Although some of these studies have demonstrated such dif-

ferences—for instance, altered electroencephalographic (EEG) activity (greater slow-wave, reduced fast-wave), reduced cerebral blood flow to the striatum, or diminished orienting galvanic skin responses (see Chapter 5, this volume)—none of these laboratory measures are of value in the diagnostic process as yet. The quantitative EEG (QEEG) is showing some promise in accurately distinguishing children with ADHD from nondisabled children, but has not yet demonstrated sufficient classification accuracy among disorders (a more stringent test) to merit an unqualified endorsement for diagnostic purposes at this time (see Loo & Barkley, 2005). Parents, teachers, or even other mental health professionals are sometimes misled by reports of such findings or by the conclusion that ADHD is a biologically based disorder, and they frequently ask for their children to be tested medically to confirm the diagnosis. At this moment, no such tests exist. Consequently, laboratory studies such as blood work, urinalysis, chromosome studies, EEGs, averaged evoked responses, magnetic resonance imaging, or computerized tomography (CT scans) should not be used routinely in the evaluation of children with ADHD. Only when the medical and developmental history or physical exam suggests that a treatable medical problem (such as a seizure disorder) exists, or that a genetic syndrome is a possibility, should these laboratory procedures be recommended, and such cases are quite rare.

When children with ADHD are being placed on the stimulant drug pemoline (Cylert), routine liver function studies need to be done at baseline and again periodically during the use of this drug, because of an apparently greater risk of hepatic complications from this medication. This is not the case for the more popular stimulants, methylphenidate (Ritalin), D-amphetamine (Dexedrine), or Adderall. Blood assays of levels of stimulant medication have so far proven unhelpful in determining appropriate dosage, and therefore are not recommended as part of routine clinical titration and long-term management of these medications. The use of the tricyclic antidepressants for treating children with ADHD, especially those with greater anxiety or depressive symptoms, requires that a baseline routine electrocardiogram be done and then repeated several weeks after beginning drug treatment, given the greater potential for changes in cardiac rhythm and cardiotoxicity of these drugs. The same is true if antihypertensive agents are considered for use in those rare cases of severe ADHD and typically aggression where they may be indicated. Whether blood levels of the tricyclics are useful in titrating them for maximum clinical response is debatable at this time, as there is little standardized information to serve as a guide in the matter.

THE FEEDBACK SESSION

The feedback session with parents concludes the diagnostic evaluation. This session should take place after all the direct testing with the child is completed and scored, and after the clinician has reviewed all the data and drawn diagnostic conclusions (the family may need to wait while the clinician makes any necessary collateral phone calls to the school, current therapist, etc.). As with the parent interview, we generally do not include a child under the age of 16 in the feedback session, but the child may be invited in at the end of the session to be given diagnostic conclusions at a level appropriate to his or her age and cognitive development.

The first step in the feedback session is to give parents some information about ADHD. We generally explain to parents that ADHD is defined as a developmental disorder, not a mental illness or the result of stress in families. The developmental delay affects the child's ability to regulate behavior, control activity level, inhibit impulsive responding, or sustain attention. In other words, a child with ADHD will be more active, impulsive, and less attentive than other children of the same age.

We then explain that there is no direct test for ADHD—no lab test, X-ray, or psychological test that definitely tells us that a child has ADHD. What we have to do instead is collect a lot of information and analyze it statistically. Therefore, everything that has been learned about their child has been scored, and these scores have been compared with the scores that have been collected on hundreds if not thousands of children of the same age. If their child's scores are consistently placing him or her at or above the 93rd percentile in the areas of activity level, impulse control, or attention span, this suggests ADHD, because it suggests that the child is having more difficulty than 93

of 100 children of the same age. This is the level of "developmental deviance" that must be established.

The second step is to establish a history consistent with the notion of a "developmental" problem. Do these symptoms have a longstanding history that stretches back over time, for at least the past year—not something that cropped up last week or last month, or something that only came about after a trauma occurred in the child's life?

The third step is to rule out any other logical explanation for the problem. Is there anything else going on that would overrule ADHD as a diagnosis or be a better explanation than ADHD for the problems the child is having?

We then walk parents through the data obtained about their child, step by step, so they can see clearly how the diagnostic conclusion was reached. These steps include the following:

1. Explanation and results of the ADHD Rating Scale–IV

   • Parent interview responses
   • Parent ADHD Rating Scale–IV
   • Teacher ADHD Rating Scale–IV

2. Broad-band scale results

   • Parent versions, especially scales for attention problems and/or hyperactivity
   • Teacher version

3. Teacher rating scales (such as the Conners Rating Scales or ADHD Rating Scale–IV)
4. Parenting Stress Inventory
5. Social Skills Rating System
6. Academic Performance Rating Scale
7. Clinic-based testing results (such as IQ and achievement testing)

Before any discussion of a treatment plan occurs, parents are asked whether they have any questions about the diagnostic process or any comments about the conclusions that were drawn. Parents are always asked whether they are surprised that their child was (or was not) diagnosed with ADHD.

When parents are walked through the data this way, any confusion can be quickly clarified. Parents should leave the diagnostic interview with the impression that the evaluation has been comprehensive and that the clinician has been compassionate and competent. This sense of security will help them cope with the grief and disappointment they may experience at being told that their child has a developmental disability, as well as the confidence to follow any treatment recommendations that are made.

In closing, a number of implications for clinical practice seem evident from the earlier chapters of this text, particularly that on parent–child relations (Chapter 4):

1. The clinical assessment of children with ADHD must incorporate measures that assess not only child behavior and adjustment but also parent–child interactions, parental psychological status, and marital/couple functioning, if a thorough picture of the children's social ecology is to be obtained.

2. Reference must be made to the developmental context in which the findings from this assessment were obtained. The manner in which the levels of the social-ecological system have interacted to result in a family as it now presents must be appreciated. Determining "fault" within such reciprocal systems is often difficult and needlessly judgmental. A clinician can identify those problems within the family that seem primarily attributable to separate child and parent characteristics, without the "witch hunt" atmosphere that sometimes occurs in such clinical assessments. Great compassion and empathy are far more useful both in discovering these sources of maladjustment and in understanding their direction of effects.

3. In counseling the parents of children with ADHD, it is necessary to separate the causes and mechanisms for the children's ADHD from that of hostile/defiant behavior or ODD/CD (Barkley, 1997b). The former is clearly a developmental disorder of behavioral disinhibition associated with neuromaturational immaturity and having a strong hereditary predisposition. Parents therefore cannot be held liable for this developmental disorder. The ODD or CD, however, is likely to arise within and be maintained by family characteristics, particularly parental psychiatric factors and conditions of social adversity. These characteristics permit the modeling of aggressive social exchanges with others, as well as the success of garden-variety aggression in escaping these attacks and unwanted task demands made by others. Consequently, parents can and should be held accountable (not blamed) for many (though not all) of these circumstances, and should be

strongly encouraged to accept this responsibility and seek mental health services to change them. The treatments for ADHD and ODD/CD are clearly distinct.

4. The clinical treatment of ADHD when it coexists with ODD/CD must involve more comprehensive interventions that focus as needed on parental beliefs and attitudes, psychological distress, communication and conflict resolution skills, and family systems, rather than simply using medication or training parents in child management skills alone. Training in child management, when provided, must concentrate on the inconsistent and often noncontingent use of social consequences within these families, and on increasing the availability of rewards and incentives for prosocial conduct. It must also strive to increase parental involvement and particularly monitoring of child behavior, both at home and in the neighborhood, if it is to prevent the escalation to more serious stages of antisocial behavior. Exemplar programs for each of these approaches are described in the chapters of this text dealing with treatment.

5. The families of children with both ADHD and ODD/CD are likely to require more frequent and periodic monitoring via follow-up visits and periodic reintervention (as each case dictates) than the families of children with other types of psychological disorders, if a significant impact is to be made on the long-term outcome of the former children.

KEY CLINICAL POINTS

✓ The ultimate goal of the evaluation of a child with ADHD is the determination of the interventions that may be needed to address the child's presenting complaints.

✓ The evaluation itself is a process driven by the issues that must be addressed, not necessarily by the methods with which the clinician is most comfortable.

✓ The key issues involved in most cases will be (1) evaluating presenting complaints, (2) taking a history of those complaints, (3) making a differential diagnosis, (4) establishing developmental deviance, (5) determining domains of impairment (major life activities affected), (6) clarifying possible comorbidities, (7) evaluating the integrity of the information, (8) documenting parental psychological adjustment and motivation to change, and (9) assessing child and family strengths (and weaknesses) and community resources.

✓ The evaluation requires integrating information from multiple sources (parents, teachers, other caregivers, and professionals); using multiple means of collecting that information (semistructured and structured interviews, standardized behavior rating scales, the medical exam, and psychological testing as indicated); and surveying multiple domains of major life activities (family, peer, school, and community functioning, among others).

✓ Useful psychological testing involves screening of intelligence and academic achievement skills, with subsequent more thorough testing if patients fail the screens. Other psychological tests (e.g., neuropsychological tests) are not currently able to diagnose ADHD accurately, but may in some cases remain useful for helping define impaired cognitive processes.

✓ The medical examination will prove useful when (1) prior physical exams are unavailable or outdated, (2) history implies a treatable medical condition, (3) another medical disorder may better account for the presenting complaints, and/or (4) drug treatment of the child is anticipated.

✓ Laboratory tests or other medical procedures are usually unnecessary for purposes of diagnosing ADHD.

✓ The parental feedback session that concludes the evaluation is the first step in treatment, providing parents with useful scientific information on the nature, course, outcomes, and causes of ADHD, as well as the treatments that are empirically established or that are unproven and to be avoided.

REFERENCES

Abidin, R. R. (1995). *Parenting Stress Index* (3rd ed.). Lutz, FL: Psychological Assessment Resources.

Achenbach, T. M. (2001). *Child Behavior Checklist.* Burlington, VT: Research Center for Children, Youth, and Families.

Achenbach, T. M., McConaughy, S. H., & Howell, C. T. (1987). Child/adolescent behavioral and emotional problems: Implications of cross informant correlations for situational specificity. *Psychological Bulletin, 101,* 213–232.

Adams, G. L. (1984). *Normative Adaptive Behavior Checklist.* Portland, OR: Author. (Available from G. L. Adams, 2000 NE 42nd Avenue, Portland, OR 97213)

Altepeter, T. S., & Breen, M. J. (1992). Situational variation in problem behavior at home and school in attention deficit disorder with hyperactivity: A factor analytic study. *Journal of Child Psychology and Psychiatry, 33,* 741–748.

American Academy of Child and Adolescent Psychiatry. (1997). Practice parameters for the assessment and treatment of children, adolescents, and adults with attention-deficit/hyperactivity disorder.. *Journal of the American Academy of Child and Adolescent Psychiatry, 36*(10, Suppl.), 085S–121S.

American Psychiatric Association. (2000). *Diagnostic and statistical manual of mental disorders* (4th ed., text rev.). Washington, DC: Author.

Angold, A., Erklanli, A., Costello, E. J., & Rutter, M. (1996). Precision, reliability, and accuracy in the dating of symptoms onsets in child and adolescent psychopathology. *Journal of Child Psychology and Psychiatry, 37,* 657–664.

Applegate, B., Lahey, B. B., Hart, E. L., Waldman, I., Biederman, J., Hynd, G. W., et al. (1997). Validity of the age of onset criterion for ADHD: A report from the DSM-IV field trials. *Journal of the American Academy of Child and Adolescent Psychiatry, 36,* 1211–1221.

Atkins, M. S., & Pelham, W. E. (1992). School-based assessment of attention deficit-hyperactivity disorder. In S. E. Shaywitz & B. A. Shaywitz (Eds.), *Attention deficit disorder comes of age: Toward the twenty-first century* (pp. 69–88). Austin, TX: PRO-ED.

Barkley, R. A. (1981). *Hyperactive children: A handbook for diagnosis and treatment.* New York: Guilford Press.

Barkley, R. A. (1988). Child behavior rating scales and checklists. In M. Rutter, H. Tuma, & I. Lann (Eds.), *Assessment and diagnosis in child psychopathology.* (pp. 113–155). New York: Guilford Press.

Barkley, R. A. (1990). *Attention-deficit hyperactivity disorder: A handbook for diagnosis and treatment.* New York: Guilford Press.

Barkley, R. A. (1997a). *ADHD and the nature of self-control.* New York: Guilford Press.

Barkley, R. A. (1997b). *Defiant children: A clinician's manual for assessment and parent training* (2nd ed.). New York: Guilford Press.

Barkley, R. A. (2001). Accidents and ADHD. *The Economics of Neuroscience, 3,* 64–68.

Barkley, R. A., & Biederman, J. (1997). Towards a broader definition of the age of onset criterion for attention deficit hyperactivity disorder. *Journal of the*

American Academy of Child and Adolescent Psychiatry, 36, 1204–1210.

Barkley, R. A., DuPaul, G. J., & McMurray, M. B. (1990). A comprehensive evaluation of attention deficit disorder with and without hyperactivity. *Journal of Consulting and Clinical Psychology, 58,* 775–789.

Barkley, R. A., & Edelbrock, C. S. (1987). Assessing situational variation in children's behavior problems: The Home and School Situations Questionnaires. In R. Prinz (Ed.), *Advances in behavioral assessment of children and families* (Vol. 3, pp. 157–176). Greenwich, CT: JAI Press.

Barkley, R. A., Fischer, M., Edelbrock, C. S., & Smallish, L. (1991). The adolescent outcome of hyperactive children diagnosed by research criteria: III. Mother–child interactions, family conflicts, and maternal psychopathology. *Journal of Child Psychology and Psychiatry, 32,* 233–256.

Barkley, R. A., & Macias, M. (2005). Attention deficit hyperactivity disorder. In R. David (Ed.), *Child and adolescent neurology* (3rd ed.). New York: Blackwell.

Barkley, R. A., & Murphy, K. R. (2006). *Attention-deficit hyperactivity disorder: A clinical workbook* (3rd ed.). New York: Guilford Press.

Barkley, R. A., Shelton, T. L., Crosswait, C., Moorehouse, M., Fletcher, K., Barrett, S., et al. (2002). Preschool children with high levels of disruptive behavior: Three-year outcomes as a function of adaptive disability. *Development and Psychopathology, 14,* 45–68.

Beck, A. T., Steer, R. A., & Brown, G. K. (1996). *Beck Depression Inventory–II.* San Antonio, TX: Psychological Corporation.

Biederman, J., Keenan, K., & Faraone, S. V. (1990). Parent-based diagnosis of attention deficit disorder predicts a diagnosis based on teacher report. *American Journal of Child and Adolescent Psychiatry, 29,* 698–701.

Breen, M. J., & Barkley, R. A. (1988). Child psychopathology and parenting stress in girls and boys having attention deficit disorder with hyperactivity. *Journal of Pediatric Psychology, 13,* 265–280.

Campbell, S. B. (1990). *Behavior problems in preschool children: Clinical and developmental issues.* New York: Guilford Press.

Campbell, S. B., & Ewing, L. J. (1990). Follow-up of hard to manage preschoolers: Adjustment at age 9 and predictors of continuing symptoms. *Journal of Child Psychology and Psychiatry, 31,* 871–889.

Conners, C. K. (2001). *Conners Rating Scales—Revised.* North Tonawanda, NY: Multi-Health Systems.

Conners, C. K., Erhardt, D., & Sparrow, E. (2000). *Conners Adult ADHD Rating Scales.* North Tonawanda, NY: Multi-Health Systems.

Costello, E. J., Edelbrock, C. S., Costello, A. J., Dulcan, M. K., Burns, B. J., & Brent, D. (1988). Psychopathology in pediatric primary care: The new hidden morbidity. *Pediatrics, 82,* 415–424.

Derogatis, L. R. (1995). *Manual for the Symptom Checklist 90—Revised (SCL-90-R).* Minneapolis: Pearson Assessments.

Dodge, K. A., McClaskey, C. L., & Feldman, E. (1985). A situational approach to the assessment of social competence in children. *Journal of Consulting and Clinical Psychology, 53,* 344–353.

DuPaul, G. J., & Barkley, R. A. (1992). Situational variability of attention problems: Psychometric properties of the Revised Home and School Situations Questionnaires. *Journal of Clinical Child Psychology, 21,* 178–188.

DuPaul, G. J., & Ervin, R. A. (1996). Functional assessment of behaviors related to attention-deficit/hyperactivity disorder: Linking assessment to intervention design. *Behavior Therapy, 27,* 601–622.

DuPaul, G. J., Power, T. J., Anastopoulos, A. D., & Reid, R. (1998). *The ADHD Rating Scale-IV: Checklists, norms, and clinical interpretation.* New York: Guilford Press.

DuPaul, G. J., Rapport, M. D., & Perriello, L. M. (1991). Teacher ratings of academic skills: The development of the Academic Performance Rating Scale. *School Psychology Review, 20,* 284–300.

DuPaul, G. J., & Stoner, G. (2003). *ADHD in the schools: Assessment and intervention strategies (2nd ed.).* New York: Guilford Press.

Evans, S. W., Vallano, G., & Pelham, W. (1994). Treatment of parenting behavior with a psychostimulant: A case study of an adult with attention-deficit hyperactivity disorder. *Journal of Child and Adolescent Psychopharmacology, 4,* 63–69.

Faraone, S. V., Biederman, J., & Milberger, S. (1995). How reliable are maternal reports of their children's psychopathology?: One-year recall of psychiatric diagnoses of ADHD children. *Journal of the American Academy of Child and Adolescent Psychiatry, 34,* 1001–1008.

Faraone, S. V., Monuteaux, M. C., Biederman, J., Cohan, S. L., & Mick, E. (2003). Does parental ADHD bias maternal reports of ADHD symptoms in children? *Journal of Consulting and Clinical Psychology, 71,* 168–175.

Fischer, M., Barkley, R. A., Fletcher, K., & Smallish, L. (1993). The stability of dimensions of behavior in ADHD and normal children over an 8 year period. *Journal of Abnormal Child Psychology, 21,* 315–337.

Gadow, K. D., Drabick, D. A. G., Loney, J., Sprafkin, J., Salisbury, H., Azizian, A., et al. (2004). Comparison of ADHD symptom subtypes as source-specific syndromes. *Journal of Child Psychology and Psychiatry, 45,* 1135–1149.

Gresham, F., & Elliott, S. (1990). *Social Skills Rating System.* Circle Pines, MN: American Guidance Service.

Hinshaw, S. P. (1994). *Attention deficits and hyperactivity in children.* Thousand Oaks, CA: Sage.

Hinshaw, S. P., Han, S. S., Erhardt, D., & Huber, A. (1992). Internalizing and externalizing behavior problems in preschool children: Correspondence among parent and teacher ratings and behavior observations. *Journal of Clinical Child Psychology, 21,* 143–150.

Hinshaw, S. P., & Nigg, J. (1999). Behavioral rating scales in the assessment of disruptive behavior disorders in childhood. In D. Shaffer, C. P. Lucas, & J. Richters (Eds.), *Diagnostic assessment in child and adolescent psychopathology* (pp. 91–126). New York: Guilford Press.

Kentgen, L. M., Klein, R. G., Mannuzza, S., & Davies, M. (1997). Test–retest reliability of maternal reports of lifetime mental disorders in their children. *Journal of Abnormal Child Psychology, 25,* 389–398.

Lahey, B. B., Applegate, B., McBurnett, K., Biederman, J., Greenhill, L., Hynd, G. W., et al. (1994). DSM-IV field trials for attention deficit/hyperactivity disorder in children and adolescents. *Journal of the American Academy of Child and Adolescent Psychiatry, 151,* 1673–1685.

Lahey, B. B., Pelham, W. E., Schaughency, E. A., Atkins, M. S., Murphy, H. A., Hynd, G. W., et al. (1988). Dimensions and types of attention deficit disorder with hyperactivity in children: A factor and cluster-analytic approach. *Journal of the American Academy of Child and Adolescent Psychiatry, 27,* 330–335.

Latham, P., & Latham, R. (1992). *ADD and the law.* Washington, DC: JKL Communications.

Locke, H. J., & Wallace, K. M. (1959). Short marital adjustment and prediction tests: Their reliability and validity. *Journal of Marriage and Family Living, 21,* 251–255.

Loeber, R., Green, S., Lahey, B. B., & Stouthamer-Loeber, M. (1991). Differences and similarities between children, mothers, and teachers as informants on disruptive behavior disorders. *Journal of Abnormal Child Psychology, 19,* 75–95.

Loo, S. K., & Barkley, R. A. (2005). Clinical utility of EEG in attention deficit hyperactivity disorder. *Applied Neuropsychology, 12,* 64–76.

Mash, E. J., & Barkley, R. A. (Eds.). (2003). *Child psychopathology* (2nd ed.). New York: Guilford Press.

Mash, E. J., & Barkley, R. A. (Eds.). (in press). *Treatment of childhood disorders* (3rd ed.). New York: Guilford Press.

Matson, J. L., Rotatori, A. F., & Helsel, W. J. (1983). Development of a rating scale to measure social skills in children: The Matson Evaluation of Social Skills with Youngsters (MESSY). *Behavior Research and Therapy, 21,* 335–340.

McGee, R., Williams, S., & Feehan, M. (1992). Attention deficit disorder and age of onset of problem behaviors. *Journal of Abnormal Child Psychology, 26,* 487–502.

McMurray, M. B., & Barkley, R. A. (1997). The hyperactive child. In R. B. David (Ed.), *Child and adolescent neurology* (2nd ed., pp. 561–571). St. Louis, MO: Mosby.

Mitsis, E., McKay, K. E., Schulz, K. P., Newcorn, J. H., & Halperin, J. M. (2000). Parent-teacher concordance for DSM-IV attention-deficit/hyperactivity disorder in a clinic-referred sample. *Journal of the American Academy of Child and Adolescent Psychiatry, 39,* 308–313.

Murphy, K., & Barkley, R. A. (1996). Prevalence of DSM-IV symptoms of ADHD in adult licensed drivers: Implications for clinical diagnosis. *Journal of Attention Disorders, 1,* 147–161.

Newcomb, A. F., Bukowski, W. M., & Pattee, L. (1993). Children's peer relations: A meta-analytic review of popular, rejected, neglected, controversial, and average sociometric status. *Psychological Bulletin, 113,* 99–128.

Palfrey, J. S., Levine, M. D., Walker, D. K., & Sullivan, M. (1985). The emergence of attention deficits in early childhood: A prospective study. *Journal of Developmental and Behavioral Pediatrics, 6,* 339–348.

Piacentini, J. C., Cohen, P., & Cohen, J. (1992). Combining discrepant diagnostic information from multiple sources: Are complex algorithms better than simple ones? *Journal of Abnormal Child Psychology, 20,* 51–63.

Reeves, J. C., Werry, J., Elkind, G. S., & Zametkin, A. (1987). Attention deficit, conduct, oppositional, and anxiety disorders in children: II. Clinical characteristics. *Journal of the American Academy of Child and Adolescent Psychiatry, 26,* 133–143.

Reich, W. (1997). *Diagnostic Interview for Children and Adolescents—revised DSM-IV version.* Toronto, Ontario: MultiHealth Systems.

Reynolds, C., & Kamphaus, R. (2004). *Behavioral Assessment System for Children* (2nd ed.). Circle Pines, MN: American Guidance Service.

Roizen, N. J., Blondis, T. A., Irwin, M., & Stein, M. (1994). Adaptive functioning in children with attention-deficit hyperactivity disorder. *Archives of Pediatric and Adolescent Medicine, 148,* 1137–1142.

Shaffer, D., Fisher, P., Lucas, C., Dulcan, M., & Schwab-Stone, M. (2000). NIMH Diagnostic Interview Schedule for Children version IV (NIMH DISC-IV): Description, differences from previous versions, and reliability of some common diagnoses. *Journal of the American Academy of Child and Adolescent Psychiatry, 39,* 28–38.

Shaywitz, S. E., & Shaywitz, B. A. (1984). Diagnosis and management of attention deficit disorder: A pediatric perspective. *Pediatric Clinics of North America, 31,* 429–457.

Shelton, T. L., Barkley, R. A., Crosswait, C., Moorehouse, M., Fletcher, K., Barrett, S., et al. (1998). Psychiatric and psychological morbidity as a function of adaptive disability in preschool children with high levels of aggressive and hyperactive-impulsive-inattentive behavior. *Journal of Abnormal Child Psychology, 26,* 475–494.

Sleator, E. K., & Ullmann, R. K. (1981). Can the physician diagnose hyperactivity in the office? *Pediatrics, 67,* 13–17.

Sonuga-Barke, E. J. S., Daley, D., & Thompson, M. (2002). Does maternal ADHD reduce the effectiveness of parent training for preschool children's ADHD? *Journal of the American Academy of Child and Adolescent Psychiatry, 41,* 696–702.

Sparrow, S. S., Cicchetti, D. V., & Balla, D. A. (2005).

Vineland Adaptive Behavior Scales (2nd ed.). Circle Pines, MN: American Guidance Service.

Wahler, R. G. (1980). The insular mother: Her problems in parent–child treatment. *Journal of Applied Behavior Analysis, 13,* 207–219.

Wolf, S. M., & Forsythe, A. (1978). Behavior disturbance, phenobarbital, and febrile seizures. *Pediatrics, 61,* 728–731.

Wolraich, M. L., Lambert, E. W., Bickman, L., Simmons, T., Doffing, M. A., & Worley, K. A. (2004). Assessing the impact of parent and teacher agreement on diagnosing attention-deficit hyperactivity disorder. *Journal of Developmental and Behavioral Pediatrics, 25,* 41–47.

CHAPTER 9

Tests and Observational Measures

MICHAEL GORDON
RUSSELL A. BARKLEY
BENJAMIN J. LOVETT

Over the past several decades, researchers have made substantial progress in developing objective tools for assessing Attention-Deficit/Hyperactivity Disorder (ADHD) symptoms in children. Some tests boast robust normative data and detailed psychometrics. A rough consensus is also emerging about the proper role these measures should play in the overall diagnostic process. Our review attempts to place psychological testing in context and to provide a general road map for making decisions regarding their inclusion and interpretation.

Incorporating information based on a child's actual behavior has strong intuitive appeal, especially for a diagnostic process so heavily founded upon perception and opinion. The essential attraction of objective measures is that they seem to provide a beacon of reality when the diagnostic seas are cluttered by inconsistent reports and unreliable information. Indeed, research regarding the nature of subjective reports (whether formatted through a rating scale or gathered via semistructured interviews) discourages complete confidence in their reliability. Although they represent the heart of the diagnostic process, they nonetheless are subject to a full spectrum of distorting influences of the

sort detailed in a previous edition of this book (Barkley, 1990).

Despite advances in our knowledge about the role of psychological testing and the allure of numbers over perception, the search for accurate and reliable measures of ADHD symptoms has not yielded a litmus test. The absence of a gold standard for the diagnosis, as well as the heterogeneity of the disorder itself, precludes any one test (and, for that matter, any one rating scale or interview format) from claiming pinpoint accuracy. At best, research in this arena has produced techniques that can have some clinical utility, but cannot supplant other sources of information. Perhaps their strongest contributions are in identifying comorbid conditions or in substantiating alternative diagnoses.

THE POTENTIAL CONTRIBUTIONS OF PSYCHOLOGICAL TESTING

In our view, psychological testing can help the clinician address the three fundamental questions that lie at the heart of all evaluations for ADHD:

1. *Is the diagnosis of ADHD justified?* Clinicians often seek psychological testing for help in ruling ADHD in or out. Because no one source of information is free from potential error, inclusion of additional data may be indicated, especially when disagreements among other sources are wide or there are concerns about the credibility of other clinical information. Also, clinicians hope to gather information that will refine the diagnosis by providing evidence regarding severity, potential responsiveness to therapy, and outcome. Clinicians also may value the opportunity to observe a patient in a setting likely to elicit ADHD-type behavior.

2. *If the diagnosis of ADHD is not justified, are there alternative explanations that better account for the symptoms?* A competent evaluation for ADHD works hard to rule out the possibility that presenting complaints either are variants of typical development or are better tied to other diagnostic entities. Psychological testing can play an important role in this process, because it can compare one child's functioning to that of nonreferred children with similar demographic characteristics. Therefore, it can place a youngster at points along population distributions for multiple traits and abilities. Such a profiling of scores for a particular patient often becomes indispensable for determining the potential role of intellectual and socioemotional factors.

3. *If the ADHD diagnosis is justified, are there comorbid conditions that should be identified and treated?* Because of the high rates of comorbidity (see Chapter 4, this volume), it is likely that a child with ADHD will exhibit other problems. Psychological testing is typically regarded as key in documenting such coexisting disorders, such as mental retardation or learning disabilities. Clinicians hope that this information will put them in a better position to develop a comprehensive treatment program that best addresses each child's full mosaic of needs.

Our review of psychological testing is organized around these three domains: identifying ADHD, exploring alternative diagnoses, and documenting comorbidity. By way of overview, we make the following points:

• Psychological testing is usually most productive when the goals of the assessment are clearly established from the beginning. Is testing necessary primarily to document ADHD, to rule out alternative explanations, or to identify comorbid conditions? Or is it some combination of all three domains? Psychodiagnostic "fishing expeditions" are often inefficient and counterproductive.

• The goals of testing (and its potential contribution) vary widely, depending on the nature of the clinical setting. In an ADHD subspecialty clinic, testing aimed at documenting the disorder may be less useful, because the likelihood of identifying a youngster as having ADHD is already high. For example, in a clinic previously operated by Barkley at the University of Massachusetts Medical Center, an average of 86% of referred children were eventually given a diagnosis of ADHD. With such a high base rate, few if any tests are likely to be more accurate than just guessing this base rate. Testing might be more important for establishing levels of severity or for identifying comorbid conditions. In most clinic settings, a test's ability to discriminate nondisordered from disordered children will also be less relevant, because most referred children do have some disorder. For example, at the University of Massachusetts Medical Center ADHD Clinic, fewer than 6% of referred children are without any disorder. Therefore, the greatest need in this type of setting is for a test that aids in differential diagnosis. Unfortunately, none of the specific tests reviewed in this chapter have been thoroughly evaluated from this perspective. A study by Matier-Sharma, Perachio, Newcorn, Sharma, and Halperin (1995) did evaluate a research version of the continuous-performance test, or CPT (discussed later in this chapter). Although they found that this CPT accurately classified children with nonaverage scores as having ADHD in comparison to children with average scores (90–96%!), it accurately classified those same children with average scores as having ADHD or some other psychiatric disorder at a level of only 50–60%. The accuracy of the test in predicting children with average scores as not having ADHD in that same comparison (ADHD vs. other psychiatric disorders) was 62–73%. If these data are replicated across a variety of clinic settings and populations, it may be that psychological or neuropsychological testing is at its most limited utility in the domain that many clinicians would find it most relevant. In other settings with lower base rates of disorder—for example, in speech and language clinics or schools—a test's ability to discriminate nondisordered from disordered children may be more germane.

• Although data generated by psychological testing may contribute to the diagnostic process, *they cannot be considered in isolation.* Data from such testing are never conclusive (although, to be fair, no source of information has a lock on reality). With the possible exception of mental retardation, testing data alone cannot point directly to a psychiatric or learning disorder. In our view, problems with psychological tests derive not from their use per se, but from their potential for overinterpretation. Testing is most abused when scores are judged out of the context of a child's history and current functioning. A diagnosis based entirely on test scores is a diagnosis to doubt.

• Psychological testing is at its weakest in determining etiology. To the best of our knowledge, no index from a psychological test can determine why a particular child suffers from a particular disorder or set of disorders. Proclamations of causality are especially risky in the ADHD arena, because of the disorder's high degree of heritability. Clinicians should be especially careful about making assumptions about the presence of some specific neurological syndrome based on psychological testing.

• The patina of scientific credibility afforded by the standardization and, at times, computerization of tests does not obviate the need for credible psychometric data (Gordon, 1987). Advertising claims, testimonials, or justifications based on clinical experience or theoretical speculation cannot substitute for scientific information. The administration of psychological testing should enhance diagnostic rigor, not cloud matters further. At the same time, evaluating the validity of psychological testing for ADHD is inherently daunting, because the field lacks a gold standard for diagnosis. Unfortunately, most studies purporting to explore test validity draw conclusions as if such a benchmark existed. But, in essence, it is hard to establish whether an arrow hits the mark when the mark's location is itself uncertain. Nonetheless, any measure employed should offer credible information regarding its psychometric properties. Specifically, a test or battery of tests should boast the following characteristics based on published research:

Ample standardization (manualized, representative norms, etc.)
Reliability of administration
Test–retest reliability
Validity, or evidence that it can discriminate among diagnostic groups (ADHD vs. no disorder, ADHD vs. other clinical entities, or other clinical entities from no disorder or other clinical entities)
Proof that it enhances diagnostic accuracy and treatment planning (even if it does not have high predictive value)
Demonstrated practicality

The last two points on our list warrant some elaboration. Much of the scientific focus on psychological testing falls, appropriately, on the capacity of a test to predict group status. Most studies explore the degree of agreement among various clinical measures, often with a selected combination established as the benchmark. However, a psychological test can be of significant value even if it does not wholly agree with other measures. For example, a test may provide unique information regarding the severity of a child's pathology or the child's amenability to certain treatments. A test may also have value in predicting outcome (e.g., drug response), ascertaining a cognitive process (e.g., working memory), or confirming a diagnosis in unique populations or age groups (e.g., mental retardation). Therefore, a single-minded focus on discriminative power may overlook other possible contributions of testing (Fischer, Newby, & Gordon, 1995). Nevertheless, when test developers argue for the value of their tests in making diagnostic classifications, data must be provided from peer-reviewed scientific studies that the test in fact achieves those aims.

The requirement that tests should be practical to administer and interpret reflects the realities of modern clinical practice. As demands for cost efficiency mount, practitioners cannot afford to use measures that are unwieldy, time-consuming, or complicated. The ever-increasing focus on practicality has influenced our recommendations for psychological testing and observational techniques. Simply put, it makes little sense to consider approaches that are impractical, even if they might offer meaningful information.

A REVIEW OF PSYCHOLOGICAL TESTS

Our review of commonly administered psychological tests would be enhanced if we actually knew from current survey data which tests were commonly administered by clinicians who conduct ADHD evaluations. Aside from one survey of practitioners who use a particular CPT (Gordon, 1994), the only available data come from a recent polling of school psychologists (Demaray, Schaefer, & Delong, 2003). Although most respondents administered IQ tests (73.1%) and achievement tests (67.4%) as part of an ADHD assessment, far fewer respondents administered personality tests (28.8%), neuropsychological measures (22.5%), or CPTs (13.3%).

Our impression is that many clinicians, especially psychologists, administer a wide variety of psychological and neuropsychological tests, from IQ screening measures to inkblots. The various tests incorporated into ADHD-related evaluations tend to fall into four categories: (1) intelligence/achievement tests, (2) general neuropsychological batteries, (3) individual neuropsychological tests, and (4) projective/personality tests. We review measures in each category for the extent to which they have been documented as valid and useful for clinical determinations.

Intelligence/Achievement Tests

Information from intelligence and achievement testing is often considered central to differential diagnosis. Most clinicians routinely request prior evaluations from the school, so that such information can be incorporated into the ADHD assessment. If such testing is not available, practitioners usually suggest that it be pursued. Indeed, some form of psychoeducational testing is often administered as a matter of course within a comprehensive ADHD evaluation, even if previous testing is available.

Are intelligence/achievement tests useful in the identification of ADHD? There is no doubt that children with ADHD, as a group, routinely demonstrate lower intellectual ability than children in nondisabled or community comparison groups; their average score is often 7–10 points or about 0.61 standard deviations below the mean of the comparison group (see Frazier, Demaree, & Youngstrom, 2004, for a meta-analysis). But general cognitive deficits are also characteristic of other disorders (e.g., mental retardation), making them a rather nonspecific finding. To date, these tests have not been shown to be of value in detecting

ADHD characteristics specifically, or in accurately classifying cases of this disorder relative to no disorder or to other psychiatric disorders. In other words, no subtest or configuration of subtests is sensitive or specific to ADHD.

We arrive at this conclusion based largely on studies investigating the Freedom from Distractibility (FFD) factor of the Wechsler Intelligence Scale for Children (WISC). In the most recent edition of this test, the subtests constituting this factor have been resorted into other factors, such as Working Memory or Perceptual Reasoning. The FFD factor has been widely touted as a measure of attention and distractibility in children, and has been adopted by many as a clinical measure of ADHD. It consists of the scores on the Arithmetic, Digit Span, and Coding subtests, and was given the FFD label "because of research with hyperactive children showing that drug therapy leads to decreased distractibility and improved memory and arithmetic skills in these youngsters" (Kaufman, 1980, p. 179). Scores on this factor have been found to correlate to a low but significant degree with other tests of attention (Klee & Garfinkel, 1983).

Evidence is conflicting, however, as to whether the tests forming this factor can adequately discriminate groups of children with ADHD from groups with no disability or with reading disabilities (Brown & Wynne, 1982; Milich & Loney, 1979). A large-scale study of WISC profiles of 465 Dutch children suggested that both mood disorders and ADHD in children may be associated with lower scores on this factor than other psychiatric disorders in children may be (Rispens et al., 1997). Yet several other studies found that this factor was unable to distinguish children who had Attention Deficit Disorder (ADD) with Hyperactivity from children with ADD without Hyperactivity, from those with learning disabilities, or from those with no disability (Anastopoulos, Spisto, & Maher, 1994; Barkley, DuPaul, & McMurray, 1990; Golden, 1996). Others, however, found group differences on these tests (see Chapter 3, this volume). These subtests appear to assess short-term or verbal working memory, facility with numbers, perceptual–motor speed, visual–spatial skills, and arithmetic calculation. Consequently, poor performances on this factor do not indicate in any straightforward way that deficits in attention account for them. Moreover, a number of investigators urged caution in interpreting these subtests as measures of distractibility, believing the FFD label to be an oversimplification and misleading (Ownby & Matthews, 1985; Stewart & Moely, 1983; Wielkiewicz, 1990; Wielkiewicz & Palmer, 1996). Studies using the WISC-III to assess depressed third-factor scores have not found them to be reliably associated with the diagnosis of ADHD. Very poor rates of classification were noted, such that between 48% and 77% of children with ADHD would be classified as nondisabled (false negatives) if this factor were used for diagnostic purposes (Anastopoulos et al., 1994; Golden, 1996). Indeed, Greenblatt, Mattes, and Trad (1991), in a study of 526 clinic-referred children, found that although 11% had depressed third-factor scores, this fact was relatively nonspecific to any disorder. Only 4.8% of the children with a diagnosis of ADD according to the third edition of the *Diagnostic and Statistical Manual of Mental Disorders* (DSM-III; American Psychiatric Association, 1980), had depressed third-factor scores. For these and other reasons, we do not recommend that the FFD factor or the more recent subset of Wechsler factors be used in establishing evidence for or against a diagnosis of ADHD.

Perhaps the best indication that the FFD factor should not be considered as a diagnostic tool for ADHD is that it no longer emerges as a factor on the latest edition of the WISC. Indeed, Digit Span and Coding on the WISC-IV load on separate factors; Arithmetic has been made an optional test (Wechsler, 2003). This is not to say that children with ADHD may not perform poorly on these tests, or that groups of children having ADHD may not be found to be significantly more impaired on them than non-disabled children; indeed, both may be the case (see Frazier et al., 2004). It is to say that these tests or factors cannot accurately classify sufficient numbers of children with ADHD relative to control children to recommend their use for clinical diagnosis of ADHD.

IQ and achievement data can contribute to establishing the ADHD diagnosis in more indirect ways, because the determination hinges in part on documenting severity of impairment. The argument that a youngster's deficits are significant and meaningful can be bolstered by evidence of serious problems in acquiring age-appropriate skills. Well-normed tests can provide evidence of impairment relative both to the general population and also to the child's own innate abilities. The argument is, of course, most compelling if evidence also exists from teacher reports that skill attainment has been heavily affected by ADHD-type symptoms.

Such tests also contribute to the diagnosis of ADHD by generating information that may help to rule in or out other possible explanations for presenting complaints. Consider the following scenario: A girl is referred because of inattention, poor concentration, and underachievement. The teachers report that she is especially unfocused during assignments that involve reading and creative thinking. Furthermore, although the parents indicate that their daughter can be somewhat fidgety and avoidant when frustrated by school demands, they do not paint a picture of severe impulsivity across most settings. Because the symptoms of inattention and poor concentration are relatively circumscribed, the clinician becomes suspicious that learning problems may be more at the heart of this girl's difficulties than ADHD per se. In this instance, administration of IQ and achievement testing may be instrumental in ruling out the possibility that the girl's inattention is secondary to problems handling grade-appropriate academic tasks as a function of low achievement abilities or even a frank learning disorder.

More generally, IQ/achievement data help the clinician determine cognitive factors that might contribute to a youngster's inattention and academic underachievement (e.g., poor working memory). As we have indicated, they are especially valuable in ensuring that the child's symptoms are not largely a reaction to being overwhelmed by academic demands. Because specific learning disabilities so commonly coexist with ADHD (see Chapter 3), cognitively oriented testing can also play a key role in their identification.

Should IQ/achievement testing be conducted in every case? Our opinion is that clinicians should routinely have access to some estimate of overall intellectual functioning, whether the information is gleaned from past records or from current administration of a screening measure. Without some documentation that a youngster's abilities fall within the average range, the possibility that this youngster is either unusually limited or gifted cannot be eliminated. Because parent and teacher estimation of a child's intellectual level is not always accurate, some formal assessment may be necessary even when all involved are convinced that the youngster's abilities are average. We suggest that one of the brief IQ screening tests be used initially, followed by a more complete intellectual test should the scores fall well outside the average range.

Although clinicians should have at least a rough estimate of a child's intellectual abilities, we do not feel that comprehensive psychoeducational assessment should necessarily be a routine component of all ADHD evaluations. If sufficient information is not often already available in the child's record, the testing can usually be administered by the school at no cost to the family. At the least, we feel that parents should be advised that they can have their child tested free of charge through their local school district, although the time delay in doing so in some districts can be considerable.

If evidence from parent and teacher reports indicate that the youngster may suffer from some specific learning weakness (beyond the general academic underachievement common to all children with ADHD), a comprehensive psychoeducational evaluation may be warranted. Data from such an evaluation might identify a specific learning disability as either the primary condition or as comorbid with the ADHD symptoms. Of course, it may also rule out learning disabilities altogether. In any of these scenarios, data from testing would ultimately affect not only the diagnosis but also treatment planning.

Although complete psychoeducational testing may be justified in certain cases, clinicians often find it hard to interpret the data, especially for youngsters who have a highly impulsive style. The meaning of low test scores can be unclear if a youngster has spent much of the session grabbing test materials, hiding under the table, and running to the bathroom. For highly distractible and active children, the gulf between competence and performance is large. A study by Aylward, Gordon, and Verhulst (1997), for example, demonstrated that subtest scores from psychoeducational testing (including IQ and achievement scores) were pervasively, albeit moderately, correlated with measures of attention and self-control. Similar findings were reported by Billings (1996) and Gordon, Thomason, and Cooper (1990). Thus, for a child with ADHD symptoms, testing for cognitive abilities and achievement may more accurately reflect actual competence if it is administered while the child is on a therapeutic dose of medication.

General Neuropsychological Batteries

As noted in earlier chapters (particularly Chapter 7) of this volume, it is increasingly evident that ADHD is associated with deficits in executive functioning (see Frazier et al., 2004, for a meta-analysis of such tests). This has led some clinicians to incorporate neuropsychological tests, particularly those that presumably assess such functions, in the evaluation of children with ADHD. Such an approach has sometimes included administration of formal and comprehensive neuropsychological test batteries, such as the Halstead–Reitan (H-R) and the Luria–Nebraska Neuropsychological Battery (LNNB). These core batteries consist of various subtests that assess a broad range of neuropsychological functions. Their inclusion is typically justified by the compelling evidence of a strong neurobiological basis for ADHD symptoms. The rationale is as follows: If neurobiological factors, particularly frontal lobe dysfunction, heavily contribute to ADHD symptom formation, and if ADHD is associated with diminished executive functioning, then neuropsychological testing should be particularly useful in testing for the presence and strength of those functions.

Unfortunately, the fact that a series of tests is characterized as neuropsychological does not guarantee that it actually taps into relevant neuropsychological processes, or that it is capable of detecting more subtle developmental deficits in these abilities (as opposed to the more gross deficiencies evident in frank brain damage for which the tests may have been originally intended). In our review of the literature, we can establish no basis for suggesting routine administration of neuropsychological batteries within an ADHD evaluation (we cover individual tests in the next section). As for identification purposes, no single subtest or combination of subtests within the LNNB or the H-R has demonstrated predictive value. For example, Shaughency et al. (1989) showed that none of the subtests on the LNNB were related in any meaningful way to ADHD symptoms. And, to our knowledge, there has been no further research since the preceding edition of this book on the utility of such comprehensive test batteries in the evaluation of ADHD.

We have also been unable to justify core neuropsychological testing for highlighting alternative explanations for symptoms or for identifying comorbid conditions. Convincing data simply have not been presented to demonstrate that neuropsychological testing of a child contributes to the understanding of the child's functioning in a manner that is more predictive or prescriptive than a standard psychoeducational assessment. Although general neuropsychological testing may indicate significant and relevant weaknesses (especially if the battery includes IQ and achievement measures), those deficits often either will be clear from the child's academic functioning, or will be reflected on IQ or academic testing itself without the need to pursue further specialized neuropsychological testing.

We are concerned about two other issues related to routine administration of extensive, multitest batteries. First, the inclusion of many measures raises the possibility of false-positive errors. Because of sequential error, the probability is high that at least several test scores from an array of 30 or 40 will be atypical. The likelihood of overidentification of problems increases further because the psychometric properties for these tests have not been well established for child populations. Therefore, the scattershot quality of comprehensive neuropsychological testing almost guarantees some indication of abnormality.

Our other concern is tied more to economics than to methodology: If one accepts the proposition that most if not all the tests administered in a neuropsychological battery are of dubious diagnostic benefit for ADHD-related decisions, routine testing could fairly be judged by third-party payers as frivolous. Given the nature of the U.S. health care system, it is not unlikely that psychological testing in general will be unfairly painted with the same brush. Because psychodiagnostic assessment certainly has a legitimate role in the diagnosis of other childhood disorders, we are concerned that the entire enterprise will be tarnished because of overtesting for ADHD. The exceptions may be those instances in which evidence from history and imaging studies are suggestive of brain injury.

Individual Neuropsychological Measures

Although routine administration of core neuropsychological batteries is hard to justify, certain individual tests may have a role in the evaluation process. These tests are often subsumed under the construct of "executive functioning." There is no doubt now that ADHD is associated with deficits in executive neuropsychological tasks (average effect size difference is 0.59 standard deviations from control groups; Frazier et al., 2004). Before we actually review the most common of these techniques, we want to discuss the current state of the testing art: With the exception of certain computerized tests, remarkably little is actually known about many of the tests developed or adapted for the assessment of ADHD. For most, the totality of relevant published data might involve 50 clinic-referred children selected by somewhat idiosyncratic criteria. The scientific literature is often so sparse regarding a given measure that we are hesitant to comment either way about the test's utility. One or two studies should not be the basis on which a test is praised or damned, especially in light of the well-documented vagaries of clinical research. Therefore, the real conclusion to be drawn from an overview of this literature is that entirely too little empirical study has been conducted for a clinical activity that is so common, time-consuming, and costly. Indeed, if clinicians are seeking the most ecologically valid index of executive functioning in ADHD, they would do better to employ the Behavior Rating Inventory of Executive Functioning, as it provides parent and teacher ratings of the major dimensions of executive functioning based on considerably longer observation periods of children (weeks to months) in more natural settings (home, school) than is the case for these neuropsychological measures (just minutes of observation in an unnatural clinical setting). With these sentiments as a backdrop, we review the individual measures most often employed.

Wisconsin Card Sort Test

The Wisconsin Card Sort Test (WCST; Grant & Berg, 1948) is one of the most commonly used measures of adult frontal lobe or executive dysfunction (Lezak, 1995). An examiner presents a series of cards with various colored geometric shapes and numbers of shapes on them. The subject is to sort these cards based on a categorizing rule known only to the examiner (color, number, shape). The examiner gives the subject feedback after each effort to sort a card, indicating whether the sort is correct or incorrect. From this feedback, subjects must deduce the categorizing rule as quickly as possible to limit their number of sorting errors. After a certain number of such trials, the examiner shifts the sorting rule to a different category, and the subject must again deduce the rule from the limited feedback provided. Norms for children were reported by Chelune and Baer (1986). Test–retest reliability appears to be satisfactory (Lezak, 1995). Chelune, Ferguson, Koon, and Dickey (1986) reported significant differences between children with ADHD and nondisabled children on the WCST. However, subsequent efforts have failed to replicate these findings or have produced highly inconsistent results (Fischer, Barkley, Edelbrock, & Smallish, 1990; Grodzinsky & Diamond, 1992; see also Chapter 3, this volume). A recent meta-analysis revealed that effect size differences from control groups involving 14–25 studies ranged from 0.15 to 0.35, being of only small to moderate magnitude (Frazier et al., 2004). More important for clinical diagnosis are the findings that positive and negative predictive power are also rather modest. For instance, Barkley and Grodzinsky (1994) found that the WCST accurately predicted the presence of ADHD in only 50–71% of true cases, while accurately predicting the absence of the disorder in only 49–56% of cases. False-negative rates were 61–89%, and overall accuracy of classification ranged from 49% to 58%, depending on which score from the WCST was used. *Such findings do not encourage the diagnostic use of this test for ADHD.*

Stroop Word–Color Test

The Stroop Word–Color Test (Stroop, 1935) is a timed test measuring the ability to suppress or inhibit automatic responses. Children must read the names of colors, although the names are printed in a different-colored ink from the color specified in the name (e.g., the word "red" is printed in blue ink). Test–retest reliability is well established as is sensitivity to frontal lobe functions in adults (Lezak, 1995). Most studies employing this test have found groups of children with ADHD to perform

more poorly than control groups of children (see Chapter 2, this volume). And one recent meta-analysis revealed an effect size of 0.56 for the interference portion of this test, relative to comparison groups (Frazier et al., 2004). But a meta-analysis specific to this test (Homack & Riccio, 2004) concluded that the specificity of impaired scores on this test as an indicator of ADHD has not been well established. Studies that compared the performance of children with ADHD to that of children with other types of psychopathology typically showed small effect sizes. This finding, along with the lack of compelling evidence concerning positive and negative predictive power, clearly indicate that *this test cannot be used to accurately diagnose children as having ADHD.*

Hand Movements Test

The Hand Movements Test, part of the Kaufman Assessment Battery for Children (Kaufman & Kaufman, 1983), is a well-standardized and well-normed test for children based on a traditional measure of frontal lobe function in adults. Children are presented with progressively longer sequences of three hand movements, which they must imitate. The test has acceptable reliability and normative data, and three studies have shown it to differentiate groups of children with ADHD from groups of nondisabled children (Grodzinsky & Diamond, 1992; Mariani & Barkley, 1997) and from children who have ADD without Hyperactivity (Barkley, Grodzinsky, & DuPaul, 1992). Its sensitivity to ADHD may rest in the well-known fine motor coordination difficulties often seen in these children, as well as in their inattention to the task itself or deficits in nonverbal working memory, especially as sequences of movements become progressively longer. Yet, once again, when subjected to appropriate analysis of its classification accuracy, this test suffers from many of the same problems as those mentioned earlier. Among children with abnormal scores, 88% were found to have ADHD (positive predictive power), which seems impressive. However, the test had a 66% rate of accurately classifying children without the disorder (negative predictive power), a false-negative rate of 63%, and an overall classification accuracy of only 70%. Thus, as with the other neuropsychological tests reviewed here, its major problem is in misclassifying children as nondisabled who actually have ADHD (false negatives). *Again, we must caution against the use of this test for the diagnosis of ADHD.*

Rey–Osterrieth Complex Figure Drawing

The Rey–Osterrieth Complex Figure Drawing (see Lezak, 1995) is a paper-and-pencil task requiring planning and visual–spatial–constructional abilities, and is sensitive to deficits from frontal lobe injuries. The task requires the subject to copy a complex geometric shape. The Waber and Holmes (1985) scoring procedure is often used, yielding scores for organization age (five levels) and style (four categories). Several studies of children with ADHD have shown that they perform this test more poorly on average than do nondisabled children (see Chapter 3, this volume). However, effect size differences from control groups are a mere 0.24–0.26 (Frazier et al., 2004). And once again, Barkley and Grodzinsky (1994) found that although nonaverage test scores accurately predicted the presence of ADHD 100% of the time, average test scores accurately predicted the absence of disorder only 50% of the time, and the false-negative rate was a stunning 96%. Overall, the test accurately classified only 52% of the children. *Therefore, we urge clinicians not to employ this test for diagnostic purposes concerning ADHD.*

Trail Making Test (Parts A and B)

The Intermediate version of the Trail Making Test from the H-R is frequently used with children. It comprises two parts: A and B (Reitan & Wolfson, 1985). In Part A, the subject connects a series of numbered circles distributed arbitrarily on a page. Part B comprises circles that contain letters or numbers scattered randomly across the page; the subject is to alternate connecting numbers and letters in ascending order until the end of the sequences. The scores are the time taken to complete each part by the subject. Some studies have found this test to be useful for differentiating groups of children with ADHD from control groups (Barkley et al., 1992). The average effect size for Part A in 13 studies was 0.40, while that for Part B in 14 studies was slightly higher, being 0.59 (Frazier et al., 2004). Barkley and Grodzinsky (1994) found that the test as a whole accurately predicted presence of disorder 68–71% of the time, accurately predicted

absence of disorder just 51% of the time, and had false-negative rates of 80–82%. Overall classification accuracy was just 54%. Here, then, is another test that *we must recommend against for diagnosing ADHD in children.*

Continuous-Performance Tests

The most popular and widely studied form of testing for use in ADHD evaluations is based on a paradigm called the CPT (Rosvold, Mirsky, Sarason, Bransome, & Beck, 1956). Although the CPT has been administered with many variations (e.g., visual, auditory, numbers, and characters), the most common one requires the youngster to observe a screen while individual letters or numbers are projected onto it at a rapid pace (typically at one per second). The child is told to respond (e.g., to press a button) when a certain stimulus or pair of stimuli in sequence appears. The scores derived from the CPT are the number of correct responses, number of target stimuli missed (omission errors), and number of responses following nontarget or incorrect stimuli (commission errors). The latter score is presumed to tap both sustained attention and impulse control, whereas the two former measures are believed to assess sustained attention only (Sostek, Buchsbaum, & Rapoport, 1980).

Researchers have been examining versions of the CPT paradigm for almost 40 years. A wide-ranging literature has shown it to be the most reliable of psychological tests for discriminating groups of children with ADHD from nondisabled children (Corkum & Siegel, 1993). Average effect size across 40 studies using the commission error score was 0.55, while that for omissions was 0.66 (33 studies), and that for correct hits was 1.00 (19 studies) (Frazier et al., 2004); these were nearly twice the effect sizes found for other tests, such as the Rey–Osterrieth or the WCST (see above). CPTs are also sensitive to stimulant drug effects among children and adolescents with ADHD (Coons, Klorman, & Borgstedt, 1987; Fischer, 1996; Garfinkel et al., 1986). Although concerns abound about its actual discriminative ability and ecological validity (Barkley, 1991), the CPT nonetheless is the only psychological measure that seems to directly assess the core symptoms of the disorder—namely, impulsivity and inattention. Moreover, the CPT assesses these dimensions without undue contamination from other cognitive factors, such as conceptual ability, visual scanning, and so on. In all its embodiments, the CPT places relatively little demand on subjects other than to sustain attention and to refrain from responding except in special circumstances. Finally, use of the CPT may be especially important when clinicians are assessing adults or those suspected of malingering. Quinn (2003) found that college undergraduates asked to simulate malingering were able to do so easily on rating scales, but not on a CPT.

The CPT serves as the paradigm for several commercially available performance measures, including the Conners CPT (Conners, 1995) and Conners CPT II (Conners & MHS Staff, 2000); the Gordon Diagnostic System (GDS; Gordon, 1983); the Test of Variables of Attention (Greenberg & Kindschi, 1996); and the Intermediate Visual and Auditory Continuous Performance Test (Sandford, Fine, & Goldman, 1995). Each format requires the child to respond to certain signals embedded in a series of irrelevant targets. Whereas each measure is a CPT, the tasks vary considerably along what would seem to represent important dimensions, including the length of the task, the type of stimulus, the duration between stimuli, and the instructions to the subject. For example, one measure requires the child to respond based on the position of a certain graphic for 23 minutes; another presents numbers on a screen for 9 minutes; and still another presents a combination of numbers both visually and auditorily. Typically, children sit passively observing (or listening) to the presentation of nontarget stimuli and then must respond (often manually) to the occasional target stimulus. The CPT that differs most from the traditional paradigm was developed by Conners (1995). In this test, the child is told to press a button on each trial until the target appears, at which time the child is to inhibit responding; a different form of response inhibition is thus required.

Which CPT should a clinician choose? Because no data have been published on head-to-head comparisons for reliability, validity, or clinical utility, we cannot offer an empirically based opinion. It is therefore unclear whether these measures would differ from one another in their contributions to accurate identification, ruling out alternative explanations, or confirming comorbid conditions. It is also uncertain whether diagnosis would be more accurate or productive if some combination of these

tests were administered. For example, some investigators say that attention should be assessed both in visual and in auditory modalities. Although some data suggest that children generally find auditory versions more difficult than visual ones (Aylward & Gordon, 1997), no one has presented data that show a superiority of one format over the other. Parenthetically, based on Barkley's theory of ADHD (see Chapter 7, this volume), it would be unlikely that a child would suffer problems with response inhibition in just one sensory modality.

In the absence of *Consumer Reports*-type comparisons, decisions must be based on the sort of parameters mentioned earlier in this chapter: practicality, robustness of standardization, reliability of administration, and the extent to which the technique has been scrutinized scientifically for its potential contributions (or lack thereof). Unfortunately, here again we are constrained by a literature that is limited in scope and depth. Although the past several years have witnessed more research examining the psychometric properties of CPTs, a review by Nichols and Waschbusch (2004) concludes that still more evidence of validity is needed before CPTs can reach their potential for high clinical utility. Limiting progress has been diversity among studies in criterion measures. Also, not all studies have assessed reliability, practicality, and standardization.

One measure that has published information available on all these relevant dimensions was developed by one of us (Gordon). The GDS has been used extensively in research and clinical practice. It is a portable, solid-state, childproofed computerized device that administers a 9-minute vigilance task wherein the child must press a button each time a specified, randomly presented numerical sequence (e.g., a 1 followed by a 9) occurs. Another version of this task presents random distracters on either side of the center target. Normative data are available for more than 1,000 children on the mainland United States ages 3–16 years (Gordon & Mettelman, 1988) and for Puerto Rican children (Bauermeister, Berrios, Jiminez, Acevedo, & Gordon, 1990). Norms are also available for an auditory version of this task (Gordon, Lewandowski, Clonan, & Malone, 1996). Gordon's CPT has been found to have satisfactory test–retest reliability (Gordon & Mettelman, 1988), to correlate modestly but significantly with other laboratory measures of attention (Barkley, 1991), to discriminate groups of children with ADHD from nondisabled children (Barkley, DuPaul, & McMurray, 1991; Gordon, 1987; Grodzinsky & Diamond, 1992; Mariani & Barkley, 1997), and to be sensitive to moderate to high doses of stimulant medication (Barkley, Fischer, Newby, & Breen, 1988; Barkley, DuPaul, & McMurray, 1990; Fischer & Newby, 1991; Fischer, 1996; Rapport, Tucker, DuPaul, Merlo, Stoner, 1986). The GDS is useful in the assessment of children with hearing impairment (Mitchell & Quittner, 1996). A body of literature also suggests that poor GDS performance is tied to other neuropsychological measures (Grant, Ilai, Nussbaum, & Bigler, 1990) and to general academic underachievement (Aylward et al., 1997; Billings, 1996; Gordon, Mettelman, & Irwin, 1994).

One study (Mayes, Calhoun, & Crowell, 2001) investigated the clinical validity of the GDS, using a DSM-based assessment as the criterion measure. Large differences were found between groups with and without ADHD in GDS composite standard scores (d = .92) and IQ-GDS discrepancies (d = 1.08). More importantly, a discrepancy score cutoff formula (a 13-point discrepancy between GDS composite and IQ) resulted in a sensitivity of 90% and a specificity of 70%.

As with the interpretation of any psychological test for the diagnosis of ADHD, interpreting the data from traditional validity studies of CPTs can be vexing, because no gold standard is available to use for comparison with these tests (Gordon, 1993). Nonetheless, if we use either a high score on ADHD-related behavior rating scales or DSM clinical diagnoses as benchmarks, the GDS appears to accurately classify 83–90% of children with abnormal scores as having ADHD (Barkley & Grodzinsky, 1994). Its classification accuracy for children with average scores as not having the disorder is, however, 59–61%. Moreover, a range of 15–52% has been found for its false-negative rate (i.e., children who are rated by parents or teachers as having ADHD, but who obtain average scores on the test) (Gordon, Mettelman, & DiNiro, 1989; Barkley & Grodzinsky, 1994; Trommer, Hoeppner, Lorber, & Armstrong, 1988). Therefore, as with all the neuropsychological tests discussed here, if a child performs well on this measure, it does not indicate that the child is nondisabled or without ADHD. But it may have some diagnostic significance when a child otherwise considered to have ADHD exhibits average performance on the GDS. Research by Fischer et al. (1995) shows that these children are typically rated as less impaired, more likely to show comorbid internalizing problems, and less likely to be prescribed stimulant medications. Data such as these suggest that, if anything, GDS performance might represent an indication of severity.

The false-positive rate of the instrument is good to excellent, with 2–17% of nondisabled children being classified as having ADHD (Gordon et al., 1989; Barkley & Grodzinsky, 1994). These kinds of data may be helpful in cases for which objective confirmation of the diagnosis is important. But even here, the GDS cannot be used for objective *disconfirmation* of the disorder, given the rate of false negatives found in some studies. Once again, the presence of a nonaverage score probably (but not necessarily) indicates the presence of disorder, whereas the presence of an average score must go uninterpreted, as it may not indicate the absence of disorder. As with rating scales, the test provides one source of information to be integrated with other sources in reaching a final diagnostic decision.

Another popular measure, the Conners CPT (Conners, 1995), has enjoyed some scientific attention. Two such studies focused specifically on its diagnostic utility in ADHD assessments—one study with children (McGee, Clark, & Symonds, 2000) and another with adults (Epstein, Conners, Sitarenios, & Erhardt, 1998).

McGee et al. (2000) investigated associations between Conners CPT scores and several other measures, including parent and teacher ratings as well as neuropsychological and achievement tests. These researchers reported several positive findings concerning the Conners CPT, including its lack of relation to age, order and fatigue effects, or peripheral motor skill. However, the Conners test's overall index failed to relate to parent and teacher ratings, and only slightly over half of those participants who met criteria for ADHD "failed" this CPT (i.e., obtained a total index score of over 11). Furthermore, the test demonstrated poor discriminant validity, in that children with a reading disability actually performed more poorly than children with ADHD.

Epstein et al. (1998) conducted a similar study, using adult participants who were given a semistructured interview to classify them as having ADHD or not, and who then were administered the Conners CPT. Importantly, these investigators created dependent variables from this CPT using signal detection theory (e.g., d'), and also used raw scores such as reaction time, rather than using cutoff scores or total index scores. Even so, none of the Conners CPT scores correlated significantly with ADHD symptoms as measured by the semistructured interview. When scores on the three most discriminating aspects of this CPT were compared with initial classifications, the test's sensitivity was only 55%, although its specificity was somewhat better (76.4%).

A more recent study assessed the newly revised version of the Conners CPT (the Conners CPT II; Conners & MHS Staff, 2000) in a school-based sample by Weis and Totten (2004). Like McGee et al. (2000) and Epstein et al. (1998), Weis and Totten's results cast doubt on the utility of the Conners CPT II, extending previous findings to the new version. These investigators found mostly nonsignificant relationships between CPT II performance and three other kinds of measures (parent ratings, teacher ratings, and classroom observations). Furthermore, Weis and Totten questioned the discriminative validity of the CPT II, due to a significant negative correlation between IQ (as assessed by the Kaufman Brief Intelligence Test) and omission scores on the CPT II. The authors interpret this finding, in the context of other results, as suggesting that the CPT II may measure letter recognition skills or phonological awareness rather than impulsivity or inattention per se.

Two recent studies by Conners and his colleagues contain interesting information about the properties of the Conners CPT II as well as newer normative data, but neither paper allows for direct inferences concerning diagnostic utility. Conners, Epstein, Angold, and Klaric (2003) present interesting analyses of this CPT, looking at age × gender interactions, and also varying the interstimulus interval. Epstein et al. (2003) used generalized estimating equation statistics to show strong associations between various indices of Conners CPT II performance and ADHD symptoms, but since the latter variable is continuous, we are not able (given only the published data) to calculate easily the sensitivity and specificity or the positive and negative predictive power of this CPT for ADHD status.

Other Motor Inhibition Tasks

Two other motor inhibition tasks show promise as aids in diagnostic assessment. In the go/no-go task, an individual responds to a certain class of stimuli (e.g., leftward-pointing arrows flashed on a screen) by making some motor response (e.g., pressing a button, squeezing a dynamometer), but withholds any response to another class of stimuli (e.g., upward- and downward-pointing arrows flashed on a screen). In a similar second task, the stop signal task (SST), an individual is asked to press one of two computer keys, depending on which of two stimuli is shown on the screen—except when a certain tone sounds before the stimulus is presented, in which case neither key should be pressed. These two tasks are both presumed to measure executive functioning in the motoric domain (Zelazo & Müller, 2002).

Recent meta-analyses (Frazier et al., 2004; Hervey, Epstein, & Curry, 2004) have found moderate to large effect sizes (0.55–0.66) when groups with ADHD and control groups are compared on the SST paradigm. In their review, Nichols and Waschbusch (2004) singled out the SST as one of the "most promising" developments in ADHD assessment, but noted that much of the convergent validation has related SST performance to other laboratory measures, rather than to tasks in more naturalistic settings. Furthermore, Nichols and Waschbusch found inconsistency across studies comparing the performance of individuals with ADHD to those in other clinical groups; the differences tended to be small and not always in the same direction.

The go/no-go task, though it comes from a rich intellectual heritage (e.g., Luria, 1966), boasts less research in clinical populations. Most of that research has dealt either with schizophrenia or with the electrophysiological underpinnings of performance on the task. The one recent study examining the discriminative validity of the go/no-go task in ADHD assessments (Berlin, Bohlin, Nyberg, & Janols, 2004) combined performance on this measure with results from eight other neuropsychological measures. There was a statistically significant difference between participants with ADHD and controls on the go/no-go task, but in a logistic regression model used to predict group status, performance on the go/no-go task did not contribute significantly, and the predictive power of the regression model did not decline when the go/no-go task was dropped as a variable.

Cancellation Tasks

Several paper-and-pencil versions of CPTs have been used as methods of assessing attention. These tasks typically involve having a child scan a series of symbols (letters, numbers, shapes) presented in rows on sheets of paper. The child is typically required to draw a line through or under the target stimulus, using a pencil. One such task, which has shown promise in discriminating children with ADHD from nondisabled children, is the Children's Checking Task (CCT; Margolis, 1972). The CCT consists of seven pages with a series of 15 numerals per row printed in 16 rows on a page. A tape recorder reads off the numbers in each row, and the child is required to draw a line through each number as it is read. Discrepancies between the tape and printed page are to be circled by the child. There are seven discrepancies between the tape and printed pages. The CCT takes about 30 minutes to complete. Scores are derived for errors of omission (missed discrepancies) and errors of commission (numbers circled that were not discrepancies). Brown and Wynne (1982) found that the task discriminated groups of children with ADHD from those with reading disabilities. The CCT correlates modestly but significantly with other measures of attention (Keogh & Margolis, 1976), often to a larger degree than any of the other laboratory measures (see Barkley, 1991). Perhaps this is because it is somewhat similar to the academic accuracy demands made during work that children must do in the classroom. *Nevertheless, its sensitivity to ADHD symptoms requires more research and replication of these initially promising results before it can be recommended for clinical practice.*

Matching Familiar Figures Test

This Matching Familiar Figures Test (MFFT; Kagan, 1966) has a lengthy history of use in research studies investigating impulse control in both nondisturbed and disturbed children and adolescents. This match-to-sample test involves the examiner's presenting a picture of a recognizable object to the youngster, who must choose the identical matching picture from among an array of six similar variants. The test includes 12 trials, with scores derived for the mean time taken to the initial response (latency) and the total number of errors (incorrectly identified pictures). A longer version of the MFFT employing 20 stimulus trials (MFFT-20) has been developed (Cairns & Cammock, 1978); it is purported to achieve greater reliability among older children and adolescents (Messer & Brodzinsky, 1981). Unfortunately, more recent research on the original test has often failed to find significant differences between children with ADHD and nondisabled children (Barkley et al., 1991; Fischer et al., 1990; Milich & Kramer, 1984). A meta-analysis of 11 studies found an average effect size of 0.27 for the timing score, but a more satisfactory result of 0.60 for the errors score (Frazier et al., 2004). The MFFT has also shown conflicting and often negative results in detecting stimulant drug effects in children with ADHD (Barkley, 1977; Barkley et al., 1991). Furthermore, norms for the adolescent population are not currently available for either the MFFT or the MFFT-20, thus limiting their use as diagnostic measures. Evidence for acceptable positive and negative predictive power is lacking, and no new research on this measure could be located since the publication of the preceding edition of this text that would alter these conclusions. The MFFT appears to have fallen into both clinical and scientific disuse. *Consequently, we do not endorse this instrument for use in clinical practice in making diagnostic decisions about ADHD in children.*

GDS Delay Task

The GDS Delay Task, a part of the GDS discussed above (Gordon, 1983), is a measure of response inhibition. It utilizes a paradigm of direct reinforcement of low rates of behavior. The child sits before the portable, computerized GDS device and is told to wait a while before pressing a large blue button on the front panel of the device. Children are told that if they have waited long enough, they will earn a point when they push the button. If they press it too early, they must wait a while before pushing the button again. Cumulative points are scored on a digital counter on the face of the device. The child is not informed of the actual delay required to earn reinforcement (6 seconds). The test lasts 8 minutes and has normative data for more than 1,000 children. Initial evidence (Gordon, 1979; Gordon & McClure,

1983; McClure & Gordon, 1984) indicated that the test discriminated groups of children with ADHD from children with no disorder or with other disorders, correlated significantly with parent and teacher ratings of hyperactivity and other lab measures of impulsivity, and had adequate test–retest reliability (Gordon & Mettelman, 1988). However, others (Barkley et al., 1988) have found the task to be insensitive to stimulant drug effects in children with ADHD, and to correlate poorly if at all with ratings of hyperactivity by parents and teachers (Barkley, 1991). One benefit of such measures is that it allows a clinician to observe a youngster in a situation requiring inhibition and sustained attention. *But the test has not been examined for its classification accuracy with regard to discriminating either ADHD from no disorder or ADHD from other psychiatric disorders, and so its role in a diagnostic evaluation remains to be established..*

Measures of Activity

The measurement of activity level was discussed in a prior edition of this chapter (Barkley, 1990). Given that there have been no clinically meaningful advances in this field of study since that time, no further comment about such measures is made here. Although advances have been made in various technologies for the measurement of activity levels in children with ADHD (see Matier-Sharma et al., 1995; Teicher, Ito, Glod, & Barber, 1996), such improvements are more useful in conducting research investigations of activity level than in making clinically accurate diagnoses. For instance, Matier-Sharma et al. (1995) examined the classification accuracy of a solid-state activity recording device (the actigraph) in judging children as having either ADHD or no disability and then as having either ADHD or another psychiatric disorder. In the first comparison, the activity measure accurately classified 91% of children with high activity scores as having ADHD. But it accurately classified children with low activity scores as having no disability at a level of just 36%. The situation for the comparison of ADHD to other psychiatric disorders was worse. The presence of a high activity level predicted the presence of ADHD in this case with only 77% accuracy; the presence of an average score predicted the presence of a non-ADHD disorder with an accuracy of just

63%. Such figures do not support a recommendation to use the activity measurement in the differential diagnosis of children with ADHD from either nondisabled children or children with other disorders. A parent and teacher rating scale of hyperactive–impulsive behavior would be a more economical and ecologically valid means of assessing this dimension of behavior than would the use of laboratory activity-recording devices.

Projective Measures

No published studies demonstrate the predictive validity of projective tests (such as drawings, inkblots, or storytelling techniques) for the identification of ADHD. However, there is some indication of differences between children with ADHD and nondisabled children on the Rorschach inkblots (Bartell & Solanto, 1995; Gordon & Oshman, 1981; Cotungo, 1995). Indices of impulsivity on the Rorschach may correlate with an objective measure of impulsivity (Ebner & Hynan, 1994); however, this does not necessarily make the Rorschach useful in evaluating ADHD, as no evidence is available for the positive and negative predictive power of this test for ADHD, especially relative to other clinical disorders. Some evidence is also available that children with ADHD may differ from nondisabled children on the Thematic Apperception Test (Costantino, Collin-Malgady, Malgady, & Perez, 1991). But the data do not support use of this test, either, for judging whether a child suffers from this disorder. The gist of these studies is that children with ADHD are indeed more impulsive and easily frustrated than controls. Groups with ADHD also demonstrate more intense feelings of loneliness and dependence, and come across as more avoidant and socially uncomfortable. Yet much of this information could have been more economically obtained, and probably with greater ecological validity, from the broad-band parent and teacher rating scales and/or from the parent and teacher clinical interviews discussed in Chapter 8 (this volume).

Projective measures might be useful when questions are raised about the possibility of serious thought or emotional disturbance. In our opinion, most of the best diagnostic indicators for ADHD are only valid for children who do not otherwise display the more devastating forms of psychiatric impairment. This holds especially true for judging the quality and onset of socially impulsive behavior, because deeply disturbed children (i.e., those suffering from a pervasive developmental disorder, from schizophrenia or another psychotic disorder, or from an acute trauma) are also likely to act out with some consistency. Yet even here, poor inhibition seems to be relatively specific to ADHD (Pennington & Ozonoff, 1996). In these cases, administration of a reliable and valid test of cognitive coping skills may steer the clinician in the right diagnostic direction. For children and adolescents, the Rorschach inkblots administered and scored according to the comprehensive system (Exner, 1993) can provide meaningful data regarding levels of psychopathology and stress. Yet, as noted above, it is also possible that this information could have been gleaned more economically from a structured psychiatric interview that reviews the major child psychiatric disorders with parents, in combination with parent and teacher behavior rating scales, as recommended in Chapter 8. The utility of projective tests in the routine clinical evaluation of children with ADHD remains doubtful, *warranting us to conclude that they should not be routinely used in the examination of children for ADHD.*

OBSERVATIONAL MEASURES

Although a number of studies support the benefit of incorporating structured classroom observations of children into the diagnostic process (see DuPaul & Stoner, 2003), they are not enough to justify the considerable cost and effort they involve. For most clinicians, formal behavior coding is simply impractical; even if clinicians desired to observe a child in a school setting, insurance carriers are not likely to cover this cost, which would leave it to parents to foot the bill out of pocket. Thus we do not review classroom observation methods here. Readers who want to consider instituting an informal observational protocol should refer to Gordon (1995). A more formal approach to behavior coding is available in a previous edition of this book (Barkley, 1990).

Another observational setting that may have merit is the clinician's office during the psychological testing session itself. Clinicians have long recorded test session behavior while administering standardized tests, but the behavior assessments themselves have rarely been standardized. The newly developed Test Observation Form (TOF; McConaughy, 2005; McConaughy & Achenbach, 2004) is part of the Achenbach System of Empirically Based Assessment (ASEBA; Achenbach & Rescorla, 2003). It asks clinicians to write narrative observations of specific behaviors during the test administration and then to rate the child on 125 items (e.g., "fidgets"), based on the narrative observations. As in the other ASEBA instruments (e.g., the Child Behavior Checklist), item scores are summed to make subscale scores, which together form a profile of the child's test session behavior. The TOF's syndrome scales are (a) Withdrawn/Depressed, (b) Language/Thought Problems, (c) Anxious, (d) Oppositional, and (e) Attention Problems. In addition, item scores can be used to obtain scores on Internalizing and Externalizing subscales, as well as on a DSM-based ADHD scale. For each subscale, the child's scores are compared with a national sample of normative data to derive standardized *T* scores. Although the TOF may hold promise as a method of enhancing the number and quality of data from a psychological test session, at this point few data are yet available to support its use as a tool in the diagnosis of ADHD. As noted in Chapter 8, ratings of child behavior during clinical testing are significantly associated with school behavioral problems and so may have some predictive validity.

In a study of 158 children ages 6–11 years, McConaughy, Volpe, and Eiraldi (2005) found that children with ADHD scored significantly higher than typically developing control children on all TOF scales except the Withdrawn/Depressed syndrome. Children with ADHD scored significantly higher than clinically referred children without ADHD on 8 of 11 TOF scales. Children with ADHD, Combined Type, scored significantly higher than referred children without ADHD on the TOF Oppositional and Attention Problems syndromes, Externalizing, and Total Problems, plus the DSM-based ADHD total score and two ADHD subscales measuring Inattention and Hyperactivity–Impulsivity. Children with ADHD, Predominantly Inattentive Type, scored significantly higher than referred children without ADHD on the TOF Language/Thought Problems, Attention Problems, Externalizing, and Total

Problems, plus the DSM-based ADHD total score and Inattention subscale. Children with ADHD, Combined Type, scored significantly higher than children with ADHD, Predominantly Inattentive Type, on the TOF ADHD total score and the Hyperactivity–Impulsivity subscale, plus the TOF Oppositional syndrome, Externalizing, and Total Problems. These findings show good discriminative validity of the TOF for differentiating children with ADHD from nondisabled controls and clinically referred children without ADHD, as well as differentiating two ADHD subtypes from each other.

CONCLUSION

Our review places psychological testing somewhere in a middle ground of clinical utility. Although no evidence exists to support performance measures as pristinely diagnostic, data do justify their use under certain conditions and within a context of respect for their limitations. We therefore disagree with the extreme position that such measures are so inaccurate as to be always irrelevant to clinical evaluations of children with ADHD. Because markers for the disorder have been elusive, assessment and identification continue to rest on the integration of data derived from multiple yet inherently imperfect sources. Therefore, any meaningful information that can help a clinician judge the nature and severity of a child's deficits can be of potential benefit. As we have indicated, psychological test data may be of particular help when information from parents or teachers is unavailable or of questionable credibility.

Although we disagree with positions that completely reject psychological testing within ADHD evaluations under all circumstances, we are equally uncomfortable with the opposite stance. Psychological test data should not be oversold either as a basis for diagnosis or as a unitary standard for assessing treatment effects. The empirical basis for championing that level of confidence is far from solid. In our view, the most sensible advice is to target psychological testing to discrete issues that the particular tests may have some validity to address, such as impairment in various cognitive processes, rather than using them to make diagnostic decisions.

KEY CLINICAL POINTS

✓ Data from psychological testing or direct observational methods, when considered in isolation, have not been established as sensitive or specific markers for ADHD. Therefore, identifying an individual as having ADHD primarily on the basis of psychological testing or classroom observations is inappropriate.

✓ Although psychological testing is not diagnostic of ADHD per se, it can play a meaningful role in the diagnostic enterprise. Such measures can establish levels of intellectual/academic functioning, contribute behavior-based data to a process that is based primarily on opinion, and aid in the pursuit of alternative explanations for presenting complaints.

✓ Continuous-performance tests (CPTs) are the most evidence-based of the currently available psychological tests. They have demonstrated reasonable sensitivity and specificity, as well as promising positive predictive power. As for almost all such measures, however, a high false-negative rate can limit the validity of CPTs in certain clinical settings.

✓ Some psychological tests, because they may document deficits in children with ADHD, can be informative for treatment (particularly educational planning). Yet, again, such information should be regarded with caution, because it may have low ecological validity.

REFERENCES

Achenbach, T. M., & Rescorla, L. A. (2003). *Manual for the ASEBA Adult Forms and Profiles*. Burlington, VT: University of Vermont, Research Center for Children, Youth, and Families.

American Psychiatric Association. (1980). *Diagnostic and statistical manual of mental disorders* (3rd ed.). Washington, DC: Author.

Anastopoulos, A. D., Spisto, M. A., & Maher, M. C. (1994). The WISC-III Freedom from Distractibility factor: Its utility in identifying children with attention deficit hyperactivity disorder. *Psychological Assessment, 6*, 368–371.

Aylward, G. P., & Gordon, M. (1997). Visual and auditory CPTs: Comparisons across clinical and nonclinical samples. *ADHD Newsletter, 24*, 2–4.

Aylward, G. P., Gordon, M., & Verhulst, S. J. (1997).

Relationships between continuous performance task scores and other cognitive measures: Causality or commonality? *Assessment, 4*(4), 313–324.

Barkley, R. A. (1977). A review of stimulant drug research with hyperactive children. *Journal of Child Psychology and Psychiatry, 18,* 137–165.

Barkley, R. A. (1990). *Attention-deficit hyperactivity disorder: A handbook for diagnosis and treatment.* New York: Guilford Press.

Barkley, R. A. (1991). The ecological validity of laboratory and analogue assessment methods of ADHD symptoms. *Journal of Abnormal Child Psychology, 19,* 149–178.

Barkley, R. A., DuPaul, G. J., & McMurray, M. B. (1990). A comprehensive evaluation of attention deficit disorder with and without hyperactivity. *Journal of Consulting and Clinical Psychology, 58,* 775–789.

Barkley, R. A., DuPaul, G. J., & McMurray, M. B. (1991). Attention deficit disorder with and without hyperactivity: Clinical response to three dose levels of methylphenidate. *Pediatrics, 87,* 519–531.

Barkley, R. A., Fischer, M., Newby, R., & Breen, M. (1988). Development of a multi-method clinical protocol for assessing stimulant drug responses in ADHD children. *Journal of Clinical Child Psychology, 17,* 14–24.

Barkley, R. A, & Grodzinsky, G. (1994). Are tests of frontal lobe functions useful in the diagnosis of attention deficit disorders? *Clinical Neuropsychologist, 8,* 121–139.

Barkley, R. A., Grodzinsky, G., & DuPaul, G. J. (1992). Frontal lobe functions in attention deficit disorder with and without hyperactivity: A review and research report. *Journal of Abnormal Child Psychology, 20,* 163–188.

Bartell, S. S., & Solanto, M. V. (1995). Usefulness of the Rorschach inkblot test in the assessment of attention deficit hyperactivity disorder. *Perceptual and Motor Skills, 80*(2), 531–541.

Bauermeister, J. J., Berrios, V., Jimenez, A. L., Acevedo, L., & Gordon, M. (1990). Some issues and instruments for the assessment of attention-deficit hyperactivity disorder in Puerto Rican children. *Journal of Clinical Child Psychology, 19,* 9–16.

Berlin, L., Bohlin, G., Nyberg, L., & Janols, L. (2004). How well do measures of inhibition and other executive functions discriminate between with ADHD and controls? *Child Neuropsychology, 10,* 1–13.

Billings, R. (1996). *The relationship between the Gordon Diagnostic System and measures of intelligences and achievement.* Poster presented at the Eighth Annual International Conference of CHADD, Chicago.

Brown, R. T., & Wynne, M. E. (1982). Correlates of teacher ratings, sustained attention, and impulsivity in hyperactive and normal boys. *Journal of Clinical Child Psychology, 11,* 262–267.

Cairns, E., & Cammock, T. (1978). Development of a more reliable version of the Matching Familiar Figures Test. *Developmental Psychology, 11,* 244–248.

Chelune, G. J., & Baer, R. A. (1986). Developmental norms for the Wisconsin Card Sort Test. *Journal of Clinical and Experimental Neuropsychology, 8,* 219–228.

Chelune, G. J., Ferguson, W., Koon, R., & Dickey, T. O. (1986). Frontal lobe disinhibition in attention deficit disorder. *Child Psychiatry and Human Development, 16,* 221–234.

Conners, C. K. (1995). *The Conners Continuous Performance Test.* North Tonawanda, NY: Multi-Health Systems.

Conners, C. K., Epstein, J. N., Angold, A., & Klaric, J. (2003). Continuous performance test performance in a normative epidemiological sample. *Journal of Abnormal Child Psychology, 31,* 555–562.

Conners, C. K., & MHS Staff. (2000). *Conners Continuous Performance Test II.* Tonawanda, NY: Multi-Health Systems.

Coons, H. W., Klorman, R., & Borgstedt, A. D. (1987). Effects of methylphenidate on adolescents with a childhood history of ADD: II. Information processing. *Journal of the American Academy of Child and Adolescent Psychiatry, 26,* 368–374.

Corkum, P. V., & Siegel, L. S. (1993). Is the continuous performance task a valuable research tool for use with children with attention-deficit-hyperactivity disorder? *Journal of Child Psychology and Psychiatry, 34,* 1217–1239.

Costantino, G., Collin-Malgady, G., Malgady, R. G., & Perez, A. (1991). Assessment of attention deficit disorder using a thematic apperception technique. *Journal of Personality Assessment, 57,* 87–95.

Cotungo, A. (1995). Personality attributes of ADHD using a Rorschach inkblot test. *Journal of Clinical Psychology, 5,* 554–562.

Demaray, M. K., Schaefer, K., & Delong, L. K. (2003). Attention-deficit/hyperactivity disorder (ADHD): A national survey of training and assessment practices in the schools. *Psychology in the Schools, 40,* 583–597.

DuPaul, G. J., & Stoner, G. (2003). *ADHD in the schools: Assessment and intervention strategies* (2nd ed.). New York: Guilford Press.

Ebner, D. L., & Hynan, L. S. (1994). The Rorschach and the assessment of impulsivity. *Journal of Clinical Psychology, 50,* 633–638.

Epstein, J. N., Conners, C. K., Sitarenios, G., & Erhardt, D. (1998). Continuous performance test results of adults with attention deficit hyperactivity disorder. *The Clinical Neuropsychologist, 12,* 155–168.

Epstein, J. N., Erkanli, A., Conners, C. K., Klaric, J., Costello, J. E., & Angold, A. (2003). Relations between continuous performance test performance measures and ADHD behaviors. *Journal of Abnormal Child Psychology, 31,* 543–554.

Exner, J. E. (1993). *The Rorschach: A comprehensive system* (Vol. 1). New York: Wiley.

Fischer, M. (1996). Erratum regarding medication response of the Gordon Diagnostic System. *Journal of Clinical Child Psychology, 25*(1), 121.

Fischer, M., Barkley, R. A., Edelbrock, C. S., & Small-ish, L. (1990). The adolescent outcome of hyperactive children diagnosed by research criteria: II. Academic, attentional, and neuropsychological status. *Journal of Consulting and Clinical Psychology, 58,* 580–588.

Fischer, M., & Newby, R. F. (1991). Assessment of stimulant response in ADHD children using a refined multimethod clinical protocol. *Journal of Clinical Child Psychology, 20,* 232–244.

Fischer, M., Newby, R. F., & Gordon. M. (1995). Who are the false negatives on continuous performance tests? *Journal of Clinical Child Psychology, 24,* 427–433.

Frazier, T. W., Demaree, H. A., & Youngstrom, E. A. (2004). Meta-analysis of intellectual and neuropsychological test performance in attention-deficit/hyperactivity disorder. *Neuropsychology, 18,* 543–555.

Garfinkel, B. D., Brown, W. A., Klee, S. H., Braden, W., Beauchesne, H., & Shapiro, S. L. (1986). Neuroendocrine and cognitive responses to amphetamine in adolescents with a history of attention deficit disorder. *Journal of the American Academy of Child Psychiatry, 25,* 503–508.

Golden, J. (1996). Are tests of working memory and inattention diagnostically useful in children with ADHD? *ADHD Report, 4*(5), 6–8.

Gordon, M. (1979). The assessment of impulsivity and mediating behaviors in hyperactive and non-hyperactive children. *Journal of Abnormal Child Psychology, 7,* 317–326.

Gordon, M. (1983). *The Gordon Diagnostic System.* DeWitt, NY: Gordon Systems.

Gordon, M. (1987). How is a computerized attention test used in the diagnosis of attention deficit disorder? In J. Loney (Ed.*), The young hyperactive child: Answers to questions about diagnosis, prognosis, and treatment* (pp. 53–64). New York: Haworth Press.

Gordon, M. (1993). Do computerized measures of attention have a legitimate role in ADHD evaluations? *ADHD Report, 1*(6), 5–6.

Gordon, M. (1994). A survey of GDS users. *ADHD Newsletter, 20,* 4.

Gordon, M. (1995). *How to operate an ADHD clinic or subspecialty practice.* Syracuse, NY: GSI.

Gordon, M., Lewandowski, L., Clonan, S., & Malone, K. (1996). *Standardization of the Auditory Vigilance Task.* Paper presented at the Eighth Annual International Conference of CHADD, Chicago.

Gordon, M., & McClure, F. D. (1983, August*). The objective assessment of attention deficit disorders.* Paper presented at the 91st Annual Convention of the American Psychological Association, Anaheim, CA.

Gordon, M., & Mettelman, B. B. (1988). The assessment of attention: I. Standardization and reliability of a behavior based measure. *Journal of Clinical Psychology, 44,* 682–690.

Gordon, M., Mettelman, B. B., & DeNiro, D. (1989,

August). *Are continuous performance tests valid in the diagnosis of ADHD/hyperactivity?* Paper presented at the 97th Annual Convention of the American Psychological Association, New Orleans, LA.

Gordon, M., Mettelman, B. B., & Irwin, M. (1994). Sustained attention and grade retention. *Perceptual and Motor Skills, 78,* 555–560.

Gordon, M., & Oshman, H. (1981). Rorschach indices of children classified as hyperactive. *Perceptual and Motor Skills, 52,* 703–707.

Gordon, M., Thomason, D., & Cooper, S. (1990). To what extent does attention affect K-ABC scores? *Psychology in the Schools, 27,* 144–147.

Grant, D. A., & Berg, E. A. (1948). *The Wisconsin Card Sort Test: Directions for administration and scoring.* Odessa, FL: Psychological Assessment Resources.

Grant, M. L., Ilai, D., Nussbaum, N. L., & Bigler, E. D. (1990). The relationship between continuous performance tasks and neuropsychological tests in children with attention-deficit hyperactivity disorder. *Perceptual and Motor Skills, 70,* 435–445.

Greenberg, L. M., & Kindschi, C. L. (1996). *T.O.V.A. Test of Variables of Attention: Clinical guide.* St. Paul, MN: TOVA Research Foundation.

Greenblatt, E., Mattis, S., & Trad, P. V. (1991). The ACID pattern and the Freedom from Distractibility factor in a child psychiatric population. *Developmental Neuropsychology, 7,* 121–130.

Grodzinsky, G. M., & Diamond, R. (1992). Frontal lobe functioning in boys with attention-deficit hyperactivity disorder. *Developmental Neuropsychology, 8,* 427–445.

Hervey, A. S., Epstein, J. N., & Curry, J. F. (2004). Neuropsychology of adults with attention-deficit/hyperactivity disorder: A meta-analytic review. *Neuropsychology, 18,* 495–503.

Homack, S., & Riccio, C. A. (2004). A meta-analysis of the sensitivity and specificity of the Stroop Color and Word Test with children. *Archives of Clinical Neuropsychology, 19,* 725–743.

Kagan, J. (1966). Reflection–impulsivity: The generality and dynamics of conceptual tempo. *Journal of Abnormal Psychology, 71,* 17–24.

Kaufman, A. S. (1980). Issues in psychological assessment: Interpreting the WISC-R intelligently. In B. B. Lahey & A. E. Kazdin (Eds.), *Advances in clinical child psychology (*Vol. 3, pp. 177–214). New York: Plenum Press.

Kaufman, A. S., & Kaufman, N. L. (1983). *Kaufman Assessment Battery for Children.* Circle Pines, MN: American Guidance Service.

Keogh, B. K., & Margolis, J. S. (1976). A component analysis of attentional problems of educationally handicapped boys. *Journal of Abnormal Child Psychology, 4,* 349–359.

Klee, S. H., & Garfinkel, B. D. (1983). The computerized continuous performance task: A new measure of attention. *Journal of the American Academy of Child Psychiatry, 11,* 487–496.

Lezak, M. D. (1995). *Neuropsychological assessment* (3rd ed.). New York: Oxford University Press.

Luria, A. R. (1966). *Higher cortical functions in man.* New York: Basic Books.

Mariani, M., & Barkley, R. A. (1997). Neuropsychological and academic functioning in preschool children with attention deficit hyperactivity disorder. *Developmental Neuropsychology, 13,* 111–129.

Margolis, J. S. (1972). *Academic correlates of sustained attention.* Unpublished doctoral dissertation, University of California–Los Angeles.

Matier-Sharma, K., Perachio, N., Newcorn, J. H., Sharma, V., & Halperin, J. M. (1995). Differential diagnosis of ADHD: Are objective measures of attention, impulsivity, and activity level helpful? *Child Neuropsychology, 1,* 118–127.

Mayes, S. D., Calhoun, S. L., & Crowell, E. W. (2001). Clinical validity and interpretation of the Gordon Diagnostic System in ADHD assessments. *Child Neuropsychology, 7,* 32–41.

McClure, F. D., & Gordon, M. (1984). Performance of disturbed hyperactive and nonhyperactive children on an objective measure of hyperactivity. *Journal of Abnormal Child Psychology, 12,* 561–572.

McConaughy, S. H. (2005). The Test Observation Form (TOF): A new observation tool for school psychologists. *NASP Communique, 33*(5), 36–38.

McConaughy, S. H., & Achenbach, T. M. (2004). *Manual for the Test Observation Form for Ages 2 to 18.* Burlington, VT: University of Vermont, Research Center for Children, Youth, and Families.

McConaughy, S. H., Volpe, R. J., & Eiraldi, R. B. (2005). *Discriminant validity of the Test Observation Form for attention deficit-hyperactivity disorder and the combined versus inattentive subtypes.* Manuscript submitted for publication.

McGee, R. A., Clark, S. E., & Symonds, D. K. (2000). Does the Conners' Continuous Performance Test aid in ADHD diagnosis? *Journal of Abnormal Child Psychology, 28,* 415–424.

Messer, S., & Brodzinsky, D. M. (1981). Three year stability of reflection–impulsivity in young adolescents. *Developmental Psychology, 17,* 848–850.

Milich, R., & Kramer, J. (1984). Reflections on impulsivity: An empirical investigation of impulsivity as a construct. In K. Gadow & I. Bialer (Eds.), *Advances in learning and behavioral disabilities* (Vol. 3, pp. 57–94). Greenwich, CT: JAI Press.

Milich, R., & Loney, J. (1979). The role of hyperactive and aggressive symptomatology in predicting adolescent outcome among hyperactive children. *Journal of Pediatric Psychology, 4,* 93–112.

Mitchell, T. V., & Quittner, A. L. (1996). Multimethod study of attention and behavior problems in hearing-impaired children. *Journal of Clinical Child Psychology, 25*(1), 83–96.

Nichols, S. L., & Waschbusch, D. A. (2004). A review of the validity of laboratory cognitive tasks used to assess symptoms of ADHD. *Child Psychiatry and Human Development, 34,* 297–315.

Ownby, R. L., & Matthews, C. G. (1985). On the meaning of the WISC-R third factor: Relations to selected neuropsychological measures. *Journal of Consulting and Clinical Psychology, 53,* 531–534.

Pennington, B. F., & Ozonoff, S. (1996). Executive functions and developmental psychopathology. *Journal of Child Psychology and Psychiatry, 37,* 51–87.

Quinn, C. A. (2003). Detection of malingering in assessment of adult ADHD. *Archives of Clinical Neuropsychology, 18,* 379–395.

Rapport, M. D., Tucker, S. B., DuPaul, G. J., Merlo, M., & Stoner, G. (1986). Hyperactivity and frustration: The influence of control over and size of rewards in delaying gratification. *Journal of Abnormal Child Psychology, 14,* 181–204.

Reitan, R. M., & Wolfson, D. (1985). *The Halstead–Reitan Neuropsychological Test Battery.* Tucson, AZ: Neuropsychology Press.

Rispens, J., Swaab, H., van den Oord, E. J. C. C., Cohen-Kettenis, P., van Engeland, H., & van Yperen, T. (1997). WISC profiles in child psychiatric diagnosis: Sense or nonsense? *Journal of the American Academy of Child and Adolescent Psychiatry, 36,* 1587–1594.

Rosvold, H. E., Mirsky, A. F., Sarason, I., Bransome, E. D., & Beck, L. H. (1956). A continuous performance test of brain damage. *Journal of Consulting Psychology, 20,* 343–350.

Sandford, J. A., Fine, A. H., & Goldman, L. (1995). *Validity study of IVA: A visual and auditory CPT.* Paper presented at the 103rd Annual Convention of the American Psychological Association, New York.

Schaughency, E. A., Lahey, B. B., Hynd, G. W., Stone, P. A., Piacentini, J. C., & Frick, P. J. (1989). Neuropsychological test performance and the attention deficit disorders: Clinical utility of the Luria–Nebraska Neuropsychological Battery—Children's Revision. *Journal of Consulting and Clinical Psychology, 57,* 112–116.

Sostek, A. J., Buchsbaum, M. S., & Rapoport, J. L. (1980). Effects of amphetamine on vigilance performance in normal and hyperactive children. *Journal of Abnormal Child Psychology, 8,* 491–500.

Stewart, K. J., & Moely, B. E. (1983). The WISC-R third factor: What does it mean? *Journal of Consulting and Clinical Psychology, 51,* 940–941.

Stroop, J. R. (1935). Studies of interference in serial verbal reactions. *Journal of Experimental Psychology, 18,* 643–662.

Teicher, M. H., Ito, Y., Glod, C. A., & Barber, N. I. (1996). Objective measurement of hyperactivity and attentional problems in ADHD. *Journal of the American Academy of Child and Adolescent Psychiatry, 35,* 334–342.

Trommer, B. L., Hoeppner, J. B., Lorber, R., & Armstrong, K. (1988). Pitfalls in the use of a continuous performance test as a diagnostic tool in attention deficit disorder. *Journal of Developmental and Behavioral Pediatrics, 9,* 339–346.

Waber, D., & Holmes, J. M. (1985). Assessing children's copy productions of the Rey–Osterrieth Complex Figure. *Journal of Clinical and Experimental Neuropsychology, 7,* 264–280.

Wechsler, D. (2003). *Wechsler Intelligence Scale for Children—Fourth Edition.* San Antonio, TX: Psychological Corporation.

Weis, R., & Totten, S. J. (2004). Ecological validity of the Conners' Continuous Performance Test II in a school-based sample. *Journal of Psychoeducational Assessment, 22,* 47–61.

Wielkiewicz, R. M. (1990). Interpreting low scores on the WISC-R third factor: It's more than distractibility. *Psychological Assessment, 2,* 91–97.

Wielkiewicz, R. M., & Palmer, C. M. (1996). Can the WISC-R/WISC-III third factor help in understanding ADHD? *ADHD Report, 4*(3), 4–6.

Zelazo, P. D. & Müller, U. (2002). Executive functions in typical and atypical development. In U. Goswami (Ed.), *Handbook of childhood cognitive development* (pp. 445–469). Oxford: Blackwell.

Integrating the Results of an Evaluation

Ten Clinical Cases

WILLIAM L. HATHAWAY
JODI K. DOOLING-LITFIN
GWENYTH EDWARDS

This chapter contains the results of 10 actual clinical cases seen by clinicians who are specialists in ADHD assessment. Six of the case examples represent the most common types of presentations seen in ADHD clinics: "pure" ADHD, Combined Type; ADHD with Oppositional Defiant Disorder (ODD); ADHD with Conduct Disorder (CD); ADHD, Predominantly Inattentive Type; ADHD, Predominantly Inattentive Type with sluggish cognitive tempo (SCT); and ADHD Not Otherwise Specified (NOS). A seventh case is described in which Bipolar I Disorder was comorbid with ADHD. Three ADHD-"negative" clinical presentations are also included, to illustrate the types of problems sometimes mistakenly conceptualized as ADHD: an anxiety disorder, Generalized Anxiety Disorder; a mood disorder, Dysthymic Disorder; and a pervasive developmental disorder, Autistic Disorder. The case examples reflect common evaluation practices used by specialists in ADHD: the types of information gathered, the tests administered, some of the diagnostic issues considered in con-

ceptualizing the clients, and the sorts of recommendations generated.

We utilize a multimethod, multiinformant assessment approach like that outlined in the foregoing chapters on assessment. First, this approach incorporates a diagnostic interview with the parents and a brief interview with the child. Telephone interviews with teachers or other key informants are pursued when needed. Careful history taking is vital to an adequate ADHD assessment (see Chapter 8). Parents and teachers typically complete an ADHD symptom rating scale based on the symptom indicators from the *Diagnostic and Statistical Manual of Mental Disorders*, fourth edition, text revision (DSM-IV-TR; American Psychiatric Association [APA], 2000); general measures of child psychopathology and social competence, such as the Child Behavior Checklist (CBCL) or Behavior Assessment System for Children (BASC), which are general measures of social competence and child psychopathology; and various other instruments as indicated by the presenting problems. Some of these instruments are chosen to screen for potential impairments arising from the ADHD symptoms, such as the Social Skills Rating System (SSRS) or the Parenting Stress Index (PSI).

In addition to key informant data, some direct testing of the child is performed. The direct testing typically includes some brief screening test of intellectual functioning (often a vocabulary subtest from an intelligence scale) and a measure of executive functioning related to attention and response inhibition, such as the Conners Continuous Performance Test (CPT) or the Das–Naglieri Cognitive Assessment System (CAS). The direct testing batteries will otherwise vary, based on the presenting problem profile. For instance, complete intelligence and achievement tests may be administered when the child's pattern of intellectual functioning creates a challenge for differential diagnosis.

ADHD, COMBINED TYPE, NO COMORBID CONDITIONS

Jimmy's parents, Mr. and Mrs. N., thought they had a busy job raising Jimmy's "rambunctious" older brother. By comparison, Jimmy made his brother look calm and controlled. Mr. and Mrs. N. emphasized that Jimmy was not a "bad" child. He was not oppositional, aggressive, stubborn, or ill-tempered. Rather, he was difficult to keep up with because he was "always in motion." Mrs. N. recalled that "as soon as Jimmy learned to walk, he seemed to be wandering off and getting into things." Jimmy's active style was particularly problematic, because he often made poor choices with seemingly little forethought (e.g., running out into the road without looking or putting keys into an electric outlet).

Jimmy seemed eager to please his parents, but he frequently did not follow through on things they asked of him (e.g., picking up his toys or making his bed). His parents explained that Jimmy was easily "sidetracked" by more interesting things and consequently failed to complete requested tasks. They did not feel this was due to a deliberate refusal to comply. For example, when they reminded Jimmy about uncompleted tasks, he would seem surprised and say, "Oh, I forgot." He would quickly restart uncompleted tasks when reminded, but would again become distracted if left to his own devices. Mr. and Mrs. N. had developed a very active parenting style to get Jimmy to fin-

ish tasks more consistently. They found it necessary to give short commands and always to be ready to check up on Jimmy's progress in carrying out instructions. They used immediate consequences, such as praise for compliance and privilege removal or time out for noncompliance, to motivate Jimmy. Even with this added structure, they found it necessary to give frequent prompts and reminders to keep Jimmy directed to assigned tasks.

Although Jimmy's inattentive, impulsive, and overactive behaviors required his parents to be very active in his management, it was not until Jimmy entered preschool that Mr. and Mrs. N. became aware of the magnitude of these behaviors. When Jimmy was 3 years old, his parents placed him in a Montessori preschool program. This program met for 2–3 hours 5 days a week and involved many structured, developmentally appropriate learning activities. Jimmy was unable to adjust to the "structure" of the program. For instance, he frequently talked out during quiet times, quickly lost interest in group activities, and did not persist with preacademic tasks. His parents switched Jimmy to another preschool program after 3 months, but similar problems arose in this setting. Jimmy was asked to leave the second preschool program after 1 month of attendance because he "engaged in too much imagination play," would not participate adequately in directed activities, and consequently distracted other students. Jimmy spent the remainder of his preschool time with a home day care provider who was trained as an education consultant for children with special needs. The home day care provider used a variety of behavioral strategies, such as a token system, to manage Jimmy's behavior.

Jimmy's kindergarten teacher noted that he had problems with "not being focused," being unable to work independently, and being too "active." These problems became disruptive to the class unless the teacher gave Jimmy a great deal of individualized attention—for example, redirecting him back to school activities and reminding him about appropriate behavior when he was blurting out comments or interrupting others. Jimmy also had some difficulty with academic tasks that required attention to detail, such as letter writing. Although Jimmy did not "fall far below grade level" in his academics, his teacher expressed concerns that Jimmy seemed to be performing "beneath his potential." Because of his difficulties in kindergarten, Jimmy's parents requested an evaluation to determine whether Jimmy was eligible for government-mandated individualized education services. The school psychologist administered the Wechsler Intelligence Scale for Children—Third Edition (WISC-III) and the Woodcock–Johnson Psycho-Educational Battery—Revised (WJ-R). He obtained a WISC-III Full Scale IQ of 111 (77th percentile), which fell in the high-average range of overall intellectual functioning. His achievement scores on the WJ-R were somewhat mixed, ranging from the low-average to high-average range. The school psychologist stated that Jimmy had the intellectual ability to do better in school, but "attentional factors seemed to be a key factor contributing to underachievement for Jimmy." Although Jimmy was not found eligible for government-mandated services based on his psychoeducational testing, the school psychologist recommended further evaluation of Jimmy's attentional problems.

Jimmy's impulsivity created problems in his social functioning that became increasingly evident as he made the transition into the elementary grades. Jimmy was described as often "immature" or "silly" in his interpersonal style. By first grade, his peers were frequently complaining that Jimmy "bothered them" by "grabbing," "pulling," or otherwise "touching" them. Jimmy's difficulties regulating his social behavior did not stand out as a problem in earlier years, because few of his peers acted differently. As his peers started to develop greater restraint, Jimmy's social progress lagged further and further behind. Although Jimmy was typically engaging or "friendly," he was unable to maintain friendships. He also had difficulty in organized activities such as seasonal sports. His coaches frequently complained that Jimmy was "too off task" and that his "silly" behavior sometimes led to conflicts with teammates.

Jimmy's first-grade teacher continued to note many of the problems that had surfaced in preschool and kindergarten: Jimmy frequently failed to follow through on instructions, did not complete work within an appropriate amount of time, and was often disruptive due to his "constant activity and noise making." By the end of the first grade, Jimmy had fallen behind in his reading and writing skills because of his difficulty persisting on these tasks. His teacher frequently had to prompt Jimmy to return to assigned tasks and to cease off-task behaviors, such as playing with his pencil or "drumming" on his desk. Although Jimmy's teacher used a behavior management plan to reduce Jimmy's off-task behavior and increase his productivity, she stated that he continued to complete only a "minimum" of the required work. During a parent–teacher conference, his teacher reiterated the school psychologist's recommendation to have Jimmy evaluated for his attentional difficulties.

Jimmy's parents discussed the school's recommendation to have Jimmy evaluated with his pediatrician during a physical examination in the spring of his first-grade school year. The pediatrician referred Jimmy to our clinic for evaluation. Table 10.1 summarizes the results of the testing. Mr. and Mrs. N. reported a significant number of both the inattentive and hyperactive–impulsive symptoms of ADHD for Jimmy during an interview and on rating scales. His first-grade teacher also reported significant levels of both inattention and hyperactivity–impulsivity on rating scales. Both Jimmy's parents and his first-grade teacher rated him as having significantly fewer-than-average social skills. Despite describing Jimmy as a very "bright" boy, his teacher rated him as low-average in productivity compared to other first-grade boys on the Academic Performance Rating Scale (APRS). No evidence of other psychiatric difficulties, such as depression or anxiety, was obtained from the evaluation results. During the interview, Jimmy's parents explained that their son's ADHD characteristics had caught them "off guard." They denied any previous family history of ADHD, learning disabilities, or other psychiatric problems. Although Jimmy's brother was also very active, they pointed out that Jimmy's difficulties seemed to be substantially greater.

Jimmy participated willingly in the interview and testing, but shifted in his seat and fidgeted a great deal. He mentioned that he was often "daydreaming" in school and found reading very boring. He also reported having great difficulty listening to the teacher when she was talking. He often made noises in the classroom, "for no particular reason." Jimmy's performance on the Conners CPT provided some evidence of problems with attention. Although Jimmy only infrequently responded to inappropriate test items (commissions), he frequently failed to respond to appropriate items (omissions) and was highly variable in his speed of response. This pattern suggested difficulties with sustaining his level of attention.

The clinical impression of Jimmy that

TABLE 10.1. Results for a Case of ADHD in a 6-Year-Old Boy

Mother		Father		Teacher	
Interview report of ADHD symptoms		**Interview report of ADHD symptoms**			
Inattention	9	Inattention	9		
Hyperactivity–impulsivity	7	Hyperactivity–impulsivity	8		
ADHD Rating Scale–IV (Symptoms rated >2)		**ADHD Rating Scale–IV** (Symptoms rated >2)		**ADHD Rating Scale–IV** (Symptoms rated >2)	
Inattention	9	Inattention	7	Inattention	8
Hyperactivity–impulsivity	6	Hyperactivity–impulsivity	6	Hyperactivity–impulsivity	9
BASC		**BASC**		**BASC**	
Subscale	Percentile	Subscale	Percentile	Subscale	Percentile
Hyperactivity	95*	Hyperactivity	95*	Hyperactivity	96*
Aggression	58	Aggression	58	Aggression	72
Conduct Problems	78	Conduct Problems	67	Conduct Problems	72
Anxiety	82	Anxiety	64	Anxiety	80
Depression	89	Depression	74	Depression	73
Somatization	45	Somatization	9	Somatization	84
Atypicality	90	Atypicality	79	Atypicality	92
Withdrawal	44	Withdrawal	44	Withdrawal	53
Attention Problems	97*	Attention Problems	95*	Attention Problems	96*
Social Skills	3*	Social Skills	39	Social Skills	30
				Learning Problems	90
PSI-SF		**DBRS**		**SSRS**	
Total stress	85	Number of defiant behaviors	1	Total score	26 (below average)

Testing data			
Test	Raw score	Standard/scaled score	Percentile
WISC-III Vocabulary	19	15	95*
Conners CPT			
Hits	279 (86%)		91
Omissions	51 (16%)		72
Commissions	21 (58%)	44	28
Hit rate	508	43	27
Hit rate standard error (*SE*)	22	67	96*
Variability of *SE*	28	50	50

Note. An asterisk indicates a clinically significant elevation (≥ 95th percentile or ≤ 5th percentile). BASC, Behavior Assessment System for Children; PSI-SF, Parenting Stress Index—Short Form; DBRS, Defiant Behavior Rating Scale; SSRS, Social Skills Rating System; WISC-III, Wechsler Intelligence Scale for Children—Third Edition; CPT, Continuous Performance Test.

emerged from the evaluation was of a 6-year, 9-month-old boy of above-average intelligence who had a significant, chronic, and pervasive history of the inattentive and hyperactive–impulsive symptoms of ADHD. These features had been evident since Jimmy's early childhood years and significantly impaired his school behavior and social functioning. No other psychiatric difficulties were detected for Jimmy.

Consequently, Jimmy was diagnosed as having ADHD, Combined Type.

We made a number of recommendations to Jimmy's parents:

1. We emphasized parent education about ADHD through follow-up consultation, suggested readings, websites (*www.chadd.org*), and participation in a support group.

2. We suggested a trial of stimulant medication.

3. We developed a variety of beneficial environmental modifications, such as those described in later chapters in this volume.

4. We advised the development of a home-based reinforcement program to increase appropriate school behavior and academic productivity. This program made use of the daily school behavior report card (see Chapter 15, this volume).

Jimmy's case highlights a number of important observations about individuals who have ADHD, Combined Type, but who do not have comorbid conditions. Because of the high comorbidity of ADHD and ODD, it is common for individuals to confuse the two disorders. Jimmy was not viewed as an oppositional child either at home or at school. Although Jimmy required a more active, structured, and deliberate management style in both of these settings, he was not viewed as having "conduct problems" by his parents or his teachers. Adults generally regarded Jimmy as a well-meaning boy who too often allowed his impulses to "get the better of him." Jimmy's inappropriate and disruptive behavior appeared to stem from disinhibition, rather than from the intentional misbehavior, coercive defiance cycles, or deliberate aggression associated with ODD.

Jimmy's case also illustrates the pervasive and chronic nature of the ADHD features required for the diagnosis. Although Jimmy's ADHD characteristics had been present since his preschool years, they did not create a substantial problem in his functioning until Jimmy entered a setting that taxed his weak self-regulation skills. Jimmy's ADHD created problems primarily in his social functioning and school behavior. Although his ADHD appeared to be interfering with his educational functioning, Jimmy's academic performance was not substantially impaired by his ADHD, relative to that typical for same-age peers. Whereas Jimmy may have been underachieving in school relative to his intellectual ability, it was his inappropriate school behavior that first raised concerns about him. Although intelligence cannot completely buffer the impact of ADHD, it is likely that Jimmy would have displayed greater academic difficulties due to his ADHD if his level of intellectual functioning had been significantly lower.

ADHD WITH OPPOSITIONAL DEFIANT DISORDER

Sam was difficult-tempered from birth. Although he displayed no developmental problems as an infant or toddler, he was overactive, stubborn, and colicky. It seemed impossible to maintain Sam on a consistent eating and sleeping schedule. Sam always had a "mind of his own," and consequently everything was a battle: If he did not want to be dressed as a toddler, he would take off his shoes immediately after his parents dressed him and hide them. Once Sam began to speak, he incessantly demanded things from his parents and forcefully shouted "No!" when he did not want to comply with their requests. When Sam's parents, Mr. and Mrs. G., pushed him to finish a task (such as eating his dinner or picking up after himself), Sam often displayed intense outbursts of anger. His parents dreaded taking him to public locations, such as grocery stores or malls, because Sam typically threw tantrums during these outings.

By early childhood, Sam's behavior had become increasingly aggressive. His defiance escalated to include hitting his mother, throwing objects, and screaming "I hate you!" at his parents. Sometimes his outbursts turned destructive: For instance, he once impulsively threw a wrench through his mother's windshield, and on another occasion he smashed a toy through a glass coffee table when he was upset. Sam always seemed to be in an irritable mood, but he was difficult to manage even when he was not being aggressive. Once Sam learned to walk, he was "always on the go." He was constantly climbing and running in inappropriate places, such as through the clothing racks at department stores. If Sam was around, it seemed impossible to carry on a conversation because of his frequent interrupting and noisy play. Although he was difficult for both parents to manage, he seemed to be much more challenging for his mother. His parents often argued over how to handle Sam. His mother tried to be much more appeasing, while his father was stern. Despite their disagreement over how to handle Sam, neither parent felt they knew how to manage him well.

Sam was placed in a day care program when he was 9 months of age. Even at this early age, his teachers often made comments about Sam's being obstinate, overactive, and disruptive. As Sam entered the toddler years, he was often aggressive with his peers. He rarely shared toys with other children and often grabbed toys away from them. Although new children at the day care center often played with Sam, they soon learned to avoid him because of his "bossy" and physically aggressive style. Sam was very short-tempered at the day care program; he was easily provoked and would hit, push, or bite when upset. Consequently, Sam was typically rejected by his peers. By the time Sam was 5 years old, Mr. and Mrs. G. had attempted to involve Sam in several organized recreational activities, such as baseball or skating. However, he was asked to stop participating in these activities because he was "unable to wait his turn."

Halfway through Sam's 4th year, he started attending an integrated preschool program run by the public school system in his community. Sam attended the preschool for 2–3 hours, 3 days a week. All the children in this program had special needs or were viewed as "at risk" for educational problems. Sam stood out from his preschool classmates as a much more "moody," "argumentative," and "angry" child. Sam seemed unable to persist with preacademic tasks and frequently displayed inappropriate behaviors in the classroom, such as running around the desks, yelling out, interrupting, not staying seated during group time, and grabbing other people or their things.

Sam responded to teacher cues to behave appropriately, but he required many such cues to maintain a minimal level of acceptable behavior throughout the day. When corrected for misbehavior, Sam typically talked back or covered his ears in defiance. However, Sam's inappropriate behavior improved somewhat after he had been in the program for several months, secondary to an intense behavior management plan initiated by his teacher. The plan involved clearly delineated rules for specific activities, such as circle time or using the rest room. The class would often recite the rules. Consequences for breaking the rules, including time out, were described in advance. Engaging in desired activities, such as using the computer or doing crafts, was used as an incentive for compliance. In addition to this general management plan, Sam's teacher seated Sam immediately next to her, frequently prompted him to behave appropriately, and gave him abundant praise for efforts at appropriate behavior. During special events or anticipated blocks of unstructured time, such as performing a school

play, Sam's teacher often asked his father to attend the class to provide additional support in managing Sam. Sam's teacher observed that Sam was able to behave in a modestly appropriate manner with this amount of management, but that it was very taxing for him. At a parent–teacher conference, she expressed concerns about Sam's ability to engage in the level of "academic listening" that would be required in elementary school. For instance, she noted that during the "language circle," all of Sam's efforts seemed to be invested in trying to behave appropriately. Consequently, his performance seemed to be far below his conversational language skills displayed at other times. His teacher questioned whether Sam should be placed in a regular kindergarten program the following year, and also recommended that his parents have Sam evaluated for ADHD.

Mr. and Mrs. G. brought Sam to the ADHD clinic for an assessment of his impulsive, restless, and aggressive behavior. His parents requested assistance in identifying any disorder that might be contributing to Sam's problems and advice on how to manage Sam more successfully both at home and at school. Table 10.2 summarizes the results of this evaluation. Both Sam's parents and preschool teacher reported all of the hyperactive—impulsive features of ADHD either on rating scales or during an interview. His mother also reported significant levels of the inattentive features of ADHD. Both Sam's mother and his teacher rated him as having significantly below-average levels of social skills. Although his teacher also rated Sam as displaying significant levels of "depression" on the BASC, the significant elevation seemed to be due to items reflecting his "irritable," "moody," or "negative" demeanor. In terms of his oppositional behaviors, Sam's parents reported all eight of the defiant behaviors required for a diagnosis of ODD as frequently displayed by Sam. His mother described very high levels of stress arising from parenting Sam.

During the interview, Sam's parents stated that they had hoped Sam would "grow out of his problems, but they only seemed to get worse." They had had some experience dealing with "psychiatric problems" in the past: Mr. G. had been treated for both alcohol abuse and depression. He had been sober for 5 years by the time of the evaluation, but continued to attend Alcoholics Anonymous. Sam's paternal grandfather also had chronic difficulties with

TABLE 10.2. Results for a Case of Comorbid ADHD and ODD in a 5-Year-Old Boy

Mother	Father	Teacher

Interview report of ADHD symptoms		Interview report of ADHD symptoms		
Inattention	7	Inattention	5	
Hyperactivity–impulsivity	9	Hyperactivity–impulsivity	9	

ADHD Rating Scale–IV			ADHD Rating Scale–IV	
(Symptoms rated >2)			(Symptoms rated >2)	
Inattention	7		Inattention	2
Hyperactivity–impulsivity	9		Hyperactivity–impulsivity	9

BASC			BASC	
Subscale	Percentile		Subscale	Percentile
Hyperactivity	97*		Hyperactivity	96*
Aggression	97*		Aggression	95*
Anxiety	85		Anxiety	80
Depression	80		Depression	95*
Somatization	20		Somatization	14
Atypicality	68		Atypicality	54
Withdrawal	30		Withdrawal	59
Attention Problems	97*		Attention Problems	90
Social Skills	5*		Social Skills	41

PSI-SF			SSRS	
Total stress	98*		Total score	25 (below average)

	Testing data		
Test	Raw score	Standard/scaled score	Percentile
PPVT-III	78	110	75
Conners CPT			
Hits	273 (84%)		
Omissions	51 (16%)		72
Commissions	29 (81%)	54	69
Hit rate	453	59	82
Hit rate *SE*	33	71	98*
Variability of *SE*	64	66	95*

Note. An asterisk indicates a clinically significant elevation (≥ 95th percentile or ≤ 5th percentile). PPVT-III, Peabody Picture Vocabulary Test—Third Edition; other abbreviations as in Table 10.1.

alcohol abuse and had been diagnosed with Bipolar Mood Disorder. His grandfather had been hospitalized on several occasions due to his mood disability and had been on a "full-disability" pension since he was 50.

Sam separated easily from his parents and spontaneously engaged with the evaluator during the interview. His speech appeared to be typical in tone, rate, and volume; however, he talked constantly throughout the interview. Sam appeared to understand the directions for testing tasks, but was able to complete these tasks only with frequent prompting and encouragement. He frequently fidgeted and appeared to be very restless. His affect and thought process appeared within typical limits. Again, Table 10.2 summarizes direct testing results obtained during the evaluation. Because psychoeducational testing had never been performed with Sam, he was given the Peabody Picture Vocabulary Test—Third Edition (PPVT-III) to obtain a brief estimate of his verbal intelligence. On the PPVT-III, Sam obtained a raw score of 78, which corresponded to a scaled score of 110 and fell at the 75th percentile. His performance on this receptive vocabulary test suggested that Sam had a high-average level of verbal intelligence. Although he did not fail to respond to appropriate items (omissions) or mistakenly respond to inappropriate items (commissions) to an unusual degree on the Conners CPT, he was very inconsistent in his speed and pattern of response. This response pattern provided evidence of difficulties with sustained attention.

Based on the results of the evaluation, Sam was viewed as a 5-year, 1-month-old boy of presumably above-average intelligence who had chronic and pervasive difficulties with noncompliance, excessive inappropriate activity, aggression, and poor sustained attention. Significant levels of the hyperactive–impulsive features of ADHD were reported both at home and at school. Although only Sam's mother rated him as displaying significant levels of the inattentive features of ADHD, his teacher also described many problems with inattention in written comments about Sam. Sam was given the diagnosis of ADHD, Combined Type. Sam's ADHD was complicated by a significant pattern of defiant behavior, both at home and at school, which met the criteria for ODD. Sam's combination of ADHD and ODD substantially impaired his social functioning, school adjustment, and family relationships.

Following the evaluation, we made a number of recommendations to Sam's family:

1. We emphasized parent education about the nature of both ADHD and ODD through follow-up consultation, suggested readings, and participation in a support group. The importance of implementing an adequate treatment plan to reduce the chances of negative outcomes, such as school failure or CD, was stressed.

2. We advised parent participation in a 9-week course of behavior management training, identical to that described in Chapter 12.

3. We suggested a trial of stimulant medication.

4. We gave Sam's parents information about legal rights relevant to the education of children with ADHD. We encouraged the parents to request an evaluation by Sam's school to determine whether an individualized education plan should be established for Sam.

5. We suggested a variety of environmental modifications/accommodations for implementation during Sam's kindergarten year.

Sam's case illustrates the characteristics of an ADHD subtype researchers have described as an early-onset "aggressive type" (Hinshaw, 1987; Hinshaw & Lee, 2003). This subtype is discussed in Chapter 4 (this volume). Children with ADHD and aggression tend to have irritable temperament, poor sustained attention, and high activity level, all of which are quite evident by an early age. Sam's difficult temperament had been recognized from birth, and concerns about his ADHD symptoms had been recognized since his toddler years. Also common for children with the aggressive subtype of ADHD, Sam was rated as significantly below average in his social functioning both at home and at school. His aggressive and overly impulsive behavior frequently resulted in Sam's being rejected by his peers.

There has been some discussion in recent years about a higher rate of Bipolar Mood Disorder in children with ADHD (again, see Chapter 4). Biederman (1995) and his associates (Faraone et al., 1997; Wozniak et al., 1995, Wilens et al., 1999) have argued that children who present with features such as those in the early-onset aggressive subtype of ADHD may actually be suffering from Bipolar I Disorder. A chief difficulty in evaluating this claim is the substitution of persistent irritable moods for the manic or hypomanic phase of the disorder. DSM-IV-TR lists Criterion A for a Manic Episode as "a distinct period of abnormally and persistently elevated, expansive, or irritable mood, lasting at least 1 week" (APA, 2000, p. 362). However, a number of the diagnostic indicators for ODD reflect frequent or persistent patterns of irritability, such as "often loses temper," "is often touchy or easily annoyed by others," and "is often angry and resentful" (APA, 2000, p. 102) The primary differences between the expressions of irritability in the two disorders may be both history and severity. Manic irritability is characterized in DSM-IV-TR as tied to a "distinct period" or phase (Carlson, 2002). It is therefore episodic, although the phase itself may last for more than just a week or two. The irritability characteristic of children with aggression and ADHD reflects a general temperament and is less tied to distinct periods. The irritability manifested in Bipolar I Disorder is often severe, characterized by irrational levels of hostility and rage (emotional storms), explosive destructive behavior, and sometimes violence. That of ODD is often less severe; is typically provoked by parental commands to shift from a child-chosen activity (e.g., watching TV) to doing work (e.g., picking up toys); and is characterized more by verbal defiance, stubbornness, refusal to obey, and a gradually escalating use of oppositional behavior as the parent and child engage in a coercive spiral around the child's obeying the command.

It is possible that an individual may meet the criteria for both ADHD and Bipolar I Disorder. In Sam's case, there was a positive family history of Bipolar I Disorder in a paternal grandfather. However, his temperamental difficulties were not expressed in a phasic manner. Furthermore, he did not meet Criterion B for a Manic Episode. Although he might be at increased risk for Bipolar I Disorder, he did not meet the criteria for this condition at the time of the evaluation.

ADHD WITH CONDUCT DISORDER

Jeff's mother used to joke that he "shot out of the womb" and never stopped moving. As an infant, he was quite demanding, and as soon as he could walk, he was into everything. It was always a challenge to manage his behavior, and given that the family lived in a cramped apartment in an unsafe neighborhood, there were a lot of dangerous things he could get into. By the time he was 4, he had suffered numerous bruises and one broken bone, sustained when he climbed up a ladder some workmen had left outside the apartment building. After Mrs. R. (and the emergency room staff) had endured 5 hours of trying to control Jeff during the wait to set his broken arm, she brought him to the pediatrician and asked for some help. Mrs. R. asked the doctor whether Jeff was "retarded." The doctor reassured her that his cognitive skills were developing typically, but shared her concern about Jeff's hyperactivity. He skipped from toy to toy in just a few seconds, ran out into the street without looking where he was going, and was constantly climbing on things and running about. The pediatrician prescribed a stimulant medication, which seemed to help. However, Mrs. R.'s mother "read her the riot act" when she found out Jeff was "taking drugs," and Mrs. R. soon discontinued treat-

ment. Jeff's father had left home when he was 3, and Mrs. R. worked long hours to make ends meet. She was constantly frustrated by Jeff's behavior; she often told him that he needed to "shape up" and that he was likely to turn out like his father (who had many difficulties with the law).

Perhaps because of his defiant behavior, Jeff's kindergarten teachers barely commented on his hyperactivity. His behavior was quite disruptive to the class, despite the frequent time outs used. He took other children's toys, hit, and bit. When punished, he seemed to get even more defiant. This pattern continued throughout elementary school. Consequently, Jeff's peers rejected him. Jeff struggled academically, but mainly because it was almost impossible to get him to do anything. His teachers felt that he was underachieving, and it seemed as if he was deliberately sabotaging himself. As elementary school progressed, he was involved in physical fights with his peers, often as the instigator. He seemed to interpret even neutral social situations negatively, and responded with aggression. Jeff spent a great deal of time in the principal's office. He blamed others for the problems; nothing was ever his fault. By the time he reached middle school, he had been suspended from school three or four times for fighting. He also used foul language with his teachers. In early middle school, Jeff became involved in serious rule violations. He often skipped school with a couple of his friends; they would go to the mall and shoplift CDs and baseball caps. Jeff was quite good at forging his mother's signature on excuses. Despite this, he was caught skipping school on a number of occasions, which led to detention and suspensions.

As Jeff entered early adolescence, he became less involved in fighting, but more covert problem behaviors increased in frequency and severity. He experimented with alcohol and marijuana, and stayed out late at night. His mother felt she couldn't control him; his father had long been out of the picture, and there wasn't much Mrs. R. could do to discipline her son. She also worked the night shift at a local factory, and wasn't always able to track Jeff's whereabouts. When she did confront him, he simply told her to "get out of my face." Jeff continued to perform poorly in school; his sixth-grade teacher even referred him for evaluation for possible learning disabilities. The results indicated that his IQ was low-average and his academic achievement was commensurate with this, with no sign of learning disability. It appeared that he had the ability to perform his schoolwork adequately, but was simply refusing to put forth effort.

The summer before he started high school, Jeff's behavior problems escalated. He had failed eighth-grade English, and was supposed to be making it up in summer school. However, his attendance was sporadic, and he spent most of his time smoking marijuana down by the river with the few friends who would tolerate him, all of whom had significant behavioral problems themselves. One day, they saw a car that had been left unlocked while the owners were biking along the bike trail. Jeff impulsively jumped in and hot-wired the car; he had seen this done in a movie. When he was able to start it, he and his friends drove the car out to a suburb to look for some girls from school. How-

ever, the owners had returned and called the police, and Jeff and his friends were soon caught. This incident resulted in juvenile court charges; ultimately Jeff ended up with a sentence of probation and mandated community service. By this time, he was in high school, was failing two courses, and was barely hanging on in the others. His teachers all complained about his "attitude," and his mother was at her wits' end.

When Jeff violated his probation by staying out all night, he was ordered by the court to undergo psychological evaluation to determine whether he required any mental health services. He was referred to our clinic. Table 10.3 summarizes the results of the evaluation. Mrs. R. reported a significant number of both inattentive and hyperactive–impulsive symptoms of ADHD for Jeff during an interview and on rating scales. His algebra and English teachers

TABLE 10.3. Results for a Case of Comorbid ADHD and CD in a 15-Year-Old Male

Mother		Math teacher		English teacher	
Interview report of symptoms					
ADHD					
Inattention	7				
Hyperactivity–impulsivity	7				
Conduct Disorder	7				
BASC		**BASC**		**BASC**	
Subscale	Percentile	Subscale	Percentile	Subscale	Percentile
Hyperactivity	98*	Hyperactivity	99*	Hyperactivity	99*
Aggression	92	Aggression	96*	Aggression	96*
Conduct Problems	99*	Conduct Problems	98*	Conduct Problems	96*
Anxiety	81	Anxiety	58	Anxiety	50
Depression	30	Depression	73	Depression	58
Somatization	39	Somatization	50	Somatization	68
Atypicality	50	Attention Problems	>99*	Attention Problems	>99*
Withdrawal	27	Learning Problems	84	Learning Problems	58
Attention Problems	97*	Atypicality	79	Atypicality	73
Social Skills	1*	Withdrawal	63	Withdrawal	63
		Social Skills	2*	Social Skills	<1*
		Leadership	16	Leadership	31
		Study Skills	1*	Study Skills	4*
CPRS-R:S		**CTRS-R**		**CTRS-R**	
Oppositional	>99*	Oppositional	96*	Oppositional	97*
Inattention	98*	Inattention	99*	Inattention	98*
Hyperactivity	98*	Hyperactivity	96*	Hyperactivity	98*
ADHD Index	96*	ADHD Index	96*	ADHD Index	99*
PSI-SF		**SSRS**		**SSRS**	
Total stress	99*	Total score (30)	3*	Total score (33)	5*

Note. An asterisk indicates a clinically significant elevation (≥ 95th percentile or ≤ 5th percentile). CPRS-R:S, Conners Parent Rating Scale—Revised: Short Form; CTRS-R, Conners Teacher Rating Scale—Revised; other abbreviations as in Table 10.1.

both also reported significant levels of inattention and hyperactivity–impulsivity on rating scales. Moreover, his teachers and his mother rated him as having fewer-than-average social skills, in addition to having significant symptoms of aggressive behavior and conduct problems on rating scales. During the parent interview, Jeff's mother reported that his behavior had gotten worse over the years, and that she felt terrible about her inability to control him. She described him as being quite similar to his father, who she explained was now in prison in another state after seriously injuring another man in a bar fight. No evidence of any depression or anxiety was apparent from the evaluation results.

Jeff was initially quite hostile and guarded during the interview. He stated that he didn't "need any shrink," but when reminded that he was court-ordered to participate in the evaluation, he did agree to participate in the evaluation activities. After he was given information regarding the evaluation and the psychologist's role, he relaxed somewhat, and she was able to develop a rapport with him. Jeff had difficulty sitting in the evaluation room, and asked to take frequent breaks to "stretch his legs." Once he began talking, he talked a great deal, and it was difficult to keep him on topic. He reported feeling bored frequently, and stated that much of the time when he got into trouble, it was because he just decided to do something for fun. He did not show much remorse for his activities; he stated that the people whose car he had stolen were just "rich folks who probably have two more cars at home." When asked about his fighting, he stated that other people had provoked him, and they "deserved what they got." Jeff defended his violations of house rules by stating that he should be able to come home whenever he wanted to, and that it was none of his mother's business where he was. He reported having difficulty concentrating on his schoolwork, and admitted that this had always been a problem for him. He also stated that it felt "like torture" to remain seated in school all day, and acknowledged that it had always been hard for him to wait when he wanted something.

The clinical impression of Jeff that emerged from the evaluation was that of a 15-year-old boy of low-average intelligence who had a chronic and pervasive pattern of problems with both inattention and hyperactivity–impulsivity, the two primary areas associated with ADHD. He failed to give close attention to details,

had difficulty sustaining his attention, had difficulty following through on instructions, had difficulty organizing tasks and activities, avoided tasks requiring sustained mental effort, lost things, was easily distracted, fidgeted frequently, left his seat when remaining seated was expected, acted as if driven by a motor, talked excessively, blurted out answers, had difficulty waiting his turn, and frequently interrupted. These features were evident from a very young age, and significantly impaired his social and academic functioning. In addition, he displayed a pattern of behavior in which major age-appropriate rules and societal norms were violated, including initiating physical fights, property destruction, theft, frequent lying, staying out late at night, and truancy. Therefore, Jeff met DSM-IV-TR criteria for diagnoses of both ADHD, Combined Type and CD.

We made a number of recommendations to the court system, Jeff, and his mother:

1. We emphasized the need for a chemical dependency evaluation to clarify the extent of Jeff's substance usage.

2. We strongly recommended intensive therapy that would assist Jeff's mother in better monitoring and managing his behavior, as well as to help him improve his social problem-solving skills. It would be important for therapy to teach Mrs. R. how to use contingency management effectively. Other targets for therapy included improving communication and problem solving between Jeff and his mother. Given the severity of some of Jeff's conduct problems, as well as his mother's difficulty in managing his behavior, we strongly recommended that therapy include systemic supports, so that school and the court system would be involved in his care as well. We recommended multisystemic therapy (Borduin et al., 1995) as the treatment of choice for Jeff; this approach combines elements of family therapy, parent training, and cognitive-behavioral therapy. We also felt that education about ADHD should be part of the therapy for both Jeff and his mother. An additional target of therapy would be to increase Jeff's association with models of prosocial behavior through activities involving his interests, such as organized sports or music, and to restrict his interaction with other peers demonstrating delinquent behavior.

3. We suggested that a trial of stimulant medication *not* be considered at the present,

due to Jeff's conduct problems and potential for substance abuse. We did, however, recommend consideration of a medication that would address his impulsivity and inattention but with less potential for abuse, such as atomoxetine (Strattera).

4. We gave Jeff's mother information about legal rights relevant to the education of adolescents with ADHD. We encouraged her to request an evaluation by the school to determine whether an individualized education plan or a Section 504 plan should be established for Jeff. We also gave her information about a group that provided advocates to assist parents in determining their children's legal rights within the educational system.

5. We suggested a variety of environmental modifications/accommodations for implementation in school. We also recommended that Jeff's mother ask the school to conduct a functional behavior assessment of his disruptive behavior within the school setting.

Jeff's case demonstrates the complexity of intervening with older adolescents who have a combination of ADHD and CD. Although international consensus guidelines (Kutcher et al., 2004) suggest that the first-line treatment of comorbid ADHD and CD should include a combination of psychosocial interventions and psychostimulant medication, the risk of stimulant abuse in adolescents with this combination of disorders makes the use of stimulant medication a less clear choice. On the one hand, psychosocial intervention alone typically produces less pronounced effects than those obtained with the use of stimulant medication. Therefore, the decision as to whether to use stimulant medication is one that involves carefully weighing the risks and benefits. Moreover, those consensus guidelines were developed at a time when less was known about the value of a new medication, atomoxetine. The research now available is impressive and suggests that this medication may be considered a front-line treatment for ADHD alongside the stimulants.

This case also illustrates the common clinical problem of focusing on the symptoms that are most distressing, with the potential of missing more subtle deficits. In a case such as Jeff's, the CD symptoms of aggression, serious rule violations, and property destruction are typically more distressing to adults than the ADHD symptoms of hyperactivity and poor attention. However, given that the majority of adolescents with CD also meet diagnostic criteria for ADHD, the clinician assessing or treating an adolescent with CD should always address the possibility of comorbid ADHD. Without an understanding of the comorbid conditions, treatment may not be as effective.

ADHD WITH COMORBID BIPOLAR DISORDER

Kenny had just had his 6th birthday when he was referred by his pediatrician for an evaluation due to his aggressive behavior, hyperactivity, and sleep disturbance. Since age 3, he had displayed hyperactivity and impulsivity to such a degree that his pediatrician had diagnosed him with ADHD, Predominantly Hyperactive–Impulsive Type. His symptoms had been both persistent and cross-situational since that time, with no noticeable difference in behavior at home, at preschool, or in the community. When Kenny reached age 5, however, his parents began to have difficulty managing his severe, physically aggressive behavior. He would often fight with other children and with his siblings at home. Sometimes this fighting would take place with weapons such as kitchen knives.

Kenny's parents described temper outbursts that were severe, occurring multiple times per day, and extremely difficult for either parent to manage. These anger attacks had not improved with any of the medications his pediatrician had tried, including clonidine, methylphenidate (Ritalin), guanfacine, and hydroxyzine (Atarax). His mother said that Kenny's behavior seemed to cycle. Kenny could have "wild periods" that could last anywhere from 4 to 14 days, alternating with periods of 4–5 days of relative calm. During these wild periods, he would demonstrate even more extreme violent ideation. He would often hold his head and complain that his thoughts were going too fast. This cycling took place in the context of chronic hyperactivity and was not exacerbated by the Ritalin trial.

In addition, Kenny displayed a significant sleep disturbance. His mother felt that his sleep was very fragmented. He was often up all night and had a history of walking in his sleep. He had also experienced classic night terrors from the time he was a toddler. Two to 4 hours after falling asleep, he would wake up screaming and quite frantic. These episodes could last anywhere from a few minutes to half an hour, and Kenny would have no recollection of them when he woke up in the morning. His pediatrician had prescribed clonazepam (Klonopin), 0.25 to 0.5 mg in the evenings; this was initially very effective, but had become less effective over time. Kenny had also begun to complain of nightmares, and for the past several months he had been reluctant to fall asleep because of his nightmares.

Further complicating Kenny's initial presentation was his history of severe asthma. His hyperactivity had actually precipitated several asthma attacks, which resulted in emergency room visits and one hospitalization. His mother reported that it was extremely difficult for her to administer his breathing treatments for the asthma, due to his activity level and aggression. A recent neurological workup was reported to be within typical limits, as was a recent electroencephalogram. There were no known drug allergies.

Kenny's family history included ADHD diagnosed for both his older brother and two paternal cousins. Kenny's mother had a history of both alcohol and other substance abuse, as did extended maternal and paternal relatives. His father, older sister, and several members of his mother's family had been diagnosed with unipolar depression. According to Kenny's mother, several members of her extended family had been diagnosed with schizophrenia. Kenny's father had a past history of seizure disorder, and his mother required frequent hospitalization for severe asthma.

Kenny had been asked to leave kindergarten in order to have an additional year of preschool, due to his behavioral and social difficulties. Following a psychoeducational evaluation, he was found to have average cognitive abilities but was nonetheless deemed eligible to receive speech therapy and occupational therapy. His parents expected that he would be enrolled in a special education kindergarten classroom with a great deal of structure and a low student-to-teacher ratio.

Along with various medication trials, multiple attempts at psychosocial and family therapy had been attempted and abandoned because of the absence of any perceived benefit. At the time of the evaluation, there was no treatment taking place at all apart from clonidine hypocholoride, 0.1 mg twice daily, and Klonopin at bedtime.

Kenny had no difficulty separating from his mother for the evaluation. Although his receptive language appeared to be within typical limits, he did demonstrate some articulation problems. He related well to the examiner, displaying appropriate social interaction skills and a nice ability to play in a symbolic fashion. His play, however, revealed repetitive themes of aggression and protection. Although Kenny reported that he often felt fearful at night, there were no obvious symptoms of anxiety or depression observed during the evaluation. No psychotic symptoms were noted, nor did he display any hyperactivity or impulsivity.

Table 10.4 summarizes the assessment results for Kenny. His teacher completed the CBCL. Results revealed elevations in the domains of Attention Problems, Aggressive Behavior, Social Problems, and Somatic Complaints. A brief behavioral rating scale, the Conners Global Index—Teacher Form (CGI-T), also revealed that in the classroom Kenny had significant difficulty with overactivity, impulsivity, fidgeting, distractibility, temper outbursts, explosive and unpredictable behavior, needing his demands to be met immediately, and becoming easily frustrated. His mother's CBCL revealed elevated scores for Attention Problems, Social Problems, Thought Problems, and Aggressive Behavior. Maternal ratings on the ADHD Rating Scale–IV indicated that seven out of nine symptoms of hyperactivity–impulsivity were typical of Kenny, but only two out of nine symptoms of inattention.

In summary, Kenny presented with a history of early-onset aggression within the context of ADHD, complicated by a significant sleep disturbance. His hyperactivity and noncompliance with breathing treatments raised medical concerns about his asthma. He was considered to be an at-risk child requiring long-term medical and psychological follow-up, given his multiple risk factors. There was an extensive family history of ADHD and mood disorders in first-, second-, and third-degree maternal and paternal relatives. Kenny also displayed a history of cycling behavior accompanied by psychomotor and sleep changes. We therefore diagnosed Kenny with both ADHD, Predominantly Hyperactive–Impulsive Type, and Bipolar I Disorder. The following recommendations were provided to his parents:

1. Kenny's medications needed adjustment. Medications for ADHD were recommended, including D-amphetamine (Dexedrine) or perhaps combined pharmacotherapy

TABLE 10.4. Results for a Case of Comorbid ADHD and Bipolar Disorder in a 6-Year-Old Male

Mother		Teacher	
ADHD Rating Scale–IV			
(Symptoms rated >2)			
Inattention	2		
Hyperactivity–impulsivity	8		

CBCL—Parent		CBCL-TRF	
Subscale	Percentile	Subscale	Percentile
Withdrawn	50	Withdrawn	69
Somatic Complaints	87	Somatic Complaints	98*
Anxious/Depressed	70	Anxious/Depressed	55
Social Problems	99*	Social Problems	95*
Thought Problems	98*	Thought Problems	84
Attention Problems	98*	Attention Problems	95*
Delinquent Behavior	90	Delinquent Behavior 70	
Aggressive Behavior	99*	Aggressive Behavior	95*

CGI-T	
6 out of 10 items rated as "very much"	

Note. An asterisk indicates a clinically significant elevation (≥ 95th percentile or ≤ 5th percentile). CBCL, Child Behavior Checklist; TRF, Teacher's Report Form; CGI-T, Conners Global Index—Teacher Form.

with Dexedrine and medications that would down-regulate arousal. In addition, tricyclic antidepressants were suggested to improve Kenny's sleep, decrease his nightmares, and treat his ADHD in combination with stimulants.

2. Night terrors can be responsive to benzodiazepines. These medicines are generally given on a short-term basis. Night terrors are a developmental disorder and usually get better with age. If Klonopin did not prove effective, diazepam (Valium) at night might help Kenny's night terrors.

3. This evaluation supported a highly structured, therapeutic, educational placement for Kenny. If his ADHD symptoms improved with medication, he should received cognitive testing to determine his IQ and any possible learning disabilities that might affect educational treatment planning.

4. In addition to medication, Kenny's parents were referred to a parent management training program to assist them in managing Kenny's aggression at home. Rather than recommend a behaviorally based program, we suggested a program that was more cognitive in nature, such as that described by Ross Greene (1998) in *The Explosive Child: Understanding and Parenting Easily Frustrated, "Chronically Inflexible" Children.* This program emphasizes a nonconfrontational approach to child management, a reduction of unnecessary commands and instructions by parents, and a more measured and cautious approach to discipline so as not to provoke explosive episodes during irritable phases.

LOW-AVERAGE INTELLECTUAL FUNCTIONING AND POSSIBLE ADHD NOS

Lakeshia was a quiet and polite girl whose academic problems tended to "fly under the radar" of her teachers. She had always been considered a "slow learner" in school. She started attending a preschool when she was 2½ years old. Her mother voiced some concerns during these years that Lakeshia did not seem to be picking up preparatory academic skills as quickly as her peers. Because she was a well-behaved and compliant child whose learning difficulties did not seem to be drastically below the typical but highly variable range of development seen in preschool, her teachers were not overly concerned with her progress. However, Lakeshia was placed in a readiness program at her mother's prompting prior to kindergarten. She moved from this program through her first year or so of elementary school uneventfully, apart from her teachers' noting some weak or slow learning of academic skills across a variety of subjects. By second grade, however, her teacher became convinced that this was a greater difficulty than had been previously recognized. Lakeshia was placed in a remedial reading problem, which provided some help, but she continued to experience delayed progress. Consequently, her mother requested a child study team to determine whether her daughter might require special education services.

At the time of the second-grade team evaluation, the school observed that Lakeshia was making only "slow progress." They noted that she was below grade level in all of her subjects, despite the fact that she "works well in groups and likes to help others." Achievement testing by a school psychologist found her to be in an "average skill range" on all subjects, despite her poorer graded performance at school. The child study team reported that Lakeshia was a cooperative child without a history of behavioral problems. She was somewhat reserved, but would participate when called upon in class. The team concluded that Lakeshia did not qualify for an individualized education plan under special education law. Yet they did recommend that Lakeshia be retained in second grade, to allow her more time to "catch up" with her peers.

Lakeshia did better during her repeated attempt at second grade, but still was struggling to keep up. This lag again became more pronounced in third grade, and she fell behind in several subjects. When this pattern continued in the fourth grade, her mother switched Lakeshia to another school halfway into the year. But this was to no avail; her grades continued to deteriorate, despite her mother's also arranging tutorial assistance. By the end of the fall in the fifth grade, Lakeshia was failing all of her subjects. Her mother sought help from a pediatrician, who referred Lakeshia for a psychological evaluation.

According to her mother, Lakeshia's development seemed quite typical until she encountered problems in school. She was born full-term, with no prenatal or neonatal complications. Her health had always been good, and she had no sensory problems. She was the middle of three children whose biological father had died of complications from diabetes when Lakeshia was 2 years old. Her mother was a homemaker, and the family was supported by the father's military pension. No learning, behavioral, or psychological problems were reported for Lakeshia's siblings. Her mother stated that she herself had been a "slow reader" in school. Lakeshia's mother described herself as "running a tight ship" at home. The children all had daily chores, which they completed without difficulty.

Lakeshia seemed to be doing well in social settings outside of school. She was active in dance classes, where she studied ballet and tap. She also participated in a dance team during the worship services at her family church. She enjoyed doing arts and crafts for a pastime. She had recently started to participate in youth cheerleading classes and found this quite fun. In all of these situations, she got along well with her peers.

Lakeshia accompanied her mother to the first evaluation appointment. She was quiet and offered only brief responses when questions were directed to her. She never spontaneously engaged the examiner in conversation. Yet she was otherwise respectful and compliant. During the individual testing, Lakeshia appeared somewhat sad. She appeared to be genuinely trying to perform the testing tasks, but she would frequently give up—stating "I don't know" to verbal queries, or proceeding very slowly indeed on visual–motor tasks. As the test items became more difficult, Lakeshia became tearful at times, but stated that she wanted to "keep trying." This pattern of self-doubt was also acknowledged by Lakeshia's fifth-grade teacher, who stated that the student appeared "nervous" during tests and frequently made comments about "not being good at school." Lakeshia's mother wanted to clarify the causes of her daughter's academic problems. She wondered whether attention problems might be contributing to these difficulties. She reported five out of the nine inattentive features of ADHD as frequently displayed by Lakeshia, including poor focus on detail, failing to finish work, disorganization, task avoidance, and forgetfulness. Lakeshia was often fidgety, but none of the other hyperactive–impulsive features of ADHD were noted for her.

The results of Lakeshia's evaluation are summarized in Table 10.5. Her teacher reported the same symptoms of ADHD mentioned by her

TABLE 10.5. Results for a Case of Low IQ and Possible ADHD NOS in an 11-Year-Old

Mother		Teacher	

Interview report of ADHD symptoms			
Inattention	5		
Hyperactivity–impulsivity	1		

ADHD Rating Scale–IV		ADHD Rating Scale–IV	
(Symptoms rated >2)		(Symptoms rated >2)	
Inattention	5	Inattention	5
Hyperactivity–impulsivity	1	Hyperactivity–impulsivity	1

CBCL		BASC	
Subscale	Percentile	Subscale	Percentile
Withdrawn	77	Hyperactivity	45
Somatic Complaints	50	Aggression	38
Anxious/Depressed	50	Conduct Problems	54
Social Problems	77	Anxiety	83
Thought Problems	80	Depression	26
Attention Problems	93	Somatization	66
Delinquent Behavior	50	Attention Problems	92
Aggressive Behavior	50	Learning Problems	93
		Atypicality	52
Vineland—mother interview		Withdrawal	37
Communication	42	Adaptability	51
Daily Living Skills	91	Social Skills	67
Socialization	70	Leadership	57
Motor Skills	81	Study Sills	50
Composite	71		
	(above average)		

Testing data			
Test	Raw score	Standard/scaled score	Percentile
WISC-IV			
Full Scale IQ		75 (71–81)	5*
Verbal Comprehension Index		79	8
Similarities		7	16
Vocabulary		5	5*
Comprehension		7	16
Perceptual Reasoning		79	8
Block Design		9	37
Picture Concepts		6	9
Matrix Reasoning		5	5*
Working Memory		86	18
Digit Span		8	25
Letter–Number Sequencing		7	16
Processing Speed		80	9
Coding		6	9
Symbol Search		7	16
WJ III Tests of Achievement			
Total Achievement		86	18
Oral Expression		92	30
Listening Comprehension		88	21
Written Expression		107	67
Basic Reading		93	31
Mathematics Calculation		79	8
Mathematics Reasoning		86	17

Note. An asterisk indicates a clinically significant elevation (≥ 95th percentile or ≤ 5th percentile). Vineland, Vineland Adaptive Behavior Scales; WISC-IV, Wechsler Intelligence Scale for Children—Fourth Edition; WJ III, Woodcock–Johnson III; other abbreviations as in earlier tables.

mother. Although none of the behavior ratings of Lakeshia fell into a clinical range, both the teacher ratings on the BASC and the maternal CBCL ratings placed Lakeshia in a borderline clinical range on Attention Problems (92nd to 93rd percentile). In addition, her teacher's BASC ratings were in the borderline range on Learning Problems.

Lakeshia was given the WISC-IV and the Woodcock–Johnson III (WJ III) Tests of Achievement to screen for cognitive patterns that could be contributing to her difficulties. Her WISC-IV Full Scale IQ fell at the 5th percentile and in the borderline range of overall intellectual functioning. Her performance on the four index factors of the WISC-IV all fell at either the high end of the borderline range or in the low-average range. There were no significant differences between the composite scores or across the subtests, indicating a fairly consistent picture of a low-average to high-borderline level of intellectual ability. The achievement testing on the WJ III was less consistent. Although it reflected a low-average overall achievement performance, Lakeshia displayed somewhat stronger performance on Oral Expression, Written Expression, and Basic Reading. Maternal ratings of Lakeshia's adaptive behavior on the Vineland Adaptive Behavior Scales reflected average or better adjustment across all domains of adaptive functioning.

Based on the results of the testing, we gave Lakeshia a provisional diagnosis of ADHD NOS. This diagnosis indicates that ADHD-type difficulties are present, but that the full criteria are not met for the disorder. Although Lakeshia was rated as nearly meeting the symptom requirement for the Predominantly Inattentive Type of ADHD, her low-average to borderline intellectual performance prevented a clear attribution of her academic performance problems to inattention alone. Consequently, we stressed that the diagnosis of ADHD NOS was provisional and could not be made with certainty. The following recommendations were given to Lakeshia's mother:

1. We advised the mother to continue to work closely with Lakeshia's school to develop an appropriate education plan. It was possible that the diagnosis of ADHD NOS would qualify Lakeshia to receive special accommodations under a Section 504 plan. We suggested that Lakeshia's mother should request a meeting with the appropriate school officials to determine whether this was the case. Regardless of whether a formal plan was implemented, careful structuring of Lakeshia's educational experience through the use of techniques such as horizontal deceleration would be important to maximize her progress. Greater care would also need to be taken to encourage her for any investment she displayed in her schooling, signs of academic demoralization were beginning to emerge.

2. A number of environmental modifications were recommended to minimize the consequences of Lakeshia's attentional problems, such as those described in Chapters 12 and 15 (this volume).

3. The importance of keeping Lakeshia involved in nonacademic activities that she found self-affirming, such as her dance classes, was noted. This would help compensate for the blows to her self-esteem that she was experiencing from her ongoing academic difficulties.

4. Periodic reevaluation of Lakeshia's psychoeducational functioning was recommended (approximately every 3 years). The importance of appropriate technical or other less academic occupational training in high school and beyond was discussed, should this same pattern of intellectual performance persist. The importance of keeping expectations realistic, while also not handicapping Lakeshia by setting expectations too low, was discussed.

This case illustrates the complexity of the issue of "caseness" in making diagnostic decisions. Mulder, Frampton, Joyce, and Porter (2003) point out that the research diagnostic criteria informing the DSM-IV(-TR) involve somewhat arbitrary decisions about diagnostic thresholds. One can still encounter professional debates over whether ADHD constitutes a true, discrete condition or a socially constructed pathological reification of a typical variant in a functional trait (Timimi, Taylor, Cannon, McKenzie, & Sims, 2004). Although we do not share the nihilism inherent in the latter view, we do accept ADHD as a dimensional disorder along the same lines as mental retardation, learning disabilities, and language disorders. As Chapter 2 in this volume discusses, ADHD difficulties are experienced by individuals on a continuum of severity. Some individuals who display a borderline clinical level of the symptoms may suffer many of the same problems as others who exceed the clinical threshold. Those with borderline symptoms would be likely to benefit significantly from many of the same interventions that have been shown effective for those with clear ADHD. The ADHD NOS label provides a diagnostic recourse for clinicians who want to provide assistance to individuals with such subthreshold, borderline symptoms. Lakeshia's case highlights the issue that clinicians are in the business of ultimately relieving suffering, not engaging in verbal parlor games about whether or not a single symptom or two changes a child from being in the borderline range to being in the clearly disordered range of behavior. Treatment is to be provided whenever sufficient evidence of impairment is documented, in spite of the precise level of symptom expression that may be evident and whether or not it surpasses formally stated diagnostic criteria. Diagnosis is a means to an end, not an end in itself; treatment (the relief of suffering) is the endpoint that society expects from mental health professionals.

In Lakeshia's case, even this less clear diagnosis could only be made provisionally, because her borderline to low-average intellectual functioning may have been the sufficient cause of her academic problems. Still, even after we considered the lower mental age suggested by the WISC-IV performance, it was not clear that all of Lakeshia's attention problems could be explained as a result of lower intellectual ability. A real possibility of an independent attention problem persisted. No foreseeable adverse consequences would arise from giving a provisional ADHD NOS diagnosis, and some possible benefit might be obtained. Lakeshia would perhaps now qualify for special accommodations at school. It is important to note that we did not decide to give this diagnosis just to qualify her for school services. This would be an unethical practice that would undercut our professional credibility and potentially result in client harm. Rather, we believed ADHD NOS to be a real diagnostic possibility for Lakeshia, and then qualified our diagnosis with comments indicating our degree of confidence. We also made treatment recommendations that were tailored to helping with Lakeshia's particular pattern of presenting problems, but were not strictly dependent upon whether she fully qualified for an ADHD diagnosis or not. A primary function of diagnosis for a clinician is the facilitating of effective treatment planning. In cases such as Lakeshia's, the ADHD NOS label may help to achieve that goal.

ADHD, PREDOMINANTLY INATTENTIVE TYPE

Daniel was the youngest of three children; his parents had a stable marriage. Daniel's father had a high school education and owned a limousine service. His mother had an associate's degree and worked as an occupational therapy assistant.

Daniel was a healthy infant who was difficult to put on a schedule. Subsequent major developmental milestones were achieved at typical ages. As a toddler, he was very stubborn and always quite active. Because the family was a very busy and active one, these traits were not identified as deviant. Daniel attended public schools, where he was seen as very active beginning in kindergarten. Throughout his elementary school years, his teachers commented on his distractibility, inattention, overactivity, impulsivity, and failure to complete assignments. When he completed his work, it was usually of high quality; however, he frequently forgot to turn in his assignments, rushed through them, or simply did not complete them. Thus his grades were generally C's, with his poor work habits partially compensated for by his excellent test performance. Daniel was always seen as a happy child, with no behavioral or emotional concerns. However, because he appeared so inattentive and distractible and was not putting forth the expected amount of effort in school, school personnel conducted a psychoeducational evaluation in the fifth grade. The results of the evaluation indicated that Daniel was of above-average intelligence and had no specific learning disabilities. School personnel determined that he was ineligible for any special services.

As Daniel entered middle school, his behavior at home became more difficult to manage. He was frequently argumentative with his parents and refused to comply with their requests. He also threw tantrums when he did not get his way. His parents found that the traditional parenting techniques they had used successfully with their older children did not work with Daniel. They found themselves engaging in increasingly negative interactions with him, and giving in when they got tired of arguing. Finally, they consulted a behavior therapist for parenting suggestions. The use of these resulted in some improvement in Daniel's behavior in the home setting.

In school, however, Daniel was experiencing greater difficulty as the workload and responsibilities increased. His grades began to drop. His teachers, aware of his cognitive abilities, reprimanded him frequently for being "lazy" and "unmotivated." Finally, Daniel failed the eighth grade. His parents took Daniel to see a counselor to determine why he was not working up to his potential. Daniel did not want to go to therapy, and his parents finally gave up the struggle to make him attend, as they did not see any improvement. Daniel appeared to stop trying in school after the eighth-grade failure, and his mood became more noticeably subdued. Although he continued to enjoy spending time with a few close friends, he appeared sad or irritable at home. He appeared to worry about school and continued to perform poorly. He also began experimenting with marijuana and alcohol at about this time. He failed the 10th grade as well. After repeating the 10th grade, Daniel failed all but one of his courses in the first semester of 11th grade. Art classes were the only courses in which he consistently performed well; he rarely completed the work in any other courses.

School personnel conducted another psychoeducational evaluation after Daniel failed the first semester of 11th grade. On the Wechsler Adult Intelligence Scale—Revised (WAIS-R), Daniel obtained a Full Scale IQ of 129. Behavior rating scales completed by his parents and teachers noted the presence of inattentiveness. A self-report measure completed by Daniel noted the presence of depressive symptoms. Despite a clear history of academic underachievement dating back to the first grade and no evidence of depressive symptoms prior to Daniel's junior high school years, the school psychologist attributed Daniel's school failure to depression and recommended a medication evaluation. Daniel's parents were not convinced that this was the root of Daniel's problems and brought him into our clinic for an evaluation.

At the time of the evaluation, Daniel was 17 years, 10 months old. His health was very good, although he was nearsighted and had poor handwriting skills. His most recent medical examination had been completely unexceptional. A review of family psychiatric history indicated that one of Daniel's paternal uncles had experienced school difficulties, alcohol abuse, and depression. There was no history of any other psychiatric or learning difficulties on either side of the family.

Throughout the interview, Daniel was quite fidgety and active. He tapped his feet throughout the evaluation and shifted in his chair frequently. He occasionally got up and walked around the room. This activity did not appear to be motivated by anxiety, as Daniel appeared very comfortable during the evaluation. His answers were clear and informative. He reported having no problems at home, but did indicate that he did not enjoy spending time with his family. He reported that he preferred to spend time with his friends skateboarding and playing music. He admitted to occasional marijuana and alcohol use in the past 2–3 years. He reported that he did not enjoy school, because he did not like the rules and found most of the work boring. He did enjoy his art classes. He reported some worries about his school performance, but denied that these symptoms interfered with his life. Daniel indicated that he had been depressed in the past, but denied any current depressive symptoms or suicidal ideation. He indicated that he felt he had been depressed because he was not doing well in school, despite trying. He viewed many of his difficulties as being the results of distractibility and inattentiveness. Daniel reported that he displayed nine of nine symptoms of inattention and four of nine symptoms of hyperactivity–impulsivity on a frequent basis.

Similarly, Daniel's parents endorsed nine of nine symptoms of inattention and three or four of nine symptoms of hyperactivity–impulsivity as being typical of Daniel. They also reported Daniel to display five of eight behaviors associated with ODD to a significant degree for his age, including irritability and noncompliance with adult requests. No symptoms of CD were endorsed, nor did Daniel currently meet criteria for any other psychiatric condition.

Table 10.6 shows the results of the parent and teacher rating scales and psychological testing. Daniel's mother completed the CBCL, which indicated clinically significant problems on the Attention Problems, Withdrawal, Social Problems, Delinquent, and Anxious/Depressed factors. On the ADHD Rating Scale–IV, Daniel was rated as having all symptoms of inattention occurring on a frequent basis within the home setting. Results of the Defiant Behavior Rating Scale (DBRS) revealed significant symptoms of ODD occurring on a frequent basis within the home setting. SSRS results revealed below-average peer socialization skills.

Teacher ratings also revealed significant attention problems. These rating scales were

TABLE 10.6. Results for a Case of ADHD, Predominantly Inattentive Type, in a 17-Year-Old

Mother		Father		Teachers	
Interview report of ADHD symptoms		Interview report of ADHD symptoms			
Inattention	9	Inattention	9	Inattention	6 and 7
Hyperactivity–impulsivity	4	Hyperactivity–impulsivity	4	Hyperactivity–impulsivity	2 and 4
ADHD Rating Scale–IV					
(Symptoms rated >2)					
Inattention	9				
Hyperactivity–impulsivity	1				

CBCL			CBCL-TRF	
Subscale	Percentile		Subscale	Percentile
Withdrawn	>99*		Withdrawn	91
Somatic Complaints	83		Somatic Complaints	50
Anxious/Depressed	98*		Anxious/Depressed	61
Social Problems	99*		Social Problems	73
Thought Problems	75		Thought Problems	80
Attention Problems	99*		Attention Problems	96*
Delinquent Behavior	99*		Delinquent Behavior	86
Aggressive Behavior	89		Aggressive Behavior	50

DBRS			SSRS	
Number of ODD symptoms	5		Total raw score (29)	2* (below average)

	Testing data		
Test	Raw score	Standard/scaled score	Percentile
SB-IV			
Vocabulary	36	108	70
Conners CPT			
Hits	324 (100%)		18
Omissions	0 (0%)		18
Commissions	8 (22%)	40	15
Hit rate	525	18	1*
Hit rate *SE*	9	63	91
Variability of *SE*	10	53	65

Note. An asterisk indicates a clinically significant elevation (≥ 95th percentile or ≤ 5th percentile). SB-IV, Stanford–Binet Intelligence Scale: Fourth Edition; other abbreviations as in earlier tables.

completed by Daniel's English and algebra teachers, based on their observations of him in 45-minute classes with 30 other students, over the course of a semester. On the Teacher's Report Form of the CBCL, Daniel obtained scores in the clinically significant range on the Attention Problems scale. His teachers' ADHD Rating Scale–IV results revealed six or seven of nine symptoms of inattention, and two to four of nine symptoms of hyperactivity–impulsivity occurring on a frequent basis within the classroom setting. (These ratings of ADHD behaviors in the classroom are quite high for high school teachers. Because their interactions with students are much more limited than those of elementary or even middle school teachers, they are less likely to notice and report significant symptoms of ADHD.) Results of the DBRS revealed that in the classroom, zero or one of eight behaviors associated with ODD occurred on a frequent basis. SSRS results revealed below-average peer socialization skills in the areas of cooperation, assertiveness, and self-control.

Daniel was administered psychological tests, the results of which appear in Table 10.6 as well. Daniel's Stanford–Binet Intelligence Scale: Fourth Edition (SB-IV) Vocabulary test performance yielded a total score of 36 and a corresponding standardized score of 108, which was within the average range. Although Daniel's Conners CPT performance was slow and inconsistent, this test did not provide strong evidence of attention difficulties.

The results of this evaluation supported a diagnosis of ADHD and ODD. According to both Daniel and his parents, he did not meet DSM-IV-TR criteria for any other psychiatric disorder. His marijuana and alcohol use was experimental at this time, rather than indicative of full-fledged substance dependence or abuse. Daniel's depressive symptoms were subclinical, based on his report and that of his parents. Furthermore, it appeared to be secondary to the years of school failure, rather than primary (as the school psychologist had believed). The chronological onset of the depression was much later than the onset of ADHD symptoms. Daniel's ODD behaviors were much more significant in the home than in school. In fact, his teachers did not see him as defiant at all.

Evidence of impairment was found in Daniel's history of academic underachievement and school failure, as well as his parent- and teacher-reported peer socialization difficulties.

We made several recommendations to the family:

1. We emphasized education about ADHD and its associated features for Daniel, his parents, and his teachers.
2. We recommended a course of family therapy, focused on problem-solving and communication training for Daniel and his parents. The therapy described in Chapter 13 (this volume) would be ideal.
3. We referred Daniel to a psychiatrist for consideration of a trial of stimulant or atomoxetine medication.
4. We recommend a number of educational modifications for Daniel's ADHD difficulties in the school setting, including a guidance counselor or other school personnel to play a coaching role, a modified homework load, and additional time to complete assigned tasks.
5. We suggested supportive counseling for Daniel to help him adjust to his ADHD diagnosis and plan for his future, considering his

ADHD as part of his pattern of strengths and weaknesses.

Daniel refused to participate in any form of family therapy, but readily agreed to the other interventions.

This case illustrates a number of issues in assessing ADHD in older adolescents. First of all, because ADHD is a developmental disorder, there must be a history of preadolescent onset of ADHD characteristics. This history is often difficult to ascertain in an older adolescent. In Daniel's case, school report cards from his entire academic career were available and clearly confirmed his mother's report of early ADHD symptoms. It is important to attempt to obtain such objective data. Second, it is interesting to note that other mental health professionals had attributed Daniel's difficulties to depression. Although he did display depressive symptoms and had possibly been clinically depressed at the time of the previous evaluation, a diagnosis of Major Depressive Disorder or Dysthymic Disorder does not necessarily rule out comorbid ADHD. In Daniel's case, careful interviewing revealed that the ADHD symptoms predated the onset of the depression by at least 5 years. Third, this case illustrates some points about the developmental course of ADHD. Although Daniel was given the diagnosis of ADHD, Predominantly Inattentive Type, this type often does not involve pure inattention. If he had been evaluated as a child, it is quite possible that Daniel might have met diagnostic criteria for ADHD, Combined Type. He had a history of impulsivity and continued to be fidgety and impulsive even now. However, in the course of development, symptoms of hyperactivity are likely to decline (see Chapter 2), whereas the inattention and impulsivity may continue. The DSM-IV(-TR) items were selected and normed on children 4–16 years of age, and the items do not necessarily apply as well to the manifestation of ADHD in adolescents or adults. Thus it is entirely possible for older adolescents or adults to meet DSM-IV-TR criteria for ADHD, Predominantly Inattentive Type, when they actually display a pattern of symptoms characteristic of ADHD, Combined Type—namely, difficulties with response inhibition. In short, children with ADHD, Combined Type can easily move into the Predominantly Inattentive Type by late adolescence merely as a function of declines in some symptoms of hyperactivity, and not because of a qualitative change in typology. Such cases should actually be considered borderline or subthresholds cases of ADHD, Combined Type for the sake of treatment planning, rather than as a qualitatively different type. But see the next case for an instance of what we believe to be a form of *pure* inattention.

ADHD, PREDOMINANTLY INATTENTIVE TYPE WITH SLUGGISH COGNITIVE TEMPO

Tim was a quiet and somewhat introverted child who readily "faded into the crowd." Apart from his quiet demeanor, his early development was unremarkable. He reached the developmental milestones at appropriate times and was not a behavior problem for his mother, who had raised Tim and his younger brother alone. Tim's father and mother had split up before Tim was born, and Tim had no contact with his father.

Tim attended a parochial elementary school, where he performed "adequately" both academically and behaviorally. However, he never volunteered information and often seemed to be "off in a daze." His teachers frequently had to repeat questions when they called on him, because he did not seem to catch what they asked. Although Tim did not have problems with reading decoding, he had some difficulty staying with a train of thought when he began to read passages. This pattern created problems in his ability to comprehend what he read, and consequently Tim received some individual assistance from his teachers for his weak reading skills. Tim's family moved prior to his entering the third grade, resulting in a transfer to another parochial school. About this time, Tim began to display greater difficulties in school because of the increased amount of independent work expected of him. Tim typically failed to complete his work in an appropriate amount of time and had trouble finishing assigned readings. His teachers often made comments that Tim seemed unable to "focus" on his work and consequently made very inefficient use of his time.

Because of these difficulties, Ms. P. requested that the local public school system evaluate Tim prior to his entering fourth grade, to determine whether he was eligible for government-mandated individualized education services. The school evaluation team detected some weaknesses in reading skills, but Tim was not found eligible for such services. Tim's problems with "attentional lapses," "poor focusing," and low productivity continued to be problems as he moved into middle school in fifth grade. His grades became much more inconsistent in middle school, ranging from B's to D's. Although Tim was on a rotating schedule in middle school and consequently had much briefer contact with his teachers, school personnel continued to comment about Tim's "spacey" demeanor and frequent tendency to get lost in "daydreams." Tim's productivity continued to decline in seventh and eighth grades as a result of uncompleted homework, inadequate preparation, and slow completion of classroom work. Tim obtained passing grades, but his greatest difficulties were in reading-intensive subjects, such as English and history.

Tim's social adjustment was generally uneventful. He had no problems forming or maintaining friendships and was typically well received by his peers. Tim's interpersonal style was often described as "reserved" or "somewhat withdrawn"; he never showed an interest in organized recreational activities and did not usually initiate social contacts with his peers. Yet he often was included by his friends in informal activities, such as playing basketball or going to the mall. Despite Tim's tendency to "keep to himself," his friends seemed to enjoy having him around.

During his freshman year in high school, Tim's attention problems and poor study habits had a more significant impact on his academic performance. He failed three classes because of low test scores and uncompleted work. He was able to pass on to the 10th grade because he retook the failed classes in summer school. Tim's academic difficulties became a larger point of contention between him and his mother at about this time. They frequently argued about Tim's poor performance, and his mother often accused Tim of "not trying hard enough." Tim expressed frustration over these accusations and typically retorted that he was doing his best. Despite the increased pressure from his mother, Tim failed his 10th-grade English class and had to take the class over in summer school to enter the 11th grade. Although his 10th-grade teachers did not view Tim as having conduct problems, they frequently complained about his failure to complete work, weak ability to focus, distractibility, and disorganization. Because of Tim's persistent difficulty displaying appropriate study skills in academic subjects, his mother and school officials decided to transfer him to a vocational high school for 11th grade. Although he still faced academic demands, they were interspersed with more applied activities. He spent every other week in an auto mechanic program. Despite this alternative school placement, Tim was clearly failing a literature course 3 months into the school year, and his teachers commented about his frequent "zoning out in class."

Ms. P. decided to take Tim to a psychiatrist for an evaluation of his "attention problems" halfway through his 11th-grade year. Based on an interview with Tim and his mother, the psychiatrist diagnosed Tim with provisional ADHD. He placed Tim on a trial of pemoline (Cylert), which produced some subjective improvement in Tim's ability to focus, but his teachers noted no objective improvement. (This case occurred at a time before Cylert had received a "black-box" warning for rare instances of hepatoxicity.) Consequently, the medication was stopped until a more extensive evaluation could be accomplished. Tim's psychiatrist referred him to the ADHD clinic for further evaluation and consultation. Table 10.7 presents the results of this evaluation. Tim's mother and two teachers all reported a significant number of the inattentive features of ADHD; however, none of the hyperactive–impulsive symptoms of ADHD were reported for Tim. Although Tim's teachers rated him as displaying an average number of social skills, his mother also rated Tim as significantly "withdrawn."

During the interview, Ms. P. described Tim as a frequently "sullen" youth. Yet she pointed out that Tim had never displayed any prolonged periods of depression or excessive anxiety. She stated that their relationship had become tense and periodically conflict-ridden over the few years prior to the evaluation, with the focus of their disagreements being Tim's inconsistent academic performance. Ms. P. indicated that Tim was often irritable around her, often blamed others for his mistakes, and frequently "talked back." However, she denied any substantial problems with Tim's complying with her wishes in other areas. For example, she indicated that Tim typically completed chores around the house when asked or expected to do so.

Tim appeared very calm during the interview and readily cooperated with the examiner. Again, Table 10.7 summarizes Tim's test re-sults. Because no recent cognitive testing had been completed with Tim, he was given the SB-IV Vocabulary subtest to obtain a brief estimate of his verbal intelligence. Tim obtained a raw score of 32 and a corresponding Verbal Reasoning standard score of 96 on this subtest. His performance fell at the 39th percentile and in the average range, suggesting that Tim had at least an average level of verbal intelligence. Consequently, comparisons of test results with chronological age norms were deemed appropriate. Tim displayed a good performance on the Conners CPT. He responded to target items with an average level of accuracy (omissions) and only infrequently responded to inappropriate test items (commissions), indicating an average performance on this measure of inattention and impulsivity.

Tim acknowledged seven inattentive symptoms of ADHD but denied any impulsive or overactive symptoms. He mentioned that his attention problems were most significant on reading tasks. Tim explained that he had problems "focusing" on what he was reading; when asked to elaborate on these problems, he described them as being unable to tune out distractions. Tim often had to read and reread literature in a very quiet area to comprehend what he was reading. Although his inattentive difficulties had been present since his elementary school years, Tim felt that they became most intense in high school.

Based on the evaluation, an impression was formed of Tim as a 17-year, 9-month-old young man of presumably average intelligence who had a chronic history of inattentiveness, distractibility, and underachievement on academic tasks since kindergarten. A significant number of the inattentive symptoms of ADHD were consistently reported for Tim, but he had no history of any of the hyperactive–impulsive symptoms of this condition. Based on the DSM-IV-TR criteria, Tim's pattern of symptoms and associated difficulties supported a diagnosis of ADHD, Predominantly Inattentive Type. No other clinical diagnoses emerged from the evaluation. The pattern of conflict between Tim and Ms. P. was classified as Parent–Child Relational Problem. Tim's difficulties were complicated by a history of weaknesses on reading-related tasks. Psychoeducational testing completed by the school had reportedly ruled out any substantial specific learning disabilities, which would account for his reading-related weaknesses. Yet it was unclear whether

TABLE 10.7. Results for a Case of ADHD, Predominantly Inattentive Type with Sluggish Cognitive Tempo, in a 17-Year-Old Male

Mother		English teacher		Math teacher	
Interview report of ADHD symptoms					
Inattention	6				
Hyperactivity–impulsivity	0				
ADHD Rating Scale–IV		ADHD Rating Scale–IV		ADHD Rating Scale–IV	
(Symptoms rated >2)		(Symptoms rated >2)		(Symptoms rated >2)	
Inattention	5	Inattention	9	Inattention	7
Hyperactivity–impulsivity	0	Hyperactivity–impulsivity	0	Hyperactivity–impulsivity	0
CBCL		CBCL		CBCL	
Subscale	Percentile	Subscale	Percentile	Subscale	Percentile
Withdrawn	95*	Withdrawn	84	Withdrawn	50
Somatic Complaints	50	Somatic Complaints	76	Somatic Complaints	50
Anxious	93	Anxious	55	Anxious	73
Social Problems	50	Social Problems	84	Social Problems	63
Thought Problems	50	Thought Problems	50	Thought Problems	50
Attention Problems	95*	Attention Problems	95*	Attention Problems	88
Delinquent Behavior	86	Delinquent Behavior	61	Delinquent Behavior	60
Aggressive Behavior	84	Aggressive Behavior	70	Aggressive Behavior	50
SSRS		SSRS		SSRS	
Total score (40)	16	Total score (52)	63	Total score (46)	37
DBRS					
Number of ODD symptoms	3				

	Testing data		
Test	Raw score	Standard/scaled score	Percentile
SB-IV Verbal Reasoning (prorated from Vocabulary score)	32	96	39
Conners CPT			
Hits	324 (100%)		18
Omissions	0 (0%)		18
Commissions	13 (36%)	46	35
Hit rate	348	47	38
Hit rate *SE*	4	43	25
Variability of *SE*	4	43	26

Note. An asterisk indicates a clinically significant elevation (≥ 95th percentile or ≤ 5th percentile).

subtle processing problems, such as a central auditory processing deficit, had been fully ruled out as a contributing factor in Tim's inconsistent academic performance.

We made several recommendations to Ms. P. and Tim following the evaluation:

1. Parent and patient education about ADHD through directed readings, follow-up consultation, and participation in a support group were suggested. However, we distin-guished the Predominantly Inattentive Type of ADHD from the Combined and Predominantly Hyperactive–Impulsive Types, and we also explained our belief that Tim had a *purely* inattentive subtype of ADHD (see below).

2. A neuropsychological evaluation was recommended, to more definitively rule out the possibility that a language-related learning disability or working memory disorder might be contributing to Tim's academic difficulties.

3. Vocational assessment to help establish

appropriate career goals for Tim was emphasized.

4. Participation in family counseling by Tim and his mother was stressed.

5. Various organizational and compensatory behavior strategies for Tim were discussed.

6. The option of treatment with stimulant medication or atomoxetine was discussed. The possibly lower efficacy of stimulant medication for the treatment of the purely inattentive form of ADHD was noted, however.

Tim's case illustrates the differences between the more common form of ADHD, which seems to be primarily a problem of response control, and a *purely* inattentive type of the condition that some researchers are now calling "sluggish cognitive tempo" (SCT) (Milich, Ballentine, & Lynam, 2001). No current DSM-IV-TR category explicitly outlines the *purely* inattentive type of the condition. The most closely related DSM-IV-TR classification for this group is ADHD, Predominantly Inattentive Type, which was the diagnosis Tim received. Yet although many individuals may not display a significant number of the hyperactive–impulsive symptoms of ADHD, particularly by adolescence, problems with impulsivity or self-regulation are often present. Pure inattention or SCT, discussed in Chapter 4 (this volume), is a much rarer condition that may account for approximately 30–50% of children currently diagnosed with the Predominantly Inattentive Type of ADHD. It appears to have distinct attention problems and associated difficulties. This subgroup is characterized by a history of inattentive problems devoid of any significant difficulties with impulsivity or overactivity. Such individuals tend to be described as "daydreamy," "spacey," "staring," "confused," or "in a fog." They tend to be viewed more as lethargic and slow-moving, even hypoactive. Socially, they are characterized as reticent, passive, or even withdrawn. Individuals with all types of ADHD tend to have academic problems, such as failing to complete work, but such problems are often due to different reasons for these types. Individuals with SCT typically have trouble completing work because they struggle to process competing sources of information. Individuals with ADHD, Combined Type, tend either to rush through their work impulsively or to have difficulty holding themselves to the task. The difference is one of accuracy (SCT) versus productivity (Combined Type). Although individuals with SCT are more frequently anxious, depressed, and withdrawn, they typically have fewer social problems than do children with other forms of ADHD. They also carry a much lower risk for comorbid ODD or CD (and hence probably substance use disorders).

Tim's case illustrates many of these differences. There was no evidence of the substantial problems with response control characteristic of ADHD, Combined Type. Although some difficulty in his interactions with his mother was reported, no significant behavioral disorder was evident at home. Tim had been rated as significantly "withdrawn," but no substantial problems in his social functioning were reported. His academic difficulties appeared to be due to his problems in focusing attention, particularly on reading tasks, rather than due to problems with sustaining attention. It is possible that a neurocognitive problem, such as a subtle learning disability or a central auditory processing deficit, may have been the source of Tim's *purely* inattentive form of ADHD.

GENERALIZED ANXIETY DISORDER WITHOUT ADHD

Fifteen-year-old Vanessa was the elder of two sisters. Her mother had been treated for "nerves" early in her marriage to Vanessa's father. From the time Vanessa was born, she was difficult to comfort and appeared to display greater difficulty adjusting to new situations than Vanessa's mother had seen her friends' children display. However, her early development was not unusual.

In addition to her own history of probable anxiety, Vanessa's mother was somewhat anxious and protective with Vanessa. She discouraged exploration and risk taking. Vanessa's father was much more impulsive, and Vanessa's mother did what she could to make certain Vanessa did not take after him. When Vanessa was 3, her sister was born. It became clear early that the two girls had very different temperaments. People often said that Vanessa was the image of her mother, and her sister took after her father.

Vanessa had a great deal of difficulty separating from her mother when she began school. She would cling to her mother and cry each day when her mother left her at kindergarten. After a few weeks, Vanessa was able to tolerate the separation, but she was a very shy child who hung back and did not initiate interactions with the other children. Academically, however, Vanessa did extremely well. She was an A student throughout her school years, and the only concerns teachers ever expressed had to do with her social reticence.

Vanessa's parents, however, noticed that she was a "worrier." Although she consistently performed well in school, she spent a great deal of time on her schoolwork and expressed anxiety regarding tests and her academic performance. She also worried about making friends, as well as any number of possible things that might go wrong with her family members. She complained of frequent headaches and stomachaches when tests were coming up or when she had to give a presentation in class.

When Vanessa entered middle school in the sixth grade, she moved to a bigger school and did not have classes with many of her friends. She appeared very sad, and withdrew from activities in which she had been interested. Her mother noted that she seemed easily fatigued and somewhat distracted. She saw a counselor, and her mood seemed to improve by the time she entered seventh grade. Soon thereafter, Vanessa's father went to see a psychologist after he was fired from a job because he could not keep up with his paperwork. He was diagnosed with ADHD and successfully treated with a stimulant. As Vanessa's mother began reading about ADHD, she wondered whether Vanessa's symptoms of inattention and distractibility might be explained by this disorder. She learned that it was hereditary and felt that Vanessa might meet the profile for the Predominantly Inattentive Type.

Vanessa was in the 10th grade at the time of the evaluation. Her health was reported to be very good, though she did experience environmental allergies. She also had difficulty falling asleep at night, which had been true for much of her life; she experienced related difficulty waking in the morning. Her appetite was unexceptional. Her speech, hearing, vision, and motor coordination skills were also within typical limits.

The review of childhood and adolescent psychiatric symptoms with Vanessa's mother indicated that Vanessa displayed four of nine symptoms of inattentiveness and no symptoms of hyperactivity–impulsivity. She frequently failed to pay close attention to details, was easily dis-

tracted, and appeared forgetful in her daily activities. No ODD or CD behaviors were endorsed. Her mood was described as typically worried or sad, and many symptoms of Generalized Anxiety Disorder and Dysthymic Disorder were endorsed. She was reported to have a withdrawn peer interaction style and difficulty making friends. Vanessa had done well academically throughout her school years, and no teacher had ever reported any behavioral problems or difficulty with inattention or distractibility. A review of the family psychiatric history revealed depression and anxiety on the maternal side. Vanessa's sister had recently been diagnosed with ODD.

The interview with Vanessa revealed a neatly groomed adolescent who participated willingly in the interview and testing, but appeared reserved and bit her nails throughout the session. No obvious signs of ADHD were observed. Vanessa responded to the interviewer's questioning in a clear and informative manner. She was generally aware of the reasons for her being evaluated. She reported that she liked school overall, especially seeing her friends and going to gym class. She reported that did not like some of her peers and did not enjoy much of the schoolwork. She admitted that she was somewhat shy, but reported that she did have a group of friends with whom she went to the mall and to see movies. She described a variety of additional recreational activities she enjoyed, such as playing with the computer and playing pool. Vanessa reported positive family relationships. She indicated that she was generally worried about a lot of things and had been at least since late elementary school. She stated that she was worried more days than not, and her worries interfered with her social life as well as with her schoolwork. She had difficulty controlling the worry. Vanessa endorsed five of the nine symptoms associated with inattention in the DSM-IV-TR ADHD symptom list, but reported that those symptoms were primarily present when she was worried about something.

Table 10.8 shows the behavior rating scales and results of psychological testing. The results of the parent rating scales revealed average scores on all scales except the BASC Withdrawal subscale. Results of the parent version of the ADHD Rating Scale–IV revealed borderline significant symptoms of inattention occurring on a frequent basis within the home setting and no symptoms of hyperactivity–impulsivity.

TABLE 10.8. Results for a Case of Generalized Anxiety Disorder without ADHD in a 15-Year-Old Female

Mother		Math teacher	
Interview report of ADHD symptoms			
Inattention	4		
Hyperactivity–impulsivity	0		
ADHD Rating Scale–IV		**ADHD Rating Scale–IV**	
(Symptoms rated >2)		(Symptoms rated >2)	
Inattention	6	Inattention	0
Hyperactivity–impulsivity	0	Hyperactivity–impulsivity	0
CBCL		**CBCL**	
Subscale	Percentile	Subscale	Percentile
Withdrawn	50	Withdrawn	55
Somatic Complaints	74	Somatic Complaints	78
Anxious	50	Anxious	78
Social Problems	50	Social Problems	50
Thought Problems	50	Thought Problems	50
Attention Problems	87	Attention Problems	50
Delinquent Behavior	50	Delinquent Behavior	50
Aggressive Behavior	50	Aggressive Behavior	50
DBRS		**DBRS**	
Number of ODD symptoms	0	Number of ODD symptoms	0

	Testing data		
Test	Raw score	Standard/scaled score	Percentile
WISC-III Vocabulary	46	11	63
Conners CPT			
Hits	324 (100%)		14
Omissions	0 (0%)		14
Commissions	28 (78%)	73	99*
Hit rate	287	64	92
Hit rate *SE*	4	39	15
Variability of *SE*	5	42	22

Note. An asterisk indicates a clinically significant elevation (≥ 95th percentile or ≤ 5th percentile).

None of the scores on the various teacher rating scales were clinically elevated. The teacher endorsed no symptoms of either inattention or hyperactivity–impulsivity on the ADHD Rating Scale–IV.

Vanessa's WISC-III Vocabulary scaled score of 11 suggested that her overall verbal abilities were within the average range. The Conners CPT provided no evidence for problems with inattention or impulsivity.

The results of this evaluation did not support a diagnosis of ADHD. The only significant ratings of ADHD symptoms came from Vanessa's mother, and even those were merely in the borderline range or even lower on most of the rating scales. In addition, there was no evidence of any impairment due to her inattention in any domain of Vanessa's life. She performed very well in school. Vanessa's difficulties lay more clearly in the emotional domain. She and her mother both reported that she had been experiencing, at least since late elementary school, a pattern of excessive anxiety of sufficient frequency and severity to warrant a DSM-IV-TR diagnosis of Generalized Anxiety Disorder. Given the paternal history of ADHD, it is understandable that Vanessa's parents identified her attentional difficulties as possibly being related to ADHD. However, distractibility and difficulty in concentrating can also be symptoms of anxiety, and in this case, the evidence pointed much more clearly in that direction as an explanation for Vanessa's difficulties. We made the following recommendations to the family members, and they planned to follow through on these:

1. We stressed cognitive-behavioral therapy and relaxation training for Vanessa, aimed at ameliorating her emotional difficulties. We also recommended social skills training.

2. We emphasized the development of organizational strategies for Vanessa, as well as coping strategies to help manage her anxiety regarding school projects.

3. We referred the family to a therapist in the family's home community.

Although we did not recommend any medication for Vanessa, it is possible that cases like this one may be appropriate for a trial on atomoxetine (Strattera), in view of very recent findings that this medication may greatly reduce symptoms of anxiety in inattentive children (see *www.strattera.com*).

In this case, Vanessa's symptoms of inattention were different in quality from the inattention typically found in ADHD. For instance, she was distracted by her own intrusive thoughts rather than being impulsively drawn off task, as someone with ADHD would experience. Her inattentiveness cut across all activities, whereas someone with ADHD would not display attention problems when the task at hand was interesting. She was more preoccupied, was more easily fatigued, and had difficulty *focusing* on tasks, whereas an adolescent with ADHD would display more problems with *vigilance* or *sustained* attention.

This case illustrates the importance of viewing inattention as a symptom or set of symptoms, rather than a disorder in and of itself. Inattention and distractibility can be symptoms of many things, from anxiety to ADHD to learning disabilities to a hearing impairment. It is important for the evaluating clinician to consider all possible explanations for inattention, rather than simply assuming that inattention in and of itself is evidence of ADHD.

DYSTHYMIC DISORDER WITHOUT ADHD

Claudia was 17 when she was referred by her therapist for an evaluation of possible ADHD. Her early developmental history was unremarkable. Her health had been good over the course of her life. She had been taking bupropion (Wellbutrin) for the past year and had been in therapy to treat depression; she had a history of Bulimia Nervosa. She lived with her two siblings and her biological parents in a single-family home where the family had resided for 18 years. Her parents were in good health and were both college-educated. There was a reported family history of diagnosed ADHD, as well as Bipolar I Disorder, depression, and alcohol abuse. Claudia's youngest sibling had died suddenly and unexpectedly when Claudia was 11.

Claudia had experienced no difficulties in preschool or elementary school. Her grades were excellent, and there were no teacher concerns about her behavior, work habits, or effort. Following entry into seventh grade, however, Claudia was hospitalized for an eating disorder, and her grades deteriorated. She entered high school in ninth grade, where she had difficulty getting along with teachers and did not consistently do her work. This continued in 10th grade, when she also left class without permission and lost interest in sports. At the time of the evaluation, Claudia was in the 11th grade in a private day school. She attended a franchised learning center for help with reading, received extra help from her teachers to improve her academics, and was able to take quizzes in a one-on-one setting to avoid distractions. Her grades had been variable.

During the diagnostic interview, Claudia and her mother both reported that Claudia displayed a significant number of attentional problems. She made careless errors in schoolwork, was forgetful, procrastinated, had poor organizational skills, and had difficulty following through on instructions. However, these had been typical of Claudia only since seventh grade. She was also fidgety at times and had trouble staying seated. Since seventh grade Claudia had displayed significant symptoms of oppositional and defiant behavior, such as difficulty managing her temper, argumentativeness, and defiance of adult requests. She also displayed problems associated with CD, such as frequently lying, running away from home, and shoplifting. She denied any significant substance abuse, although she had experimented with both alcohol and marijuana within the past year.

Claudia reported that her mood was often irritable, although this had improved since she entered therapy. For at least the past year, she had been increasingly worried about her appearance, her peer relationships, and her future. She had frequent stomachaches, although no physical illness had been identified. She picked at her skin, bit her nails, and twirled her hair. Her sleep was restless, and she often lay in bed at night obsessing about her boyfriend. She also reported that she had a very low opinion of herself and often felt hopeless about her future. Although she denied any suicidal thoughts, she said she had considered cutting her arms when she was very upset, having observed this behavior in her peer group. She had played basketball and soccer throughout middle school, but had given up team sports in high school. She had worked at summer jobs since ninth grade, and generally performed successfully in employment situations. She had some friends, although she was somewhat dissatisfied with her peer relationships.

Table 10.9 summarizes the assessment results for Claudia. One of Claudia's teachers completed the BASC. All scales fell in the average range, including Attention, Hyperactivity, and Learning Problems. Claudia's mother also completed the BASC. In contrast to Claudia's school functioning, in the home setting several BASC scales fell into a clinically significant range, including Attention Problems, Anxiety, Depression, Conduct Problems, Somatization, and Social Skills.

Claudia was a willing participant in the interview and testing. She was well groomed and appropriately dressed. She displayed no problems in her ability to understand or to follow directions. Her eye contact, emotional affect, and thought processing were within typical limits.

Results of the Conners CPT, a computerized measure of sustained attention and impulse control, provided evidence for problems with sustained attention but not impulsivity. Results of the Das–Naglieri CAS indicated that Claudia's ability to focus her attention was in the average range (scaled score on Attention of 109). Planning and organizational skills as assessed by the CAS were also in the average range (scaled score of 100 on Planning).

Claudia was administered the WAIS-III. Her Full Scale IQ (98) was in the average range, as were her Verbal IQ (96) and Verbal Comprehension Index (93). The Working Memory Index also fell in the average range (94), and Claudia obtained her highest score on the Arithmetic subtest, which is a measure of the ability to perform mental calculations. Claudia's Performance IQ was in the average range as well (99), as were her Perceptual Organization Index (95) and Processing Speed Index (96).

Evidence for the specific criteria for ADHD—obtained from the interview with Claudia and her mother, teacher rating scale results, and testing results—were insufficient to provide a convincing case that Claudia's attentional and academic difficulties could not be more readily explained by her adolescent-onset behavioral and emotional problems. Although her symptoms of depression had improved with therapy and medication, Claudia met the diagnostic criteria for Dysthymic Disorder. Claudia and her parents were advised to discuss an alternative medication with her psychiatrist, such as Strattera (which is an antidepressant that improves attentional abilities), or else to suggest increasing her dose of Wellbutrin. Claudia was also advised to continue in psychotherapy to address symptoms of anxiety, which might help to improve her ability to concentrate on academics.

Claudia's case demonstrates the importance of carefully identifying the specific types of difficulties lumped together under descriptions of "poor attention." Mood or anxiety disorders can interfere with a student's academic productivity, concentration, and motivation. A prolonged, moderate depressive condition such as Dysthymic Disorder often leads to reduced productivity, increased apathy, and a subjective loss of mental efficiency. What was particularly notable about Claudia's case was the referral from her therapist, who was clearly aware of Claudia's mood difficulties. When queried after the ADHD diagnosis was ruled out, the therapist explained that it was her understanding that many girls with ADHD were overlooked as youngsters, because of their tendency to be quiet and less disruptive in the classroom than hyperactive boys. The therapist had therefore questioned, particularly with Claudia's family history of diagnosed ADHD, whether this had happed to Claudia.

We certainly agree that there are younger students, both boys and girls, whose ADHD may be overlooked—particularly if they have mild symptoms, cognitive strengths, and no comorbid ODD. In Claudia's case, however, not only did she display increasing academic difficulties in middle school, but she also had a

TABLE 10.9. Results for a Case of Dysthymic Disorder without ADHD in a 17-Year-Old Female

Mother		English teacher	

Interview report of ADHD symptoms

Inattention	6
Hyperactivity–impulsivity	1

BASC		BASC	
Subscale	Percentile	Subscale	Percentile
Hyperactivity	75	Hyperactivity	81
Aggression	70	Aggression	10
Conduct Problems	87	Conduct Problems	52
Anxiety	90	Anxiety	66
Depression	99*	Depression	12
Somatization	93	Somatization	18
Atypicality	60	Attention Problems	82
Withdrawal	63	Learning Problems	68
Attention Problems	90	Atypicality	69
Social Skills	5*	Withdrawal	8
		Social Skills	79
		Leadership	50
		Study Skills	29

Test	Testing data		
	Raw score	Standard/scaled score	Percentile
WISC-III			
Full Scale IQ		98	45
Verbal IQ		96	39
Vocabulary		10	59
Similarities		8	25
Arithmetic		14	91
Digit Span		6	9
Information		8	25
Comprehension		11	63
Letter–Number Sequencing		7	16
Performance IQ		99	47
Picture Completion		8	25
Digit Symbol-Coding		9	37
Block Design		11	63
Matrix Reasoning		9	37
Picture Arrangement		13	84
Symbol Search		11	63
Verbal Comprehension Index		93	32
Perceptual Organization Index		95	37
Working Memory Index		94	34
Processing Speed Index		96	39
CAS			
Planning		100	50
Matching Numbers		11	63
Planned Codes		9	37
Attention		109	73
Expressive Attention		14	91
Number Detection		9	37
Conners CPT			
Omissions	29 (80.6%)	68	97*
Commissions	6 (1.9%)	50	54
Hit rate	318.60	38	12
Hit rate *SE*	10.03	61	88
Variability of *SE*	24.50	64	93

Note. An asterisk indicates a clinically significant elevation (≥ 95th percentile or ≤ 5th percentile). CAS, Cognitive Assessment System (Das–Naglieri); other abbreviations as in earlier tables.

very clear simultaneous onset of behavioral and emotional difficulties. In the case of a student whose early history was much less clear, though, we might recommend that the child return for a reevaluation once the mood disorder was resolved, to confirm the rule-out of the ADHD diagnosis.

AUTISTIC DISORDER WITHOUT ADHD

Jesse was difficult from birth. He was colicky, impossible to comfort, and resistant to physical contact. His mother was concerned about his lack of babbling from the time he was an infant; she had many nieces and nephews, and recognized that he was babbling much later than they had. He had a number of ear infections, and finally pressure equalizing (PE) tubes were placed when he was about 1 year old. This resulted in some babbling, but about 6 months later, his mother noticed that he rarely made a sound. Jesse was also difficult to feed, because he resisted nursing and vomited frequently. He also responded quite negatively to any changes in routine; when the family visited an unfamiliar place, Jesse cried until they left, even if it was hours later. He appeared quite attached to a Phillips screwdriver, and insisted on carrying it everywhere the family went, screaming and sometimes even banging his head on the floor if his mother tried to remove it from his grip.

From very early on, Jesse's mother shared her concerns with the pediatrician. He initially reassured her that the language delay was due to Jesse's frequent ear infections, and that he would catch up after the tubes were placed. Initially, it appeared that he was right, as Jesse began babbling almost immediately. However, when he had stopped babbling completely by age 18 months, Jesse's mother felt a sense of dread. She took him back to the pediatrician, who encouraged her to wait and see, stating that children develop at different rates. Finally, 6 months later, she convinced him to make a referral to a speech/language pathologist, who began treating Jesse's language delay. He made progress, and said his first word around 28 months. He began putting phrases together by age 4, and by age 5, he tested in the average range on measures of speech and language and had been discharged from speech/language therapy as a success. Although they were encouraged by the improvement in his language,

Jesse's parents remained concerned about his temperament. He still reacted violently to changes in routine, insisted on carrying around odd objects (although his preferred objects changed over time), and seemed "difficult to connect with." He also preferred being alone to playing with his cousins, and his play was repetitive. Sometimes when he thought he was alone, his parents caught him tensing and flicking his fingers in an odd way. Even as his speech developed, he seemed to use it in a strange way, repeating words and phrases almost as if he simply liked the sound of them. He continued to have severe temper tantrums, yelling and even hitting, well beyond the age at which their older two children had persisted in their tantrums.

When Jesse began seeing the speech/language therapist, she referred the family to their local school district's Birth-to-Three program. He began to receive services through that program, which included three mornings a week in a classroom with two other children with language delays. His teacher commented on his lack of interest in his peers; while the other two children played together during free-play time, Jesse was content to sit in the corner by himself and repeatedly put together puzzles. When his peers approached him, he didn't seem bothered, but also didn't engage with them. If they tried to pick up a puzzle piece he had laid out, however, he was easily provoked and would push or hit. His teacher often commented on the difficulty she had getting him to attend during circle time; he seemed off in his own world and often didn't even respond to her calling his name in an attempt to gain his attention. When Jesse graduated from the Birth-to-Three program, he continued in an early childhood special education program, where similar concerns were noted.

When Jesse was 5, he started attending kindergarten in a regular classroom in the public schools, without any special educational support. His expressive and receptive language skills were age-appropriate now, and although he was seen as shy and somewhat "spacey," his cognitive development appeared unexceptional. Jesse's district had full-day rather than half-day kindergarten. While Jesse was able to perform the preacademic tasks adequately, and even excelled at puzzles and learning his letters and numbers, he stood out from his preschool classmates as inflexible in his habits. For example, he insisted on sitting on the same carpet square each circle time, although the rest of the children changed places regularly. He also seemed unable to change course if he was interrupted during a task; for instance, if the class was copying letters, and the teacher told the students it was time to put their work away for milk break, he insisted on continuing until he had finished the task. His teacher quickly learned that if she insisted he move on, he would have a tantrum and become inconsolable, to the point that she had to call his mother to come get him. Oddly, though he seemed overfocused on some tasks, it was extremely difficult to get his attention in other tasks, particularly in group activities. He also seemed to have difficulty with organization; when presented with a new task, he couldn't seem to figure out how to approach it, and would often become overwhelmed. Once he was taught a strategy, however, he tended to apply it rigidly, and then became upset if a peer or adult tried to get him to do the activity in another way.

Jesse began to respond to peer initiations during his kindergarten year. The peers he interacted with tended to be children he was familiar with from his neighborhood. He still did not initiate interaction with them, but would engage in chase, tag, and other physical games when they approached him. Jesse tended to keep to himself when his peers were engaged in make-believe play. As he continued into first grade, he appeared to gain more interest in his peers and began approaching those with whom he was most familiar. However, he still seemed "different" to both adults and peers. Although his vocabulary was by now quite good, he tended to interact with people by asking them repetitive questions—often about odd topics, such as what time they went to bed at night and what time all of their family members went to bed. When peers tried to engage him in conversation about an area of interest to them, such as Harry Potter, he would abruptly change the subject to Martha Stewart, whose television show he preferred. However, if he were talking about video games (a particular interest of his), he would list the ratings of various video games for as long as a conversational partner would listen to him, ignoring obvious signs of boredom. He also liked to recite the farm reports, and went on in great detail. Jesse's vocabulary was quite large, but not always supported by knowledge; for instance, he knew the technical names for all of the dinosaurs, but he didn't seem to understand that they no longer existed on earth.

In second grade, it became apparent that Jesse could work well alone or in small groups, but it was almost impossible to keep his attention in the classroom setting. However, when the teacher prompted him to move to a small group for reading or math instruction, he often became quite upset during the transition. She found it helpful to tape a schedule to his desk, but if an assembly or other activity caused the class to deviate from that routine, Jesse became tense and overwhelmed. Sometimes he even yelled or screamed. Jesse typically remained alone on the playground, but occasionally he abruptly joined a group of children, interrupting in a way the peers found intrusive. He continued to talk about video games incessantly; his teacher often had to remind him to be quiet during seatwork. He also developed a strong aversion to the popular cartoon character Arthur, and when other children would talk about this character, he impulsively yelled for them to stop. Jesse had a great deal of difficulty with creative writing and storytelling, and would often insist that someone else's story was stupid because it wasn't true. He couldn't seem to produce any imaginative work of his own. He rarely completed language arts worksheets and seemed to take significantly longer than the other children to do his reading work. On the other hand, he performed quite well on tasks that required rote memory, and showed an amazing fount of very specific knowledge about dinosaurs in the different eras when the class did a dinosaur unit in science.

Jesse's second-grade teacher was very concerned about his inattentiveness, excessive talking, disorganization, and social skills deficits from the beginning of the year. When she attended a teacher education workshop on ADHD during the fall break, she wondered whether that might be Jesse's problem, and whether stimulant medication would be helpful for him. She shared her concerns with Jesse's parents, who were especially concerned about the social skills deficits. When the teacher reported how common such deficits were in children with ADHD, they agreed to have Jesse evaluated. After contacting Jesse's pediatrician, the family was referred to our clinic for evaluation. Their chief presenting concerns included Jesse's severe problems with behavior and self-regulation, school work completion problems, and social skills.

Jesse's assessment results are summarized in Table 10.10. Teacher reports indicated concerns about his fidgeting with particular items in his desk, talking during work and instruction time, difficulty listening in group settings, minimal concentration, pouting and refusing when asked to do a nonpreferred activity, difficulty with conversation with peers, and poor work completion. Jesse was endorsed by his teacher as meeting all inattention criteria for ADHD, and four of nine hyperactivity–impulsivity criteria. She also endorsed some oppositional and defiant behaviors, and some reactivity (but otherwise no internalizing behavior problems). She endorsed many items compatible with atypical behavior problems. On the BASC, Jesse's father rated him as being in the top 3% of boys his age in displaying atypical behaviors, attention problems, and rule-violating behaviors. On the Conners Parent Rating Scale—Revised: Short Form (CPRS-R:S), he rated him in the clinically significant range for Oppositional, Cognitive Problems/Inattention, and the ADHD Index. Jesse's mother rated him quite similarly. Intellectual testing with the WISC-IV yielded a Verbal Comprehension Index of 91, a Perceptual Organization Index of 88, a Working Memory Index of 80, and a Processing Speed Index of 69. The Conners CPT revealed an elevated number of commission errors, but was otherwise unexceptional. Due to concerns raised by the rating scale results and behavioral observations, the team decided also to administer the Autism Diagnostic Observation Schedule (ADOS, Module 3). This is a standardized interview/behavioral observation designed to press for behaviors associated with autism spectrum disorders (ASDs) (Lord et al., 2000). Results of the ADOS provided strong evidence of atypical communication style and deficits in reciprocal social interaction. Jesse displayed poor use of eye contact in regulating social interaction, difficulty describing his role in social relationships, limited social overtures and response, difficulty describing emotions, lack of initiation of social "chat," limited insight and empathy, and poor creativity—all often seen in individuals with ASDs.

During the interview, Jesse was generally unaware of the reasons for his being evaluated. He denied any significant problems, and named a number of friends (almost all of whom his parents later reported were people in his class who occasionally were assigned to eat lunch at his table). He used sentences in a largely correct fashion, but tended to use stereotyped words and phrases unusual for his age, such as "Shall we move on now?" when he wanted to change topics. Jesse could not identify many emotions in a story; for instance, when asked how a man might feel, he said "mad" when the character was clearly surprised or scared. He talked in great detail about his video games, and was quite preoccupied with the ratings of each video game; when asked to tell about how the games were played, he simply listed the ratings. When asked to make up a story with action figures, he enacted a scene from one of his favorite video games. He did not describe any significant school problems, nor did he report any depression or anxiety. When asked about the problems his parents had reported, he simply stated that it was all better now, or that his teacher had been wrong about some things.

In general, it was our opinion that although some of Jesse's inattentive and disorganized behavior might be explained by ADHD, Predominantly Inattentive Type, that diagnosis would not account for his severe social deficits and atypical behaviors. In fact, the preponderance of evidence indicated that Jesse met DSM-IV-TR criteria for a diagnosis of Autistic Disorder (his presentation might commonly be thought of as high-functioning autism, or HFA). Evidence of impairment was found in both parent- and teacher-reported below-average peer socialization skills, as well as the disruption in the home environment caused by the need to adjust family routines for Jesse's idiosyncracies. While Jesse's parents and teacher reported significant attention and behavior problems, those were found to occur secondary to his symptoms of autism. Therefore, no additional DSM-IV-TR diagnoses were given. We made the following recommendations to the parents:

1. We recommended selected readings to educate the parents about HFA and its associated features. During our feedback session, we explained how the way Jesse interpreted situations might lead him to become overwhelmed and have difficulty generating appropriate coping responses, so that his parents would understand that his outbursts came from skill deficits and not defiant behavior. We also recommended that Jesse's parents consider participating in a local support group for parents of children with ASDs.

TABLE 10.10. Results for a Case of Autistic Disorder without ADHD in a 7-Year-Old-Male

Mother		Father		Teacher	
Interview report of ADHD symptoms		Interview report of ADHD symptoms		ADHD Rating Scale–IV (Symptoms rated >2)	
Inattention	9	Inattention	9	Inattention	9
Hyperactivity–impulsivity	4	Hyperactivity–impulsivity	4	Hyperactivity–impulsivity	4
BASC		BASC		BASC	
Subscale	Percentile	Subscale	Percentile	Subscale	Percentile
Hyperactivity	96*	Hyperactivity	89	Hyperactivity	96*
Aggression	97*	Aggression	95*	Aggression	99*
Conduct Problems	99*	Conduct Problems	99*	Conduct Problems	93
Anxiety	27	Anxiety	67	Anxiety	93
Depression	43	Depression	50	Depression	92
Somatization	39	Somatization	31	Somatization	80
Atypicality	>99*	Atypicality	99*	Atypicality	>99*
Withdrawal	7	Withdrawal	84	Withdrawal	86
Attention Problems	>99*	Attention Problems	99*	Attention Problems	>99*
Social Skills	2*	Social Skills	<1*	Adaptability	1*
Leadership	27	Leadership	5*	Social Skills	<1*
				Leadership	5*
				Study Skills	18
CPRS-R:S		CPRS-R:S		CTRS-R:S	
Oppositional	95*	Oppositional	97*	Oppositional	93
Inattention	95*	Inattention	91	Inattention	93
Hyperactivity	53	Hyperactivity	30	Hyperactivity	30
ADHD Index	91	ADHD Index	97*	ADHD Index	90
PSI-SF				SSRS	
Total stress	76			Total score	15 (below average)

	Testing data		
Test	Raw score	Standard/scaled score	Percentile
WISC-IV			
Full Scale IQ	80	85	16
Verbal Comprehension	25	91	27
Perceptual Reasoning	24	88	21
Working Memory	13	80	9
Processing Speed	9	69	2*
ADOS, Module 3			
Communication	3 (autism cutoff)		
Reciprocal Social Interaction	7 (autism range)		
Total score	10 (autism cutoff)		
Imagination/Creativity	2		
Stereotyped Behaviors/Restricted Interests	2		

Note. An asterisk indicates a clinically significant elevation (≥ 95th percentile or ≤ 5th percentile). ADOS, Autism Diagnostic Observation Schedule; other abbreviations as in earlier tables.

2. We recommended that the parents ask school personnel to evaluate whether Jesse would meet educational eligibility criteria for special educational services under the category of ASDs. He would benefit from support and help in the regular classroom. In addition, he would benefit from individualized instruction on social skills from the speech/language pathologist or an autism specialist.

3. We recommended a number of educational modifications for Jesse's autism-related difficulties in the school setting, including breaking tasks down into steps for him and providing him with cues prior to transitions.

4. We referred Jesse to a developmental/behavioral pediatrician for consideration of a trial of a selective serotonin reuptake inhibitor, which might address his cognitive rigidity and overfocusing. We felt that a physician who was experienced in pharmacological treatment of children with ASDs would be able to determine the appropriate medication or combination thereof to address Jesse's specific problems.

5. We suggested cognitive-behavioral therapy for Jesse to help him notice and respond to nonverbal cues, incorporate visual strategies into his daily life, reduce compulsive behavior, increase his tolerance for transitions, and teaching him organizational strategies. We thought that these goals might best be met through a combination of individual therapy and parent guidance in implementation of environmental modifications and behavioral strategies.

This case illustrates a number of issues in differentiating HFA from ADHD. It is quite common for individuals with Asperger syndrome or HFA to be referred for evaluation of possible ADHD, prior to the identification of their ASD. Because these children have intact cognitive functioning and often exhibit some degree of social interest, adults often don't think of autism as a possible source of their problems. Moreover, their problems overlap with those of individuals with ADHD. For instance, many individuals with ASDs have difficulties with sustained attention, don't appear to be listening when spoken to, have difficulty following through on instructions, have difficulty organizing tasks and activities, dislike tasks that require sustained mental effort, appear forgetful in daily activities, are fidgety, out of their seats, talk excessively, have difficulty waiting their turn, interrupt frequently, and so on. However, often the nature of the difficulties is different. For instance, individuals with HFA are often described as having somewhat different attentional difficulties. They have problems with planning and flexibility of their attention, rather than the sustained attention and distractibility problems seen in ADHD. "Fidgeting" may actually be related to stereotyped movements in autism, whereas in ADHD it is often motor overflow. Excessive talking is usually related to a specific area of interest in autism, rather than social chatting. People with autism exhibit behaviors that look impulsive (e.g., interrupting), but these are more likely to be caused by their poor understanding of social cues and difficulty with perspective taking than by the behavioral inhibition problems seen in ADHD. Although children with both ASDs and ADHD have problems with social skills, the nature of the problems is somewhat different. A child with ADHD is likely to be seen as intrusive, noisy, and overwhelming due to excessive talking and touching objects and people, while a child with an ASD is likely to be seen as odd and possibly intrusive (if he or she is socially interested), due to perseverative talking about unusual subjects and lack of understanding of social norms. Although these problems can look similar, the child with an ASD has more pervasive deficits in social understanding that will not be solved by motivation alone.

Both children with ASDs and those with ADHD are seen to perform poorly on neuropsychological tests measuring executive functioning. In general, findings indicate that the children with ASDs exhibit more severe impairment, but some findings also indicate that there may be a difference in profile. The children with ASDs perform more poorly on tasks measuring planning ability (although the children with ADHD also have difficulty on these tasks). The children with ADHD exhibit more impairment on tasks measuring inhibition than do those with ASDs; children with ASDs do not typically show impairment on these tasks relative to their overall ability. The children with ASDs do show more impairment in tasks measuring cognitive flexibility, on which the children with ADHD are not significantly impaired. These findings do not indicate that neuropsychological testing is required to make either diagnosis, but it can be helpful in determining a child's strengths and weaknesses, and especially in developing an educational plan.

REFERENCES

American Psychiatric Association (APA). (2000). *Diagnostic and statistical manual of mental disorders* (4th ed., text rev.). Washington, DC: Author.

Biederman, J. (1995). Developmental subtypes of juvenile bipolar disorder. *Sexual and Marital Therapy, 3*(4), 227–230.

Borduin, C. M., Mann, B. J., Cone, L. T., Henggeler, S. W., Fucci, B. R., Blaske, D. M., et al. (1995). Multisystemic treatment of serious juvenile offenders: Long-term prevention of criminality and violence. *Journal of Consulting and Clinical Psychology, 63*, 569–578.

Carlson, G. A. (2002). Bipolar disorder in children and adolescents: A critical review. In D. Shaffer & B. Waslick (Eds.), *The many faces of depression in children and adolescents* (pp. 105–128). Washington, DC: American Psychiatric Press.

Faraone, S. V., Biederman, J., Wozniak, J., Mundy, E., Mennin, D., & O'Connell, D. (1997). Is comorbidity with ADHD a marker for juvenile-onset mania? *Journal of the American Academy of Child and Adolescent Psychiatry, 36*(8), 1046–1055.

Greene, R. (1998). *The explosive child: A new approach to understanding and parenting easily frustrated, "chronically inflexible" children.* New York: HarperCollins.

Hinshaw, S. P. (1987). On the distinction between attentional deficits/hyperactivity and conduct problems/aggression in child psychopathology. *Psychological Bulletin, 101*, 443–463.

Hinshaw, S. P., & Lee, S. S. (2003). Conduct and oppositional defiant disorders. In E. J. Mash & R. A. Barkley (Eds.), *Child psychopathology* (2nd ed., pp. 144–198). New York: Guilford Press.

Kutcher, S., Aman, M., Brooks, S. J., Buitelaar, J., van Daalen, E., Fegert, J., et al. (2004). International consensus statement on attention-deficit/hyperactivity disorder (ADHD) and disruptive behavior disorders (DBDs): Clinical implications and treatment practice suggestions. *European Neuropsychopharmacology, 14*, 11–28.

Lord, C., Risi, S., Lambrecht, L., Cook, E. H., Jr., Bennett, L., Leventhal, P. C., et al. (2000). The Autism Diagnostic Observation Schedule—Generic: A standard measure of social and communication deficits associated with the spectrum of autism. *Journal of Autism and Developmental Disorders, 30*, 205–223.

Milich, R., Ballentine, A. C., & Lynam, D. R. (2001). ADHD/combined type and ADHD/predominantly inattentive type are distinct and unrelated disorders. *Clinical Psychology: Science and Practice, 8*, 463–488.

Mulder, R. T., Frampton, C., Joyce, P. R., & Porter, R. (2003). Randomized controlled trials in psychiatry. Part II: Their relationship to clinical practice. *Australian and New Zealand Journal of Psychiatry, 37*, 265–269.

Timimi, S., Taylor, E., Cannon, M., McKenzie, K., & Sims, A. (2004). ADHD is best understood as a cultural construct. *British Journal of Psychiatry, 184*, 8–9.

Wilens, T. E., Beiderman, J., Millstein, R. B., Wozniak, J., Hahesy, A. L., & Spencer, T. J. (1999). Risk for substance use disorders in youths with child- and adolescent-onset bipolar disorders. *Journal of the American Academy of Child and Adolescent Psychiatry, 38*, 680–685.

Wozniak, J., Biederman, J., Kiely, K., Ablon, J., Faraone, S., Mundy, E., et al. (1995). Mania-like symptoms suggestive of childhood-onset bipolar disorder in clinically referred children. *Journal of the American Academy of Child and Adolescent Psychiatry, 34*(7), 867–876.

CHAPTER 11

Assessment of Adults with ADHD

KEVIN R. MURPHY
MICHAEL GORDON

The idea that the core symptoms of Attention-Deficit/Hyperactivity Disorder (ADHD) might persist into adulthood is relatively new on the clinical scene. In fact, the first edition of this handbook focused largely on childhood variants and contained little information on adult manifestations. This focus reflected the state of the art at that time. Until the late 1980s, ADHD was generally considered a childhood disorder that was typically outgrown by adolescence and always by adulthood (Ross & Ross, 1976). Clinicians routinely told parents that if they survived their hyperactive child's elementary school years, the future would be rosy.

We now have clear evidence that ADHD symptoms do not usually diminish with the onset of puberty. Numerous prospective and retrospective studies of children diagnosed with ADHD followed into adulthood have demonstrated that from 50% to 80% continue to experience significant ADHD symptoms and associated impairment into their adult lives (see Chapter 6, this volume; see also Barkley, Fischer, Edelbrock, & Smallish, 1990; Barkley, Fischer, Smallish, & Fletcher, 2002; Weiss, Minde, Werry, Douglas, & Nemeth, 1971; Mendelson, Johnson, & Stewart, 1971; Menkes, Rowe, & Menkes, 1967; Borland &

Hechtman, 1976; Feldman, Denhoff, & Denhoff, 1979; Loney, Whaley-Klahn, Kosier, & Conboy, 1981; Weiss, Hechtman, Perlman, Hopkins, & Wener, 1979; Hechtman, Weiss, & Perlman, 1978, 1980; Hechtman, Weiss, Perlman, & Tuck, 1985; Weiss, Hechtman, Milroy, & Perlman, 1985; Satterfield, Hoppe, & Schell, 1982; Gittelman, Mannuzza, Shenker, & Bonagura, 1985; Mannuzza, Gittelman-Klein, Bessler, Malloy, & LaPadula, 1993; Wender, 1995; Weiss & Hechtman, 1993). Although there is some question about the actual percentage of children with ADHD who will still suffer from the disorder when they become adults, little doubt remains that it is a substantial number. For instance, a recent study by Barkley et al. (2002) found that up to 66% of cases diagnosed in childhood continued to be rated as placing in the top 2% of control adults in the severity of their symptoms, and 46% still met DSM criteria for the full disorder. Estimates place the prevalence of adult ADHD at 4–5% (Kessler et al., 2005; Murphy & Barkley, 1996).

Why did it take so long for researchers and clinicians to realize that ADHD is a disorder that, more often than not, endures across the lifespan? Much of the blame can be assigned to the natural life history of the disorder itself.

ADHD's most visible and disruptive feature, physical overactivity, often diminishes with age. Research has established that most children with ADHD are somewhat less motoric by the time they reach adolescence (Hart, Lahey, Loeber, Applegate, & Frick, 1995). Although they may still suffer from profound problems associated with the more cognitive manifestations of impulsivity, these symptoms are often more subtle and more difficult to detect. Poor planning, self-regulation, time management, and disorganization are not quite as obvious a set of symptoms as ill-conceived flights from the tops of trees or headlong bursts into traffic.

The other reason for the delayed emergence of recognition of adult ADHD relates to the time and expense involved in the conduct of longitudinal research. The most empirically sophisticated studies are just now evaluating the life circumstances and clinical functioning of children once diagnosed as hyperactive who are now entering young adulthood. At least another decade will pass until more data are available regarding the nature of ADHD in individuals who are squarely into adulthood. Complicating matters is that criteria for the disorder change (sometimes often) over the years while children are slowly aging. Therefore, conclusions are often based on subject selection criteria that have long since been supplanted.

Although the concept of ADHD in adulthood was late in arriving, it has certainly gained visibility with lightning speed. What was unheard of just 15–20 years ago has now become a popular topic within the conversations of our society. Stories or editorials about the disorder appear in the mass media regularly. Bookstore shelves are filled with volumes for both professionals and the general public. Even the cartoon pages are apt to carry references to ADHD in adults, so thoroughly has the label found its way into everyday parlance.

In our view, the explosion of interest in adult ADHD has been the most mixed of blessings. On the positive side, the widespread exposure has resulted in scores of adults benefiting from accurate diagnosis and treatment—for many, after years of failure and frustration. The quality of life for these adults has surely improved, as they have found it easier to lead more productive and satisfying lives. At the least, they can take comfort from knowing that their struggles have a legitimate explanation, and that this explanation rests more on neuro-genetics than on attributions to poor character. The popularity of this disorder has therefore heightened awareness of its existence, forced clinicians to take adult variants of symptoms seriously, and promoted the beginnings of scientific exploration.

Although the benefits of the widespread publicity about the disorder are tangible, so too are the disadvantages. Simply put, the public interest in ADHD and the attendant pressures for services have completely outstripped the pace and volume of scientific inquiry. We cannot emphasize enough how extraordinarily few sound empirical data are available to guide clinical management. From a scientific standpoint, the field of ADHD in adults is still in its infancy. For the most part, what many purvey as common knowledge is based on clinical impression, anecdote, and extrapolations from the more robust child literature. Among the unfortunate by-products of limited scientific information are that myths become entrenched, speculations and impressions pass for "truths," and diagnostic conclusions emerge based on hunches and pet theories rather than on well-established evidence.

The fervor that has accompanied the adult ADHD movement seems to have given rise to more folklore than fact. For example, many popular books and speakers claim as truth that adults with ADHD are often more creative, intelligent, or entrepreneurial than others. In reality, not a particle of data supports these contentions. The gulf between speculation and what is actually known about ADHD in adults is wide. Therefore, we advise clinicians to hold a sincere and healthy respect for the paucity of sound scientific information.

Although the popularity and visibility of adult ADHD has continued to increase since the preceding edition of this book, allusions to clinical experience and anecdote still far outpace data-based conclusions. All the intense focus on ADHD in adults, and even the meager body of scientific literature, would of course be far more manageable if this were a less elusive disorder to identify. If clinicians could point to a unique set of symptoms, a configuration of test scores, or a specific etiological event, and identify the disorder with some certainty, we would not be nearly as concerned about the current frenzy. But the length of this book alone serves as testament to the challenges inherent in identifying and treating ADHD across the lifespan.

Why is ADHD at any age so difficult to diagnose? The answer goes directly to the very nature of the disorder itself (see, e.g., Gordon, 1995; Gordon & McClure, 1995; Gordon & Irwin, 1996). First, the core symptoms of the disorder are also core symptoms of human nature. All of us are prone toward inattention and impulsivity at one time or another, especially if we are under some physical or mental distress. The mere fact that an individual may be inattentive or impulsive is of little diagnostic value, because these are such ubiquitous human proclivities. Whereas some symptoms of mental illness (e.g., hallucinations) are pathognomonic, the same cannot be said for the characteristics of ADHD. The symptoms alone do not necessarily demarcate abnormal functioning. To be fair, of course, ADHD is not unique in this regard; almost all mental illnesses, from depression to mania, represent normal human tendencies gone awry.

Parenthetically, the nonspecific nature of some ADHD symptoms accounts for much of ADHD's current popularity as a presenting complaint. Metaphorically, these symptoms fashion a suit of clothes that most of us can fit ourselves (or our children) into, especially if we are experiencing a setback or if we have the sense that we are somehow underperforming. The ease with which individuals can don the ADHD label is further promoted by a culture that often seeks psychiatric explanations for failures that might better be accounted for in other terms.

The second barrier to easy identification is that some ADHD symptoms are typical not only of normal behavior, but also of the full range of psychiatric abnormalities. Nearly every listing of criteria in the *Diagnostic and Statistical Manual of Mental Disorders*, fourth edition, text revision (DSM-IV-TR; American Psychiatric Association, 2000) contains at least one symptom associated with poor concentration and disorganization. In fact, inattention is so universal a symptom of mental illness that, in isolation, it provides little diagnostic direction. If anything, it is a global marker for distress, regardless of origin.

The third characteristic of ADHD that ensures a degree of diagnostic complexity is its dimensionality. As already mentioned in this textbook (see Chapter 2) and elsewhere (Gordon & Murphy, 1998), ADHD is not an all-or-nothing condition like pregnancy. Instead, most cases represent the extreme end of a continuum or normal curve, while others (most likely acquired cases) comprise a smaller and more severe bell curve within this lower tail. Because ADHD is defined as a point along a continuum, its identification inherently involves some degree of subjectivity and even arbitrariness in establishing cutoff points. How inattentive or impulsive one has to be to qualify for a diagnosis is therefore a matter of some judgment, especially when the intensity of problems falls within those gray zones between normal and abnormal. Whenever opinion forms the basis for important aspects of diagnostic decision making, the door is left open for a measure of uncertainty and inconsistency. Beyond these three elemental features of ADHD at any age, the diagnosis is especially difficult in adulthood for the following reasons:

• The diagnosis of ADHD in adulthood hinges primarily on reports of functioning during childhood. Most patients provide this historical information from memory rather than from actual records. Despite some suggestion that symptoms self-reported either directly or via rating scales can be valid (Wilens, Faraone, & Biederman, 2004; Murphy & Schachar, 2000), much of the evidence points to the opposite conclusion. Retrospective data are notoriously vulnerable to historical inaccuracy, incompleteness, and distortion (Henry, Moffitt, Caspi, Langley, & Silva, 1994; Hardt & Rutter, 2004). Our own study (Murphy, Gordon, & Barkley, 2002) demonstrated how common it was for normal adults in the community to endorse having a high frequency of ADHD symptoms at least some of the time during both childhood and as adults. For example, almost 80% of a sample of 719 normal adults who came to two Department of Motor Vehicles locations to renew their licenses endorsed six or more ADHD symptoms as occurring "at least sometimes" during their childhood. Seventy-five percent of this sample endorsed experiencing six or more ADHD symptoms "at least sometimes" currently in their adult lives. Even when more stringent criteria for symptom frequency were applied (endorsing "often" or "very often" as opposed to "sometimes"), a full 25% of this sample endorsed having six or more symptoms occur during childhood, and 12% during current adult functioning. In another study (Mannuzza, Klein, & Klein, 2002), many of the subjects in the control group (used as a comparison group to a cohort of 176 subjects diagnosed with ADHD in childhood and followed into adulthood) recalled having ADHD symptoms in childhood, and 11% were incorrectly classified as having ADHD by interviewers unaware of the subjects' diagnostic status. These data suggest that it is common for adults to perceive they have exhibited ADHD symptoms at least some of the time throughout their lives; they add further support that mere symptom endorsement on ADHD rating scales is not sufficient to diagnose this disorder reliably.

• Although ADHD is often joined by other disorders at all ages, adults are especially prone to suffer from a wide range of comorbid conditions, some of which are probably secondary to the years of ADHD-related frustration and failure. Outcome studies have established that individuals diagnosed with ADHD in childhood are at risk for developing comorbid conditions, including anxiety and mood disorders, substance abuse, Antisocial Personality Disorder, and Intermittent Explosive Disorder as adults (Biederman et al., 1987; Weiss & Hechtman, 1993; see also Chapter 6, this volume). Therefore, adults referred for ADHD commonly display a complex interweaving of psychiatric disorders. Ironically, although some comorbid conditions represent fallout from years of ADHD-type functioning, they can often develop a life of their own and can actually come to predominate the clinical picture.

• Many psychiatric disorders have their typical onset in late adolescence or young adulthood. Thus clinicians evaluating adults have a broader range of disorders to rule out than those working with children do. Furthermore, many of these later-onset disorders have symptoms that can, at least in part, mimic ADHD characteristics. Patients with Borderline Personality Disorder, some other personality disorders, Bipolar I or II Disorder, Cyclothymic Disorder, various forms of depression, Obsessive–Compulsive Disorder, Generalized Anxiety Disorder, some forms of schizophrenia, substance abuse, chronic pain, precursors of Alzheimer disease, or head injury may all endorse many DSM-IV-TR symptoms of ADHD.

• Adults are more prone to suffer from medical conditions that can produce ADHD-like symptoms. Hypo- or hyperthyroidism, malnutrition, diabetes, certain heart problems, perimenopause, and other adult physical disorders can all affect attention and working memory. The heightened possibility that ADHD symptoms in adults can have a medical cause underscores the importance of ruling out medical conditions before arriving at a final diagnostic determination. This may require a comprehensive physical exam in some cases.

• A longer life also means more opportunities to suffer from stressful or traumatic life events. Divorce, grief, financial problems, health concerns, or other major lifestyle changes can affect an individual's ability to concentrate. The performance-impairing effects of stress are therefore important to rule out prior to assigning an ADHD diagnosis.

• It can be more difficult to determine degree of impairment in adults than in children. Because all children are in classrooms, teacher input and ratings are not especially difficult to obtain. Adult jobs vary in demands for attention, planning, listening, structure, or attention to detail. Obtaining supervisor input or ratings is much more difficult and potentially risky.

• A growing problem in the diagnosis of ADHD in adults is informant bias. With the bounty of publicity, patients are savvy about formal characterizations of the disorder. Consciously or otherwise, this knowledge can affect the accuracy of information that patients present to clinicians.

One final, clinically relevant caveat: Findings from outcome studies often differ, depending on whether the subjects were first identified as having ADHD during childhood or adulthood (see Barkley & Gordon, 2002). The general conclusion is that adults diagnosed during childhood as having ADHD are a more impaired group than those individuals who were identified or self-referred later in life. For example, the prevalence of learning disabilities in adults diagnosed with ADHD is well below that found in children with ADHD (Barkley, Murphy, & Kwasnik, 1996; Biederman et al., 1993; Matochik, Rumsey, Zametkin, Hamburger, & Cohen, 1996), while the presence of anxiety disorders is markedly higher in self-referred adults than in children followed to adulthood (Barkley & Gordon, 2002).

Why might this be? First, children referred early in life showed enough maladjustment such that adults (usually parents and teachers) referred them for services. In contrast, most adults that seek evaluation for the first time as adults presumably did not evidence sufficient impairment to warrant a childhood referral.

For whatever reason, most of them were able to avoid being identified as maladjusted because they were (1) truly unimpaired; (2) normal enough to develop compensations for any ADHD-type weaknesses; or (3) living in circumstances that were extraordinarily unusual for the extent to which they were either insensitive to pathology or able to provide external support sufficient to mask problems. Second, the diagnostic criteria at the time may have differed from the current conceptualization of the disorder. The development of the more recent DSM-IV(-TR) Predominantly Inattentive Type of ADHD, in combination with the increased awareness and media attention on adult ADHD, has resulted in more adults seeking assessment today than a generation ago—and perhaps for different reasons (i.e., inattention vs. problems with hyperactivity/impulsivity/behavioral self-control). Furthermore, there is no guarantee that adults receiving their first diagnosis as adults would have met the prevailing clinical criteria for ADHD during their childhood. Third, although ADHD causes consistent types of impairments, their impact will be quite different across developmental stages of life. For example, many of the differences between childhood and adult ADHD are associated with the differences between childhood and adult expectations for independence and self-management (Barkley & Gordon, 2002). During childhood, the major adaptive functioning tasks include self-care, peer relationships, academics, family functioning, and participation in extracurricular activities (e.g., sports, clubs, and Scouts). In adulthood, these domains have expanded to include such areas as occupational functioning, marital/couple relations, child rearing, driving, sexual activity, and financial management. The consequences of the ADHD symptoms in adulthood can be far more problematic with the "higher-stakes" tasks of adulthood.

Those who seek evaluation for the first time as adults may not have experienced a degree of disruption that would result in pursuing professional treatment during their earlier lives, and this phenomenon may suggest a milder magnitude of impairment. Hence any differences that are found between longitudinal and cross-sectional studies may be explained at least in part by the kinds of subjects represented in the studies (i.e., adult subjects identified with ADHD as children vs. those first identified as adults). Future research will be needed to shed additional light on whether there may be differences in comorbidity, educational and occupational attainment, driving performance, marital/couple satisfaction, treatment response, or other variables between these two groups.

Why are we presenting this onslaught of cautions and admonitions about ADHD in adults? Are we suggesting that the assessment process is hopelessly difficult, or that the diagnosis itself should even be abandoned? Not at all. All the potential pitfalls notwithstanding, ADHD is not a phantom disorder that defies proper diagnosis. Clear evidence exists that it is a legitimate diagnostic entity that trained clinicians can identify efficiently and accurately. But it absolutely requires a comprehensive and thoughtful assessment that fairly considers critical aspects of history and current functioning, the degree of impairment, and the possible validity of alternative explanations.

We have presented this litany of warnings about the diagnostic process simply to encourage a careful and conservative approach to diagnosis. Our sense is that some clinicians are overly enthusiastic about encouraging individuals to seek a label of ADHD. This observation stems in part from watching changing trends in our own clinics. When we began our adult ADHD clinics some 15 years ago, more than 85% of adults referred for evaluations (usually from mental health practitioners or primary care physicians) ultimately received the diagnosis of ADHD. Due in part to the public's increased recognition of ADHD symptoms, that percentage has plummeted to 50% or lower, even though at least as many patients are referred by other professionals. Nowadays, it is far more likely that a patient will leave our respective clinics either with no diagnosis at all or with a diagnosis other than ADHD.

Our concern about the potential for misdiagnosis or overdiagnosis is more than an exercise in academic hand wringing. Beyond lost opportunities for appropriate treatment (or for staying free of treatment), inaccurate identification diminishes the credibility of the disorder itself. If individuals receive a diagnosis even though they do not meet criteria for it, skepticism about ADHD will quickly mount. Those who truly suffer from the disorder will not benefit from the serious consideration they deserve. Also, given the nationwide shortages of mental health services, allocating resources to those who are actually unimpaired limits access for those who are more truly in need. Therefore, the ADHD label should be assigned only to those individuals with a lifelong history of serious inattention and poor self-control. It should not be diluted to cover what amount to normal variations of human personality.

The emphasis on careful adherence to diagnostic standards is also heightened by the impact of antidiscrimination laws, such as the Americans with Disabilities Act of 1990 (ADA; Public Law 101-336). This body of legislation is intended to level the playing field for those individuals with substantial disabilities (see Gordon & Keiser, 1998; Murphy & Gordon, 1996; Gordon, Barkley, & Murphy, 1997). According to federal regulations and case law, ADHD is considered a legitimate disability. Employers, educational institutions, and testing organizations are therefore required to provide reasonable accommodations to those who suffer from this disorder. If clinicians are overly liberal in assigning the diagnosis, people who actually function within a normal or average range will receive benefits and advantages that are not warranted.

CORE DIAGNOSTIC CONSIDERATIONS

Before plunging into the intricacies of the assessment of ADHD in adults, we want to outline a general strategy for the diagnostic process. Our focus here is on those concepts that underlie formal criteria for the disorder. We subsequently discuss clinical interviews, rating scales, psychological testing, and other methods for gathering information, but we begin here by highlighting our diagnostic quarry.

The evaluation for ADHD should be designed to answer four fundamental questions:

1. Is there credible evidence that the patient experienced ADHD-type symptoms in early childhood, and that at least by the middle school years, these led to substantial and chronic impairment across settings?
2. Is there credible evidence that ADHD-type symptoms currently cause the patient substantial and consistent impairment across settings?
3. Are there explanations other than ADHD that better account for the clinical picture?
4. For patients who meet criteria for ADHD, is there evidence for the existence of comorbid conditions?

In questions 1 and 2, by "credible" we mean evidence that can be corroborated by some other means than just the patient's verbal self-report.

Presence of Symptoms Since Childhood

Of the four questions, the first one, concerning a childhood history of ADHD is the most critical—and, unfortunately, it is the most often overlooked or sidestepped. *To qualify for the diagnosis of adult ADHD, the patient must have suffered from ADHD as a child.* This does not mean that the individual must have been formally diagnosed in childhood; it only means that sufficient symptoms were present to make it plausible that the condition existed at that stage of development. Although some debate exists concerning the specific age by which symptoms must appear (Barkley & Biederman, 1997), the consensus is that the symptoms must cause meaningful impairment no later than the early teenage years. In support of this assertion, consider that all children with ADHD included in the DSM-IV field trial had developed symptoms producing impairment by 12 years of age (Applegate et al., 1997). The only exceptions come in rare instances in which an adult acquires ADHD symptoms because of brain injury or some other medical condition. Therefore, any credible evaluation for ADHD in adults must provide compelling evidence of early-appearing and long-standing problems with attention and self-control. Without such evidence, the diagnosis of ADHD is likely to be inappropriate even in the face of other clinical information that might appear consistent. For example, atypical or below average scores on psychological testing are never diagnostic unless they coincide with a childhood history of ADHD-type impairment—and possibly not even then, if other comorbid disorders better account for the test results.

Although documentation of a childhood history is essential, we recognize that it is no easy task. Parents may be unavailable or deceased, school report cards may be hard to obtain, and many adults attended school at a time when ADHD was not commonly identified. Nevertheless, every effort should be made to gather as many hard historical data as possible, because they can substantiate self-reported recollections and improve reliability.

In establishing an early ADHD onset, it is important to make a distinction between symptoms and impairment. The DSM-IV(-TR) states that symptoms *producing impairment* must be present by age 7. The patient must therefore show some traits or characteristics of the disorder from early in life that led to impairment before age 7. This criterion implies that onset of impairing symptoms after age 7 is the result of some difficulty or disorder other than ADHD, whereas onset before 7 represents the true disorder. We are aware of no evidence that supports this criterion; indeed, we know of some that undercuts such an idea (Barkley & Biederman, 1997). Clinicians should focus on the onset of symptoms producing impairment sometime during childhood, broadly construed, as the criterion for diagnosis, and should not insist on an onset of impairment before age 7. Certainly, signs of impairment from the symptoms must be evident for the diagnosis to be granted, but this impairment need not predate 7 years of age. Onset of impairing symptoms by puberty or roughly 12–14 years of age would be sufficient. It is extraordinarily rare for someone with bona fide ADHD not to show signs of impairment by at least the middle school years. Those who display no observable signs of disruption until college, graduate school, or later may have valid symptoms and impairment, but it is highly unlikely that their current problems stem from having ADHD. Again, the basic premise is that those suffering from ADHD virtually always leave a trail of evidence of impairment in their wake as they go through life. Because ADHD is defined by impairment, there should be markers (some sort of paper trail) along the way that reflect impairment. The rare exceptions are those in which the individual operated within a family or educational environment that was extraordinarily unusual for the extent of supervision and support it provided.

In the absence of a convincing early history of impairment, clinicians often offer a series of explanations that too often lack credibility. The most common is that high intelligence masked symptoms and allowed for successful compensation throughout childhood and even adolescence. Accordingly, the individual was able to hide deficits because he or she was so swift at managing the material and devising ways to compensate. Although this argument may make intuitive sense, in reality no evidence supports it. Although IQ is related to academic achievement, it is not associated in a meaningful way with ADHD symptom presentation. If

anything, the presence of ADHD appears to diminish intellectual functioning by as much as 7 to 10 points (an average effect size of 0.39) (Hervey, Epstein, & Curry, 2004) and certainly diminishes executive functioning as well (see Chapter 3, this volume; see also Frazier, Demaree, & Youngstrom, 2004). Those with high IQs can still exhibit the full range of ADHD symptoms, and, of course, people with average or low IQs can have normal attention. High intelligence may reduce the level of academic impairment, but it does not serve as a protective factor that shuts down the expression of ADHD symptoms across settings. For instance, Fischer, Barkley, Fletcher, and Smallish (1993) found that childhood IQ in children with ADHD was significantly predictive of levels of academic achievement skills in adolescence, but accounted for less than 14% of the variance in that outcome. Moreover, IQ was unrelated to any other domain of functioning at outcome, including the extent to which the subjects might have repeated a grade, been suspended or expelled, suffered from other disorders, committed antisocial acts, or experienced peer rejection. All this suggests that IQ is not as much of a protective factor from the developmental risks of impairments associated with ADHD as some have believed. If an individual meets criteria for ADHD, those symptoms will become manifest throughout childhood, even in the context of high intelligence. In essence, no amount of intellectual power can overcome the impact of ADHD-level disinhibition and poor self-regulation. Cognitive capacity may allow for quicker learning, but it does not guarantee efficient self-control, organization, time management, or the exercise of good judgment.

Another common explanation for the absence of a childhood history is based on the notion of compensation. The argument is made that a patient showed no symptoms because he or she was able to compensate sufficiently to graduate from high school without any discernible impairment. In our view, the capacity to compensate successfully reflects healthy functioning and belies clinically significant impairment. We base this view on the notion that all children have a profile of relative strengths and weaknesses. One of the tasks of childhood is to learn ways to compensate for abilities that are less well developed. Children who are able to master all the challenges of schooling without any meaningful problems have adequately adapted to any weaknesses. Their ability to manage the many demands of school, home, and neighborhood reflects intact psychological functioning. If problems first surface after secondary school, they are more likely to be the results of circumstance, inappropriate career choice, other psychiatric disorder, or factors not related to the core features of ADHD. Indeed, the disorder is defined by poor compensation during the childhood years.

Having stated a firm rule, we acknowledge the possibility of exceptions. As we already mentioned, some individuals may have been enrolled in unique educational environments—ones entailing so much supervision and structure that only the most desperately impulsive children would experience problems. Others may have gone to school in extraordinarily chaotic environments, in which grossly impulsive behavior was the norm. And still others may have been able to compensate, but only with massive amounts of special educational services, tutoring, extraordinary time and effort, and psychological support. It may be that a person also paid a high psychological price for compensation, to the extent that a formal psychiatric disorder emerged (as opposed to common reactions to daily stress). In other words, a particular patient may have compensated generally, but at such great personal strain that formal symptoms of depression or anxiety were documented.

Evidence of Current Impairment across Settings

The second fundamental question that lies at the heart of an evaluation concerns the degree of current impairment. Are the patient's ADHD symptoms still present and sufficiently disruptive to warrant a current diagnosis of ADHD? This question may seem easy or obvious, but it often is not. Who among the general population would not like to be more attentive, organized, efficient, focused, or productive? It is part of the human condition to be fallible, and there is always room for improvement. How does the clinician differentiate the threshold of impairment necessary to justify a clinical diagnosis from symptoms or behavior falling within the "normal" range?

As we have stressed, the diagnosis of ADHD in adulthood requires a body of evidence that establishes a long-standing pattern of serious life disruption because of impulsive and inattentive behavior. Isolated instances of minor setbacks of the "welcome to the human race" variety do not constitute the kind of impairment that should qualify for a diagnosis. Bona fide ADHD is a serious disorder that affects daily adaptive functioning and causes a chronic and pervasive pattern of impairment in academic, vocational, and social arenas. Individuals with ADHD can provide evidence of poor adjustment with rather serious consequences: loss of jobs due to ADHD-related problems, a history of severe academic underachievement relative to ability, unsatisfactory marital/couple or other interpersonal relationships, disruption of employment and daily adaptive functioning due to impulsivity, forgetfulness, disorganization, and generally inadequate day-to-day adjustment.

Does this mean that a patient has to fail miserably in all academic or vocational settings to qualify for a diagnosis? No. However, we believe that the nature and degree of impairment need to be robust and documented by objective records attesting to lifetime struggles—not transient ones, such as failing a particular exam or having problems in a particular class or course of study. These objective records could be in the form of elementary, junior high, and high school report cards; college or graduate school transcripts; performance reviews from prior jobs held; past psychological/educational test reports; notes or letters from past treatment providers and/or tutors; evidence of being granted academic accommodations in prior schooling; copies of prior individualized education plans; standardized test scores; or any documents attesting to academic or behavioral problems in earlier functioning. These kinds of supporting documents can be extraordinarily helpful in understanding the nature, chronicity, and degree of disruption the symptoms caused. They can also serve either to validate or to refute self-reported recollections of prior symptoms. Again, in order to meet DSM-IV-TR criteria for an ADHD diagnosis, clinicians should be looking beyond mere symptom counts. The ADHD symptoms must result in adverse impact to the patient in major life activities to qualify for a clinical diagnosis. When there is no significant impairment arising from the symptoms, there is no disorder.

What about those who report or complain about a subjective sense of never achieving the goals of which they believe they are capable? Their "internal barometer" tells them they should be doing better, and they may feel an inner sense of dissatisfaction and/or frustration around not meeting all their aspirations. Is this enough "impairment" to qualify for a diagnosis? We feel that in most instances, self-perceptions of underattainment are not the basis for declaring a psychiatric disorder. "Perceived" impairment is not always synonymous with "real" impairment. We have encountered countless patients who come in completely convinced that having ADHD is responsible for their perceived underachievement—despite an almost complete absence of a childhood history of symptoms, current impairment that is nowhere near clinically significant, and a failure and/or unwillingness to consider other possible reasons for their difficulties.

A multitude of reasons besides ADHD can account for why people do not achieve as much as they would like. Many are quick to conclude that ADHD may be the culprit, despite much evidence to the contrary. In fact, we have our most difficult and contentious feedback sessions when we inform people that they do not have the diagnosis. Such patients are often angry and defensive, because they feel we have dismissed the seriousness of their problems. However, once they hear our rationale for why they do not meet the criteria, they usually have a better understanding and acceptance of our diagnostic conclusion.

We understand that in the heat of clinical "battle," making these kinds of diagnostic judgments and distinctions can be difficult. A significant number of cases may fall along the margins and can be particularly hard calls to make. Clinicians need to determine their own thresholds for what constitutes clinically significant impairment and make every attempt to apply their decision-making paradigm in an objective and consistent manner across cases. To assist in making diagnostic judgments, it may be helpful for diagnosticians to picture themselves on the stand being cross-examined by an opposing attorney regarding what evidence substantiates the ADHD diagnosis. If diagnosticians sense that they are on thin ice regarding the quality, quantity, and credibility of the data, we would recommend against rendering the diagnosis—at least at this time. If additional objective historical information that sufficiently substantiates an ADHD-like pattern is provided at a later time, the diagnostic conclusion can be changed.

To determine the degree to which someone is impaired, a clinician must establish the benchmark for comparison. For example, if a person functions well enough to gain entry to law school but fails several courses, is impairment indicated? Some clinicians may argue that relative to other law students, the patient has demonstrated relatively poor functioning. But comparison to an educational cohort can lead to the slippery slope. This person may have at least average or even above-average abilities across the board, but may be declared disordered simply because of failure to perform as well as others in a chosen (or perhaps ill-chosen) training program. We believe that an individual is not necessarily psychiatrically impaired simply because he or she achieves less well than others who are high achievers.

The retort to this position is that disability can be defined by the relative discrepancy between what someone should be able to achieve (usually defined by IQ) and what someone actually manages to attain. The flaw in this argument is that IQ, although it may predict academic achievement through high school, is a poor indicator of overall occupational, social, or psychiatric adjustment. The extent to which an individual achieves, even in college or graduate settings, is determined by far more than intellectual factors. IQ is therefore not a birthright guaranteeing that an individual should be able to achieve a certain academic level. Put another way, it is not a reliable indicator of what an individual should be able to attain, because so many other psychological, motivational, and environmental factors are involved. Anxiety, inadequate social skills, personality style, unrealistic goals, a mismatch between demands and abilities, socioeconomic status, accessibility to educational/vocational opportunities, cultural issues, motivation, substance abuse, and/or having a relative weakness in a selected area are just some of the possible reasons that could explain discrepancies between measured intelligence and real-world performance. Our inclination, then, is to use the population mean as the basis for determining discrepancies in important dimensions of functioning, consistent with the interpretation of the ADA by the Equal Opportunity Employment Commission.

For determinations of disability under antidiscrimination laws such as the ADA, the "average person" as a basis for comparison has been well established. An individual can only be qualified as disabled if he or she is functionally impaired relative to the general population. Under the ADA, for example, a person is not disabled if he or she functions at least as well as or better than most people. Clinicians who evaluate patients seeking legally sanctioned accommodations, such as those required by the ADA, must keep this standard in mind.

An obvious but again often neglected aspect of an adult ADHD evaluation is to review and document which and how many of the official DSM-IV-TR criteria for ADHD the patient (and parent, spouse, or significant other, if possible) endorses both currently and retrospectively to determine whether diagnostic thresholds are met. Strictly speaking, without reviewing the formal criteria with the patient to see if the criteria are met, there is no way to rule in or rule out the disorder. We highly recommend using the DSM-IV-TR symptom list, because it is considered to be the "gold standard" in our current conceptualization of this disorder. Although other symptom lists/rating scales are often used (most notably the Wender Utah Rating Scale and the Brown Attention–Activation Disorder Scale), the DSM-IV-TR items should be included because they remain the most commonly recognized, accepted, and scientifically verified set of criteria.

Are Symptoms Better Explained by a Condition Other Than ADHD?

The third key area in the assessment of adult ADHD has already been alluded to several times, but it bears repeating. It is to make sure that the presenting symptoms are not better explained by some other psychiatric diagnosis, personality factors, learning problem, or situational stressor. Documenting an attempt in the written report of the evaluation to rule out other conditions as being responsible for the ADHD-like symptoms is another critical but often overlooked component of an evaluation. The rationale for arriving at the ADHD diagnosis should be clearly spelled out, and a discussion or statement as to why other possible diagnoses do not fit should be included in the report. It seems that many clinicians get caught up trying to "make ADHD fit" when they should be considering the range of alternative hypotheses that could account for the symptoms. Administering the Structured Clinical Interview for DSM-IV (SCID; First, Spitzer, Gib-

bon, & McWilliams, 1997), which surveys all the major Axis I diagnoses, can be helpful in both ruling out other reasons for the symptoms and establishing comorbid conditions.

Documenting Comorbidity

The last goal of the evaluation is to identify any conditions that might be joining ADHD as part of the clinical picture. Adult patients often have comorbid psychiatric diagnoses, which in some cases may be far more problematic and impairing than their ADHD. Clinicians need to prioritize any comorbid conditions by their degree of impact on functioning. For example, it is more important to treat and stabilize a current Major Depressive Episode, Manic Episode, or alcohol dependence before treating the ADHD component. Patient outcomes can be seriously compromised if clinicians look only for ADHD and fail to consider or treat other potentially more serious conditions first.

In summary, the major aim of the evaluation process is to garner enough data and evidence to reliably answer the four core considerations we have been discussing. Figure 11.1 offers a pictorial diagram summarizing what we believe are the essential steps in the assessment of ADHD in adults.

How clinicians gather their data in support of these four key questions, and what methods they use in the process, are in our view not as important as ensuring that at the end of the evaluation these questions can be answered as validly and reliably as possible. It may be helpful to view the four core considerations as the "process" or the "thinking/judgment/intellectual" part that underlies a credible assessment. The methodology employed is more the mechanical or "content" part of the evaluation and should be considered tools in the service of helping answer these four core questions. As Chapter 8 of this volume has noted, assessment is an issues-driven and not a methods-driven process. A clinician should articulate the issues to be addressed in any particular evaluation, and only then should select the most appropriate methods for collecting the information that addresses those issues. The methods or tools used can be considered data-gathering mechanisms that help to enhance the reliability and validity of the diagnostic conclusions drawn. There are many ways to pursue this information, but no one right way.

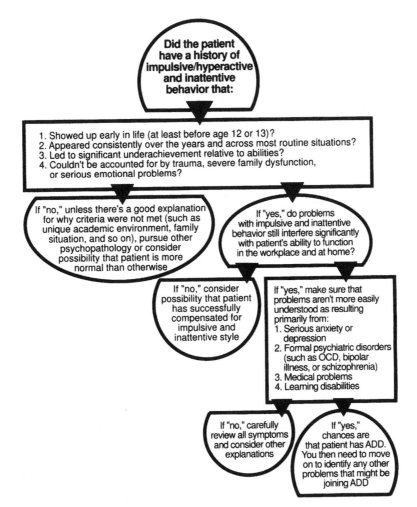

FIGURE 11.1. The road to a diagnosis of adult ADHD.

SUGGESTED PROTOCOL FOR AN ADULT ADHD EVALUATION

Relatively little has occurred with respect to new assessment instruments or empirical research in the assessment of ADHD in adults since the preceding edition of this book. The assessment protocol described below was used at the Adult ADHD Clinic at the University of Massachusetts Medical Center for several years and is one way to conduct a comprehensive evaluation (although not necessarily the best and certainly not the only way). Clinicians need to tailor their methods depending on the time and resources available to them. But all evaluations should attempt to address the four questions at the heart of an adult ADHD evaluation. A comprehensive, practical, and easy-to-

use set of interviews and rating scales that readers may wish to use in their evaluations is provided in the workbook accompanying this text (see Barkley & Murphy, 2006). Included are DSM-IV-TR symptom rating scales for patients, spouses/significant others, and parents; impairment ratings; sample diagnostic interviews for both child and adult ADHD evaluations; and an ADHD Fact Sheet that can be used as a handout for patients/families.

When patients call the clinic, an administrative assistant conducts a brief intake interview over the phone; gathers demographic and insurance information, reason for the referral, and referral source; explains costs; and asks a set of questions to ensure that it is an appropriate referral. A packet of rating scales and questionnaires (described below) is then mailed out to the patient and to the spouse/significant other and/or parent if appropriate. These questionnaires and rating scales are completed at home and are returned to the clinic in a self-addressed stamped envelope. At this point, an appointment date is scheduled. We strongly encourage a spouse/significant other or parent who knows the patient well to participate in the evaluation. Also, patients are emphatically asked to search for and bring with them (or mail) any and all kinds of objective records that attest to their prior history and behavior. These records include report cards, past testing evaluations, individualized education plans, performance evaluations from prior jobs, college transcripts, and the like. Our typical adult evaluation lasts approximately 3 hours. It consists of a comprehensive interview with the patient, spouse/significant other, and/or parent; an intellectual assessment/screening; and a detailed feedback session. In most cases, we also administer a continuous-performance test (CPT), and in some cases the Wide Range Achievement Test–3 (Wilkinson, 1993) to screen for the presence of learning disabilities.

Patient Rating Scales

DSM-IV-TR Based ADHD Symptom Rating Scales

As previously discussed, it is crucial to determine the number of DSM-IV-TR symptoms of ADHD endorsed both currently and retrospectively during childhood. Therefore, we ask the patient, spouse/significant other, and parent to complete the ADHD portion of the Adult Interview (see Barkley & Murphy, 2006), which lists the DSM-IV-TR criteria for current functioning (Current Symptom Scale). The parent and patient also complete the retrospective version for childhood (ages 5–12). Each item is rated on a scale from 0 to 3 ("rarely or never," "sometimes," "often," or "very often," respectively). An item endorsed as "often" or "very often" indicates the presence of a symptom.

A new rating scale entitled the Adult ADHD Self-Report Scale—version 1.1 (ASRS-v1.1) was recently published by the World Health Organization, along with a companion rating scale called the ASRS-v1.1 Screener (Adler, Kessler, & Spencer, 2003). Most ADHD rating scales were designed and standardized for clinician administration to patients. In contrast, the

ASRS-v1.1 is a self-administered instrument that is currently being studied to determine how valid and reliable it is compared to clinician-administered ADHD rating scales. Like other DSM-IV-TR based rating scales (e.g., the Current Symptom Scale described above and the ADHD Rating Scale–IV), it is based on the 18 Criterion A symptoms for ADHD from the DSM-IV-TR, but measures only the frequency of these symptoms (Murphy & Adler, 2004). The decision to assess frequency-based ratings was made to avoid confusing patients with questions of severity. The features of the ASRS-v1.1 that differentiate it from other adult ADHD rating scales include the following:

1. It has an expanded range of 0–4, in which the "never or rarely" rating from the ADHD Rating Scale–IV and Current Symptom Scale has been separated: 0 = "never," 1 = "rarely," 2 = "sometimes," 3 = "often," and 4 = "very often." The thinking here was that "never" and "rarely" are too different to be viewed as part of the same response.
2. The wording of items is designed to be suitable for adults rather than children or adolescents. For example, references to "play" and "schoolwork" were eliminated.
3. The wording of the items provides a context for some symptoms that adults can relate to. For example, the item "Loses things necessary for tasks or activities" from the ADHD Rating Scale–IV was changed to "how often do you misplace or have difficulty finding things at home or work?" in the ASRS-v1.1.
4. It eliminates questions that ask about more than one symptom. For example, "Fails to give close attention to details or makes careless mistakes in schoolwork" from the ADHD Rating Scale–IV became "How often do you make careless mistakes when you have to work on a boring or difficult project?" for the ASRS-v1.1.

The ASRS-v1.1 Screener (Adler, Kessler, & Spencer, 2003) is intended for people age 18 or older and is an initial screening instrument to help determine whether a more comprehensive evaluation for ADHD is warranted. The Screener comprises the first 6 items of the larger 18-item ASRS-v1.1. Four or more checkmarks in the darkly shaded areas of the scoring grid indicates that a person's symptoms may be consistent with ADHD and that a more comprehensive evaluation may be beneficial. Although the psychometric properties of the ASRS-v1.1 have not yet been established, a validation study on a pilot version of the ASRS-v1.1 versus the clinician administered ADHD Rating Scale–IV (Adler, Spencer, & Faraone, 2003) found high internal consistency between the scales, and the kappa coefficients for all items were significant ($p < .001$). Copies of the current version of the ASRS-v1.1 and the ASRS-v1.1 Screener are available online at (*www.med.nyu/psych/training/adhd.html*).

We anticipate some significant changes when the DSM-V is published in the not-too-distant future. It is likely that a new and different set of diagnostic criteria specifically for adults will be included, and that this set will be better at capturing the manifestations of the disorder in adulthood than the current DSM-IV-TR criteria. These two different sets of symptoms will more accurately reflect the developmental changes that occur in the natural history of the disorder over time, and will also more clearly illuminate the impact of the disorder on adult functioning. New DSM-V-based rating scales similar to the ASRS-v1.1 will then need to be constructed and validated to reflect this latest conceptualization of the disorder in adults.

Developmental History Questionnaire

The patient also completes a developmental history questionnaire. This asks about neonatal and birth complications; mood and temperament difficulties; early peer relationships; developmental milestones and whether these were reached at age-appropriate times; and any significant developmental or behavioral problems that occurred early on. Again, during the evaluation we attempt to gather as many data as possible, beginning with neonatal development and continuing up to the present. Parents sometimes describe their sense of knowing that this child was different from other siblings and indicate early concerns about behavior, temperament, mood, or activity level. However, because many children diagnosed with ADHD experience relatively normal early developmental histories, clinicians should not overinterpret or place too much emphasis on developmental history as being necessarily diagnostic or not diagnostic of ADHD.

Health History Questionnaire

The health history questionnaire asks about current and past medical problems, current and past medications (including dosages and efficacy), prior head injuries, allergies to any medications, or the presence of any other serious conditions (e.g., epilepsy, high blood pressure, thyroid problems, chronic pain, and heart conditions). This information can help to rule out possible medical reasons for ADHD-like symptoms and may also have implications for treatment decisions, especially medication choices.

Employment History Questionnaire

The employment history questionnaire asks about current employment status and job title; the number of past jobs held; the types of difficulties encountered in past jobs; the number and reasons for prior terminations; military experience and any problems encountered in the service; and the kinds of coping strategies the patient has employed to manage symptoms in the past. Employment history is pursued in more depth during the interview, in an effort to determine the exact nature of the symptoms and difficulties the patient has experienced, the types of work that have been most successful, and the patient's current and future vocational goals. A major goal is to shed light on the nature and degree of vocational impairment (and success) experienced over the course of the patient's life. Probing for specific examples regarding strengths and weaknesses can help to illuminate the nature and degree of impairment stemming from a patient's symptoms. This is an often overlooked area of assessment that can also have important implications for treatment—regarding optimal job choices in the future.

Social History Questionnaire

The social history questionnaire inquires about the patient's ability to make and maintain friendships, typical moods, temper problems, and perceived reasons for any social skills difficulties during childhood and currently. Two additional open-ended questions are included on this questionnaire: (1) "In what ways do your ADHD symptoms interfere in your life?" (2) "In what ways have you tried to compensate for or cope with your deficits?" How patients answer these questions can offer valuable clues regarding the nature of their most troublesome symptoms, the scope of impairment, and prior attempts to manage their symptoms. The clinical interview can explore the realm of social functioning in greater detail if necessary.

Michigan Alcohol Screening Test

The Michigan Alcohol Screening Test (Selzer, 1971) is a screen for assessing substance abuse problems that previous research has shown to be reliable and valid. It consists of 27 yes–no questions about substance use behavior and can be used as necessary in conjunction with the clinical interview to explore past and present substance use/abuse. This test is also given to the spouse/significant other and parent when possible, to determine the degree of their agreement with the patient's views.

Symptom Checklist 90—Revised

The Symptom Checklist 90—Revised (Derogatis, 1986) is a self-report screening instrument that provides a measure of current psychological distress. It assesses a variety of symptoms of psychological maladjustment using 90 items, each rated on a 5-point scale. Scores for nine subscales are obtained (Anxious, Phobic, Paranoia, Depression, Somatization, Obsessive–Compulsive, Interpersonal Sensitivity, Psychoticism, Hostility), as well as a Global Severity Index.

Spouse/Significant Other Forms

The patient's spouse or significant other is mailed a DSM-IV-TR-based ADHD symptom scale and the Michigan Alcohol Screening Test for current functioning, and is asked to mail the completed forms back to the clinic if he or she is unable to attend the assessment. The spouse/significant other is strongly encouraged to participate in the diagnostic interview as well, preferably in person or via telephone. Additional informants (parents and siblings, as well as spouse/significant other) are often crucial in obtaining a full picture of the patient's overall life functioning.

Parent Rating Scales

At least one parent should also be administered a DSM-IV-TR-based ADHD symptom scale for both current functioning and retrospective childhood functioning, and the Michigan Alcohol Screening Test for another view of the patient's substance use/abuse. It may also be helpful for a parent to complete a developmental history questionnaire, to capture any additional developmental issues, behaviors, or concerns from the parent's perspective that the patient may be unaware of or may not remember.

The Clinical Interview

A comprehensive clinical interview should be conducted that surveys past and present ADHD symptoms; developmental and medical history; school history; work history; psychiatric history, including any medications prescribed, dosages, and responses; social adjustment; family history of ADHD or any psychiatric or medical conditions that are evident in the family bloodlines; any arrests or trouble with the law; and general day-to-day adaptive functioning (i.e., how the patient is doing in meeting the demands of daily life). In our view, this is the most crucial component of the assessment. It should not simply be a brief, cursory, surface-level exam. To accomplish the appropriate rule-outs and to truly understand the patient's life history in all the necessary domains, the interview usually requires a minimum of 1–2 hours. Ideally, the interview should rely on several informants (a parent and spouse/significant other, if possible) and survey behavior over time and across multiple settings (work, school, social, home).

In most cases, interviews with the patient, parent, and/or spouse/significant other are conducted jointly. Only in rare cases (severe animosity or defensiveness between the patient and one of the other parties) have we found it necessary to do separate interviews. However, we also find it valuable to offer some private time to each party participating in the assessment, to elicit any data that the individual may have been reluctant to share in the presence of others. It is also during the clinical interview that the clinician must attempt to rule in or rule out other psychiatric diagnoses that may be a more accurate explanation for the presenting symptoms. As noted earlier, we suggest using the SCID, which asks standardized questions surveying criteria for all Axis I diagnoses. This instrument not only helps in the differential diagnosis of ADHD, but may also help to establish the existence of comorbid conditions that may accompany ADHD.

Psychological Testing

Our views on the role of psychological testing in adult evaluations are consistent with those expressed for children and adolescents in Chapter 9 (this volume). Psychological testing can play a meaningful role in clinical assessment, but practitioners should be highly circumspect when interpreting such data. Such caution is especially justified when dealing with adults, because the scientific literature on the classification accuracy of psychological testing in the diagnosis of ADHD in adults is wafer-thin. Prior research has demonstrated that no single test or battery of tests has adequate predictive validity or specificity to reliably make an ADHD diagnosis.

Unfortunately, we have often seen evaluations that consist almost entirely of psychological testing, usually incorporating measures of marginal relevance or validity to the identification of this disorder. *Under no conditions should psychological testing be offered as a sole basis for the diagnosis of ADHD.* We particularly discourage evaluations that focus too broadly on neuropsychological test performance in the absence of other clinical data. In the adult arena, psychological testing is most helpful when it is used to support conclusions derived from childhood history, rating scales, and a careful analysis of current functioning.

Beyond the sentiments expressed in Chapter 9, we offer the following observations:

• We routinely administer a brief IQ screening measure, such as the Shipley Institute of Living Scale, the Kaufman Brief Intelligence Test, or the Peabody Picture Vocabulary Test—Third Edition, if no prior or recent intelligence test results are available. In this way we can screen for any gross cognitive weaknesses. We can also get a sense of a discrepancy between measured intelligence and academic performance. For example, it is quite common (but not diagnostic) for an adult with ADHD to score in the average to above-average or even superior range of intelligence, and yet to have a school history of extreme grade variability with mostly C's, D's, and F's.

• Routine administration of a complete IQ test, such as the Wechsler Adult Intelligence Scale—Third Edition (WAIS-III; Wechs-

ler, 1997) is not necessary, in our view, unless there are specific questions about the possibility of specific cognitive deficits. In most cases, a brief screening measure is sufficient.

• Significant differences between Verbal and Performance subscale scores on the WAIS-III are often offered as evidence of ADHD. Clinical lore aside, no evidence exists that such discrepancies are at all meaningful for this diagnosis. The same conclusion holds for specific patterns of subtest scores or for disparities between IQ test scores and indices of achievement.

• We usually administer a computerized measure of sustained attention and distractibility, such as the Conners CPT II (Conners & MHS Staff, 2000), Conners CPT (Conners, 1995), the Test of Variables of Attention (Greenberg & Kindschi, 1996), or the Gordon Diagnostic System (Gordon, 1983). Although the last of these offers published normative data (Saykin et al., 1995) and some validity data (Rasile, Burg, Burright, & Donovick, 1995), none of the measures yet boasts sufficient data to justify much reliance. (Part of the reason for the absence of good data is because criteria for subject inclusion in the adult arena are still highly uncertain.) So why do we administer them? Simply because these tests provide the opportunity to observe the patient coping with a task that requires sustained attention and impulse control. We have noticed that many who ultimately receive the diagnosis struggle with these tasks. For example, it is not uncommon for some patients with ADHD to develop a headache or to appear worn or tired after just a few minutes of testing, even if their scores ultimately fall in the average range. These observations, although never unilaterally diagnostic, can be informative. Also, when an adult fares poorly on a CPT, we have found that this often confirms other clinical data supportive of the ADHD diagnosis.

The Medical Examination

As noted earlier, instances are likely to arise in which potential medical problems may better account for the complaints of inattention expressed by clients. These will obviously require referral to the appropriate medical specialist to rule in or out these possible medical comorbidities. More likely, the clinician anticipates that the client is likely to require medication management as part of the treatment plan being considered. If the client has not already had a recent medical examination, this will need to be added to the evaluation in order to rule out any conditions that may contraindicate the medication(s) under consideration. The details of the medical examination have been addressed in the chapter on the evaluation of ADHD in children (Chapter 8) and will not be reiterated here, except to note that issues more relevant to adulthood may also need to be covered in this examination (e.g., sexual functioning, age-related conditions such as perimenopause, etc.). As indicated in Chapter 8, there are no lab or medical tests that are useful for the diagnosis of ADHD in adults, just as there are none yet established for child ADHD.

ASSESSMENT DILEMMAS

Discrepancies among Informants

In clinical practice, assessment data are not always consistent across sources. Significant discrepancies may exist among the patient's, the parent's, and the spouse/significant other's reports on symptom rating scales or on perceptions of severity of impairment. For example, in our experience, it is not uncommon for the parent of an adult patient with ADHD to endorse far fewer DSM-IV-TR ADHD symptoms (current and retrospective) than the patient does. Why might this be so? A number of reasons are possible, ranging from simply forgetting behavior that occurred long ago to parental psychopathology ("My parents had their own problems and were unable or unwilling to tune in to mine"). Other possible explanations for lack of symptom endorsement by parents include cultural factors, guilt ("Maybe I should have sought help during childhood, but because I did not, the behavior must not have been that bad"), relative impairment compared to other siblings ("He was not nearly as bad as his brother"), or simply a general reluctance to view one's offspring as impaired. Whose version is the most reliable or valid? How do clinicians resolve such apparent discrepancies?

Assessing the credibility of each source is crucial. Although this is not always the case, we have found that the patient is often the most credible reporter. If the preponderance of the assessment data point to a robust history of ADHD, and the only piece that does not seem to fit is a parent's or spouse's/significant other's endorsement of fewer DSM-IV-TR symptoms,

the clinician may want to weigh this piece less heavily and consider potential explanations for the differing viewpoints. For example, does the patient have a contentious marriage? Has the parent been absent for many years? How mentally healthy is the parent, and how involved has the parent been? Is there a cultural or generational barrier against psychiatric labels that lowers the probability of positive symptom endorsement?

In other cases, a discrepancy may go in the opposite direction. For example, sometimes adolescents and younger adults tend to deny their ADHD symptoms, and their parents' reports may be more accurate. Clinicians need to carefully consider these types of issues and exercise sound clinical judgment in their attempts to resolve these discrepancies.

ADHD, Predominantly Inattentive Type

Patients who present primarily with complaints of inattention, but who do not offer a history of poor self-control and overactivity, are often the most difficult to evaluate. Although early-appearing, chronic, and pervasive disinhibition is associated almost uniquely with ADHD, the same cannot be said about inattention when it presents outside the context of poor self-control. As we have indicated, inattention is an omnipresent item on symptom lists for most psychiatric and many medical conditions. It can also be a result of situational or environmental stressors. It is therefore hard to justify a diagnosis of ADHD, Predominantly Inattentive Type, unless convincing evidence is presented to rule out the full range of other psychiatric and medical possibilities.

We clearly distinguish here those patients with a clear history of ADHD, Combined Type who, by virtue of marked and typical declines in hyperactivity, no longer have sufficient symptoms to meet the full criteria for that type in adulthood. Such patients would be reclassified in the DSM as having the Predominantly Inattentive Type. Clinicians, however, should continue to conceptualize such patients as having the Combined Type; these patients have not actually changed types of ADHD so much as they have moved to having borderline or subthreshold Combined Type, merely as a consequence of declines in hyperactivity.

Such cases aside, we generally approach the diagnosis of ADHD, Predominantly Inattentive Type as a process of elimination. If a patient presents with symptoms that fall almost entirely into a cognitive realm (inattention, poor concentration, lack of focus, distractibility), we first rule out the possibility that other psychiatric problems are at play, especially those related to Generalized Anxiety Disorder, Obsessive–Compulsive Disorder, and various forms of depression or schizophrenia. If those explanations prove inappropriate, we next consider learning problems, such as intellectual limitations, specific learning disabilities, or a poor match between abilities and the patient's educational program or occupation. If learning problems fail to account for the patient's presenting complaints, the diagnosis of ADHD, Predominantly Inattentive Type may be indicated. However, this diagnosis still requires evidence that the patient's ability to attend is limited to such a degree that it causes clinically significant impairment. We again remind the reader that inattention is a common outcropping of human nature. Pathological inattention therefore requires an uncommon degree of underperformance and poor adjustment.

In our experience, the inattentive-only variant of ADHD is a relatively rare phenomenon. Most of the patients referred to us who have already been assigned this diagnosis exit our evaluation either with a different diagnosis or with none at all. In many cases, our impression is that other clinicians, hearing complaints of inattention, sometimes jump too quickly to the ADHD, Predominantly Inattentive Type diagnosis without exploring other possibilities. We suggest that this diagnosis be applied judiciously and only after all other diagnostic avenues have been pursued.

Substance Abuse/Dependence and ADHD

The high degree of comorbidity between substance abuse and ADHD can offer another set of challenges to the clinician. The most frequent drugs of choice in our clinic populations are alcohol, marijuana, and (to a lesser extent) cocaine. The kinds of questions that routinely arise include the following: Are the ADHD symptoms due to substance abuse, ADHD, or both? Is it appropriate to prescribe a stimulant to someone with substance abuse? Does the patient need to stop using substances completely before beginning medication treatment for ADHD? If so, how long must the patient remain sober before attempting a medication trial? Will medication for ADHD jeopar-

dize the patient's sobriety or make the patient worse?

In the case of alcohol abuse, when a clinician is attempting to make a differential diagnosis, it is important to consider the following: When did alcohol abuse begin? Was there clear evidence of ADHD symptoms during childhood before the onset of the alcohol abuse? How would the patient's life be different if he or she was able to maintain sobriety for a significant length of time? Would the ADHD symptoms then remit? Or is there evidence of ongoing ADHD symptoms even after a period of sustained sobriety (at least several months)? Answering questions such as these will give valuable clues in differentiating ADHD from substance abuse.

What about the issue of substance abuse versus substance dependence? In our view, those who meet criteria for substance dependence should always be referred to primary addiction treatment to stabilize their condition before any ADHD medication treatment is attempted. Even if ADHD is present in a patient with substance dependence, we believe that the first step in his or her ADHD treatment is to get the substance problem under control. Once this is accomplished, assessment of any residual ADHD symptoms can be more reliably made. In our experience, we usually require at least 1–2 months of sobriety before prescribing any stimulant medication to treat comorbid ADHD symptoms.

In the case of episodic substance abuse of alcohol or marijuana, where the patient is not physiologically addicted or out of control, we sometimes take a more liberal stance. If the assessment yields a clear history of ADHD with comorbid substance abuse, we do not routinely disqualify these patients from a medication trial for their ADHD. In some of our cases, concurrent treatment for ADHD (with stimulant medication) and substance abuse has resulted in significant improvement of both the substance abuse and the underlying ADHD symptoms. In other individuals, this has not been the case. All instances of ADHD and comorbid substance abuse require close vigilance and monitoring to ensure safety and optimal treatment outcome. In most cases, a reasonable course to follow in differentiating ADHD from substance dependence or abuse is to (1) determine the age of onset of the substance use, (2) determine whether there was a childhood history of ADHD predating the substance use, and (3) require a significant period of sobriety with reassessment of any residual ADHD symptoms before assigning the ADHD diagnosis.

Differential Diagnosis from Other Psychiatric Disorders

As we have repeatedly emphasized, it is critical for a clinician to attempt to rule out other psychiatric conditions before assigning the ADHD diagnosis. In addition to substance abuse, other conditions that can mimic ADHD that need to be ruled out include mood disorders (see especially the discussion of the bipolar disorders, below); anxiety disorders, especially Generalized Anxiety Disorder and Obsessive–Compulsive Disorder; head injury; some personality disorders, especially Borderline Personality Disorder; and some types of schizophrenia. The SCID can help determine whether criteria are met for these other disorders. Generally speaking, most other psychiatric disorders have a later onset of symptoms (after age 7); a childhood school history that does not indicate disruptive behavior or teacher complaints concerning inattentive, hyperactive, or impulsive behavior; and a different symptom profile and course. Again, paying close attention to age of onset, any clear evidence of ADHD symptoms from early childhood, and the qualitative description and nature of the presenting symptoms/impairment will offer important clues in differentiating ADHD from other psychiatric conditions. Clinicians will need to have the requisite training, skills, and experience to do the necessary rule-outs and to recognize and assess the range of adult psychiatric disorders that can either mimic ADHD or coexist with it.

ADHD versus the Bipolar Disorders

The differential diagnosis between ADHD and the various forms of Bipolar Disorder can be an especially tricky task. Impulsivity, hyperactivity, distractibility, increased talkativeness, agitation, and emotional lability can be characteristic of both ADHD and bipolar disorders. Furthermore, the DSM-IV-TR criteria for ADHD and for a Major Depressive Episode both have symptoms related to concentration and agitation. Given this significant symptom overlap, it is not surprising that these two types of disorders can be commonly confused.

In our view, it is not particularly difficult to differentiate ADHD from Bipolar I Disorder. True mania, with its associated symptoms of severe emotional lability, the perception of possessing special powers or abilities, insomnia for long periods, and in some cases psychotic symptoms, is clearly different from ADHD. However, it can be far more difficult to distinguish a severe form of ADHD from Bipolar II Disorder or Cyclothymia. A hyperactive child or adult with pronounced impulsivity, disinhibition, hyperactivity, and emotional overreactivity can be very difficult to distinguish from a person with one of these lower-magnitude bipolar disorders.

The following guidelines may assist in distinguishing the two types of disorders:

1. The age of onset is typically earlier in ADHD than in a bipolar disorder. In our clinical experience, it is quite rare in particular for a child to be diagnosed with Bipolar I Disorder, which typically tends to have an onset in the late teenage or early adult years. However, recent research (Wozniak & Biederman, 1994; Wozniak et al., 1995) has challenged the view that childhood-onset Bipolar I Disorder is rare. Further research may shed additional light on this issue in the future.

2. ADHD results in a chronic and pervasive pattern of impairment over time and across situations. Bipolar disorders tend to be characterized by more of an episodic and cyclical nature, with wide mood swings and grandiosity. The person with a bipolar disorder is clearly not his or her normal self and may engage in reckless behavior, such as spending sprees, excessive speeding, or other dangerous and uncharacteristic behavior. Such people may believe they have special powers or abilities and exhibit enormous energy. Bipolar disorders may also be characterized by bursts of productivity, where the person accomplishes a great deal in a short amount of time and sleeps very little over the course of several days. ADHD is relatively free from these bursts of productivity and tends to have a more chronic and consistent presentation, with less variability in behavior, mood, energy, and productivity.

3. There is an absence of psychotic features and abnormally expansive or elevated mood in ADHD, whereas these features can be evident in a bipolar disorder. Furthermore, Bipolar I Disorder (except for the Single Manic Episode

type) requires meeting criteria for both a Major Depressive Episode and a Manic Episode, which is not the case for ADHD.

4. An examination of the extended family bloodlines for psychiatric illness may offer important clues. For example, if several first-degree relatives have a history of bipolar disorders and ADHD is absent from the family bloodlines, this could be considered supportive evidence for a bipolar disorder. Conversely, if there is a family pattern of ADHD and no bipolar (or other mood) disorders in the extended family, the possibility of ADHD is stronger.

5. Evaluating responses to prior medication trials may offer clues as to whether the patient has ADHD or a mood disorder. For example, those with ADHD (and not a bipolar disorder) typically respond rather poorly to lithium but rather well to a stimulant. Conversely, those with a bipolar disorder may describe a history of positive responses to antidepressant medication or lithium and would typically not respond as well to a stimulant.

Part of the difficulty in differentiating these two disorders is also related to the possibility that both disorders can occur together. Hence, it is not always an either–or proposition. A thorough and careful assessment is essential to adequately address this potential comorbidity. Although both disorders can occur together, in our population this has proven to be quite rare.

THE PHENOMENOLOGY OF ADULT ADHD

Another aspect of the evaluation is to pay attention to how the person behaves, responds, or comes across over the course of the evaluation. How a person responds to certain questions may offer important clues in determining whether this person has lived with or experienced true ADHD. Rating scales, testing, input from a parent and/or a spouse/significant other, and inspection of past records are all important parts of the evaluation, but it is also important to consider the overall behavior of the person throughout the course of the evaluation. Although not scientific or diagnostic, these subjective impressions can be invaluable in helping to make diagnostic decisions and bolstering one's confidence in those decisions. As a result of listening to many hundreds of adult ADHD patients share their lifetime struggles, we have

developed a "sixth sense" of sorts regarding how people who have lived with clinically significant ADHD all their lives behave in the context of an evaluation.

The clinician should be aware of the "tone" of the interview. Those who have lived with ADHD almost always communicate a sense of long-standing pain, frustration, and underachievement, and they display a certain emotional "heaviness" regarding the type and degree of lifelong impairment they have experienced. Often these patients display episodic tears and express despair, intense frustration, anger, a sense of lost opportunities, regret, low self-esteem, defensiveness, and sometimes a sense of learned helplessness. On the other hand, patients who do not turn out to have ADHD may display a relative lack of pain and come across simply desiring to do better in a particular life domain. They are reasonably satisfied with their lives, are experiencing no obvious impairment, and seem to be seeking performance enhancement—not help for a disability. The tone of the evaluation for someone who turns out not to have ADHD is often lighter and relatively free from significant frustration or impairment. These patients may laugh about their foibles and imply that their behavior is seen as cute or funny instead of causing bona fide problems. When the overall tone is lighthearted, flippant, and full of laughter, and the degree of disruption/pain/impairment seems minimal, a patient is not likely to be describing ADHD. This is not to say that a heavy pall must be cast over the entire course of the evaluation, and that a patient who does have ADHD cannot display a sense of humor. We are not here confusing ADHD with Major Depressive Episodes. We simply mean that ADHD is defined by significant impairment, which by definition is disruptive to one's life. People who seek evaluations for ADHD are usually in some pain or distress. If this is not evident during the evaluation, the person is unlikely to have ADHD. Put another way, if a diagnostician has to struggle with the question, "Where's the impairment?", chances are that he or she is not dealing with ADHD.

Semantics

During the course of the evaluation, we take note of both qualitative and quantitative responses offered to certain key questions. For example, at the outset of an evaluation we routinely ask this question: "What are some of the symptoms you have experienced that make you think you have ADHD?" How the person responds to this question can be telling and may yield valuable information. Often those who truly have the disorder respond to that question in a robust and compelling way. They are usually not at a loss for words and have no difficulty answering this question. They frequently express a litany of symptoms, with an overall tone of intense exasperation or frustration. They may well describe numerous examples of not finishing tasks, of frustrations and failures in school, of social/interpersonal difficulties, and of problems in the workplace. The quality of their response to this question may assist clinicians to better determine whether these persons have "walked the walk" and know firsthand what it is like to live with ADHD day in and day out. Those who do not have the disorder, or who may have another psychiatric problem instead of ADHD, often provide a response to this question that comes across as more hollow and far less compelling and robust with respect to capturing the experience of living with ADHD.

A useful follow-up to the previous question is to ask, "And how long have these symptoms been going on for you?" Again, those who truly have the disorder often answer this question with statements clearly suggesting that their symptoms have been long-standing—that these have been present over time and across situations throughout their lives. Those who turn out not to have ADHD may answer this question by describing an onset of problems at some point in their adult lives and identifying a situational stressor, such as a divorce or death in the family, job termination or change, lifestyle change (e.g., a new baby), onset of a Major Depressive Episode, or the beginnings of a substance abuse problem.

Another question we frequently ask toward the end of an evaluation is this: "If I had a magic wand and could make two or three things much better for you, what would you want me to fix or help you improve upon?" The purpose of this question is to determine whether the patient's response is consistent with or magnifies/reinforces the "impairment themes" that have emerged over the course of the evaluation. Does the patient immediately and unflinchingly come back to themes that are reflective of typical ADHD disruption?

Or is the patient confused by the question or having a difficult time coming up with an answer? More often than not, those with bona fide ADHD respond with a variation of the following: "I just want to be able to focus and concentrate," "I just want to finish something," "I want to be able to sustain my effort and motivation long enough to complete something," "I want to be less impulsive or be able to think before I act," "I want to have better control of my temper," "I just want to slow down and relax," "I want to be able to do the routine things in life more efficiently," or "I want to be able to read, study, and remember more effectively." The person who turns out not to have ADHD usually answers this question in a qualitatively different way, which gives the diagnostician the sense that his or her core problems have little to do with attention, concentration, distractibility, hyperactivity, or impulse control.

Because underachievement in school relative to native potential is so common in those with ADHD, we often ask and take note of the response to the following question: "What is your best guess as to why you did not perform as well as you should have in school?" Those with ADHD frequently pause, make a halfhearted attempt at an explanation, and finally may express frustration and exasperation and impatiently say, "I just don't know." They usually struggle with and do not have a good answer for this question, or they may say something like "I was not interested in school," "I was lazy," or "It was too boring."

Another question we routinely ask the patient (and spouse/significant other or parent, with appropriate rewording) at the end of the evaluation is this: "On an impairment scale ranging from 1 to 10 (1 being extremely mild and 10 being severe impairment), how would you rate yourself in terms of how impairing your symptoms are to you in your overall life, and why?" The rating and reasoning for their choices can help to illuminate the degree of perceived impairment and add another piece of data in determining whether the patient truly meets the threshold for a clinical diagnosis of ADHD.

Recognition Responses

Being cognizant of both verbal and affective responses to certain symptom items is another nonscientific but potentially useful piece of information to consider. We have noticed some fairly common behavioral and affective reactions (which we call "recognition responses") in many of our bona fide adult ADHD cases. For example, when asked about the symptom of losing things frequently, the person with ADHD (and usually his or her spouse/significant other) may disgustedly recite a litany of examples clearly indicating that the person's degree of forgetfulness and losing items is far different from that of the "average person" in the population. It often has a "you wouldn't believe how bad it is" quality, and the person or spouse/significant other may display a sense of humor about it as well. When this information is followed up by asking what specifically the person loses, someone who turns out to have ADHD may well offer a series of items—keys, wallet, cell phones, license, credit cards, bills, clothes, books—and then, with obvious exasperation, say, "Everything!" Clearly, none of these examples alone is sufficient to substantiate the diagnosis, but in combination with other objective and reliable historical information, they can provide additional support for the diagnosis.

The patient or the parent may also relate childhood nicknames of the patient that reflected his or her behavioral/symptom pattern ("Calamity Jane," "space cadet," "absentminded professor," "Dennis the Menace," "dream girl"). Parents may also relate childhood stories that are legendary in the family circle, detailing instances of impulse control problems or hyperactivity. There is often a rich cache of stories and events attesting to the patient's consistently annoying or disruptive behavior. These memories or stories are not simply isolated instances of misbehavior; they represent a consistent pattern clearly illustrating that "Johnny has always been Johnny" over time and across situations. Conversely, as evidence for ADHD, some of our adult patients who turn out not to receive the diagnosis offer recollections of an isolated example of behavior that may have occurred once or twice in third grade. They may offer such statements as "I remember when my fourth-grade teacher said I looked out the window too much," or "I remember that time when Mr. Smith gave me a detention for not handing in my homework." What is important to remember is that in most cases of bona fide ADHD, a behavioral pattern is quite evident to teachers and parents and is not difficult to identify. Such persons usually

leave a trail of evidence in their wake as they move on in school/life.

Related questions we routinely ask include "Did your parents ever take you to see anyone about these problems when you were a child?" and "How old were you when you first sought any treatment or professional help? For what reasons?" Those with clinically significant ADHD usually (although by no means always) either sought help or were referred for assistance relatively early in life. In our experience, it is relatively rare (although not impossible) for an adult who has never sought or received any prior treatment to be diagnosed with ADHD.

Yet another useful question to ask is "Did you have any trouble doing homework?" Both the content and the affect inherent in the response are important to consider. If students with ADHD have one universal Achilles heel, most would agree it is in consistently doing homework. Almost all adults with ADHD (and children, for that matter) report histories of problems completing homework. Many of our adult patients scoff and say one of the following: "I never did homework," "I always copied someone else's," "I did it 5 minutes before class," "I only did it when I had to," "I did it in school," "I never took books home," "I could never sit still and focus long enough to get it done," "There was always something better or more fun/interesting to do," "I was great at pulling a rabbit out of my hat at the last minute," "I was a good schmoozer and was always able to get teachers to cut me some slack," or "I was in the lower group and was never given homework." Careful questioning on this issue often uncovers that their choice not to do homework was not usually deliberate—at least initially. What may be more accurate is that despite their best efforts, these patients were unable to focus, concentrate, or sustain their effort/motivation long enough to get it done. Homework is so often a frustrating and emotionally charged issue for both parents and children. If an adult reports no history of homework difficulty or does not remember whether it was a problem, we would seriously question an ADHD diagnosis.

In summary, taking into account not just what patients say in response to assessment questions, but how they say it in terms of tone, affect, and robustness, can offer useful clues in assessing ADHD.

A WORD ABOUT ADHD AS A BASIS FOR DISABILITY

Over the past decade, increasing numbers of students and employees have been pursuing ADHD evaluations to document requests for accommodations under the ADA. This law is designed to prevent discrimination against individuals with physical, mental, or learning disabilities. Under ADA-related regulations and case law, ADHD is considered a legitimate disability.

Providing documentation for ADA requests is a complicated undertaking, which requires special knowledge about the law. A comprehensive book on this general topic (Gordon & Keiser, 1998) contains a chapter specifically on legal documentation for the ADHD diagnosis (Gordon & Murphy, 1998). We have also summarized the essential steps and requirements in this process in three articles (Murphy, 2004; Murphy & Gordon, 1996; Gordon et al., 1997). Table 11.1 summarizes the gist of these articles.

Although a full discussion of disability determination falls outside the scope of this book, we offer the following comment: This is a highly specialized and poorly understood area of clinical practice, and many clinicians have a fundamental misunderstanding of the rigorous documentation requirements that are necessary to secure testing (or workplace) accommodations for their patients. Many diagnosticians fully believe that their reports are more than adequate to justify awarding accommodations, when in fact they often fall short in several key areas. The standard evaluation reports routinely done by most clinicians are almost always inadequate to satisfy ADA-level documentation requirements. The burden of proof

---

TABLE 11.1. Documenting Requests for Accommodations under the Americans with Disabilities Act (ADA)

1. Show that DSM-IV-TR symptoms occur to a degree that is significantly greater than the normal population (state that DSM-IV-TR was employed; report number of symptoms endorsed for current functioning).
2. Show that DSM-IV-TR symptoms arose in childhood (state that DSM-IV-TR was employed retrospectively; report number of symptoms endorsed for childhood; report approximate age of onset of symptoms [onset before age 12 is acceptable—cite Barkley & Biederman, 1997, to support this adjustment to age of onset if need be]).
3. Present evidence of impairment since childhood. Indicate how disorder has significantly interfered with the individual's social, educational, or occupational functioning.
4. Present evidence of cross-setting symptoms/impairment. Provide history of symptoms producing impairment in home and school settings in childhood.
5. Demonstrate corroboration of symptoms in childhood from someone who knew the patient well (parents, siblings, long-time friend, etc.).
6. Demonstrate corroboration of current symptoms of ADHD from someone who knows the patient well (spouse, significant other, parent, sibling, employer, etc.).
7. Show evidence of current impairment in a major life activity (education, occupation, social, etc.). Impairment has been defined in the ADA as being relative to the average person or the majority of the population—*not* relative to a high-achieving, highly intelligent, or high-functioning peer group (undergraduate, graduate, professional, or medical students, etc.). State the evidence and how it has reduced the person's functioning well below that of the average person.
8. State that a differential diagnosis was conducted and other disorders were ruled out that might have better accounted for this person's performance problems or current symptoms and impairment.
9. Describe the history of prior treatment and its success.
10. Describe any history of prior accommodations for the disorder and their success. If no prior accommodations were ever provided for the disorder, explain why not.
11. State the accommodations being recommended *and* why: What is the rationale for each, and why are they reasonable for this disorder in this person?
12. If the diagnostician does not hold a terminal degree in clinical psychology or psychiatry, indicate what training qualifies the professional to conduct a differential diagnosis of mental illness.

for these legal determinations is far greater than that for everyday clinical diagnosis. Institutions and employers have the right to request that individuals supply full and convincing documentation of disability. These reports are often reviewed by other professionals, who pay close attention to evidence that the individual is truly impaired. According to the bulk of case law, the standard for judging impairment is the functioning of the average American. Therefore, to be qualified as disabled under the ADA requires evidence that in a major life activity, the individual demonstrates substantial impairment relative to most people (not, e.g., a cohort of other students in a professional program). In the case of ADHD, the clinician has to supply evidence that the patient fully meets DSM-IV-TR criteria for both early and current impairment. Also required is a clear rationale for why the accommodations requested are in keeping with both the nature of the disorder and the circumstances in which the person functions.

Why is it so important for diagnosticians to understand the documentation requirements to substantiate a diagnosis and a disability (and how these are different)? The answer is that a lack of such understanding can end up causing great harm to patients. For example, clinicians may be overly confident about patients' chances for approval, leading them not even to consider the possibility of a denial of accommodations. Patients may then avoid altogether preparing for the possibility that they may have to take tests or meet other academic or vocational requirements without accommodations. Denial at the last minute in scenarios like this can cause great anxiety and anger, and can influence test or other results. Even those with legitimate disabilities who are deserving of accommodations may be denied, because their clinicians produce documentation that is incomplete or otherwise fails to adequately address the crucial points that the organizations or testing boards are looking for. For a more detailed discussion of the full range of issues related to ADHD, documentation requirements, and the ADA, interested readers are encouraged to consult the references listed above.

FUTURE RESEARCH DIRECTIONS

For over 100 years, our understanding of and knowledge base on what we now refer to as ADHD have constantly evolved and changed as a result of scientific study. The future will be no different, because there will continue to be changes in our view of this disorder as new scientific findings emerge. Some of the assessment-related issues that need further study include better ways of measuring impairment in the major life activities of adults; development of separate diagnostic criteria and rating scales for adults that are more sensitive and specific to adult functioning than the existing criteria; developing a better understanding of whether the Predominantly Inattentive Type of ADHD should be considered an entirely separate disorder from the Combined and Predominantly Hyperactive–Impulsive Types; exploring any gender differences that may exist in the adult population with ADHD; expanding our knowledge of structural and functional brain differences in ADHD via neuroimaging studies; attempting to find biological markers for the disorder; and exploring differences in course and outcome between adults who were diagnosed with ADHD during childhood and those who were first diagnosed as adults.

CONCLUSION

It should be quite clear by now that the assessment of adult ADHD is a formidable challenge. Our current state of scientific knowledge has improved somewhat, and our technology and assessment measures have matured a bit, but all are still quite primitive. Furthermore, the relative lack of well-normed rating scales for adults, the fact that everyone experiences the symptoms of ADHD to some degree, the high degree of comorbidity, the myths and confusion perpetuated in part by widespread media exposure, and the lack of a "litmus test" for diagnosing the disorder all contribute to making ADHD a most difficult disorder to diagnose accurately in adults. The major goals of this chapter have been (1) to communicate the complexities of this disorder; (2) to show that the diagnosis should be reserved only for those who meet full clinical criteria (early onset, current and historical evidence of clinically significant impairment in major life domains, and not better explained by another condition); (3) to show that having ADHD is disruptive and impairing to lives and is not advantageous; and (4) to show that ADHD is not simply the identification of certain personality characteristics or a simple matter of symptom endorsement. It is our hope that this "tighter" conceptualization of ADHD will help to uphold the legitimacy and integrity of the disorder, help to reduce some of the current confusion and skepticism surrounding ADHD in adults, and assist clinicians in better understanding and diagnosing this often misunderstood disorder.

KEY CLINICAL POINTS

✓ Approximately 4–5% of adults may have ADHD, with referrals to clinicians seeking a diagnosis of the disorder rising markedly during the past 15 years.

✓ The evaluation of adults for ADHD, like that for children, is a process that is organized around and directed at addressing the issues of a particular case. It is not a process solely determined by a rigid set of methods with which the clinician feels comfortable, but which may not address the issues related to diagnosis for the individual case. The most appropriate and valid methods must be selected to address the particular issues in each case.

✓ Four issues are central to the evaluation:

- Establishing the presence of developmentally inappropriate and chronic symptoms producing impairment dating back to childhood (before 12–14 years of age).
- Documenting evidence of impairment across several domains of current major life activities.
- Determining whether symptoms are better explained by another psychiatric disorder, life events, or a medical condition (differential diagnosis).
- Clarifying the existence and nature of likely comorbid disorders, if any.

The evaluation is likely to involve the following:

- The collection of rating scales and referral information prior to the evaluation.
- A semistructured interview with the client.
- Review of previous records that may document impairment.
- Psychological testing to rule out general cognitive delay or learning disabilities.
- Corroboration of patient reports through

at least one other source who knows the patient well.
- A general medical examination in cases where medication management is anticipated, or where coexisting medical conditions warrant further evaluation and management.

Although the diagnosis of ADHD should always adhere closely to professional criteria, evaluations aimed at documenting disabilities for legal entitlements (such as those afforded under the Americans with Disabilities Act) require special rigor. These assessments should build a particularly tight case for the presence of significant impairment.

✓ Impairment is defined relative to the average person, and not to the individual's general cognitive ability (intelligence) or to some special group of peers (e.g., other graduate students).

REFERENCES

Adler, L. A., Kessler, R. C., & Spencer, T. (2003). *The Adult ADHD Self-Report Scale (ASRS-v1.1) Symptom Checklist.* Geneva, Switzerland: World Health Organization.

Adler, L. A., Spencer, T., & Faraone, S. V. (2003, May). *Validity of patient administered Adult ADHD Self-Report Scale v1.1 to rate adult ADHD symptoms.* Poster presented at the 43rd annual meeting of the New Clinical Drug Evaluation Unit, Boca Raton, FL.

American Psychiatric Association. (2000). *Diagnostic and statistical manual of mental disorders* (4th ed., text rev.). Washington, DC: Author.

Applegate, B., Lahey, B. B., Hart, E. L., Waldman, I., Biederman, J., Hynd, G. W., et al. (1997). Validity of the age-of-onset criterion for ADHD: A report of the DSM-IV field trials. *Journal of American Academy of Child and Adolescent Psychiatry, 36,* 1211–1221.

Barkley, R. A., & Biederman, J. (1997). Toward a broader definition of the age-of-onset criterion for attention-deficit hyperactivity disorder. *Journal of the American Academy of Child and Adolescent Psychiatry, 36*(9), 1204–1210.

Barkley, R. A., Fischer, M., Edelbrock, C. S., & Smallish, L. (1990). The adolescent outcome of hyperactive children diagnosed by research criteria: I. An 8-year prospective follow-up study. *Journal of the American Academy of Child and Adolescent Psychiatry, 29,* 546–555.

Barkley, R. A., Fischer, M., Smallish, L., & Fletcher, K. (2002). The persistence of attention-deficit/hyperactivity disorder into young adulthood as a function of reporting source and definition of disorder. *Journal of Abnormal Psychology, 111,* 279–289.

Barkley, R. A., & Gordon, M. (2002). Research on comorbidity, adaptive functioning, and cognitive impairments in adults with ADHD: Implications for a clinical practice. In S. Goldstein & A. T. Ellison (Eds.), *Clinicians' guide to adult ADHD: Assessment and intervention* (pp. 43–68). San Diego, CA: Academic Press.

Barkley, R. A., & Murphy, K. R. (2006). *Attention-deficit hyperactivity disorder: A clinical workbook* (3rd ed.). New York: Guilford Press.

Barkley, R. A., Murphy, K. R., & Kwasnik, D. (1996). Motor vehicle driving competencies and risks in teens and young adults with ADHD. *Pediatrics, 98,* 1089–1095.

Biederman, J., Faraone, S. V., Spencer, T., Wilens, T. E., Norman, D., Lapey, K. A., et al. (1993). Patterns of psychiatric comorbidity, cognition, and psychosocial functioning in adults with attention deficit hyperactivity disorder. *American Journal of Psychiatry, 150,* 1792–1798.

Biederman, J., Munir, K., Knee, D., Armentano, M., Autor, S., Waternaux, C., et al. (1987). High rate of affective disorders in probands with attention deficit disorders and their relatives: A controlled family study. *American Journal of Psychiatry, 144,* 330–333.

Borland, B. L., & Heckman, H. K. (1976). Hyperactive boys and their brothers: A 25-year follow-up study. *Archives of General Psychiatry, 33,* 669–675.

Conners, C. K. (1995). *The Conners Continuous Performance Test.* North Tonawanda, NY: Multi-Health Systems.

Conners, C. K., & MHS Staff. (2000). *Conners Continuous Performance Test II.* Tonawanda, NY: Multi-Health Systems.

Derogatis, L. R. (1986). *Manual for the Symptom Checklist 90—Revised (SCL-90–R).* Baltimore: Author.

Feldman, S. A., Denhoff, E., & Denhoff, J. I. (1979). The attention disorders and related syndromes: Outcome in adolescence and young adult life. In L. Stern & E. Denhoff (Eds.), *Minimal brain dysfunction: A developmental approach.* New York: Masson.

First, M. B., Spitzer, R. L., Gibbon, M., & Williams, J. B. W. (1997). *Structured Clinical Interview for DSM-IV Axis I Disorders—Clinical Version (SCID-CV).* Washington, DC: American Psychiatric Press.

Fischer, M., Barkley, R. A., Fletcher, K. E., & Smallish, L. (1993). The adolescent outcome of hyperactive children: Predictors of psychiatric, academic, social, and emotional adjustment. *Journal of the American Academy of Child and Adolescent Psychiatry, 32,* 324–332.

Frazier, T. W., Demaree, H. A., & Youngstrom, E. A. (2004). Meta-analysis of intellectual and neuropsychological test performance in attention-deficit/hyperactivity disorder. *Neuropsychology, 18,* 543–555.

Gittelman, R., Mannuzza, S., Shenker, R., & Bonagura, N. (1985). Hyperactive boys almost grown-up. *Archives of General Psychiatry, 42,* 937–947.

Gordon, M. (1983). *The Gordon Diagnostic System.* DeWitt, NY: Gordon Systems.

Gordon, M. (1995). *How to operate an ADHD clinic or subspecialty practice.* Syracuse, NY: GSI.

Gordon, M., Barkley, R. A., & Murphy, K. (1997). ADHD on trial. *ADHD Report, 5*(4), 1–4.

Gordon, M., & Irwin, M. (1996). *ADD/ADHD: A nononsense guide for the primary care physician.* Syracuse, NY: GSI.

Gordon, M., & Keiser, S. (Eds.). (1998). *Accommodations in higher education under the Americans with Disabilities Act (ADA): A no-nonsense guide for clinicians, educators, administrators, and lawyers.* New York: Guilford Press.

Gordon, M., & McClure, F. D. (1995). *The down and dirty guide to adult ADD.* Syracuse, NY: GSI.

Gordon, M., & Murphy, K. R. (1998). Attention-deficit/hyperactivity disorder. In M. Gordon & S. Keiser (Eds.), *Accommodations in higher education under the Americans with Disabilities Act (ADA): A nononsense guide for clinicians, educators, administrators, and lawyers* (pp. 98–129). New York: Guilford Press.

Greenberg, L. M., & Kindschi, C. L. (1996). *T.O.V.A. Test of Variables of Attention: Clinical guide.* St. Paul, MN: TOVA Research Foundation.

Hardt, J., & Rutter, M. (2004). Validity of adult retrospective reports of adverse childhood experiences: Review of the evidence. *Journal of Child Psychology and Psychiatry, 45*(2), 260–273.

Hart, E. L., Lahey, B. B., Loeber, R., Applegate, B., & Frick, P. J. (1995). Developmental changes in attention-deficit hyperactivity disorder in boys: A four-year longitudinal study. *Journal of Abnormal Child Psychology, 23,* 729–750.

Hechtman, L., Weiss, G., & Perlman, T. (1978). Growth and cardiovascular measures in hyperactive individuals as young adults and in matched normal controls. *Canadian Medical Association Journal, 118,* 1247–1250.

Hechtman, L., Weiss, G., & Perlman, T. (1980). Hyperactives as young adults: Self-esteem and social skills. *Canadian Journal of Psychiatry, 25,* 478–483.

Hechtman, L., Weiss, G., Perlman, T., & Tuck, D. (1985). Hyperactives as young adults: Various clinical outcomes. *Adolescent Psychiatry, 9,* 295–306.

Henry, B., Moffitt, T. E., Caspi, A., Langley, J., & Silva, P. A. (1994). On the "remembrance of things past": A longitudinal evaluation of the retrospective method. *Psychological Assessment, 6,* 92–101.

Hervey, A. S., Epstein, J. N., & Curry, J. F. (2004). Neuropsychology of adults with attention-deficit/hyperactivity disorder: A meta-analytic review. *Neuropsychology, 18,* 495–503.

Kessler, R. C., Adler, L., Ames, M., Barkley, R. A., Birnbaum, H., Greenberg, P., et al. (2005). The prevalence and effects of adult attention deficit/hyperactivity disorder on work performance in a nationally representative sample of workers. *Journal of Occupational and Environmental Medicine, 47*, 565–572.

Loney, J., Whaley-Klahn, M. H., Kosier, T., & Conboy, J. (1981). *Hyperactive boys and their brothers at 21: Predictors of aggressive and antisocial outcomes.* Paper presented at the meeting of the Society for Life History Research, Monterey, CA.

Mannuzza, S., Gittelman-Klein, R. G., Bessler, A. A., Malloy, P., & LaPadula, M. (1993). Adult outcome of hyperactive boys: Education achievement, occupational rank, and psychiatric status. *Archives of General Psychiatry, 50*, 565–576.

Mannuzza, S., Klein, R. G., & Klein, D. F. (2002). Accuracy of adult recall of childhood attention deficit hyperactivity disorder. *American Journal of Psychiatry, 159*, 1882–1888.

Matochik, J. A., Rumsey, J. M., Zametkin, A. J., Hamburger, S. D., & Cohen, R. M. (1996). Neuropsychological correlates of familial attention-deficit hyperactivity disorder in adults. *Neuropsychiatry, Neuropsychology, and Behavioral Neurology, 9*, 186–191.

Mendelson, W. B., Johnson, N. E., & Stewart, M. A. (1971). Hyperactive children as teenagers: A follow-up study. *Journal of Nervous and Mental Disease, 153*, 273–279.

Menkes, M. M., Rowe, J. S., & Menkes, J. H. (1967). A twenty-five-year follow-up study on the hyperkinetic child with minimal brain dysfunction. *Pediatrics, 39*, 393–399.

Murphy, K. R. (2004). ADHD documentation requirements for test accommodations under the ADA: Clarifying the confusion. *ADHD Report, 12*(5), 1–5.

Murphy, K. R., & Adler, L. A. (2004). Assessing attention-deficit/hyperactivity disorder in adults: Focus on rating scales. *Journal of Clinical Psychiatry, 65*(Suppl. 3), 12–17.

Murphy, K. R., & Barkley, R. A. (1996). Prevalence of DSM-IV symptoms of ADHD in adult licensed drivers: Implications for clinical diagnosis. *Journal of Attention Disorders, 1*(3), 147–161.

Murphy, K. R., & Gordon, M. (1996). ADHD as a basis for test accommodations: A primer for clinicians. *ADHD Report, 4*(6), 10–11.

Murphy, K. R., Gordon, M., & Barkley, R. A. (2002). To what extent are ADHD symptoms common?: A reanalysis of standardization data from a DSM-IV checklist. *ADHD Report, 8*(3), 1–5.

Murphy, P., & Schachar, R. (2000). Use of self-ratings in the assessment of symptoms of attention deficit hyperactivity disorder in adults. *American Journal of Psychiatry, 157*, 1156–1159.

Rasile, D. A., Berg, J. S., Burright, R. G., & Donovick, P. J. (1995). The relationship between performance on the Gordon Diagnostic System and other measures of attention. *International Journal of Psychology, 30*(1), 35–45.

Ross, D. M., & Ross, S. A. (1976). *Hyperactivity: Research, theory, and action.* New York: Wiley.

Satterfield, J. H., Hoppe, C. M., & Schell, A. M. (1982). A prospective study of delinquency in 110 adolescent boys with attention deficit disorder and 88 normal adolescent boys. *American Journal of Psychiatry, 139*, 795–798.

Saykin, A. J., Gur, R. C., Gur, R. E., Shtasel, D. L., Flannery, K. A., Mozley, L. H., et al. (1995). Normative neuropsychological test performance: Effects of age, education, gender, and ethnicity. *Applied Neuropsychology, 2*(2), 79–88.

Selzer, M. L. (1971). The Michigan Alcoholism Screening Test (MAST): The quest for a new diagnostic instrument. *American Journal of Psychiatry, 127*, 1653–1658.

Wechsler, D. (1997). *Wechsler Adult Intelligence Scale—Third Edition.* San Antonio, TX: Psychological Corporation.

Weiss, G., & Hechtman, L. T. (1993). *Hyperactive children grown up* (2nd ed.). New York: Guilford Press.

Weiss, G., Hechtman, L., Milroy, T., & Perlman, T. (1985). Psychiatric status of hyperactives as adults: A controlled 15-year follow-up of 63 hyperactive children. *Journal of the American Academy of Child Psychiatry, 24*, 211–220.

Weiss, G., Hechtman, L., Perlman, T., Hopkins, J., & Wener, A. (1979). Hyperactive children as young adults: A controlled prospective 10-year follow-up of the psychiatric status of 75 children. *Archives of General Psychiatry, 36*, 675–681.

Weiss, G., Minde, K., Werry, J. S., Douglas, V. I., & Nemeth, E. (1971). Studies on the hyperactive child: VIII. Five year follow-up. *Archives of General Psychiatry, 24*, 409–414.

Wender, P. (1995). *Attention-deficit hyperactivity disorder in adults.* New York: Oxford University Press.

Wilens, T. E., Faraone, S. V., & Biederman, J. (2004). Attention-deficit hyperactivity disorder in adults. *Journal of the American Medical Association, 292*(5), 619–623.

Wilkinson, G. S. (1993). *Wide Range Achievement Test-3.* Wilmington, DE: Wide Range.

Wozniak, J., & Biederman, J. (1994). Prepubertal mania exists and co-exists with ADHD. *ADHD Report, 2*, 5–6.

Wozniak, J., Biederman, J., Kiely, K., Ablon, S., Faraone, S. V., Mundy, E., et al. (1995). Mania-like symptoms suggestive of childhood-onset bipolar disorder in clinically referred children. *Journal of the American Academy of Child and Adolescent Psychiatry, 34*, 867–876.

PART III

TREATMENT

CHAPTER 12

Counseling and Training Parents

ARTHUR D. ANASTOPOULOS
LAURA HENNIS RHOADS
SUZANNE E. FARLEY

Since the publication of the preceding edition of this text, a shift has taken place in the way child health care professionals think about treating children with Attention-Deficit/Hyperactivity Disorder (ADHD). In large part influenced by findings from the Multimodal Treatment of ADHD Study (MTA) (Jensen et al., 2001; Pelham, 1999; Swanson et al., 2002), many clinicians now adhere to the view that using multiple treatments in combination is the most effective way to address the clinical management needs of child populations with ADHD. Although a large number and variety of new medications (see Chapters 17–19, this volume) have arrived on the scene for use in such multimodal interventions, relatively fewer advances have been made with respect to parent training (PT) interventions. That is not to say that PT research has not occurred, or that clinicians have stopped using this approach. On the contrary, PT is alive and well within both research and clinical practice circles. Numerous research studies have established its efficacy and effectiveness for the management of disruptive child behavior in the home (Kazdin, 1997), and specifically ADHD-related behavioral problems (Chronis, Chacko, Fabiano, Wymbs, & Pelham, 2004; Pelham, Wheeler, &

Chronis, 1998). But, as was the case when the preceding edition of this text appeared, the PT research that has been published since that time has been anything but systematic. Consequently, substantive changes in how PT is conceptualized and incorporated into clinical practice have not occurred.

Despite this limitation, most researchers and practitioners continue to regard PT as a treatment option that should be given serious consideration for inclusion in any multimodal intervention program for ADHD. This bias has been, and continues to be, readily apparent in our clinical management approach. To provide a better understanding of why we advocate for this position, we begin by discussing the rationale for including PT as a treatment for children with ADHD. We will first consider a number of theoretical factors that enter into our decision to use PT. We then review many of the clinical circumstances that influence choosing this form of treatment. Further justification for using PT is then provided in the context of a review of pertinent empirical findings. Against this background, we enumerate the details of the PT/parent counseling program that we have employed for a number of years. We subsequently provide a brief case study to illustrate how this program is implemented in a real-world context. At the conclusion of this chapter, we speculate on future directions that PT research may take. In so doing, our hope is to encourage further discussion of how PT interventions can be enhanced to better serve the clinical management needs of the child population with ADHD.

RATIONALE

For any mental disorder, there are usually many different options available for treating the condition. ADHD is no exception. A perusal of the relevant treatment outcome literature quickly reveals that there are many ways to address ADHD-related problems. When faced with a new child referral, many clinicians, especially those early in their training, have a difficult time sorting through the myriad of possible treatments. So how does one decide which treatment or treatments to use? As would be the case for any disorder, determining whether or not to use a particular treatment should be guided by careful consideration of several factors, including (1) the clinician's conceptual understanding of how the disorder arises and is maintained; (2) the manner in which the disorder presents itself clinically across development; and (3) the degree to which research findings support its use. With these parameters in mind, we now discuss the various theoretical, clinical, and empirical considerations that we believe provide justification for including PT in the overall clinical management of ADHD.

Theoretical Considerations

As noted elsewhere in this text, various neurochemical, neurophysiological, and neuroanatomical abnormalities have been implicated in the etiology of ADHD. Genetic mechanisms are thought to be the main pathway by which brain structure and functioning are altered in most cases, while acquired injuries to these pathways may exist in a minority of cases. Working from the assumption that this neurobiological explanation is valid, one could reasonably argue that medical treatments, especially those involving stimulant medications or atomoxetine, are perhaps best suited to treating ADHD. If such is indeed the case, then why would anyone want to consider using PT (or

any other psychosocial treatment, for that matter)?

Ironically, part of the answer to this question may be inferred from recent neuropsychological perspectives that have been taken on this issue. In particular, Barkley and many other experts now view ADHD as a condition characterized by neurologically based deficits in the process known as "behavioral inhibition" (Barkley, 1997a; see also Chapter 2, this volume). There is also accumulating evidence that deficits in executive functioning and self-regulation may also be present (see Chapter 7). To the extent that deficits in behavioral inhibition and executive functioning are central to understanding this disorder, this suggests that children with ADHD will not be very adept at thinking through the consequences of their actions. Such a limitation arises because children with ADHD have less proficient working memory skills, which limit their capacity to reflect back on their learning experiences or to think ahead with respect to future consequences that may follow their behavior. This impaired capacity to regulate behavior relative to time and to anticipate future consequences is of particular relevance here. To the extent that children's awareness of the connection between their behavior and its probable consequences can be increased, greater external control, as well as self-control, over their behavior can be achieved. More so than many other forms of treatment, PT lends itself especially well to meeting this therapeutic objective.

Further theoretical justification stems from a consideration of the apparent relationship that exists among ADHD, Oppositional Defiant Disorder (ODD), and Conduct Disorder (CD) (see Figure 12.1). More specifically, recent findings from the field of developmental psychopathology have implicated the possibility of a developmental pathway leading from ADHD to these comorbid conditions (Loeber, Keenan, Lahey, Green, & Thomas, 1993). If having ADHD greatly increases the risk for developing ODD or CD at a later time, then it would seem to be of utmost clinical importance to begin treatment as soon as possible, to reduce this risk among children not yet affected by these comorbid conditions. Although research of this sort has yet to be conducted, the fact that PT has worked so well with noncompliant children (Forehand & McMahon, 1981) and children with CD (Patterson, 1982) provides an empirical basis for considering its use in such a

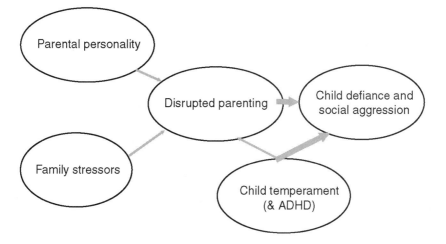

FIGURE 12.1. The four-factor model of child behavior problems. Disrupted parenting is a final common pathway through which parental characteristics, family stress, and even child defiance may further fuel child social aggression and disruptive behavior. ADHD may also make a direct contribution to risk for child defiance and social aggression.

preventive role. Further justification for using PT to target comorbid ODD and CD features stems from a consideration of the fact that environmental factors (e.g., coercive parenting, parental psychopathology, family stress), more so than biological factors, are thought to be intimately involved in the etiology of both conditions. Thus, using PT to address comorbid ODD and CD features is on solid theoretical footing.

Although not yet widely recognized, another conceptually based reason for using PT is that it has the potential to help address problems that exist in attachment security, or emotional bonding between parent and child. Preliminary findings from our own research program (Gerrard & Anastopoulos, 2005) have indicated that children with ADHD display less secure attachment across early childhood than nondisabled controls do. According to many attachment theorists (Ainsworth, Blehar, Waters, & Wall, 1978), such attachment problems, left unchecked, place a child at increased risk for developing a host of psychological problems. Because PT interventions teach parents how to interact with children in more effective and less stressful ways, PT may contribute to improvements in the emotional bonding between a parent and child. This in turn may enhance the overall emotional climate within the family and reduce the likelihood of the child developing the types of long-term problems that have been associated with insecure attachment.

Family systems theory (Minuchin & Fishman, 1981) also seems to have bearing on the use of PT in populations with ADHD. According to this viewpoint, having a child with ADHD places a family at increased risk for disrupted family relationships. These might include, for example, strained alliances between mothers and fathers or between brothers and sisters who treat the sibling affected by ADHD as an outcast. When such circumstances arise, family systems theory would predict that changes in the structure of the family need to occur if family functioning is to improve. To this end, PT may strengthen the alliance between parents by teaching them common ways to parent the child with ADHD. Similarly, cognitive therapy strategies, which are often embedded in PT programs, may be used to alter the way other family members view the child with ADHD—that is, to make them more accepting and tolerant, both of which are necessary conditions for interacting in a more positive fashion.

Clinical and Developmental Considerations

Having ADHD places individuals at risk for a multitude of psychosocial difficulties across the lifespan (Anastopoulos & Shelton, 2001). For example, preschoolers with ADHD place enormous caretaking demands on their parents and frequently display aggressive behavior when interacting with siblings or peers. Difficulties in acquiring academic readiness skills may be evident as well, but these tend to be of less clinical concern than the family or peer problems that preschoolers present. As children with ADHD move into the elementary school years, academic problems take on increasing importance. Together with their ongoing family and peer relationship problems, such school-based difficulties set the stage for the development of low self-esteem and other emotional concerns. Similar problems persist into adolescence, but on a much more intense level. New problems may develop as well (e.g., traffic violations, experimentation with alcohol and drugs), stemming from the increased demands for independence, self-regulation, and self-control that teenagers with ADHD face.

In addition to being affected by its primary symptoms, individuals with ADHD are at increased risk for having secondary or comorbid diagnoses (Jensen, Martin, & Cantwell, 1997). As noted above, ODD is especially common early on, affecting approximately 40% of the preschoolers and elementary school-age children who have ADHD. From 20% to 30% of these children will eventually display secondary features of CD. When ADHD is accompanied by either ODD or CD, there is also an increased risk for depression and anxiety disorders to be present, especially during adolescence. Antisocial Personality Disorder, Major Depressive Disorder, and substance abuse are just a few of the many comorbid problems that may be found among adults with ADHD. In combination with ADHD, such comorbid conditions increase the severity of an individual's overall psychosocial impairment, thereby making the prognosis for such an individual less favorable.

Whether alone or in combination with various comorbid conditions, ADHD can also have a significant impact on the psychosocial functioning of parents and siblings (see Chapter 4). Research has shown, for example, that parents of children with ADHD very often become overly directive and negative in their parenting style. In addition to viewing themselves as less skilled and less knowledgeable in their parenting roles, they may also experience considerable stress in their parenting roles, especially when comorbid features of ODD are present. Parental depression and marital discord may arise as well. Whether these parent and family complications result directly from the child's ADHD is not entirely clear at present. Clinical

experience would suggest that they probably do, at least in part, given the increased caretaking demands that children with ADHD impose on their parents. These include more frequent displays of noncompliance, related to these children's difficulties in following through on parental instructions. In addition, parents of these children often find themselves involved in resolving various school, peer, and sibling difficulties, which occur throughout childhood and into adolescence as well.

In view of its chronicity, pervasiveness, and comorbidity, ADHD is clearly not a condition that lends itself to single treatment approaches. To address all of the problems that children with ADHD so often present, clinicians must employ multiple treatment strategies in combination, each of which addresses a different aspect of these children's psychosocial difficulties.

Although stimulant medication therapy is by far the most commonly used treatment in the clinical management of children with ADHD, 10–20% of those who take such medication do not show clinically significant improvements in their primary ADHD symptomatology (Greenhill, Halperin, & Abikoff, 1999; see also Chapter 17, this volume). Even when a favorable response is obtained, some children experience side effects that are of sufficient frequency and severity to preclude continued use of stimulant medication. Independent of these issues, many parents prefer not to use any form of medication in treating their children. To the extent that there are children with ADHD for whom stimulant medication therapy (or the use of other medications) is not a viable treatment option, alternative treatments must be used. Among these, PT is certainly worthy of further consideration.

PT can also be helpful to children with ADHD who do respond to stimulant medication. For example, in an effort to reduce the risks for insomnia and various other side effects, most physicians limit their stimulant prescriptions to daily dosages whose therapeutic benefits wear off prior to dinnertime. For similar reasons, some physicians further limit children's medication regimens to school days only. What this means from a practical standpoint is that there are substantial portions of any given day, usually in the late afternoon and early evening, when children are not deriving any therapeutic benefits from stimulant medication. For parents and other caretakers, this necessitates finding other means for handling their children's behavioral difficulties in the home. Here again, PT can play a useful role.

Additional justification for utilizing PT stems from a consideration of the potential for comorbidity. As was noted earlier, children with ADHD often display oppositional defiant behavior, aggression, conduct difficulties, and other externalizing problems. Because such secondary features cannot be fully addressed through the use of medication, alternative treatment approaches need to be considered. In view of its highly successful track record with noncompliant children (Kazdin, 1997) and children with CD (Patterson, 1982), PT is well suited to this purpose.

Of additional clinical importance is the fact that raising a child with ADHD can place enormous strains on family functioning. In particular, levels of parenting stress can be quite high, along with a diminished sense of parenting competence (Mash & Johnston, 1990). Such circumstances are not usually due to faulty parenting. On the contrary, the parents of a child with ADHD often use parenting strategies that work just fine for nondisabled siblings in the family. Alerting the parents to this reality begins the process of alleviating their distress. Teaching them more effective ways of dealing with their difficult child, through the use of PT, can also go a long way toward facilitating their own personal adjustment.

Empirical Support

As was true at the time our chapter appeared in the preceding edition of this text, systematic examination of PT's effects on populations with ADHD has continued to be lacking. Across studies, enormous variability exists with respect to the manner in which ADHD has been defined. Even in samples with well-defined ADHD, little attention has been directed to controlling for the many types of comorbid conditions that may be present within this population. Sample sizes have all too often been small in many of the reported studies. In addition to these sampling issues, much variability exists across studies with respect to the PT interventions themselves. By and large, most of these programs trained parents in the use of specialized contingency management techniques, such as positive reinforcement, response cost, and/or time-out strategies. The exact manner in which they implemented these interventions, however, was highly variable. Whereas some adhered to the Barkley (1997b) program, others followed the programs outlined by Cunningham (see Chapter 13, this volume), Patterson (1982), or Forehand and McMahon (1981), for example. Still others combined contingency management training with cognitive therapy strategies and ADHD counseling, aimed at increasing parental acceptance, knowledge, and understanding of ADHD (Anastopoulos, Shelton, DuPaul, & Guevremont, 1993). Most of these interventions utilized weekly therapy sessions. Some were delivered in group formats, while others dealt with individual families. The manner in which PT outcomes has been assessed has also been highly variable, ranging from measuring changes in child behavior, to changes in parenting stress, to changes in other areas of family functioning. Also conspicuously absent from this literature are studies examining the long-term impact of PT. For example, little is known about the extent to which PT-induced changes in parental perceptions of their children serve as a long-term protective factor, reducing the likelihood of any further deterioration in the parent–child relationship. Many other methodological shortcomings and variations could be mentioned as well (see Chronis et al., 2004). The main point to be made, however, is that such methodological differences seriously complicate the process of comparing findings across studies. Consequently, definitive conclusions about what PT can and cannot do are not possible at this time.

Bearing these limitations in mind, we can now state, as we did in our previous chapter, that there is reason to be cautiously optimistic about the efficacy of PT for children with ADHD. Recent reviews of this literature have come to this very same conclusion (Chronis et al., 2004; Farmer, Comptom, Burns,, 2002; McGoey, Eckert, & DuPaul, 2002; Pelham et al., 1998). Along with traditional group-based approaches, many well designed case study reports have appeared in the recent literature, lending further support to the efficacy of PT interventions (Chronis et al., 2001; Danforth, 1999). In addition to producing changes in child behavior, PT interventions have contributed to improvements in various aspects of parental and family functioning, including decreased parenting stress and increased parenting self-esteem (Anastopoulos et al., 1993; Sonuga-Barke, Daley, Thompson, Laver-

Bradbury, & Weeks, 2001; Weinberg, 1999). Following the lead of Pisterman and her colleagues (Pisterman, McGrath, Firestone, & Goodman, et al., 1989; Pisterman et al., 1992), many recently published studies have examined the impact of PT on preschoolers with ADHD (Sonuga-Barke, Daley, & Thompson, 2002; Shelton et al., 2000), thereby emphasizing a more preventive approach. Sonuga-Barke et al. (2002) have also added a new dimension to the PT literature by noting the negative impact that adult ADHD can have on a parent's capacity to benefit from PT interventions.

Information about the efficacy of PT also comes from studies in which this form of treatment was combined with other interventions, such as school-based modifications and social skills training (Shelton et al., 2000). Findings from the recently completed MTA study have further shown that the efficacy of psychosocial treatment depends in large part upon the type and context of the outcome being assessed (Jensen et al., 2001; Pelham, 1999; Swanson et al., 2002). When using changes in primary ADHD symptomatology as a yardstick for therapeutic change, the MTA found that a rigorously controlled medication regimen was equal to or better than either a psychosocial treatment package that included a PT-inclusive component or the combination of medication and the PT-psychosocial treatment package. However, in subsequent analyses that utilized indices of functional impairment (e.g., family functioning) and other ecologically valid measures (e.g., consumer satisfaction) to assess outcome, the combination of medication and the psychosocial treatment package containing PT did produce therapeutic benefits above and beyond those from medication alone. Moreover, certain types of children with ADHD, such as those with comorbid anxiety, also seemed to benefit more from the combination of medication and PT-inclusive psychosocial treatment versus medication alone.

Although the MTA findings are encouraging, many questions about PT remain. Particularly limited is our understanding of how PT works. Most PT programs are multifaceted in nature, typically including some combination of various contingency management techniques and counseling about ADHD. Which of these components might be responsible for the observed therapeutic benefits of PT is not at all clear. Also limited is our knowledge of the scope of PT benefits. Although research has shown that PT brings about improvements in child behavior, parent–child relations, and parent functioning, little is known about its impact on a child's emotional functioning. Even less information is available regarding the role of fathers. What little research there is implies that father involvement in treatment may not enhance the initial benefits of parent training with mothers, but may result in greater maintenance of treatment gains after treatment ends than in father-absent families (Bagner & Eyberg, 2003).

Although not yet published, our own research has produced some interesting preliminary findings pertaining to these unanswered questions. In particular, a therapeutic component analysis was conducted, comparing the effects of a complete PT program (i.e., contingency management plus ADHD counseling; Anastopoulos & Barkley, 1990) versus ADHD counseling alone. It was predicted that both forms of treatment would produce benefits, with the complete PT program clearly being the superior of the two. This study also included child emotional indices as outcome measures, based on the assumption that PT would improve this area of functioning as well. Input from fathers was obtained, with the expectation that their ratings would reflect relatively less therapeutic change than those of mothers.

The sample for this study was drawn from a larger group of 138 clinic-referred children participating in a federally funded project examining comorbidity and ADHD PT outcome. All children carried a diagnosis of ADHD, with half also displaying ODD. Sample selection was further determined by parental psychopathology, with relatively equal numbers of mothers displaying either low or high levels. For the current project, a subsample of 59 children (47 boys, 12 girls) and their parents served as participants. The children ranged in age from 6 to 11 years, with a mean of 106 months. All were of at least average intelligence, with 49% receiving special education services. None was taking medication for behavior management purposes during the active portion of the study. Most were from two-parent (71%), middle-class, European American homes.

Participants were randomly assigned either to a group receiving the complete PT program (n = 35) or ADHD counseling (AC; n = 24).

The PT program followed the 10 steps outlined later in this chapter. The therapeutic goal of the AC program was threefold: to provide basic information about ADHD; to give parents an opportunity to describe how ADHD affected their child and family; and to encourage parents to generate solutions to their child management problems, based on the knowledge they gained. No contingency management training was offered. Both groups received 10 weekly 1-hour individually delivered treatment sessions over the course of 3–4 months. Experienced PhD-level psychologists delivered the treatments in accordance with treatment manuals that had been developed for the project. Treatment integrity was further addressed via expert review of randomly selected audiotapes of the treatment sessions. For both treatment conditions, all of the reviewed tapes met the minimum criteria for adherence (i.e., covering at least 85% of the session outline). Assessment data were gathered prior to, immediately following, and 6 months after treatment.

As expected, knowledge of ADHD increased over time for mothers and fathers in both groups. Also in line with expectations, posttreatment knowledge of behavior management principles was significantly greater for mothers and fathers receiving PT than for parents receiving AC. Mothers and fathers receiving PT also reported using more effective parenting strategies at posttreatment, but these differences were not maintained at follow-up. Contrary to expectations, repeated-measures analyses of the various child, parent, and marital outcome data failed to show significantly better outcomes for PT than for AC. However, a number of nonsignificant trends did emerge, consistently favoring PT over AC. For example, mothers and fathers in PT reported lower rates of ODD symptoms at posttreatment but not at follow-up. Coded observations of mothers in PT interacting with their children revealed lower levels of child inattention and anger at posttreatment. Fathers in PT also reported lower rates of hyperactivity–impulsivity and internalizing symptoms in their children, along with lower levels of parenting stress and greater parenting alliance. Of additional interest is that children in PT reported greater improvement in their self-esteem.

Except for the parental depression and marital satisfaction indices, both groups showed posttreatment improvements on all other par-

ent rating scale measures. The same was true for child self-esteem and for two of the coded behaviors from the mother–child observations (i.e., appropriate parenting, mutual enjoyment). Although the difference was not statistically significant, fewer parents in PT (6%) than in AC (17%) dropped out of treatment.

The obtained findings provided partial support for the study's hypotheses. As expected, PT and AC increased parental knowledge of ADHD. But PT was clearly superior to AC in terms of increasing parents' knowledge of behavior management principles and improving their parenting effectiveness. Although such changes indicated that the experimental manipulation was in fact successful, statistically significant group differences were not evident on any of the child, parent, or family functional outcome measures. Because both treatment groups produced a number of significant improvements over time, it would appear that giving parents' knowledge of ADHD is far more therapeutically beneficial than previously thought. That said, it would be premature to conclude that AC alone is sufficient. Numerous trends in the data consistently pointed toward contingency management training as an important component of PT.

In addition to reducing child behavior problems, there was evidence to suggest that PT produced anticipated changes in the children's emotional functioning. This was seen in terms of parent-reported reductions in internalizing symptomatology and child-reported improvements in self-esteem. We speculate that such changes may stem from increased parental use of positive attending and positive reinforcement strategies, which are emphasized throughout PT.

Contrary to expectations, input from fathers revealed more treatment-related changes in home functioning than did similar input from mothers. The basis for this discrepancy is unclear. At the very least, this difference of parental opinion highlights the need for including fathers' perspectives in subsequent treatment research.

Expectations for Therapeutic Change

Based on the preceding discussion, it should come as no surprise that the therapeutic objective of PT is multifaceted in nature. Not only is the child with ADHD a target for change; so too are his or her parents and other family members.

In terms of child objectives, it would be unreasonable to think that neurologically based ADHD symptoms could be eliminated through the use of an environmentally based treatment such as PT. More realistically, what can be accomplished is greater parental control over such symptoms as they occur in the home. In addition to targeting primary ADHD symptoms, PT can also prevent, reduce, or eliminate secondary features of oppositional defiant behavior or conduct problems that the child may be displaying. To the extent that such behavior problems come under better control, a child with ADHD is likely to be exposed to less failure, frustration, correction, and criticism. Thus, improvements in the child's self-esteem and mood may also ensue.

Parents who receive PT learn a great deal about ADHD. Such knowledge has great potential for altering faulty perceptions of their child and of themselves. Parents also receive supervised instruction and detailed information about behavior management principles, which makes it possible for them to tailor their parenting style to their child's special needs. Together, these changes in parental knowledge of ADHD and contingency management skills can set the stage for greater control over child behavior. This in turn can lead to changes in the emotional quality of the parent–child relationship and in parental psychological adjustment. In two-parent families, there may also be less disagreement over parenting issues, thereby reducing marital/couple tensions. Other tensions within the family (e.g., sibling problems) may lessen as well.

THE PARENT TRAINING PROGRAM

Although there are many ways to conduct PT programs for children with ADHD (Chronis et al., 2004), little is known about their relative efficacy (Newby, Fischer, & Roman, 1991). Thus, it would not be unreasonable to present any one of them to illustrate how PT is applied in clinical practice. For the purposes of this chapter, the one presented here is the one that we have used for a number of years. Originally developed by Barkley (1987), this particular program later underwent minor modifications (Anastopoulos & Barkley, 1990; Barkley, 1997b), a summary of which will be presented below.

Child and Family Considerations

PT is not necessarily appropriate for all children who receive an ADHD diagnosis. At the very least, there needs to be some indication that a child's ADHD is contributing to family difficulties. This need not be limited to hard-to-manage child behavior. It may also encompass elevated levels of parenting stress and other types of family disruption that would benefit from PT intervention. Another limitation is that PT is best suited for parents of children with ADHD between 4 and 12 years of age. Although elements of the program can be adapted for use with adolescents, many teenagers with ADHD do not respond well to PT, primarily because parental control over the meaningful contingencies in their lives decreases dramatically. For teens with ADHD, alternative psychosocial treatments, such as problem-solving communication training (Robin & Foster, 1989; see also Chapter 14, this volume), need to be considered.

A parent's capacity for undergoing PT also needs to be taken into account. Parents who are troubled by significant levels of psychological distress or marital/couple discord may not be good candidates for this form of treatment. Depending on the situation, some parents may need to defer starting PT until such clinical matters are resolved. Others may find it more appropriate to address such problems at the same time that they are participating in PT.

Therapist Qualifications

Delivering PT to parents of children with ADHD might seem to be a relatively easy task. If all that is done is didactic in nature—that is, simply presenting the program to attentive and cooperative parents—then it can be. More often than not, this is not the case. Thus, its delivery typically requires the skills of a qualified therapist.

A professional degree is perhaps the least important of these qualifications. What is of utmost relevance is the depth of a therapist's understanding of ADHD, as well as his or her familiarity with and expertise in using behavior management strategies. Having these skills is especially critical to the success of the program, because a one-size-fits-all approach just doesn't work. Finding ways to tailor PT to fit the needs of individual parents requires a great deal of flexibility and creativity, and these attributes typically come from extensive experience and in-depth knowledge.

Possessing cognitive therapy skills can also play an important role in delivering this form of treatment. Such skills can be used to overcome parental difficulties in utilizing recommended PT strategies and in setting realistic expectations for therapeutic change.

Clinical and Stylistic Considerations

Being cognitive-behavioral in nature, the PT program routinely and systematically incorporates the use of highly specific between-session assignments, which are generally carried out within the home setting. Such assignments in part facilitate parents' acquisition of various observational and monitoring techniques pertinent to their child's behavior. Of additional clinical significance is that they increase the likelihood that acquired parenting skills will generalize from the clinic, where they are learned, to the home setting. Between-session assignments may also serve as a vehicle for indirectly accessing clinically relevant thoughts and feelings, which parents may experience in the process of employing recommended child management tactics. Such information may then be used for cognitive restructuring purposes or for any other aspect of the counseling that is conducted.

Because satisfactory completion of between-session assignments is a critical factor in the outcome of the program, clinicians must take steps to ensure that it occurs. One such step is to send parents home with written handouts, which summarize important in-session and between-session information. At times, it may also be appropriate to have them audiotape treatment sessions. Such recorded information may then be reviewed as often as necessary to clarify clinical points pertinent to the between-session assignment. Should insurmountable problems arise in implementing a particular assignment, parents can also contact the therapist by telephone to solve problems prior to the next regularly scheduled treatment session.

At the start of every session, time is set aside for reviewing parental efforts to carry out between-session assignments. Special attention is typically focused on those assignments related to parental implementation of recommended child management strategies. Refinements in the parents' application of such strategies are made as necessary. When clinicians begin to

sense that parents have acquired a certain level of skill mastery, they shift therapeutic attention to the next treatment step. In this regard, the PT program follows a building-block model, with each step dependent upon successful completion and mastery of the preceding step. Use of such a model affords clinicians ample flexibility in proceeding with treatment at a pace meeting the needs of individual children and their families.

Successful passage through the treatment program also requires close collaboration and cooperation between parents and clinicians. Several clinical and stylistic considerations must be taken into account in achieving this goal. As is the case for any other treatment, clinicians must convey to parents a sense of genuine understanding, caring, respect, and support. At the same time, they must present therapeutic information in ways that are clear and easy to understand. Everyday language should be employed, rather than professional jargon, which may be confusing to many parents. For similar reasons, daily life experiences commonly encountered by children with ADHD and their families should be used as a context for illustrating clinical points that need to be made. Given that parenting children with ADHD can be a very trying and stressful experience, it is sometimes helpful as well to incorporate humor into sessions. Not only does humor allow parents a welcome moment of relief; it can also help them understand and remember clinical information more effectively.

A Socratic style of questioning is also routinely used throughout treatment to foster close collaboration and cooperation. Such questioning generally makes it easier for clinicians to avoid succumbing to professional lecturing, which some parents may find condescending and offensive. It also forces parents to become more actively involved in the treatment process. By responding to questions that lead to therapeutically desirable solutions, parents gain a sense of having reached such solutions on their own. This in turn increases parents' self-esteem and decreases parental dependence on clinicians. Such decreased dependence increases the likelihood that treatment gains will generalize across situations, even when they have not specifically been covered in treatment. Decreased dependence on the therapist can also increase the chances that treatment gains will remain stable after the active portion of the PT program is completed.

Although implementation of these clinical and stylistic considerations can facilitate the therapy process, it does not necessarily guarantee a successful outcome. Even with ongoing clinical supervision, some parents may continue to experience child management difficulties. Such difficulties frequently stem from complications that parents encounter in practicing recommended treatment strategies. These complications might include family illnesses or job schedule changes that arise unexpectedly and interfere with PT efforts. As long as these sorts of complications are not chronic in nature, their impact on the treatment program is minimal, and therefore they do not need to be addressed as a clinical issue. If, on the other hand, they occur more regularly, it may become necessary to postpone completion of the treatment program until after such complications have been resolved.

Forgetfulness, procrastination, and even adult ADHD symptoms can contribute to parental difficulties in practicing recommended parenting skills. When these sorts of problems arise, clinicians may wish to impose appropriate contingencies upon parents as a way of increasing their motivation to incorporate prescribed child management tactics. Withholding treatment sessions until greater compliance is achieved is one method for dealing with this kind of difficulty. Other creative solutions to this type of problem may be used as well (see Barkley, 1997b):

- Proceed no further with training; allow 1 missed assignment if in a group.
- Focus on reasons for noncompliance.
- Consider whether parent needs treatment first.
- Reevaluate parent readiness for change (motivation to participate).
- Establish a "breakage fee" if need be (monetary fines for missed assignments).
- Terminate training if absenteeism is persistent (defined as more than three missed assignments).

As noted earlier in this chapter, parents who maintain negative perceptions of themselves and of their children may find it difficult to employ recommended treatment PT strategies. To the extent that this occurs, counseling should be initiated to help them identify the basis of their faulty thinking. Once they do so, alternative perceptions should be generated and tested.

Presumably, this will lead parents to more accurate appraisals of themselves and of their children, which eventually should facilitate their implementation of prescribed home management strategies.

There are times, of course, when parental difficulties in utilizing specialized child management techniques are not related to improper motivation or to faulty perceptions. Instead, they may be the result of parenting skill deficiencies. An especially effective way of pinpointing such deficiencies is through clinic-based observations of parent–child interactions. Specifically, parents may be asked to implement the intervention strategy in question while being observed through a one-way mirror. This observation allows the clinician to identify any problems that parents may be having in using a particular technique. Feedback about such problems may then be given to parents after the session is completed. Or the clinician may choose to demonstrate proper application of the strategy with the child and then ask the parents to try once again before they depart. In an extension to this approach, parents can wear a "bug-in-the-ear" device (a hearing aid with a radio receiver) while being observed, often from behind a one-way mirror. This device enables clinicians to provide discreet feedback, which parents can use immediately to facilitate their management of their child. As might be expected, such close clinical supervision is usually highly effective in bringing about desired improvements in targeted parenting skills.

Use of any of the supervisory tactics described above does not have to be limited to problematic situations. In some cases, they may be employed throughout all phases of treatment to enhance parental acquisition of the various child management techniques that are part of the program. For many clinicians, this may not be a feasible option, because they do not have access to one-way mirrors or bug-in-the-ear devices. If these resources are not available, other therapeutic strategies may be utilized to enhance parental learning of new child management procedures. For example, clinicians may include in-session modeling and role-playing exercises as part of their therapeutic contact with parents. In addition, they may choose to amplify clinical points by representing them pictorially or graphically, either on a dry-erase board or on a piece of paper; the latter may then be taken home for review.

Treatment Objectives

In broad terms, the therapeutic goals of our PT program are twofold. The first of these involves laying down a foundation of knowledge that will support and enhance the specific skills to be taught; the second of these objectives is to supervise parental acquisition of a wide array of specialized child management skills, tailored to the needs of children with ADHD.

Consistent with the notion that parents' understanding of a disability enhances their ability to manage it, part of our initial objective is to provide parents with a conceptual yet practical foundation of ADHD knowledge. For similar reasons, we also seek to increase parental understanding of behavior management principles, so as to enhance their maintenance of such skills over time and across settings. Upon this knowledge base, the remainder of the program is designed to teach parents in a step-by-step, building-block fashion a number of empirically supported contingency management strategies for dealing with child behavior problems more effectively. To the extent that these objectives are achieved, improvements in child behavior should follow.

Specific Training Steps

Although the PT program typically can be completed in 8–12 sessions in either a group or individual format, it does not confine clinicians to a specific number of treatment sessions that must be followed inflexibly. Instead, it allows clinicians to guide parents through the 10 phases of treatment in a step-by-step fashion, taking as many sessions as necessary to bring about desired therapeutic change. When the program is delivered to individual families, each session typically lasts 1 hour. When it is delivered to multiple families in a group format, 90-minute sessions are commonly used. Regardless of whether an individual or a group format is employed, the same sequence of treatment steps is followed. A summary of these 10 steps appears in Table 12.1.

Before we elaborate on the specifics of each step, it is important to keep in mind that many features of the current program have been discussed in great detail elsewhere (see Barkley, 1997b). Consequently, it is not our intent to provide the equivalent of a technical manual. Instead, what we plan to do is to present summary descriptions of these procedures, so as to give readers a better understanding of the framework that guides us in our implementation of the program.

Step 1: Program Orientation and Overview of ADHD

Following a detailed orientation to the program, an overview of ADHD is presented. This begins with a brief discussion of how ADHD has evolved from earlier diagnostic conceptualizations and labels with which parents may be more familiar (e.g., "ADD," "hyperactivity," "minimal brain dysfunction"). Against this historical background, the core symptoms of ADHD and its currently accepted diagnostic criteria are presented next. Also covered are many of the commonly encountered associated features of ADHD. This is generally followed by a discussion of what is known about the immediate and extended families of children with ADHD. Up-to-date information about the developmental course of this disorder is presented as well. Attention is then directed to etiological concerns. In the context of this discussion, emphasis is placed on the view that for most children, ADHD is a biologically based inborn temperamental style that predisposes them to be inattentive, impulsive, and physically restless. Special efforts are also made to clarify the confusion surrounding the situational variability of this disorder's primary symptoms. The importance of using a multimethod assessment approach is discussed next. In the ensuing treatment discussion, emphasis is placed on the need for taking a multimodal intervention approach.

Presentation of this information should be as brief as possible. This allows parents to focus more attentively upon the main points that need to be made. It is also helpful for clinicians to limit their references to summary statistics and percentages obtained from the population with ADHD as a whole. As so many parents have frankly stated, they are not interested in facts and figures that have little to do with their own child. The more that the presentation relates to a parent's own child, the more likely it is that they will grasp the clinical and theoretical points that need to be made. Another precaution for clinicians to bear in mind as they describe the general population with ADHD is that some parents will incorrectly infer that their child is doomed to a life filled with comorbidity, failure, and misery. For this rea-

TABLE 12.1. Major Components of Barkley's Parent Training (PT) Program

Step 1: Program Orientation and Overview of ADHD

Session Goal and Content:
Present parents with detailed information on ADHD—causes, course, risks, and effective and ineffective treatments.

Step 2: Understanding Parent–Child Relations

Session Goals:
1. Teach parents the causes of disruptive child behavior.
2. Correct misinformation.
3. Identify causes in each family.
4. Address these causes, if possible.
5. Discuss principles of behavior management via antecedent–behavior–consequence model.

Session Content:
• Review events since last contact.
• Have parents discuss their views of causes of disruptive child behavior.
• Introduce four-factor model (see Figure 12.1):
  • Child characteristics.
  • Parent characteristics.
  • Family stress events.
  • Disrupted, coercive parenting.
• Note that the aim of PT is to ameliorate factor 4.

Step 3: Improving Positive Attending Skills

Session Goals:
1. Teach parents the power of positive attending in human relationships.
2. Improve parental methods of attending to child behavior.
3. Encourage parental use of these attending skills at home.
4. Improve parent–child relationship.

Session Content:
• Focus discussion on adult work relations and how powerful the nature of attention can affect those relations.
• Then shift discussion to the way parents currently interact with the child.
• Review handout on attending skills and special time.
• Discuss initial reactions to handout.
• Demonstrate attending skills.
• Have parents practice skills.
• Discuss parental reactions and concerns.

Homework:
• Practice attending skills and "catching child being good" during "special time" play periods.
• Record information on the practice periods.
• Try using attending skills at other times.

Step 4: Extending Positive Attending Skills and Improving Child Compliance

Session Goals:
1. Teach parents to extend positive attending.
2. Teach parents to give effective commands.
3. Teach parents to pay more attention to nondisruptive child behavior (introduce concept of shaping to parents).
4. Increase parental monitoring.

(continued)

TABLE 12.1. *(continued)*

Session Content:
- Review homework.
- Explain extending positive attending to work situations so as to increase compliance.
- As in play, attention should be immediate, genuine, and given throughout the task.
- Discuss situations in which the child interrupts the parents' activities (telephone use, visitors in home, etc.).
- Note how child gets attention for disruption, but not for good behavior.
- Present and discuss handout on increasing independent play.
- Give examples of how to use it.
- Review and discuss parent handout on attending to compliance.
- Then discuss handout on giving effective commands:
  - Heavily praise high compliance to commands initially.
  - Use imperatives, not questions.
  - Go to child, touch, and use eye contact.
  - Have child repeat request.
  - Make complex tasks simpler ones.
  - Make chore cards for multistep tasks.
  - List all steps involved in task on 3×5 file card.
  - Stipulate a time period on the card.
  - Reduce time delays for consequences.
  - Use timers at points of performance.
  - Don't assign multiple tasks at once.
  - Praise the initiation of compliance.
  - Reward throughout the task.
- Discuss parental reactions to handouts.

Homework:
- Continue special play periods.
- Institute giving effective commands.
- Utilize positive attending for compliance to commands and tasks.
- Implement compliance training periods.
- Practice attending to independent play.

Step 5: Establishing a Home Token/Point System

Session Goals:
1. Create a more systematic, predictable, and motivating way for parents to reinforce child compliance.
2. Make child privileges contingent on work.
3. Teach parents the mechanics of setting up a home token or point system.

Session Content:
- Review homework.
- Discuss the need to create an artificial reward program:
  - Reduced intrinsic motivation in ADHD.
  - Need to establish clarity and certainty.
- Review advantages of tokens/points: Powerful, convenient, versatile (rewards can be varied to avoid satiation), systematic.
- Present and review handout.
- Construct list of privileges.
- Create list of chores and tasks; choose some social behaviors as well.
- Choose range of tokens (or points).
- Assign point values to tasks.
- Use two-thirds rule for setting prices.
- Don't forget "bonuses" for extra effort.

(continued)

TABLE 12.1. *(continued)*

- Review important reminders:
  - No use of fines this week.
  - Reward for obeying first commands.
  - No credit or borrowing.
  - Praise when giving tokens/points.
  - Give tokens/points prolifically.

Homework:
- Set the system up within 3 days (use it 8 weeks).
- Bring all charts/notebooks next week.

Step 6: Adding Response Cost
Session Goal:
1. Introduce fines (response cost) for misbehavior.

Session Content:
- Review homework.
- Make adjustments to token/point system.
- Explain use of fines within system.
  - Payment for task is now the fine amount.
  - Explain the 2:1 ratio of rewards to fines.
  - Be careful of punishment spirals.
  - Don't go to fines if child is depressed.

Homework:
- Continue rewarding with poker chips/points.
- Begin taking away poker chips/points for minor misbehavior.

Step 7: Using Time Out
Session Goals:
1. Teach parents to use time out from reinforcement for more serious forms of misbehavior.
2. Determine a backup method if child tries to escape from time out.
3. Select one or two misbehaviors for time out.

Session Content:
- Review handout for time-out methods.
- Prepare parents for impending power struggle.
- Explain the three-step method for giving commands:
  - Give initial command.
  - Give warning.
  - Take child immediately to time out.
- Post a list of household rules.
- Have parents choose a time-out location.
- Explain the three criteria for ending the time-out period:
  - Child has served minimum sentence (1–2 min. × age).
  - Child becomes quiet.
  - Child agrees to comply with the command.
- Have parents select a consequence for escape:
  - Hefty fine within the token system.
  - Increasing time-out period (doubtful).
  - Isolation in a bedroom free of play material.
  - Locking door if escape is attempted.
- Discuss ploys to expect from child in time out.
- Discuss parental reactions to methods.
- Have parents select one or two misbehaviors for time out.

(continued)

TABLE 12.1. *(continued)*

- Role-play time out with child (if available).
- Have parents rehearse with child.
- Discuss whether siblings are to receive time out for misbehavior.

Homework:
- Review time-out restrictions:
  - Only parents implement time out.
  - Parents stay near enough to monitor time out.
  - One parent does not interfere with the other one.
- Employ time out for one or two problems.
- Keep a diary of all time-out use and bring it to next session.

Step 8: Managing Behavior in Public Places

Session Goals:
1. Teach parents "transition planning."
2. Review adjustments to previously taught methods for use in public places.
3. If need be, assist parents in coping with their own emotional reactions that may interfere with managing child in public places (via cognitive restructuring techniques).

Session Content:
- Review homework.
- Discuss kinds of public places in which child is likely to misbehave.
- Note that with this information, parents can become more proactive around public misbehavior—anticipate and plan.
- Distribute and discuss handout on "transition planning."
- Present the four "transition plan" steps to be done before entering a public place:
  1. Set up your three rules.
  2. Establish your incentives.
  3. Review your penalties.
  4. Assign the child something to do.
- Give parents some examples of situations (stores and malls, church/synagogue/mosque, restaurants, car trips, etc.).
- Review the methods to be used in the public place:
  - Identify time-out location.
  - Start rewarding at entry into building.
  - Use praise, touch, and tokens.
- Review substitutes for time out.
- Discuss parental reactions; if needed, introduce cognitive therapy strategies.

Homework:
- Continue using prior methods.
- Take two "training trips" to a store.
- Record trips in a diary.
- Bring the diary to the next session.
- Consider in what other transitions in the home or elsewhere it would be good to use "transition planning."

Step 9: School Issues and Preparing for Termination

Session Goals:
1. Review with parents the nature of any school behavior problems.
2. Train parents in the use of a daily school behavior report card linked to their home token/point system.
3. Extend "transition planning" to other possible problem situations.
4. Encourage parents to consider how to use parenting skills for future problems.
5. Prepare parents for termination.

(continued)

TABLE 12.1. *(continued)*

Session Content:
- Review homework.
- Discuss how to extend "transition planning" to other public and home situations (visitors in the home, car trips, etc.).
- Have parents review any school behavioral problems of this child.
- Review children's rights to special education services and related issues.
- Decide whether using a daily school behavior report card would be helpful.
- If so, give parents the handout, then explain the system.
- Review how to fade out the system when child has succeeded for 4 weeks.
- Review and discuss parental reactions to card system.
- Distribute handout on managing future problems and review.
- Discuss parental reactions.
- Quiz parents about some behavior problems they have not had before. What would they do?
- Schedule booster session.

Homework:
- Meet with the child's teachers to explain the card system, if needed.
- Then explain system to child.
- Institute report card system.
- Continue all prior methods of behavior management.
- Bring in used cards for review at booster session.

Step 10: Booster Session

Session Goals and Content:
- Review status of child and family.
- Discuss problems that remain and how to address.
- Terminate parent training.

son, clinicians must be sure to clarify that (1) what applies to the population with ADHD as a whole does not necessarily apply to any one individual; and (2) outcome is determined by a large number and variety of factors, of which ADHD is just one influence (albeit an important one).

Although it is certainly possible to conduct this first session in a lecture format, most clinicians would agree that its therapeutic impact is much greater when parents have an opportunity to ask questions, to voice their emotional reactions to what they have just heard, and to discuss expectations for the program. Should parents feel overwhelmed by the sheer volume of new information about ADHD, they are reminded that processing such information will occur gradually over time. Should they wish to facilitate their acquisition of such knowledge, they are also alerted to the availability of pertinent texts and websites, and encouraged to review videotaped presentations on the topic. To the extent that parental feelings of shock, guilt, sadness, or anger arise, therapeutic attention must then be directed to addressing such

negative emotions. For this purpose, cognitive restructuring and other cognitive therapy techniques are especially helpful. Similar therapeutic efforts can be utilized to address unrealistic parental expectations for treatment outcome— unrealistic in the sense that changes in child behavior are expected to occur in a rapid, continuous fashion. As an alternative to this viewpoint, clinicians might instead suggest that therapeutic change will occur in a gradual and variable manner. Moreover, they must remind parents that what they learn needs to become part of their everyday parenting style, not just what they do during the treatment program. To the extent that a child's parents can continue to use these skills after the program ends, their chances for bringing about improvements in their child's behavior increase dramatically.

Step 2: Understanding Parent–Child Relations

After reviewing carryover concerns from the previous session, clinicians provide parents with a conceptual framework for understanding deviant parent–child interactions and their therapeutic management. In this context, parents are alerted to four major factors that, in various combinations, can contribute to the emergence and/or maintenance of children's behavioral difficulties. The first of these consists of child characteristics. Along with these characteristics, various parent characteristics are cited as circumstances that can place children at risk for conflict with their parents; additional attention is directed to the goodness of fit between various child and parent characteristics. Stresses impinging upon the family are recognized as well. The way that parents respond to child behavior is also discussed. In particular, attention is directed to explaining how certain parenting styles (e.g., excessive or harsh criticism, inconsistency), though not the cause of ADHD, nevertheless can complicate the management of this disorder and its associated features.

At this point in the session, clinicians provide parents with an overview of general behavior management principles as a way of preparing them for later coverage of specific behavioral techniques. This overview may be introduced with a discussion of how antecedent events, as well as consequences, can be altered to modify children's behavior. Included as part of this discussion are different types of positive reinforcement, ignoring, and punishment strategies; the need for using such consequences in combination; and the advantages of dispensing them in a specific, immediate, and consistent fashion. Special attention is also directed to the role played by negative reinforcement via the request–noncompliance cycle—that is, the cycle of multiple parental requests following multiple instances of child noncompliance, which generally leads to escalating emotions and coercive interactions, not to mention an increased likelihood of further noncompliance from the child.

Step 3: Improving Positive Attending Skills

The third step begins with a discussion of the importance of attending positively to individuals of any age. Because children with ADHD frequently engage in aversive behaviors, many parents prefer not to interact with them. When parent–child interactions do occur, parents often assume that negative child behavior will arise and therefore adopt a parenting style that is overly directive, corrective, coercive, or unpleasant. This in turn contributes to the chil-

dren's becoming even less willing to behave in a compliant manner. For reasons such as these, the "special time" assignment is presented. Unlike other types of special time, which simply involve setting aside time with a child, special time in this program requires that parents remain as nondirective and as noncorrective as possible. Doing so allows them to see their child's behavior in a different light—in particular allowing them the opportunity to "catch the child being good." This, of course, leads to opportunities to attend positively to the child, which in turn helps to rebuild positive parent–child relations. Those who have tried special time are well aware of how difficult it is to do. This difficulty, along with various other complications (e.g., busy daily schedules), is called to the attention of parents for the purpose of setting realistic expectations for its implementation. To be sure that parents get sufficient practice, they are encouraged to catch their children being good, not just during special time, but throughout the day as well. Such spontaneous opportunities can be used for increasing the amount of positive attention that children receive.

Step 4: Extending Positive Attending Skills and Improving Child Compliance

Once it is clear that parents have become sufficiently adept at using positive attending strategies in the context of special time, it becomes possible to expand these skills to other situations. In particular, parents are taught how to use positive attending to increase independent play while the parents are engaged in home activities, such as talking on the telephone, preparing dinner, or visiting with company. Positive attending skills may also be applied to parental command situations. Although most parents have little trouble pointing out the various ways in which children with ADHD do not comply with their requests, it is much harder for them to identify request situations that elicit compliance. Some even get to the point of believing that their child "does nothing that I ask him [or her] to do." Although it is certainly true that children with ADHD are frequently noncompliant, it is equally important for parents to recognize an unintentional tendency on their part to ignore instances of compliance when they occur. In cognitive therapy terms, parents are selectively attending to the negative aspects of their child's responses to their requests. In behavior therapy terms, they are discouraging compliance through their ignoring, and encouraging noncompliance through their attention to it. Against this background, clinicians point out the importance of paying positive attention to children whenever they are compliant. In addition, parents are advised to set the stage for practicing their use of such positive attending skills, by issuing brief sequences of simple household commands that have a high probability of eliciting compliance from their child.

The final topic for this step is the manner in which commands are given. Verbal and nonverbal parameters of how parents communicate commands to children are examined. This includes coverage of the following recommendations: that parents only issue commands they intend to follow through on; that commands take the form of direct statements rather than questions; that commands be relatively simple; that they be issued in the absence of outside distractions, and only when direct eye contact is being made with the child, so as to increase the likelihood of the child's attending to such instructions; and that commands be repeated back to the parents, so as to give them an opportunity to clarify any misunderstanding before the child responds.

Step 5: Establishing a Home Token/Point System

Setting up a reward-oriented home token system is the focus of this step. Such a system provides children with ADHD with the external motivation they need to complete parent-requested activities that may be of little intrinsic interest and/or may provide a trigger for their defiance. Another reason for using such a system is that positive attending and ignoring strategies are often insufficient for managing children with ADHD, who generally require more concrete and meaningful rewards.

Following review and refinement of the therapeutic skills taught in steps 3 and 4, clinicians embark on a somewhat philosophical, yet practical, discussion of children's rights versus their privileges. Such a discussion often serves to alert parents to how they have inadvertently been treating many of their child's privileges as if they were rights. This in turn makes it easier to set up the home-based poker chip or point system described below.

Parents are initially asked to generate two lists: one list of daily, weekly, and long-range privileges that are likely to be interesting and motivating to the child; the other list pertaining to regular chores and/or household rules that parents would like done better. Such target behaviors should include not only instances of noncompliance and defiance, but also those situations where a child doesn't follow through because of loss of interest, distractions, and other ADHD symptoms. Upon returning home, parents may wish to incorporate input from the child as to any other items that should be included in these lists.

Point values are then assigned to items on each list. For children 9 years old and under, plastic poker chips are used as tokens. Earned poker chips are collected and stored in a home "bank" that a child has set aside specifically for that purpose. For 9- to 11-year-old children, points are used in place of chips and are monitored in a checkbook register or some other type of notebook of interest to a youngster. Generally speaking, children can earn predetermined numbers of poker chips or points for complying with initial parent requests and for completing assigned tasks, which previously may have been left incomplete due to lack of interest in or motivation for doing them. In addition, parents can dispense bonus chips or points for especially well-done chores or independent displays of appropriate behavior. At no time, however, should chips or points be taken away for noncompliance in this phase of the training program. Instead, encountered noncompliance should be handled in the same way that parents have dealt with such situations previously.

Parental motivation, which may have been quite high up until now, may begin to waver for several reasons. Some parents may once again tell us, "I've done something like this before, and it doesn't work." As described earlier, cognitive therapy strategies may be used to correct this type of faulty thinking, which has the potential to interfere with parental efforts to institute a home token system.

Step 6: Adding Response Cost

The sixth session begins with a careful review of parental efforts to implement the home token system. Because problems inevitably arise, most of this session is set aside for clarifying confusion where needed and for making suggestions for increasing the effectiveness of this system.

Following this discussion, the response cost technique is introduced, which represents the first time in the treatment program that a penalty or punishment approach has been considered for use. More specifically, parents are instructed to begin deducting poker chips or points for noncompliance with one or two particularly troublesome requests on the list. Similar penalties may be used for one or two "don't" behaviors—for instance, "don't hit," "don't talk back"—that may be added to the program. At this stage, not only does a child with ADHD fail to earn chips or points that would have resulted from compliance; previously earned chips or points are now also removed from the bank for displays of noncompliance. The number of chips or points lost is equal to the number of chips or points that would have been gained, had compliance occurred. For many children with ADHD, who over the past week may have learned how to expend minimal effort to get the privileges that they desire, adding a response cost component to their token system often increases their overall level of compliance with parental requests, because they now have the additional incentive of trying not to lose what they have already earned. Clinicians also routinely caution parents to avoid getting into punishment spirals, whereby so many chips are taken away that a debt is incurred. If needed, backup penalties, such as time out, can be employed instead.

Step 7: Using Time Out

After reviewing the home token system and making whatever adjustments are deemed necessary, clinicians begin discussing "time out from reinforcement," or simply "time out." Although most types of noncompliance will continue to be handled via response cost, parents are encouraged to identify one or two especially resistant or serious types of noncompliance or rule violations (e.g., hitting a sibling) that may become the targets of time out. Once these are identified, attention is then focused on teaching the mechanics of implementing the time-out procedure. Like the token system, time out is a rather difficult technique to employ. Its use must be explained very carefully before parents are asked to practice it at home.

Critical to the success of this technique is that three conditions must be met prior to releasing a youngster from time out. First, the child must serve a minimum amount of time,

generally equal in minutes to the number of years in his or her age. Once this condition is met, parents may approach the time-out area only when the child has been quiet for a brief period of time. This, of course, avoids the problem of inadvertently dispensing parental attention for inappropriate behavior. Next, and perhaps most importantly, parents must reissue the request or command that initially led the youngster to be placed into time out. In cases where the child does not comply with the reissued directive, the entire three-step time-out cycle is repeated as many times as is necessary, until compliance is achieved. In other words, under no circumstances does the child avoid doing what was asked.

In addition to covering these facets of time out, clinicians routinely address other aspects of this procedure, including how to select a location for serving time out and what to do if the child defiantly leaves the time-out area. Because time out is a strategy that usually has been tried in one form or another, many parents have firm beliefs about its potential for success or lack thereof. Such biases therefore will need to be addressed via cognitive restructuring techniques.

Step 8: Managing Behavior in Public Places

Once the home-based program is running relatively smoothly, attention is then directed to a discussion of settings outside the home in which problem behaviors arise. Among the many settings that are often identified by parents as problematic are grocery stores, department stores, malls, movie theaters, restaurants, and places of worship (churches, synagogues, mosques, etc.). Disciplinary strategies previously employed in such settings are reviewed and analyzed in terms of their overall ineffectiveness.

Against this background, the importance of anticipating such problems in public is discussed. In particular, parents are advised to have a plan of action before entering a predictably problematic public situation. This may be accomplished as follows. First, parents must review their expectations for the child's behavior in this setting. Next, they must establish some incentive for compliance with these rules. Finally, they must specify what types of punishment will be applied, should noncompliance with these rules ensue. Of equal importance to the success of this plan is to have the child state his or her understanding of these rules and consequences prior to entering the public situation. This allows parents an opportunity to clarify any misunderstanding on the child's part that may result from confusion or from inattentiveness.

Generally speaking, modified versions of the strategies used successfully within the home are incorporated into this plan. Unfortunately, many parents are less than enthusiastic about experimenting with these techniques in public places. The perceived threat of public embarrassment is often cited: After all, "what will people think?" The mind-reading aspects of this particular situation are highlighted as the basis for the parents' jumping to such a conclusion. Alternative viewpoints of what people might think, and the relative importance of what others think when it pertains to their child's welfare, are discussed. Addressing parental perceptions of this situation in this manner generally makes it possible to reduce their uneasiness and to increase their motivation for trying such a new and challenging approach.

Step 9: School Issues and Preparing for Termination

The ninth step serves many purposes: to increase parental knowledge of relevant school issues; to discuss how to handle future problems that might arise; and to begin preparing for termination, including instructions on how to fade out the home-based program. In addition to reviewing and fine-tuning parental efforts to deal with problem behavior in public places, clinicians review and refine all other aspects of the training program. Parental feedback about the training program may be elicited at this time as well. Such comments often serve as a backdrop against which handling of future behavior problems may be discussed.

An important feature of this session is to discuss the child's current school status, including what modifications (if any) are being employed to deal with his or her ADHD. This is followed by a description of the legal rights of children with ADHD within the school system. Emphasis is placed on the child's being placed in the least restrictive educational environment. How and when to consider special education accommodations is covered as well. Independent of placement issues, parents receive numerous suggestions for modifying their child's classroom environment to accommodate the ADHD. Throughout this discussion, parents are strongly encouraged to work with school personnel in as collaborative and cooperative a manner as possible. It is in this spirit that particular attention is directed to the mechanics of setting up a daily report card system, in which home-based consequences are used in conjunction with written daily feedback from the teacher. Figure 12.2 is one example of such a card (see Barkley, 1997b, for several other versions; see also Chapter 14). The card is then reviewed at home, and points are awarded for the various ratings that the teachers have pro-

Subjects	1	2	3	4	5	6	7
Participates in class							
Performs assigned classwork							
Follows class rules							
Gets along well with others							
Completes homework assignments							
Teacher's initials							

FIGURE 12.2. An example of a daily behavior report card for monitoring behavior at school. Each teacher rates each behavior at end of each class: 1 = "excellent" (+25); 2 = "good" (+15); 3 = "fair" (+5); 4 = "poor" (−15); 5 = "terrible" (−25).

vided. These points can then be spent within the home point system discussed above.

Parents also discuss what they believe might be problematic for them in the future and how they might handle such problematic situations. Attention is then directed to the various ways in which many parents slip away from adherence to this program. Although some degree of slippage or departure from the protocol is acceptable, and in fact encouraged, too much may lead to increased behavioral difficulties. For this reason, parents are informed how to run a check on themselves to ascertain where fine-tuning of their specialized child management skills is required. A written handout summarizing this self-check system is distributed at this time.

The final portion of this session is used to address termination and/or disposition issues. In addition to agreeing upon an appropriate booster session date, clinicians discuss with parents whether any other types of clinical services are needed. These might include, for example, adding a medication component or scheduling school consultation visits to address classroom management concerns directly with school personnel.

Step 10: Booster Session

Although any length of time may be deemed acceptable, it is customary to meet with parents for a booster session approximately 1 month after conducting step 9. One objective of this session is to readminister pertinent child behavior and parent self-report rating scales and questionnaires, which serve as indices of any posttreatment changes that may have occurred. Further review and refinement of previously learned intervention strategies are conducted as well. Also established at this time is a mutually agreed-upon final clinical disposition. If desired, this may include scheduling of additional booster sessions.

CASE EXAMPLE: DAVID G.

A case example is now presented to illustrate how this empirically supported PT approach can be implemented in a real-world setting. To ensure confidentiality, fictitious names have been used, and all information that potentially could identify the child and his family has been either removed or altered.

Reason for Referral

At the time clinical services were sought, David G., a European American male, was 9 years old and enrolled in a regular fourth-grade classroom. He was initially referred for services by his parents who, along with his teachers, were concerned about his long-standing home and school difficulties. These included problems getting along with his family and friends, diminished self-esteem, and not working up to his academic potential.

Background Information

David's developmental history was unremarkable. He had been in good health throughout his lifetime. He had not taken any prescription medications for behavior management purposes or for any other reason. He and his two younger half-siblings lived with their parents in a home where the family had resided for more than a year. David maintained typical relations with his siblings, neither of whom had any major medical, behavioral, or learning problems. Mr. and Mrs. G. had been together for nearly 7 years but married for only the past 3. Their relationship was generally stable, with no history of major marital difficulties. No recent psychosocial stressors had occurred. Although there was no extended family history of ADHD, several maternal relatives had displayed conduct problems and antisocial behavior, as well as learning disorders. Throughout his schooling, David's performance had varied from grade level to somewhat below grade level in all facets of his academic work. Moreover, the quality and quantity of his work were highly variable from day to day. Both his parents and his teachers believed that his academic achievement was well below his intellectual potential.

Despite such long-standing concerns, David had never undergone school based testing or received psychological testing. He carried no prior diagnoses and had never received any ongoing psychotherapy or special education assistance.

Assessment Process

Prior to embarking on a course of treatment, David underwent a formal psychological evaluation. In particular, a comprehensive multimethod assessment was performed (Anastopoulos & Shelton, 2001) to capture the situational variability of David's ADHD, as well as its comorbid features and impact on home, school, and social functioning. This included not only the traditional methods of parent and child interviews, but also standardized child behavior rating scales, parent self-report measures pertaining to personal and family functioning, clinic-based psychological testing, and a review of prior medical and school records.

Diagnostic Conceptualization

David met *Diagnostic and Statistical Manual of Mental Disorders*, fourth edition, text revision (DSM-IV-TR) criteria for a diagnosis of ADHD, Combined Type. In addition, it was quite clear that he met DSM-IV-TR criteria for a secondary diagnosis of ODD. Together, these conditions were very likely to be responsible for the elevated parenting stress reported by his parents, his diminished academic productivity, the significant gap between his predicted and actual levels of educational achievement, and his peer relationship difficulties. No other major diagnostic concerns emerged from this evaluation. However, there was evidence to suggest that symptoms of depression and anxiety might be emerging. In addition to these child concerns, there was reason to believe that Mrs. G. might be having adult ADHD difficulties, as well as mild depressive symptoms and other types of psychological distress.

Treatment Plan

Given the multiple problems inherent in David's clinical presentation, it was quite clear that no one treatment could address all of his clinical management needs. Thus, a multimodal treatment plan, incorporating a combination of intervention strategies that has recently received empirical support (Jensen et al., 2001), was adopted. This plan included a trial of stimulant medication, classroom modifications, and home management strategies, as well as individual counseling for Mrs. G.

In view of the fact that David was also displaying mild symptoms of depression and anxiety, as well as peer relationship problems, Mr. and Mrs. G. were advised to monitor his status in these areas. Direct treatment of these problem areas was deferred, however, because there was reason to believe that these difficulties might be secondary manifestations of David's primary ADHD and ODD symptoms. More specifically, it was assumed that as the above-described treatments brought his primary ADHD and ODD symptoms under better control, concomitant improvements in his emotional and social functioning would be likely to ensue.

Course of Treatment

To deal with David's ADHD symptoms both at home and in school, a trial of stimulant medication was recommended. Concurrent with David's medication trial, numerous school-based changes were introduced to create classroom conditions that would further reduce the impact of his ADHD, thereby maximizing his academic performance. In order to deal with David's ADHD and ODD problems in the home, which were identified by his parents as a priority for treatment, Mr. and Mrs. G. began receiving training in the use of specialized behavior management strategies tailored to the needs of children with ADHD. This was accomplished in the context of our 9-week, clinic-based PT program.

Goals during the first session were to acquaint Mr. and Mrs. G. with the mechanics of participating in the treatment program, to increase their knowledge of ADHD, and to set appropriate expectations for therapeutic change. During the second session, Mr. and Mrs. G. learned about the four-factor model for understanding parent–child conflict and gained knowledge of behavior management principles as they apply to children with ADHD.

The main objective of session 3 was to begin teaching Mr. and Mrs. G. positive attending and ignoring skills in the context of special time. In particular, they were encouraged to "catch David being good" as often as possible, so as to see him in a different, more realistic, and more positive light. Doing so, of course, helped establish more positive parent–child relations.

During the next session, Mr. and Mrs. G. learned how to extend positive attending skills to other situations, including times when David was displaying appropriate behavior that allowed Mr. and Mrs. G. to engage in activities without interruption. Like many other children with ADHD, David often became disruptive when his parents were engaged in home activities, such as talking on the telephone, preparing dinner, or visiting with company. Why? Presumably because children with ADHD have trouble waiting for things and delaying gratification, they frequently interrupt. After calling attention to the fact that most parents generally do not hesitate to stop an ongoing activity to address these disruptions, the following questions were posed: Should Mr. and Mrs. G. stop what they were doing to attend positively to David when he was engaged in independent play that was not disruptive? Like most parents, Mr. and Mrs. G. did not think so, citing a "let sleeping dogs lie" philosophy as their rationale. This assumption was first examined from a cognitive therapy perspective—as an example of jumping to conclusions (in this case, predicting a negative outcome). Mr. and Mrs. G. were then asked how certain they were that dispensing positive attention in this manner would be disruptive. They stated that they were pretty sure, but not 100%. While acknowledging that they might in fact be correct in their prediction, the clinician also pointed out that they might not be. Until their "sleeping dogs" philosophy was empirically tested against an alternative hypothesis, it could neither be confirmed or disconfirmed. Additional justification for testing these competing assumptions was inferred from what was learned earlier in the review of general behavior management principles—namely, that when any behavior is ignored, this decreases its probability of occurring. This in turn increases the likelihood that various disruptive behaviors will develop inadvertently. If attended to positively, however, independent play is much more likely to reappear in the future. With some degree of trepidation, Mr. and Mrs. G. agreed to test these competing hypotheses. As so often happens, they came back the following week with good news to report. Illustrative of their success, Mr. G. reported that he had actually read the newspaper uninterrupted for the first time in many years!

Establishing a reward-oriented home token system was the major focus of session 5. The intent of such a system was to provide David with the external motivation he needed to complete parent-requested activities that might be of little intrinsic interest to him and that served to trigger his defiance. Mr. and Mrs. G.'s confidence and motivation, which had been increasing, began to waver at the start of this session. Like many parents, they believed that they had "already done something like this before, and that it just doesn't work." These overgen-

eralizations were addressed by asking them to provide a detailed description of the techniques they had used. Against this background, the details of the current home token system were presented, and the differences between it and their previous attempts were emphasized. Although this information did not immediately convince Mr. and Mrs. G. that this new approach would work, they became more receptive to the idea that alternative approaches might exist. Consequently, they were willing to try the recommended home token system, which ultimately brought about major improvements in David's home behavior.

The primary purpose of session 6 was to refine the home token system, including the addition of response cost strategies for minor misbehavior. More specifically, Mr. and Mrs. G. were instructed to begin deducting poker chips for noncompliance with one or two requests. Similar penalties were introduced to address problematic behaviors, including physical aggression and talking back. Another punishment strategy was added during the seventh therapy session: Mr. and Mrs. G. learned how to use a version of time out for dealing with more serious forms of noncompliance. As had been the case for the home token system, Mr. and Mrs. G. had unsuccessfully used a variation of the time-out strategy in the past. Their negative expectations were addressed via the same type of cognitive restructuring techniques that had been used to deal with their reluctance to using the home poker chip system.

Although David's behavior had improved, treatment effects rarely generalize to new settings without planning and effort. With this in mind, the purpose of session 8 was to begin expanding Mr. and Mrs. G.'s use of the behavior management program to settings outside the home. Among the settings that were identified as problematic for David were department stores and restaurants. Modified versions of the strategies that had been used successfully at home were incorporated into this plan. In contrast to their eagerness to use behavior management techniques at home, Mr. and Mrs. G. were much less enthusiastic about implementing these techniques in public. After all, they noted, "what will people think?" Such mind reading, a common cognitive distortion, was highlighted as the basis for their reaching a negative conclusion. Alternative viewpoints as to what people might think, and the importance they were attaching to others' opinions as these pertained to David's welfare, were discussed. Addressing the parents' perceptions in this manner reduced their uneasiness, thereby increasing their motivation for trying such a new and challenging approach.

The ninth session served many purposes: to increase Mr. and Mrs. G.'s knowledge of relevant school issues; to discuss how to handle future problems that might arise, and to begin preparing for termination, including instructions on how to fade out the home-based behavior management program. Given how well they had acquired the knowledge and skills of this program, Mr. and Mrs. G. agreed that termination from this phase of the multimodal treatment program was in order.

Although the contingency management system worked well for several weeks following termination, David eventually began to display some resistance, and his behavior began to deteriorate. This led Mr. and Mrs. G. to the erroneous conclusion that the program had not worked. During a follow-up telephone consultation, it was pointed out that this was not an unusual occurrence for children with ADHD, given the facts that they tend to become bored easily and that specific rewards may lose their salience over time. The parents were encouraged to make minor modifications in David's contingency management system, so as to increase its novelty, salience, and meaningfulness. It was hypothesized that doing so would increase his interest in the program. When put to the test, this prediction was supported.

After several months, it was clear that the combination of stimulant medication therapy, parent training, and school-based modifications had brought about many improvements in David's psychosocial functioning. Of additional importance was that David's parents reported feeling less stress and guilt in their roles as parents. Moreover, both parents indicated that they had learned to view and to accept David's ADHD in a different light. This in turn reduced the disagreements they themselves had over parenting issues. Equally important, David seemed to be happier and more involved in social activities with peers. Had the opposite outcome scenario unfolded—that is, had there been no concomitant improvements in his emotional and social functioning—it would then have been necessary to consider targeting these emotional and social areas more directly

through the use of individual therapy and school-based social skills training, respectively.

Although not directly related to the management of David's ADHD, one last aspect of this case bears mentioning. Because there was evidence that Mrs. G. might be experiencing mild depression, as well as adult ADHD problems, these possibilities too needed to be addressed. Thus, a recommendation was made for her to undergo further evaluation and to begin receiving treatment as needed. To her credit, she followed through on these recommendations. Through a combination of cognitive therapy and stimulant medication, she was able to bring about improvements in her depression and ADHD symptoms. This not only served to alleviate her personal distress, but also allowed her to implement her newly acquired PT techniques and other aspects of David's treatment plan more effectively.

CONCLUSIONS

PT is frequently used in the treatment of children with ADHD. Although many variations of PT exist, all share a common therapeutic objective—namely, to teach parents specialized child management techniques. Some PT programs, such as the one described in this chapter, incorporate additional therapeutic components that systematically provide parents with factual information about ADHD and utilize cognitive therapy techniques to facilitate parental acceptance, understanding, and management of the disorder.

One of the major advantages of using PT is that it can be used to target not only the child's primary ADHD symptoms, but also many comorbid features that may be present or emerging, including oppositional defiant behavior and conduct problems. Moreover, because PT interventions utilize parents as co-therapists, many parents themselves derive indirect therapeutic benefits from their involvement in treatment. Although it remains to be seen what the long-term impact of PT interventions may be, preliminary evidence would seem to suggest that treatment-induced improvements in psychosocial functioning can be maintained in the absence of ongoing therapist contact, at least in the short run.

As noted earlier, much of the research to date has focused on the clinical efficacy of PT interventions when used alone. One benefit of pursuing this type of research is that it has allowed for a better understanding of the unique impact this form of treatment can have on outcome in a population with ADHD. Examining PT by itself has also provided important insight into its therapeutic limitations, including the fact that not everyone benefits from PT.

Although early multimodal treatment studies suggested that PT does not produce therapeutic benefits above and beyond that accounted for by medication, the recently reported MTA findings have shown that the combination of medication and psychosocial treatment that includes a PT component is superior to medication alone for certain types of outcomes (e.g., family functioning) and for certain types of children (e.g., with comorbid anxiety) and families (of lower socioeconomic status). Thus, what remains to be clarified is not so much whether PT is an efficacious treatment for ADHD. Rather, it would seem timely for the field to begin conducting research that addresses this question: For which children and for which outcomes is the combination of medication and PT best suited? (Chronis et al., 2004).

As suggested by our own preliminary findings and those of others (Sonuga-Barke et al., 2001), one fruitful area for future research would be to continue exploring the beneficial impact that PT has so far been shown to have on the emotional climate in a family. In addition to addressing the emotional well-being of the parent and child, such research could potentially examine changes in the emotional well-being of other family members, particularly in terms of the emotional connection that characterizes the parent–child relationship. Anecdotal clinical evidence consistently suggests that parents and children like each other much more after PT interventions. The long-term benefits of such improved parent–child relations cannot be underestimated. Therefore, efforts to determine empirically whether PT produces changes in the emotional bonding between parents and children would appear to be in order.

In sum, much remains to be learned about the role that PT can play in multimodal intervention programs for treating ADHD. In the meantime, based upon a consideration of the various clinical, theoretical, and empirical issues presented in this chapter, there should be little doubt that PT does have a place in the overall clinical management of ADHD.

KEY CLINICAL POINTS

✓ Parent training (PT) is an effective treatment for the reduction of parent–child conflict, child defiance, related disruptive behavior, and (to a lesser extent) ADHD symptoms in clinically referred children diagnosed with ADHD.

✓ PT may add some benefit to medication treatments for selective subsets of the general population with ADHD, including families of low socioeconomic status, families of children whose ADHD is comorbid with anxiety, and families of children whose ADHD symptoms are more severe than usual.

✓ Parenting stress is often reduced by PT, and some evidence now suggests that both parents' and children's sense of well-being may also be enhanced.

✓ Father involvement in PT does not seem to result in enhancement of training effects, but does appear to increase the maintenance of those effects after treatment termination.

✓ PT also enhances parental knowledge about ADHD, which can result in significant beneficial changes in child and parent behavior in its own right.

✓ Most PT programs involve various methods of contingency management, including proactive tactics such as improving the effectiveness of commands, transition planning, and altering tasks and settings to be more conducive to performance by children with ADHD. Reactive tactics are also included, such as positive attending, token or point systems, response cost, and time out from reinforcement. Monitoring programs, such as daily school behavior report cards, can also be included for tracking and responding to child behavior when away from home.

✓ Parental ADHD may have an adverse impact on PT, and may require treatment prior to or commensurate with PT for child ADHD and related disruptive behavior to enhance the effectiveness of PT.

REFERENCES

Ainsworth, M., Blehar, M., Waters, E., & Wall, S. (1978). *Patterns of attachment: A psychological study of the Strange Situation.* Hillsdale, NJ: Erlblaum.

Anastopoulos, A. D., & Barkley, R. A. (1990). Counseling and training parents. In R. A. Barkley, *Attention deficit hyperactivity disorder: A handbook for diagnosis and treatment.* New York: Guilford Press.

Anastopoulos, A. D., & Shelton, T. L. (2001). *Assessing attention-deficit/hyperactivity disorder.* New York: Kluwer Academic/Plenum.

Anastopoulos, A. D., Shelton, T. L., DuPaul, G. J., & Guevremont, D. C. (1993). Parent training for attention-deficit hyperactivity disorder: Its impact on parent functioning. *Journal of Abnormal Child Psychology, 21,* 581–596.

Bagner, D. M., & Eyberg, S. M. (2003). Father involvement in parent training: When does it matter? *Journal of Clinical Child and Adolescent Psychology, 32,* 599–605.

Barkley, R. A. (1987). *Defiant children: A clinician's manual for parent training.* New York: Guilford Press.

Barkley, R. A. (1997a). *ADHD and the nature of self-control.* New York: Guilford Press.

Barkley, R. A. (1997b). *Defiant children: A clinician's manual for parent training* (2nd ed.). New York: Guilford Press.

Chronis, A. M., Chacko, A., Fabiano, G. A., Wymbs, B. T., & Pelham, W. E., Jr. (2004). Enhancements to the behavioral parent training paradigm for families of children with ADHD: Review and future directions. *Clinical Child and Family Psychology Review, 7,* 1–27.

Chronis, A. M., Fabiano, G. A., Gnagy, E. M., Wymbs, B. T., Burrows-MacLean, L., & Pelham, W. E. (2001). Comprehensive, sustained behavioral and pharmacological treatment for attention deficit/hyperactivity disorder: A case study. *Cognitive and Behavioral Practice, 8,* 346–358.

Danforth, J. S. (1999). The outcome of parent training using the Behavior Management Flow Chart with a mother and her twin boys with oppositional defiant disorder and attention-deficit hyperactivity disorder. *Child and Family Behavior Therapy, 21,* 59–80.

Farmer, E. M., Compton, S. N., Burns, J. B., & Robertson, E. (2002). Review of the evidence base for treatment of childhood psychopathology: Externalizing disorders. *Journal of Consulting and Clinical Psychology, 70,* 1267–1302.

Forehand, R. L., & McMahon, R. J. (1981). *Helping the noncompliant child: A clinician's guide to parent training.* New York: Guilford Press.

Gerrard, L., & Anastopoulos, A. D. (2005, August). *The relationship between AD/HD and mother–child attachment in early childhood.* Paper presented at the annual meeting of the American Psychological Association, Washington, DC.

Greenhill, L. L., Halperin, J. M., & Abikoff, H. (1999). Stimulant medications. *Journal of the American Academy of Child and Adolescent Psychiatry, 38*(5), 503–512.

Jensen, P. S., Hinshaw, S. P., Swanson, J. M., Greenhill, L. L., Conners, C. K., Arnold, L. E., et al. (2001). Findings from the NIMH Multimodal Treatment Study of ADHD (MTA): Implications and applications for primary care providers. *Journal of Developmental and Behavioral Pediatrics, 22,* 60–73.

Jensen, P. S., Martin, D., & Cantwell, D. P. (1997). Comorbidity of ADHD: Implications for research, practice, and DSM-V. *Journal of the American Academy of Child and Adolescent Psychiatry, 36,* 1065–1079.

Kazdin, A. E. (1997). Parent management training: Evidence, outcomes, and issues. *Journal of the American Academy of Child and Adolescent Psychiatry, 36,* 1349–1356.

Loeber, R., Keenan, K., Lahey, B. B., Green, S. M., & Thomas, C. (1993). Evidence for developmentally based diagnoses in oppositional defiant disorder and conduct disorder. *Journal of Abnormal Child Psychology, 21,* 377–410.

Mash, E. J., & Johnston, C. (1990). Determinants of parenting stress: Illustrations from families of hyperactive children and families of physically abused children. *Journal of Clinical Child Psychology, 19,* 313–328.

McGoey, K. E., Eckert, T. L, & DuPaul, G. J. (2002). Early intervention for preschool-age children with ADHD: A literature review. *Journal of Emotional and Behavioral Disorders, 10,* 14–28.

Minuchin, S., & Fishman, H. C. (1981). *Family therapy techniques.* Cambridge, MA: Harvard University Press.

Newby, R. F., Fischer, M., & Roman, M. A. (1991). Parent training for families of children with ADHD. *School Psychology Review, 20,* 252–265.

Patterson, G. R. (1982). *Coercive family process.* Eugene, OR: Castalia.

Pelham, W. E. (1999). President's message: The NIMH Multimodal Treatment Study for ADHD: Just say yes to drugs? *Clinical Child Psychology Newsletter, 14,* 1–10.

Pelham, W. E., Wheeler, T., & Chronis, A. (1998). Empirically supported psychosocial treatments for attention deficit hyperactivity disorder. *Journal of Clinical Child Psychology, 27,* 190–205.

Pisterman, S., Firestone, P. McGrath, P., Goodman, J., Webster, I., Mallory, R., et al. (1992). The effects of parent on parenting stress and sense of competence. *Canadian Journal of Behavioural Science, 24,* 41–58.

Pisterman, S., McGrath, P., Firestone, P., & Goodman, J. T. (1989). Outcome of parent-mediated treatment of preschoolers with attention deficit disorder with hyperactivity. *Journal of Consulting and Clinical Psychology, 57,* 636–643.

Robin, A. L., & Foster, S. (1989). *Negotiating parent–adolescent conflict.* New York: Guilford Press.

Shelton, T. L., Barkley, R. A., Crosswait, C., Moorehouse, M., Fletcher, K., Barrett, S., et al. (2000). Multimethod psychoeducational intervention for preschool children with disruptive behavior: Two-year post-treatment follow-up. *Journal of Abnormal Child Psychology, 28,* 253–266.

Sonuga-Barke, E. J. S., Daley, D., & Thompson, M. (2002). Does maternal ADHD reduce the effectiveness of parent training for preschool children's ADHD? *Journal of the American Academy of Child and Adolescent Psychiatry, 41,* 696–702.

Sonuga-Barke, E. J. S., Daley, D., Thompson, M., Laver-Bradbury, C., & Weeks, A. (2001). Parent-based therapies for preschool attention-deficit/hyperactivity disorder: A randomized, controlled trial with a community sample. *Journal of the American Academy of Child and Adolescent Psychiatry, 40,* 402–408.

Swanson, J. M., Arnold, L. E., Vitiello, B., Abikoff, H. B., Wells, K. C., Pelham, W. E., et al. (2002). Response to commentary on the Multimodal Treatment Study of ADHD (MTA): Mining the meaning of the MTA. *Journal of Abnormal Child Psychology, 30,* 327–332.

Weinberg, H. A. (1999). Parent training for attention-deficit hyperactivity disorder: Parental and child outcome. *Journal of Clinical Psychology, 55,* 907–913.

CHAPTER 13

COPE

Large-Group, Community-Based,
Family-Centered Parent Training

CHARLES E. CUNNINGHAM

Although the diagnosis of Attention-Deficit/ Hyperactivity Disorder (ADHD) emphasizes problems with sustained attention, activity level, and impulse control, it is the impact of these difficulties on a child's social relationships that often prompts parents to seek professional assistance. The difficulties experienced by children with ADHD may adversely affect their relationships with parents (Cunningham & Barkley, 1979; Gerdes, Hoza, & Pelham, 2003; Mash & Johnston, 1982), peers (Clark, Cheyne, Cunningham, & Siegel, 1988; Cunningham & Siegel, 1987; Cunningham, Siegel, & Offord, 1985, 1991), and teachers (Campbell, Endman, & Bernfield, 1977; Whalen, Henker, & Dotemoto, 1980). With their parents, children with ADHD are more active, less cooperative, and less likely to sustain their attention to play or task-related activities (Cunningham & Barkley, 1979; DuPaul, McGoey, Eckert, & VanBrakle, 2001; Gomez & Sanson, 1994; Mash & Johnston, 1982); these difficulties are associated with problems in virtually all daily activities (Barkley & Edelbrock, 1987). Parents of chil-

dren with ADHD report low self-esteem (Cunningham & Boyle, 2002; Mash & Johnston, 1983), a limited sense of control over the children's difficulties (Sobol, Ashbourne, Earn, & Cunningham, 1989), higher parenting stress (Anastopoulos, Guevremont, Shelton, & DuPaul, 1992; DuPaul et al., 2001; Podolski & Nigg, 2001), poorer coping (Keown & Woodward, 2002), and more depressive symptoms (Byrne, DeWolfe, & Bawden, 1998; Cunningham, Benness, & Siegel, 1988; Cunningham & Boyle, 2002).

In studies using a wide range of sampling frames, diagnostic strategies, and measures, parents of children with ADHD often show a more controlling, less positive approach to child management (Cunningham & Barkley, 1979; DuPaul et al., 2001; Johnston, 1996; Keown & Woodward, 2002; Mash & Johnston, 1982; Woodward, Taylor, & Dowdney, 1998). Although controlled studies show that this approach to child management is to some extent elicited by the active, poorly regulated behavior of children with ADHD (Barkley & Cunningham, 1979; Barkley,

Karlsson, Pollard, & Murphy, 1985; Cunningham & Barkley, 1978; Cunningham & Boyle, 2002), it is associated with poorer long-term adjustment (Campbell, 1990; Earls & Jung, 1987; Patterson, 1982; Patterson, Reid, & Dishion, 1992; Weiss & Hechtman, 1986) and less positive treatment outcome (Hoza et al., 2000; Webster-Stratton, Reid, & Hammond, 2001).

Parent training programs of the type described in Chapters 12 and 14 have emerged as an important component in the management of children with ADHD. Parent training improves child management skills (Bor, Sanders, & Markie-Dadds, 2002; Chronis, Chacko, Fabiano, Wymbs, & Pelham, 2004; Pisterman et al., 1989), enhances parental confidence (Anastopoulos, Shelton, DuPaul, & Guevremont, 1993; Bor et al., 2002; Pisterman et al., 1992), reduces stress (Anastopoulos et al., 1993; Pisterman et al., 1992), and improves family relationships (Anastopoulos et al., 1993; Bor et al., 2002). Improvements in parenting skills are accompanied by a reduction in symptoms of inattention, overactivity, and impulsivity (Anastopoulos et al., 1993; Dubey, O'Leary, & Kaufman, 1983; Freeman, Phillips, & Johnston, 1992; Sonuga-Barke, Daley, Thompson, Laver-Bradbury, & Weeks, 2001), noncompliance (Pisterman et al., 1989; Pollard, Ward, & Barkley, 1983), aggression (Anastopoulos et al., 1993; Freeman et al., 1992), and general management problems (Bor et al., 2002). The gains established in parent training programs are maintained at both short-term (Anastopoulos et al., 1993; Bor et al., 2002; Dubey et al., 1983; Freeman et al., 1992; Pisterman et al., 1989; Sonuga-Barke et al., 2001) and longer-term (McMahon, 1994) follow-ups.

A systems perspective implies that parenting will influence and be affected by structural and transactional relationships within the child's nuclear family, extended family, and community. From such a perspective, parent training would be conducted most effectively with reference to a wider family and community framework. Several lines of evidence suggest that a more systemic approach to parent training might be particularly useful with families of children with ADHD. First, during the course of children's development, families of children with ADHD confront a substantially larger number of behavioral, developmental, and educational problems than those of children without ADHD. The time, logistical demands, and energy required to cope with these difficulties is associated with an enormous burden of stress on marital/couple and family functioning (Anastopoulos et al., 1992; DuPaul et al., 2001; Podolski & Nigg, 2001), as well as with poorer coping (Keown & Woodward, 2002).

Secondly, although referrals to parent training programs are often prompted by child management difficulties, parents of children with ADHD frequently report problems in related areas of individual adjustment, marital/couple relationships, and family functioning. These include a lack of confidence in their parenting skills (Cunningham & Boyle, 2002; Johnston, 1996; Mash & Johnston, 1983), adult ADHD (Harvey, Danforth, McKee, Ulaszek, & Friedman, 2003; Sonuga-Barke, Daley, & Thompson, 2002), depression (Befera & Barkley, 1985; Breen & Barkley, 1988; Cunningham et al., 1988; Cunningham & Boyle, 2002), marital/couple conflict (Stormont-Spurgin & Zentall, 1995), family dysfunction (Cunningham & Boyle, 2002; DuPaul et al., 2001), and fewer social supports (Cunningham et al., 1988; DuPaul et al., 2001; Woodward et al., 1998). These factors are associated with negative perceptions of child behavior (Chi & Hinshaw, 2002), ineffective child management strategies (Harvey et al., 2003; Mash & Johnston, 1983; Panaccione & Wahler, 1986), and a reduction in the effectiveness of parenting programs (Sonuga-Barke et al., 2002).

Third, from 40% to 60% of children with ADHD also evidence oppositional or conduct problems (Szatmari, Offord, & Boyle, 1989). Children with both ADHD and oppositional or conduct disorders confront parents with more management difficulties (Barkley, Fischer, Edelbrock, & Smallish, 1990; Cunningham & Boyle, 2002) and are at greater long-term risk than children with either type of disorder alone (Taylor, Chadwick, Heptinstall, & Danckaerts, 1996). Whereas epidemiological evidence suggests that ADHD is correlated with developmental variables, conduct problems in children are associated with an increase in the likelihood of marital/couple conflict between parents and more general family dysfunction (Cunningham & Boyle, 2002; Stormont-Spurgin & Zentall, 1995; Szatmari et al., 1989).

REDESIGNING PARENT TRAINING PROGRAMS

In the preceding edition of this text, I described a family-systems-oriented program for couples of children with ADHD. Although our own experience and accumulating evidence (Webster-Stratton, 1994) supports a combined emphasis on parenting and family functioning, several limitations to this clinic-based approach to individual families prompted the development of the program described here.

First, ADHD is among the most prevalent childhood psychiatric disorders (Offord et al., 1987) and the most common reasons for referrals to outpatient clinics. Utilization studies in both North America (Offord et al., 1987; U.S. Department of Health and Human Services, 1999; Zahner, Pawelkiewicz, DeFrancesco, & Adnopoz, 1992) and Europe (Pihlakoski et al., 2004), however, suggest that a significant majority of children with psychiatric difficulties do not receive professional assistance. To extend the availability of parent training programs for families of children with ADHD, my colleagues and I have developed a large-group version of our individual family programs (Barkley, 1990)—a model we call the Community Parent Education (COPE) program (Cunningham, Bremner, & Secord-Gilbert, 1998).

Second, clinic-based parent training programs often pose barriers preventing potentially interested parents from participating. Work schedules that do not allow daytime attendance, extracurricular activities, travel time, or transportation costs may prevent parents from enrolling in or consistently attending parent training programs (Cunningham et al., 2000; Cunningham, Bremner, & Boyle, 1995; Kazdin, Holland, & Crowley, 1997; Prinz & Miller, 1994). These factors may pose particular difficulties to families whose children are at higher risk. Specifically, younger, economically disadvantaged parents with limited education, who are more socially isolated or depressed are least likely to enroll in or complete intervention programs (Cunningham et al., 2000; Firestone & Witt, 1982; Kazdin, 1990; Kazdin, Mazurick, & Bass, 1993; Kazdin, Mazurick, & Siegel, 1994). Consumer preference modeling studies suggest that locations reducing travel time and providing a choice of daytime, evening, and Saturday morning workshops exert an important influence on the decision to enroll

in parent training (Cunningham, Buchanan, Deal, & Miller, 2003). To reduce barriers and increase accessibility, therefore, COPE workshops are conducted in conveniently located schools at morning, evening, and Saturday morning times.

Families interested in a parenting program may also have difficulty securing reliable child care. Child care may pose a special problem to socially isolated or economically disadvantaged families who might benefit from a parenting course (Cunningham et al., 2003). The COPE program's on-site social skills activity group for children, therefore, allows parents who are unable to obtain child care to participate.

The psychological or cultural implications of seeking professional mental health assistance may represent barriers to other families (McMiller & Weisz, 1996). Immigrant families or parents using English as a second language, for example, are less likely to enroll in parent training programs conducted at children's mental health centers (Cunningham et al., 1995). COPE addresses the needs of culturally diverse communities in several ways. First, locating parenting workshops in community settings, such as neighborhood schools, increases utilization by parents from different cultural backgrounds (Cunningham et al., 1995). Second, COPE uses a coping-modeling/problem-solving approach (Cunningham, Davis, Bremner, Dunn, & Rzasa, 1993), which encourages participants to formulate solutions to common child management problems. Participants often comment that this approach is more respectful of their cultural perspective than programs in which leaders teach skills more didactically. Third, COPE's discussions encourage parents to formulate rationales supporting the strategies developed by the group. These explanations reflect the unique perspective different cultural communities bring to COPE workshops. Finally, manuals and leader training workshops encourage professionals from different cultural, ethnic, and linguistic groups to adopt COPE (Lakes et al., 2004).

Families of children with ADHD move more frequently (Barkley et al., 1990), report fewer contacts with relatives, consider these contacts less helpful (Cunningham et al., 1988), and have more difficulty acquiring other sources of social support (DuPaul et al., 2001). Accordingly, social isolation may compromise parenting and limit the effectiveness of individual parent training programs (Wahler, 1980). COPE's large-group, community-based model encourages the development of supportive personal contacts and the exchange of knowledge regarding local resources useful to parents of children with ADHD.

Access to mental health services may be limited by financial constraints (Boyle & Offord, 1988). The availability of parent training may be restricted when programs are located in expensive clinic or hospital settings, when professionals devote a disproportionate percentage of their time to extensive preprogram diagnostic assessments, or when children's mental health services are delivered exclusively to individual families. The COPE program reduces per family costs by offering parenting workshops in large groups, using a model that does not require a coleader, and providing manuals and training programs that allow the program to be conducted successfully by leaders from a wide range of professional backgrounds (Cunningham et al., 1998).

In addition to increasing the cost of parent training, waiting for the assessments required in many clinic-based programs may delay access to parent training and reduce the readiness for participation that is often evident when families first seek help (Cunningham, 1997). COPE workshops are offered as a universal program (Offord, Kraemer, Kazdin, Jensen, & Harrington, 1998) available to all parents in the community (Cunningham et al., 2000). Parents may enroll without a referral to a children's mental health assessment service, while they are on waiting lists for assessment and treatment services, or as a component of a more comprehensive service plan. To reduce waiting times, COPE workshops begin on consecutive weeks in the fall, winter, spring, and summer terms of the year.

STRUCTURE AND PROCESS OF THE LARGE-GROUP PROGRAM

The processes of COPE parenting workshops is based on an integration of principles, techniques, and goals from social-learning-based parenting programs, social-cognitive psychology, family systems theory, small-group interventions, and models for larger support groups.

Social Learning Contributions to Large-Group Process

The parenting component of this program is based on the social learning approach developed by Connie Hanf (Hanf & Kling, 1973) at the University of Oregon Health Sciences Center. Many of the child management strategies introduced in the COPE program are based on social learning principles common to related parenting programs (Barkley, 1997c, 1997d; Eyberg, Boggs, & Algina, 1995; McMahon & Forehand, 2003; Sanders, Markie-Dadds, Tully, & Bor, 2000; Webster-Stratton, 1994). Social learning models also contribute to the COPE program's large-group training process, in which leaders use modeling, role playing, homework goal setting, and self-monitoring to introduce new strategies, strengthen skills, and encourage transfer to functionally important situations at home.

Cognitive and Social-Psychological Contributions

Successful parent training often requires a shift in established expectations and beliefs regarding child behavior, discipline, and family relationships. The COPE program, therefore, incorporates a number of principles from cognitive and social-psychological models of attitude change (Leary & Miller, 1986). Social-psychological research suggests that optimal shifts in attitudes and behavior will be obtained when parents devise their own solutions and rationales (Leary & Miller, 1986; Meichenbaum & Turk, 1987). Indeed, more didactic instructional strategies may increase resistance to skill acquisition (Cunningham et al., 1993; Patterson & Forgatch, 1985). This program incorporates a coping-modeling/problem-solving approach, in which participants collaborate in the formulation of solutions to common problems (Cunningham et al., 1993). COPE group leaders present videotaped vignettes depicting exaggerated versions of common child management errors. During small-subgroup discussions, participants identify errors, discuss their consequences, develop alternative strategies, and formulate supporting rationales. Leaders model the solutions developed by the group, dyads rehearse the strategy in role-playing exercises, and individual parents transfer the skill to relevant home or community settings via daily homework projects.

There are several advantages to this large-group coping-modeling/problem-solving approach. First, videotaped models simplify child management problems by breaking complex interactions into segments and allowing large groups to develop solutions in a cohesive, step-by-step manner.

Second, "COPEing models" depict the longer-term consequences of common errors that may be less evident in daily interaction. Exploring the consequences of both positive and negative approaches to management helps participants understand the relationship between parenting and child behavior.

Third, formulating alternative strategies and devising supporting rationales in the program's small- and large-group discussions enhances adherence and commitment (Greenwald & Albert, 1968; Janis & King, 1954; King & Janis, 1956; Meichenbaum & Turk, 1987). Developing solutions to complex child management problems promotes a sense of personal accomplishment, encourages a sense of ownership, and enhances commitment to the success of homework projects (Cunningham et al., 1993).

Fourth, the coping-modeling/problem-solving approach elicits less resistance and yields a more positive large group process than more didactic instructional strategies do (Cunningham et al., 1993; Patterson & Forgatch, 1985). COPE leaders adopt a neutral, facilitative approach to group discussions, which encourages participants to explore the potential advantages and disadvantages of alternative approaches to child management. COPE leaders pose "attributional questions" encouraging the group to discuss the consequences of common parenting errors and the relative advantages of alternative parenting strategies. Social learning attributional questions, for example, encourage participants to consider the lessons different parenting strategies teach their children. Relational/communicative attributional questions invite the group to explore the messages different management strategies communicate to children. Long-term outcome attributional questions anticipate the impact that using a strategy consistently over time might have on a child and family.

Fifth, although the COPE program described here is designed for families of children with ADHD, there is considerable heterogeneity in the age, severity, and associated problems experienced by the children of parents participating

in the group. Moreover, the cultural, ethnic, and sociodemographic composition of groups may vary considerably. The combination of coping modeling with problem solving yields child management solutions that have greater validity for individual members of the group.

Sixth, in coping-modeling discussions, participants break complex problems into smaller components; discuss potential errors; generate alternative strategies; consider the relative advantages and disadvantages of different approaches; select promising alternatives; and evaluate the efficacy of potential solutions in modeling, role-playing, and homework exercises. The large group process, therefore, builds the collaborative problem-solving skills that constitute an important family systems goal of the program.

In addition to their contributions to the design of COPE's large-group process, cognitive and social-psychological models suggest a number of goals for the parenting program. Because the problems of many children with ADHD reflect deficits in self-regulation (Barkley, 1997a, 1997b), COPE encourages parents to prompt and reinforce their children's planning and self-regulatory efforts. Attributional research suggests that parental explanations regarding the causes of children's behavior (e.g., "He's doing this intentionally") exert an important impact on their emotional (Harrison & Sofronoff, 2002) and disciplinary (Baden & Howe, 1992; Johnston & Freeman, 1997) responses. The COPE program's large- and small-group discussions encourage participants to collaborate in the formulation of cognitive strategies that promote an accurate interpretation of the child's behavior, an appreciation of the limits of parental influence, and a realistic longer-term sense of personal control over child management problems.

Contributions from Family Systems Theory

This program's systemic goals are derived from the McMaster model of family functioning (Epstein, Bishop, & Levine, 1978). Although family dysfunction is more closely related to oppositional disorders or conduct problems (Cunningham & Boyle, 2002; Schachar & Tannock, 1995; Szatmari et al., 1989), the long-term difficulties of managing a child with ADHD may erode a family's coping skills. This program does not represent a comprehensive approach to intervention with families of children with ADHD; however, formulating, mastering, implementing, and maintaining parenting skills provide an opportunity for parents to develop more effective problem-solving skills, achieve a more balanced distribution of child care and child management responsibilities, build more consistent family routines, and increase supportive communication among family members. The association between oppositional disorders and family dysfunction suggest that these systemic goals are particularly important for families of children with both ADHD and oppositional disorders (Cunningham & Boyle, 2002; Szatmari et al., 1989)

Contributions from Group Theory

Feedback from many parents who have participated in COPE programs suggests that the large-group and subgroup processes in COPE workshops make an important contribution to the outcome of the program (MacKenzie, 1990). Groups provide a sense of universal parenting experiences that places the problems facing individual families in greater perspective. Participants have an opportunity to share helpful child management skills, coping strategies, and information regarding children's development. Groups can assist in the solution of complex problems and provide the emotional support parents need to implement solutions consistently. Indeed, the opportunity to support and assist other parents is a source of considerable altruistic satisfaction (MacKenzie, 1990). In addition to the skill-building, cognitive, and systemic dimensions of the program, COPE leaders facilitate the development of a cohesive working group, capitalize on the contributions of different membership roles, and encourage completion of the tasks critical to each stage of the group's development (MacKenzie, 1990).

ORGANIZATION OF LARGE-GROUP COPE WORKSHOPS

The organization of a typical "COPEing with ADHD" parenting workshop is summarized in Table 13.1.

Advertising and Recruiting Participants

Although COPE is often conducted as a universal service for all parents interested in improving their skills (Cunningham et al., 2000), COPEing with ADHD workshops are designed specifically for parents of children with ADHD. Realizing the service delivery potential of large groups; catching parents during critical windows, when readiness for parent training is high and family schedules permit participation; and increasing utilization among families who are less likely to use available mental health services—all these require a comprehensive, long-term advertising program. Schools are points of virtually universal contact with families of children with ADHD. The COPE program, therefore, sends flyers via schools advertising upcoming workshops to all parents, includes reminders in school newsletters, places posters on parent information boards, and encourages educators to speak directly to parents who might benefit from a parenting workshop.

TABLE 13.1. Curriculum of a 10-Session COPE Workshop for Parents of 4- to 12-Year-Olds with ADHD

I. Advertising and recruiting participants
II. Parent training curriculum
    Session 1: Information Night and Introduction to ADHD
    Session 2: Attending, Balanced Attending, and Rewards among Siblings
    Session 3: Planned Ignoring
    Session 4: Token Incentive Systems 1
    Session 5: Transitional Warnings and "When–Then"
    Session 6: Planning Ahead
    Session 7: Token Incentive Systems 2 (Response Cost)
    Session 8: Time out from Positive Reinforcement 1
    Session 9: Time out from Positive Reinforcement 2
    Session 10: Closing Session
III. Optional one-session workshop electives

Community physicians provide alternative points of contact with families who might benefit from parent training. Using general practice, family medicine, or pediatric office visits to contact parents allows more preventive programs during children's preschool years, when child management problems often emerge (Cunningham & Boyle, 2002; DuPaul et al., 2001; Keown & Woodward, 2002) and when parent training may be more effective (Dishion & Patterson, 1992). In addition to notifying community physicians of upcoming workshops, COPE advertises directly to parents by placing flyers announcing workshops in the waiting rooms of local physicians. Finally, COPE advertises via CHADD groups, children's mental health centers, and the local cable and print media's community service announcements.

Information Night

Parents considering enrolling in a COPE workshop begin with a 2-hour information session. The leader asks participants to introduce themselves, outlines the goals of the program, discusses the format of individual sessions, and presents the time and location of alternative COPE workshops. Because many parents anticipate the short-term resolution of chronic child management difficulties, the leader provides a more realistic estimate of the incremental changes that may be expected in parenting courses. Leaders encourage participants to discuss the potential benefits of consistent attendance, active participation, and conscientious completion of homework projects. Finally, parents discuss solutions to obstacles (e.g., transportation difficulties, child care, or work schedules) that might limit participation.

The decision to participate in parent training requires accurate information regarding the etiology of ADHD, factors influencing the course of the disorder, and the relative benefits of different interventions. Information night sessions, therefore, feature a videotaped introduction to ADHD (Barkley, 1993a, 1993b). These very popular videotapes give groups a common theoretical and empirical framework that provides a rationale for each of the strategies introduced in the program. Andrews, Swank, Foorman, and Fletcher (1995) confirmed that this type of videotaped information by itself increases service utilization and improves outcome—findings consistent with a larger body of evidence regarding the effectiveness of media-based interventions for child mental health problems (Montgomery, 2002).

Readiness-for-change research (Cunningham, 1997; Prochaska, DiClemente, & Norcross, 1992) suggests that parents attending information night will be at different stages in the process of change. Some (e.g., those attending on the advice of health or educational professionals), may be at a "contemplative" stage—simply considering the possibility of change. Others may be at a "preparatory" or "action" stage, ready to initiate a change in child management skills. Research in this area suggests that a shift to the preparatory or action stage occurs when the anticipated benefits of change outweigh the logistical costs of change (Prochaska et al., 1994). To enhance readiness, participants are encouraged to share their goals for the course and discuss the benefits participation might provide parents, children, and families. Accurate information regarding the long-term course of ADHD, familiarity with the format of the program, and large-group discussions regarding the many potential benefits of participation all enhance readiness for change and increase the proportion of information night attendees who enroll and attend subsequent sessions.

Parenting Workshop

COPE parenting workshops are typically organized into a curriculum of approximately 10 weekly 2-hour sessions. The curriculum of a 10 session COPEing with ADHD workshop is presented in part II of Table 13.1 and discussed in a later section.

Children's Social Skills Activity Group

Participants have the option of enrolling their children in a social skills activity group scheduled during the parenting course. Children observe leaders or competent members of the group modeling a weekly curriculum of social skills, and rehearse new skills in role-playing exercises. Leaders prompt children to apply new skills during in-session games, art projects, physical activities, and snack times; reinforce follow-through with a token incentive system; and help plan homework projects (Cunningham, Clark, Heaven, Durrant, & Cunningham, 1989). This group solves child care problems, familiarizes children with strategies parents will use (e.g., planning ahead and point systems), allows parents an immediate opportunity to rehearse new strategies during the transition home, and may contribute to social skills development.

Maintaining Gains and Preparing for Adolescence

The COPE program is part of a community educational service providing large-group, skill-building workshops on a wide range of topics. We encourage parents to attend a series of one-session workshops (e.g., COPEing with Sibling Conflict, COPEing with Homework, COPEing with Bedtime) that strengthen the skills developed in the COPE program, encourage the application of COPE strategies to functionally important daily activities, and build social networks. Parents are encouraged to prepare for the challenges of parenting an adolescent with ADHD (Edwards, Barkley, Laneri, Fletcher, & Metevia, 2001; Fletcher, Fischer, Barkley, & Smallish, 1996) by enrolling in a version of the COPE program designed specifically for parents of adolescents (McCleary & Ridley, 1999).

Structure of Large Group Sessions

The structure of COPE sessions is summarized in Table 13.2 and discussed below.

TABLE 13.2. Structure of Large-Group Sessions

Phase 1: Informal social activities.
Phase 2: Leader outlines session plan.
Phase 3: Subgroups review homework successes.
Phase 4: Large-group discussion of homework projects.
Phase 5: Subgroups discuss errors made by videotaped coping model.
Phase 6: Large-group discussion of errors.
Phase 7: Subgroups formulate alternatives to videotaped errors.
Phase 8: Large-group discussion of proposed solutions.
Phase 9: Leader models group's solution.
Phase 10: Subgroups brainstorm application.
Phase 11: Dyads rehearse strategies.
Phase 12: Homework planning.
Phase 13: Leader closes session.

Social Networking and Community Resources

Each COPE session begins with a brief social phase, encouraging supportive interaction among participants. A resource table features books and videos providing information about ADHD, local support groups, and useful services for families of children with ADHD. Parents are encouraged to add resources, borrow videotapes or books, and request information on topics of special interest.

Subgrouping

To allow active participation in workshops that may average 25 members (Cunningham et al., 1995), parents are seated in 5-member subgroups. Each week, each subgroup selects a leader responsible for encouraging participation and keeping members on task, recording discussions, and sharing the subgroup's conclusions with the larger group.

Subgroup Homework Reviews

After a large-group review of the preceding session's strategy, each subgroup member describes one situation where he or she used the strategy. To minimize unrealistic short-term outcome expectations and to build self-efficacy, parents are encouraged to focus on successful application, small gains, and the longer-term impact of strategies on parent–child relationships or social conduct. The workshop leader prompts participants to give supportive feedback regarding homework efforts to partners or subgroup members. Following homework discussions, parents acting as subgroup leaders describe an example of a successful homework project to the larger group. The workshop leader summarizes these examples, demonstrates a brief example, and encourages a larger-group attributional discussion to increase the group's commitment to the strategy (e.g., the lessons different strategies might teach, the messages they communicate, or their impact if used consistently over a longer period of time).

Problem Solving: Identifying Videotaped Parenting Errors

In the initial phase of problem solving, leaders play a videotape depicting errors in the management of potentially problematic situations (e.g., getting ready for school or starting homework). In subgroups, parents identify the mistakes observed on the tape and discuss potential consequences. Each subgroup leader summarizes his or her group's conclusions for the larger group. COPE leaders prompt a large-group attributional discussion of the lessons parents inadvertently teach, the message these errors may communicate to the children, and the long-term consequences if this pattern of interaction persists (Cunningham et al., 1993, 1995).

Problem Solving: Discussing Alternative Strategies

Next, each subgroup discusses alternatives to the errors depicted on tape, considers their relative merits, and presents their conclusions to the larger group. Leaders complete this phase by summarizing and integrating the suggestions of the respective subgroups and prompting a large-group attributional discussion.

Modeling Proposed Strategies

To facilitate the application of new skills to situations that are most relevant to participants, the larger group suggests three common problems to which the session's strategy might be applied (e.g., completing chores or getting ready for bed). The large group selects one problem and develops a detailed, step-by-step plan as to how the session's strategy might be applied. The course leader summarizes the plan proposed by the group, poses questions to refine the strategy, and models the solution with a member of the group playing the role of a child. The leader prompts the large group to describe each component of the strategy demonstrated and prompts an attributional discussion to increase the group's commitment. This is repeated for the two additional problems identified by the group.

Brainstorming the Application of New Skills

To encourage a more generalized application of the session's strategies, each subgroup develops a list of different situations, behaviors, or problems to which the session's strategy might be applied. Subgroup leaders summarize these suggestions for the larger group.

Rehearsing

To strengthen skills, build confidence, and prepare for the application of new skills at home, subgroups divide into dyads, determine who will play the roles of parent and child, and develop a plan for how the session's strategy might be applied to a homework problem of interest to the participant playing the role of the parent. Next, participants find a comfortable spot in the room and rehearse the session's strategy. After each exercise, role-playing partners give positive feedback regarding the effective use of new skills. The partners then switch roles and repeat this exercise. Parents whose children are enrolled in the social skills activity group may be given an opportunity to rehearse these strategies in structured interactions with their children.

Planning Homework

Using a homework monitoring sheet, parents set goals to apply new strategies to specific situations, discuss where to post monitoring sheets to ensure an effective visual reminder of homework plans, and check off daily application. Parents whose children are in the social skills activity group review the social skill introduced during the session, consider how strategies developed in the workshop might be used to encourage their children to apply newly learned social skills, and plan how the session's strategy might be applied on the way home.

Closing the Session

To enhance participation and strengthen social networks, COPE leaders prompt members to contact participants who were unable to attend the session. The larger group discusses solutions to obstacles (e.g., car pooling) that might prevent members from attending the next session.

Strengthening Family Functioning

COPE workshops provide an opportunity for participants to build the family-system-level skills needed to manage children with ADHD effectively. Large-group sessions build collaborative problem-solving skills, encourage members of couples to share child management responsibilities, and prompt parents to provide each other with supportive feedback. COPE leaders use behavioral and social-psychological strategies to enhance commitment to these changes. Prior to homework reviews, problem solving, brainstorming, and role-playing exercises, COPE leaders prompt participants to give supportive feedback to their partner or another member of their subgroup. Once participants exchange positive feedback comfortably, the leader fades prompts by gradually reducing the amount of detail provided in each instruction. Over the course of the COPE program, the amount of spontaneous supportive feedback increases gradually. In each session, leaders label a group transaction that is a positive example of one of the COPE program's systemic goals: problem solving, shared management responsibility, supportive communication, or the use of social networks. Leaders prompt a large-group attributional discussion exploring lessons learned from, messages communicated by, or longer-term impact of these approaches to family relationships.

Leaders prompt the group to consider whether child management strategies discussed in the session are applicable to interactions with younger siblings, older children, or adults—a strategy we term "prompting generational transfer." Given the aggregation of child mental health problems in families (Szatmari, Boyle, & Offord, 1993), many parents of children with ADHD have children with other difficulties. Conversational skills, strategies for balancing time and attention, giving compliments, avoiding escalating arguments, and planning solutions to potential problems may prove useful in a variety of contexts.

As the group's commitment to new approaches to problem solving, communication, and shared child management responsibility increases, these systemic goals are included in weekly homework assignments. Participants plan how specific changes might be implemented, anticipate obstacles, develop reminders, and monitor application at home. These projects are included in the next session's homework review.

Curriculum of the Program

The curriculum of a 10-session COPE workshop for families of children with ADHD is outlined in part II of Table 13.1. It's main points are discussed below.

Encouraging Positive Behavior and Improving Parent–Child Relationships

Although children with ADHD seem to respond favorably to more immediate, frequent, and salient reinforcement (Barkley, 1997b; Haenlein & Caul, 1987), their poorly regulated oppositional behavior sometimes elicits a less positive parental response (Barkley et al., 1985; Cunningham & Barkley, 1979; Cunningham & Boyle, 2002). In early sessions, therefore, participants develop strategies for attending to and rewarding positive behavior, identify situations to which attending skills might be applied, and target behaviors for reinforcement. These strategies strengthen positive behavior, reduce coercive interactions, and may support the development of language and social skills. They are prerequisite components of the strategies developed in later sessions, and foster parent–child relationships that facilitate the collaborative solution of more complex problems.

Balancing Family Relationships

While difficult children often demand a disproportionate amount of attention, siblings are often upset by unequal allocations of parental time. Parents develop strategies for balancing time and attention among siblings, and for attending to several children simultaneously (e.g., "You've both been very helpful this morning"). This general principle is used to examine balance in dimensions of family life that may affect child management and coping skills (e.g., time for children vs. spouse or time for family vs. self).

Avoiding Conflicts

The active, impulsive, poorly regulated behavior of children with ADHD is often irritating or provocative. In session 3, therefore, parents formulate strategies for ignoring the minor issues that may precipitate the coercive cycles leading to an escalation in parent–child conflict. Because parental cognitions may intensify anger (e.g., "He's doing this intentionally to irritate me"), the group develops cognitive coping strategies. Homework assignments encourage parents to identify situations where ignoring strategies are appropriate, to agree on behaviors that are best ignored, and to rehearse the application of new coping skills.

Point Systems

Children with ADHD have difficulty mediating intervals between positive behavior and delayed consequences (Barkley, 1997a, 1997b). Session 4, therefore, introduces a simple home-based token incentive system. Parents identify behaviors to encourage, construct a menu of rewards, assign a cost to each reward, and select an age-appropriate token (e.g., marbles in a jar, stars, or points). If indicated, parents develop a daily report card allowing points earned at school to be exchanged for home-based rewards. The tangible qualities of token incentive systems help children with ADHD bridge intervals between positive behavior and more distant rewards while menus allow parents to leverage more effective consequences. Introducing point systems on session 5 provides an opportunity for parents to share successful examples on subsequent homework reviews, allows time to solve the logistical problems parents inevitably encounter in implementing token systems, and ensures that a positive incentive system is functioning for several weeks before token loss is introduced as a potential consequence for negative behaviors.

Managing Transitions

Children with ADHD often fail to anticipate transitions, have difficulty modulating their reaction to the termination of reinforcing activities, or resist the start of more effortful tasks. Session 5, therefore, focuses on the development of more effective transitional strategies. Parents shift a child's attention by reinforcing positive behaviors, present a transitional prompt ("At the end of this game, it will be bedtime"), discourage arguments by ignoring protests, and reward follow-through. "When–then" strategies encourage compliance via the application of the Premack principle, where low-probability behaviors (e.g., homework completion) are rewarded with higher-probability behaviors (e.g., watching television). During brainstorming and homework planning, parents organize daily activities into transitional prompts (e.g., "In 5 minutes, it will be time to start your homework") and "when–

then" sequences (e.g., "When you finish your homework, then you can watch television").

Planning Ahead

Children with ADHD often fail to anticipate problematic situations, review relevant rules, consider alternative strategies, or reflect on the consequences of their behavior. As a result, they approach social interactions, academic activities, and daily tasks in a poorly planned, impulsive manner (Barkley, 1997a, 1997b). Because children with ADHD have great difficulty internalizing these skills, short-term interventions may not yield generalized improvements (Abikoff, 1991). COPE, therefore, integrates preparatory and planning strategies (e.g., transitional warnings, "when–then," and planning ahead) into daily parent–child interactions. Session 6 focuses on planning ahead: Parents identify situations where children act impulsively or fail to regulate their behavior according to rules ("I'm expecting an important phone call"), and prompt the children to develop a prosocial plan ("What could you do to help?"). To encourage the application of well-intentioned but easily forgotten goals, parents ask the children to review plans immediately prior to target situations ("There's my phone call. What was your plan?"), reward successful follow-through, ignore minor errors, and prompt the child to review plans as necessary. Prompting and reinforcing collaborative planning during the preadolescent years should build the collaborative planning skills parents will need to manage the conflicts that are common in adolescence (Edwards et al., 2001; Fletcher et al., 1996).

Dealing with More Serious Problems: Response Cost

Although the positive parenting strategies developed during the first several sessions of the program encourage prosocial behavior and solve problems, parents of many children with ADHD require effective responses to more persistent difficulties. A response cost strategy, in which tokens or points are deducted for agreed-upon infractions, is introduced in session 7. Response cost provides a logistically simple but effective consequence for negative behaviors, represents an alternative to time out, and can be used flexibly in public settings.

Dealing with More Serious Problems: Time Out from Positive Reinforcement

Groups typically formulate a strategy for time out from positive reinforcement, which includes (1) the presentation of firm, emotionally neutral commands; (2) a quick neutral warning if noncompliance occurs; and, if necessary, (3) the application of an effective consequence (e.g., time on a chair or loss of privileges). Groups explore the social consequences of harsh physical discipline and its association with poor social adjustment and aggressive behavior (Weiss, Dodge, Bates, & Pettit, 1992).

Problem Solving

Although parents solve a significant number of problems over the course of a 10-session COPE workshop, many benefit from an opportunity to address unresolved difficulties. Problem solving is often added as an optional session or elective workshop for dealing with outstanding issues. In this session, parents formulate a general approach to the solution of child management problems ("PASTEing problems"). This typically includes scheduling problem solving at a time when discussion can proceed without interruption, and then (P) picking a soluble problem, (A) analyzing the advantages and disadvantages of alternative solutions, (S) selecting the most promising option, (T) trying it out, and (E) evaluating outcome. This general approach to problem solving is then applied to the solution of selected management difficulties.

COPE Plus

COPE Plus is a small-group (four-family), four-session program developed by two senior COPE group leaders, Rita Harrison and Randi Knight. COPE Plus gives parents an opportunity to strengthen newly acquired skills and solve outstanding problems. Parents who have completed a standard COPE program and have unusually challenging children are eligible for COPE Plus. Parents bring unsolved problems from home, formulate a solution using COPE strategies, and rehearse these during role-playing exercises with the leader. Children participate in an abbreviated version of the social skills activity group discussed above. Using a scenario simulating the problem they have

identified, each parent practices the solution with his or her child while receiving feedback from the leader through an FM earphone. Other members of the group observe through a one-way mirror and provide supportive feedback.

Dissemination and Training

To ensure successful dissemination, COPE leaders conduct the program according to a detailed manual (Cunningham et al., 1998). In addition to a leader's manual, COPE offers supporting videotapes and a four-level leader training program, which includes a 2-day introductory workshop, supervised coleading opportunities, a 1-day advanced leader training session, and a videotaped leader certification process.

BENEFITS OF LARGE-GROUP COMMUNITY BASED WORKSHOPS

Service Utilization

Community COPE workshops appear to reduce the barriers that clinic-based programs may pose. We (Cunningham et al., 1995), for example, demonstrated that parents from economically disadvantaged backgrounds, immigrants, parents using English as a second language, and families of children with more severe problems were more likely to utilize parenting workshops conducted in community settings. Subsequent studies suggest that COPE programs boost enrollment by providing a choice among day, evening, and Saturday morning courses; providing child care; and reducing the time required to travel to parenting programs (Cunningham et al., 2003). Several factors that have been linked to poor treatment adherence in clinic-based trials (Kazdin et al., 1993, 1994; Webster-Stratton & Hammond, 1990) are less likely to influence the utilization of this school-based program. Economic disadvantage, family stressors, family dysfunction, and parental depression, for example, do not predict participation in large-group community-based programs (Cunningham et al., 1995, 2000). Together, these studies suggest that large-group COPE workshops in community settings pose fewer logistical and psychological demands for parents than do programs for families conducted in outpatient clinics.

Large-Group Process

Social-psychological research suggests that formulating solutions, devising supporting rationales, and setting personal goals in a group context should improve commitment and adherence to new strategies (Janis, 1983; Leary & Miller, 1986; Meichenbaum & Turk, 1987). We (Cunningham et al., 1993) demonstrated that participants in coping-modeling conditions, in which strategies were formulated by the group, attended significantly more training sessions, arrived late to fewer sessions, completed significantly more homework assignments, interacted more positively during training sessions, reported significantly higher personal accomplishment scores, and rated the program more favorably than those who were introduced to new skills in a more didactic mastery-modeling condition.

Informal interactions, subgroup exercises, and larger-group discussions allow parents to exchange information regarding typical child development and behavior, problems common at different stages in child development, and potentially useful management strategies. As a result, data from our own trials suggest that larger groups generate more potential solutions to child management problems than individual parenting programs do (Cunningham et al., 1995).

A problem-based model in which parents explore a range of optional child management strategies emphasizes a flexible approach that may better meet the diverse temperamental and developmental needs of this population (Grusec & Goodnow, 1994). In addition, a learning process encouraging participants to formulate their own solutions and generate their own rationales is more likely to yield parenting strategies respecting the diverse cultural backgrounds of the participants enrolling in these community-based programs (Cunningham et al., 1995).

Parents of children with ADHD sometimes find themselves isolated from potentially important social supports (Cunningham et al., 1988). Formal feedback suggests that school-based COPE workshops provide an important sense of membership in a group sharing common problems, provide a perspective regarding the severity of child management problems, and "normalize" the experience of parent training. The opportunity to assist other parents in the solution of common problems provides an important source of altruistic satisfaction (MacKenzie, 1990) and encourages the development of the supportive contacts that sometimes elude parents of children with ADHD (Cunningham et al., 1988; DuPaul et al., 2001). Although COPE sessions focus on a relatively standard curriculum of child management skills, the group provides a forum to discuss other issues of concern—an opportunity that appears to enhance the efficacy of parent training (Prinz & Miller, 1994).

The large-group format of the COPE program yields a process with several advantages. First, large-group activities generate energy and create momentum that motivates parents to implement and sustain challenging changes in their parenting skills. Second, large groups are able to generate solutions to problems that often frustrate individual parents. Third, the consensus-building capabilities of large groups allow participants to resolve divergent opinions and disagreements. Finally, large groups appear less vulnerable to the potentially disruptive effects of inconsistent attendance and dropouts (MacKenzie, 1990).

Cost Efficacy

We (Cunningham et al., 1995) compared the cost of large-group COPE workshops with that of clinic-based services for individual families. Even with leader travel times, longer sessions, and additional preparation, the COPE workshops remained more than six times as cost-effective as clinic-based programs. Community-based workshops reduced the time and travel costs incurred by participants, and did not increase the secondary costs resulting from contacts with other medical, mental health, or educational professionals (Cunningham et al., 1995).

Utilization studies suggest that when COPE is offered universally to all families, many parents of children with less severe problems enroll (Cunningham et al., 2000). Although providing individualized or small-group services to families of lower-risk children in clinic-based programs may increase costs or limit access by families of children with more severe difficulties, including parents of lower-risk children in large COPE groups results in small incremental costs (Cunningham et al., 1995). In addition to the potential preventive advantages of including families of lower-risk children (Offord et al., 1998), these parents often represent a valuable resource to the group.

Outcome

To examine the effectiveness of this larger-group COPE model, we prospectively screened a community sample of 4-year-olds entering junior kindergarten programs; identified children more than 1.5 standard deviations above the mean on a measure of behavior problems at home (Barkley & Edelbrock, 1987); and randomly assigned 150 participants to either a large neighborhood school-based COPE course, an individual family clinic-based parent training program, or a waiting-list control group (Cunningham et al., 1995). Larger groups yielded better performance on objectively measured parental problem-solving tasks, greater reductions in reported child management problems, and improved maintenance at 6-month follow-up. Although this type of efficacy study is promising, it is also important to determine whether these outcomes can be obtained in clinical practice—an approach Margison et al. (2000) have termed "practice-based evidence." Figure 13.1 shows data from a sample of 117 families of 3- to 12-year-olds who participated in either community-based COPE or COPEing with ADHD programs. In order to compare these results to the benchmarks of our clinical trials, we selected children according to the same enrollment criteria (Home Situations Questionnaire *T* scores of 65 or greater) used in our previous study (Cunningham et al., 1995) of the COPE program. Parents completing both COPE and COPEing with ADHD workshops reported significant reductions in Home Situations Questionnaire *T*

scores. These large effect sizes are comparable to those in earlier clinical trials and substantially larger than the changes occurring in untreated control groups (Cunningham et al., 1995).

LIMITATIONS OF PARENT TRAINING?

The robustness of parent training is evident in the number of different variations on the social learning paradigm that have proven effective for families of children with ADHD (Anastopoulos et al., 1993; Bor et al., 2002; Chronis et al., 2004; Pisterman et al., 1989; Sonuga-Barke et al., 2001). An even larger number of trials have proven the effectiveness of parent training for families of children with the oppositional and conduct problems that often accompany ADHD (Eyberg et al., 1995; Sanders et al., 2000; Schumann, Foote, Eyberg, Boggs, & Algina, 1998; Webster-Stratton & Hammond, 1997). Nonetheless, there are limitations to parent training. First, as noted previously, many families do not have access to the professional services described here (Offord et al., 1987; Pihlakoski et al., 2004; Zahner et al., 1992). Second, utilization studies suggest that even when services are available, a significant percentage of parents fail to enroll in or to complete these programs (Barkley et al., 2000; Cunningham & Boyle, 2000). Third, reliable change indices or measures of clinically meaningful change (Evans, Margison, & Barkham, 1998) suggest that parent training is not helpful to all families of children with ADHD

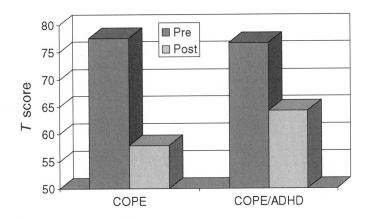

FIGURE 13.1. Home Situation Questionnaire *T* scores before and after participating in a COPE parenting program for children with ADHD or without ADHD.

(Bor et al., 2002; Sonuga-Barke et al., 2001). Finally, children with ADHD whose parents evidence symptoms of adult ADHD may show more limited improvement in parent training programs (Sonuga-Barke et al., 2002). These studies emphasize the importance of a continuing program of research to develop parenting services that better meet the needs of families of children with ADHD, while providing a range of evidence-based treatment options.

KEY CLINICAL POINTS

✓ Large groups increase the availability of parent training programs for families of children with ADHD.

✓ Conducting COPE groups in accessible community locations, scheduling groups at convenient times, and offering a children's social skills activity group increases utilization by families of children with more severe problems, families from cultural minorities, and families who are economically disadvantaged.

✓ COPE employs a problem-solving approach to skill acquisition that respects the views and experiences of parents from different cultural backgrounds. This approach enhances participation, attitude change, and adherence.

✓ COPE includes the social learning parenting skills that are the active components of all evidence-based parenting programs.

✓ COPE's focus on conflict reduction, transitional preparation, planning ahead, and contractual incentives are especially useful for impulsive children.

✓ COPE emphasizes the importance of supportive communication, problem solving, and balance in parent–child and family relationships.

✓ Large groups normalize the experience of parent training, build supportive social networks, generate a range of solutions to common problems, and support the process of parenting change.

✓ In clinical practice, COPE yields effects sizes comparable to other social learning parent-training programs. COPE, however, can be offered at a substantially lower cost per participant than individual parenting programs.

REFERENCES

Abikoff, H. (1991). Cognitive training in ADHD children: Less to it than meets the eye. *Journal of Learning Disabilities, 24,* 205–209.

Anastopoulos, A. D., Guevremont, D. C., Shelton, T. L., & DuPaul, G. J. (1992). Parenting stress among families of children with attention deficit hyperactivity disorder. *Journal of Abnormal Child Psychology, 20,* 503–520.

Anastopoulos, A. D., Shelton, T. L., DuPaul, G. J., & Guevremont, D.C. (1993). PT for attention deficit hyperactivity disorder: Its impact on child and parent functioning. *Journal of Abnormal Child Psychology, 21,* 581–596.

Andrews, J. A., Swank, P. R., Foorman, B., & Fletcher, J. M. (1995). Effects of educating parents about ADHD. *ADHD Report, 3,* 12–13.

Baden, A., & Howe, G. W. (1992). Mothers' attributions and expectancies regarding their conduct-disordered children. *Journal of Abnormal Child Psychology, 20,* 467–485.

Barkley, R. A. (1990). *Attention deficit hyperactivity disorder: A handbook for diagnosis and treatment.* New York: Guilford Press.

Barkley, R. A. (1993a). *ADHD—What do we know?* [Videotape]. New York: Guilford Press.

Barkley, R. A. (1993b). *ADHD—What can we do?* [Videotape]. New York: Guilford Press.

Barkley, R. A. (1997a). Behavioral inhibition, sustained attention, and executive functions: Constructing a unifying theory of ADHD. *Psychological Bulletin, 121,* 65–94.

Barkley, R. A. (1997b). *ADHD and the nature of self control.* New York: Guilford Press.

Barkley, R. A. (1997c). *Defiant children: A clinician's manual for assessment and parent training* (2nd ed.). New York: Guilford Press.

Barkley, R. A. (1997d). *Managing the defiant child: A guide to parent training.* New York: Guilford Press.

Barkley, R. A., & Cunningham, C. E. (1979). The effects of methylphenidate on the mother child interactions of hyperactive children. *Archives of General Psychiatry, 36,* 201–208.

Barkley, R. A., & Edelbrock, C. (1987). Assessing situational variation in children's problem behaviors: The Home and School Situations Questionnaires. In R. J. Prinz (Ed.), *Advances in behavioral assessment of children and families* (Vol. 3, pp. 157–176). Greenwich, CT: JAI Press.

Barkley, R. A., Fischer, M., Edelbrock, C. S., & Smallish, L. (1990). The adolescent outcome of hyperactive children diagnosed by research criteria: I. An 8–year prospective follow-up study. *Journal of the*

American Academy of Child and Adolescent Psychiatry, 29, 546–557.

Barkley, R. A., Karlsson, J., Pollard, S., & Murphy, K. (1985). Developmental changes in the mother–child interactions of hyperactive children: Effects of two doses of Ritalin. *Journal of Child Psychology and Psychiatry, 13,* 631–638.

Barkley, R. A., Shelton, T. L., Crosswait, C., Moorehouse, M., Fletcher, K., Barrett, S., et al. (2000). Multimethod psychoeducational intervention for preschool children with disruptive behavior: Preliminary results at post-treatment. *Journal of Child Psychology and Psychiatry, 41,* 319–332.

Befera, M., & Barkley, R. (1985). Hyperactive and normal boys and girls: Mother–child interaction, parent psychiatric status, and child psychopathology. *Journal of Child Psychology and Psychiatry, 26,* 439–452.

Bor, W., Sanders, R. M., & Markie-Dadds, C. (2002). The effects of the Triple P-Positive Parenting Program on preschool children with co-occuring disruptive behavior and Attentional/Hyperactive difficulties. *Journal of Abnormal Child Psychology, 30,* 571–587.

Boyle, M. H., & Offord, D. R. (1988). Prevalence of childhood disorder, perceived need for help, family dysfunction, and resource allocation for child welfare and children's mental health services in Ontario. *Canadian Journal of Behavioural Science, 20,* 374–388.

Breen, M., & Barkley, R. A. (1988). Parenting stress and child psychopathology in ADHD boys and girls. *Journal of Pediatric Psychology, 13,* 265–280.

Byrne, J. M., DeWolfe, N. D., & Bawden, H. N. (1998). Assessment of attention-deficit hyperactivity disorder in preschoolers. *Child Neuropsychology, 4,* 49–66.

Campbell, S. B. (1990). *Behavior problems in preschool children.* New York: Guilford Press.

Campbell, S. B., Endman, M., & Bernfield, G. (1977). A three year follow-up of hyperactive preschoolers into elementary school. *Journal of Child Psychology and Psychiatry, 18,* 239–249.

Chi, T. C., & Hinshaw, S. P. (2002). Mother–child relationships of children with ADHD: The role of maternal depressive symptoms and depression-related distortions. *Journal of Abnormal Child Psychology, 30,* 387–400.

Chronis, A. M., Chacko, A., Fabiano, G. A., Wymbs, B. T., & Pelham, W. E., Jr. (2004). Enhancements to the behavioral parent training paradigm for families of children with ADHD: Review and future directions. *Clinical Child and Family Psychology Review, 7,* 1–27.

Clark, M. L., Cheyne, A. J., Cunningham, C. E., & Siegel, L. S. (1988). Dyadic peer interaction and task orientation in attention-deficit disordered children. *Journal of Abnormal Child Psychology, 16,* 1–15.

Cunningham, C. E. (1997). Readiness for change: Applications to the management of ADHD. *ADHD Report, 5,* 6–9.

Cunningham, C. E., & Barkley, R. A. (1978). The effects of Ritalin on the mother–child interactions of hyperactive identical twins. *Developmental Medicine and Child Neurology, 20,* 634–642.

Cunningham, C. E., & Barkley, R. A. (1979). The interactions of hyperactive and normal children with their mothers during free play and structured tasks. *Child Development, 50,* 217–224.

Cunningham, C. E., Benness, B., & Siegel, L. S. (1988). Family functioning, time allocation, and parental depression in the families of normal and ADHD Children. *Journal of Clinical Child Psychology, 17,* 169–178.

Cunningham, C. E., & Boyle, M. (2002). Preschoolers at risk for attention deficit hyperactivity disorder and oppositional defiant disorder: Family, parenting, and educational correlates. *Journal of Abnormal Child Psychology, 30,* 555–569.

Cunningham, C. E., Boyle, M., Offord, D., Racine, Y., Hundert, J., Secord, M., et al. (2000). Tri Ministry Project: Diagnostic and demographic correlates of school-based parenting course utilization. *Journal of Consulting and Clinical Psychology, 68,* 928–933.

Cunningham, C. E., Bremner, R. B., & Boyle, M. (1995). Large group community-based parenting programs for families of preschoolers at risk for disruptive behaviour disorders: Utilization, cost effectiveness, and outcome. *Journal of Child Psychology and Psychiatry, 36,* 1141–1159.

Cunningham, C. E., Bremner, R. B., & Secord-Gilbert, M. (1998*). COPE, the Community Parent Education Program: A school based family systems oriented workshop for parents of children with disruptive behavior disorders (Leader's manual).* Hamilton, Ontario, Canada: COPE Works.

Cunningham, C. E., Buchanan, D., Deal, K., & Miller, H. (2003). *Modeling client-centred children's services using discrete choice conjoint analysis.* Poster presented at the annual meeting of the American Psychological Association, Toronto.

Cunningham, C. E., Clark, M. L., Heaven, R. K., Durrant, J., & Cunningham, L. J. (1989). The effects of group problem solving and contingency management procedures on the positive and negative interactions of learning disabled and attention deficit disordered children with an autistic peer. *Child and Family Behavior Therapy, 11,* 89–106.

Cunningham, C. E., Davis, J. R., Bremner, R., Dunn, K. R., & Rzasa, T. (1993). Coping modeling problem solving versus mastery modeling: Effects on adherence, in-session process, and skill acquisition in a residential PT program. *Journal of Consulting and Clinical Psychology, 61,* 871–877.

Cunningham, C. E., & Siegel, L. S. (1987). Peer interactions of normal and attention-deficit disordered boys during free-play, cooperative task, and simulated classroom situations. *Journal of Abnormal Child Psychology, 15,* 247–268.

Cunningham, C. E., Siegel, L. S., & Offord, D. R.

(1985). A developmental dose response analysis of the efforts of methylphenidate on the peer interactions of attention deficit disordered boys. *Journal of Child Psychology and Psychiatry, 26,* 955–971.

Cunningham, C. E., Siegel, L. S., & Offord, D. R. (1991). A dose–response analysis of the effects of methylphenidate on the peer interactions and simulated classroom performance of ADD children with and without conduct problems. *Journal of Child Psychology and Psychiatry, 32,* 439–452.

Dishion, T. J., & Patterson, G. R. (1992). Age effects in parent training outcome. *Behavior Therapy, 23,* 719–729.

Dubey, D. R., O'Leary, S., & Kaufman, K. F. (1983). Training parents of hyperactive children in child management: A comparative outcome study. *Journal of Abnormal Child Psychology, 11,* 229–246.

DuPaul, G. J., McGoey, K. E., Eckert, T. L., & Van Brakle, J. (2001). Preschool children with attention-deficit/hyperactivity disorder: Impairments in behavioral, social, and school functioning. *Journal of the American Academy of Child and Adolescent Psychiatry, 36,* 1036–1045.

Earls, F., & Jung, K. G. (1987). Temperament and home environment characteristics as causal factors in the early development of childhood psychopathology. *Journal of the American Academy of Child and Adolescent Psychiatry, 26,* 491–498.

Edwards, G., Barkley, R. A., Laneri, M., Fletcher, K., & Metevia, L. (2001). Parent–adolescent conflict in teenagers with ADHD and ODD. *Journal of Abnormal Child Psychology, 29,* 557–572.

Epstein, N. B., Bishop, D. S., & Levine, S. (1978, October). The McMaster model of family functioning. *Journal of Marriage and Family Counseling,* pp. 19–31.

Evans, C., Margison, F., & Barkham, M. (1998). The contribution of reliable and clinically significant change methods to evidence-based mental health. *Evidence-Based Mental Health, 1,* 70–72.

Eyberg, S. M., Boggs, S., & Algina, J. (1995). Parent–child interaction therapy: A psychosocial model for the treatment of young children with conduct problem behaviour and their families. *Psychopharmacology Bulletin, 31,* 83–91.

Firestone, P., & Witt, J. (1982). Characteristics of families completing and prematurely discontinuing a behavioral PT program. *Journal of Pediatric Psychology, 7,* 209–221.

Fletcher, K. E., Fischer, M., Barkley, R. A., & Smallish, L. (1996). A sequential analysis of the mother-adolescent interactions of ADHD, ADHD/ODD, and normal teenagers during neutral and conflict discussions. *Journal of Abnormal Child Psychology, 24,* 271–297.

Freeman, W., Phillips, J., & Johnston, C. (1992, June). *Treatment effects on hyperactive and aggressive behaviours in ADHD children.* Paper presented at the meeting of the Canadian Psychological Association, Québec City.

Gerdes, A. C., Hoza, B., & Pelham, W. E. (2003). Attention-deficit/hyperactivity disordered boys' relationships with their mothers and fathers: Child, mother and father perceptions. *Development and Psychopathology, 15,* 363–382.

Gomez, R., & Sanson, A. V. (1994). Mother–child interactions and noncompliance in hyperactive boys with and without conduct problems. *Journal of Child Psychology and Psychiatry, 35,* 447–490.

Greenwald, A. G., & Albert, R. D. (1968). Acceptance and recall of improvised arguments. *Journal of Personality and Social Psychology, 8,* 31–35.

Grusec, J. E., & Goodnow, J. (1994). Impact of parental discipline methods on the child's internalization of values: A reconceptualization of current point of view. *Developmental Psychology, 30,* 40–19.

Haenlein, M., & Caul, W. F. (1987). Attention deficit disorder with hyperactivity: A specific hypothesis of reward dysfunction. *Journal of the American Academy of Child and Adolescent Psychiatry, 26,* 356–362.

Hanf, C., & Kling, J. (1973). *Facilitating parent–child interactions: A two stage training model.* Unpublished manuscript, University of Oregon Medical School.

Harrison, C., & Sofronoff, K. (2002). ADHD and parental psychological distress: Role of demographics, child behavioural characteristics, and parental cognitions. *Journal of the American Academy of Child and Adolescent Psychiatry, 41,* 703–711.

Harvey, E., Danforth, J. S., McKee, T. R., Ulaszek, W. R., & Friedman, J. L. (2003). Parenting of children with attention-deficit/hyperactivity disorder (ADHD): The role of parental ADHD symptomatology. *Journal of Attention Disorders, 7,* 31–42.

Hoza, B., Owens, J. S., Pelham, W. E., Swanson, J. M., Conners, C. K., Hinshaw, S. P., et al. (2000). Parent cognitions as predictors of child treatment response in attention-deficit/hyperactivity disorder. *Journal of Abnormal Child Psychology, 28,* 569–583.

Janis, I. L. (1983). The role of social support in adherence to stressful decisions. *American Psychologist, 38,* 143–160.

Janis, I. L., & King, B. T. (1954). The influence of role-playing on opinion change. *Journal of Abnormal and Social Psychology, 49,* 211–218.

Johnston, C. (1996). Parent characteristics and parent–child interactions in families of nonproblem children and ADHD children with higher and lower levels of oppositional-defiant behavior. *Journal of Abnormal Child Psychology, 24,* 85–104.

Johnston, C., & Freeman, W. (1997). Attributions for child behavior in parents of children without behavior disorders and children with attention deficit-hyperactivity disorder. *Journal of Consulting and Clinical Psychology, 65,* 636–645.

Kazdin, A. E. (1990). Premature termination from treatment among children referred for antisocial behavior. *Journal of Child Psychology and Psychiatry, 31,* 415–425.

Kazdin, A. E., Holland, L., & Crowley, M. (1997). Family experience of barriers to treatment and premature termination from child therapy. *Journal of Consulting and Clinical Psychology, 65,* 453–463.

Kazdin, A. E., Mazurick, J. L., & Bass, D. (1993). Risk for attrition in treatment of antisocial children and families. *Journal of Clinical Child Psychology, 22,* 2–16.

Kazdin, A. E., Mazurick, J. L., & Siegel, T. C. (1994). Treatment outcome among children with externalizing disorder who terminate prematurely versus those who complete psychotherapy. *Journal of the American Academy of Child and Adolescent Psychiatry, 33,* 549–557.

Keown, L. J., & Woodward, L. J. (2002). Early parent–child relations and family functioning of preschool boys with pervasive hyperactivity. *Journal of Abnormal Child Psychology, 30,* 541–553.

King, B. T., & Janis, I. L. (1956). Comparison of the effectiveness of improvised versus nonimprovised role-playing in producing opinion changes. *Human Relations, 9,* 177–186.

Lakes, K., Tamm, L., Childress, C., Simpson, S., Nguyen, A. S., Cunningham, C. E., et al. (2004, April). *Early intervention for preschoolers at risk for ADHD: The CUIDAR for attention and learning program.* Poster presented at the Society for Pediatric Psychology's Conference on Child Health Psychology, Charleston, SC.

Leary, M. R., & Miller, R. S. (1986). *Social psychology and dysfunctional behavior.* New York: Springer-Verlag.

MacKenzie, K. R. (1990). *Introduction to time limited group psychotherapy.* Washington, DC: American Psychiatric Press.

Margison, F., Barkham, M., Evans, C., McGrath, G., Mellor-Clark, J., Audin, K., et al. (2000). Measurement and psychotherapy: Evidence-based practice and practice-based evidence. *British Journal of Psychiatry, 177,* 123–130.

Mash, E. J., & Johnston, C. (1982). A comparison of the mother–child interactions of younger and older hyperactive and normal children. *Child Development, 53,* 1371–1381.

Mash, E. J., & Johnston, C. (1983). Parental perceptions of child behavior problems, parenting self-esteem, and mothers' reported stress in younger and older hyperactive and normal children. *Journal of Consulting and Clinical Psychology, 51,* 68–99.

McCleary, L., & Ridley, T. (1999). Parenting adolescents with ADHD: Evaluation of a psychoeducation group. *Patient Education and Counseling, 38,* 3–10.

McMahon, R. J. (1994). Diagnosis, assessment, and treatment of externalizing problems in children: The role of longitudinal data. *Journal of Consulting and Clinical Psychology, 62,* 901–917.

McMahon, R. J., & Forehand, R. (2003). *Helping the noncompliant child: Family-based treatment for oppositional behavior* (2nd ed.). New York: Guilford Press.

McMiller, W. P., & Weisz, J. R. (1996). Help-seeking preceding mental health clinic intake among African-American, Latino, and Caucasian youths. *Journal of the American Academy of Child and Adolescent Psychiatry, 35,* 1086–1097.

Meichenbaum, D., & Turk, D. C. (1987). *Facilitating treatment adherence: A practitioner's guidebook.* New York: Plenum Press.

Montgomery, P. (2002). Media-based behavioural treatments for behavioural disorders in children. *Cochrane Database of Systematic Reviews, 2.*

Offord, D. R., Boyle, M. H., Szatmari, P., Rae-Grant, N., Links, P. S., Cadman, D., et al. (1987). Ontario Child Health Study: II. Six month prevalence of disorder and rates of service utilization. *Archives of General Psychiatry, 44,* 832–836.

Offord, D. R., Kraemer, H. C., Kazdin, A. E., Jensen, P. S., & Harrington, M. D. (1998). Lowering the burden of suffering from child psychiatric disorder: Trade-offs among clinical, targeted, and universal interventions. *Journal of the American Academy of Child and Adolescent Psychiatry, 37,* 686–694.

Panaccione, V. F., & Wahler, R. G. (1986). Child behavior, maternal depression, and social coercion as factors in the quality of child care. *Journal of Abnormal Child Psychology, 14,* 263–278.

Patterson, G. R. (1982). *Coercive family process.* Eugene, OR: Castalia.

Patterson, G. R., & Forgatch, M. S. (1985). Therapist behaviour as a determinant for client noncompliance: A paradox for behaviour modification. *Journal of Consulting and Clinical Psychology, 53,* 846–851.

Patterson, G. R., Reid, J. B., & Dishion, T. J. (1992). *Antisocial boys.* Eugene, OR: Castalia.

Pihlakoski, L., Aromaa, M., Sourander, A., Rautava, P., Helenius, H., & Sillanpaa, M. (2004). Use of and need for professional help for emotional and behavioral problems among preadolescents: A prospective cohort study of 3 to 12–year old children. *Journal of the American Academy of Child and Adolescent Psychiatry, 43,* 974–983.

Pisterman, S., Firestone, P., McGrath, P., Goodman, J. T., Webster, I., Mallory, R., et al. (1992). The effects of parent training parenting stress and sense of competence. *Canadian Journal of Behavioural Science, 24,* 41–58.

Pisterman, S., McGrath, P. J., Firestone, P., Goodman, J. T., Webster, I., & Mallory, R. (1989). Outcome of parent-mediated treatment of preschoolers with attention deficit disorder with hyperactivity. *Journal of Consulting and Clinical Psychology, 57,* 636–643.

Podolski, C. L., & Nigg, J. T. (2001). Parent stress and coping in relation to child ADHD severity and associated child disruptive behavior disorders. *Journal of Clinical Child Psychology, 30,* 503–513.

Pollard, S., Ward, E. M., & Barkley, R. A. (1983). The effects of PT and Ritalin on the parent–child interactions of hyperactive boys. *Child and Family Therapy, 5,* 51–69.

Prinz, R. J., & Miller, G. E. (1994). Family-based treatment for childhood antisocial behavior: Experimental influences on dropout and engagement. *Journal of Consulting and Clinical Psychology, 62,* 645–650.

Prochaska, J. O., DiClemente, C. C., & Norcross, J. C. (1992). In search of how people change. Applications to addictive behaviors. *American Psychologist, 47,* 1102–1114.

Prochaska, J. O., Velicer, W. R., Rossi, J. S., Goldstein, M. G., Marcus, B. H., Rakowski, W., et al. (1994). Stages of change and decisional balance for 12 problem behaviors. *Health Psychology, 13,* 39–46.

Sanders, M. R., Markie-Dadds, C., Tully, L. A., & Bor, W. (2000). The Triple P-Positive parenting program: A comparison of enhanced, standard, and self-directed behavioral family intervention for parents of children with early onset conduct problems. *Journal of Consulting and Clinical Psychology, 68,* 624–640.

Schachar, R., & Tannock, R. (1995). Test of four hypotheses for the comorbidity of attention-deficit hyperactivity disorder and conduct disorder. *Journal of the American Academy of Child and Adolescent Psychiatry, 34,* 639–648.

Schumann, E., Foote, R., Eyberg, S., Boggs, S., & Algina, J. (1998). Efficacy of parent–child interaction therapy: Interim report of a randomized trial with short-term maintenance. *Journal of Clinical Child Psychology, 27*(1), 34–45.

Sobol, M. P., Ashbourne, D. T., Earn, B. M., & Cunningham, C. E. (1989). Parents' attributions for achieving compliance from attention-deficit disordered children. *Journal of Abnormal Child Psychology, 17,* 359–369.

Sonuga-Barke, E. J., Daley, D., & Thompson, M. (2002). Does maternal ADHD reduce the effectiveness of parent training for preschool children's ADHD? *Journal of the American Academy of Child and Adolescent Psychiatry, 41,* 696–702.

Sonuga-Barke, E. J., Daley, D., Thompson, M., Laver-Bradbury, C., & Weeks, A. (2001). Parent-based therapies for preschool attention-deficit/hyperactivity disorder: A randomized, controlled trial with a community sample. *Journal of the American Academy of Child and Adolescent Psychiatry, 40,* 402–408.

Stormont-Spurgin, M., & Zentall, S. S. (1995). Contributing factors in the manifestation of aggression in preschoolers with hyperactivity. *Journal of Child Psychology and Psychiatry, 36,* 491–509.

Szatmari, P., Boyle, M. H., & Offord, D. R. (1993). Familial aggregation of emotional and behavioral problems of childhood in the general population. *American Journal of Psychiatry, 150,* 1398–1403.

Szatmari, P., Offord, D. R., & Boyle, M. H. (1989). Correlates, associated impairments and patterns of service utilization of children with attention deficit disorder: Findings from the Ontario Child Health Study. *Journal of Child Psychology and Psychiatry, 30,* 205–217.

Taylor, E., Chadwick, O., Heptinstall, E., & Danckaerts, M. (1996). Hyperactivity and conduct problems as risk factors for adolescent development. *Journal of the American Academy of Child and Adolescent Psychiatry, 35*(9), 1213–1226.

U.S. Department of Health and Human Services. (1999). *Mental health: A report of the Surgeon General.* Washington, DC: U.S. Government Printing Office.

Wahler, R. G. (1980). The insular mother: Her problems in parent–child treatment. *Journal of Applied Behaviour Analysis, 13,* 207–219.

Webster-Stratton, C. W. (1994). Advancing videotape parent training: A comparison study. *Journal of Consulting and Clinical Psychology, 62,* 583–593.

Webster-Stratton, C. W., & Hammond, M. (1990) . Predictors of treatment outcome in parent training for families with conduct problem children. *Behavior Therapy, 21,* 319–337.

Webster-Stratton, C. W., & Hammond, M. (1997). Treating children with early-onset conduct problems: A comparison of child and parent training interventions. *Journal of Consulting and Clinical Psychology, 65*(1), 93–109.

Webster-Stratton, C. W., Reid, J., & Hammond, M. (2001). Social skills and problem-solving training for children with early-onset conduct problems. Who benefits? *Journal of Child Psychology and Psychiatry, 42,* 943–952.

Weiss, B., Dodge, K. A., Bates, J. E., & Pettit, G. S. (1992). Some consequences of early harsh discipline: Child aggression and a maladapted social information processing style. *Child Development, 63*(6), 1321–1335.

Weiss, G., & Hechtman, L. T. (1986). *Hyperactive children grown up: Empirical findings and theoretical considerations.* New York: Guilford Press.

Whalen, C. K., Henker, B., & Dotemoto, S. (1980). Methylphenidate and hyperactivity: Effects on teacher behaviours. *Science, 208,* 1280–1282.

Woodward, L., Taylor, E., & Dowdney, L. (1998). The parenting and family functioning of children with hyperactivity. *Journal of Child Psychology and Psychiatry, 39,* 161–169.

Zahner, G. E. P., Pawelkiewicz, J., Defrancesco, J. J., & Adnopoz, J. (1992). Children's mental health service needs and utilization patterns in an urban community: An epidemiological assessment. *Journal of the American Academy of Child and Adolescent Psychiatry, 31,* 951–960.

CHAPTER 14

Training Families with Adolescents with ADHD

ARTHUR L. ROBIN

Adolescence is a challenging developmental period for families, because children are undergoing exponential physiological, cognitive, behavioral, and emotional changes. The typical problems of adolescence are magnified exponentially for the individual with Attention-Deficit/Hyperactivity Disorder (ADHD) and the family, because the core symptoms and associated features of ADHD interfere with successfully mastering the developmental tasks of adolescence. As a result, teens with ADHD suffer academic failure, social isolation, depression, and low self-esteem, and become embroiled in many unpleasant conflicts with their families. They experience a lower quality of life than their peers without ADHD (Topolski et al., 2004).

Parents encounter a variety of home management problems with their adolescents who have ADHD, including noncompliance with rules; conflicts over issues such as chores, curfew, friends, driving, and general attitude; and school-related issues such as homework. These conflicts usually reflect independence-related themes; for example, the adolescent desires to make his or her own decisions about chores, homework, or whatever the issue may be, and the parents desire to retain decision-making authority. Such conflicts take the form of unpleasant verbal exchanges characterized by shouting, yelling, name calling, and other hurtful and coercive communication styles.

THEORY

A comprehensive biobehavioral–family systems model is helpful in understanding the factors that determine the degree of conflict concerning home management issues experienced by the family with an adolescent who has ADHD. Within this model, my colleagues and I postulate that the biological/genetic factors underlying ADHD interact with the developmental tasks of adolescence and environmental/family contingencies to influence the frequency and intensity of home management problems. Teenagers are expected to accomplish five major developmental tasks: (1) individuate from their parents, (2) adjust to sexual maturation, (3) develop new and deeper peer relationships, (4) form a self-identity, and (5) plan for a career. Parent–teen relations undergo radical restructuring punctuated by periodic perturbation and conflict as adolescents become more independent, necessitating a shift from a more authoritarian to a more democratic parental decision-making structure and communication process.

Three major dimensions of family relations determine the degree of clinically significant conflict likely to occur as teenagers individuate from their parents (Robin, 1998; Robin & Foster, 1989): (1) deficits in problem solving, communication, and contingency management skills; (2) cognitive distortions; and (3) family structure problems. Families that are unable to solve problems through a process of mutual problem definition, brainstorming alternative solutions, solution evaluation and negotiation, and careful implementation planning are likely to develop excessive independence-related disputes. When a family also communicates in an accusatory, defensive, or sarcastic manner, members become enraged and act on the basis of hot emotions rather than cool logic, precluding rational problem solving. Parents' inability to implement consistently positive reinforcement, response cost, and other contingency management techniques contributes to the escalation of oppositional, coercive adolescent behavior.

"Cognitive distortions" are unreasonable expectations and malicious attributions that elicit angry affect and sidetrack solution-oriented communication. A parent, for example, may fear the ruinous consequences of giving too much freedom to an adolescent; demand unflinching loyalty or obedience; or incorrectly attribute innocent adolescent behavior to malicious, purposeful motives. An adolescent may jump to the conclusion that the parents' rules are intrinsically unfair and likely to ruin any chance of having fun in peer relations, and that teenagers should have as much autonomy in decision making as they desire. In crisis situations, unreasonable beliefs color judgment and add emotional overtones to behavioral reactions. A father who demands obedience, is concerned about ruination, and believes that the adolescent is purposely misbehaving will have a difficult time, for example, remaining rational at 2:00 A.M. when his daughter comes home 2 hours past the agreed-upon curfew. If the daughter thinks her father's midnight curfew is unfair because it prevents her from ever having any fun with her friends, and that her father has no right to dictate her curfew, she will also be less than rational. Such unrealistic cognitive reactions mediate emotional overreactions, which spur continued conflict.

"Family structure problems" are difficulties in the organization of the family. All families have a hierarchy or "pecking order," and in Western civilization parents are typically in charge of children. Adolescence is a transitional period when parents are supposed to be upgrading the children's status in the hierarchy, culminating in an egalitarian relationship between adult children and their parents. It is easy for a coercive child to overwhelm the parents, and by adolescence such a child may have too much power in the family—a situation we call "hierarchy reversal." In an earlier edition of this book (Barkley, 1990), Patterson's (1982) coercion theory was integrated with Barkley's research findings on family interaction between children with ADHD and their parents to illustrate how the oppositional behavior of school-age children with ADHD may develop into a pattern of severe hierarchy reversal. Such a pattern often meets criteria according to the current version (fourth edition, text revision) of the *Diagnostic and Statistical Manual of Mental Disorders* (DSM-IV-TR; American Psychiatric Association, 2000) for Oppositional Defiant Disorder (ODD) or Conduct Disorder (CD) by adolescence. Sometimes one parent and the adolescent may also take sides against the other parent, forming a cross-generational coalition. Two family members may place the third in the middle of a conflict, forcing the third to take sides. This pattern, called "triangulation," often occurs with adolescents who have ADHD. For example, the father comes home to find that the mother and son have had a major battle earlier that afternoon. The mother and son both turn to the father, presenting their sides of the argument and appealing for support, and the father is triangulated or caught in the middle. Sometimes the father sides with his wife, other times with his son. Each of these structural problems may result in a "divide and conquer" situation, where the adolescent can continue to engage in some antisocial or inappropriate behavior because the parents are not able to work well as an executive team on setting and enforcing limits.

It is also useful to view ADHD symptoms within a broader context of executive functions of the brain. Barkley's (1997a) executive function model of ADHD, for example, conceptualizes behavioral inhibition as the core executive function in deficit for individuals with ADHD (see also Chapter 7, this volume). Deficits in four other executive functions—nonverbal working memory, verbal working memory, self-control over affect, and reconstitution—follow from poor behavioral inhibition. Poor nonverbal working memory may make it difficult for the adolescent with ADHD to stay on task and solve problems in a planful way when resolving conflicts during family discussions; to carry out agreements with parents; and to complete schoolwork, chores, or other responsibilities. The distorted sense of time associated with poor nonverbal working memory may spur increased conflict, because impatient adolescents badger their parents to meet their demands right away, however unreasonable or inappropriate those demands may be (e.g., "Buy me a car," "Take me to my friend's house right now," "Let me get my license today").

Poor internalization of language (verbal working memory) may impede learning from past parental consequences and following parental rules, which frustrates parents tremendously and often leads them to form excessively malicious attributions that the adolescent is purposely failing to meet their expectations. Poor self-regulation of affect/motivation/arousal may account for the emotional overreactivity, poor frustration tolerance, poor intrinsic motivation, and explosiveness of many adolescents with ADHD, fueling family conflict. Poor reconstitution may contribute to poor interpersonal problem solving and the tendency to select the first solution that comes to mind, rather than dissembling the problem into its component parts and attempting to creatively reassemble the parts into a new solution. Researchers have begun to compare these executive functions in adolescents with and without ADHD, finding partial support for the model given here (Barkley, Edwards, Laneri, Fletcher, & Metevia, 2001a; Frazier, Demaree, & Youngstrom, 2004).

Individual psychopathology in the parents, such as depression, substance abuse, anxiety, personality disorders, or schizophrenia, adds even more complexity and stress to the home-based problems of an adolescent with ADHD. As the genetic basis for ADHD is becoming more widely known and accepted, therapists are diagnosing many of the parents of children with ADHD as having ADHD themselves. Indeed, the risk to the parents is between 20% and 40%. The stress of having two or more distractible, hot-tempered, impulsive, restless

members in a single family exponentially raises the probability of clinically significant conflict. Such a view is supported by a longitudinal study of twins in which the majority of family conflict experienced in families of teens 15 and older was found to be heritable; that is, it was accounted for by genetic factors (Braungart-Rieker, Rende, Plomin, DeFries, & Fulker, 1995; Pike, McGuire, Hetherington, Reiss, & Plomin, 1996). How can family conflict be so heavily influenced by genetics? Because by the teen years, many of the purely psychosocial factors contributing to conflict have often remitted, diminished, or resolved. If conflicts persist, it is usually because of the increasing role of genetic effects (via personality factors and executive functioning or self-control) in the teens (Elkins, McGue, & Iacono, 1997) and parents that predispose to conflict. And those factors are largely inherited, ADHD being one among them. Finally, extrafamilial factors, such as the school and peer environments, have an impact on the overall family relationships.

Figure 14.1 summarizes this biobehavioral–family systems model. Prior to the adolescence of its children, a family has developed a homeostatic pattern or system of "checks and balances" regulating its members' interactions. The developmental changes of adolescence disrupt homeostatic patterns, spurring an acute period of "typical parent–teen conflict" between ages 12 and 14. Most families emerge from this stage with new homeostatic patterns and methods of resolving home-based conflicts. Deficits in problem solving, communication skills, contingency management skills, cognitive distortions, family structure problems, and individual or marital/couple pathology promote clinically significant conflict during early adolescence. These five factors interact with the executive functions rendered less efficient by impaired behavioral inhibition to create a clinical presentation of severe, moderate, or mild ADHD with or without associated ODD or CD. Although there has been no comprehensive research validating this entire model, researchers have examined its problem-solving communication skills component, demonstrating that families with teens who have ADHD plus ODD exhibit more specific disputes, more negative communication, and more aggressive tactics and hostile affect than families with typical adolescents (Edwards, Barkley, Laneri, Fletcher, & Metevia, 2001).

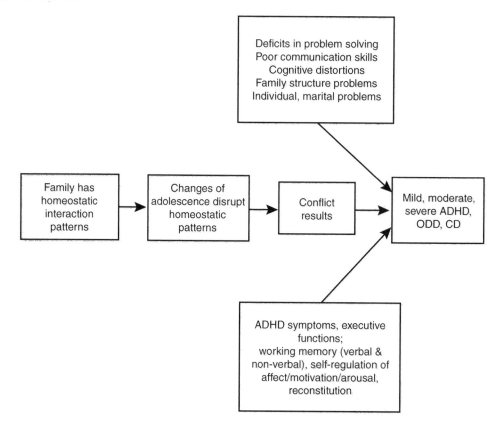

FIGURE 14.1. A biobehavioral–family system model of ADHD.

INTERVENTION

At the point of diagnosis and/or referral, most adolescents with ADHD are (1) experiencing difficulty completing their schoolwork and making satisfactory academic progress; and (2) getting into frequent conflict with their parents not only about their poor school performance, but also about a variety of compliance-related issues (e.g., chores, curfew, dating, bedtime, fighting with siblings, negative voice tone, and general disrespect). Some are also having significant difficulties with peer relationships and behavior in the community, as well as low self-esteem, depression, anxiety, and other comorbid conditions. A minority are actively antisocial and aggressive; in trouble with the legal authorities; and/or abusing marijuana, alcohol, or other substances. To make matters worse, many of the younger adolescents (ages 12–15) vehemently deny that there is anything wrong with them and strongly resist taking medication or participating in any other interventions.

A multidimensional intervention approach is therefore essential to address these complex issues. We need to keep in mind that ADHD is a chronic condition with a neurobiological underpinning. At the point of referral, an adolescent's immediate problems may be at the crisis level in school and at home. As a result, the majority of adolescents with ADHD and their parents benefit from an intensive burst of approximately 25 sessions of a flexible combination of family and individual therapy, held two to four times per month spaced over several months. Many families look upon this burst of intervention as a "cure" or "correction" and don't expect to have to continue interventions indefinitely. However, chronic conditions require far more than intensive, brief interventions. After putting out the immediate fires, the clinician will need to educate the adolescent and the family about the implications of ADHD as a chronic condition, help them accept and adjust to the notion that it is a chronic condition, and establish systems for ongoing monitoring and reintervention throughout adolescence and into adulthood.

The clinician must always remember and must repeatedly remind the adolescent and the parents that ADHD is primarily a neurobiological condition that affects behavior and emotions. To address the neurobiological aspects of ADHD, it is useful to borrow a conceptual framework from the cognitive rehabilitation field. Cognitive rehabilitation models approach the rehabilitation of a neurologically impaired individual with three broad strategies (Nadeau, 2002): (1) improve cognitive function; (2) develop internal and external compensatory strategies; and (3) restructure the physical and social environment to maximize functioning. The use of medication is the most effective example we have at present of directly improving cognitive functioning. The use of behavioral interventions with parents combined with teaching the adolescent effective compensatory strategies assist with restructuring the home environment. Educational accommodations (seating the adolescent close to the teacher, keeping a second set of textbooks at home, allowing extended time to complete examinations, making use of home–school reports, etc.) exemplify restructuring the physical and social environment at school to maximize functioning. The clinician is urged to explain this framework to families and keep it in mind as specific interventions are reviewed in this chapter.

Overview of the Phases of Intervention

Table 14.1 outlines the phases of this initial burst of intervention. The practitioner first needs to decide whether the adolescent is out of control in an antisocial, aggressive, and/or substance-abusing manner (i.e., whether a comorbid diagnosis of CD or substance abuse is warranted). If either or both of these conditions apply, they become the highest-priority treatment goals. In the case of substance abuse, the clinician decides whether the severity of the problem merits immediate referral to a substance abuse specialist, or whether it will be possible to proceed with the treatment program while monitoring substance use through, for example, random urine or Breathalyzer testing. If an adolescent is using marijuana or alcohol on a recreational basis on weekends or even once or twice a week, and he or she makes a genuine commitment to work toward curtailing drug use, I usually keep the case but arrange for urine or Breathalyzer testing. More frequent marijuana or alcohol use, or any use of cocaine, heroin, hallucinogens, or other drugs, is cause for an immediate referral to a substance abuse specialist, who triages the patient to either an inpatient or outpatient substance abuse program.

In the case of out-of-control behavior that warrants a diagnosis of CD, the practitioner should undertake an intensive outpatient intervention designed to restore reasonable parental controls through the use of strategic/structural family interventions. Home-based interventions such as multisystemic therapy (Henggeler, Schoenwald, Borduin, Rowland, & Cunningham, 1998) have proven useful in such cases. If several months of intensive intervention such as multisystemic therapy fail to restore parental controls, the practitioner should consider out-of-home placements for the adolescent. Such placements might include inpatient psychiatric hospitalization, therapeutic foster care, specialized residential schools or treatment centers, or even military school in certain cases.

In the majority of cases, the adolescent and his or her family are next provided with comprehensive ADHD education, designed to instill the attitudes and expectations necessary to cope with a chronic condition and benefit from the remainder of the interventions. Because the natural developmental changes of adolescents render many youngsters highly resistant to acceptance of chronic conditions such as ADHD and their treatments, ADHD education assumes a very important role. Such education takes place over several weeks through conducting direct discussions in family and individual sessions; providing bibliotherapy, videotapes, and referrals to local and national support groups; and putting the adolescent in touch with peers who have ADHD and can

TABLE 14.1. Phases of Intervention

Sessions 1–2	Family ADHD education
Session 3	Preparing for medication
Sessions 4–9	Enhancing academic success
Sessions 10–22	Home-based interventions
Sessions 23–25	Consolidation, termination

Note. At any point where the therapist becomes aware of substance abuse and/or severely out-of-control conduct, the ongoing course of intervention is interrupted. The adolescent is referred for substance abuse treatment, intensive multisystemic intervention, or both, as needed.

serve as positive role models. Of course, like many facets of a comprehensive intervention, ADHD education continues for a long time beyond the initial efforts made by the practitioner.

Getting medication started is the next phase of intervention. If medication is to be prescribed, it is important to begin it early in the overall intervention—to help break the cycle of past failure and conflict abruptly, and to have time to adequately titrate the dose and maximize the synergistic potential of medication plus educational and behavioral/psychological interventions. However, it is crucial to start medication after family ADHD education; a common error is to start medication immediately upon diagnosis, without taking adequate time to make sure that the adolescent understands and accepts medication. Such an error is likely to result in premature rejection of medication, because it sometimes leads the adolescent to feel that the practitioner is not truly interested in him or her as a person, but rather only interested in pleasing the parents by drugging the adolescent into compliance.

Targeting school performance is the next phase of intervention. After assessing the specific reasons why the adolescent is doing poorly at school, the clinician (1) teaches the adolescent and the parents compensatory strategies to work around these problems; (2) educates the teachers and other school personnel about ADHD in general and the patient's specific problems; and (3) helps the family advocate effectively with the school to obtain accommodations, special education, and any other educational interventions that modify the school environment to increase the adolescent's chances of succeeding in school.

As the adolescent begins to experience success at school, the therapist continues to the next phase of intervention—targeting problems at home. Using a combination of behavioral parent training, contingency management, and problem-solving communication techniques, the therapist helps the family members reduce parent–adolescent conflict and integrate solution-oriented communication and effective parenting principles into their natural response styles.

Afterward, the therapist assesses the need to address any residual problems. Such residual problems often include peer relationship issues, anxiety or depression, possible ADHD in the parents or siblings, or parental marital/couple

and/or personal problems. Individual cognitive-behavioral and supportive interventions are helpful for addressing adolescent or parent anxiety, depression, or related issues. Social skills group interventions may be used for peer relationship problems, as long as the practitioner keeps in mind the lack of evidence for generalizability and builds in procedures to spur generalization. Conjoint marital/couple therapy is sometimes needed for the parents' dyadic conflicts.

In the last few sessions of the initial burst of intervention, the therapist lengthens the interval between sessions to 3 and then 4 weeks, helps the family consolidate the gains they have made, and shifts into the "dental checkup" model of follow-up care. Most families enthusiastically appreciate the idea of periodic ADHD "checkups" several times per year.

Typically, the 25 sessions are divided as follows: Sessions 1–2 cover family ADHD education; session 3 covers medication issues; sessions 4–9 cover school success interventions; sessions 10–22 cover home-based interventions; and sessions 23–25 focus on other issues, gradually fading out to a follow-up mode. In the following sections of the chapter, each "module" of this multidimensional intervention is reviewed. Restoring parental control over an adolescent with severely disordered behavior is discussed after home-based interventions, even though the therapist may need to implement this intervention earlier.

Family ADHD Education

The goals of family ADHD education are to deal with the full spectrum of reactions to the ADHD diagnosis; to spur understanding and acceptance of the ADHD diagnosis; and to develop in the adolescent and his or her family the kind of coping, positive attitudes compatible with active participation in the multifaceted treatments discussed in this book. Typically, this is more challenging with the adolescent than with the parents. The practitioner begins this process at the feedback session, where the results of the diagnostic evaluation are conveyed to the adolescent and the parents, and continues it over the course of the first few therapy sessions. Of course, emotional acceptance takes time; thus ADHD education becomes an ongoing issue throughout the entire course of therapy.

We find it helpful to conceptualize the family ADHD education process as having four broad, somewhat overlapping stages: (1) giving the facts about ADHD and stating the treatment options; (2) listening to the reactions to the presentations of the facts and the treatment options; (3) applying cognitive restructuring and reattributional techniques to correct myths and false beliefs and to instill positive, coping attitudes toward ADHD; and (4) collaboratively establishing the specific treatment goals and tailoring the treatment options to the particular adolescent and his or her family. It is usually better to go through these steps separately with the adolescent and the parents, because (1) parents and adolescents have very different reactions and issues to be dealt with, and some steps are more applicable to parents, whereas others are more applicable to adolescents; (2) separate meetings signal to the adolescent that the practitioner respects him or her as an individual whose opinions and ideas are important and worthwhile apart from the parents' ideas; (3) family interaction problems are removed as a source of variance from ADHD education; and (4) the adolescent may open up more fully in the absence of the parents.

Giving the Facts

We usually start by making a clear statement that ADHD applies to the adolescent; giving a brief definition of ADHD, discussing its neurobiological/genetic etiology with the aid of concrete information, such as a photograph of the positron emission tomography (PET) scans from Zametkin's classic study (Zametkin et al., 1990); and highlighting how it impairs the quality of the adolescent's life in practical ways to which the teenager can relate. We talk in simple sentences that the teenager can understand, incorporate things the teenager has previously told us into our explanations, and pause often to check for understanding and questions. If the adolescent does not spontaneously bring up the most common myths about ADHD and its treatment, we bring them up and debunk them.

The following points, briefly illustrated here in the language used with teenagers, need to be covered throughout this presentation, although not necessarily all in one meeting or in the order given here:

1. "ADHD is a disorder involving difficulty paying attention, controlling the urge to act before thinking, and sometimes feeling or acting restless."
2. "You are not crazy or sick if you have ADHD. It is an invisible disability that represents the extremes of traits or characteristics that all people exhibit to a greater or lesser degree."
3. "ADHD usually lasts a lifetime, but it changes as you mature and grow older. In particular, the restlessness changes from more physical to more mental, but the inattention and impulsivity remain."
4. "ADHD affects all areas of your life, not just school. It may influence how you get along with other people, how you relate in intimate interpersonal situations, how organized you are at home, how you do in sports and hobbies, how easily you fall asleep and wake up, how you feel about yourself, and how you do on the job in the future."
5. "ADHD is not your fault, your parents' fault, or anyone's fault. It is a physical disorder, usually inherited, and is caused by a difference in brain chemistry."
6. "Chemicals called 'neurotransmitting chemicals,' which pass signals for self-control throughout the brain, aren't operating efficiently in people with ADHD. It would be like having too little brake fluid in your car; when you press the brake pedal, you can't stop. When an idea to do something pops into these persons' minds, they can't stop and think whether it is good or bad before they do it, because the chemicals that help the brain stop and think aren't working properly."
7. "Because ADHD is usually inherited, it is possible that your parents, brothers or sisters, or other relatives also have ADHD, even if they don't know it. If you have kids some day, they may also have ADHD. This could make family life like a real roller coaster!"
8. "ADHD is also influenced by your environment—for example, your parents, your school, and your friends. A good family, a good school, and good friends can make life a lot easier for the person with ADHD."
9. "ADHD is a challenge, not an excuse.

You are still responsible for your actions, even though you have a physical disorder that makes it harder for you to control your actions."

10. "ADHD is influenced by your physical health. It will be easier to deal with ADHD if you take proper care of yourself—for example, get enough sleep, maintain good nutrition, don't smoke or put drugs or alcohol in your body, and exercise regularly."

11. "Because ADHD is inherited and physical, we can't totally cure or eliminate it. Instead, we can help you learn to cope so life goes well for you. There are three general methods for learning to cope: (a) medical, (b) behavioral/psychological, and (c) educational. We will talk about these in detail as time goes on."

Listening to the Reactions to the Presentation

After presenting the facts, the practitioner listens carefully to the adolescent's reactions—using active listening to clarify how he or she is feeling, but not challenging or being confrontational. It is very important for adolescents to feel that they have been listened to and understood, and that their opinions have been taken seriously, because in the past their ideas may have often been discounted by adults. Let us look at an example of 15-year-old Bill, voicing his concerns about the diagnosis of ADHD:

BILL: So if I have ADHD, does this mean I am dumb and have a bad brain?

DR. ROBIN: You're feeling like having ADHD means you're stupid.

BILL: All the retards on the special education bus have ADHD. The whole football team whips their butts at gym.

DR. ROBIN: You feel like a retard, and you think your friends on the football team would give you a hard time about having ADHD.

BILL: Yeah, this is the kiss of death for me. My parents are going to freak out and take me to a million doctors, tutors, and shrinks. I'll probably miss football practice and get kicked off the team! And they will make me take medicine that will make me weird.

DR. ROBIN: So ADHD is going to mess up your whole life, take away all your free time and fun, and make you into a zombie?

BILL: Yeah, and just when Jennifer was starting to like me, too. Now Mike will get her for sure.

DR. ROBIN: You will also strike out with girls? This all sounds like a nightmare.

BILL: Yeah.

As Bill voices his fears and anxieties about peer ridicule, feeling stupid, having to go to a lot of doctors, getting kicked off the football team, losing his freedom, and never having a girlfriend, I empathetically clarify them but do not yet deal with them. Many adolescents may be thinking what Bill has verbalized, but it may take many sessions before they become comfortable confiding their worries in the therapist—although an advantage of their being impulsive is that they often blurt out their worries, despite their desire to hide them.

Dealing with Reactions: Application of Cognitive Restructuring

Cognitive restructuring and reattributional techniques, two of the mainstays of cognitive-behavioral therapy (Braswell & Bloomquist, 1991), are applicable techniques for dealing with adolescents' negative reactions to the ADHD diagnosis. Typically, one or more of the following types of distorted beliefs underlies the negative reaction:

1. "ADHD is a life sentence; my life is over. I'll never amount to anything."

2. "This means I am really dumb, stupid, crazy, or a bad person. All the bad things my parents and teachers have said about me are really true."

3. "I'll never have any friends any more; they will all think I'm a total nerd."

4. "I'll never have any fun, because I will have to spend all my time with tutors, doctors, and therapists."

5. "Medication will change my personality in bad ways. I like being wild, loud, and crazy. This is me, who I am, and no one is going to change me."

6. "I'm different from my friends, and I'll never be normal."

7. "I've really messed up now. It's all my fault."
8. "This whole ADHD thing is bull; it's just one more way my parents are trying to control my life."

These beliefs are really variations on three underlying extreme belief themes to which adolescents commonly adhere (Robin & Foster, 1989): (1) ruination ("This ADHD diagnosis is going to ruin my life, fun, and friends"); (2) autonomy ("Having ADHD will take away or limit my freedom"); and (3) perfectionism ("Now the world will know I'm less than a perfect person, and that's terrible"). We will revisit these beliefs later within the context of parenting and family conflict.

In cognitive restructuring with an adolescent, the therapist tactfully collaborates with the patient to (1) identify the distorted belief, (2) provide a logical challenge to it, (3) suggest a more reasonable belief, and (4) help the patient discover through collection of evidence that the reasonable belief is more valid than the unreasonable belief (Robin & Foster, 1989). Often, reframing negatively valenced ideas or thoughts to more positive motives or connotations is used along with cognitive restructuring.

Let us see how cognitive restructuring might proceed with Bill:

DR. ROBIN: I understand how you feel that ADHD will mess up your whole life, but before we jump to any quick conclusions, let's look at the evidence.

BILL: What evidence? I'm done, finished, all washed up!

DR. ROBIN: Let's start with the idea that you are dumb. On the IQ test I just gave you, you received a score of 115, which is above average. You may feel like you are dumb, but in fact you are smart. ADHD has nothing to do with being smart or dumb.

BILL: If I'm so smart, why do I do dumb things like spray paint on the garage?

DR. ROBIN: Good question. Your brain is like an expensive sports car without any brake fluid. We all get crazy ideas popping into our minds. People without ADHD press the brake pedal and it works; they don't act on their crazy ideas. People with ADHD press the brake pedal and nothing happens. They just keep on acting. This has nothing to do with IQ. You have a high IQ, just as the sports car has a great engine. But without brake fluid, the car won't stop, no matter how good the engine is. Now let's take your worry about having to go to the office to take pills and your friends teasing you. First of all, not everyone with ADHD takes medication. You would only take medication if you agree to, after you fully understand it. But let's say you did agree. We now have medicines that you take once in the morning and they last all day, so the only way your friends will know about it is if you tell them.

BILL: Great! Those drugs would make me into a weird zombie all day, then.

DR. ROBIN: The truth is, most people don't feel any different on medicine for ADHD, except they are not as hungry while it is in their bodies. Are any of your good friends on medicine for ADHD?

BILL: You wouldn't catch me hanging out with those retards.

DR. ROBIN: Do you know a kid named Danny Jones?

BILL: Danny Jones? Sure. The whole school knows him. He is captain of the football team, Mr. Cool. Every girl in school goes nuts over him. But he is really a great guy.

DR. ROBIN: He has ADHD and takes medicine for it every morning.

BILL: No way. Not Danny. He's too cool. Doc, you're kidding, right?

DR. ROBIN: Nope. Don't take my word for it. Ask him. He is glad to talk about it privately, and he gave me permission to tell other teens with ADHD about it, but he has no reason to announce it on the overhead speaker system in school. And don't forget to ask him whether medicine makes him feel weird.

The steps of cognitive restructuring flow together in this case example. The discussion of the IQ test illustrates challenging a distorted belief with the introduction of a more reasonable alternative and clear-cut evidence to back it up. The introduction of the highly regarded positive peer model who happens to have ADHD is the most potent type of evidence for changing beliefs about ADHD in teenagers, because peers are such an important part of their lives. It behooves clinicians who work with adolescents to develop a referral list of such positive peer models with ADHD in the local areas in which they work. Of course, the peers must consent in writing to have their names released. Clinical experience strongly suggests that adolescents will be more convinced to accept and cope with ADHD by their peers than by adults.

The use of books and audiovisual materials on ADHD written by adolescents for adolescents, and the orchestration of teen forum group sessions directed by adolescents, are additional techniques for fostering understanding and acceptance of ADHD. Several such books and videos are commercially available (Gordon, 1993; Quinn, 1995; Schubiner, 1995; Zeigler Dendy, 1999; Zeigler Dendy & Dendy, 2003). In addition, organizations such as Children and Adults with Attention-Deficit/Hyperactivity Disorder (CHADD) and the Attention Deficit Disorder Association (ADDA) schedule teen-directed sessions for adolescents at their national conferences and through their regional chapters.

Collaborative Treatment Planning

The last phase of the family ADHD education process with the adolescent is collaborative treatment planning. Let us return to Bill as I directly approach him about participating in treatment.

DR. ROBIN: We have one last thing to talk about—exactly what you are going to do, and how your parents, teachers, and I am going to help you deal with ADHD. For one, are you now willing to consider medication as one way to deal with ADHD?

BILL: I guess so.

DR. ROBIN: I'm not asking you to take it for sure, but just to go talk to a friend of mine, Dr. Jones, who specializes in medicine for teens with ADHD. Agreed?

BILL: OK. What else?

DR. ROBIN: Do you want your parents off your case at home? And your teachers off your case at school?

BILL: Sure. How?

DR. ROBIN: You've got to be willing to learn some new habits. I am willing to be like a coach and give you ideas and guide you, if

you will come in several times, but you will have to do the work.

BILL: Will I have to come at this time? I'm missing one of my favorite TV shows.

DR. ROBIN: Absolutely not. We can find another time.

BILL: I'll try.

The therapist continues to discuss and formulate the treatment goals with the adolescent, interacting in this informal manner. Now that the therapist has taken the time to listen to and deal with the adolescent's reactions, the teenager is more cooperative. Most of the time, this strategy works. But the practitioner needs to be prepared to be patient in those cases in which the adolescent's resistance lasts a longer time. With some 12- to 14-year-old adolescents, it is very difficult to enlist them collaboratively in the treatment process. Occasionally, the only reasonable strategy to follow is to decide to treat the case as if the young teenager were an 8- or 9-year-old and work with the parents on a management approach, without regularly involving the adolescent. This is clearly the less preferred approach, but nonetheless it is sometimes necessary.

Getting Medication Started

The Multimodal Treatment Study of ADHD (MTA Cooperative Group, 1999) demonstrated that in school-age children medication was the most effective treatment for ADHD symptoms, and that in some cases the combination of medication and behavioral interventions was superior to medication alone for changing other variables (e.g., ODD behavior, social interactions, and family interactions). Although this study was conducted with younger children, we have no reason to doubt that similar findings would occur with adolescents. Thus it is important to consider including medication in a comprehensive intervention for helping adolescents with ADHD. As mentioned earlier, within a neurocognitive rehabilitation model for treating ADHD, medication is the only intervention we have to date that reliably produces direct changes in the cognitive functions underlying ADHD.

However, adolescents must "buy into" medication as a potentially helpful intervention before it can be initiated. Clinically, we find that adolescents have negative attitudes toward medication. This section first reviews the research on adolescents' attitudes toward medication, and then provides clinical recommendations.

Three studies have asked children and adolescents currently receiving stimulant medication for ADHD to self-report their attitudes toward the medication and the impact of the medication on them. These studies pooled the results for teenagers and younger children, although in two of the studies all of the subjects were in middle or high school. Bowen, Fenton, and Rappaport (1991) interviewed 45 children and teenagers ages 8–18 with ADHD who were currently taking stimulant medication; it is important to note that they were interviewed in the presence of their parents. Eighty-nine percent felt that medication was helpful; 89% indicated that they would keep taking the medication if it was completely up to them, but 85% reported various side effects. Doherty, Frankenberg, Fuhrer, and Snider (2000) anonymously surveyed 924 middle and high school students, 86 of whom were taking stimulant medication for ADHD. Nearly the same number of students reported that they would stop taking the medication right now as reported they would really like to keep taking it. When asked how medication helped them, the students reported that it had positive effects on paying attention in school and earning better grades, but lesser effects on tests, homework, or paying attention to things they liked to do. They reported that the greatest effect of the medicine was that their parents and teachers liked them better when they were taking it. Such findings occurred prior to the widespread use of once-a-day delivery systems for methylphenidate or amphetamine-based stimulants, which may last 9–12 hours, or new nonstimulants such as atomoxetine. These newer medicines eliminate the need for school-time dosing and may provide benefits later into the day when homework may be accomplished. Even so, the fact that half of these teens would give up their medication shows that many are not very invested in continuing their medication management without parental or teacher pressure to do so.

Moline and Frankenberger (2001) asked 651 students ages 11–18 to complete an anonymous questionnaire regarding ADHD and medication; 50 of the students who reported currently taking medication for ADHD responded regarding their attitudes and the impact of the medication. Thirty-three percent of these students indicated that they would stop taking it right away, and 43% indicated that they would continue taking their medication if it were completely up to them; 23% were undecided. Although the students reported that medication helped their behavior, attention span, and social interactions with friends, parents, and teachers, they did not feel that the medication helped improve their academic achievement. As in the Doherty et al. (2000) study, the adolescents' perceptions of the greatest impact of the medication was that their parents and teachers liked them better on medication. Eighty-six percent reported experiencing side effects, with the following specific breakdown: (1) not feeling like eating lunch, 57%; (2) headaches, 48%; (3) difficulty getting to sleep, 44%; (4) stomachaches, 40%; and (5) tics, 40%.

These authors also collected data from 611 subjects who did not have ADHD, but who knew peers taking stimulant medication for ADHD, regarding their attitudes toward these peers. The students without ADHD thought that the students taking medication for ADHD were not very different from other students and did not act differently as a function of taking their medication. Furthermore, they reported that they did not treat students who took medication for ADHD differently than they treated anyone else.

Finally, Moline and Frankenberger (2001) collected data regarding the inappropriate diversion of stimulant medication. They found that 34% of the students taking medication reported being approached to sell or trade their medication, and 53% of the students without ADHD reported that some peers with ADHD gave away or sold their medication.

Taken together, these three studies paint a picture of mixed attitudes by children and adolescents toward taking stimulant medication for ADHD. Although the vast majority of participants reported a positive impact of stimulant medication on their functioning, the studies with anonymous self-reports found that over one-third were ready to give up taking the medication; not surprisingly, when parents were in the room, most children and adolescents reported that they wanted to continue taking their medication. Interestingly, the students reported greater effects of their medication on attention and social functioning than on academic achievement; this is consistent with the conclusions of double-blind placebo studies on the effects of stimulant medication (see Chapter 17). The evidence that adolescents without ADHD do not hold negative views of their peers who take medication for ADHD provides important information for clinicians to use in reassuring adolescents concerned about negative peer reactions to their taking medication. The data on the high rate of giving away or selling the medication reinforce the need for every clinician to prepare their adolescent patients to resist peer pressure to divert their stimulant medication.

It is important to note that the subjects in these three studies were already taking stimulant medication at the time they responded to the surveys; a clinician is faced with a newly diagnosed adolescent with ADHD who has not yet experienced the positive effects of medication. It is not at all clear whether the results of the research discussed here would generalize to medication-naïve adolescents at the point of initial diagnosis. Research is needed that assesses attitudes toward medication at the point of initial diagnosis.

We understand the reluctance of many adolescents with ADHD to take medication within a developmental context. During a time of identity exploration marked by a fierce desire to be different from their parents but carbon copies of their peers, adolescents do not want to do anything that makes them feel different from their friends. Nor do they wish to follow regimens they perceive as imposed by adults—either parents or physicians. They believe they know what is best for themselves and look on medication as a source of "external control" from which they need to "individuate." Teenagers who took stimulant medication as younger children often complain that it calms them down too much, or, as one athletic youngster said, "Medicine takes away my killer instinct." What they mean is that they enjoy being wild and impulsive, which medication curbs. They also often attribute a variety of extraneous somatic complaints to the medication, even though most of these bear little relation to the side effects of psychostimulants. Thus their resistance stems from basic developmental needs, as well as a history of poor parent–child relations.

A sensitive professional must present the use of medication to an adolescent within a context that takes these developmental factors into account. The traditional "doctor knows best" au-

thoritarian presentation often backfires. A Socratic approach that permits the adolescent to be in control and make decisions for him- or herself about the use of medication eliminates resistance and activates motivation to take medication (Schubiner, Robin, & Young, 2003). The following excerpt from a discussion between a physician and an adolescent illustrates this approach:

DR. JONES: I understand that things are pretty rotten at school. Tell me about it.

BILL: Yeah. I'm getting lousy grades. And the teachers get on my case about talking out.

DR. JONES: How would you like your grades to be?

BILL: C's, B's, but at least passing.

DR. JONES: It seems like keeping your mind on the work in school and at homework time has been tough, right?

BILL: Sure has. School's so boring. I can't make myself study, even if I want to. And all the noise in class bugs me.

DR. JONES: This is all part of the ADHD thing you've talked about with Dr. Robin. Your body won't let your mind stay with things, through no fault of yours. Say, I've got an idea I'd like to run by you. You and I both wear glasses. When we take our glasses off, what happens?

BILL: Things look foggy.

DR. JONES: Right! We need glasses to see clearly. We didn't choose to need glasses. That's the way our bodies and eyes are, right?

BILL: I guess so.

DR. JONES: ADHD is similar. You didn't choose to have trouble with concentrating and thinking before acting. Your body is just that way. I don't have any glasses for concentration, but I do know of some medications that act on your concentration like glasses do on your eyes.

BILL: What do you mean? I'm not taking any smart pills! Only retards need that.

DR. JONES: You feel like I think you're a retard because I'm suggesting medication?

BILL: All my friends make fun of those special ed kids on the bus who take pills.

DR. JONES: Bill, you have plenty of smarts. Remember how Dr. Robin explained that you got a high score on the IQ tests?

BILL: Yeah.

DR. JONES: And as for kids making fun of you, no one is going to know about the pills unless you tell. By the way, does wearing glasses make either of us retards?

BILL: I guess not.

DR. JONES: I prescribe medication for ADHD frequently because it helps most people. I think medication might help you, but it is totally up to you. I don't have stock in medication companies, and I don't really care if you take medication or not. But I do care if you do well in school. If you want to see if this medication can help you do better in school, I will help you find the best medicine.

BILL: But what if this medicine makes me feel weird?

DR. JONES: I won't ask you to put up with any bad side effects. If the medicine makes you feel weird, we will change it right away—either the amount or the type of medicine.

BILL: What if I get hooked on the stuff and can't stop taking it?

DR. JONES: You can stop "cold turkey" any time you want. You won't get hooked on it. You would use the medicine on a trial basis, to see if you focus better, organize better, and get things done more efficiently. If it doesn't work, you stop.

BILL: How do I know my parents won't trick you into making me take medicine for longer than I want? Or taking so much medicine that I turn into a wimp?

DR. JONES: I give you *my word* that you have *the last word* on all decisions about medication. I will not make any decisions about medication that you do not agree with, no matter what your parents want. We will discuss it just between ourselves, and tell your parents afterwards what we decided.

BILL: OK, I will give it a try, but just for 1 month.

DR. JONES: You're the boss. One month it will be, and then you can tell me what you think.

Dr. Jones first establishes that Bill wishes to improve his school performance and that increased concentration is essential. Then he uses the analogy of visual impairment to provide a rationale for stimulant medication. When Bill objects, he empathizes with Bill's concerns but provides accurate information about medica-tion. He makes it clear to Bill that he does not have a personal investment in whether Bill takes medicine or not, but that he cares about helping Bill do better in school. He debunks several myths Bill mentions about the medication and reiterates that Bill is going to be in control of all medication decisions. He "puts his money where his mouth is" by agreeing to Bill's request for a 1-month trial on medication.

When using this approach, we need to be prepared to accept the decisions of some adolescents to forgo medication at one point in time, and we need to convince their parents that they also need to accept this decision. We explain to parents that if they try to force an adolescent to take medication now, they may ruin any chances that the adolescent will ever agree to take medication; it is better to use other interventions and see whether the adolescent comes to his or her own decision later to try medication. In such cases, we help the adolescent develop other approaches to improving school performance. However, we ask the adolescent to make a contract with us that if school grades improve, medication will not be mentioned again, but if other interventions prove insufficient to improve school grades, the adolescent will consent to reconsider medication at the end of the next marking period. If the adolescent later decides to try medication, the physician is usually perceived as an ally rather than an enemy. The adolescent also learns how to use a problem-solving approach to dealing with important life issues: He or she makes a decision, tries one alternative solution, and then comes back and tries another alternative if the first one does not work.

The clinical use of stimulant, antidepressant, and other medications is discussed in detail in Chapters 17, 18, and 19 of this volume, respectively. When prescribing medication for adolescents, a physician must pay particular attention to ensure an adequate dose level, careful titration of doses to particular academic activities, clear-cut criteria for evaluating outcome, careful attention to minimizing side effects, and adjustment of timing to provide adequate length of medication coverage throughout the day. Long-acting stimulants or atomoxetine are clearly the medications of first choice, since they eliminate the noon dose and often give a more even release of medication across the day. However, many adolescents are working on homework into the evening, after even the longest-acting stimulants have worn off. They may need to supplement their morning long-acting medication with a dose of a short-acting version of their stimulant in the late afternoon or early evening.

It is important to work directly with the adolescent, in addition to obtaining teacher and parent feedback, to judge the effectiveness of the medication and determine the optimal dose. Schubiner et al. (2003) recommend a rapid titration schedule when first starting a stimulant. The physician starts with 18 mg of Concerta or 10 mg of the other long-acting medicines, and increases the dose by that same increment every week for at least 4 weeks (e.g., 36, 54, and 72 mg of Concerta or 20, 30, and 40 mg of the other long-acting stimulants during weeks 2, 3, and 4). The teenager returns after 1 month and tells the physician which dose worked best. If the physician titrates the dose of medicine for 1 month at each level (as pediatricians often do with younger children), the adolescent is likely to become impatient with the lower, ineffective doses and give up completely on the medication trial. With the rapid titration schedule, an effective dose can usually be determined within a month. The physician should help the adolescent pinpoint a medicine-sensitive behavior to use as a yardstick to judge the effectiveness of various doses. For example, reading a boring textbook or doing math problems is often medication-sensitive. The teen is asked to read the boring book several times on each dose of medicine and report the results to the physician. Together, the teen and the physician decide upon the optimal dose of medication. When physicians follow the suggestions given here, they encounter a relatively low rate of adolescents' refusing to try medication.

Enhancing Academic Success

Common Academic Difficulties

As youngsters make the transitions into middle and high school, secondary education places increased demands on them in eight areas (Mercer & Mercer, 1993): (1) gaining information from printed materials; (2) gaining information from lectures; (3) demonstrating knowledge through tests; (4) expressing information in writing; (5) working independently; (6) demonstrating a broad set of cognitive and metacognitive strategies; (7) interacting appropriately with both same-sex and opposite-sex

peers and adults; and (8) demonstrating motivation to learn. The core symptoms of ADHD and the associated deficits in executive functions impair an adolescent's ability to meet these eight demands. In addition, many adolescents with ADHD have learning disabilities in reading, mathematics, and/or writing, which further complicate their school difficulties.

As a result, adolescents with ADHD commonly present to the clinician with one or more of the following school difficulties: (1) failure to complete and turn in their homework; (2) superficial quality of homework; (3) poor test performance; (4) inadequate study habits; (5) disorganization, forgetfulness, and memory problems; (6) inconsistent listening and poor note taking during classes; (7) difficulty writing essays and papers; (8) sloppy or illegible handwriting; (9) poor reading comprehension; (10) poor understanding of the material; (11) lack of classroom participation and failure to ask teachers for needed help; (12) disrupting the classroom and/or socializing instead of working; (13) getting in conflicts with peers; and (14) tardiness and/or truancy.

Establishing Goals for Change

In this phase of treatment (sessions 4–9) the therapist meets with the adolescent and the parents together, identifies which of these 14 difficulties apply, and establishes goals for change. Then the therapist and the family decide which goals can be addressed in the therapy sessions and which goals require action in the school. The therapist coaches the parents to approach the appropriate school officials to arrange for informal accommodations or set in motion either a Section 504 Plan or a special education plan. The therapist backs up the parents' approach to the school by telephoning the principal and sending written reports and recommendations. The therapist may also attend school meetings and take an active role in advocating for accommodations and school-based interventions. More information about the public school's legal responsibilities to provide services for adolescents with ADHD can be found in DuPaul and Stoner (2003) and Zeigler Dendy (2000).

A word should be said about the status of empirically effective interventions for enhancing academic performance in adolescents with ADHD. DuPaul and Stoner (2003) have reviewed research on the effectiveness of various school-related interventions for students with ADHD. There is relatively little empirical research in this area. Existing studies strongly support the effectiveness of token reinforcement systems, contingency contracts, response cost, time out, and home–school report systems—and, to a lesser extent, self-management interventions. DuPaul and Stoner (2003) only located two studies using secondary education students; the rest involved elementary school children. Thus many of the suggestions below are deduced from well-validated behavioral principles and clinical experience rather than empirically effective interventions.

The therapist begins by reviewing the checklist in Figure 14.2 with the adolescent and the parents to pinpoint specific school problems. Each item is rated on a 1–5 Likert scale, with higher numbers representing more positive ratings. Any items rated 3 or less are considered potential targets for change. All such items are highlighted and discussed with the family. Also taken into consideration are recent report cards, ability and achievement testing, recent teacher conferences, current special education or Section 504 services offered to the student by the school, teacher rating scales, and the adolescent's own perceptions of which classes are difficult or easy. Over the course of sessions 4–9, the therapist develops and implements a flexible plan for remediating the areas found deficient in Figure 14.2. This plan clearly delineates the responsibilities of the student, the parents, the teachers, and the therapist, working as a collaborative team to enhance the student's academic success. Here I will discuss the core elements of the plan for enhancing academic success that are needed by virtually every adolescent with ADHD. Readers interested in a comprehensive discussion of interventions for many of the other school issues facing adolescents with ADHD should consult Davis, Sirotowitz, and Parker (1996), DuPaul and Stoner (2003), Greenbaum and Markel (2001), Markel and Greenbaum (1996), Robin (1998), Zeigler Dendy (2000), and Zentall and Goldstein (1999).

Core Academic Intervention

Virtually every adolescent with ADHD has difficulties with homework, long-term assignments, organization, listening in class, note taking, sloppy handwriting, studying, and taking tests. Designed to address these difficul-

ties, the core academic intervention involves a weekly home–school communication system; effective use of the student planner; teachers' informing parents of recently assigned long-term assignments; breaking long-term assignments down into shorter units; an effective homework contract; backpack organization; and a number of classroom modifications in teaching methods, assignments, test taking, and level of supervision.

Home–School Communication. First, the therapist establishes a weekly home–school communication system in order to provide the therapist and the adolescent's parents with (1) timely information about the status of the adolescent's assignments; (2) a list of upcoming tests and assignments, particularly long-term projects; and (3) a basis to provide positive reinforcement to the adolescent for timely task completion. Such information is essential, so that parents can monitor their adolescent's task completion independently of the student planner and enforce consequences for completing or not completing the homework. After talking to the teachers at a school meeting, by phone, or by e-mail, the therapist defines a small set of daily target behaviors that each teacher will rate the student on. Because of the difficulty of talking with all of the adolescent's teachers, the therapist often identifies a key person (such as a teacher consultant, guidance counselor, or school social worker) who talks to the teachers on the therapist's behalf. The therapist provides a form such as that in Figure 14.3, or uses a preexisting form constructed by the school. This form provides a place for the teachers to record assignment completion, list test grades, rate behavior, and list any upcoming major projects.

There are three methods to get the form completed and home, listed in order of decreasing preference:

1. Ideally, since many teachers now have e-mail at their desks, every Thursday a parent e-mails a blank form to the teachers. On Friday, the teachers fill it out and e-mail it back to the parents.
2. Alternatively, a teacher consultant, social worker, or counselor collects the forms from each teacher and faxes them to the parent, or the parent calls the identified case manager and obtains a report by phone.
3. Under the old-fashioned approach, the ado-

The therapist should review each item on this checklist with the parents and adolescent, determining whether it applies. Most of the items refer to the behavior of the adolescent; some refer to the actions of the teachers and school personnel. Rate each item on a 1–5 scale:

1 = Never 2 = A little 3 = Sometimes 4 = Often 5 = Always

HOMEWORK

_____ 1. Uses an assignment book
_____ 2. Does homework in nondistracting, quiet environment
_____ 3. Has an planful approach to the order for doing homework
_____ 4. Completes homework on time
_____ 5. Hands in homework on time
_____ 6. Spends sufficient time on homework
_____ 7. Keeps and follows a written plan with calendar for long-term assignments
_____ 8. Is currently up-to-date on homework

ORGANIZATION

_____ 9. Comes to class prepared with materials
_____ 10. Keeps notebooks, papers, study area organized and accessible
_____ 11. Uses calendar, schedule, planner to manage time
_____ 12. Keeps track of grades regularly/knows grading criteria
_____ 13. Brings home materials needed for homework
_____ 14. Keeps locker organized

TEST PREPARATION AND TEST TAKING

_____ 15. Spends sufficient time studying (e.g., doesn't cram at last minute)
_____ 16. Matches study to the type of questions on exam
_____ 17. Uses old tests to help prepare for upcoming exams
_____ 18. Has an organized approach to studying (e.g., SQ4R)
_____ 19. Has an organized approach to taking tests
_____ 20. Reads and follows directions carefully and doesn't respond impulsively
_____ 21. Writes legibly or uses word processor
_____ 22. Pays attention adequately during tests
_____ 23. Receives passing or higher grades on tests
_____ 24. Does not cheat
_____ 25. Remembers information during the test
_____ 26. Finishes the test within the allotted time
_____ 27. Manages anxiety effectively during tests

NOTE TAKING

_____ 28. Takes notes during lectures
_____ 29. Gets main points in notes
_____ 30. Notes are legible
_____ 31. Uses notes for studying
_____ 32. Notes are accurate

READING COMPREHENSION

_____ 33. Uses organized method such as SQ4R
_____ 34. Can identify topics, main ideas, and details
_____ 35. Understands what has been read
_____ 36. Underlines text effectively
_____ 37. Can answer questions about text

(continued)

FIGURE 14.2. Diagnostic checklist for school success.

FIGURE 14.2. *(continued)*

_____ 38. Can summarize what was read
_____ 39. Has method for learning new vocabulary in readings
_____ 40. Can pay attention while reading

MEMORIZING

_____ 41. Plans strategies for memorization
_____ 42. Selects facts to memorize accurately from notes, books, handouts
_____ 43. Knows own learning style (auditory, visual, kinesthetic, combined)
_____ 44. Matches memorization techniques to learning style
_____ 45. Rehearses sufficiently to memorize material
_____ 46. Distributes rehearsal over time (e.g., doesn't cram)
_____ 47. Uses acrastrics (silly sentences)
_____ 48. Uses acronyms
_____ 49. Uses charting, graphing
_____ 50. Uses visualization
_____ 51. Uses word, sentence association techniques
_____ 52. Recalls information when needed

CLASSROOM PARTICIPATION AND CONDUCT

_____ 53. Attends all classes
_____ 54. Gets to class on time
_____ 55. Participates in discussion
_____ 56. Volunteers answers to questions
_____ 57. Is with the class when called on by the teacher
_____ 58. Cooperates with teacher
_____ 59. Raises hand and doesn't call out of turn
_____ 60. Follows classroom rules
_____ 61. Talks respectfully to teachers
_____ 62. Relates positively to peers
_____ 63. Asks for help when needed

UNDERSTANDING/PROCESSING PROBLEMS

_____ 64. Student understands material
_____ 65. Student decodes accurately
_____ 66. Student comprehends what is read
_____ 67. Handwriting is legible
_____ 68. Student can express thoughts in writing
_____ 69. Student can express thoughts orally
_____ 70. Student understands mathematical concepts
_____ 71. Mathematical calculation is accurate

SCHOOL RESPONSIBILITIES

_____ 72. Individualized education program or Section 504 plan exists in writing
_____ 73. Written plan meets needs outlined above
_____ 74. Written plan is adequately implemented
_____ 75. Content area teachers are familiar with plan
_____ 76. Case manager appointed to monitor plan
_____ 77. Teachers are accountable for providing accommodations
_____ 78. Informal accommodations (not in writing)
_____ 79. School keeps parents informed of student progress

SOCIAL SCENE

_____ 80. Adolescent has close friends at school
_____ 81. Friends encourage academic success and prosocial behavior
_____ 82. Student is satisfied with his or her social life

Name _____   Date _____

Math: Homework up to date   Yes   No   N.A.
               Student planner accurate   Yes   No   N.A.
               Behavior appropriate   Yes   No   N.A.
               Test grades this week   _____

    Any incomplete assignments:

    Any long-term assignments due soon:

    Teacher signature: _____

English: Homework up to date   Yes   No   N.A.
               Student planner accurate   Yes   No   N.A.
               Behavior appropriate   Yes   No   N.A.
               Test grades this week   _____

    Any incomplete assignments:

    Any long-term assignments due soon:

    Teacher signature: _____

French: Homework up to date   Yes   No   N.A.
               Student planner accurate   Yes   No   N.A.
               Behavior appropriate   Yes   No   N.A.
               Test grades this week   _____

    Any incomplete assignments:

    Any long-term assignments due soon:

    Teacher signature: _____

FIGURE 14.3. Sample weekly school–home report.

lescent carries the form around and asks each teacher to complete it at the end of class, then brings it home.

Obviously, there are many more pitfalls to the third approach than the other two, but some schools insist on the third approach.

Next, the therapist coaches the parents and the adolescent to write a behavioral contract specifying how the student gains and/or loses privileges, depending upon the teacher's evaluation of the task completion, use of the student planner, and behavior. The parents use the home–school report as a vehicle to prevent the student from falling too far behind, to monitor the accuracy of the student planner, to become aware of recently assigned long-term projects, and to extrinsically motivate the student to complete assignments. Readers interested in more discussion of home–school reports might consult Kelley's (1990) book on this topic.

When a long-term project appears on the weekly home–school report, a parent initiates a planning discussion with the adolescent. During this discussion, the parent coaches the adolescent to break the assignment into several shorter units, select times to complete each unit, and put these times on the calendar. Positive incentives may be negotiated to be earned contingent upon completion of each step, and punishments may be negotiated for failure to comply. When the designated time arrives, the parent gives a single reminder to the adolescent to complete the agreed-upon task.

Homework. The therapist conducts a logical analysis of where in the homework process there is a breakdown and aims the interventions at these weak links. The logical analysis is translated directly into a homework contract specifying how these points of breakdown will be overcome. Each of the following questions leads directly to components of this contract. Does the adolescent reliably and accurately write down the homework assignments in a student planner or an assignment book? Does the adolescent bring the student planner home from school, along with the textbooks, notebooks, and other materials needed to complete homework? Do the parents monitor the planner? Is there a backup plan for getting the assignment if the adolescent forgets to bring it home? Does the adolescent have a quiet, nondistracting, well-lit, and comfortable place in which to do the homework? Are pens, pads, in-

dex cards, a computer, and other needed resources easily accessible and neatly organized in the room? Is there an agreed-upon time for starting homework, and does the adolescent have difficulty getting started at the agreed-upon time? Is there consistency in time and location for doing homework over days and weeks? Will a parent be in the house when the adolescent is supposed to be doing homework, to monitor and "keep the adolescent honest"? Does the adolescent have an organized plan of attack to sequence multiple homework assignments in one evening? To what extent does the adolescent become easily distracted and unable to concentrate and persist for the time it takes to get homework done? Is it taking inordinate amounts of time, despite good concentration, because of a slow cognitive tempo or reading/writing difficulties? Is medication prescribed so that it covers the adolescent during homework time?

Are the parents actively involved in tracking completion of homework, and have they learned to achieve the delicate balance between confrontational intrusiveness and disengagement? How does the adolescent divide the time between doing the next day's assignments and working on long-term projects? What steps does he or she take after completing the assignment to make sure that it will get to school and be handed in on time? How severe are the conflicts between the parent and adolescent about homework, and has homework become a battleground for adolescent independence seeking?

The homework contract clearly delineates the adolescent's, parents', teachers', and therapist's own role in the homework process (Markel & Greenbaum, 1996). The teachers' role is to give the student a rationale for doing homework, base homework on skills that have already been learned and need reinforcement or practice (not to ask students to learn new skills on their own or to ask parents to teach new skills), clearly give the assignment and outline expectations for its completion, give a clear prompt for the student to turn in the assignment, grade the assignment and give feedback to the students about their homework in a timely manner, and keep parents informed when students fall behind on homework for more than 2 or 3 days. In addition, secondary education teachers need to keep in mind that there is life after school and to make the amount of homework realistic. When there is an accommodation plan, the teachers are also expected to implement the accommodations relevant to homework. A student's role is certainly to complete the homework, but it goes beyond this. Students are expected to keep track of what homework is assigned, develop a homework plan with assistance from their parents, decide when and where to do their homework with input from their parents, follow the homework plan without needing to be nagged, ask for help when they need it, complete their homework to the best of their ability, check it over for mistakes and legibility, and hand it in on time.

The parents' role is to stay involved in the structuring of their youngster's homework. (Even though most teenagers should take full responsibility for their own homework, this is not usually possible for teenagers who have ADHD.) Specifically, parental involvement includes helping the student develop a homework plan; providing the student with a nondistracting, comfortable location for doing homework; providing the student with the basic materials; being in the house to monitor compliance with the homework plan when they expect homework to be done; helping the student analyze homework problems when the student asks for help; expecting the adolescent to adhere to the plan; administering any agreed-upon positive or negative consequences for doing or not doing homework; and communicating regularly with the teachers to track whether homework has been completed and discuss any homework problems that arise. The therapist's role is to guide the adolescent and family in determining where the breakdown in the homework process is, to provide guidance and direct instruction for fixing the breakdown, and to help coordinate efforts between the school and family around homework issues.

Figure 14.4 illustrates such a very detailed homework contract for Michael Adams. Michael's contract includes sections related to keeping track of assignments, bringing home materials, setting and scheduling homework, prioritizing, medication, turning in assignments, feedback, and consequences. All of the homework problems outlined earlier are addressed in this contract. Many students require much shorter contracts, targeting only one or two of these areas. The therapist helps the family enlist the teachers in carrying out their part of the contract; assigns the family members the task of carrying out their parts;

and, over several sessions, follows up to see whether everyone complies with his or her roles in the contract, fine-tuning the details and dealing with implementation problems and resistance.

In those cases where the high level of negativity in parent–adolescent relations precludes using parents to structure the adolescent's homework completion, I usually recommend that the parents hire a homework tutor, who may be an ADHD coach, a professional tutor, or an older honors student. The homework tutor comes to the home three to five times per week and coaches the adolescent in the completion of his or her homework.

Backpack Organization. I believe that undue emphasis on an adolescent's room or locker as the central area for organization is misguided and misplaced. Adolescents do not spend most of the day in their rooms, and they hardly spend any time at their lockers. By contrast, a backpack travels to and from school every day, and where permitted, travels to each classroom with an adolescent. Both the therapist and the parents can have complete access to the backpack, permitting the use of modeling, guided practice, and feedback in organizing it. The backpack should be the primary focus of our organizational efforts.

The therapist stages the "Big Dump." The adolescent brings the backpack to a session and dumps everything out on a table. This should be done in a light-hearted and humorous way, to defuse resistance. The therapist explains that the goal is to find a simple, efficient organizational plan for the backpack. Together, the therapist and the adolescent look at each item on the table, sorting them into the following types of categories: (1) alive or smelly (trash it); (2) paper no longer needed (trash it); (3) notice or paper for Mom or Dad (put it in a section of a notebook or binder labeled "Papers for parents"); (4) homework not yet handed in (put it in a section of the notebook or binder labeled "Papers to hand in"); (5) homework to complete (put it in a section of the notebook or binder labeled "Papers to complete"). Sections of the backpack are labeled for various functions, and everything is placed in the correct sections.

The parents are called into the session, and the adolescent is asked to explain the "Big Dump" to them. Then the adolescent is assigned the task of dumping and reorganizing

I, Michael Adams, and my parents, my teachers, my guidance counselor, and Dr. Jones agree to carry out to the best of our ability the following homework plan:

I. Keeping track of assignments
   A. My teachers will write the assignments on the board every day. They will also give a copy of all the assignments for the week to Mrs. Smith, my guidance counselor, each Monday. She will keep a copy and e-mail a copy to my parents.
   B. I will write down the assignment from the board every day before I leave each class. I will write it in the section of my assignment book for that subject. I will read over what I have written down to make sure I understand it. I will ask the teacher to explain any assignment I do not understand.
   C. During my last-period study hall, I will read over each assignment I have written down and make sure I understand what I am being asked to do. I will make a list of all of the materials I need to bring home and gather them from my locker. My study hall teacher agrees to give me a hall pass to go to my locker and find any materials I need during last period.

II. Bringing home materials
   A. I will bring home all the materials I have gathered and my assignment book.
   B. My mother agrees to ask me nicely one time without nagging to see my list of assignments. I agree to show it to her without a big hassle or an attitude.
   C. As a backup in case I forget to write the assignment down, I will pick a study buddy in each of my classes, get that person's phone number, and post those phone numbers on the refrigerator door.

III. Schedule and setting for doing homework
   A. From Sunday through Thursday, I agree to work on homework from 6:00 P.M. to 8:00 P.M. If I finish early, I will show my completed work to a parent, and if he or she agrees that it is completed, I can do whatever I want.
   B. I will do my homework at the big desk in the den. I can listen to soft music with headphones, but no loud rock. If I find myself getting distracted, I will take a short break, do something physical (not telephone), and start working again.
   C. My mother will remind me once without nagging to start on my homework at 6:00 P.M. I will start without an attitude.

IV. Daily plan for organizing homework completion
   A. With help from my mother, I will make an organized plan for each night's homework. This plan will guide me in what subject I will do first, second, etc. It will also divide up homework time between assignments due tomorrow and long-term assignments. My mother agrees to permit me to determine the order of doing homework.
   B. In my plan, I will estimate the time needed to complete each assignment, as well as how I will check each assignment over for accuracy, completeness, and legibility.
   C. The plan will specify how often I will take breaks during homework time, how long the breaks will be, and how large assignments will be divided into smaller units.
   D. The plan will specify where I will put the completed assignments and how I will make sure I turn the work in.

V. Medication. I agree to supplement my long-acting medicine with a dose of short-acting medicine at 5:00 P.M. on Sunday through Thursday, to help me concentrate on homework.

VI. Turning in assignments
   A. As I finish an assignment, I will put it in the section of my binder for that class.
   B. I will do my best to remember to hand in each assignment.
   C. I will back up all assignments typed on my computer to a disk or CD.

VII. Feedback. My teachers agree to tell me how I did within 2 days after I hand in an assignment. They also agree to e-mail my parents feedback about how many of the last week's assignments were turned in on time when they send the next week's assignment list.

VIII. Rewards. My parents agree to let me make 20 minutes of cell-phone calls to my girlfriend each night that I do my homework. If I do my homework for 5 nights in a row, they agree to let me freely use my cell phone on the weekend.

Signed,   *Michael Adams*   *Robert Adams*   *Barbara Adams*   *Bill Jones, Principal*
          Brenda Smith, Guidance Counselor   *Millie Broadbent, Algebra*   *Tom Jones, English*
          Darla Breeze, French   *William Sonoma, Chemistry*   *F.A.O. Schwartz, Gym*
          Neiman Marcus, History

FIGURE 14.4. The homework plan for Michael Adams.

the backpack, under parental supervision, at home three to four times per week. If needed, positive incentives are specified for the adolescent to earn contingent upon successfully reorganizing the backpack.

In those cases where schools do not permit backpacks to be brought into the classroom, the therapist helps the adolescent develop a simple organizational system for the locker and plan for how many trips the student will make to the locker during school.

Classroom Modifications and Accommodations. Several accommodations made by the teacher and school personnel are central to this core academic intervention plan. First, adolescents with ADHD should be given access to computers or word processors for all substantial written work completed in school, including quizzes, exams, essays, and miscellaneous writing. It is pointless to struggle with trying to improve their often illegible handwriting. Second, extra time to take examinations in a distraction-free environment should be made available, even though the teenagers will not need this modification on all exams. Some adolescents with severe reading or writing disabilities may also need to have examinations administered orally. Third, teachers should routinely distribute copies of their lecture notes and tactfully arrange for a student with ADHD to receive a copy of another student's notes, selecting a student with strong note-taking skills as the source. Most teenagers with ADHD are unable to take notes effectively and listen to the lecture attentively at the same time. Fourth, the school should issue a second set of textbooks to the adolescent, so that it is no longer necessary to bring the books to and from school. Fifth, teachers should reduce the amount of rote, written homework for youngsters who have deficits in processing speed.

Sixth, alternative approaches to handing in the homework should be considered when an adolescent is forgetting to turn in completed assignments. Possibilities include e-mailing assignments from home; handing all the homework for the day to the school secretary in the morning, to be placed in teachers' mailboxes; or handing all the homework for the day to a counselor or teacher consultant, who distributes it to the various teachers. Seventh, teachers should break large assignments down into a number of small sections and hold the student accountable for completing each section by a specified deadline; this prevents procrastination. Innovative approaches to teaching writing, such as the self-regulated strategy development method (De La Paz, 2001), may be employed for those students who have serious writing deficiencies. Eighth, parents should have input into the selection of each year's classes and teachers, through a meeting with the guidance counselor. Finally, a single member of the school staff should be designated as a case manager who will oversee the implementation of the accommodations, either informally or under a Section 504 plan or an individualized education plan. Schwiebert, Sealander, and Dennison (2002) have argued that the guidance counselor is often the best person to fulfill this function.

For those students who are certified to receive special education, an afternoon resource center is a useful intervention. Ideally, the special education teacher proctors the students while they complete their homework and/or obtain help understanding material taught earlier in the day. Direct instruction in study strategies is also a valuable activity during resource center time. During the last 15 minutes of this time, the teacher should ask the student to organize the books and materials needed for homework, and should review the student planner to make sure all of the homework assignments are recorded. The teacher might send the student to his or her locker to obtain additional books and papers needed for homework. Upon return from the locker, the student shows the teacher the books and materials that have been gathered. In some schools, a class with a title such as "Learning Strategies" replaces the resource center. Making the grade in this class contingent upon correct use of the student planner, backpack and binder organization, and timely completion of homework during class time is a particularly effective strategy. For other suggestions on academic interventions, see Chapter 15 of this volume.

Home-Based Interventions

Research

Over the course of sessions 10–22, we target problems between the parents and the adolescents through the use of contingency management, parent training, and family problem-solving communication training (PSCT). These therapeutic interventions have been subjected to empirical scrutiny in two outcome studies. A review of these two studies and the lessons learned from this research sets the context for a clinical discussion of home-based interventions.

In the first study, Barkley, Guevremont, Anastopoulos, and Fletcher (1992) compared three family therapy programs for treating family conflicts in adolescents with ADHD. Sixty-one 12- to 18-year-olds were randomly assigned to 8–10 sessions of behavior management training (BMT), PSCT, or structural family therapy (SFT). To be eligible, the adolescents had to (1) be referred to the investigators' ADHD clinic; (2) meet DSM-III-R (American Psychiatric Association, 1987) criteria for ADHD and have parent or teacher complaints of inattention, impulsivity, and restlessness; (3) if receiving psychoactive medication, be willing to remain on this medication during the active phase of treatment in the study; and (4) have T scores greater than 65 on the Hyperactivity scale of the Child Behavior Checklist (CBCL). The treatments were conducted by two licensed clinical psychologists trained and supervised by senior clinicians expert in each treatment. The adolescent and at least one parent (usually the mother) participated in each SFT and PSCT session; the parent(s) participated in the BMT sessions without the adolescent.

The BMT approach followed Barkley's (1997b) manual, with several modifications. The session on developing parental positive attention was modified slightly for adolescents, and the session on time out was changed so that brief groundings at home replaced the use of the time-out chair. Successive sessions focused on the use of positive parent attention, point systems or token reinforcement, daily home–school report cards linked with the home token system, groundings for unacceptable behavior, and instructions for parents on how to anticipate impending problem situations and establish plans in advance to deal with them. Regular homework was assigned following Barkley's (1997b) protocol.

The PSCT approach followed our (Robin & Foster's, 1989) approach, outlined later in this chapter, and included three main activities: (1) problem-solving training, (2) communication training, and (3) cognitive restructuring of extreme beliefs and unreasonable expectations. Homework assignments were given in later sessions; these involved applications and practice of problem-solving and communication skills.

The SFT approach helped families identify and alter maladaptive family systems or interaction patterns, such as transgenerational coalitions, scapegoating, and triangulation. The therapists focused on creating transactions, joining with each family's transactions, and helping to restructure maladaptive transactions; they relied on analysis and targeting of family boundaries, alignments, and power. Homework assignments typically involved instructions to replace ineffective transactions with novel strategies.

Each family was assessed before and after treatment and at a 3-month follow-up on the following dependent measures: (1) the CBCL Parent and Youth Self-Report versions—social competence scales and broad-band Internalizing and Externalizing psychopathology scales; (2) the Conflict Behavior Questionnaire (CBQ); (3) the Issues Checklist (IC); (4) the Locke–Wallace Marital Adjustment Test; (5) the Beck Depression Inventory; and (6) videotaped interactions during a neutral and a conflict topic discussion coded with the Parent–Adolescent Interaction Coding System—Revised (PAICS-R). The PAICS-R yields summary scores for the frequency of two negative communication categories (Puts Down/Commands, Defends/Complains), and four positive communication categories (Problem-Solves, Defines/Evaluates, Facilitates, and Talks). The Family Beliefs Inventory (FBI) was given at pre- and postassessment, and a five-item consumer satisfaction survey was given at the end of treatment. The therapists rated family cooperation on a five-item scale at the end of each session.

Analyses revealed that all three treatments resulted in significant improvements on most measures from before to after treatment, with further gains in many cases from postassessment to follow-up. There were very few differences between treatments. Specifically, parents and adolescents reported improvement on parent-reported school adjustment, externalizing and internalizing behavior problems, maternal depression, parent- and adolescent-reported communication, number of specific disputes, and the anger/intensity level of specific disputes. The results were much more variable and difficult to interpret on the videotaped interaction measures and the FBI. In some cases there were no improvements, and in others there were changes in the opposite direction from that predicted. In general, very few positive changes occurred on these measures.

But mean changes in scores of these treated groups provide only limited information on clinical effectiveness. The percentage of individuals showing reliable change is more informative. So Barkley et al. (1992) determined the clinical significance of the results, following Jacobson and Truax's (1991) recommendations by computing the index of Reliable Change (magnitude of the improvement) and the Recovery Index (is client within the normal range?), using the maternal-reported IC quantity and weighted anger intensity scores. For the number of conflicts, the percentages of subjects showing a reliable change were 10% for BMT, 24% for PSCT, and 10% for SFT; none showed deterioration. For the Recovery Index, the percentages of subjects who moved into the normal range were 5% for BMT, 19% for PSCT, and 10% for SFT. Comparable percentages were obtained for the weighted anger intensity score. There were no significant differences between treatments on these indices, but the sample sizes were so small that the power to do so may not have been adequate.

Consumer satisfaction ratings were high and did not vary significantly across the three treatments. However, therapist ratings of family cooperation did differ significantly. The therapists rated the families receiving PSCT as significantly less cooperative than those receiving either BMT or SFT; this was one of the only differences between groups on any of the measures. PSCT makes greater demands on families for practicing new interaction tasks between sessions; perhaps the greater amount of effort required from the families receiving PSCT influenced the cooperation ratings.

The results of this study were promising, in that they did indicate that all three treatment approaches resulted in statistically significant amelioration of mother- and adolescent-reported parent–adolescent conflicts and negative communication, decreases in externalizing and internalizing behavioral problems and maternal depression, and a high degree of consumer satisfaction with the treatments. At the same time, the results were very sobering when the stringent criteria of reliable change and movement into the normal range were applied: 80–95% of the families with adolescents who had ADHD did not make any clinically significant improvements through any of these family-based interventions. Nonetheless, the high degree of parental satisfaction suggested that even if clinically significant results were not ob-

tained for the majority of families on the dependent measures, the families felt they benefited. Barkley et al. (1992) speculated that perhaps the parents felt better prepared to cope with the problems inherent in raising adolescents with ADHD, even if they continued to have conflicts with their adolescents.

In the second study, Barkley, Edwards, Laneri, Fletcher, and Metevia (2001b) attempted to increase the efficacy of the family-based treatments by doubling the length of treatment and combining two of the treatments, BMT and PSCT. Ninety-seven teens with ADHD and ODD ages 12–18 and their parents were assigned in a quasi-random manner to receive 18 sessions of either PSCT alone or nine sessions of BMT followed by nine sessions of PSCT (BMT/PSCT). In 90% of the group receiving PSCT and 87% of the group receiving BMT/PSCT, the adolescents were males. As in the first study, the adolescents either were not currently receiving psychoactive medication or, if receiving medication, agreed to remain at a stable dose through the 18 sessions of therapy. At the start of the study, 62% of the teens in the PSCT condition and 49% of those in the BMT/PSCT condition received some form of psychoactive medication; for those teens completing the study, 53% in the PSCT condition and 47% in the BMT/PSCT condition received medication. No details were provided about the type and dosing of the psychoactive medications.

The interventions followed the identical manuals used in the first study. For PSCT, the parents and adolescents participated in all sessions together; for BMT/PSCT, the parents participated in the first nine sessions, and the parents and teens participated in the next nine sessions. Dependent measures were collected before treatment, at the midpoint of treatment, after treatment, and at a 2-month follow-up interval. Measures included mother, father, and adolescent reports of conflict/communication; the number and anger intensity levels of specific disputes; conflict tactics; ADHD and ODD symptoms; and videotapes of neutral and conflict discussions coded for positive and negative mother, father, and adolescent communication with a global/inferential coding system. Parents and adolescents also completed treatment effectiveness and consumer satisfaction ratings at postassessment.

Interestingly, there was a highly significant differential rate of dropout from the two treatment conditions. At midpoint, 23% of the families receiving PSCT versus 8% of those receiving BMT/PSCT had dropped out; at post-assessment, 38% of those receiving PSCT versus 18% of those receiving BMT/PSCT dropped out. At follow-up, 46% of the families in PSCT condition versus 23% of those in the BMT/PSCT condition failed to attend this assessment. The investigators carefully examined whether there were any differences at pre-assessment between the families dropping out of and completing treatment. In those families that dropped out, the teens had more mother-reported ODD symptoms than in those families who completed the study.

Both of the treatment conditions demonstrated significant improvements on mean group ratings of parent teen conflict, the number and anger intensity level of specific disputes, and conflict tactics, as reported by mothers, fathers, and adolescents. For the videotaped interaction measures, mothers demonstrated significantly increased positive and significantly decreased negative communication. There were no differences between treatment conditions on any of these measures. Consumer satisfaction and treatment effectiveness ratings were equally high in both treatment conditions. Most of the improvements were maintained at the 2-month follow-up, with the exception of a decrease in father positive and an increase in father negative communication in the BMT/PSCT condition from postassessment to follow-up.

As in the Barkley et al. (1992) study, the percentages of families reporting reliable changes were computed for the number of conflicts, the anger intensity level of specific disputes, and communication. These were computed separately as reported by mothers and fathers. At postassessment, a maximum of 20–24% of each treatment group showed reliable changes, depending upon the measure and source of information; there were no differences between groups on these measures. The percentages of families within the normal range were also computed. At postassessment, as reported by mothers, 34–78% of the families were within the normal range; as reported by fathers, 25–91% of the families were within this range. There were no differences between groups for mother reports, but for the number of specific disputes reported by fathers, more families in the PSCT condition than in the BMT/PSCT condition were within the normal range.

The Barkley et al. (2001b) study partially replicated and extended the results of the 1992 study in demonstrating the strengths and limitations of BMT and PSCT interventions in helping adolescents with ADHD and their parents reduce conflict and improve their relationships. Taken together, these two studies clearly demonstrated that BMT and PSCT, alone or in combination, can help some families with teens who have ADHD/ODD improve communication, reduce specific conflicts, and ameliorate ADHD and ODD symptoms; most of the significant changes were on parent- or teen-reported measures, rather than direct observations of family interaction during neutral or conflict tasks. Parents were highly satisfied with the outcomes and judged the interventions to be highly effective. Very few differences between the efficacy of BMT and that of PSCT emerged.

However, high percentages of the families did not make clinically significant changes and/or move from the abnormal to the normal range on the dependent measures. In Study 1, 80–95% of the families did not make clinically significant changes. In Study 2, with double the length of therapy, 76–80% of the families failed to make reliable changes and 22–64% were still in the abnormal range at the end of the study. Interestingly, doubling the length of therapy did not increase the percentage of families making reliable changes, but did increase the percentage of families moving from the abnormal to the normal range of the dependent measures.

In Study 1, the families receiving PSCT cooperated less with the therapists than those receiving BMT or SFT. In Study 2 more families dropped out of the PSCT-alone condition than the BMT/PSCT combined condition. Having a greater number of teen ODD symptoms was associated with dropping out of treatment in Study 2. Taken together, these findings suggest that PSCT alone is a more stressful intervention for families with adolescents who have ADHD and moderately severe ODD. As Barkley et al. (2001b) pointed out, PSCT thrusts a family into more immediate and frequent confrontations from the start of therapy, whereas the BMT/PSCT combination first prepares the parents to cope with a defiant teenager before thrusting them into direct confrontations during family therapy sessions. Perhaps parents are better able to deal with confrontations with their adolescent after having a number of prior sessions with the therapist, and this was why the dropout rate was lower in the BMT/PSCT condition.

A very important variable in these two studies was the medication status of the adolescents. In both studies, adolescents were either not on medicine or remained on their prior medication regimens throughout the study. There was no attempt to assess the extent to which the teenagers in the two studies complied with their prescribed medication regimens, and no data were presented regarding the types or doses (doses to cover the evenings and/or weekends, holidays, etc.) of medication. Thus we cannot regard medication as having been optimized in the two Barkley et al. (1992, 2001b) studies, and we must interpret the results of the studies as assessments of the psychosocial interventions without systematic medication conditions.

The MTA (MTA Cooperative Group, 1999) has clearly demonstrated for school-age children that medication has a greater impact on ADHD symptoms than behavioral interventions do, and that there are modest advantages to the combination of medication and behavioral interventions over medication alone. Medication administered by the physicians in the MTA also had a greater impact on ADHD symptoms than medication obtained by subjects from their community physicians did. The community physicians tended to use lower, less frequent dosing of the stimulants, and to monitor the effects of medication less frequently and without teacher feedback; these differences in prescribing and monitoring practices probably accounted for the differences in the effectiveness of the medication. In addition, the combined intervention in the MTA had a greater impact than either medication alone or behavioral interventions on outcomes such as ODD symptoms and family interactions. Although no comparable study exists with adolescents, we have little reason to expect that behavioral interventions would be equal or superior to medication in adolescents with ADHD, compared to younger children. The medication taken by some of the teens in the Barkley et al. (1992, 2001b) studies most closely resembles medication as administered by nonstudy physicians in the community control condition of the MTA. Given the MTA findings, it should not, therefore, come as a huge surprise that behavioral interventions without an optimized medication condition only resulted in positive outcomes for a modest percentage of the families in the Barkley et al. research. Future investigators should conduct double-blind placebo trials of long-acting stimulants to assess their impact on parent–teen relations; existing medication studies with adolescents primarily examine ratings of ADHD symptoms. Then investigators should evaluate the incremental effectiveness of BMT/PSCT plus medication compared to medication alone, to better determine the role of short-term behavioral interventions in supplementing medication in an overall treatment regimen for adolescents with ADHD.

These studies have a number of implications for us as clinicians intervening to help parents and adolescents with ADHD deal with problems at home:

1. The therapist should meet with the parents first for at least several sessions before conducting meetings with the parents and adolescents together. This becomes especially important in a case where an adolescent displays high rates of oppositional behavior, because conjoint family sessions at the outset of therapy might lead to angry confrontations; when such confrontations occur before the therapist has strong rapport with the family, there is an increased risk that the family will drop out of treatment.

2. PSCT needs to be embedded within a broader context of other family and parent management interventions, rather than used as the sole intervention for home-based problems of adolescents with ADHD.

3. At the outset of therapy, parents need to be given realistic expectations for the amount of homework involved in behavioral interventions and the likely effectiveness of such interventions. This will help prevent dropping out due to the perception that the therapist is assigning too much homework.

4. Since ADHD is a neurobiological disorder, we must remember to take a cognitive rehabilitation approach to intervention. Therapies such as BMT and PSCT both alter the environment and teach families ways to compensate for the deficits of ADHD. However, they do not directly alter ADHD symptoms. At present, medication is the only intervention known to alter ADHD symptoms directly.

5. The findings of the MTA indicate that it is essential to optimize medication for the adolescent with ADHD at the start of psychosocial

interventions. This will provide the greatest synergistic effect of the combination of medication and behavioral interventions.

6. When the teen is also taking medication, parents can be given higher expectations for the likely positive outcomes of a combined behavioral and medical intervention than when behavioral intervention alone is being undertaken. We often summarize the MTA results to help parents understand the relative effectiveness of behavioral and medical interventions, alone or combined.

Parenting Principles

Keeping in mind the results and implications of the two Barkley et al. (1992, 2001b) outcome studies, my colleagues and I target problems between the parents and the adolescent at home by meeting first with the parents in sessions 10–16, then inviting the adolescents to join in family meetings for sessions 17–22. We also meet with the adolescent individually for 15–20 minutes during session 11. During the sessions with the parents, we (1) present a set of principles for parenting the teen with ADHD; (2) use cognitive restructuring to instill reasonable expectations for parent–teen relationships; and (3) teach behavior management skills. During the family sessions, we teach problem-solving communication skills and address other issues, such as the need to restore parental control.

Session 10 consists of a discussion of principles of parenting the teen with ADHD and establishment of reasonable expectations and beliefs about parent–teen relationships. Table 14.2 summarizes these principles. We tell parents that these principles won't always work, but that they are based upon sound behavioral research. It is helpful to derive a course of action from one of these principles when a parent does not know how to respond to a problem situation with an adolescent who has ADHD. We give examples and solicit feedback from the parents as we present these principles.

1. *Shift your parenting style away from authoritarian control or permissiveness, and more in a democratic direction to foster responsible independence-seeking behavior.* The extremes of authoritarian control or permissiveness are not effective with adolescents. Parents run out of power and can't possibly control all of their adolescent's behavior. At the

TABLE 14.2. Principles for Parenting the Adolescent with ADHD

1. Shift your parenting style away from authoritarian control or permissiveness, and more in a democratic direction.
2. Divide the world of issues into those than can be negotiated and those that cannot.
3. Give explanations for the stated rules regarding the non-negotiable issues.
4. Give the adolescent more immediate feedback and consequences.
5. Give the adolescent more frequent feedback.
6. Use more powerful consequences.
7. Use incentives before punishments.
8. Strive for consistency.
9. Act, don't yak.
10. Plan ahead for problem situations.
11. Actively encourage and shape responsible independence-related behavior.
12. Involve the adolescent in decision making regarding negotiable issues.
13. Maintain good communication.
14. Actively monitor the adolescent's behavior outside the home.
15. Maintain structure and supervision for longer than you think you should.
16. Be the adolescent's cheerleading squad.
17. Encourage the adolescent to build on his or her strengths.
18. Keep a disability perspective.
19. Don't personalize the adolescent's problem or disorders.
20. Practice forgiveness.

other extreme, failure to exercise sufficient authority leads to the adolescent's experimenting with dangerous behavior.

2. *Divide the world of issues into those that can be negotiated and those that cannot.* There is an important distinction between issues that can be handled democratically and those that cannot. This is our basic framework for disciplining adolescents. Each parent has a small set of bottom-line issues that relate to basic rules for living in civilized society, values, morality, and legality, which are not subject to negotiation. Such issues usually include drugs, alcohol, aspects of sexuality, religion, and perhaps several others. These are the non-negotiable issues. The remainder of issues can be negotiated between parents and their adolescent. Each parent needs to clearly list and present to

the teenager those issues that are nonnegotiable.

3. *Give explanations for the stated rules regarding non-negotiable issues.* Adolescents are more likely to accept non-negotiable rules if they are legitimized with a compelling rationale, rather than presented through pure power assertion ("Do it because I'm your mother," or "Do it because I told you to"). Parents show respect for the adolescent's emerging identity as an independent being by taking the time to give him or her reasons for decisions.

4. *Give the adolescent more immediate feedback and consequences.* Adolescents with short attention spans and impaired behavioral inhibition are more likely to stay on task when given immediate positive feedback contingent upon performance of boring and tedious tasks, coupled with mild negative consequences for shifting off task. Punishments given long after misbehavior was committed are ineffective.

5. *Give the adolescent more frequent feedback.* Adolescents with ADHD benefit from frequently hearing nice things said about their actions and appearances, as well as from receiving frequent feedback and corrections for their errors. Because there are so many factors in the life of the average adolescent with ADHD that pull down his or her self-esteem, the adolescent desperately needs to hear frequently what he or she did right.

6. *Use more powerful consequences.* Because those with ADHD satiate easily on any one stimulus and respond best to highly salient stimuli, effective parenting involves using a wide variety of highly salient consequences, ranging from physical affection to verbal praise to material reinforcers.

7. *Use incentives before punishments.* Parents commonly load on immense punishments until they have used up all their ammunition and the adolescent has little else to lose by misbehaving. When parents wish to modify a behavior, we need to train them to ask first what positive behavior they wish to see the adolescent perform, and next how they can reinforce that positive behavior. Only after taking this step should they select a punishment for the negative behavior.

8. *Strive for consistency.* Parents of adolescents with ADHD often give up easily on behavior change interventions at the first sign of failure. These adolescents incessantly bicker with their parents, sometimes wearing them down to the point where the parents back off.

We need to help parents to stick with their interventions and demands (i.e., to maintain consistency over time).

9. *Act, don't yak.* Many parents repeat themselves incessantly when their adolescents fail to comply with their requests. Adolescents quickly learn that Mom, Dad, or both are "all talk, no action." We need to help parents learn that the time to talk is during family meetings and when negotiating solutions to disagreements, but after the rules have been stated and the consequences decided, it is the time to act, not yak.

10. *Plan ahead for problem situations.* Because many conflicts between parents and adolescents are highly predictable, it behooves therapists to help parents learn to anticipate and plan in advance to handle these situations.

11. *Actively encourage and shape responsible independence-related behavior.* Because becoming independent from the family is the primary developmental task of adolescence, and because individuals with ADHD need extra guidance and learning trials to acquire new behaviors, parents need to look for opportunities to gradually give their adolescent more freedom in return for demonstrating responsibility. A parent might break the terminal independence response into small units and shape each behavior, moving on to the next step after the teenager has demonstrated responsibility on the last step.

12. *Involve the adolescent in decision making regarding negotiable issues.* Teenagers are more likely to comply with rules and regulations they have helped to create. Furthermore, they may have novel and creative perspectives on issues because of their youth and unique position in the family. Often, their perspectives lead them to suggest novel solutions. PSCT, discussed later in the chapter, is the primary technique for involving adolescents in decision making.

13. *Maintain good communication.* Parents need to make themselves available to listen when their adolescents wish to talk, but not to expect their adolescents to confide regularly in them. Parents and adolescents need to learn effective skills for listening to each other and expressing their ideas and feelings assertively, but without putting down or hurting each other.

14. *Actively monitor an adolescent's behavior outside the home.* Parents should always know the answer to four basic questions: (a) Whom are your adolescents with? (b) Where

are they? (c) What are they doing? (d) When will they be home? Research has shown that parents who cannot consistently answer these four questions have adolescents who are at risk for drifting into deviant peer groups, substance abuse, and delinquency (Patterson & Forgatch, 1987).

15. *Maintain structure and supervision for longer than you think you should.* Parents often ask when they can relax the increased structure they have created to monitor their adolescent's academic performance and home behavior. Individuals with ADHD need to be more closely monitored for their entire lives, but we expect them to learn to do some of their own monitoring and/or to enlist the help of spouses or significant others in monitoring their actions by adulthood.

16. *Be the adolescent's cheerleading squad.* Adolescents with ADHD need unconditional positive regard from their parents and focused positive time with their parents. Follow-up studies (Weiss & Hechtman, 1993) have found that successful adults with ADHD say that the single most important thing during their adolescence was having at least one parent (or, in some cases, an adult outside the family) who truly believed in their ability to succeed. Adolescents with ADHD need their parents to believe in them, to applaud their every positive achievement, and generally to be their cheerleading squad.

17. *Encourage the adolescent to build on his or her strengths.* Many adolescents with ADHD receive so much criticism they actually begin to believe that they are lazy and unmotivated. We need to teach their parents to help these teenagers identify those interests, hobbies, artistic pursuits, sports, and activities that are pockets of strength, and help them pursue and succeed at these pursuits to build on their strengths.

18. *Keep a disability perspective.* This principle has to do with expectations and beliefs, which will be considered in depth later. Briefly, therapists need to help parents remember that their adolescents with ADHD have a neurobiologically based disability, and that there is a "can't do" as well as a "won't do" component to their unthinking actions. Thus parents can keep from overreacting with anger when their adolescents inevitably make mistakes.

19. *Don't personalize the adolescent's problems or disorder.* Closely aligned to the preceding principle, this principle is designed to help parents keep from blaming themselves or losing their personal sense of self-worth over their adolescent's problems.

20. *Practice forgiveness.* Parents need to forgive themselves for the mistakes they will inevitably make raising an adolescent with ADHD, and to forgive their adolescent for his or her mistakes. Adolescents should, however, be held accountable for their actions, and consequences should be administered as planned, but parents should not "hold a grudge" afterward.

At the end of this session, the parents are given the assignment to make a list of their non-negotiable rules for their adolescent and bring it to the next session.

Fostering Realistic Beliefs and Expectations

At the beginning of session 11, the therapist reviews the list of non-negotiable rules that the parents have brought in and gives them feedback. Then the therapist focuses on the beliefs, expectations, and attitudes of the parents and the adolescent. This focus continues to be interwoven amidst other material throughout the remainder of the therapy. The parents and adolescent are seen separately, each for 20–30 minutes.

The parents are given a "crash course" in the basics of adolescent development to help foster realistic expectations. From a cognitive restructuring point of view, the crash course also represents a "normalizing," or reframing with a positive intent, of much of the negative behavior adolescents inevitably emit. By presenting this information within the context of adolescent development, the therapist makes it easier for the parents to accept it without activating any natural defensive reactions they might otherwise have. The therapist is helping the parents learn to apply principle 19 ("Don't personalize the adolescent's problems or disorder") by distancing from the constant barrage of strange teenage behavior, understanding it within a developmental framework, and learning to prioritize what to respond to and what to ignore. The sensitive therapist will be cognizant of this attitudinal portion of the agenda and will monitor the parents' level of defensiveness and reactivity during the crash course, pacing his or her statements to shape their responses in productive directions.

The therapist reviews the five developmental

tasks of adolescence discussed earlier in the chapter and points out that becoming a productive, happy, and personally fulfilled adult depends on successful accomplishment of these tasks. The adolescent is supposed to accomplish these tasks while getting along with the family and doing his or her schoolwork. The therapist helps the parents to realize that the adolescent has a great deal of work to do.

The nature of independence seeking or individuation from parents is explored in more depth. We find it useful to present the metaphor of a nation establishing its independence:

"Imagine a nation establishing its independence, going from a dictatorship to a democracy. What often happens? This process does not typically go smoothly. There may be a bloody revolution with a great deal of fighting. Or if there isn't physical fighting, there are certainly a lot of verbal rhetoric and power plays. Why should you expect your family to make it through the independence seeking of your adolescent without a disturbance of the peace? A certain amount of conflict is inevitable and even healthy. I worry more about adolescents who never do anything rebellious than I do about those who do rebel. This rebellion typically happens in early adolescence, between ages 12 and 14. In order to become independent, teenagers need to push against something, and parents are the something that they push against. Usually, teenagers typically rebel more strongly against their mothers than their fathers. Wise parents learn how to channel their conflicts into more innocuous areas that have no ultimate impact on life. It is much better, for example, to have conflicts with your adolescent over how clean the room is than over sexuality and drugs."

We go on to help parents understand that it is natural for adolescents to reject established parental and other adult societal values during this process of individuation, and to be embarrassed about being seen with their parents. To begin to establish their own identity, adolescents need to experiment with a variety of alternative ideas and values, usually those of their peers, and decide what they are comfortable with. At the same time this is happening, their bodies are changing very rapidly, and their minds are maturing to the point where they now can think more abstractly. The multiple influences of rapid physical maturation, cognitive development, and emotional change are very unsettling to adolescents, leading them to have a fragile self-image. One response to this fragile self-image is to project an air of omnipotence or, put another way, to shy away from anything that or anyone who suggests they are less than perfect physically or mentally. Thus it is natural for a developing adolescent to be less than enthusiastic about disabilities, psychiatric diagnoses, chronic physical illnesses, or any other condition that could be seen as a further insult to an already fragile self-image. We help parents to understand that this is the basis for resistance to accepting the diagnosis of ADHD and its treatments.

The therapist then turns to the question of how ADHD interacts with these natural developmental tendencies during adolescence. Adolescents with ADHD undergo the same physical changes and face the same developmental challenges as other teenagers. They experience the same desires for independence and freedom as other teenagers. Yet their social and emotional maturity may lag behind that of other teenagers. They may be less ready to assume the responsibilities that accompany more independence.

Specifically, teenagers with ADHD may lag behind other teenagers in the overall development of self-control and organization. Because of inefficient verbal and nonverbal working memory, they may be less able to exercise hindsight, forethought, and planning, or to engage in future-oriented, goal-oriented behavior. Given the difficulties with self-regulation of affect, they may remain more likely to be victims of the moment—acting on impulse, self-centered, and insensitive to the needs of others. Poor attention and follow-through make it more difficult for them to stick to discussions with their parents, carry out agreements with their parents, and finish homework. Impulsivity translates into increased moodiness (which is augmented by severe PMS for many teenage girls), hypersensitivity to criticism, emotional overreactivity, and poor judgment and low resistance to temptations. Hyperactivity often continues more as minor motor restlessness and mental restlessness than as overt physical overactivity. Such restless behavior is easily misinterpreted as "disrespect" by parents. Repeatedly badgering parents to get their way is another manifestation of hyperactivity in some adolescents with ADHD.

The ADHD symptoms become inextricably intertwined with the developmental changes of adolescence. Many parents ask the therapist whether a particular adolescent behavior is a result of ADHD or "just adolescence." They may be wondering whether to excuse or to punish the behavior. Did Stephanie really "forget" to put away the dishes, or was she just being "oppositional"? The answer usually is that the behavior is both an example of ADHD and the developmental changes of adolescence. We usually advise that the parent should hold the adolescent accountable for his or her actions and apply whatever consequence is warranted, but that the parent might temper his or her affective response and avoid attributing the adolescent's behavior to malicious motives. We often use the example of a teenager who gets stopped by a policeman for going through a red light shortly after getting his or her driver's license. The adolescent may tell the policeman, "I didn't notice the red light because I have a disability, and I'm protected under the Americans with Disabilities Act," but the policeman is not going to care. The adolescent will be held accountable for adherence to the traffic laws, regardless of his or her ADHD.

Next, we move on to address expectations and beliefs, reminding the parents of principle 18 ("Keep a disability perspective"), 19 ("Don't personalize the adolescent's problems or disorder"), and 20 ("Practice forgiveness"), and pointing out that we are now going to discuss the beliefs and attitudes underlying these principles in more depth. Then we might ask the parents to engage in the following mental imagery exercise, which vividly teaches people the connection between extreme thinking, negative affect, and behavioral overreactions:

"Close your eyes, and imagine you are opening the mail. You find a progress report from your son's [or daughter's] school. The progress report indicates that he is failing English and math, and has fifteen late assignments in history. Suddenly you can feel your blood begin to boil and the tension mount throughout your body. Your son lied to you again! He said he was up to date on homework and passing all of his courses. This is one more example of irresponsible behavior. He is always irresponsible. You told him to keep an assignment book and get help from the teachers. He never does what he is told. He is so disobedient. If he keeps on going this way in school, he is going to fail. He will never graduate, never go to college, and never get a good job. You will be supporting him until the day you die. And the thought of confronting him is not appealing at all. He will deny it all at first, then blame it all on the teachers, showing you total disrespect. He is just doing all of this to get you mad and upset. He has no consideration for your feelings. Now open your eyes, and tell me how you feel and what you are thinking. And also, tell me: How would you react if your son walked through the door at this very moment?"

Through a Socratic discussion, we help the parents to realize how the extreme thinking evokes extreme affect and how difficult it would be to deal with the adolescent rationally, as a principle-centered parent is advised to do, in such a strong state of negative affect. Afterward, we suggest to the parents that they need to strive toward adherence to the following overall coping expectation: "We will encourage our adolescent with ADHD to go for the stars, to do his or her best, but we will accept that it is not a catastrophe when he or she fails to achieve perfection, and it does not mean that he or she is headed for certain ruination or that he or she is purposely trying to anger us."

After discussing this rationale and the more positive coping attitude, we then distribute a copy of Table 14.3 to each parent, and review the most common unreasonable beliefs. As we go through each unreasonable belief, we ask the parents to rate their own adherence to this belief and ask them for examples of particular situations that activated the belief. We look at the reasonable alternative beliefs and expectations in the right-hand column and ask the parents whether they find them credible. If they do find the reasonable beliefs credible, we continue; otherwise, we review the evidence for each unreasonable versus reasonable belief and suggest experiments the parents can do to test this evidence on their own after the session is over. A therapist does not usually have time to review every belief; he or she may quickly survey the table and concentrate on the beliefs that seem most salient for a particular family.

Most teenagers with ADHD feel that their parents are unfair and restrictive of their freedom, and that the restrictions are interfering with their lives. In the portion of the session with the adolescent, the therapist's goals are (1) to assess the rigidity of these beliefs, (2) to de-

TABLE 14.3. Parents' Expectations and Beliefs

Unreasonable beliefs	Reasonable beliefs
I. Perfection/obedience: Teens with ADHD should behave perfectly and obey their parents all the time without question.	I. It is unrealistic to expect teens with ADHD to behave perfectly or obey all of the time; we strive for high standards, but accept imperfections.

A. School

1. He should always complete homework on time
2. She should study 2 hours every night, even when she has no homework.

3. He should always come to class prepared.
4. She should do papers for the love of learning.

1. I will encourage him to complete homework all the time, but I recognize this won't always happen.
2. If your attention span is short, you are lucky to get your basic homework done. Extra study is just unrealistic. These kids need a break after all the effort it takes to do basic homework.
3. He will sometimes come to class unprepared, but I will help him learn good organizational techniques.
4. Research shows that teens with ADHD need salient, external reinforcers to motivate their behavior. That's the way it is.

B. Driving

1. He should never get any speeding tickets.

2. She will never have an accident.

3. He shouldn't adjust the radio tuner while driving down the highway.
4. She will always stop completely for stop signs.

1. All teens with ADHD get at least one speeding ticket. He should be responsible for paying it and take his medicine.
2. Research shows that most teens with ADHD will get in at least one accident. She should take her medicine and do her best. She should drive an old car.
3. He should avoid tuning the radio while driving as much as possible, but this may occasionally happen.
4. I should stop completely at stop signs, to model good behavior when my teen is in my car. I should only expect my teen to do as well as I do.

C. Conduct

1. He should be a perfect angel in church.

2. She will impress all the relatives with her love for family gatherings.

3. He should never treat us disrespectfully.

4. She should get out of a bad mood when we tell her to change her attitude.

1. This is unrealistic. As long as there are no major disturbances, I'm satisfied. Perhaps I should find a youth group service of more interest for him anyway.
2. Give her space. Teens just don't want to be with their families that much. This is typical. She should attend some family functions, but that is all I can reasonably expect.
3. You can't become your own person without some rebellion. Some backtalk is natural. He shouldn't curse or ridicule severely and might be expected to apologize occasionally.
4. People with ADHD are just moody and can't stop it. She should let us know when she is in a bad mood and wants to keep to herself. We should not make a lot of demands on her at such times.

D. Chores

1. She should put away the dishes the first time I ask.

2. He should always get the room spotless.
3. She should not waste electricity by leaving the lights on.
4. He shouldn't be on his cell phone when I've sent him to his room to clean it up.

1. It won't always happen the first time, but after several reminders, I should act, not yak (i.e., apply consequences).
2. He should get it generally neat. Spotless isn't realistic.
3. She is just forgetful. We could work out a reminder system. But this is the least of my worries with a teen with ADHD.
4. Teens with ADHD will get off task; I will redirect him back to the task, and if it happens too much, I will assume it is opposition and take away the cell phone.

(continued)

TABLE 14.3. *(continued)*

Unreasonable beliefs	Reasonable beliefs
II. Ruination: If I give my teen too much freedom, she will mess up, make bad judgments, get in big trouble, and ruin her life.	II. She will sometimes mess up with too much freedom, but this is how teenagers learn responsibility: a bit of freedom and a bit of responsibility. If they backslide, no big deal. I just pull back on the freedom for a while, and then give her another chance.
A. Room incompletely cleaned: He will grow up to be a slovenly, unemployed, aimless welfare case.	A. The state of his room has little to do with how he turns out when he grows up.
B. Home late: She will have unprotected sex, get pregnant, dump the baby on us, take drugs, and drink alcohol.	B. I have no evidence that she would do all these things. She is just self-centered and focused on having fun.
C. Fighting with siblings: He will never learn to get along with others, have friends, have close relationships, or get married. He will end up a loser, and be severely depressed or commit suicide.	C. There is no scientific evidence that sibling fighting predicts later satisfaction in relationships. Siblings always fight. They will probably be closer when they grow up.
III. Malicious intent: My adolescent misbehaves on purpose to annoy me, or get even with me for restricting him.	III. Most of the time adolescents with ADHD just do things without thinking. They aren't planful enough to connive to upset parents on purpose.
A. Talking disrespectfully: She mouths off on purpose to get even with me for punishing her.	A. Impulsive teenagers just mouth off when frustrated. I'll try not to take it to heart.
B. Doesn't follow directions: He doesn't finish mowing the grass on purpose to get me angry.	B. Teens with ADHD are allergic to effort. They don't take the time to plan to upset parents.
C. Restless behavior: She shuffles her feet and plays with her hair to get on my nerves.	C. Teens with ADHD just can't contain themselves. I'll try not to attach meaning to her restlessness and ignore it.
D. Spending money impulsively: She bought $100 of CDs just to waste our money.	D. She probably just saw the CDs and had to have them. Poor delay of gratification is part of ADHD. She won't get any extra money for lunch or gas.
IV. Love/appreciation: My teen should love and appreciate all the great sacrifices I make; if she really loved me, she would confide in me more.	IV. Teens with ADHD are so self-centered that they don't easily show appreciation until they grow up and have their own children with ADHD. Only then will they realize what you did for them.
A. Money: "What do you mean you want more allowance? You should be grateful for all the money I spend on you now. Some kids are not so lucky."	A. "You will have to earn more allowance. I'd appreciate a thank-you, even though I understand you don't really think about what I do for you."
B. Communication: She never tells me anything any more; she must not love me.	B. It's natural as teens individuate to keep more to themselves. As long as I am available when she wants to talk that's all I can expect.
C. Spending time: If he really loved us, he wouldn't spend so much time alone in his room.	C. Spending time alone has nothing to do with love. It has to do with wanting privacy as he becomes more independent.

termine how the amount of freedom given to the adolescent compares to the local norms for other adolescents of a similar age in the same schools and neighborhood, and (3) to correct any wildly unrealistic expectations that the adolescent may have. The therapist should distribute Table 14.4 to the adolescent and use it as a springboard for discussion. He or she should carry out the discussion in a lighthearted, tongue-in-cheek style, trying to remain animated and to keep the adolescent's attention. The therapist should make liberal use of exaggerations for effect. The therapist should abbreviate the session or shift gears if the adolescent seems to be drifting; the therapist must not conduct a monologue and should not worry too much if the adolescent misses the subtleties of his or her points. The extent to which the therapist will be able to accomplish these goals will vary greatly from adolescent to adolescent, depending on the adolescent's attention span, level of resistance, and general maturity.

Let us look in on Dr. Sam as he conducts a discussion of beliefs with Abe, a 15-year-old recently diagnosed as having ADHD.

DR. SAM: Look at the first thing on the list—the idea that your parents' rules are totally unfair and will mess up your life. Have you ever felt that way?

ABE: Yep. Just like the curfew one. They made me come home early from the homecoming dance. My friends probably thought I was a real nerd.

DR. SAM: If you keep thinking, "my parents are unfair, my parents are unfair, they're going to mess me up," and so on, how are you going to feel?

ABE: Pissed off at them. I do feel that way.

DR. SAM: So if you are pissed as hell at them and go to try to get a later curfew, are you going to have a nice, calm discussion?

ABE: We always have a yelling match. And I get grounded.

DR. SAM: So maybe you can do something to keep from getting so pissed off at them that you lose your cool and then your privileges. If I were you, I'd try thinking to myself something like this: "Yes, I don't like coming home early from the dance, but parents always worry too much about what could happen. Yes, it's unfair, but it's not the end of the world. My friends are loyal and will understand. There will be more dances, and maybe I can get a later curfew. I'm going to tell myself to stay cool and calm when I approach them to discuss this. I'm not going to blow it and get grounded again."

ABE: Do you really think I can convince them to change my curfew for the Halloween dance?

DR. SAM: I don't know, but if you stay calm and don't think the worst, you might. I'll help you and your parents to try to work it out to everyone's liking. What about the idea that you should have as much freedom as you want all the time? Do you ever feel that way?

ABE: Yes, it's like they are always bossing me around. Especially about homework. My mother keeps bugging me to start my homework.

DR. SAM: So your mom is the big bad slave driver on homework. Now I want you to be totally honest, and I will never tell, but do you really think you would get your homework done without your mother bugging you?

ABE: Well, I don't know. . . . Doc, probably you're right. Nope.

DR. SAM: People with ADHD need structure to get things done. So how can we get you the structure around homework without you feeling like she is taking away your freedom? Any ideas?

ABE: I could set an alarm clock to go off when it's time to do homework.

DR. SAM: Great idea. We can talk that over with your parents.

ABE: Can we talk that over next week? How much longer till we stop?

DR. SAM: You've done a great job with this discussion. Let's stop right now.

Here, Dr. Sam discusses unfairness/ruination and autonomy with Abe. The therapist uses practical motivations—for example, the possibility of a later curfew and getting Abe's parents to stop nagging him about homework—to help reinforce the utility of considering more reasonable beliefs. Teenagers respond better to such tangible contingencies than to an abstract discussion, such as why the world is intrinsically unfair or why unlimited autonomy is bad

TABLE 14.4. Adolescents' Expectations and Beliefs

Unreasonable beliefs	Reasonable beliefs
I. Unfairness/ ruination: My parents' rules are totally unfair. I'll never have a good time or any friends. My parents are ruining my life with their unfair rules. They just don't understand me.	I. Yes, I don't like my parents' rules, and maybe they are sometimes unfair. But who said life is supposed to be fair? And how many other teenagers have gone through the same thing? They turned out OK. So will I. I'll just have to put up with it the best I can.
A. Curfew: Why should I have to come home earlier than my friends? They will think I'm a baby. I'll lose all my friends.	A. My friends are loyal. They will understand that my parents are creeps about curfew. I won't lose any friends.
B. Chores: Why do I get stuck doing all of the work? Sam [brother] doesn't have to do anything. That's unfair!	B. Sam has some chores too. I'll count them up, and if I have more, I'll talk nicely to my parents about it.
C. School: My teacher is unfair. She picks on me all the time. I always get stuck doing extra homework. I'll never have time for fun. Life is one big homework assignment.	C. Maybe she does pick on me. There could be a reason. I never am with the class or know the answer when she calls on me. Maybe if I kept up with the work, she wouldn't call on me so much.
II. Autonomy: I ought to have complete and total freedom. My parents shouldn't boss me around or tell me what to do. I'm old enough for freedom now.	II. No teen has complete freedom. No adult really does, either. Sometimes I need my parents, like for money, or God forbid, even to talk to in times of trouble. I want a lot of freedom, but not total freedom.
A. Chores: I don't need any reminders. I can do it totally on my own.	A. I have not been getting them done on my own. I need to stop being an idiot and accept a little help.
B. Medicine: I don't need medicine any more. I'm grown up now and can handle everything on my own.	B. Maybe I need to see whether I do better or worse on or off medicine. I'll keep an open mind about it.
C. Smoking: It's my body. I can do whatever I want with it. You have no right to tell me not to smoke.	C. It's my body. But do I really want to mess it up? My friends have gotten hooked on smoking. It costs a lot. And it tastes terrible when you kiss.
III. Love/appreciation: Getting material things is a sign that your parents love you. Getting your way is a sign that your parents really love you.	III. Material things don't tell you whether someone really cares about you. Neither does getting your way all the time. It's how you are inside that makes the difference.
A. Clothes: If my parents really loved me, they would let me buy those designer clothes.	A. I would like designer clothes, but that's not how I tell whether my parents love me. I can tell from how they act toward me and the affection they show.
B. Concert: If my parents really loved me, they would let me go to the rock concert with my friends.	B. If they really love me and think it is dangerous to go to the concert, they would try to stop me. I won't use this to judge how they feel.
C. Sexuality: If I have sex with my boyfriend, then he will really love me forever and marry me.	C. Love does not equal sex. I need to judge from how my boyfriend acts and expresses his feelings to me whether he loves me. All boys want sex. So this tells me nothing about love.

for adolescents. After a reasonable effort, when Abe indicates he is losing interest in the discussion, the therapist stops the session. Covering one or two of the expectations and beliefs may be as much as it is reasonable to expect in a session with an inattentive adolescent.

Behavior Management Training

In sessions 12–16, parents are taught a series of behavior management tactics to employ in their interactions with their teens. Parents attend these sessions without their adolescent. These tactics include (1) building positive parent–teen interactions; (2) using praise, ignoring, and commands effectively; (3) establishing behavioral contracts; and (4) using response cost and grounding effectively. The therapist explains to parents that they should apply behavior management to the task of enforcing the non-negotiable rules that they have formulated for their adolescent. The therapist indicates that the parents will be helped to develop enforcement plans for the non-negotiable rules as they learn behavior management. This chapter gives an overview of the procedures for training parents in behavior management; readers can find more details elsewhere (Barkley, Edwards, & Robin, 1999; Forgatch & Patterson, 1989; Patterson & Forgatch, 1987; Robin, 1998).

Building Positive Parent–Teen Interactions: One-on-One Time. The therapist explains to the parents that it is important to break the seemingly endless cycle of negativity between them and their adolescent by starting with some positive interventions. The teenager is used to criticism, correction, direction, and punishment, to the point where he or she may feel demoralized, depressed, and helpless to change things. Until there is a more positive atmosphere, behavior management techniques are unlikely to work.

The therapist asks the parents to do something that is very simple, but dramatically different from what they have recently been doing with their adolescent. A parent is to spend 15–20 minutes of "one-on-one time" with the teenager, five times per week; the parents take turns. During this time, the teen selects an activity that he or she enjoys doing, and the parent and adolescent participate in the activity together. The teen needs to experience the parents as totally nondemanding, noncritical, attentive,

and positive. Therefore, the parents are to refrain from giving commands, asking questions, giving directions, suggesting changes, criticizing, or organizing the activity; the parents are to be totally accepting and make only neutral to positive remarks. The teen is completely in charge of the activity. If the teen cheats or doesn't follow the rules of a game, the parents are to go along with the deviation from the rules during "one-on-one time," but indicate that the rules do apply at other times.

The therapist explains that the goal is for the parent and adolescent to have fun together during "one-on-one time," as perhaps they did at some time in the past before conflict escalated. Hopefully, the teen will rediscover that parents can be fun, at least some of the time. The therapist relates this task to parenting principle 16 ("Be the adolescent's cheerleading squad").

Clinicians have found that there is a distinct advantage for a parent's carrying out the "one-on-one time" at the beginning of the largest chunk of time during the day that the parent and adolescent are together (Kaufman, 2003). The positive feeling created by experiencing a parent as totally accepting and noncritical often persists for several hours after the completion of the "one-on-one time." As a result, the adolescent is more cooperative and respectful toward the parent during those hours.

Developing Parental Attending Skills. At the beginning of session 13, the therapist reviews the homework assignment of "one-on-one time." If any problems arose, the therapist helps the parents find solutions to those difficulties; afterward, the therapist prescribes continued practice of "one-on-one time" five times per week.

Session 13 involves instructions in praising positive behaviors, ignoring minor negative behaviors, and giving effective commands. First, the therapist asks the parents to identify common situations in which the teenager misbehaves. The therapist inquires as to how they now handle such situations. Often the parents will describe taking away privileges, grounding, or using other punishments to handle misbehavior. Then the therapist asks the parents to imagine the same scene, except that the adolescent now behaves appropriately. What would the parents do then? Often they respond, "Nothing." The therapist points out how misbehavior results in parental attention, while appropriate behavior receives no attention. Reminding parents of parenting principle 7 ("Use incentives before punishments"), the therapist suggests that parents should praise the teen for positive behavior as often as feasible. Minor negative behaviors should be ignored; the goal is to shift parental attention from negative to positive behavior. Parents are then assigned the homework task of identifying a minor misbehavior of their adolescent to use for practicing praise and ignoring. They are instructed to ignore the minor misbehavior and praise all instances of the opposite, positive behavior.

Second, the therapist focuses on spontaneous praise for compliance with commands. The parents are asked to consider the last 100 commands that they gave their teenager. How many times did the teen refuse to comply or delay compliance? What percentage of these times did they attend to the noncompliant behavior? How many times did their teen comply with the commands? What percentage of these times did the parents praise the positive behavior? Parents are assigned the task of increasing their praise for the adolescent's compliance with their commands.

Third, the therapist models effective commands for the parents, following these guidelines:

1. Make sure that you mean it when you give a command. That is, only give those commands that you intend to follow up on.
2. Do not present a command as a question or favor; state it simply, directly, and in a business-like tone.
3. Do not give more than one command at a time.
4. Make sure you have your teen's attention before giving a command.
5. Reduce all distractions (TV, computer, video games) before giving a command.
6. Ask your teen to repeat commands right after you give them.

Parents are assigned the task of practicing effective commands at home over the next week.

Establishing Behavioral Contracts. A behavioral contract is simply a written agreement between a parent and an adolescent specifying an exchange of behavior for privileges. Spelling out an agreement in writing underscores each party's commitment to change and prevents later misunderstanding of the terms of the agreement. The contract can be short or long,

simple or complex; it can cover one specific exchange or many different exchanges, depending upon the therapist's judgment of the family's interaction style. In session 14, parents are taught to develop behavioral contracts.

First, the therapist asks the parents to make a list of the behaviors that they want the adolescent to do more often; if the parents focus on negative behaviors to be stopped, the therapist helps them refocus on the positive behaviors that are the opposites of the negative behaviors they bring up. Second, the parents are asked to rank-order the target behaviors, based upon how difficult it would be for their teen to comply, in terms of time, effort, and the likelihood of compliance. Third, the therapist asks the parents to make a list of potential privileges that the teen can earn; parents are asked to review this list with the adolescent at home and modify it according to the adolescent's input. Fourth, the therapist prompts the parents to select a target behavior of relatively low difficulty and a privilege of moderate value to the adolescent. Fifth, a brief contract is written up specifying that the adolescent will only gain access to the privilege by completing the target behavior. The written contract should clearly specify the behavior to be performed, the date and time the behavior is to be performed, the consequences for compliance, and the consequences for noncompliance. Sixth, the parents are instructed to present this contract to the adolescent, ask the adolescent to sign it, and then implement it.

Here are several examples of contracts:

I, Bill Peterson, agree to take the trash cans from the garage to the street every Tuesday night by 8:00 P.M. If I carry this out, I will earn $3.00.

Jenny Jones agrees to clean up her room every Sunday by noon. We, John and Jane Jones, consider the room clean if:

a. The bed is neatly made.
b. The clothes are off the floor and in the drawers, the hamper, or hanging in the closet.
c. All books, papers, CDs, makeup, etc., are off the floor and in a container.
d. The carpet has been vacuumed (i.e., we heard the vacuum cleaner running for at least 6 minutes and there is no visible dirt on the floor).

One of us will inspect the room at noon at Sunday. If the room meets all of the criteria above, Jenny can go to the movies with two friends that afternoon. We will pay for the movie and give her $5.00 spending money.

Parent often say that there are no privileges that their teenagers want—that they "already have it all." We explain to parents that teenagers have come to regard access to television, computers, the Internet, video games, and the car (for those who are driving) as their "birthright." In many families, a teen has access to all of these privileges unless they have been taken away as a punishment for misbehavior. However, there is no written law that adolescents should be in charge of access to these activities. The therapist asks the parents to recall their own childhood and what they had access to. Most parents will admit that they had to work to earn access to such privileges. The therapist points out that the parents have the right to make all of these privileges contingent upon compliance and work.

By the end of this session, the parents should have written a behavioral contract, with the therapist's coaching. They are assigned for homework the task of explaining the contract to their adolescent and implementing it.

Using Response Cost and Grounding. At the beginning of session 15, the therapist reviews the implementation of the behavioral contract written during the previous session. If the contract was effectively implemented, the therapist praises the parents and continues to the new material. If the parents encountered difficulties implementing the contract, the therapist helps the parents plan to work around those difficulties and try to implement the contact again. In accordance with parenting principle 7 ("Use incentives before punishments"), the therapist does not introduce the material on response cost and grounding until the parents have experienced success implementing a positive incentive system in the form of a behavioral contract.

"Response cost" refers to taking away a privilege as a punishment for a problem behavior. Parents can creatively remove an infinite variety of privileges when the teen emits a problem behavior. Examples include telephone/cell phone usage, television time, CD player use, computer use, video games, having a friend over, borrowing things, special foods, bicycle, skateboard, sports equipment, access to playing various sports, use of the car, various types of privacy (e.g., having a door on the teen's room), parental transportation to special events, and monetary fines. The therapist should ask the parents to list all

of the meaningful privileges the adolescent has. Then the therapist should give the parents examples of how to "fit the punishment to the crime"—that is, to come up with a loss of privileges of appropriate intensity and duration for the problem behavior that it is designed to decrease. The therapist should give correct versus incorrect examples, explaining to the parents the rationale for each case. A few examples follow:

1. *Misbehavior*: Alice refuses to clean up her room. *Appropriate response cost*: Alice loses all her electronics (TV, radio, computer, video games, cell phone) for 1 evening. *Too mild*: Alice loses 1 hour of TV. *Too severe*: Alice loses all her electronics for one week.
2. *Misbehavior*: Peter curses frequently at his younger sister. *Appropriate response cost*: A monetary fine of 50 cents per cursing episode. *Too mild*: A monetary fine of 1 cent per cursing episode. *Too severe*: Peter loses TV for 1 week.
3. *Misbehavior*: Sharon lies about not having homework. *Appropriate response cost*: Sharon loses cell phone privileges for 4 days. *Too mild*: Sharon can't use her cell phone for 1 hour. *Too severe*: Sharon loses the cell phone until the next report card comes out.

Parents should only remove those privileges that they can control. For example, it is not effective for a mother who works until 6:00 P.M. to tell her 15-year-old daughter that she cannot watch television after school, if the daughter is home alone.

Grounding the adolescent (i.e., confining him or her to the house for a period of time) is also a common and effective punishment, often reserved for more serious misbehavior. However, it is easy for parents to pile on long groundings, one after another, until it becomes more of a punishment for the parent who has to stay home to enforce the grounding than for the adolescent. Then the parent is also backed into a corner, with no more punishments left to give. Many adolescents decide that they have nothing more to lose by acting very disrespectful at such times; severely negative verbal behavior occurs, and the overall level of conflict escalates rapidly. Grounding the adolescent for one weekend or 2–3 days is usually as effective as grounding for a week or longer.

Parents do need to be present to monitor and enforce groundings; if a parent cannot be present, the grounding should be postponed.

After discussing response cost and grounding, the therapist should coach the parents to select a problem behavior that the parents are already working on through positive incentives and add a punishment to it. For example, Mr. and Mrs. Smith had implemented a behavioral contract to reduce fighting and teasing between their 13- and 12-year-old sons, both of whom had ADHD. The contract divided the school day into three intervals: before school in the morning, after school until dinner, and after dinner until bedtime. The contract stipulated that for each interval that the boys cooperated with each other or left each other alone, they each earned a quarter. Over the first two weeks of the contract, fighting decreased from four episodes per day to two episodes per day. Nonetheless, two physical fights per day were still excessive, so response cost was added. For every fight, no matter who started it, both boys were deprived of all electronics for the rest of that day and the next day. Over the next 3 weeks, fighting stopped completely.

Concluding Comment on Behavior Management. In one last session focused on behavior management, the therapist should review all of the behavioral interventions started by the parents, assess their progress, help the parents troubleshoot any difficulties that have arisen, and help them decide where to go next with these interventions.

Problem-Solving Communication Skill Training

In sessions 17–22, families are taught to follow the four-step model of problem solving in Table 14.5 when discussing parent–child disagreements over negotiable issues (Robin & Foster, 1989). First, each family member *defines the problem* by making a clear, short, nonaccusatory "I statement," which pinpoints the others' problem actions and describes why these are problems. As each person gives his or her definition, the therapist teaches the others to verify their understanding of the definition by paraphrasing it to the speaker. This phase ends with a statement by the therapist acknowledging that there may be several different "problems" defined, but that if all agree on the same definition, there would be no disagreement.

Second, the family members take turns *generating a variety of alternative solutions* to the problem. Three rules of brainstorming are enforced by the therapist to facilitate free exchange of ideas:

1. List as many ideas as possible—quantity breeds quality.
2. Don't evaluate the ideas at this point; criticism stifles creativity.
3. Be creative, knowing that just because you say it doesn't mean you will have to do it.

The therapist has the family members take turns recording the ideas on a worksheet. At first, the adolescent may be asked to record the ideas—a strategy that helps maintain a minimal level of attention to the task. Usually, parents and adolescents begin by suggesting their original positions as solutions. Gradually, however, new ideas emerge. If the atmosphere is very tense or the family runs out of ideas, the therapist may suggest ideas too, but usually the therapist suggests outlandish ideas to lighten the atmosphere and spur creativity. When the therapist judges that there are one or two "workable" ideas (i.e., ideas that may achieve mutual acceptance), the family is asked to move to the next phase of problem solving.

Third, the family is asked to *evaluate the ideas and decide on the best one*. The members take turns evaluating each idea, projecting the consequences of implementing it and rating it "plus" or "minus." The therapist teaches family members to clarify each others' projections of the consequences of particular ideas, but to refrain from critical cross-talk, which could sidetrack the discussion. The ratings are recorded in separate columns for each member on the worksheet. Here the therapist prompts members to consider carefully whether the ideas address their perspectives on the original problem. When the ideas have all been rated, the family reviews the worksheet to determine whether a consensus was reached (all "plus") for any ideas. Surprisingly, a consensus is reached about 80% of the time. The family then selects one of the ideas rated positively by everyone, or combines several such ideas into the solution.

If a consensus was not reached on any idea, the therapist teaches the family negotiation skills. The therapist looks for the idea on which the family came closest to a consensus, and uses it as a catalyst for generating additional al-

TABLE 14.5. Problem-Solving Outline for Families

I. Define the problem.
  A. Tell the others what they do that bothers you and why. "I get very angry when you come home 2 hours after the 11 P.M. curfew we agreed upon."
  B. Start your definition with an "I"; be short, clear, and don't accuse or put down the other person.
  C. Did you get your point across? Ask the others to paraphrase your problem definition to check whether they understood you. If they understood you, go on. If not, repeat your definition.

II. Generate a variety of alternative solutions.
  A. Take turns listing solutions.
  B. Follow three rules for listing solutions:
    1. List as many ideas as possible.
    2. Don't evaluate the ideas.
    3. Be creative; anything goes since you will not have to do everything you list.
  C. One person writes down the ideas on a worksheet (See Figure 14.5).

III. Evaluate the ideas and decide on the best one.
  A. Take turns evaluating each idea.
    1. Say what you think would happen if the family followed the idea.
    2. Vote "plus" or "minus" for the idea and record your vote on the worksheet next to the idea.
  B. Select the best idea.
    1. Look for ideas rated "plus" by everyone.
    2. Select one of these ideas.
    3. Combine several of these ideas.
  C. If none are rated plus by everyone, negotiate a compromise.
    1. Select an idea rated "plus" by one parent and the teen.
    2. List as many compromises as possible.
    3. Evaluate the compromises (repeat steps III.A and III.B).
    4. Reach a mutually acceptable solution.
    5. If you still cannot reach an agreement, wait for the next therapy session.

IV. Plan to implement the selected solution.
  A. Decide who will do what, where, how, and when.
  B. Decide who will monitor the solution implementation.
  C. Decide upon the consequences for compliance or noncompliance with the solution.
    1. Rewards for compliance: privileges, money, activities, praise.
    2. Punishments for noncompliance: loss of privileges, groundings, work detail.

---

ternatives and conducting further evaluations, to spur agreement to a compromise position. A great deal of emphasis is placed on analyzing the factors impeding the parents and teen from reaching agreement and addressing them. Often cognitive distortions underlie intransigence in reaching a consensus, and these factors must be addressed (following suggestions provided earlier in this chapter) before a consensus can be reached.

During the fourth phase of problem solving, the family *plans to implement the selected solu-* *tion and establishes the consequences for compliance versus noncompliance.* Family members must decide who will do what, when, where, and with what monitoring, to make the solution work. For adolescents with ADHD in particular, establishing clear-cut consequences for compliance versus noncompliance is very important, because we know that their performance deteriorates in the absence of regular structure and immediate consequences. It is important to provide prompts for performing behaviors related to the solution, reinforcement for successful task completion, and punishment for noncompliance. Occasionally, a home token economy may be useful if reinforcement is needed for a number of solutions. Common reinforcers include extensions on bedtime or curfew, extra cell phone or computer privileges, video games or movies, money, or access to the family car. Common punishments include work detail around the house, groundings, and loss of video games or other privileges. Prompts must be salient and timely, because the natural distractibility and forgetfulness that are part of ADHD make it difficult for the teenager to remember effortful tasks; for example, if the adolescent needs to remember to take the trash out on Tuesday and Thursday evenings, the mother might post a bright sign as a reminder earlier those afternoons and give one verbal reminder as the evening begins. Figure 14.5 illustrates a completed worksheet for a problem with chores.

Problem-solving skills are taught through the use of instructions, modeling, behavior rehearsal, and feedback. The therapist briefly introduces problem solving at the beginning of this phase of treatment, and helps the family select an issue of moderate intensity for discussion. Moderate-intensity issues are better than hot issues in the early stages of training, because the family can concentrate on skill acquisition without excessive anger. The therapist gives instructions and models, then guides the family to rehearse each step of problem solving. As family members emit each problem-solving behavior, the therapist gives them feedback, successively approximating criterion responses by prompting them to restate their point in an improved fashion. To facilitate

---

Name of family: The Joneses

Date: 11/25/05

Topic: Household Chores

Definitions of the problem:

Mom: "I get upset when I have to tell Allen 10 times to take out the trash and clean up his room."

Dad: "It bothers me to come home and find the trash still in the house and Allen's CDs and books all over the family room, with my wife screaming at him."

Allen: "My parents tell me to take out the trash during my favorite TV show. They make me clean up my room when all my friends are out having fun."

Solutions and evaluations:

	Mom	Dad	Allen
1. Do chores the first time asked	+	+	−
2. Don't have any chores	−	−	+
3. Grounded for 1 month if not done	−	+	−
4. Hire a maid	+	−	+
5. Earn allowance for chores	+	+	+
6. Room cleaned once—by 8 P.M.	+	+	+
7. Parents clean the room	−	−	+
8. Close the door to room	+	−	−
9. Better timing when asking Allen	+	+	+
10. One reminder to do chores	+	+	+

Agreement: Nos. 5, 6, 9, 10

Implementation plan: By 9 P.M. each evening Allen agrees to clean up his room, meaning books and papers neatly stacked and clothes in hamper or drawers. Doesn't have to pass "white glove test." Will earn extra $1.00 per day on allowance if complies with no reminders or one reminder. By 8 P.M. on Tuesdays, Allen agrees to have trash collected and out by curb. Will earn $2.00 extra if complies. Punishment for noncompliance: grounding for the next day after school. Dad to monitor trash; Mom to monitor room.

FIGURE 14.5. Example of a completed problem-solving worksheet.

completion of the discussion, negative communication is interrupted and redirected rather than corrected.

At the end of the discussion, the family is asked to implement the solution at home and report back to the therapist during the next week. If the solution was effectively implemented, the therapist praises the family and begins a new problem-solving discussion. Otherwise, the reasons for failure are analyzed, and the problem is again discussed to help the family members reach a more effective agreement. Generalization of problem solving is programmed by having the family establish a regular meeting time, during which problem solving is applied to accumulated complaints or components of problem solving are practiced.

After two sessions of problem-solving practice, the therapist introduces communication training by distributing a copy of Figure 14.6 and reviewing these common negative communication patterns with the family. The therapist asks the family members to recall recent incidents of any negative communication habits that apply to them. The incidents are reviewed, identifying who said what to whom and what the impact was on the victim, as well as on the relationship between the perpetrator and the victim. The therapist is careful to note how negative communication not only produced bad feeling and a counterattack, but also sidetracked the discussion away from effective problem solving. Thus the hurtful effects of negative communication are identified, and the reciprocal escalation of negative interchanges can be highlighted. Any examples that occur during the session become prime material for discussion. Next, the therapist points out alternative, more constructive methods for communicating negative affect, disagreement, or criticism, or generally telling another person that his or her behavior is unacceptable. Family members are asked to rehearse specific positive communication interchanges that apply to

Check if people in your family do this:	*More positive way to do it.*
1. ___ Call each other names.	Express anger without hurtful words.
2. ___ Put each other down.	"I am angry that you did _____."
3. ___ Interrupt each other.	Take turns; keep it short.
4. ___ Criticize all the time.	Point out the good and bad.
5. ___ Get defensive when attacked.	Listen carefully and check out what you heard—then calmly disagree.
6. ___ Give a lecture/big words.	Tell it straight and short.
7. ___ Look away, not at speaker.	Make good eye contact.
8. ___ Slouch or slide to floor.	Sit up and look attentive.
9. ___ Talk in sarcastic tone.	Talk in normal tone.
10. ___ Get off the topic.	Finish one topic, then go on.
11. ___ Think the worst.	Keep an open mind. Don't jump to conclusions.
12. ___ Dredge up the past.	Stick to the present.
13. ___ Read the others' mind.	Ask the others' opinion.
14. ___ Command, order.	Ask nicely.
15. ___ Give the silent treatment.	Say it if you feel it.
16. ___ Throw a tantrum, "lose it."	Count to 10; take a hike; do relaxation; leave room.
17. ___ Make light of something serious.	Take it seriously, even if it is minor to you.
18. ___ Deny you did it.	Admit you did it, but say you didn't like the way you were accused.
19. ___ Nag about small mistakes.	Admit no one is perfect; overlook small things.

Your "Zap Score" (total no. of checks) _____

FIGURE 14.6. Family handout on negative communication.

them. The therapist is careful to emphasize that he or she is not urging family members to suppress their feelings and hide their anger, but rather to express their legitimate affect with intensity but nonhurtful specificity.

Following this overview of communication skills, the therapist pinpoints one or two negative communication patterns per session and intervenes to change them. Whenever the negative pattern occurs, the therapist directly stops the session, gives feedback about the occurrence of the negative communication, and asks the family to "replay the scene" using more constructive communication methods. Such corrections are frequent during this phase of intervention. To be effective, the therapist must wield a "velvet sledgehammer"—coming down consistently on each instance of the inappropriate behavior, but landing with aplomb. To program generalization, the family is assigned homework to practice positive communication skills in daily interchanges and at family meetings. Family members are taught how to correct each other's communication without spurring excessive antagonism, extending the "velvet sledgehammer" approach to the home.

Experience has suggested that the use of PSCT in families of adolescents with ADHD involves a number of special considerations. First, the therapist must maintain the adolescent's attention during crucial moments of each session—not a trivial task for many teens with ADHD. Keeping comments brief, bringing the adolescent into the discussion at crucial moments while addressing the remainder of the comments to the parents, and talking in an animated manner are three useful hints for the therapist.

Second, some younger (12- to 14-year-old) adolescents with ADHD are not able to understand the concepts of problem solving or may not be ready emotionally and/or developmentally to assume responsibility for generating and negotiating solutions. In such cases, the therapist can rely more on having the parents use the contingency management techniques taught earlier in the intervention, mainly consulting the adolescent about the choice of reinforcers.

Third, family members with ADHD may have such "short fuses" because of their deficits in behavioral inhibition that they often explode at each other during the sessions. The therapist should see Robin and Foster (1989, pp. 219–221) for advice on maintaining ses-

sion control—interrupting "runaway chains" as soon as they start, establishing nonverbal cues for "having the floor," teaching anger control and relaxation techniques, and being as directive as necessary to control the session.

Fourth, adolescents with ADHD can be so impulsive and distractible that their parents feel the need to correct everything they do or say, creating an endless series of issues and negative communication patterns. Such adolescents are not typically aware of how their behavior "drives their parents up a tree," and they react strongly, spurring endless conflict. The therapist must build on the advice given during the earlier ADHD family education and beliefs/expectations phases of treatment: The parents must realize that the adolescent did not choose to be this way and cannot help some of the forgetful, counterintuitive behavior. Parents need to learn to "pick their issues wisely," deciding on what to take a stand and what to ignore. For example, fidgety/restless adolescent behavior during family discussions is best reframed as the result of a biological tendency and then ignored, rather than treated as "another sign of disrespect for authority."

The therapist usually sequences PSCT over six to seven sessions. The first two sessions typically involve problem-solving discussion followed by a communication training session. The fourth and fifth sessions involve continued problem-solving training with correction of negative communication habits. Intense issues are handled in these sessions. The sixth and seventh sessions include a great deal of emphasis on troubleshooting the use of the skills at home and preparing the family members to continue their use without the therapist's guidance.

Restoring Parental Control: Principles and Case Example

We return here to the strategies for the therapist to use when it is necessary to restore parental control over a severely oppositional adolescent. The therapist must relate to such an adolescent in an extremely assertive manner, making it clear that although the teen's opinions will be valued and listened to, there will be certain ground rules for decent interpersonal conduct. Such ground rules usually include no physical violence during the session or at home; no vile language during the session; and all present taking a turn to express their opinions, but only one person at a time talking. The therapist helps model control for the parents by enforcing these ground rules strictly during the sessions. The therapist also moves to reestablish parental control by strengthening the parental coalition and teaching the parents to work as a team in setting limits and enforcing consequences. The power of extrafamilial sources of control, such as the juvenile justice system, the police, and the inpatient mental health system, can be used to back up parental authority. A "bottom line" for antisocial, illegal, and aggressive behavior must be set, with a clear specification of extrafamilial consequences if the adolescent crosses this line.

After the ground rules have been established, the therapist meets individually with the adolescent, then with the couple. In the session with the adolescent, the therapist has the adolescent project the positive and negative consequences of "crossing the bottom line" and being removed from the house. Graphic descriptions of juvenile settings and foster homes, with careful comparison of the material advantages and disadvantages of the adolescent's own home versus the extrafamilial setting, are given. The therapist is careful not to preach to the adolescent, but rather to develop a Socratic discussion of these points. It is important for the therapist to indicate that the adolescent—not the therapist and not the parents—must choose what is best for him or her.

In the meeting with the couple, the therapist begins the process of asking the parents to reach an agreement about appropriate limits and consequences for severe acting-out behavior. Usually the parents need a lot of support and direction from the therapist to accomplish this task, as they have been unable to reach effective agreements in the past and feel extremely "burned out" by the time of this session. The parents often have different styles of relating to the adolescent—one overinvolved and emotional, the other disengaged and harsh—and the adolescent has often been able to take advantage of these differences to "divide and conquer," transforming disciplinary efforts into marital/couple disputes. The therapist should break down the severe antisocial behaviors into small components and help the parents reach agreements to work as a team in exercising effective control over one component at a time. As each component is targeted for change, the parents are helped to anticipate

all the adolescent's possible "escape routes" to avoid compliance and close them off.

When a plan of action for controlling antisocial behavior has been reached, the therapist asks the parents to present it assertively to the adolescent in a family session—empathizing with the adolescent's anger, but insisting on the necessity for implementing the plan. At the next session, the therapist reviews the effectiveness of the plan, helps the parents make adjustments, responds to reasonable suggestions from the adolescent for modifications, and then moves on to additional components of antisocial behavior in a similar fashion.

The Nordons illustrate these procedures. In the Nordon family, 14-year-old Andrew was having impulsive temper tantrums at home, during which he engaged in destructive behavior toward his father's property or aggressive behavior toward his mother and sister. Seemingly minor provocations set off Andrew's tantrums. When his father refused to take him to the store to purchase a Halloween costume, Andrew squirted a bottle of mustard on his father's $400 suit, ruining it. When his mother refused to give him his favorite dessert, he threw a bottle of pop at her, making a hole in the wall. He terrorized his sister constantly—randomly punching her, pulling her hair, and stealing her money and possessions. Mr. and Mrs. Nordon disagreed vehemently with each other about how to handle their son. Mr. Nordon favored physical punishments ("the belt"), while his wife was afraid that Andrew and his dad would hurt each other if her husband used too many spankings. She tried to "reason" with her son, and in fact stood between her husband and son to prevent physical confrontations. Aside from reasoning, she did nothing to consequate Andrew's tantrums. The couple argued constantly about the tantrums, which occurred four to five times per week.

When the therapist met with Mr. and Mrs. Nordon, they agreed that the bottom line would be to call the police and press charges in the event of assaultive behavior, and to require financial restitution in the case of property destruction. They had a very difficult time, though, reaching an agreement about how to respond at the time of each impulsive episode. Mr. Nordon insisted on the necessity for physical punishment, and his wife insisted on doing nothing except for having a quiet discussion with her son at a later time. Each parent rigidly accused the other of perpetuating Andrew's tantrums. Andrew minimized the intensity of his tantrums and claimed he could control them at any time. He objected to his parent's "stupid" rules and perceived his destructive behavior as "getting even." Mrs. Nordon also punished her husband for hitting her son by withdrawing sexually from him for a week following each episode. However, she did this subtly, developing headaches or other somatic symptoms rather than directing refusing to have sexual relations. By the end of the week, he would move out of their bedroom and sleep on the couch in the living room.

The therapist pushed the parents to reach a number of agreements for controlling components of Andrew's tantrums. First, the father agreed to refrain from physical violence toward his son if his wife would be verbally assertive in telling Andrew to get in control or go to his room for 30 minutes until he calmed down during a tantrum. The implementation of this agreement was fraught with perils, because Mrs. Nordon either "forgot" to be assertive or, despite prior rehearsal, responded to her son in a "mousy manner." Mr. Nordon at first exercised restraint, but by the third time his wife refused to assert herself, he resorted to physical punishment. Only when her husband actually stood by and coached her every statement was Mrs. Nordon able to begin to respond to her son assertively. After a month of the therapist's pushing the parents to refine and implement their agreement, Mrs. Nordon began to assert herself. An episode where Andrew hit and taunted his sister so intensely that she huddled in the corner sucking her thumb and crying hysterically was the turning point for Mrs. Nordon. She "realized" how tyrannical her son was and began to crack down. Mr. Nordon was incredulous, but strongly supported his wife. Within 3 more weeks, the tantrums had diminished from four or five to one or two per week. Andrew attributed the change in his behavior to his own "willpower," a fantasy the therapist did not challenge. The parents were again having regular intimate relations—a change that strengthened their general resolve to work as a team. Strategic family therapists might wonder about the role of Andrew's tantrums in helping the couple avoid sexual relations, but whatever this connection might have been, from a behavioral family systems viewpoint therapy needed to focus directly on Andrew's behavior and his parents' responses to it.

A therapist may not always be able to reestablish parental control. The Nordons expressed a great deal of affection for each other, despite their anger and disagreements. Our experience suggests that these techniques for restoring parental control are less effective in families where anger and hatred predominate, rather than an underlying love and affection.

Concluding Phase of Therapy

Any residual problems (depression, anxiety, anger management, etc.) are addressed in the concluding stage of therapy, through individual sessions with the adolescent and/or the parents. The initial burst of home-management-oriented family intervention for the average adolescent with ADHD and his or her parents comes to a conclusion after 25 sessions. By this time, parental control has been restored, the adolescent's school performance has improved, the family members have acquired positive communication and effective problem-solving skills, and many of their extreme cognitions have begun to change. Crises continue to occur, but ideally the family is able to weather these storms with these newfound skills and attitudes. Therapy is gradually faded out by increasing the intervals between the last few sessions to 3, 4, and 6 weeks. In these final sessions, the therapist reviews previously acquired problem-solving skills, checks up on the continued success of solutions implemented throughout therapy, and helps the family to anticipate and plan to cope with upcoming events. When therapy ends, the family is left with an open invitation to return as needed if new ADHD-related problems occur or old problems recur.

CONCLUSION

In this chapter, I have tried to give the practitioner a feel for the type of biobehavioral–family systems intervention needed to address the issues of the adolescent with ADHD. The intervention integrates PSCT and contingency management with medication, family ADHD education, and school-related interventions. Modifications in each of these programs to deal with the special considerations of ADHD in adolescents have been incorporated into the overall protocol presented here. Recent research has begun to delineate the family relationship problems of adolescents with ADHD (Edwards et al., 2001) and to provide modest evidence for the effectiveness of at least the PSCT portions of the treatment program in populations with ADHD (Barkley et al., 1992, 2001b). Clearly, much additional research evaluating the entire treatment package outlined here is needed.

The interventions outlined in this chapter should be regarded as a starting point for such research, as well as for clinical practice. As the practitioner experiments with clinical variations on the strategies presented here, it is suggested that he or she keep in mind the major developmental differences between adolescents and younger children. Adolescents with ADHD, like all adolescents, think they know all the answers and do not typically wish to have help. The democratically oriented, problem-solving-based interventions that have been discussed are based on the notion of developing a collaborative relationship with the adolescent rather than an authoritarian approach, which is more appropriate for younger children with ADHD.

KEY CLINICAL POINTS

✔ Adolescents with ADHD can be expected to have increased family conflicts as a consequence of the weaknesses in inhibition, attention, and self-regulation (executive functioning) that accompany the disorder, making it less likely that they can successfully meet age-appropriate standards for compliance, independence, and self-responsibilities.

✔ These conflicts will be heightened in cases where ODD and/or CD may be present, given the social conflicts inherent in these comorbid disorders and their greater likelihood of arising from disrupted parenting, intrafamily conflicts, and parental psychopathology.

✔ The foregoing factors combine with the natural inclination of adolescents to seek individuation from their parents, greater self-determination in matters affecting them, closer identification with peers (some of whom may be deviant or antisocial), and less time under parental supervision—all of which may pose issues ripe for parent–teen conflict.

✔ Intervention for adolescents with ADHD therefore strives to (1) educate parents and teens on the nature of ADHD, (2) improve teens' cognitive functioning, (3) develop internal and external compensatory strategies, and (4) restructure the physical and social environment to maximize functioning.

✔ The only proven means to achieve improvements in cognitive functioning apart from maturation are medications, primarily stimulants and atomoxetine.

✔ Medications can be combined with intensive training of the adolescent and parents in methods of problem solving and communication, and, where necessary, restructuring unreasonable beliefs to assist teens with developing internal and external controls.

✔ Family training also must include instruction in behavior management methods to assist with restructuring the physical and social environment, to help teens with ADHD "show what they know," and to give parents greater influence over teen misconduct.

✔ Research indicates that a combination of behavior management training and problem-solving communication training does reduce conflict between teens with ADHD and their parents, but the effects are modest, reliably helping approximately 25% of the families. As yet, there is no research on the effectiveness of a combination of medication and these psychosocial interventions.

✔ To these treatments must frequently be added consultation with schools about the nature of ADHD, in-school behavior management programs, curriculum adjustments, formal special educational services as needed, and home-based monitoring systems (e.g., daily behavior report cards) to achieve these same goals in the educational setting.

REFERENCES

American Psychiatric Association. (1987). *Diagnostic and statistical manual of mental disorders* (3rd ed., rev.). Washington, DC: Author.

American Psychiatric Association. (2000). *Diagnostic and statistical manual of mental disorders* (4th ed., text rev.). Washington, DC: Author.

Barkley, R. A. (1990). *Attention-deficit hyperactivity disorder: A handbook for diagnosis and treatment.* New York: Guilford Press.

Barkley, R. A. (1997a). *ADHD and the nature of self-control*. New York: Guilford Press.

Barkley, R. A. (1997b). *Defiant children: A clinician's manual for assessment and parent training* (2nd ed.). New York: Guilford Press.

Barkley, R. A., Edwards, G., Laneri, M., Fletcher, K., & Metevia, L. (2001a). Executive functioning, temporal discounting, and sense of time in adolescents with attention deficit hyperactivity disorder (ADHD) and oppositional defiant disorder (ODD). *Journal of Abnormal Child Psychology, 29*, 541–557.

Barkley, R. A., Edwards, G., Laneri, M., Fletcher, K., & Metevia, L. (2001b). The efficacy of problem-solving communication training alone, behavior management training alone, and their combination for parent–adolescent conflict in teenagers with ADHD and ODD. *Journal of Consulting and Clinical Psychology, 69*, 926–941.

Barkley, R. A., Edwards, G., & Robin, A. L. (1999). *Defiant teens: A clinician's manual for assessment and family intervention*. New York: Guilford Press.

Barkley, R. A., Guevremont, D. G., Anastopoulos, A. D., & Fletcher, K. E. (1992). A comparison of three family therapy programs for treating family conflict in adolescents with attention-deficit hyperactivity disorder. *Journal of Consulting and Clinical Psychology, 60*, 450–462.

Bowen, J., Fenton, T., & Rappaport, L. (1991). Stimulant medication and attention deficit-hyperactivity disorder: The child's perspective. *American Journal of Diseases of Children, 145*, 291–295.

Braswell, L., & Bloomquist, M. L. (1991). *Cognitive-behavioral therapy with ADHD children*. New York: Guilford Press.

Braungart-Rieker, J., Rende, R. D., Plomin, R., DeFries, J. C., & Fulker, D. W. (1995). Genetic mediation of longitudinal associations between family environment and childhood behavior problems. *Development and Psychology, 7*, 233–245.

Davis, L., Sirotowitz, S., & Parker, H. G. (1996). *Study strategies made easy*. Plantation, FL: Specialty Press.

De La Paz, S. (2001). Teaching writing to students with attention deficit disorders and specific language impairment. *Journal of Educational Research, 95*, 37–47.

Doherty, S., Frankenberger, W., Fuhrer, R., & Snider, V. (2000). Children's self-reported effects of stimulant medication. *International Journal of Disability, Development and Education, 47*, 39–54.

DuPaul, G. J., & Stoner, G. (2003). *ADHD in the schools: Assessment and interventions strategies* (2nd ed.). New York: Guilford Press.

Edwards, G., Barkley, R. A., Laneri, M., Fletcher, K., & Metevia, L. (2001). Parent–adolescent conflict in teenagers with ADHD and ODD. *Journal of Abnormal Child Psychology, 29*, 557–573.

Elkins, I. J., McGue, M., & Iacono, W. G. (1997). Genetic and environmental influences on parent–son relationships: Evidence for increasing genetic influence during adolescence. *Developmental Psychology, 33*, 351–363.

Forgatch, M., & Patterson, G. (1989). *Parents and adolescents living together: Part II. Family problem solving*. Eugene, OR: Castalia.

Frazier, T. W., Demaree, H. A., & Youngstrom, E. A. (2004). Meta-analysis of intellectual and neuropsychological test performance in attention-deficit/hyperactivity disorder. *Neuropsychology, 18*, 543–555.

Gordon, M. (1993). *I would if I could: A teenager's guide to ADHD/hyperactivity*. DeWitt, NY: Gordon Systems.

Greenbaum, J., & Markel, G. (2001). *Helping adolescents with ADHD and learning disabilities: Ready-to-use tips, technique, and checklists for school success*. Paramus, NJ: Center for Applied Research in Education.

Henggeler, S. W., Schoenwald, S. K., Borduin, C. M., Rowland, M. D., & Cunningham, P. B. (1998). *Multisystemic treatment of antisocial behavior in children and adolescents*. New York: Guilford Press.

Jacobson, N. S., & Truax, P. (1991). Clinical significance: A statistical approach to defining meaningful change in psychotherapy research. *Journal of Consulting and Clinical Psychology, 59*, 12–19.

Kaufman, K. (2003, October). *How to conduct perfect special playtime: A key ingredient for improving your relationship with your ADHD child*. Breakout session presented at the 15th Annual International Conference of CHADD, Denver, CO.

Kelley, M. L. (1990). *School–home notes: Promoting children's classroom success*. New York: Guilford Press.

Markel, G., & Greenbaum, J. (1996). *Performance breakthroughs for adolescents with learning disabilities or ADD*. Champaign, IL: Research Press.

Mercer, C. D., & Mercer, A. R. (1993). *Teaching students with learning problems* (4th ed.). Columbus, OH: Merrill.

Moline, S., & Frankenberger, W. (2001). Use of stimulant medication for treatment of attention deficit/hyperactivity disorder: A survey of middle and high school students' attitudes. *Psychology in the Schools, 38*, 569–584.

MTA Cooperative Group. (1999). A 14-month randomized clinical trial of treatment strategies for attention-deficit/hyperactivity disorder. *Archives of General Psychiatry, 56*, 1073–1086.

Nadeau, K. (2002). The clinician's role in the treatment of ADHD. In S. Goldstein & A. T. Ellison (Eds.), *Clinician's guide to adult ADHD: Assessment and intervention* (pp. 107–126). San Diego, CA: Academic Press.

Patterson, G. R. (1982). *Coercive family process*. Eugene, OR: Castalia.

Patterson, G. R., & Forgatch, M. (1987). *Parents and adolescents living together: Part I. The basics*. Eugene, OR: Castalia.

Pike, A., McGuire, S., Hetherington, M. E., Reiss, D., & Plomin, R. (1996). Family environment and adolescent depressive symptoms and antisocial behavior: A multivariate genetic analysis. *Developmental Psychology, 32,* 590–603.

Quinn, P. O. (1995). *Adolescents and ADD.* New York: Magination Press.

Robin, A. L. (1998). *ADHD in adolescents: Diagnosis and treatment.* New York: Guilford Press.

Robin, A. L., & Foster, S. L. (1989). *Negotiating parent–adolescent conflict: A behavioral–family systems approach.* New York: Guilford Press.

Schubiner, H. (1995). *ADHD in adolescence: Our point of view* [Videotape]. Detroit: Children's Hospital of Michigan, Department of Educational Services.

Schubiner, H., Robin, A. L., & Young, J. (2003). Attention-deficit/hyperactivity disorder in adolescent males. *Adolescent Medicine: State of the Art Reviews, 14,* 663–676.

Schwiebert, V. L., Sealander, K. A., & Dennison, J. L. (2002). Strategies for counselors working with high school students with attention-deficit/hyperactivity disorder. *Journal of Counseling and Development, 80,* 3–10.

Topolski, T. D., Edwards, T. C., Patrick, D. L., Varley, P., Way, M. E., & Buesching, D. P. (2004). Quality of life of adolescent males with attention-deficit hyperactivity disorder. *Journal of Attention Disorders, 7,* 163–173.

Weiss, G., & Hechtman, L. T. (1993). *Hyperactive children grown up: ADHD in children, adolescents, and adults* (2nd ed.). New York: Guilford Press.

Zametkin, A. J., Nordahl, T. E., Gross, M., King, A. C., Semple, W. E., Rumsey, J., et al. (1990). Cerebral glucose metabolism in adults with hyperactivity of childhood onset. *New England Journal of Medicine, 323,* 1361–1366.

Zeigler Dendy, C. A. (1999). *Teen to teen: The ADD experience.* Atlanta, GA: Clark R. Hill.

Zeigler Dendy, C. A. (2000). *Teaching teens with ADD and ADHD: A quick reference guide for teachers and parents.* Bethesda, MD: Woodbine House.

Zeigler Dendy, C. A., & Zeigler, A. (2003). *A bird's-eye view of life with ADD and ADHD: Advice from young survivors.* Cedar Bluff, AL: Cherish the Children Press.

Zentall, S. S., & Goldstein, S. (1999). *Seven steps to homework success.* Plantation, FL: Specialty Press.

CHAPTER 15

Treatment of ADHD in School Settings

LINDA J. PFIFFNER
RUSSELL A. BARKLEY
GEORGE J. DUPAUL

Over the past decade, the quantity of information about Attention-Deficit/Hyperactivity Disorder (ADHD) and school-based interventions has increased exponentially. A number of efforts sponsored by the U.S. Department of Education have resulted in readily available written documents about recommended school-based interventions for meeting the needs of students with ADHD (see Office of Special Education Programs, 2004). Major education journals and professional education associations have focused on ADHD, and numerous texts have been written on the subject. A greater number of students with ADHD are being served by special education programs or through Section 504 accommodations in general education classrooms (Forness & Kavale, 2001). Since the 1991 memorandum from the U.S. Department of Education stipulating that ADHD or Attention Deficit Disorder (ADD) may be a qualifying condition under Part B of the "Other Health Impaired" category, the number of students with ADHD receiving services through this mechanism has increased dramatically (Forness & Kavale, 2001). Clearly, awareness and identification of ADHD are continually increasing in school districts across the country.

There remains, however, a pressing need to further develop school-based interventions and provide adequate training and resources to teachers. Several large-scale studies over the past decade have made clear some of the limitations of behavioral interventions. The largest single study of medication and psychosocial treatment effects for youth with ADHD, referred to as the Multimodal Treatment Study of ADHD (MTA), is described more fully in a later chapter, along with other combined treatment programs. Pertinent to this discussion on school-based intervention, the psychosocial treatment in that study included a package of school-based interventions received by all children in the psychosocial treatment arms, along with intensive parent management training for the parents. The school interventions included an 8-week summer treatment program (described later in the section on model interventions), 3 months of behavioral intervention in the classroom by a paraprofessional (again, described later), followed by teacher-administered behavioral interventions in the classroom for the remaining 5 months of the school year. Some improvement in ADHD and Oppositional Defiant Disorder (ODD) symptom severity occurred for those receiving this package of interventions without medication, but it was not different from the treatment-as-usual control group and was significantly less than that achieved with medication only, except that those with a comorbid anxiety disorder responded equally well to medication and psychosocial treatment (Jensen, 2002). The behavioral intervention added benefit to medication in specific areas of impairment (e.g., teacher-rated social skills, academics, parent–child relationships) (Jensen et al., 2001), and the best outcomes overall were achieved among the children receiving both behavioral interventions and medication (Conners et al., 2001; Swanson et al., 2001). Still, the lack of greater impact of the intensive behavioral intervention in the absence of medication and on ADHD/ODD symptoms generally was unexpected and could be due to a number of factors, including the well-known lack of generalization and maintenance of gains when behavioral treatments are withdrawn. Pertinent to this point, posttreatment measures were gathered at two points after the behavioral intervention had been faded and was no longer being used at its highest intensity, while medication was still being used at its most effective dose. A recent study examining school-based intervention and parent training for young children at risk for disruptive behavior disorders also found that initial treatment effects were not maintained and did not generalize to new classrooms 2 years after the treatment was terminated (Shelton et al., 2000).

These results and those from other combined treatment studies have led some to question the utility of behavioral interventions and to instead advocate for greater use of medication (Elia, Ambrosini, & Rapoport, 1999; Forness & Kavale, 2001). A number of factors, however, argue for the strong need to increase the focus on further development of nonpharmacological school-based interventions. First, despite the remarkable gains in pharmacological treatment of ADHD (i.e., new delivery systems and medications are continually coming on the market to aid in tailoring treatment to the needs of each child), not all children benefit, and even those who do still usually do not fall into a "typical" range of functioning. Second, some children show untoward side effects, and not all parents choose to use medication; in fact, parents tend to favor behavioral over pharmacological treatments (Pelham, 1999). Third, although medications are effective in reducing ADHD symptoms, pharmacological effects on associated academic and social deficits are less pronounced (Conners, 2002). Furthermore, school-based interventions can be quite powerful while they are being administered, particularly when there is confirmation that they are being administered consistently. The meta-analysis published by DuPaul and Eckert (1997) showed moderate to large effect sizes for contingency management programs, as well as academic interventions such as peer tutoring, on ADHD-related behaviors; such effect sizes can rival those achieved by medications when provided in moderate to high doses of intensity. Smaller, but still positive, effects were found on academic outcome measures.

Lest this sound like special pleading for behavioral treatments, it is important to bear in mind when one is comparing medication with behavioral interventions in schools that advances in the technology for nonpharmacological interventions have lagged well behind the advances made in psychopharmacology. Much of the work in psychopharmacology is on improving delivery systems, increasing the duration of effect, incorporating mixed (rising) dose intensities across the day, and better targeting the diverse needs of youth with ADHD. Similar issues need to be addressed for nonpharmacological interventions: how to better tailor behavioral treatments to individual child needs; how to extend the effects across time and situations; and how to improve delivery systems—in this case, how to improve the implementation of effective interventions by teachers in schools. Over the past several years, there have been some advances in these areas. Much of the recent work on school-based interventions has focused on academic interventions and use of a functional analysis in planning interventions to address individual needs. In addition, several promising new programs have been developed to facilitate implementation of behavioral interventions in school settings. This chapter reviews these advances, along with the technology as presented in previous editions of this text; this technology continues to serve as a fundamental base for the efficacy of behavioral interventions.

TEACHER EDUCATION, TRAINING, AND SUPPORT

The educational success of children with ADHD involves not only a well-documented behavioral technology (which we review later), but also the presence of teachers actively and willingly engaged in the process of working with students who have ADHD, and an administration that supports identification and intervention for ADHD. The latter two components are clearly crucial to treatment success, as behavioral technologies and curriculum modifications can only work if they are deployed regularly in classroom settings. Teachers' knowledge of and attitude toward the disorder of ADHD are critical. In a recent survey of teachers, Arcia, Frank, Sanchez-LaCay, and Fernandez (2000) found that many teachers lack basic information about the nature of ADHD or about comprehensive classroom management programs geared for these students. We have found that when a teacher has a poor grasp of the nature, course, outcome, and causes of this disorder and misperceptions about appropriate therapies, attempting to establish behavior management programs within that teacher's classroom will have little impact. On the other hand, a positive teacher–student relationship, based on teacher understanding of the student and the disorder, may improve academic and social functioning. Teachers should be aware of the following:

• ADHD is considered a biologically based, educational disability that is treatable, but not curable. Interventions can have a powerful and positive impact, because the severity of ADHD symptoms and that of comorbid conditions are very sensitive to environmental variables. However, the refractory nature of ADHD symptomatology makes it likely that these children will continue to experience at least some difficulty in their academic and social endeavors. ADHD is therefore akin to diabetes: The goals of school intervention are to contain and manage the symptoms, so as to preclude or minimize the occurrence of secondary harms that befall the child whose disorder is not well managed. In the case of ADHD, these harms include grade retention, peer rejection, suspension, expulsion, low achievement skills, and more.

• ADHD is not due to a lack of skill or knowledge, but is a problem of sustaining attention, effort, and motivation and inhibiting behavior in a consistent manner over time, especially when consequences are delayed, weak, or absent. Thus it is a disorder of performing what one knows, not of knowing what to do. That said, deficits in specific skill areas (e.g., academic, social, organizational) are common

among students with ADHD as well. These may arise in part from the high co-occurrence of learning disabilities with ADHD (as noted in earlier chapters), as well as from educational inopportunity in some instances (e.g., adoption from Third World or war-torn countries, or residing within impoverished neighborhoods). But such deficits can also arise from the direct interference of ADHD symptoms with the process of knowledge acquisition (availability for learning) and the weaknesses in executive functioning necessary to acquire information more efficiently and deploy it more effectively.

• It is harder for students with ADHD to do the same academic work and exhibit the social behavior expected of other students. Barkley (2000) has argued that students with ADHD are generally 30% or more behind typical students in social skills and organization. These students need more structure, more frequent and salient positive consequences, more consistent negative consequences, and accommodations to assigned work.

• The most effective interventions for improving school performance are those applied consistently *within* the school setting. Family therapy, individual therapy, and parent training, while often beneficial at home, rarely prove to be helpful in improving the academic and behavioral functioning of children with ADHD at school (Abramowitz & O'Leary, 1991).

• School-based interventions should include both proactive and reactive strategies to maximize behavior change (DuPaul & Stoner, 2003). Proactive interventions involve manipulating antecedent events (e.g., modifying instruction or classroom context) to prevent challenging behaviors from occurring. Alternatively, reactive strategies are characterized by implementing consequences (e.g., positive reinforcement) following a target behavior.

• Teachers should consider the use of peers, parents, or computers to deliver classroom interventions (DuPaul & Power, 2000). The acceptability and feasibility of school-based interventions may be enhanced by going beyond an exclusive reliance on teachers to deliver interventions.

Education about ADHD can be imparted through in-service presentations, as well as through brief reading materials or videotapes similar to those mentioned in Chapter 12. Prepared PowerPoint files for such purposes are also available to assist with giving such presentations (see *www.russellbarkley.com*). General education teachers also require training to implement behavioral programs, because such training is rarely provided in their education credential programs. General education teachers are less likely to use classroom accommodations and behavioral interventions than special education teachers (Zentall & Stormont-Spurgin, 1995; Forness & Kavale, 2001), and they report that a lack of training is a significant barrier to effective programming for students with ADHD (Arcia et al., 2000). Even so, many general education teachers do report using some type of behavioral intervention in their classrooms (Fabiano & Pelham, 2003), although the effects are often limited. This is probably due to the fact that the typical teacher has only cursory exposure (not training) to behavior modification and/or uses weak and untailored behavioral interventions. So, although a teacher may report using a behavioral intervention, it may not be an effective one, and the teacher may not have the training or skill needed to improve it. Training is intended to remedy this problem. At least one study found that teachers who received training reported increased confidence in setting up effective behavioral contracts and adjusting lessons and materials for students with ADHD (Arcia et al., 2000).

What type of training is most effective? It has been our experience that 1-day in-service presentations, while useful for imparting information about ADHD, are usually not sufficient for training teachers how to implement behavior modification programs. Such school-sponsored training can be effective, however, if followed up by ongoing consultation or technical support. In recent years, many schools have adopted collaborative consultation models, whereby a behavioral consultant (or school psychologist) works with educators in general and special education in a systematic manner to assess student needs and plan and implement interventions (Dunson, Hughes, & Jackson, 1994; Shapiro, DuPaul, Bradley, & Bailey, 1996). Ideally, the consultant should conduct a functional assessment of the student (discussed later), which includes an observation of the student in the classroom setting, as well as a meeting with the teacher to discuss the student and what antecedents and consequences may be related to the problems he or she is having. Once an intervention is designed and implemented, the consultant should meet with the teacher

daily or weekly to review progress. Behavioral programs usually require modification over time, so this ongoing evaluation and consultation are essential. One such program was developed at Lehigh University to serve students in middle school (Shapiro et al., 1996). The program begins with a 2-day in-service training focused on ADHD and school-based assessment and intervention. Following this basic training, intensive on-site consultation is provided for approximately 2 hours per day over a 60-day period. Consultation includes such activities as developing and implementing individual programs with students having difficulty (e.g., daily report card, self-management training), establishing methods of identifying and monitoring students with ADHD, and assisting in communicating and interacting with physicians. Advanced training in ADHD is also provided. The program has been found to substantially improve the knowledge base and service to middle school students with ADHD, and it represents a very promising approach for systematizing training efforts within school districts.

Since the preceding version of this chapter, additional models for training teachers have been developed. Atkins, Graczyk, Frazier, and Abdul-Adil (2003) have initiated several programs for improving school-based models for mental health service delivery, although these programs are not specific to ADHD. Of relevance for teacher training and support, the Teacher Key Opinion Leaders (KOL) project focused specifically on ways in which indigenous resources in urban schools could support classroom teachers in their implementation of evidence-based educational strategies for students, many of whom have ADHD. This program is based on the idea that influential peers are more likely than outside consultants to influence teachers to adopt novel classroom practices. Teachers who were highly regarded for their ability to assist with classroom issues were selected by other teachers as key opinion leaders. These leaders received training in 11 evidence-based practices (e.g., positive reinforcement, response cost, peer tutoring, home–school notes) and then served as teacher consultants at their respective schools. Preliminary data showed that KOL-supported teachers reported using significantly more of the 11 recommended strategies than teachers who did not receive such support. Consultation from other mental health providers was not associated with use of any of the strategies. Atkins et al. (2003) are also developing a program to increase service integration and sustainability in urban settings by coordinating delivery of mental health services among schools and community social service agencies. This form of "wrap-around" program has an emphasis on use of evidence-based universal, targeted, and intensive interventions, tailored to the needs of individual children and provided through close collaboration between school and mental health agencies. Funding for the program is offset by existing resources (e.g., Medicaid).

Another consideration for training teachers in school-based interventions is the extent to which these interventions are viewed as acceptable by teachers. Teachers report that they tend to prefer positive over negative consequences, behavioral interventions with medication over medication alone, and time-efficient (e.g., home–school daily report card) over time-consuming (e.g., response cost) interventions (Pisecco, Huzinec, & Curtis, 2001; Power & Hess, 1995). In actual practice, however, use of response cost also has been viewed favorably (e.g., McGoey & DuPaul, 2000). Acceptability of treatments may vary as a function of the child's gender, with medication being viewed as more acceptable for boys than for girls with ADHD (Pisecco et al., 2001). The acceptability of interventions may also differ by grade level. Teachers at the middle and secondary levels reported having tried and being more successful in using accommodations that involve students in activities and allow for alternative seating arrangements during independent work. General educators appear to show a greater resistance to making accommodations than special educators. For example, Zentall and Stormont-Spurgin (1995) found that general educators showed less willingness to use accommodations that involved varying instructional methods and providing alternative modes for teaching or responding (e.g., allowing alternative response modes, using special organizational systems, modifying tests, using prompt cards). This greater resistance may reflect poor understanding about the nature of ADHD, about individual student needs, or about how to use these interventions efficiently—all of which may be improved through in-service training.

However, it seems reasonable that special education teachers with small classes would have less difficulty implementing behavioral programs for students with ADHD than teachers

of up to 30–40 students, who may find the necessary record-keeping, close monitoring of the child, and administration of a range of rewards and/or negative consequences very time-consuming and impractical. There are several ways to help with this common situation:

- The addition of a behavioral aide in the classroom can be invaluable, even when the aide must rotate among multiple classrooms because of budget limitations.
- Teachers should be provided with ongoing consultation to help plan and troubleshoot behavioral programs.
- Teachers should be supported in their efforts to work with students with ADHD. Support may include verbal recognition for their efforts, financial compensation for special materials and books, and planning and development time. We have found that schools with effective practices for ADHD invariably have an administration that recognizes this disorder as a condition in need of specialized accommodations or interventions, and that provides the training and resources necessary to adequately serve the special needs of these students.

Unfortunately, even with adequate resources, some teachers may still be averse to working with students with ADHD or using behavior modification procedures on theoretical grounds (e.g., they may regard such procedures as dehumanizing or too mechanistic). In cases where teacher motivation or knowledge is poor, or where teacher philosophy greatly conflicts with the necessary interventions for a child with ADHD, parents should be encouraged to be assertive in pressing the school administrators for either greater teacher accountability or a transfer of the child to another classroom or school.

COLLABORATION BETWEEN HOME AND SCHOOL

An important consideration for enhancing the effectiveness of school interventions is the relationship between home and school. In cases where both teacher and parents are knowledgeable about ADHD, have realistic goals, and are motivated to work with ADHD, effective collaborations develop easily. In other cases, home–school conflicts can be significant and can ultimately compromise a student's progress. Parents may blame their child's difficulties on the school or may feel that the school system is not adequately addressing their child's needs. Teachers may believe that family problems are causing the child's symptoms or that medication should be considered in lieu of accommodations in the classroom. During recent years, conflict between home and school has escalated, as demonstrated by increased involvement of child advocates and the legal system to sort out educational placement issues. Some of the conflict is due to misinformation and can be addressed through education about ADHD. Parents and teachers need to dispel notions of blame, and to work instead toward improving the fit between the child's characteristics and the environments at school and at home. A behavioral consultant or clinician with expertise in ADHD and behavior modification can help mediate these problems by providing information regarding the nature of ADHD and its causes, as well as information regarding the role of behavioral interventions (including both their strengths and limitations) in the treatment of ADHD. The need to establish interventions in all settings in which problems occur should be stressed to parents and school personnel since changes in one setting rarely generalize without intervention to other settings. Many collaborative teams within schools routinely include parents, so that complementary programs can be designed at school and at home (Burcham et al., 1993; Colton & Sheridan, 1998; Kotkin, 1995). Recently, Atkins et al. (2003) found that an intensive parent outreach effort in urban areas—involving an extensive telephone-based engagement interview, community consultants and staff clinicians as members of school-based teams, and a flexible service delivery model including family and classroom services—resulted in a much higher rate of family participation than is typical.

To develop effective collaboration, the clinician should meet weekly or biweekly with the teacher and/or parent to provide instruction and coaching in behavioral management as well as continual monitoring and evaluation of the program. Older children should be included during some of these meetings to help set goals and determine appropriate and valuable rewards, since involving the children in this way often enhances their motivation to participate and be successful in the program.

For example, a written contract for a daily report card system (described in a later section), which indicates the different roles of teacher, parent, and child (i.e., the teacher's role in monitoring child behavior, the parent's role in dispensing rewards, and the child's role in engaging in appropriate target behaviors), is a concrete method of ensuring consistent adherence to the plan over time. It is also important for parents to understand that implementing behavior modification programs in the classroom is not an easy task for most teachers. We routinely encourage parents to be actively involved in their child's educational program, to follow through, and to use positive reinforcement liberally with their child's teacher, just as the clinician should use positive reinforcement liberally with the parent and teacher.

GENERAL BEHAVIORAL GUIDELINES

Effective management programs link the nature of the problems to specific interventions; that is, their approach is one of management by objectives. On a broad diagnostic level, interventions can be targeted to specific subtypes of ADHD and comorbid disorders. For example, there is evidence that children with the Predominantly Inattentive Type of ADHD (ADHD-PI), relative to the Combined Type (ADHD-C), show relatively slow cognitive processing; low levels of curiosity, interest, and enjoyment of learning; preference for less challenging tasks; preference for cooperative work environments; and greater reliance on external criteria for determining success (Carlson, Booth, Shin, & Canu, 2002). As a result, children with ADHD-PI may benefit from behavioral interventions that emphasize noncompetitive external incentives for meeting specific goals, as well as accommodations to tasks and assignments to address slow work style (Pfiffner, 2003). They may also be more likely to respond to as well as to worsen from inclusion in social skills training (SST), depending upon the mix of children who do and do not exhibit antisocial behavior (Antshel & Remer, 2003). With regard to comorbidity, children with ADHD and anxiety may benefit as much from behavioral interventions as from stimulant medication, whereas those with comorbid ODD or Conduct Disorder (CD) may benefit most from a combination of medication and behavioral interventions (Jensen, 2002). However, in terms of classroom management, the diagnostic level of distinction can only highlight general trends. For maximally effective behavioral interventions tailored to the specific needs of the student, one must go beyond the diagnosis and identify specific behaviors for which change is desired (e.g., deportment, academic problems, social skills), as well as the function that these behaviors serve for the student. Effective targeting of behaviors should do the following:

• *Focus on teaching children a set of skills and adaptive behaviors to replace the problems* (DuPaul & Stoner, 2003). For example, a target behavior to address organizational problems may involve teaching students to use and store materials in their desk or locker properly; aggressive children may be taught to increase good sportsmanship skills. If positive alternative behaviors are not taught and only problem behaviors are targeted for intervention, children may simply replace one problem behavior with another.

• *Include academic performance (e.g., amount of work completed accurately) rather than just on-task behavior, because improvement in classroom deportment is often not paralleled by improvement in academic functioning (e.g., children who are sitting quietly may not be any better at completing their work).* Increased attention to the development of academic skills (e.g., reading, writing, and spelling) in students with ADHD has also been stressed, to prevent the deficits in academic achievement commonly experienced by these students in their later elementary years.

• *Include common problem situations, such as transitions between classes and activities, recess, and lunch.* Teachers should consider very simple programs targeting these brief periods during the day.

Functional Assessment

DuPaul and colleagues (DuPaul & Ervin, 1996; Ervin, DuPaul, Kern, & Friman, 1998) have studied methods to better link selection of target behaviors with intervention for ADHD through use of functional assessment. A functional assessment involves the following:

1. *Carefully defining the target behavior in question, so that the teacher is able to reliably monitor the behavior.*

2. *Identifying antecedents and consequences of the behavior in the natural environment through interviews with teachers, parents, and students, and through direct observation.*

3. *Generating hypotheses about the function of the problem behavior in terms of antecedent events that set the occasion for the behavior and/or consequences that maintain it.* Potential antecedents include difficult or challenging work, a teacher direction or negative consequence, or disruption from another child. Potential consequences include teacher or peer attention, or withdrawal of a task or teacher request. Antecedent events need not immediately precede the problem behavior to be important in this analysis. Distal events, or those occurring minutes to hours before the target behavior, may have some role to play in increasing the probability of disruptive behaviors. For instance, arguments or fights with other family members at home or with other children on the bus ride to school may alter certain affective states (e.g., anger, frustration), which may make the occurrence of aggressive or defiant behavior upon arrival at school more probable.

4. *Systematically manipulating antecedents and consequences (those that can be) to test hypotheses about their functional relationship to the target behavior.* DuPaul and Ervin (1996) summarize a number of possible functions of ADHD behaviors. The most common may be to avoid or escape effortful or challenging tasks (e.g., repetitive paper-and-pencil tasks). Others include obtaining teacher or peer attention, gaining access to an activity that is more reinforcing or interested to the child (e.g., fiddling with toys rather than completing work), or accessing pleasant sensory experiences (e.g., daydreaming).

5. *Implementing interventions that alter the functional antecedents or consequences so that problem behavior is replaced with appropriate behavior.* For example, a child who is easily distracted by small toys or objects in his or her desk may be allowed access to those objects only after a specific amount of assigned work is completed.

Functional assessment provides a useful mechanism for tailoring interventions to individual children—one that goes well beyond a diagnosis of ADHD. This approach should help the clinician predict which of many behavioral interventions will have the greatest impact on changing specific problematic behaviors.

This approach can also be useful for modifying existing behavioral programs. For example, Fabiano and Pelham (2003) report a recent case study in which a teacher had been using a behavioral intervention for a student with ADHD for several weeks, yet the boy had yet to achieve his behavior goal and earn a reward. A consultant observed the boy in the classroom and, based on a functional assessment, made a few simple suggestions: provide rewards daily rather than weekly, provide immediate feedback to the boy when he violated classroom rules, and make clear the criteria for the target behaviors (fewer than three violations of each rule). These changes to the program resulted in improvement in on-task behavior and reductions in disruptive behavior.

Intervention Principles

Behavioral interventions for ADHD in the classroom include a range of modifications to the classroom environment, academic tasks, in-class consequences, homebased programs, and self-management interventions. All of these are discussed below, but before discussing specific approaches, we review a number of general principles that apply to the classroom management of children with ADHD, stemming from the model of ADHD (see Chapter 7) as an impairment in the self-regulation of behavior by its consequences and by rules, most likely owing to weaknesses in inhibition and executive functioning. These principles apply as much to classroom management as they do to parent training in child management at home (Chapters 12–14). This conceptualization of ADHD requires the following:

1. *Rules and instructions provided to children with ADHD must be clear, brief, and often delivered through more visible and external modes of presentation than is required for the management of typical children.* Stating directions clearly, having the children repeat them out loud, having the children utter them softly to themselves while following through on the instruction, and displaying sets of rules or rule prompts (e.g., stop signs, big eyes, big ears for "stop, look, and listen" reminders) prominently throughout the classroom are essential to proper management of children with ADHD. Relying on the children's recollection of the rules or upon purely verbal reminders is often ineffective.

2. *Consequences used to manage the behavior of children with ADHD must be delivered more swiftly (ideally, immediately) than is needed for typical children.* Delays in consequences greatly degrade their efficacy for children with ADHD. As will be noted throughout this chapter, the timing and strategic application of consequences for children with ADHD must be more systematic and is far more crucial to their management than in nondisabled children. This is not just true for rewards; it is especially so for punishment, which can be kept mild and still effective by delivering it as quickly after the misbehavior as possible. Swift, not harsh, justice is the essence of effective punishment.

3. *Consequences must be delivered more frequently (not just more swiftly) to children with ADHD, in view of their motivational deficits.* Behavioral tracking, or the ongoing adherence to rules after the rule has been stated and compliance initiated, appears to be problematic for children with ADHD. Frequent feedback or consequences for rule adherence seem helpful in maintaining appropriate degrees of tracking to rules over time.

4. *The type of consequences used for children with ADHD must often be of a higher magnitude, or more powerful, than that needed to manage the behavior of typical children.* The relative insensitivity of children with ADHD to response consequences dictates that those chosen for inclusion in a behavior management program must have sufficient reinforcement value or magnitude to motivate these children to perform the desired behaviors. Suffice it to say, then, that mere occasional praise or reprimands are simply not enough to effectively manage children with ADHD.

5. *An appropriate and often richer degree of incentives must be provided within a setting or task to reinforce appropriate behavior before punishment can be implemented.* This means that punishment must remain within a relative balance with rewards, or it is unlikely to succeed. It is therefore imperative to establish powerful reinforcement programs first and institute them over 1–2 weeks before implementing punishment, in order for the punishment (sparingly used) to be maximally effective. Often children with ADHD will not improve with the use of response cost or time out if the availability of positive reinforcement is low in the classroom, and hence removal from it is unlikely to be punitive. "Positives before nega-

tives" is the order of the day for children with ADHD. When punishment fails, this is the first area that clinicians, consultations, or educators should explore for problems before instituting higher-magnitude or more frequent punishment programs.

6. *The reinforcers or particular rewards that are employed must be changed or rotated more frequently for children with ADHD than for typical children, given the penchant of the former for more rapid habituation or satiation to response consequences—apparently rewards in particular.* This means that even though a particular reinforcer seems to be effective for the moment in motivating child compliance in a child with ADHD, it is likely that it will lose its reinforcement value more rapidly than in a nondisabled child over time. Reward menus in classes, such as those used to back up token systems, must therefore be changed periodically (say, every 2–3 weeks) to maintain the power of efficacy of the program in motivating appropriate child behavior. Failure to do so is likely to result in the reward program's loss of power and the premature abandonment of token technologies, based on the false assumption that they simply will not work any longer. Token systems can be maintained over an entire school year with minimal loss of power, provided that the reinforcers are changed frequently to accommodate to this problem of habituation. Such rewards can be returned later to the program once they have been set aside for a while, often with the result that their reinforcement value appears to have been improved by their absence or unavailability.

7. *Anticipation is the key with children with ADHD.* This means that teachers must be more mindful of planning ahead in managing children with this disorder, particularly during phases of transition across activities or classes, to ensure that the children are cognizant of the shifts in rules (and consequences) that are about to occur. It is useful for teachers to take a moment to prompt these children to recall the rules of conduct in the upcoming situation, repeat them orally, and recall what the rewards and punishments will be in the impending situation *before* entering the new activity or situation. "Think aloud, think ahead" is the important message to educators here. Following a three-step procedure similar to that used in parental management of children with ADHD in public places (see Chapter 12) can be effective in reducing the likelihood of inappropriate

behavior. As noted later, by themselves such cognitive self-instructions are unlikely to be of lasting benefit; when combined with contingency management procedures, however, they can be of considerable aide to the classroom management of children with ADHD.

8. *Children with ADHD must be held more publicly accountable for their behavior and goal attainment than typical children.* The weaknesses in executive functioning associated with ADHD result in children whose behavior is less regulated by internal information (mental representations) and less monitored via self-awareness than is the case in nondisabled children. Addressing such weaknesses requires that children with ADHD be provided with more external cues about performance demands at key "points of performance" in the school, be monitored more closely by teachers, and be provided with consequences more often across the school day for behavioral control and goal attainment than would be the case for typical children.

9. *Behavioral interventions, while successful, only work while they are being implemented, and even then they require continued monitoring and modification over time for maximal effectiveness.* One common scenario is that a student responds initially to a well-tailored program, but then over time, the response deteriorates; in other cases, a behavioral program may fail to modify the behavior at all. This does not mean behavioral programs do not work. Instead, such difficulties signal that the program needs to be modified. It is likely that one of a number of common problems (e.g., rewards lost their value, the program was not implemented consistently, the program was not based on a functional analysis of the factors related to the problem behavior) occurred.

A variety of effective management programs can be developed with the above-described principles in mind; the challenge lies in designing programs that can be easily integrated with classroom instruction and are practical to use. In an approach referred to as "Parallel Teaching" (Pfiffner, 1996), social behavior and academic material are taught "in parallel" throughout the day; ongoing instruction is blended with behavior management in the context of a structured classroom environment to facilitate a high state of learning readiness. The teacher carries out this blending by scanning the classroom every 1–2 minutes and inserting very brief interventions, while simultaneously delivering the lesson plan or otherwise interacting with students. Interventions may be statements of praise to students who are on task, redirections to those who are off task, nonverbal gestures (such as a thumbs-up sign or an affectionate squeeze of the shoulder), or questions about the lesson with the intention of involving students in the learning process. Managing student behavior in this manner makes it easier for the teacher to issue consequences immediately, consistently, and frequently than if consequences are only administered after behavior is out of control or only for exceptional behavior. The efficacy of embedding teachers' managerial statements into ongoing teaching was studied by Martens and Hiralall (1997) with preschool children. They demonstrated that small changes (in this case, greater use of praise in scripted sequences) could be easily incorporated into ongoing teaching interactions, with dramatic improvement in the students' behavior. In addition, once these skills are learned, they generally does not require any more time or resources than procedures the teachers are currently using. Often teachers of children with ADHD are spending a great deal of time attending to negative behavior. Parallel teaching simply involves the teachers' altering their pattern of interaction with students from attending to negative behavior to attending to positive behavior. Again, it is the timing of the attention that is so important to its success in managing behavior. A range of behavioral interventions, reviewed below, can be embedded during teaching activities; these interventions should be considered critical parts of effective teaching, rather than a time-consuming adjuncts. However, behavioral aides in the classroom will probably be necessary to implement interventions for students with more severe symptoms.

CLASSROOM STRUCTURE, TASK DEMANDS, AND ACADEMIC CURRICULA

Behavioral interventions have long emphasized consequence-based strategies (reviewed later) for ADHD, but in recent years, somewhat more attention has been paid to the importance of antecedent-based interventions for improving the school functioning of youth with ADHD (e.g., DuPaul, Eckert, & McGoey,

1997). These include modifications to the structure of the classroom environment, classroom rules, and the nature of task assignments. Section 504 accommodations commonly include these kinds of interventions, and they are often easy to implement, even in general education classrooms. Unfortunately, little research has been done to assess their actual efficacy, but our clinical experience suggests that the following kinds of interventions can be helpful.

Changing the Classroom Environment

Probably one of the most common classroom interventions involves moving a disruptive student's desk away from others to an area closer to the teacher. This procedure not only reduces the student's access to peer reinforcement of his or her disruptive behavior, but also allows the teacher to monitor the student's behavior more effectively. As a result, the teacher can provide more frequent feedback, which, as discussed earlier, is necessary for many children with ADHD. It may also be beneficial for children with ADHD to have individual and separated desks. When children sit very near one another, attention to tasks often decreases because of the disruptions that occur between children. Altering seating arrangements in this manner may sometimes be as effective as a reinforcement program in increasing appropriate classroom behavior.

Physically enclosed classrooms (with four walls and a door) are often recommended for children with ADHD over classrooms that do not have these physical barriers (i.e., "open" classrooms). An open classroom is usually noisier and contains more visual distractions, because children can often see and hear the ongoing activities in nearby classes. In light of research showing that noisy environments are associated with less task attention and higher rates of negative verbalizations among hyperactive children (Whalen, Henker, Collins, Finck, & Dotemoto, 1979), open classrooms appear to be less appropriate for children with ADHD.

The classroom should be well organized, structured and predictable, with the posting of a daily schedule and classroom rules. Visual aids have often been recommended for children with ADHD. Hand signals and brightly colored posters can reduce the need for frequent verbal repetitions of rules. Posted feedback charts regarding children's adherence to the classroom rules may also facilitate program success.

Modifying Academic Tasks

Several recommendations for altering academic tasks are as follows:

1. *As with all children, academic tasks should be well matched to each child's abilities.* In the case of children with ADHD, increasing the novelty and interest level of the tasks through use of increased stimulation (e.g., color, shape, texture) seems to reduce activity level, enhance attention, and improve overall performance (Zentall, 1993).

2. *Varying the presentation format and task materials (e.g., through use of different modalities) also seems to help maintain interest and motivation.* When low-interest or passive tasks are assigned, they should be interspersed with high-interest or active tasks in order to optimize performance. Tasks requiring an active (e.g., motoric) as opposed to a passive response may also allow children with ADHD to better channel their disruptive behaviors into constructive responses (Zentall, 1993).

3. *Academic assignments should be brief (i.e., accommodated to a child's attention span) and presented one at a time, rather than all at once in a packet or group* (Abramowitz, Reid, & O'Toole, 1994). Short time limits for task completion should also be specified and may be enforced with the use of external aids such as timers. For example, a timer may be set for several minutes, during which time the student is to complete a task. The goal for the student is to complete the task before the timer goes off. Feedback regarding accuracy of assignments should be immediate (i.e., as it is completed).

4. *Children's attention during group lessons may be enhanced by delivering the lesson in an enthusiastic yet task-focused style, keeping it brief, and allowing frequent and active child participation.* Tape-recording lectures may also be helpful.

5. *Interspersing classroom lecture or academic periods with brief moments of physical exercise may also be helpful, so as to diminish the fatigue and monotony of extending academic work periods.* Examples include having children do jumping jacks by their desks, take a quick trip outside the classroom for a brisk 2-minute run or walk, or form a line and walk around the classroom in a "conga line" fashion.

6. *Attempt to schedule as many academic subjects into morning hours as possible, leaving the more active, nonacademic subjects and lunch to the afternoon periods.* This is done in view of the progressive worsening of activity levels and inattentiveness in children with ADHD over the course of the day (see Chapter 2).

7. *Accommodations for written work may include reducing the length of a written assignment (particularly when it is repetitive), using word processors to type reports, and allotting extra time to complete work.* Allowing extra time for written tests and assignments is a frequent accommodation for students with ADHD, and some (especially those with ADHD-PI) may benefit from extra time due to slow cognitive processing speed. However, as with other accommodations, the helpfulness of this intervention should be assessed on an individual basis and used only if a student is able to benefit from having the extra time.

8. *Studies have demonstrated that providing task-related choices to students with ADHD can increase on-task behavior and work productivity* (e.g., Dunlap et al., 1994). Choice making is typically implemented by providing a student with a menu of potential tasks in a particular academic subject area from which to choose. For example, if the student is having difficulty completing independent math assignments, the child would be presented with several possible math assignments to choose from. The child would be expected to choose and complete one of the tasks listed on the menu during the allotted time period. Thus, while the teacher retains control over the general nature of the assigned work, the student is provided with some control over the specific assignment.

Increasing Computer-Assisted Instruction

Computer-assisted instruction (CAI) programs seem well-suited for engaging students with attention/distractibility problems and motivational deficits (DuPaul & Stoner, 2003). For example, these programs typically include clear goals and objectives, highlighting of important material, simplified tasks, and immediate feedback regarding accuracy; many (perhaps the more effective ones) also have a game-like format. Children with ADHD would be expected to be considerably more attentive to these types of teaching methods than to lectures. Several controlled case studies suggest that CAI methods are helpful for at least some students with ADHD (e.g., Clarfield & Stoner, 2005; Ota & DuPaul, 2002; Mautone, DuPaul, & Jitendra, in press) and may be considered as an adjunct to other behavioral interventions.

For example, Ota and DuPaul (2002) examined the on-task behavior and work productivity during math instruction for three students with ADHD and learning disabilities as a function of using computer software with a game format. Clinically significant increases in engagement and math performance were found, relative to typical classroom conditions (e.g., completion of written assignments). It appears that the instructional design features of CAI helped students to focus their attention on academic stimuli. Although they are not always present, these seemingly beneficial features of CAI include the following: Specific instructional objectives are readily presented alongside activities; essential material is highlighted (e.g., with large print and color); multiple sensory modalities are used; content material is divided into manageable bits of information; and immediate feedback about response accuracy is provided. In addition, CAI can readily limit the presentation of nonessential features that may be distracting (e.g., sound effects and animation). Clearly, more research is needed to discern the degree to which CAI is a viable classroom intervention for most children with ADHD.

Improving Academic Skills

For children with specific academic skills deficits in addition to ADHD, specialized curricula may be required; remedial instruction in skill areas such as reading, writing, spelling, and math may be recommended. For a review of instructional strategies for remediation; see DuPaul and Stoner (2003). Instructional programs for children with social skills deficits (i.e., SST are reviewed later in this chapter). Many students with ADHD also have difficulty with organizational and study skills, and may require instruction in time and materials management. Such training may include note-taking strategies (Evans, Pelham, & Grudberg, 1994), desk checks for neatness, and filing systems for organizing completed work (DuPaul & Stoner, 2003; Pfiffner, 1996).

Tutoring or educational therapy is often recommended for students with academic skills difficulties. Recently, an innovative program evaluated parent tutoring for four second- and third-grade students with ADHD (Hook & DuPaul, 1999). Parents were trained to tutor their children in reading, using the same stories covered in class. The procedure for parent tutoring involved having students read orally from a selected section of a story for 5 minutes and then having parents intervene with a set procedure when the children made reading errors. Children then read on their own for 5 minutes, followed by oral reading for one minute. Home–school communication forms were used to keep close track of homework. Results showed that reading performance generally improved for the students. As noted by the authors, this kind of intervention is probably most helpful for students who are generally compliant and have a good relationship with their parents, and for parents who are able to participate in and interested in the intervention.

TEACHER-ADMINISTERED CONSEQUENCES

Teacher-administered consequences continue to be the most well-researched and commonly used behavioral interventions for students with ADHD. A combination of positive consequences (praise, tangible rewards, token economies) and negative consequences (reprimands, response cost, time out) has been shown to be optimal. However, as noted above, their success for students with ADHD is highly dependent upon how and when they are administered. Consequences that are immediate, brief, consistent, salient, and (in the case of positive consequences) delivered frequently seem to be most effective.

Strategic Teacher Attention

"Strategic teacher attention" refers to the practice of purposely using attention to help students remain on task and redirect those who are off task. Praise and other forms of positive teacher attention (smiles, nods, pats on the back) have documented positive effects on students with ADHD. Withdrawal of positive teacher attention contingent upon undesirable behavior (i.e., active ignoring) can decrease inappropriate behavior. A teacher's approval, appreciation, and respect for a child with ADHD can go along way toward enhancing the teacher–student relationship.

Although these procedures may seem unusually simplistic, the systematic and effective use of teacher attention in this manner requires great skill. In general, praise appears to be most effective when it specifies the appropriate behavior being reinforced and when it is delivered in a genuine and personal fashion—with a warm tone of voice and varied content appropriate to the child's developmental level (O'Leary & O'Leary, 1977). Praise is also more effective when it is delivered as soon as possible following desired behavior, such as getting started on work, raising a hand to talk, and working quietly. It is this *strategic* timing in the application of teacher attention contingent upon appropriate child conduct, and attention to behaviors that are usually expected, that is so crucial to its effectiveness as a behavior change agent.

"Active ignoring" requires the complete and contingent withdrawal of teacher attention—an approach most suitable for nondisruptive minor motor and nonattending behaviors intended to gain teacher attention. Because ignored behavior often increases at first, active ignoring is generally not effective in modifying problem behavior that is not maintained by teacher attention, and should not be used for aggressive or destructive behavior. Most behavior problems exhibited by children with ADHD are not purely bids for teacher attention, and so this strategy alone is unlikely to result in dramatic changes in the behavior of these children. However, the simultaneous use of praise and ignoring can be quite effective. Thus appropriate behavior (e.g., sitting in seat) that is incompatible with ignored behavior (e.g., wandering around the class) should be consistently praised. In addition, one of the most powerful uses of teacher attention for modifying problem behavior capitalizes on the positive spillover effects of positive attention. In this procedure, the teacher ignores the disruptive student and praises students who are working quietly. Then the teacher praises the previously disruptive student once the latter begins working quietly. The student's problem behavior often improves as a result, presumably due to the vicarious learning that has occurred through this modeling procedure and the child's desire for teacher attention.

To assist teachers with remembering to attend to and reinforce ongoing appropriate child conduct, several cue or prompt systems can be recommended:

- *One such system involves placing large smiley-face stickers about the classroom in places where the teacher may frequently glance, as toward the clock on the wall for instance.* When these are viewed, they serve to cue the teacher to remember to check out what the student with ADHD is doing, and to attend to it if it is at all positive.
- *A second system relies on tape-recorded cues.* A soft tone can be taped onto a 90-minute or 120-minute cassette, so that it occurs at random intervals (see *www.addwarehouse.com*). This tape is then played during class—either openly to the class or with a pocket-size tape player, with an earpiece for private monitoring by the teacher. Whenever the tone is emitted, the teacher is to briefly note what the child with ADHD is doing and provide a consequence to the child (praise, token, or response cost) for the behavior at that point in time. We recommend that the tape contain relatively frequent tone prompts for the first 1–2 weeks, which can then be faded to less frequent schedules of prompts over the next several weeks. Such a system can then be converted to a self-monitoring program for second-grade or older students by placing two small white file cards on each child's desk. One card has a plus sign (+) or smiley face and is taped to the left side of the desk; the other has a minus sign (−) or frowning face and is taped to the right side of the desk. The teacher then instructs the children that whenever they hear the tone, if they are doing as instructed for that activity, they can award themselves a hash mark on the plus card. If they were not obeying instructions or were off task, they must place a hash mark on the negative card. The teacher's job at the sound of the tone is to rapidly scan the classroom and note the behavior of the child with ADHD, then note whether the child is delivering the appropriate consequence to him- or herself. The program can be made more effective by having an easel at the front of the classroom with a list of five or so rules that should be followed during that class period (e.g., the

five rules for deskwork might be "Stay in seat," "Stay on task," "Don't space out," "Don't bug others," "Do your work"). The teacher can then refer to the set of rules in force for that particular class period or activity by flipping to the appropriate chart when the activity begins and calling the children's attention to these rules. A controlled, within-subject experiment supports the efficacy of this procedure (Edwards, Salant, Howard, Brougher, & McLaughlin, 1995).

- *A third system for prompting strategic teacher attending and monitoring is to have the teacher place 10 or so bingo chips in his or her left pocket that must be moved to the right pocket whenever positive attention has been given appropriately to the child with ADHD.* The goal is to move all 10 chips to the right pocket by the end of that class period.

- *A fourth system is to use a small vibrating device that containing a timer that can be programmed to any interval desired by the teacher* (e.g., The Motivator, available from *www.addwarehouse.com*). Teachers can wear the device on a belt or in a pocket, and when they detect the tactile vibration, they can use this as a cue to monitor the class and briefly respond to both positive and negative student behaviors.

Tangible Rewards and Token Programs

Because of their decreased sensitivity to reward and their failure to sustain effort when reinforcement is inconsistent and weak, students with ADHD usually require more frequent and more powerful reinforcement, often in the form of special privileges or activities, to modify classroom performance (Pfiffner, Rosen, & O'Leary, 1985). Special privileges or activities may be provided for meeting certain goals. For example, a student may earn extra free time for completing assigned classwork promptly and accurately. In other cases, a token economy may be used. In this system, students earn tokens (points, numbers, or hash marks for older children; tangibles, such as poker chips, stars, or tickets, for younger children) throughout the day and then later exchange their earnings for "backup" rewards (privileges, activities). Backup rewards are typically assigned a purchase value so that rewards can be matched to the number of tokens or points earned. As will be described later, some programs also include a response cost component, where children lose points for inappropriate behavior. Some tangible or backup rewards are distributed on a daily basis, while longer periods (e.g., weekly) of appropriate behavior or academic functioning may be required for more valuable rewards.

The identification of powerful rewards and backup consequences is critical for program success and may be achieved through interviews with children regarding the kinds of activities or other rewards they would like to earn and observations of the high-rate activities normally engaged in by the children. Access to these activities can then be used as reinforcement. For instance, Legos may be an effective reward for a child who spends much of his or her free time playing with Legos. That is, the child is likely to improve his or her behavior if Lego play is made available only as a reward for appropriate behavior. Monitoring the manner in which the child spends free-time activities over a week or so may suggest what privileges or activities are especially rewarding for that particular child. We have found the following to be effective reinforcers: homework passes; removing the lowest grade or making up a missing grade; a grab bag with small toys or school supplies; free time; computer or video game (e.g., Nintendo) time; stickers/stamps; running errands; helping the teacher; earning extra recess; playing special games; and art projects.

In some cases, rewards available at school may not be sufficiently powerful to alter a child's behavior. Homebased reward programs, discussed in a subsequent section, may be considered in these cases. It is also possible to have parents provide a favored toy or piece of play equipment from home to the teacher for contingent use in the classroom as part of a classroom token or reward system. We have also been successful in approaching local civic clubs to donate reinforcement equipment to a particular classroom, or at least to offset part of its expense, by providing presentations to them on the seriousness of classroom behavioral problems and the critical need for such reinforcers in the management of disruptive (and typical!) children. Otherwise, soliciting each parent of a child in that classroom to donate a few dollars or so is often adequate to purchase these systems for reinforcement of child behavior.

Reward programs can be designed for individual children or the entire class. Individual programs or classwide programs wherein students earn rewards for their own behavior are often best for the student with ADHD. Involving the entire class may be particularly effective when peer contingencies are competing with teacher contingencies (e.g., when peers reinforce disruptive students by laughter or joining in on their off-task pursuits). Some sample programs include the following (see Pfiffner, 1996):

• *"Big Deals."* In this group contingency, stickers called "Big Deals" are earned individually and/or as a group for exhibiting target behavior/social skills (e.g., following directions, sharing, using an assertive tone of voice). Stickers are posted on a Big Deal Chart. Once the class earns a predetermined number of stickers, the class earns a group party ("Big Deal fiesta").

• *"Peg system."* In this system for younger children, the teacher sets a timer for a brief period of time (2–5 minutes). If the student follows all class rules until the timer goes off, he or she earns a peg kept in a cup. Whenever the child breaks a rule, the teacher earns a peg and resets the timer. At the end of the period, if the child has more pegs than the teacher, the child selects an activity for the class to do. Otherwise, the teacher selects the activity, and the child does not participate.

• *Visual aids (cards) taped to students' desktops serve as a way to conveniently keep track of progress toward established goals.* The cards may be divided into columns; there may be one card for positive and another for negative behavior, as described previously; or the cards may depict colorful pictures to correspond with progress. For example, a thermometer, with higher readings corresponding to greater on-task behavior, may be used with younger students. Tangible rewards are earned at the end of the day for those with high readings.

• *Lotteries and auctions.* In these popular programs, students earn tickets or "bucks" for a variety of target behaviors throughout the day and exchange them for chances in the lottery or items during class auctions offered at least once a week (daily at the beginning of the program).

• *Team contingencies.* In this variation of group programs, children are divided into competing teams and earn or lose points for their respective team, depending on their behavior.

The team with the greatest number of positive points or fewest negative points earns the group privileges. For example, teams may be divided by tables or rows. Points are given to a team for behaviors of the individual members, such as getting along and keeping the area clean. Either the team with the most points, or all teams who meet a specified criterion, earn the reward.

• *Class movies and theme parties.* To keep things interesting, we have found that posters depicting the activity to be earned and a record of class progress toward earning the activity are helpful. In one example, for every 15 minutes class members are on task, the children in the picture are moved an inch closer to a picture of a theater. When they reach the theater, the class earns the movie.

• *The Good Behavior Game* (Barrish, Saunders, & Wolf, 1969). In this approach, the class is divided into two teams. Each team receives marks for rule violations of individual team members. After a specified period of time, both teams earn a reward if their marks do not exceed a certain number; otherwise, the team with the fewest marks wins. This game has been effective in improving student behavior and has also been well accepted by teachers (Tingstrom, 1994).

Group programs targeting all students' behavior have the advantage of not singling out the child with ADHD. Given some teachers' concerns about possible stigmatization of or undue attention to children receiving treatment for behavior problems, a group procedure may be preferable. This may also be the treatment of choice when there is concern that children not involved in treatment may increase their misbehavior in order to be a part of the program and receive reinforcement. It should be noted, however, that concerns about stigmatization and escalation of problem behavior have not been substantiated in research studies. When a teacher is using group contingencies, however, care should be taken to minimize possible peer pressure and subversion of the program by one or more children. Powerful rewardonly programs may be effective in this regard.

The success of token programs in numerous studies and the utility of these programs with a wide range of problem behavior have led to their widespread use in school settings.

Tokens are portable, so they can be administered in any situation and can usually be distributed immediately following desirable behavior. Token programs also tend to be very powerful, since a wide range of backup rewards can be used to avoid satiation of any one reward. However, appropriate and realistic treatment goals are critical for the success of the program. In many typical classrooms, rewards are often reserved for exemplary performance. Although this practice may be sufficient for some children, it is unlikely to improve the performance of children exhibiting severe attentional and behavioral problems. Regardless how motivated such a child may be initially, if the criteria for a reward is set too high, the child will rarely achieve the reward and is likely to give up trying. To prevent this occurrence, rewards should initially be provided for approximations to the terminal response and should be set at a level that ensures the child's success. For instance, a child who has a long history of failing to complete work should be required to complete only a part of his or her work, not all, in order to earn a reward. Similarly, a child who is often disruptive throughout the day may initially earn a reward for exhibiting quiet, ontask behavior for only a small segment of the day. As performance improves, more appropriate behavior can be shaped by gradually increasing the behavioral criteria for rewards.

Ideally, behaviors targeted by token programs should not fail the "dead-man test for behavior" (i.e., desired behavior) articulated by Lindsley (1991). The "rule" for this test is that "if a dead boy could do it, it wasn't behavior" (Lindsley, 1991, p. 457). Treatment targets like "sitting still" and "not calling out" fail the dead-man test. Alternatively, goals such as "completing assigned work" or "participating appropriately in class discussions" not only pass this test, but encourage active, appropriate behavior rather than the simple absence of inappropriate or disruptive behavior. In our experience, teachers like the idea of targeting academic behaviors (e.g., completion and accuracy on work) because these behaviors are incompatible with disruptive behavior, are more easily monitored than classroom deportment, and tell the child exactly what is expected.

It is important to reiterate that students with ADHD typically lose interest if the same reward is used for too long. Rewards are much more effective if they are novel and change regularly. We recommend using a "reward menu" (a list of varied activities, privileges, or objects) and having a child choose his or her own rewards. The "packaging" of the reward is especially important. We strongly recommend that teachers make the reward fun and interesting by using colorful posters, creative tokens, and special words to describe the treat (e.g., "bonus," "challenges"), as well as by being enthusiastic.

Negative Consequences

Whereas use of positive approaches should be emphasized in working with students who have ADHD, negative consequences are usually necessary. In fact, some studies show that brief reprimands may be more important than praise for maintaining appropriate behavior (Acker & O'Leary, 1987). However, the effectiveness of negative consequences, particularly for students with ADHD, is highly dependent on several stylistic features as described below.

Reprimands

Reprimands and corrective statements are the most commonly used negative consequences. As is the case with praise, the effectiveness of reprimands is a function of how and when they are delivered. A number of studies (see Pfiffner & O'Leary, 1993) indicate that reprimands that are immediate, unemotional, brief, and consistently backed up with time out or a loss of a privilege for repeated noncompliance are far superior to those that are delayed, long, or inconsistent. Proximity also seems to make a difference; reprimands that are issued in close proximity to a child have an edge over those yelled from across the room. Mixing positive and negative feedback for inappropriate behavior appears to be particularly deleterious. For example, children who are sometimes reprimanded for calling out, but other times responded to as if they had raised their hands, are apt to continue (if not increase) their calling out. In addition, children respond better to teachers who deliver consistently strong reprimands at the outset of the school year (immediate, brief, firm, and in close proximity to the children) than to teachers who gradually increase the severity of their discipline over time. Finally, the practice of using encouragement ("I know you can do it") in an attempt to coax a student into good behavior is not as effective as clear, direct reprimands (Abramowitz & O'Leary, 1991).

Response Cost

"Response cost" involves the loss of a reinforcer contingent upon inappropriate behavior. Lost reinforcers can include a wide range of privileges and activities. Response cost has often been used to manage the disruptive behavior of children with ADHD in the context of a token program. This procedure involves a child's losing tokens for inappropriate behavior, in addition to earning them for appropriate behavior. It is convenient, easy to use, and readily adapted to a variety of target behaviors and situations. Furthermore, response cost has been shown to be more effective than reprimands for children with ADHD and can also increase the effectiveness of reward programs.

The classic study of response cost conducted by Rapport, Murphy, and Bailey (1980) compared the effects of response cost with stimulant medication on the behavior and academic performance of two hyperactive children. In the response cost procedure, the teacher deducted 1 point every time she saw a child not working. Each point loss translated into a loss of 1 minute of free time. An apparatus was placed at each child's desk to keep track of point totals. One child's apparatus consisted of numbered cards that could be changed to a lesser value each time a point was lost. The teacher had an identical apparatus on her desk where she kept track of point losses. The child was instructed to match the number value on his apparatus with that of the teacher's on a continual basis. The second child had a batteryoperated electronic "counter" with a number display. The teacher decreased point values on the display via a remote transmitter. Both response cost procedures resulted in increases in both ontask and academic performance, which compared favorably with the effects of stimulant medication. The immediacy with which consequences could be delivered in either procedure (the teacher was able to administer a consequence even when she was some distance away from the child) probably contributed to their efficacy.

The device used in this study, called the Attention Trainer, was designed by Mark Rapport and commercially developed and marketed by Michael Gordon (Gordon Systems, DeWitt,

NY: *www.gsi-add.com*); it continues to receive strong empirical support (DuPaul, Guevremont, & Barkley, 1992; Evans, Ferre, Ford, & Green, 1995; Gordon, Thomason, Cooper, & Ivers, 1990). Although some teachers initially believe that such a device may result in negative social stigma or excessive peer attention, we have not found this to be the case. The device can be faded out over 4–6 weeks and replaced by a less intensive class token system or self-monitoring program (e.g., the tone prompt system described above) or by a home–school report card (described later).

Response cost has been used in a variety of other formats:

• Color-coded response cost programs have been implemented in several programs across the country (Barkley et al, 1996; Kotkin, 1995). In these programs, students' behavior is reviewed every 30 minutes, and each receives a color card corresponding to how well he or she did. For example, each student starts the period with a red card (the color representing optimal behavior). Following a minor infraction, the card color changes to a yellow; following a major infraction the color changes to a blue. Color strips are either attached with Velcro to, or inserted in paper pockets on, a board containing the students' names down one side and the period listed across the top. Color earnings are totaled once or twice per day (twice for younger children, once for older children). Earnings are exchanged for graduated activities and privileges (e.g., red earns choice of most desirable activities, blue earns fewest choices). Weekly rewards based on daily earnings are also provided.

• Response cost has also been implemented in a group format. In one procedure, a self-contained class was given 30 tokens (poker chips) each day at the beginning of a 90-minute period. A token was removed contingent upon each occurrence of an interruption by any student. Tokens were counted at the end of the period; remaining tokens were exchanged for 1 minute of reading time by the teacher. Significant reductions in interruptions occurred, and most of the students rated the program very favorably (Sprute, Williams, & McLaughlin, 1990).

• A response cost raffle has also been successful in reducing mild disruptive behavior of junior high school students (Proctor & Morgan, 1991). In this system, five tickets were distributed to students at the beginning of each class period. One ticket was lost for each instance of disruptive behavior. Remaining slips were collected at the end of the period. Two tickets were labeled with the word "group." One ticket was then randomly selected. If an unlabeled ticket was chosen, the winning student chose from a list of potential rewards, including a free tardy, gum, soda, and chips. If a ticket labeled "group" was chosen, a class reward was selected (e.g., free talking, candy, a movie day).

• Response cost has also been used successfully with preschoolers. McGoey and DuPaul (2000) compared a response cost intervention wherein students lost buttons from a chart for breaking rules with a token economy wherein students earned buttons for following rules. Rewards were given at the end of preschool class for either keeping (response cost condition) or earning (token economy condition) a predetermined number of buttons. Both interventions were effective in reducing the disruptive behavior of four preschoolers with ADHD. However, the teachers had a slight preference for the response cost procedure, perhaps because it seemed easier to implement in a class of 20 students.

As with other punishment procedures, response cost is most effective when it is applied immediately, unemotionally, and consistently. When delivered in this way, response cost is as effective as token reward programs. In addition, teachers' and children's attitudes about response cost programs appear to be as positive as they are for reward programs. However, special efforts should be made to continue monitoring and praising appropriate behavior when response cost programs are in effect to avoid excessive attention to negative behavior. It is also advisable that when rewards and response cost are used together, the opportunity to earn tokens should be greater than the possibility of losing them to avoid negative earnings (i.e., below zero). Care should also be taken to avoid the use of unreasonably stringent standards, which lead to excessive point or privilege losses. In the case of aggressive or very coercive behavior, teachers may be reluctant to administer the procedure right away, because they fear that the behavior will escalate. However, response cost needs to be implemented consistently and immediately to be effective. Escalation may be minimized by reducing the amount

of the "cost" when the student does not lose control.

Time Out

Time out from positive reinforcement (i.e., "time out") is often effective for children with ADHD who are particularly aggressive or disruptive. This procedure involves the withdrawal of positive reinforcement contingent upon inappropriate behavior. Several variations of time out are used in the classroom, including these:

• Removal of the student from the classroom situation to a small empty room (i.e., "timeout room") for short periods of time (e.g., 2–10 minutes); this is referred to as "social isolation." Isolation as a time-out method has been increasingly criticized over the years, due to ethical concerns and difficulty with implementing the procedure correctly.

• Removal of adult or peer attention by removing the child from the area of reinforcement or the opportunity to earn reinforcement. This may involve having the child sit in a threesided cubicle or sit facing a dull area (e.g., a blank wall) in the classroom.

• Removal of materials, as in the case of having children put their work away (which eliminates the opportunity to earn reinforcement for academic performance) and their heads down (which reduces the opportunity for reinforcing interaction with others) for brief periods of time.

• Using a "good-behavior clock" as implemented by Kubany, Weiss, and Slogett (1971). In this procedure, rewards (e.g., penny trinkets, candy) are earned for a target child and the class, contingent upon the child's behaving appropriately for a specified period of time. A clock runs whenever the child is on task and behaving appropriately, but is stopped for a short period of time when the child is disruptive or off task.

• Instituting a "Do a Task" procedure, in which the child is instructed in how many sheets of simple academic work he or she must accomplish while seated at a time-out desk at the back of the classroom facing a wall. The teacher implements this procedure by telling the class that when the teacher says to them what they have done wrong, followed by the phrase "Give me one [or two, or three]," this means that the child has misbehaved and is to proceed immediately to the isolated desk at the back of the class, count out that many worksheets, complete them, and then put them on the teacher's desk, after which the child returns to his or her usual seat.

- The key ingredient to all variations of time out is "swift justice." That is, the speed with which teachers invoke time out immediately following misbehavior is primarily what makes it effective, rather than the length of the time-out interval to be served.

Most time-out programs set specific criteria that must be fulfilled prior to release from time out. Typically, these criteria involve the child's being quiet and cooperative for a specified period during time out. In some cases, extremely disruptive children may fail to comply with the standard procedure, either by refusing to go to time out or by not remaining in the timeout area for the required duration. To reduce noncompliance in these cases, (1) a child can earn time off for complying with the procedure (i.e., the length of the original time out is reduced); (2) the length of time out can be increased for each infraction; (3) the child may be removed from the class to serve the time out elsewhere (e.g., in another class or in the principal's office); (4) a response cost procedure can be used, wherein activities, privileges or tokens are lost for uncooperative behavior in time out; (5) work tasks, such as simple copying or marking tasks, can be made contingent on failure to follow time-out rules; and (6) the child can stay after school to serve time out for not being cooperative in following time-out rules during school hours. The use of this last procedure, however, depends on the availability of personnel to supervise the child after school.

Overall, time out appears to be an effective procedure for reducing aggressive and disruptive actions in the classroom, especially when they are maintained by peer or teacher attention. Time out may not be effective in cases where inappropriate behavior is due to a desire to avoid work or be alone, since in these cases time out may actually be reinforcing. It is important that timeout be implemented with minimal attention from teacher and peers. In cases where a child's problem behavior consistently escalates during time out and requires teacher intervention (e.g., restraint) to prevent harm to self, others or property, alternative procedures to time out may be indicated. Overall, procedural safeguards and appropriate reviews are important to ensure that time out is used in an ethical and legal way (Gast & Nelson, 1977).

Suspension

Suspension from school is sometimes used as punishment for severe problem behavior, but it may not be effective with students having ADHD. The use of suspension violates several critical features of effective punishment: It is not immediate; it is not brief; and it may not remove rewarding activities (many children may find staying at home or full day day care more enjoyable than being in school). Suspension should also not be used in cases where parents do not have the appropriate management skills needed for enforcement or in cases where parents may be overly punitive or abusive. A recent study of inner-city public school students found that detentions and suspensions were apparently ineffective for children who were aggressive, lacking social skills, and high on hyperactivity (Atkins, McKay et al., 2002).

In-school suspension programs on the other hand, may be appropriate for particularly chronic, severe, intentional infractions (serious aggressive or destructive behavior) for which response cost, time-out, and reward programs have been ineffective. For example, in-school suspension may be effective as a back-up consequence when a student fails to take time-outs or to accept a "cost," and becomes violent or seriously disruptive. If in-school suspension is used, the suspensions should be short-term (usually not more than a day or two) and have clear entry criteria, clear rules, and structured educational assignments for the student to do during the suspension period.

Minimizing Adverse Side Effects

Despite the overall effectiveness of negative consequences, adverse side effects may occur if they are used improperly. The guidelines discussed by O'Leary and O'Leary (1977) and presented in previous versions of this chapter are still timely and are reviewed here as well:

- *Punishment should be used sparingly.* Teachers who frequently use punishment to the exclusion of positive consequences may be less effective in managing children's behavior, due to a decrease in their own reinforcing value and/or due to the children's having satiated or adapted to the punishment. Excessive criticism or other forms of punishment may also cause the classroom situation to become aversive. As a result, children may begin to avoid certain academic subjects by skipping classes, or may avoid school in general by becoming truant. Frequent harsh punishment may even accelerate a child's overt defiance, especially in cases where a teacher inadvertently serves as an aggressive model.

• *When teachers use negative consequences, they should teach and reinforce children for alternative appropriate behaviors incompatible with inappropriate behaviors.* This practice will aid in teaching appropriate skills, as well as decrease the potential for the occurrence of other problem behaviors.

• *Punishment involving the removal of a positive reinforcer (e.g., response cost) is usually preferable to punishment involving the presentation of an aversive stimulus.* Use of the latter method, as exemplified by corporal punishment, is often limited for ethical and legal reasons.

Maintenance and Generalization

Maintaining treatment gains after withdrawing treatment continues to be a challenge, as does generalizing improvement made in one setting or class to another. Unfortunately, generalization does not occur automatically. The most effective approach for promoting improvement in behavior in all classes and periods (including recess and lunch) is to implement behavioral programs in all the settings in which behavior change is desired.

Technologies have also been developed to improve the probability that treatment gains will maintain over time. The most effective seems to be gradually withdrawing the classroom contingency programs. For example, a study conducted by Pfiffner and O'Leary (1987) found that the abrupt removal of negative consequences, even in the context of a powerful token program, led to dramatic deterioration in class behavior. However, when negative consequences were gradually removed, high ontask rates were maintained. Likewise, token economies should not be removed abruptly. Gradual withdrawal of token programs may be accomplished by reducing the frequency of feedback (e.g., fading from daily to weekly rewards) and substituting natural reinforcers (e.g., praise, regular activities) for token rewards. One particularly effective

procedure for fading management programs involves varying the range of conditions or situations in which contingencies are administered, in order to reduce a child's ability to discriminate when contingencies are in effect. The less the child is able to discern the changes in contingencies when fading a program, the more successful it appears to be. When a student is making the transition to a new class, it is wise to initially implement the same or a similar program in the new class and then fade it once behavior is stable.

Self-management skills such as self-monitoring and self-reinforcement (to be described in a subsequent section) have also been taught in order to improve maintenance of gains from behavioral programs and to help prompt appropriate behavior in nontreated settings. These procedures have been found to improve maintenance following withdrawal of token programs. However, they are not effective in the absence of teacher supervision, and little evidence exists to suggest that they facilitate generalization across settings.

The need to develop programs to enhance maintenance and generalization of teacher-administered interventions continues to be a critical area of need. At this time, it should be expected that specially arranged interventions for children with ADHD will be required across school settings and for extended periods of time over the course of their education, given the developmentally disabling nature of their disorder.

PEER INTERVENTIONS

Efforts to involve peers in modifying the disruptive and intrusive behavior of a child with ADHD have focused on strategies to discourage peers from reinforcing their classmate's inappropriate behavior and to encourage their attention to the classmate's positive, prosocial behavior instead. The strategies can vary considerably.

For example, group contingencies, discussed earlier, can indirectly motivate peers to encourage appropriate behavior and discourage misbehavior in their classmates. In another scenario, teachers can have peers assume roles as "behavior modifiers"; this involves their ignoring a classmate's disruptive, inappropriate behavior and praising or giving tokens for positive behavior, such as being a good sport, getting a high grade on an exam (or accepting a low grade without throwing a tantrum), contributing to a class discussion, or helping another student. To promote peers' use of reinforcement and ignoring, it is necessary that teachers reward their efforts as well—either with praise, with tangible rewards, or with tokens in a token economy. Serving as a peer monitor or dispenser of reinforcers appears to be a particularly powerful reward, and children will often purchase the privilege of distributing rewards with tokens they have earned. In similar fashion, peers can serve as social skills "tutors" in the natural environment by prompting and reinforcing the enactment of social behaviors that have been targeted in SST sessions. For example, Cunningham et al. (1998) have developed a student-mediated conflict resolution program that involves peers' acting as playground monitors. The use of this peer-mediated program was found to be associated with schoolwide reductions in playground violence and negative interactions.

This approach may be useful for several reasons. Because teachers are unable to observe every student's behavior continually, peers may be better able to monitor their classmates' behavior, and therefore may be better able to provide accurate, immediate, and consistent reinforcement. Also, training children to alter their interactions with peers not only improves peer behavior, but also directly improves the behavior of the children implementing the intervention. This would seem particularly beneficial for children with ADHD, who are at such a great risk for poor peer relations. Moreover, peer reinforcement systems may facilitate generalization, because peers may function as cues for appropriate behavior in multiple settings. In addition, peer-mediated programs may be more practical and require less time than traditional teacher-mediated programs.

Despite these advantages, several cautions are in order. A peer-mediated program is successful only to the extent that peers have the ability and motivation to learn and accurately implement the program. Peers may be overly lenient and reward too liberally, due to peer pressure, fear of peer rejection, or more lenient definitions of misbehavior. On the other hand, children may use the program in a coercive or punitive fashion. Also, recent evidence shows that involving peers by having them only correct negative behavior of students with ADHD (e.g., by using comments such as "You need

to be working") can exacerbate the problem (Northup et al., 1997), presumably due to the reinforcing value of peer attention. Because of these concerns, it is advisable that peers not be involved in implementing any punishment programs. In addition, when peers are utilized as change agents, they should be carefully trained and supervised, and contingencies should be provided for accurate ratings. (See Chapter 16 on peer mediation approaches to aggression.)

Peer tutoring represents the most recent advance in the utilization of peers as a part of the intervention process for children with ADHD. Peer tutoring focuses specifically on improving academic skills (a target that has been relatively unaffected by traditional contingency management programs), and it provides a learning environment well suited to the needs of students with ADHD (i.e., it involves immediate, frequent feedback, and active responding at a student's own pace) (DuPaul & Stoner, 2003). Classwide peer tutoring (CWPT) programs (Greenwood, Maheady, & Delquadri, 2002), tapping the "natural" resources of the classroom, have been developed; in these programs, each student is paired for tutoring with a classmate. Students are first trained in the rules and procedures for tutoring their peers in an academic area (e.g., math, spelling, reading). The student in each pair sit in adjacent, separate seats. The tutor reads a script of problems to the tutee and awards points to the tutee for correct responses. The tutor corrects incorrect responses, and the tutee can practice the correct response for an additional point. The script (problem list) is read as many times as possible for 10 minutes, and then the students switch roles, with the tutee becoming the tutor and the tutor becoming the tutee. During the tutoring periods, the teacher monitors the tutoring process and provides assistance if needed. Bonus points are awarded to pairs following all of the rules. At the end of the session, points are totaled, and those with the most points are z-declared the "winners." Studies have found CWPT to enhance the on-task behavior and academic performance of unmedicated students with ADHD in general education classrooms (DuPaul, Ervin, Hook, & McGoey, 1998; DuPaul & Henningson, 1993). Furthermore, the results of DuPaul et al. (1998) indicated that typically achieving students also showed improvements in attention and academic performance when participating in CWPT. Thus peer tutoring is an intervention that can be implemented to help *all* students; as such, it offers a practical and time-efficient strategy for meeting the needs of children with ADHD. Both teachers and students have rated peer tutoring favorably. Peer tutoring is probably most effective for students with ADHD when they are paired with well-behaved and conscientious classmates.

HOME-BASED CONTINGENCIES

Home-based contingency programs continue to be among the most commonly recommended interventions. Kelley (1990) has written a comprehensive book about school–home notes, which includes many examples and strategies for effective use. Briefly, these programs involve the provision of contingencies in the home, based on the teacher's report of the child's performance at school (see Chapter 12 for an example). The teacher's report, often referred to as a "report card," lists the target behavior(s) and a quantifiable rating for each behavior. Teacher reports should be sent home on a daily basis at first. As children's behavior improves, the daily reports may be faded to weekly, biweekly, monthly, and in some cases to the reporting intervals typically used in the school—although for many children with ADHD, report cards should be used throughout the year on a weekly basis.

The following points should be considered when teachers are tailoring report cards for students:

1. *Select important target behaviors.* In-class behavior (sharing, playing well with peers, following rules) and academic performance (completing math or reading assignments) may be targeted, along with homework—a common problem for students with ADHD, who often have difficulty remembering to bring home assignments, completing the work, and then returning the completed work to school the next day. We recommend including at least one or two positive behaviors that a child is currently reliably displaying, so that the child will be able to earn some points during the beginning of the program.

2. *The number of target behaviors may vary from as few as one to as many as seven or eight.* Targeting very few behaviors is suggested when a program is first being implemented (to maximize the child's likelihood of success), when

few behaviors require modification, or in cases where teachers have difficulty monitoring many behaviors.

3. *The daily ratings of each target behavior should be quantifiable.* Ratings may be descriptive (e.g., "poor," "fair," "good"), with each descriptor being clearly defined (e.g., "poor" = more than three rule violations). Or they may be more specific and objective, such as frequency counts of each behavior (e.g., "interrupted fewer than three times") or the number of points earned or lost for each behavior.

4. *Children should be monitored and given feedback during each period, subject, or class throughout the school day.* In this way, students' difficulties early on can be modified later in the day. School–home note cards that try to summarize the entire day in a single rating, such as with "Smileygrams" (a single smiley face for an entire day), should be avoided in favor of frequent evaluations across the day. For early success with particularly high-rate problem behaviors, children may initially be rated for only a portion of the day (say, 1 hour). As behavior improves, ratings may gradually include more periods/subjects until the child is being monitored throughout the day. In cases where children attend several different classes taught by different teachers, programs may involve some or all of the teachers, depending upon the need for intervention in each of the classes. When more than one teacher is included in the program, a single report card may include space for all teachers to sign, or different report cards may be used for each class and organized in a notebook for a child to carry between classes.

5. *The success of the program requires a clear, consistent system for translating teacher reports into consequences at home.* The student may take a new card to school each day, or the cards can be kept at school and given to the student each morning, depending upon the parents' reliability in giving the card out each day. Upon the child's return home, a parent immediately inspects the card and discusses the positive ratings first with the child. The parent may ask about any negative ratings, but the discussion should be very brief, neutral, and businesslike (not angry!). The child is then asked to formulate a plan for how to continue earning positive marks and avoid getting negative marks the next day (parents are to remind the child of this plan the next morning before the child departs for school). The parent then

provides the child with a reward dependent upon his or her earnings. Some programs involve rewards alone; others incorporate both positive and negative consequences. However, in cases where parents tend to be overly coercive or abusive, reward-only programs are preferable. At a minimum, praise and positive attention should be provided whenever a child's goals are met; however, tangible rewards or token programs are usually necessary. For example, a positive note home may translate into TV time, a special snack, or a later bedtime, or into points as part of a token economy. Both daily rewards (e.g., time with parent, special dessert, TV time) and weekly rewards (e.g., movie, dinner at a restaurant, special outing) are recommended, although parents should understand that the use of daily rewards will be more important for motivating children with ADHD. Parents should be strongly encouraged to use rewards that are basic privileges and ac-

tivities that the child enjoys—not elaborate or expensive items.

6. *Parents should be involved in planning the daily report card system from the outset, to ensure their understanding of and cooperation with the procedures.* Older children and adolescents should be included in planning the program for the same reasons. Furthermore, goals and procedures should be modified on an ongoing basis in accordance with student progress or lack thereof. Stated differently, as the child shows progress, daily/weekly goals are changed to encourage further growth.

The following are several types of home-based reward programs that rely on daily school behavior ratings. A card for one example of such a program is shown in Figure 15.1. This card contains four areas of potentially problematic behavior for a child with ADHD. Columns are provided for up to six differ-

Classroom Challenge

Name: _____   Date: _____

Please rate child in areas below according to this scale:

2 = Very good

1 = OK

0 = Needs improvement

Class period/subject

TARGET BEHAVIOR	1	2	3	4	5	6
Participation						
Classwork						
Handed in homework						
Interaction with peers						
Teacher's initials						

Total points earned: _____

Homework for tonight (list class period by assignment):

Comments:

FIGURE 15.1. A card for a home-based reward program targeting classroom behavior.

ent teachers to rate the child in these areas of behavior, or for one teacher to rate the child multiple times across the school day. The teacher initials the bottom of the column after rating the child's performance during that class period and checking for the accuracy of the copied homework, to ensure against forgery. For a particularly negative rating, we also encourage a teacher to provide a brief explanation to the parent as to what resulted in that negative mark. The teacher rates the child using a 3-point system. The parent then awards the child points for each rating on the card (0 = no points, 1 = 1 point, 2 = 2 points). The child may spend these points on activities from a home reward menu.

A similar card system may be used when a child is having problems with peers during school recess or lunch periods. This card, shown in Figure 15.2, can be completed by the recess or lunch monitor during each recess/lunch period, inspected by the class teacher when the child returns to the classroom, and then sent home for use in a home point system as described above. The class teacher can also instruct the child to use a "think aloud, think ahead" procedure just prior to the child's leaving the class for recess or lunch. In this procedure, the teacher reviews the rules for proper recess/lunch behavior with the child, notes their existence on the card, and directs the child to give the card immediately to the recess/lunch monitor.

Overall, homebased reward programs can be an effective adjunct to classroombased programs for children with ADHD:

- They offer more frequent feedback than is usually provided at school.
- They afford parents more frequent feedback regarding their child's performance than would usually be provided, and they can prompt parents when to reinforce a child's behavior (as well as when behavior is becoming problematic and requires more intensive intervention).
- The type and quality of reinforcers available in the home are typically far more extensive than those available in the classroom (a factor that may be critical for children with ADHD, as reviewed earlier).
- Virtually any child behavior can be targeted for intervention with these programs.
- School–home note programs can require somewhat less teacher time and effort than a classroom-based intervention, and may be particularly popular with teachers who are concerned that use of classroom rewards for only some students is unfair.

Recess/Lunch Challenge

Name: _____   Date: _____

Please rate this child in the following areas during recess and lunch. Use a rating of 1 = excellent, 2 = good, 3 = fair, 4 = poor.

	Recess or lunch			
	1	2	3	4
Keeps hands and feet to self—doesn't fight, push, kick, wrongly touch, or take other's belongings				
Follows rules				
Tries to get along well with others				
Recess/lunch monitor's initials				

Total points earned:

Comments:

FIGURE 15.2. A card for a home-based reward program targeting recess/lunch behavior.

However, as pointed out by Abramowitz and O'Leary (1991), effective implementation of daily report cards is not a simple procedure. All of the behavioral skills needed for developing and implementing classroom contingency programs are also needed for use of report cards; in addition, teachers need to work effectively with parents. Both teachers and parents need to understand basic behavior modification, how to select and rotate rewards, and the need for consistency (teachers need to implement the program every day, and parents need to provide rewards exactly as specified). In addition, plans should be established for handling cases where children attempt to subvert the system by failing to bring home a report, forging a teacher's signature, or failing to get certain teachers' signatures. To discourage this practice, missing notes or signatures should be treated the same way as a "bad" report (i.e., child fails to earn points or is fined privileges or points). In cases where parents may be overly punitive or lack skills to follow through with consequences, their implementation of appropriate consequences should be closely supervised (possibly by a therapist), or other adults (e.g., school counselors, principal) may implement the program.

SELF-MANAGEMENT INTERVENTIONS

Self management interventions, which include self-monitoring, self-reinforcement, and more comprehensive self-instruction and problem-solving approaches, were originally developed in order to directly treat the impulsive, disorganized, and nonreflective manner in which children with ADHD approach academic tasks and social interactions. With their emphasis on the development of self-control, it was thought that these interventions would reduce the need for extrinsic rewards and would result in better maintenance and generalization of gains made by children with ADHD than are achieved with contingency management programs. Unfortunately, these programs have fallen short of these initial expectations. However, self-monitoring and self-reinforcement strategies have had some success for students with ADHD. These approaches involve children's monitoring and evaluating their own academic and social behavior, and rewarding themselves (often with tokens or points) based on those evaluations. Training typically involves teaching chil-

dren how to observe and record their own behavior, and how to evaluate their behavior to determine whether they deserve a reward. Children may be prompted to observe their own behavior by a periodic auditory signal (tone) or visual cue (teacher's hand gesture) and trained to record instances of appropriate behavior. Accuracy of child ratings is usually assessed by comparing these ratings against the teacher's records.

Several applications of self-management interventions are now described. Barkley, Copeland, and Sivage (1980) taught hyperactive children ages 7–10 to monitor their behavior during individual seatwork. If children had been following the rules when a tone sounded, they recorded a checkmark on an index card kept at their desk. Initially, the tone sounded on a variable 1-minute schedule, but this was faded to a variable-interval 5-minute schedule. Accurate reports, defined as matching an observer's report, were rewarded with tokens that could be exchanged for privileges. With this procedure, on-task behavior improved during individual seatwork, particularly for older children, but the improvements made during individual seatwork did not generalize to the regular classroom. Thus the effectiveness of self-monitoring and self-reinforcement seemed to be limited to the context in which they were taught and where contingencies were in effect for their use. More recently, Edwards et al. (1995) implemented a similar self-monitoring procedure for students with ADHD, and also found improved on-task behavior and reading comprehension among the students.

Hinshaw, Henker, and Whalen (1984) extended the use of self-monitoring and self-reinforcement to children's peer interactions in a training program called "Match Game," designed to teach children to self-evaluate and self-reward their cooperative interactions with peers. In this procedure, trainers first taught children behavioral criteria for a range of ratings by modeling various behaviors (e.g., paying attention, doing work, cooperative behavior) and assigning each behavior from 1 to 5 points (1 = "pretty bad," 5 = "great!"). Thereafter, children participated in role plays followed by naturalistic playground games, in which trainers rated each child's behavior on the 1–5 scale and instructed children to monitor and rate their own behavior on the same scale. Children were encouraged to try to match the trainers' ratings. Initially, children were given extra points for accurate self-evaluations, regardless of the actual point value. However, once children learned the procedure, they were rewarded only when their behavior was desirable *and* matched the trainers' ratings. Results of this study revealed that reinforced self-evaluation was more effective than externally administered reinforcement in reducing negative and increasing cooperative peer contacts on the playground.

The combination of self-monitoring and self-reinforcement has also been used with success to maintain gains from a token economy with secondary-level students, for whom contingency management procedures are often not viewed favorably by either teachers or the students themselves (DuPaul & Stoner, 2003). Students are trained in evaluating their own behavior on a 6-point set of criteria ("unacceptable" to "excellent") after they have achieved success in a standard teacher-administered token economy. They earn points for positive teacher ratings and bonus points if their ratings match the teacher's ratings. Over time, teacher ratings are gradually faded to random matching checks for accuracy; students earn points for their own ratings. The "matching challenges" are increased if students' ratings become inaccurate. Although teacher involvement can be faded quite a bit with this procedure, the continued checking of student ratings and backup reinforcers appear to be important in sustaining improvement.

Hoff and DuPaul (1998) conducted a controlled case study of a contingency-based self-management program for three children exhibiting significant ADHD-related behaviors in general education classrooms. These children participated in several treatment phases, beginning with a teacher-managed token reinforcement program and proceeding through successive stages of self-evaluation and self-reinforcement (i.e., a modification of procedures first reported by Rhode, Morgan, & Young, 1983). Prior to the first stage of self-management, each student was trained by the teacher to recognize target behaviors associated with ratings from 0 ("broke one or more rules entire interval") to 5 ("followed classroom rules entire interval"). These behaviors were modeled for the children, and the latter also role-played target behaviors while stating the rating associated with each behavior. During the first stage of self-management, each student and the teacher independently rated the student's performance during one academic period. After ratings were compared, (1) if the student's rating was within 1 point of the teacher's, the student kept the points he gave himself; (2) if the student's rating matched the teacher's exactly, he received the points he gave himself plus 1 bonus point; and (3) if the student's and teacher's ratings deviated by more than 1 point, then no points were awarded. As in the token reinforcement phase, points were exchanged for preferred activities on a daily basis.

During successive stages of the treatment, the frequency of teacher–student matches was gradually reduced to 0%. For example, during the 50% match stage, a coin was flipped following each rating period, wherein the student was required to match the teacher an average of 50% of the time. Given that the outcome was random and unpredictable, the student could not assume prior to the coin flip that he didn't have to match the teacher's rating. On the occasions when he didn't have to match, the student automatically kept the points he gave himself. Generalization across school settings was programmed for and systematically evaluated. All three students were able to maintain behavioral improvements initially elicited under token reinforcement, despite the fading of teacher feedback. It is important to note that at the end of the study, the students still continued to provide written ratings of their performance and continued to receive backup contingencies. The ideal outcome would be for written ratings to be faded to oral ratings while backup contingencies are phased out.

Several studies have incorporated goal setting in addition to the self-monitoring and self-reinforcement strategies. In one study, six students were invited to participate in a tutoring class as "employees" and follow weekly employment contracts (Ajibola & Clement, 1995). Students set goals for the number of reading problems they would complete, and signed a performance contract to this effect. Thereafter, they would give themselves 1 point on a wrist counter each time they answered a reading question. At the end of tutoring class each day, students received stamps based on the points earned. Stamps were later exchanged for backup reinforcers. Self-reinforcement resulted in significant improvement in academic performance, compared to noncontingent reinforcement; it also appeared to add to the benefits of a low dose of stimulant medication. In a variant of this approach, called "correspondence training," students are trained to match their verbal behavior (promises to inhibit hyperactive behavior and conduct problems) with their later nonverbal actions. In a simulated classroom, students were reinforced with small toys when their promise to inhibit a behavior was associated with their actual inhibition of that behavior over a 10-minute period. Preliminary results showed a positive impact on child behavior (Paniagua & Black, 1992).

Barry and Messer (2003) evaluated another self-management program with five sixth-grade students having ADHD. Students set goals for their behavior and academic work, and then monitored them at 15-minute intervals during a 2-hour period of the school day. Students earned rewards for accurate self-assessment and for achieving daily goals. The intervention resulted in increases in on-task behaviors and academic performance, as well as a decrease in disruptive behavior. The authors note that the intervention took approximately 20 minutes initially with each student to go over the program, and then several additional minutes each day for checking accuracy and providing feedback about their self-assessments. Codding and Lewandowski (2003) also report benefit from a variant of the self-management approach, called "performance feedback with goal setting." In this program, students set specific goals using visual displays (graphs), evaluate the accuracy of their work, receive teacher feedback, and graph their progress. This approach was reported to result in an increase in math fluency for seven students with ADHD.

Self-management may be a particularly viable intervention for adolescents with ADHD, especially when organizational skills are a concern. For example, Gureasko-Moore, DuPaul, and White (in press) evaluated the use of a self-monitoring strategy for three seventh-grade students with ADHD. All of these participants were reported by their teachers to have significant problems with being prepared and organized for class (e.g., coming to class with correct textbook, pencils, and notebook). A checklist of preparatory behaviors was constructed for each student by his teacher. This checklist was used to determine the percentage of preparatory steps completed across experimental phases in the context of a multiple baseline across participants design. Following a baseline phase, a school psychologist provided brief training in self-monitoring to each partici-

pant. All three students showed substantial gains in the percentage of steps completed as a function of self-monitoring. In fact, several weeks later, students were observed to complete nearly 100% of required preparatory behaviors on a consistent basis, even without external prompting and reinforcement. These results were replicated and extended to include enhancement of homework completion for six middle school students with ADHD (Gureasko-Moore, DuPaul, & White, 2005).

A classwide application of self-management with a group contingency and a peer monitoring component has recently been used to decrease inappropriate verbalizations in a group of four third-grade students with ADHD (Davies & Witte, 2000). All students in the classroom were divided into groups and trained to monitor inappropriate verbalizations in their group. When an inappropriate verbalization occurred by any student, children were instructed to move one of five black dots from the green section to the blue section (or from the blue to the red section) on a chart divided into green, blue, and red sections. The group's goal was met if at least one dot was left in the green section. If children did not move the dot within 10 seconds, the teacher automatically moved the dot to the red section. Children also monitored their own verbalizations with their own tallies. During group meetings, the students discussed what they did well and what they could do better, and the entire class earned reinforcers when all students met the set criterion level. This intervention encouraged students to work together without the children with ADHD being singled out, and it seemed to help all students. Teacher monitoring, however, continued to be necessary for accurate reporting.

Many cognitive training programs or forms of cognitive-behavioral therapy (CBT) involve teaching children self-instructional and problem-solving strategies, in addition to self-monitoring and self-reinforcement (Meichenbaum & Goodman, 1971). The prototypic program involves teaching children a set of self-directed instructions to follow when performing a task. These instructions include defining and understanding the task or problem, planning a general strategy to approach the problem, focusing attention on the task, selecting an answer or solution, and evaluating performance. In the case of a successful performance, self-reinforcement (usually in the form of a positive self-statement, such as "I really did a good job") is provided. In the case of an unsuccessful performance, a coping statement is made (e.g., "Next time I'll do better if I slow down"), and errors are corrected. At first, an adult trainer typically models the self-instructions while performing a task. The child then performs the same task while the trainer provides the self-instructions. Next, the child performs the task while self-instructing aloud. These overt verbalizations are then faded to covert self-instructions. Reinforcement (e.g., praise, tokens, toys) is typically provided to the child for following the procedure, as well as for selecting correct solutions.

The provision of such forms of CBT was previously felt to hold some promise for children with ADHD (Douglas, 1980; Kendall & Braswell, 1985; Meichenbaum & Goodman, 1971). A few small-scale studies suggested some benefits for this form of treatment with such children (Fehlings, Roberts, Humphries, & Dawe, 1991). But CBT has been challenged as being seriously flawed from the conceptual (Vygotskian) point of view on which the treatment was initially founded (Diaz & Berk, 1995). Whether or not the self-statements of children with ADHD during task performance are actually deficient and in need of such correction is also open to question. And its efficacy for impulsive children or those with ADHD has been repeatedly questioned by the rather poor or limited results of empirical research (Abikoff, 1985, 1987; Abikoff & Gittelman, 1985).

Reviews of the CBT literature using meta-analyses have typically found the effect sizes to be only about a third of a standard deviation, and even less than this in many studies (Baer & Nietzel, 1991; DuPaul & Eckert, 1997; Dush, Hirt, & Schroeder, 1989). Although such treatment effects may at times rise to the level of statistical significance, they are nonetheless of only modest clinical importance and usually are to be found mainly on relatively circumscribed lab measures (Brown et al., 1986) rather than more clinically important measures of functioning in natural settings.

A large-scale, well-controlled study of CBT conducted in the Minneapolis public school system found no effect on children with ADHD. The study involved substantial training of parents, teachers, and children, and 2 years of this multicomponent intervention. But the researchers found no significant treatment effects on any of a variety of dependent measures at 1-year assessment with the exception of class observations of off-task/disruptive behavior, and no effects after 2 years of treatment (Bloomquist, August, & Ostrander, 1991; Braswell et al., 1997). Even the treatment effect on class observations was not maintained at follow-up. Therefore, given the extant research findings of limited effect sizes in most clinical studies and the absence of treatment effects in the largest study, this treatment is not recommended for ADHD. When improvement does occur, it is when external or self-reinforcement is provided for accurate and positive self-evaluations in conjunction with self-instructional training. In fact, when programs are effective, this may be more a result of reinforcement than of self-instructions.

In sum, self-monitoring and self-reinforcement strategies are the most promising of the self-management interventions, although the effects of these interventions for changing behavioral problems are not as strong, as durable, or as generalizable as was once expected and are not superior to those of traditional behavioral programs. DuPaul and Eckert (1997) report much stronger effects for contingency management and academic interventions than problem-solving training or other forms of CBT. Complete transfer of management of the program from teacher to student is unrealistic; continued teacher monitoring of the ratings is necessary to ensure honest reporting. Most gains are achieved from self-management programs when the training is of sufficient duration and when there is overlap between the skills taught during training and the requirements of the classroom or playground. Training is required in all settings in which self-control is desired, both for children and for the adult supervisors (e.g., teacher, recess monitors), and adults need to encourage children's application of the skills in day-to-day activities in each setting.

Self-management programs are best used in conjunction with teacher-administered consequences such as a token economy. In this context, self-management programs for academic and behavioral goals are relatively simple to implement, may further motivate children's participation, and may facilitate partial fading of token programs. Also, there may be some value in using self-management, particularly with older students, since these procedures may be more acceptable to teachers than token programs and therefore more likely to be used consistently (DuPaul & Stoner, 2003). In any case, children must be adequately reinforced for displaying self-management skills in order to maintain this type of behavior; the training alone is insufficient.

SOCIAL SKILLS TRAINING

SST may be conducted in either school settings or clinical settings. Given that SST has not been discussed previously in this volume, we take this opportunity to mention it here. Early reviews of SST as applied specifically to children with ADHD were quite discouraging (Hinshaw, 1992; Hinshaw & Erhardt, 1991; Whalen & Henker, 1991). Children with ADHD certainly have serious difficulties in their social interactions with peers (Bagwell, Molina, Pelham, & Hoza, 2001; Cunningham & Siegel, 1987; Erhardt & Hinshaw, 1994; Hubbard & Newcomb, 1991; Whalen & Henker, 1992). This seems to be especially so for that subgroup having significant levels of comorbid aggression (Hinshaw, 1992; Erhardt & Hinshaw, 1994), in which more than 50% of the variance in peer ratings of children whom they disliked was predicted by this behavior alone. As Hinshaw (1992) has summarized, however, the social interaction problems of children with ADHD are quite heterogeneous and are not likely to respond to a treatment package that focuses only on social approach strategies and that treats all children with ADHD as if they shared common problems in their peer relationship difficulties. Nor is it especially clear at this time what the actual sources of these peer difficulties are or by which mechanisms they operate, with the exception of aggressive behavior as noted above.. For instance, some children with ADHD may lack the knowledge of proper social skills; others may know how to act with their peers, but do not do so at the points of performance in social interactions where such skills would be useful to have performed. The theoretical model presented earlier would suggest that the latter is likely to be more of a problem than the former, at least for children having ADHD without significant aggression. Teaching them additional skills is not so much the issue as is assisting them in performing the skills they have *when* it would be useful to do so *at the point of performance*, where such skills are most likely to prove useful to the long-term social acceptance of the individual. Some investigators (e.g., Wheeler & Carlson, 1994) have suggested that the extent to which actual skill deficits are present may vary by ADHD subtype, with those children having ADHD-PI being more likely to be affected by skill deficits than those with ADHD-C.

Those children with ADHD and comorbid aggression may well have additional problems with peer perceptions—particularly in regard to the motives they attribute to others for their behavior, as well as in information processing about social interactions (Milich & Dodge, 1984). This combination of perceptual/information-processing deficits with problems performing appropriate social skills in social interactions with others may make children with ADHD and aggression particularly resistant to SST (Hinshaw, 1992).

Actual research on SST for ADHD and disruptive behavior problems has produced rather mixed results. Early studies suggested some benefit for children with aggression and conduct problems (see Hinshaw, 1992), although for ADHD, the effects of SST were not as powerful as those of other behavioral interventions (e.g., Pelham & Bender, 1982). An early meta-analysis of studies of social competence training showed that at-risk groups of children responded better (larger effect sizes) to such programs than did children with externalizing or disruptive behavioral problems (Beelmann, Pfingsten, & Losel, 1994). Frankel, Myatt, and Cantwell (1995) subsequently examined an SST program for outpatient children with peer relationship problems, most of whom met the criteria for ADHD and half met the criteria for ODD. Nearly 50% of the children in the treated and waiting-list control groups were receiving medication. Treatment assignment was not random, but associated with various factors (date of intake, class starting date, class space available). Mothers' ratings showed improved social skills in the treated compared to the waiting-list control children; teachers' ratings revealed decreased aggression and withdrawal in the treated group, but only among those who did not have ODD. A later study by this same research team (Frankel, Myatt, Cantwell, & Feinberg, 1997) provided SST to children already receiving medication. Children with ADHD ($n = 35$) were compared to a waiting-list control group ($n = 12$) of children with ADHD who were also receiving medication. Parents were trained in strategies to help with generalization to the home setting. Significant benefits on both parent and teacher ratings were found in the treated compared to the waiting-list control children, and the presence of ODD had no moderating effects, as it had in the earlier report.

A study of young children (ages 4–8 years) having either ODD or CD, some of whom had ADHD (Webster-Stratton, Reid, & Hammond, 2001), showed positive benefits of an SST and problem-solving training program on conduct problem behavior; these benefits were found both on teacher ratings and on home behavioral observations, but not on parent ratings of conduct problems (which showed improvement for both the intervention and control groups). Treatment effects remained at a 1-year follow-up. Likewise, Pfiffner and McBurnett (1997) found evidence for the efficacy of an SST program for children with ADHD, but mostly on parent ratings and not teacher ratings. Children were randomly assigned to receive SST alone, SST supplemented with parent training in generalization strategies, or a waiting-list control group. Both groups receiving SST improved in parent-rated social behavior and children's skill knowledge relative to control children, with improvements being maintained at a 4-month follow-up. But there was less evidence that these benefits generalized to the school setting, since between-group differences were not found at posttreatment. However, within-group analyses showed significant pre-to-post improvement on teacher ratings for families receiving generalization training, but not for families receiving SST alone. The addition of parent training in generalization strategies did not result in any additional benefits over SST alone, although parents in the latter group did receive written materials about the skills taught and strategies to promote the skills at home each week.

A more recent study using a clinic-referred sample of 120 children having ADHD who were all being treated with medication found significant improvement with SST on parent and child self-report measures of assertiveness, especially for the group of children with ADHD-PI (Antshel & Remer, 2003). However, parent and child reports of cooperation, responsibility, and self-control did not show treatment effects, and those with comorbid ODD did not benefit as much as those without comorbid ODD. In addition, while there was

evidence that heterogeneous groups were beneficial on some measures, 15% of parents of children having ADHD-PI who were in groups with children of both ADHD subtypes rated their children as socially worse at the end of treatment. Although it is not clear why this change in parent perception occurred (e.g., perhaps parents became more aware of their children's social problems), it could represent evidence of peer deviancy training. That is, there may have been peer reinforcement of aggressive and antisocial behavior among the children in the group, so that children increased their levels of aggressive behavior as a result of group participation. Earlier studies did not examine this possibility of a detrimental impact of group SST for some children. Such an adverse impact is certainly worthy of further examination in future research with children having ADHD.

All of these studies indicate some benefits of SST for children with conduct problems, including those with ADHD, particularly when parent ratings serve as the outcome measure. Yet important limitations in their methods are present. Two of these studies did not employ randomized assignment to treated or untreated groups (the Frankel et al. studies), and parents were aware of the intervention being received (all studies). Effects on teacher ratings of school social behavior also are not as encouraging as results from parent ratings, but imply that some children in some studies may have demonstrated reduced social withdrawal and possibly aggression in school. Treatment effects on peer sociometrics and direct observation in naturalistic settings are seldom evaluated, and when they are, the results of SST appear more sobering (e.g., Sheridan, Dee, Morgan, McCormack, & Walker, 1996). All of the studies used waiting-list control groups for their comparisons, making it difficult to discern the ingredients underlying treatment success (e.g., therapist attention, skills training, contingency management) or to determine the effects of SST relative to other treatments.

At this time, SST for children with ADHD shows promise; however, it cannot be considered a sole treatment for the social impairment associated with ADHD, and the benefit of adding SST to other treatments is not entirely clear. This reflects the somewhat inconsistent nature of the results; the limited number of studies using randomized assignment to treatment groups; parents' and teachers' awareness of treatment conditions; the absence of attention placebo or alternative treatment groups; the limited evidence of generalization to the school setting; and the fact that studies to date have mainly involved efficacy rather than effectiveness in actual clinical contexts. It is also worth noting that SST may involve some risk of accelerating antisocial behavior, or deviancy training, when delinquent youth are placed together in groups (Dishion, McCord, & Poulin, 1999). In addition, intensive environmental support at the point of performance (e.g., school, playground, home) appears to be required for optimal outcome. This level of intensity is often difficult or impractical to implement. Nevertheless, SST can have therapeutic value when this type of generalization intervention is provided and when it is tailored to specific social needs. Given the importance of social ineptitude for long-term adjustment, continued development of interventions to improve this area for youth with ADHD should be a priority. For example, programs focused on building dyadic friendships (e.g., Frankel & Myatt, 2003; Hoza, Mrug, Pelham, Greiner, & Gnagy, 2003) may prove to be more useful than programs focused on improving general social skills. Likewise, student-mediated conflict resolution programs such as the one developed by Cunningham et al. (1998; see also Chapter 16) may help in reducing the interpersonal conflict experienced by youth with ADHD.

MANAGING ACADEMIC PROBLEMS WITH ADOLESCENTS WITH ADHD

All of the recommendations described to this point apply as much to adolescents with ADHD as to children. However, implementing these recommendations becomes considerably more difficult, for several reasons: the increased number of teachers involved in middle and high school; the short duration of the class periods; the greater emphasis on individual self-control, organization, and responsibility for completing assignments; and the frequent changes that occur in class schedules across any given week. All of this is likely to result in a dramatic drop in educational performance in many children with ADHD after the elementary grades, as there is little or no accountability of teachers or students at higher levels of education until the students' behavioral offenses become sufficiently heinous to attract attention

or the academic deficiencies become grossly apparent. It is very easy for the average adolescent with ADHD to "fall through the cracks" at this stage of education unless he or she has been involved with the special educational system in elementary school. Those who have will have been "flagged" as in need of continuing special attention. But most adolescents with ADHD will not be in special education, and so are likely to be viewed merely as lazy and irresponsible. It is at this age level that educational performance becomes the most common reason adolescents with ADHD are referred for clinical services (see Chapter 4).

Dealing with large educational institutions at the middle and secondary levels can be frustrating for parents, clinicians, and teenagers with ADHD alike. Even the most interested teacher may have difficulties mustering sufficient motivation among his or her colleagues to help an adolescent with ADHD in trouble at school. Below, we have listed a number of steps that can be attempted to manage poor educational performance and behavioral adjustment problems in middle and high school. To the degree that other methods described above can also be implemented, so much the better.

1. The clinician should immediately initiate an Individuals with Disabilities Education Act (IDEA) or Section 504 evaluation of the adolescent if one has not been done before or has not been done within the past 3 years (federal law requires a reevaluation every 3 years a child is in special education). Special educational services will not be forthcoming until this evaluation is completed, and this can take up to 90 days or longer in some districts. The sooner it is initiated, the better.

2. Adolescents with ADHD invariably require counseling on the nature of their condition. Although many have certainly been previously told by parents and others that they are "hyperactive" or have ADHD, many of them still have not come to accept that they actually have a disability. In our opinion, this counseling is not intended to depress the adolescents over what they cannot do, but to help them accept that they have certain limitations and find ways to prevent their disability from creating significant problems for them. Such counseling is difficult, requiring sensitivity to the adolescents' striving to be independent and to form their own opinions of themselves and their world. It often takes more than a single session

to succeed in this endeavor, but patience and persistence can pay off. Our approach is to stress the concept of individual differences: Everyone has a unique profile of both strengths and weaknesses in mental and physical abilities, and each of us must adjust to them. We often confide about our own liabilities and use humor to get the adolescents to see that they are not the only ones who have weaknesses. It is how we all accept and cope with our weaknesses that can determine how much we all limit our successes in life. And yet we have personally sat at many school meetings where parents, teachers, school psychologists, and private tutors all had gathered to offer assistance to teenagers with ADHD only to have the teens refuse the offers while promising that they could turn things around on their own. Until adolescents with ADHD accept the nature of their disorder, they are unlikely to fully accept the help that may be offered them.

3. If an adolescent has been on medication previously and responded successfully, he or she should be counseled on the advantages of returning to the medication as a means of both improving his or her school performance and obtaining those special privileges at home that may be granted as a result of such improved performance. See Chapter 14 (this volume) for an example of such counseling with a teenager about medication. Many adolescents are concerned about others' learning that they are on medication. They can be reassured that only they, their parents, and the physician are aware of this, and that no one at school need know unless the teenagers themselves reveal it. Clinicians should be prepared in many cases, however, for the adolescents with ADHD to want to "go it alone" without the medication, believing that with extra applied effort they can correct the problem.

4. It is often essential to schedule a team meeting at the beginning of each academic year (and more often as needed) at a teen's school, at which the teachers, school psychologist, guidance counselor, principal, parents, *and the adolescent with ADHD* are to be present. The clinician should bring a handout describing ADHD to give to each participant. The clinician should briefly review the nature of the adolescent's disorder and the need for close teamwork among the school, parents, and teen if the teen's academic performance is to be improved. Each teacher should describe the current strengths and problems of the teen in their classes and make suggestions as to how they think they can help with the problem (e.g., being available after school a few days each week for extra assistance; reducing the length of written homework assignments; allowing the teen to provide oral means of demonstrating that knowledge has been acquired, rather than relying on just written, timed test grades; developing a subtle cueing system to alert the teen when he or she is not paying attention in class, without drawing the whole class's attention to the fact; etc.). At this conference, the teen should be asked to make a public commitment as to what he or she is going to strive to do to make school performance better. Once plans are made, the team should agree to meet again in 1 month to evaluate the success of the plans and troubleshoot any problem areas. Future meetings may need to be scheduled, depending upon the success of the program to date. At the least, meetings twice a year are to be encouraged even when a program is successful, so as to monitor its progress and keep the school attentive to the needs of this teen. The adolescent always attends these meetings.

5. The clinician should introduce a daily home–school report card as described above. These are often critical for teens more than any other age group, because they permit a teen and parents to have daily feedback on how well the teen is performing in each class. The back of the card can be used to record daily homework assignments, which are verified by each teacher before completing the ratings on the card and initialing the front of the card. In conjunction with this, a home point system should be set up that includes a variety of desired privileges the teen can purchase with the points earned at school. Such things as cell phone use, use of the family car, time out of the home with friends, extra money, clothes, CDs or DVDs, computer time, special snacks kept in the house, and so forth. can be placed on the program. Points can also be set aside in a savings book to work toward longer-term rewards. However, the daily, short-term, accessible privileges and not these longer-term rewards are what give the program its motivational power. Thus the reward menu should not be overweighted with too many longterm rewards. Once the adolescent is able to go for 3 weeks or so without receiving negative ratings on the card, then the card is faded to a once- or twice-per-week schedule of completion. After a month of satisfactory ratings, the card can ei-

ther be faded out or reduced to a monthly rating. The adolescent is then told that if word is received that grades are slipping, the card system will have to be reinstated.

6. Ideally, the school will provide a second set of books to the family (even if a small deposit is required to do so), so that homework can still be accomplished even if the teen forgets a book required for homework.

7. One of the teen's classroom teachers, the homeroom teacher, the school guidance counselor, or even a learning disabilities teacher should serve as the teen's "coach," "mentor," or "case manager." This person's role is to meet briefly with the teen three times a day for just a few minutes to help keep the teen organized. The teen can stop at this person's classroom or office at the start of school, at which time the manager checks to see that the teen has all the homework and books needed for the morning's classes. At lunch, the teen stops by again, again the manager checks whether the teen has copied all necessary assignments from the morning classes, helps the teen select the books needed for the afternoon classes, and then checks that the teen has the assignments to be turned in that day for these afternoon classes. At the end of school, the teen stops by once again, and the manager checks to see that the teen has all assignments and books needed to go home for homework. Each visit takes no more than 3–5 minutes, but interspersed as they are throughout the school day, these visits can be of great assistance in organizing the teen's schoolwork. Evans, Dowling, and Brown (in press) have developed a program (see discussion below) to provide ongoing coaching, monitoring, and feedback to middle school students with ADHD.

8. Getting a private tutor for the teen may be beneficial. Many parents find it difficult to do homework with a teen or to provide tutoring in areas of academic weakness. The teen often resists these efforts as well, and the tension or arguments that can arise may spill over into other areas of family functioning even after the homework period has passed. When this is the case and the family can afford it, hiring a tutor to work with the teen even twice a week can be of considerable benefit in both improving the teen's academic weakness and "decompressing" the tension and hostility that arise around homework in the family.

9. Parents should set up a special time each week to do something alone with their teen that is mutually pleasurable, so as to provide opportunities for parent–teen interactions that are not task-oriented, school-related, and fraught with the tensions that work-oriented activities can often create with teens who have ADHD. This can often contribute to keeping parent–teen relations positive and counterbalance the conflicts that school performance demands frequently create in such families.

EDUCATIONAL PLACEMENT AND MODEL PROGRAMS

Educational Placement

Most children with ADHD continue to be placed in mainstream or general education classroom settings, despite the increased accessibility to special education. For those with mild to moderate ADHD, accommodations to the general education classroom (sometimes coupled with pharmacological treatment) are sufficient; there is no need for formalized special services. There are many advantages for maintaining students in general education, including reduced social stigma and interaction with appropriate peer models. However, for teens with more severe cases of ADHD or those with accompanying problems of opposition, aggression, or learning disabilities, alternative placements should be explored. Students with ADHD and concomitant severe emotional problems or learning disabilities are likely to receive special assistance through placement in a resource program for a part of the day or in a full-day self-contained classroom. Children with ADHD and significant speech and language or motor development problems are likely to receive language interventions, occupational and physical therapy, and adaptive physical education, provided that these developmental problems are sufficient to interfere with academic performance.

The need for special education for ADHD per se has been debated over the past decade. Although ADHD is now recognized as a potentially disabling condition, it is important to know that a diagnosis of ADHD does not automatically entitle a student to special services, through either general education or special education. The educational guidelines for ADHD state that significant impairment in school performance in conjunction with a diagnosis of ADHD are necessary to qualify for special services. In the case of suspected ADHD, a number of accommodations are usually attempted in the general education classroom prior to referral for a formal evaluation. If prereferral accommodations are unsuccessful, systematic screening procedures are implemented to determine the need for specialized interventions. Currently there are two mechanisms for obtaining these services. One is through Section 504 of the Rehabilitation Act of 1973, a civil rights law prohibiting discrimination against anyone with a disability. Under Section 504, individuals who have a physical or mental impairment that substantially limits their school functioning are eligible for special accommodations. Usually these services include a number of accommodations to the general education classroom, such as using behavior management techniques, modifying homework and test delivery, using tape recorders, and/or simplifying lesson instructions. Because federal funds are not attached to Section 504, classroom adaptations may be limited in actual practice. The second mechanism is through the IDEA under the "Other Health Impaired" classification. In 1991, the definition for disability under this regulation was amended to specifically include ADD and ADHD. When children are eligible under this mechanism, they receive an individualized education plan and may be placed in small, special education classrooms. It is important that clinicians are aware that traditional special education programs were not specifically designed to serve the needs of children with ADHD. For example, "pull-out" resource programs, where a child spends a part of the day in a classroom with specialized curricula, were designed for children with specific learning problems such as reading. Because children with ADHD typically have erratic functioning throughout the day, the appropriateness of such a program to address their needs is questionable. Furthermore, children in full-day special education placements often have problems very different from those of students with ADHD, such as severe learning disabilities, speech and language problems, or severe emotional disturbance. For students with ADHD and a comorbid learning and/or emotional disorder, placement in special education classes is more common. Interestingly, since eligibility for the "Other Health Impaired" category began including ADHD, there has been a reported threefold increase in the percentage of children enrolled under this category. However, it is likely that most interventions for ADHD

continue to involve accommodations to general education classes.

The predominant practice of educating students with ADHD in mainstream settings is consistent with the established educational principle of the "least restrictive environment," and clinicians should understand this as it applies to decisions regarding special educational placement. In particular, IDEA makes it clear that special services are to be provided in such a way that children with disabilities may interact with nondisabled peers as much as possible. Hence school districts are likely to place children with ADHD in the least restrictive environment necessary to manage their academic and behavioral problems (i.e., in the program that provides the greatest contact with nondisabled students). Some teachers are not always in agreement with this, preferring that even children with mild ADHD be removed to special educational settings, rather than having to adjust their classroom curriculum and behavior management style to accommodate the maintenance of these children in regular education. Parents may be equally biased toward special education, believing that the smaller class sizes, better-trained teachers, and greater teacher attention they provide is to be preferred over regular education. School districts are likely to resist these pressures, so as not to violate the rights of the children to the least restrictive environment or risk legal action for doing so. Moreover, many students with ADHD with mild to moderate problems are likely to be best served in general education classrooms with accommodations to improve attention, work habits, and peer relations. The students with more serious problems are the ones likely to require placement in special education classrooms designed to meet their needs.

It is essential that clinicians stay up-to-date with the federal guidelines for special education as well as with their own specific state guidelines and any special or unusual local district guidelines, to advocate knowledgeably for the children in their practice. The phrase "You are only as good as your Rolodex" is a truism in dealing with educational placements for children with ADHD, as well as in locating resources within the private sector (e.g., private schools, formal and informal tutoring programs, and special summer camps for children with behavior problems). In some cases, a clinician will be contacted to provide a "second opinion" because of conflict between parents and school staff over the nature and extent of a child's problems and his or her eligibility for services. It is in such cases that the clinician must determine the precise nature of the school district's eligibility criteria and select assessment methods for addressing these criteria that are acceptable within school district policies.

Model Programs

A number of programs have been developed for serving students with ADHD. In the preceding edition of this text, a program for utilizing paraprofessionals as behavioral aides in the general education classrooms—the Irvine Paraprofessional Program (IPP; Kotkin, 1995)—was described. This program continues to be implemented at the present time. The aides' role is to assist the teachers in implementing an in-class token system and to provide collateral training in social skills. Children identified as having ADHD are initially referred to the program through the student study team. The school psychologist works with each classroom teacher to develop an initial intervention plan, which includes a number of accommodations in the classroom. If this is unsuccessful, a paraprofessional is assigned to the class for a 12-week intervention designed by the team. The intervention consists of a token economy implemented by the paraprofessional for up to 3 hours per day and by the teacher during times when the paraprofessional is not present. The school psychologist provides periodic supervision of the paraprofessional and consults with the teacher regarding implementation of the program. A child receives tokens (stamps) for up to four target behaviors every 15 minutes when the paraprofessional is in the class; time periods are longer (45 minutes) when the teacher is implementing the program. Students are also given one to three reminders during each period to do the target behavior. At the end of the day, stamp totals are exchanged for a 20-minute activity (e.g., computer games) in a schoolwide reinforcement center. The program also includes a three-level system where students earn privileges as they move up each level by consistently reaching daily and weekly goals. The three-level system also serves as a way to fade the program, since feedback intervals are increased (e.g., from 15 minutes to 1 hour) and the frequency of reminders is reduced as students achieve higher levels. The goal is to fade the program to a point where the

teacher can successfully take it over. Students also participate in an SST group led by the paraprofessionals twice per week. The IPP model has been implemented in a number of school districts, and a modified version of the program was utilized as one of several psychosocial treatments in the government-sponsored multisite study of ADHD, the MTA (Arnold et al., 1997).

The preceding edition of this text also described several programs to serve students with ADHD and more severe problems in self-contained full-day settings. A summer treatment program, initially developed by Pelham and his colleagues (Pelham et al., 1996; Pelham & Hoza, 1996), has been implemented with success for a number of years. Several sites around the country are currently providing this manualized intervention, and it too was implemented as a part of psychosocial treatment in the MTA. The program includes intensive behavioral programs (a point system with daily and weekly rewards, time out, SST) implemented by special education teachers during computer, art, and academic learning centers, and by five counselors as children participate in recreational activities (soccer, swimming) (Hoza, Vallano, & Pelham, 1995). This program was expanded to a year-round day treatment service by Swanson and his colleagues in 1986 (Swanson, 1992) and continues to be operational today. The comprehensive clinical program includes an intensive classroom behavior modification system (a token economy, schoolwide daily and weekly reinforcement, self-management training, daily behavioral report cards, and levels system), parent training, and SST. Once students achieve stable behavioral gains (usually over the course of 1–2 years), they make the transition back to their home school. This summer treatment program is associated with clinically significant gains across multiple areas of functioning (academic, social, and behavioral) for the majority of children participating in the treatment protocol (Chronis et al., 2004).

Recently, Evans et al. (in press) developed a promising comprehensive school-based treatment program for middle school students with ADHD, the Challenging Horizons Program (CHP). Two versions of the program exist: an after-school and an integrated model. In the after-school version, students attend the program for 2 hours 3 days per week. The program consists of two separate group interventions for improving social and educational skills, and 20-minute one-on-one meetings with a counselor to review progress, practice specific skills, and maintain a therapeutic relationship and connection with the program. The counselors work with each student's parents and teachers to ensure that appropriate problems are being addressed and to facilitate generalization from the after-school program to school and home. In the integrated model, school staff (teachers, administrators, counselors) implement interventions similar to those in the after-school program during the school day through consultation with study staff. A school counselor serves as a mentor to each student to review progress and practice skills, just as the counselor does for students in the after-school program. Both versions include several interventions for educational skills similar to those reviewed previously in this chapter. Every student uses an assignment notebook for homework, with school and home contingencies for its correct use. Teachers initially sign the book for accuracy, but these signatures are tapered as students become more independent. Students are also taught note-taking and study skills; they practice these first in the CHP, and then are required to show that they use the skills at school and at home. An individualized homework plan, which requires mandatory daily time for homework and use of rewards, is developed with the parents. Disruptive behavior is acknowledged within each group session; other contingencies are added if needed. Daily or weekly report cards are implemented if needed to address problem behaviors at school or home. The social skills intervention includes social problem solving, recognition of social cues, and skill development. Students view and evaluate videotapes of their own behavior during group sessions to facilitate their learning. Two pilot studies support the efficacy of the intervention, and it is currently being implemented at three sites on the East Coast.

A psychosocial treatment program called the Child Life Skills Program has been developed recently for students with ADHD-PI (Pfiffner, 2003). The program incorporates rehabilitation approaches based on similarities between those with ADHD-PI and those with mild brain injuries (e.g., sluggish cognitive tempo, forgetfulness). It emphasizes adaptive skills, functional competence, and compensatory strategies; uses cues, prompts, and routines; and involves teachers and parents to provide necessary environmental supports at school and at home. Parents and children attend eight concurrent group meetings and up to four family meetings, and teachers attend five consultation meetings with a therapist and each child's family. Children are taught a series of modules focused on independence (homework/study skills, self-care skills, getting chores done, routines, organization, and time tools), and social skills (friendship making, handling teasing, assertion, accepting, being a good sport, and problem solving). The parent group focuses on strategies to support their children's use of these skills at home and at school. Pertinent to this discussion on school-based interventions, the teacher consultation meetings are intended to provide teachers with information on behavioral interventions and classroom accommodations; the focus is on development and implementation of an individualized daily home–school report card and classroom accommodations specific to concerns of each child (e.g., additional time or "time challenges" to complete work, preferential seating, reduction in workload, use of assignment book, use of completed work folder, time limits). Target behaviors are based on the needs of each child and typically include common problem areas for ADHD-PI: academic work (e.g., completion of assigned work, completion and return of homework, accuracy of completed work); work behavior/study skills (e.g., following directions, having necessary materials to begin work, getting started on work, staying on task); and social interactions (e.g., entering peer groups, accepting consequences, being a good sport, using assertive behavior). Skills taught in the child group are shared with teachers, so that the children's use of these skills can be reinforced (often by including them as targets on the classroom challenge) in the naturalistic environment of the school. Parents are taught a set of transferable skills for working with their child's teachers in the future. Initial results support efficacy of the program (Pfiffner, Huang-Pollock, Mikami, Easterlin, & Fung, 2004).

Although efficacious academic and behavioral interventions for students with ADHD have been identified, it is unclear how best to help teachers to implement effective strategies on a consistent basis. Given that most children with ADHD are placed in general education classrooms with one teacher and many students, it is particularly challenging to design interventions that such teachers will find acceptable and feasible. DuPaul et al. (2004) have designed a teacher consultation model (Project PASS—Promoting Academic Success in ADHD Students) to address this particular issue in the general context of addressing the academic problems of students with ADHD. Initially, consultants (e.g., school psychologists or special educators) provide teachers with information about ADHD, especially in relation to school-related deficits and treatment strategies. Next, consultants follow a consultative problem-solving process (adapted from Kratochwill & Bergan, 1990) to identify the specific academic problems that students may be exhibiting, as well as the environmental conditions (i.e., antecedent and consequent events) that may be contributing to these difficulties. Direct observation and curriculum-based measurement (Shinn, 1998) data are collected on several occasions by a consultant to identify potential strategies that could directly address each student's difficulties. The teacher and consultant then collaboratively design an intervention plan that may include modifications to teacher instruction, peer tutoring, CAI, a home–school communication system, and/or self-monitoring/reinforcement. Data are then collected by the teacher and/or consultant to evaluate whether the plan is working and to identify adjustments to the plan that may be helpful. The consultant also monitors treatment integrity to provide ongoing feedback to the teacher. Over time, the consultant's involvement is faded out, and the teacher implements the plan independently. Although a controlled comparison of the Project PASS model with standard school-based intervention procedures is ongoing, initial analyses indicate that this data-based decision-making strategy is successful in promoting greater treatment integrity and more sustained gains in math and reading skills (DuPaul et al., 2004).

NEXT STEPS

Since the preceding version of this text, some advances in school-based services for ADHD have been made. The explicit recognition in 1999 by the U.S. Department of Education that ADHD may be considered a disabling condition has expanded the educational options for students with ADHD throughout the 1990s and into the new century, and more and more materials on evidence-based treatments are be-

ing widely disseminated. Several exciting new programs have been and are being developed to assist students with ADHD at varying developmental levels, and efforts are being made to develop and evaluate academic interventions and tailor the well-documented behavioral technology based on functional analyses, rather than the "one size fits all" approach. Despite this progress, the recommendations made in the preceding version of this text for advancing school-based interventions still hold. There continues to be a need for better understanding of how to match specific instructional materials and behavior management techniques to specific child characteristics, how to improve academic performance, and how to improve maintenance and generalization of intervention effects. Adequate training of teachers in the implementation of evidence-based behavioral interventions still remains elusive. Ongoing consultation models may be most helpful, but there continues to be an issue about who pays for what services. Unfortunately, while mental health insurance plans often cover non-evidence-based treatments such as play therapy, they typically do not cover evidence-based behavioral interventions in schools. Educational systems face serious challenges in funding training for teachers and the needed resources for interventions. It is increasingly recognized that ADHD is a lifelong disorder and the focus of school-based interventions need to be long-term; that is, individualized educational and behavioral plans will require ongoing evaluation, modification, and implementation across settings over the course of months and years. Further advances in helping students with ADHD achieve success at school and beyond depend upon the continued development of cost-effective evidence-based programs, and upon solving the critical problems of lack of resources and training for teachers, so that these programs can be widely available in schools across the country.

KEY CLINICAL POINTS

✓ One of the major and most common domains of major life activity impaired by ADHD in children is functioning in the educational setting. For this and other reasons, more children with ADHD are receiving services in public schools than at any previous time in history.

✓ Despite the success of medication management of ADHD in school settings, important roles for psychoeducational interventions remain. Such behavioral interventions, when given in sufficiently intensive doses, produce significant improvements in symptom management in their own right; this may lead to less need for medication or lower doses of medication in the school setting.

✓ The first goal of school-based interventions is to improve basic knowledge among educators about the nature, causes, course, and treatments for ADHD.

✓ A second goal of such interventions is to increase home and school collaboration, so as to produce a more uniform, consistent, and effective plan of management that incorporates the major caregivers.

✓ Both of these goals lead to the ultimate purpose of psychoeducational programs for ADHD, which is to increase the success and improve the academic and social effectiveness of children with ADHD in the school setting.

✓ Functional assessments of behavior in individual children with ADHD can facilitate treatment planning beyond the initial diagnostic evaluation, by revealing specific antecedent and consequent events that affect each child's academic and social functioning and that can be manipulated so as to alter that functioning.

✓ Nine principles of management have been articulated that can serve as the core premises in designing interventions for children with ADHD. Many of these derive from the understanding that ADHD disrupts executive functioning, and thus much of the extra "structure" that children with ADHD so often require is specifically aimed at redressing these executive weaknesses.

✓ Core interventions for ADHD require (1) altering the physical classroom layout, as needed; (2) modifying academic tasks to match each child's abilities and deficits; (3) increasing the use of computer-assisted instruction; (4) improving academic skills; (5) altering teacher-delivered consequences (attention, reprimands, tokens, time outs, etc.) for appropriate and inappropriate conduct, while minimizing adverse side effects; (6) in-

tentionally programming for maintenance of treatment gains and generalization outside the treatment setting; (7) using peers to facilitate academic success and behavioral control; (8) developing home-based reinforcement programs (daily behavior cards); (9) striving to enhance self-monitoring and self-management; and (10) modifying these approaches for use with teens with ADHD.

✓ Cognitive-behavioral therapies for ADHD do not appear to be effective unless combined with more publicly accountable contingency management methods, and even then they seem to add little beyond what behavioral interventions would have changed.

✓ Social skills training (SST) has shown some positive results for assisting children with ADHD in their social adjustment, but results are usually limited to settings with active behavioral programs in place to promote the skills. Grouping of children in SST is an important consideration, since aggressive behavior may increase for some children if nonaggressive and aggressive children participate together in group training.

✓ Formal special educational services under the Individuals with Disabilities Education Act and Section 504 may also be required for a child with ADHD if prereferral accommodations are not sufficient.

✓ There continues to be a need for better understanding of how to match specific instructional materials and behavior management techniques to specific child characteristics, how to improve academic performance, and how to improve maintenance and generalization of intervention effects.

REFERENCES

Abikoff, H. (1985). Efficacy of cognitive training interventions in hyperactive children: A critical review. *Clinical Psychology Review, 5,* 479–512.

Abikoff, H. (1987). An evaluation of cognitive behavior therapy for hyperactive children. In B. Lahey & A. Kazdin (Eds.), *Advances in clinical child psychology* (Vol. 10, pp. 171–216). New York: Plenum Press.

Abikoff, H., & Gittelman, R. (1985). Hyperactive children treated with stimulants: Is cognitive training a useful adjunct? *Archives of General Psychiatry, 42,* 953–961.

Abramowitz, A. J., & O'Leary, S. G. (1991). Behavioral interventions for the classroom: Implications for students with ADHD. *School Psychology Review, 20*(2), 220–234.

Abramowitz, A. J., Reid, M. J., & O'Toole, K. (1994). *The role of task timing in the treatment of ADHD.* Paper presented at the annual meeting of the Association for Advancement of Behavior Therapy, San Diego, CA.

Acker, M. M., & O'Leary, S. G. (1987). Effects of reprimands and praise on appropriate behavior in the classroom. *Journal of Abnormal Child Psychology, 15,* 549–557.

Ajibola, O., & Clement, P. W. (1995). Differential effects of methylphenidate and self-reinforcement on attention deficit hyperactivity disorder. *Behavior Modification, 19*(2), 211–233.

Antshel, K. M., & Remer, R. (2003). Social skills training in children with attention deficit hyperactivity disorder: A randomized-controlled clinical trial. *Journal of Clinical Child and Adolescent Psychology, 32,* 153–165.

Arcia, E., Frank, R., Sanchez-LaCay, A., & Fernandez, M. C. (2000). Teacher understanding of ADHD as reflected in attributions and classroom strategies. *Journal of Attention Disorders 4,* 91–101.

Arnold, L. E., Abikoff, H. B., Cantwell, D. P., Conners, C. K., Elliott, G., Greenhill, L. L., et al. (1997). NIMH collaborative multimodal treatment study of children with ADHD (the MTA): Design challenges and choices. *Archives of General Psychiatry, 54*(9), 865–870.

Atkins, M. S., Graczyk, P. A., Frazier, S. L., & Abdul-Adil, J. (2003). Toward a new model for promoting urban children's mental health: Accessible, effective, and sustainable school-based mental health services. *School Psychology Review 32*(4), 503–514.

Atkins, M. S., McKay, M. M., Frazier, S. L., Jakobsons, L. J., Arvanitis, P., Cunningham, T., et al. (2002). Suspensions and detentions in an urban, low-income school: Punishment or reward? *Journal of Abnormal Child Psychology 30*(4), 361–371.

Baer, R. A., & Nietzel, M. T. (1991). Cognitive and behavioral treatment of impulsivity in children: A meta-analytic review of the outcome literature. *Journal of Clinical Child Psychology, 20,* 400–412.

Bagwell, C. L., Molina, B., Pelham, W. E., & Hoza, B. (2001). Attention-deficit hyperactivity disorder and problems in peer relations: Predictions from childhood to adolescence. *Journal of the American Academy of Child and Adolescent Psychiatry, 40,* 1285–1292.

Barkley, R. A. (2000). *Taking charge of ADHD: The complete, authoritative guide for parents* (rev. ed.). New York: Guilford Press.

Barkley, R. A., Copeland, A., & Sivage, C. (1980). A self-control classroom for hyperactive children. *Journal of Autism and Developmental Disorders, 10,* 75–89.

Barkley, R. A., Shelton, T. L., Crosswait, C., Moorehouse, M., Fletcher, K., Barrett, S., et al. (1996). Preliminary findings of an early intervention program for aggressive hyperactive children. *Annals of the New York Academy of Sciences, 794,* 277–289.

Barrish, H. H., Saunders, M., & Wolf, M. M. (1969). Good behavior game: Effects of individual contingencies for group consequences on disruptive behavior in a classroom. *Journal of Applied Behavior Analysis, 2,* 119–124.

Barry, L. M., & Messer, J. J. (2003). A practical application of self-management for students diagnosed with attention-deficit/hyperactivity disorder. *Journal of Positive Behavior Interventions, 5*(4), 238–248.

Beelmann, A., Pfingsten, U., & Losel, F. (1994). Effects of training social competence in children: A meta-analysis of recent evaluation studies. *Journal of Clinical Child Psychology, 23,* 260–271.

Bloomquist, M. L., August, G. J., & Ostrander, R. (1991). Effects of a school-based cognitive-behavioral intervention for ADHD children. *Journal of Abnormal Child Psychology, 19,* 591–605.

Braswell, L., August, G. J., Bloomquist, M. L., Realmuto, G. M., Skare, S. S., & Crosby, R. D. (1997). School-based secondary prevention for children with disruptive behavior. *Journal of Abnormal Child Psychology, 25,* 197–208.

Brown, R. T., Wynne, M. E., Borden, K. A., Clingerman, S. R., Geniesse, R., & Spunt, A. L. (1986). Methylphenidate and cognitive therapy in children with attention deficit disorder: A double-blind trial. *Journal of Developmental and Behavioral Pediatrics, 7,* 163–170.

Burcham, B., Carlson, L., & Milich, R. (1993). Promising school-based practices for students with attention deficit disorder. *Exceptional Children, 60*(2), 174–180.

Carlson, C. L., Booth, J. E., Shin, M., & Canu, W. H. (2002). Parent-, teacher-, and self-rated motivational styles in ADHD subtypes. *Journal of Learning Disabilities 35,* 104–113.

Chronis, A. M., Fabiano, G. A., Gnagy, E. M., Onyango, A. N., Pelham, W. E., Jr., Lopez-Williams, A., et al. (2004). An evaluation of the summer treatment program for children with attention-deficit/hyperactivity disorder using a treatment withdrawal design. *Behavior Therapy, 35,* 561–586.

Clarfield, J., & Stoner, G. (2005). The effects of computerized reading instruction on the academic performance of students identified with ADHD. *School Psychology Review, 34,* 246–255.

Codding, R., & Lewandowski, L. (2003). Academic interventions for children with ADHD: A review of current options. *ADHD Report, 11,* 8–11.

Colton, D. L., & Sheridan, S. M. (1998). Conjoint behavioral consultation and social skills training: Enhancing the play behaviors of boys with attention deficit hyperactivity disorder. *Journal of Educational and Psychological Consultation, 9,* 3–28.

Conners, C. K. (2002). Forty years of methylphenidate treatment in attention-deficit/hyperactivity disorder. *Journal of Attention Disorders, 6*(Suppl. 1), S17–S30.

Conners, C. K., Epstein, J. N., March, J. S., Angold, A., Wells, K. C., Klaric, J., et al. (2001). Multimodal treatment of ADHD in the MTA: An alternative outcome analysis. *Journal of the American Academy of Child and Adolescent Psychiatry, 40*(2), 159–167.

Cunningham, C. E., Cunningham, L. J., Martorelli, V., Tran, A., Young, J., & Zacharias, R. (1998). The effects of primary division, student-mediated conflict resolution programs on playground aggression. *Journal of Child Psychology and Psychiatry, 39,* 653–662.

Cunningham, C. E., & Siegel, L. S. (1987). Peer interactions of normal and attention-deficit disordered boys during freeplay, cooperative task, and simulated classroom situations. *Journal of Abnormal Child Psychology, 15,* 247–268.

Davies, S., & Witte, R. (2000). Self-management and peer-monitoring within a group contingency to decrease uncontrolled verbalizations of children with attention-deficit/hyperactivity disorder. *Psychology in the Schools, 37*(2), 135–146.

Diaz, R. M., & Berk, L. E. (1995). A Vygotskian critique of self-instructional training. *Development and Psychopathology, 7,* 369–392.

Dishion, T. J., McCord, J., & Poulin, F. (1999). When interventions harm: Peer groups and problem behavior. *American Psychologist, 54,* 755–764.

Douglas, V. I. (1980). Higher mental processes in hyperactive children: Implications for training. In R. Knights & D. Bakker (Eds.), *Treatment of hyperactive and learning disordered children* (pp. 65–92). Baltimore: University Park Press.

Dunlap, G., dePerczel, M., Clarke, S., Wilson, D., Wright, S., White, R., et al. (1994). Choice making to promote adaptive behavior for students with emotional and behavioral challenges. *Journal of Applied Behavior Analysis, 27,* 505–518.

Dunson, R. M., III, Hughes, J. M., & Jackson, T. W. (1994). Effect of behavioral consultation on student and teacher behavior. *Journal of School Psychology, 32*(3), 247–266.

DuPaul, G. J., & Eckert, T. L. (1997). The effects of school-based interventions for attention deficit hyperactivity disorders: A meta-analysis. *School Psychology Review, 26,* 5–27.

DuPaul, G. J., Eckert, T. L., & McGoey, K. E. (1997). Interventions for students with attention-deficit/hyperactivity disorder: One size does not fit all. *School Psychology Review, 26.* 369–381.

DuPaul, G. J., & Ervin, R. A. (1996). Functional assessment of behaviors related to attention deficit hyperactivity disorder: Linking assessment to intervention design. *Behavior Therapy, 27,* 601–622.

DuPaul, G. J., Ervin, R. A., Hook, C. L., & McGoey, K. E. (1998). Peer tutoring for children with attention deficit hyperactivity disorder: Effects on classroom behavior and academic performance. *Journal of Applied Behavior Analysis, 31,* 579–592.

DuPaul, G. J., Guevremont, D. C., & Barkley, R. A. (1992). Behavioral treatment of attention deficit hy-

peractivity disorder in the classroom. *Behavior Modification, 16*(2), 204–225.

DuPaul, G. J., & Henningson, P. N. (1993). Peer tutoring effects on the classroom performance of children with attention deficit hyperactivity disorder. *School Psychology Review, 22,* 134–143.

DuPaul, G. J., Jitendra, A. K., Lutz, J. G., Volpe, R. J., Gruber, R., & Lorah, K. (2004, February). *Promoting academic success in students with ADHD: Short-term outcomes.* Paper presented at the annual Pacific Coast Research Conference, Coronado, CA.

DuPaul, G. J., & Power, T. J. (2000). Educational interventions for students with attention deficit disorders. In T. E. Brown (Ed.), *Attention deficit disorders and comorbidities in children, adolescents, and adults* (pp. 607–635). Washington, DC: American Psychiatric Press.

DuPaul, G. J., & Stoner, G. (2003). *ADHD in the schools: Assessment and intervention strategies* (2nd ed.). New York: Guilford Press.

Dush, D. M., Hirt, M. L., & Schroeder, H. E. (1989). Self-statement modification in the treatment of child behavior disorders: A meta-analysis. *Psychological Bulletin, 106,* 97–106.

Edwards, L., Salant, V., Howard, V. F., Brougher, J., & McLaughlin, T. F. (1995). Effectiveness of self-management on attentional behavior and reading comprehension for children with attention deficit disorder. *Child and Family Behavior Therapy, 17*(2), 1–17.

Elia, J., Ambrosini, P. J., & Rapoport, J. L. (1999). Treatment of attention-deficit-hyperactivity disorder. *New England Journal of Medicine, 340*(10), 780–788.

Erhardt, D., & Hinshaw, S. P. (1994). Initial sociometric impressions of attention-deficit hyperactivity disorder and comparison boys: Predictions from social behaviors and from nonbehavioral variables. *Journal of Consulting and Clinical Psychology, 62,* 833–842.

Ervin, R. A., DuPaul, G. J., Kern, L., & Friman, P. C. (1998). Classroom-based functional assessment: A proactive approach to intervention selection for adolescents with attention-deficit/hyperactivity disorder. *Journal of Applied Behavior Analysis, 31,* 65–78.

Evans, J. H., Ferre, L., Ford, L. A., & Green, J. L. (1995). Decreasing attention deficit hyperactivity disorder symptoms utilizing an automated classroom reinforcement device. *Psychology in the Schools, 32,* 210–219.

Evans, S. W., Dowling, C., & Brown, R. (in press). Psychosocial treatment for adolescents with attention deficit hyperactivity disorder. In K. McBurnett, L. Pfiffner, G. R. Schachar, G. R. Elliot, & J. Nigg (Eds.), *Attention deficit hyperactivity disorder.* New York: Marcel Dekker.

Evans, S. W., Pelham, W., & Grudberg, M. V. (1994). The efficacy of notetaking to improve behavior and comprehension of adolescents with attention deficit hyperactivity disorder. *Exceptionality, 5*(1), 1–17.

Fabiano, G. A., & Pelham, W. (2003). Improving the effectiveness of behavioral classroom interventions for attention-deficit/hyperactivity disorder: A case study. *Journal of Emotional and Behavioral Disorders, 11*(2), 122–129.

Fehlings, D. L., Roberts, W., Humphries, T., & Dawe, G. (1991). Attention deficit hyperactivity disorder: Does cognitive behavioral therapy improve home behavior? *Journal of Developmental and Behavioral Pediatrics, 12*, 223–228.

Forness, S. R., & Kavale, K. (2001). ADHD and a return to the medical model of special education. *Education and Treatment of Children, 24*(3), 224–247.

Frankel, F., & Myatt, R. (2003). *Children's friendship training.* New York: Brunner-Routledge.

Frankel, F., Myatt, R., & Cantwell, D. P. (1995). Training outpatient boys to conform with the social ecology of popular peers: Effects on parent and teacher ratings. *Journal of Clinical Child Psychology, 24*, 300–310.

Frankel, F., Myatt, R., Cantwell, D. P., & Feinberg, D. T. (1997). Parent-assisted transfer of children's social skills training: Effects on children with and without attention deficit hyperactivity disorder. *Journal of the American Academy of Child and Adolescent Psychiatry, 36*, 1056–1064.

Gast, D. C., & Nelson, C. M. (1977). Time-out in the classroom: Implications for special education. *Exceptional Children, 43*, 461–464.

Gordon, M., Thomason, D., Cooper, S., & Ivers, C. L. (1990). Nonmedical treatment of ADHD/hyperactivity: The attention training system. *Journal of School Psychology, 29*, 151–159.

Greenwood, C. R., Maheady, L., & Delquadri, J. (2002). Classwide peer tutoring programs. In M. R. Shinn, H. M. Walker, & G. Stoner (Eds.), *Interventions for academic and behavior problems II: Preventive and remedial approaches* (pp. 611–650). Bethesda, MD: National Association of School Psychologists.

Gureasko-Moore, S., DuPaul, G. J., & White, G. P. (2005). *The effects of self-management on the organizational skills of adolescents with ADHD.* Manuscript under review.

Hinshaw, S. P. (1992). Interventions for social competence and social skill. *Child and Adolescent Psychiatric Clinics of North America, 1*(2), 539–552.

Hinshaw, S. P., & Erhardt, D. (1991). Attention-deficit hyperactivity disorder. In P. C. Kendall (Ed.), *Child and adolescent therapy: Cognitive-behavioral procedures* (pp. 98–128). New York: Guilford Press.

Hinshaw, S. P., Henker, B., & Whalen, C. K. (1984). Cognitive-behavioral and pharmacological interventions for hyperactive boys: Comparative and combined effects. *Journal of Consulting and Clinical Psychology, 52*, 739–749.

Hoff, K. E., & DuPaul, G. J. (1998). Reducing disruptive behavior in general education classrooms: The use of self-management strategies. *School Psychology Review, 27*, 290–303.

Hook, C. L., & DuPaul, G. J. (1999). Parent tutoring

for students with attention-deficit/hyperactivity disorder: Effects on reading performance at home and school. *School Psychology Review, 28*(1), 60–75.

Hoza, B., Mrug, S., Pelham, W. E., Jr., Greiner, A. R., & Gnagy, E. M. (2003). A friendship intervention for children with attention-deficit/hyperactivity disorder: Preliminary findings. *Journal of Attention Disorders, 6*(3), 87–98.

Hoza, B., Vallano, G., & Pelham, W. E. (1995). Attention-deficit/hyperactivity disorder. In R. T. Ammerman & M. Hersen (Eds.), *Handbook of child behavior therapy in the psychiatric setting* (pp. 181–198). New York: Wiley.

Hubbard, J. A., & Newcomb, A. F. (1991). Initial dyadic peer interaction of attention deficit-hyperactivity disorder and normal boys. *Journal of Abnormal Child Psychology, 19*, 179–195.

Jensen, P. S. (2002). ADHD comorbity findings for the MTA study: New diagnostic subtypes and their optional treatments. In J. E. Helzer (Ed.), *Defining psychopathology in the 21st century: DSM-V and beyond* (pp. 169–192). Washington, DC: American Psychiatric Press.

Jensen, P. S., Hinshaw, S. P., Swanson, J. M., Greenhill, L. L., Conners, C. K., Arnold, L. E., et al. (2001). Findings from the NIMH Multimodal Treatment Study of ADHD (MTA): Implications and applications for primary care providers. *Journal of Developmental and Behavioral Pediatrics, 22*(1), 60–73.

Kelley, M. L. (1990). *School–home notes: Promoting children's classroom success.* New York: Guilford Press.

Kendall, P. C., & Braswell, L. (1985). *Cognitive-behavioral therapy for impulsive children.* New York: Guilford Press.

Kotkin, R. A. (1995). The Irvine Paraprofessional Program: Using paraprofessionals in serving students with ADHD. *Intervention in School and Clinic, 30*(4), 235–240.

Kratochwill, T. R., & Bergan, J. R. (1990). *Behavioral consultation in applied settings: An individual guide.* New York: Plenum Press.

Kubany, E. S., Weiss, L. E., & Slogett, B. B. (1971). The good behavior clock: A reinforcement/time-out procedure for reducing disruptive classroom behavior. *Journal of Behavior Therapy and Experimental Psychiatry, 2*, 173–179.

Lindsley, O. R. (1991). From technical jargon to plain English for application. *Journal of Applied Behavior Analysis, 24*, 449–458.

Martens, B. K., & Hiralall, A. S. (1997). Scripted sequences of teacher interaction. *Behavior Modification, 21*(3), 308–323.

Mautone, J., DuPaul, G. J., & Jitendra, A. K. (in press). The effects of computer-assisted instruction on the mathematics performance of children with attention-deficit/hyperactivity disorder. *Journal of Attention Disorders.*

McGoey, K. E., & DuPaul, G. J. (2000). Total reinforcement and response cost procedures: Reducing the disruptive behavior of preschool children with attention-deficit/hyperactivity disorder. *School Psychology Quarterly, 15*(3), 330–343.

Meichenbaum, D., & Goodman, J. (1971). Training impulsive children to talk to themselves: A means of developing self-control. *Journal of Abnormal Psychology, 77*, 115–126.

Milich, R., & Dodge, K. A. (1984). Social information processing in child psychiatric populations. *Journal of Abnormal Child Psychology, 12*, 471–490.

Northup, J., Jones, K., Broussard, C., DiGiovanni, G., Herring, M., Fusilier, I., et al. (1997). A preliminary analysis of interactive effects between common classroom contingencies and methylphenidate. *Journal of Applied Behavior Analysis, 30*(1), 121–125.

Office of Special Education Programs. (2004). *Teaching children with attention deficit hyperactivity disorder: Instructional strategies and practices.* Washington, DC: U.S. Department of Education.

O'Leary, K. D., & O'Leary, S. G. (1977). *Classroom management: The successful use of behavior modification* (2nd ed.). New York: Pergamon Press.

Ota, K. R., & DuPaul, G. J. (2002). Task engagement and mathematics performance in children with attention deficit hyperactivity disorder: Effects of supplemental computer intervention. *School Psychology Quarterly, 17*(3), 242–257.

Paniagua, F. A., & Black, S. (1992). Correspondence training and observational learning in the management of hyperactive children: A preliminary study. *Child and Family Behavior Therapy, 14*(3), 1–19.

Pelham, W. E. (1999). The NIMH multimodal treatment study for ADHD: Just say yes to drugs alone? *Canadian Journal of Psychiatry, 44*, 981–990.

Pelham, W. E., & Bender, M. E. (1982). Peer relationships in hyperactive children: Description and treatment. *Advances in Learning and Behavioral Disabilities, 1*, 365–436.

Pelham, W. E., Gnagy, B., Greiner, A., Hoza, B., Sams, S., Martin, L., & Wilson, T. (1996). A summer treatment program for children with ADHD. In M. Roberts & A. LaGreca (Eds.), *Model programs for service delivery for child and family mental health* (pp. 193–213). Hillsdale, NJ: Erlbaum.

Pelham, W. E., & Hoza, B. (1996). Intensive treatment: A summer treatment program for children with ADHD. In E. D. Hibbs & P. S. Jensen (Eds.), *Psychosocial treatments for child and adolescent disorders: Empirically based strategies for clinical practice* (pp. 311–340). Washington, DC: American Psychological Association.

Pfiffner, L. J. (1996). *All about ADHD: The complete practical guide for classroom teachers.* New York: Scholastic.

Pfiffner, L. (2003). Psychosocial treatment for ADHD—inattentive type. *ADHD Report, 11*(5), 1–8.

Pfiffner, L., Huang-Pollock, C., Mikami, A., Easterlin, B., & Fung, M. (2004). *Effects of integrated psychosocial treatment for ADHD—inattentive type.* Paper presented at the annual meeting of the American Psychological Association, Honolulu, HI.

Pfiffner, L., & McBurnett, K. (1997). Social skills training with parent generalization: Treatment effects for children with attention deficit disorder. *Journal of Consulting and Clinical Psychology, 65*, 749–757.

Pfiffner, L. J., & O'Leary, S. G. (1987). The efficacy of all-positive management as a function of the prior use of negative consequences. *Journal of Applied Behavior Analysis, 20*(3), 265–271.

Pfiffner, L. J., & O'Leary, S. G. (1993). School-based psychological treatments. In J. L. Matson (Ed.), *Handbook of hyperactivity in children* (pp. 234–255). Boston: Allyn & Bacon.

Pfiffner, L. J., Rosen, L. A., & O'Leary, S. G. (1985). The efficacy of an all-positive approach to classroom management. *Journal of Applied Behavior Analysis, 18*, 257–261.

Pisecco, S., Huzinec, C., & Curtis, D. (2001). The effect of child characteristics on teachers' acceptability of classroom-based behavioral strategies and psychostimulant medication for the treatment of ADHD. *Journal of Clinical Child Psychology, 30*, 413–421.

Power, T. J., & Hess, L. E. (1995). The acceptability of interventions for attention-deficit hyperactivity disorder among elementary and middle school teachers. *Developmental and Behavioral Pediatrics, 16*(4), 238–243.

Proctor, M. A., & Morgan, D. (1991). Effectiveness of a response cost raffle procedure on the disruptive classroom behavior of adolescents with behavior problems. *School Psychology Review, 20*(1), 97–109.

Rapport, M. D., Murphy, A., & Bailey, J. S. (1980). The effects of a response cost treatment tactic on hyperactive children. *Journal of School Psychology, 18*, 98–111.

Rhode, G., Morgan, D. P., & Young, K. R. (1983). Generalization and maintenance of treatment gains of behaviorally handicapped students from resource rooms to regular classrooms using self-evaluation procedures. *Journal of Applied Behavior Analysis, 16*, 171–188.

Shapiro, E. S., DuPaul, G. J., Bradley, K. L., & Bailey, L. T. (1996). A school-based consultation program for service delivery to middle school students with attention deficit hyperactivity disorder. *Journal of Emotional and Behavioral Disorders, 4*(2), 73–81.

Shelton, T. L., Barkley, R. A., Crosswait, C., Moorehouse, M., Fletcher, K., Barrett, S., et al. (2000). Multimethod psychoeducational intervention for preschool children with disruptive behavior: Two-year post-treatment follow-up. *Journal of Abnormal Child Psychology, 28*(3), 253–266.

Sheridan, S. M., Dee, C. C., Morgan, J. C., McCormick, M. E., & Walker, D. (1996). A multi-method introduction for social skills deficits in children with ADHD and their parents. *School Psychology Review, 25*, 401–416.

Shinn, M. R. (Ed.). (1998). *Advanced applications of*

curriculum-based measurement. New York: Guilford Press.

Sprute, K. A., Williams, R. L., & McLaughlin, T. F. (1990). Effects of group response cost contingency procedure on the rate of classroom interruptions with emotionally disturbed secondary students. *Child and Family Behavior Therapy, 12*(2), 1–12.

Swanson, J. M. (1992). *School-based assessments and interventions for ADD students*. Irvine, CA: K. C.

Swanson, J. M., Kraemer, H. C., Hinshaw, S. P., Arnold, L. E., Conners, C. K., Abikoff, H. B. et al. (2001). Clinical relevance of the primary findings of the MTA: Success rates based on severity of ADHD and ODD symptoms at the end of treatment. *Journal of the American Academy of Child and Adolescent Psychiatry, 40*(2), 168–179.

Tingstrom, D. H. (1994). The good behavior game: An investigation of teachers' acceptance. *Psychology in the Schools, 31*, 57–65.

Webster-Stratton, C., Reid, J., & Hammond, M. (2001). Social skills and problem-solving training for children with early-onset conduct problems: Who benefits? *Journal of Child Psychology and Psychiatry, 42*, 945–952.

Whalen, C. K., & Henker, B. (1991). Therapies for hyperactive children: Comparisons, combinations, and compromises. *Journal of Consulting and Clinical Psychology, 59*, 126–137.

Whalen, C. K., & Henker, B. (1992). The social profile of attention-deficit hyperactivity disorder: Five fundamental facets. *Child and Adolescent Psychiatric Clinics of North America, 1*, 395–410.

Whalen, C. K., Henker, B., Collins, B. E., Finck, D., & Dotemoto, S. (1979). A social ecology of hyperactive boys: Medication effects in structured classroom environments. *Journal of Applied Behavior Analysis, 12*, 65–81.

Wheeler, J., & Carlson, C. L. (1994). The social functioning of children with ADD with hyperactivity and ADD without hyperactivity: A comparison of their peer relations and social deficits. *Journal of Emotional and Behavioral Disorders, 2*(1), 2–12.

Zentall, S. (1993). Research on the educational implications of attention deficit hyperactivity disorder. *Exceptional Children, 60*(2), 143–153.

Zentall, S., & Stormont-Spurgin, M. (1995). Educator preferences of accommodations for students with attention deficit hyperactivity disorder. *Teacher Education and Special Education, 18*(2), 115–123.

Student-Mediated Conflict Resolution Programs

CHARLES E. CUNNINGHAM
LESLEY J. CUNNINGHAM

This chapter begins with a discussion of the social relationships of children with ADHD, in which we emphasize the long-term impact of the conflict, rejection, and social isolation that these children often experience. Next, we introduce student-mediated conflict resolution programs and discuss the potential contribution of these programs to the management of children with ADHD. Finally, we outline the implementation and maintenance of this type of school-based intervention, and we consider emerging evidence regarding the short- and longer-term effectiveness of student mediation programs.

The active, inattentive, impulsive behavior of children with ADHD exerts an adverse effect on the social relationships that influence their development and adjustment (Deater-Deckard, 2001). During interactions with their peers, for example, children with ADHD are more physically active (Madan-Swain & Zentall, 1990), engage in higher rates of social interaction (Pelham & Bender, 1982; Whalen, Henker, Collins, Finck, & Dotemoto, 1979), and are more talkative (Madan-Swain & Zentall, 1990). Children with ADHD also disrupt conversational reciprocity (Clark, Cheyne, Cunningham, & Siegel, 1988), make fewer positive social

statements (Madan-Swain & Zentall, 1990), and engage in more controlling, uncooperative interaction (Clark et al., 1988; Cunningham & Siegel, 1987; Cunningham, Siegel, & Offord, 1985, 1991). These problems appear to emerge early, with parents rating preschoolers with ADHD as more aggressive (DeWolfe, Byrne, & Bawden, 2000) and less socially skilled (Alessandri, 1992; DeWolfe et al., 2000; DuPaul, McGoey, Eckert, & VanBrakle, 2001) than peers.

Peers evaluate children with ADHD more negatively (Erhardt & Hinshaw, 1994; Hinshaw, 2002; Hodgens, Cole, & Boldizar, 2000; Johnston, Pelham, & Murphy, 1985; Milich & Landau, 1982)—an effect that emerges after even brief periods of contact (Erhardt & Hinshaw, 1994). Peers withdraw from children with ADHD (Clark et al., 1988) and adopt a less positive, less cooperative, more controlling approach to them (Cunningham & Siegel, 1987; Cunningham et al., 1985, 1991). As a result, children with ADHD have fewer friends than peers (Blachman & Hinshaw, 2002). Rejection by peers has in turn been associated with a longitudinal increase in adjustment difficulties (Ladd & Troop-Gordon,

2003), aggressive behavior (Dodge et al., 2003), conduct problems (Miller-Johnson, Coie, Maumary-Gremaud, Bierman, & Conduct Problems Prevention Research Group, 2002), and victimization by peers (Deater-Deckard, 2001). In the face of rejection, children with ADHD may affiliate with more deviant peers—a pathway to more serious antisocial behavior in adolescence (Deater-Deckard, 2001; Marshal, Molina, & Pelham, 2003).

The social behavior of children with ADHD is associated with complex attributional and attitudinal processes. Boys with ADHD, for example, overestimate their performance in social situations (Hoza, Waschbusch, Pelham, Molina, & Milich, 2000). Although an overly positive self-concept may protect their self-esteem (Ohan & Johnston, 2002), it may insulate these children from the feedback of peers and increase the risk of aggressive behavior (David & Kistner, 2000). Children with ADHD are also less likely than controls to attribute social failures to effort, and more likely to attribute failures to uncontrollable factors (Hoza et al., 2000; Kaidar, Wiener, & Tannock, 2003). Not surprisingly, these children have more difficulty adjusting their behavior to the contextual demands that characterize peer group interactions (Landau & Milich, 1988; Whalen, Henker, Collins, McAuliffe, & Vaux, 1979).

Children with ADHD tend to interpret the behavior of peers as intentionally aggressive (Milich & Dodge, 1984)—an attributional bias they may share with their parents (MacBrayer, Milich, & Hundley, 2003). They also anticipate negative responses from peers, generate fewer negotiating strategies, and propose more aggressive solutions to social vignettes (Thurber, Heller, & Hinshaw, 2002).

Epidemiological studies suggest that 40–50% of children with ADHD evidence oppositional disorders or conduct problems, which may compound relationship difficulties (Hinshaw, 1987; Offord et al., 1987). Conduct problems often manifest themselves at school as arguments, threats, and fights. Aggressive boys with ADHD seem more intent on seeking attention, less interested in fairness in their relationships than peers (Melnick & Hinshaw, 1996), and particularly reactive to minor provocations (Waschbusch et al., 2002). In recreational settings, children with ADHD and conduct problems are more likely to reinforce peers for negative behavior (Onyango et al., 2003). The aggressive, uncooperative behavior

evidenced by some children with ADHD seems to be an important predictor of rejection by peers (Erhardt & Hinshaw, 1994; McArdle, O'Brien, Macmillan, & Kolvin, 2000; Mikami & Hinshaw, 2003).

A significant number of the types of conflicts, bullying episodes, and aggressive incidents characterizing the social relationships of children with ADHD occur in recess and playground settings, where adults have difficulty monitoring peer interactions (Olweus, 1994; Rivers & Smith, 1994; Whitney & Smith, 1993). Students, for example, report that teachers intervene in fewer than 5% of the bullying episodes that occur on school playgrounds—data supported by observational studies (Craig, Pepler, & Atlas, 2000; Cunningham et al., 1998). Under typical circumstances, other students are hesitant to interrupt these types of playground conflicts. As a result, most incidents are left unresolved or are dealt with counterproductively when students avoid conflicts or react coercively to disagreements (DeCecco & Richards, 1974). On those occasions when adults detect student conflicts, solutions are typically imposed (DeCecco & Richards, 1974).

LIMITS OF TRADITIONAL TREATMENT PROGRAMS

There are significant limits to the effectiveness of clinic-based social services for children with ADHD. Utilization studies suggest that a significant majority of children with mental health problems, such as ADHD, do not receive professional assistance (Offord et al., 1987; Pihlakoski et al., 2004; U.S. Department of Health and Human Services, 1999). Indeed, many parents of children who exhibit the types of aggressive behavior common in children with ADHD do not feel that professional assistance is needed (Boyle, 1991). Moreover, the parents of those children who are at greatest risk are least likely to enroll in or complete programs that might reduce aggressive behavior (Cunningham, Bremner, & Boyle, 1995; Cunningham et al., 2000; Kazdin, Holland & Crowley, 1997). When families do participate in parent training programs that reduce problems at home, these changes may not consistently generalize to difficulties at school (McNeil, Eyberg, Eisenstadt, Newcomb, & Funderburk, 1991).

STUDENT-MEDIATED CONFLICT RESOLUTION PROGRAMS

Reducing the severity of ADHD and its associated difficulties requires effective interventions addressing problems in home, school, and community settings. These interventions need to reach children whose families do not have access to services; to address issues that limit participation in existing services (Cunningham et al., 2000); to be acceptable to parents, teachers, and students (Greenberg et al., 2003); to be sustainable across the developmental period in which these problems emerge (Greenberg, 2004); and to be affordable to service providers. School-based, student-mediated conflict resolution (Cunningham & Cunningham, 1995; Cunningham et al., 1998) is a promising component in a more comprehensive effort to improve the social relationships of children with ADHD.

Types of Mediation Programs

Mediation programs train teams of older children to help peers solve conflicts (Cunningham, Cunningham, & Martorelli, 2001). "Online mediation," which is widely used in elementary schools, helps students negotiate solutions to conflicts occurring during recess or lunch periods. Mediators intervene in interpersonal conflicts, bullying episodes, and fights; offer students the opportunity to settle disputes; help negotiate resolutions; and plan strategies to prevent future problems (Cunningham et al., 2001). This chapter focuses primarily on the online approach to mediation.

"Office mediation" is typically used in conjunction with online mediation in middle school settings and is the model of choice in secondary and postsecondary settings. In office mediation programs, conflict resolution is conducted by two mediators in a private setting (Cunningham et al., 2001). Office mediation introduces a cooling-off period, affords the confidentiality needed to deal with more personal issues, provides an atmosphere free of playground distractions, allows the time needed to deal with complex disputes, and enables teams to deal with conflicts involving groups of students. Although students may seek the assistance of the office mediation team, teachers, principals, playground supervisors, or other students typically encourage disputants to make an appointment for office mediation. Office mediation may also be available as an alternative to disciplinary actions. For example, mediators may help students solve conflicts that might have resulted in detentions, suspensions, or juvenile justice system contacts. This is a highly specialized form of mediation in which disputants negotiate a solution, sign a contract, and propose alternative consequences.

"Schoolwide mediation" programs train *all* students in mediation, negotiation, and conflict resolution strategies (Johnson, Johnson, Dudley, & Burnett, 1992; Stevahn, Johnson, Johnson, & Schultz, 2002). Students are encouraged to apply these strategies to the solution of interpersonal conflicts occurring at home or school.

Preparing for a Student Mediation Program

The implementation of an effective school-based program such as student mediation requires support from parents, teachers, school administrators, and the students themselves (Greenberg et al., 2003). All of these stakeholders must be informed and consulted prior to the implementation of the program. Key preparatory steps and policy prerequisites are summarized in Table 16.1 and discussed below.

Implementation begins with a presentation to school administrators. Representatives of the mediation program describe the program, present a simulation, summarize evidence regarding the effectiveness of student mediation teams, and respond to questions. With administrative support, the program's representatives make a similar presentation to staff members from schools considering the introduction of the program. Experienced mediators often simulate the mediation of disputes, discuss the benefits of participation, and answer staff questions (e.g., "Was it worth the time?"). Finally, potential problems are considered. Teachers are often concerned about the response of other students to mediators, the demands that the mediation program might make on staff, and the extent to which the program might compete with academic priorities. Inviting teachers from schools that have conducted successful student mediation programs provides a helpful perspective on these issues. If schools elect to implement a student mediation program, a similar presentation is scheduled for parents and interested community members.

TABLE 16.1. Benchmarks of Effective Student-Mediated Conflict Resolution Programs

Stakeholder commitment
- Administration policy supporting mediation
- Majority teacher decision supporting mediation
- Parent–Teacher Organization decision supporting mediation

Policy prerequisites
- Targets of mediation identified
- Consequences for harassing mediators

The mediation team
- Skill-focused training program (12–15 hours)
- Adequate team size (i.e., eight mediators per recess period)
- Team captains

Supportive infrastructure
- Two mediation team champions
- Assembly launching the program
- Morning announcement
- Centrally posted team bulletin board
- Two *active* playground supervisors
- Weekly team meeting

Policy Prerequisites

The success of a student mediation program is built on a series of organizational and policy prerequisites. Before launching a program, therefore, schools considering a mediation program complete a detailed program-planning process. A selection of prerequisite benchmarks is presented in Table 16.1 and summarized below:

Disagreements regarding the types of problems warranting mediation will confuse students and undermine the mediation team's effectiveness. For example, although elementary and middle school mediation teams can reliably discriminate play fighting from more serious conflicts, there may be considerable disagreement as to whether incidents warrant intervention (Costabile et al., 1991; Smith, Hunter, Carvalho, & Costabile, 1992). Teachers, parents, and students, therefore, must establish a consensus regarding behaviors that should be targeted by the team.

Before mediation begins, disputants must agree to resolve the conflict. Although a con-

siderable majority of students agree to work with mediators (Cunningham et al., 1998), schools must develop an alternative response to disputants choosing not to resolve conflicts by mediation.

Student mediators are not immune to teasing by peers. Angry disputants may on occasion subject mediators to swearing or threats of aggressive behavior. Mediators who do not feel the active support of teachers and administrators are hesitant to intervene, more inclined to leave the team, and less likely to participate in next year's mediation program (Cunningham et al., 1998). Schools must identify unacceptable behaviors (e.g., staging fake conflicts, calling mediators names, threatening mediators, etc.) and the consequences of harassing a member of the mediation team.

Recruiting Student Mediators

The impact of elementary, middle school, and secondary mediation programs depends to a considerable extent on the school's success in recruiting a large team of competent, influential students. In our studies, mediators resolve approximately 90% of the conflicts in which they intervene (Cunningham et al., 1998). Because most individual interventions are successful, the impact of a playground mediation team will be a function of the proportion of conflicts that mediators detect and respond to. Online programs must deploy a team large enough to monitor all areas of the playground where conflicts occur, deal with simultaneous disputes, allow frequent rotation, and provide a reserve of backup mediators. Most schools require at least three teams of 8–10 mediators. Smaller teams intervene in fewer conflicts and reduce the impact of the program on playground aggression (Cunningham et al., 2001).

Recruitment begins with a presentation to students, in which representatives of the program introduce the concept of mediation, experienced student mediators demonstrate the conflict resolution process, and community representatives (e.g., police officers, judges, or spiritual leaders) discuss the importance of the mediation program. At the conclusion of this presentation, students in eligible grades are invited to volunteer for the mediation team. To ensure that the program meets the needs of a culturally and linguistically diverse community (Greenberg et al., 2003), teacher, parent, and student nominations increase the pool of potential mediators; ensure that the team reflects the gender, ethnic, and social composition of the school; and identify students who might benefit from participation.

Training Student Mediators

Elementary school mediation teams, which are typically composed of students from the fourth and fifth grades, require approximately 12 hours to complete the training program. Once a program is established, the time required to train the next generation of mediators can be reduced by apprenticing prospective mediators to experienced team members. Middle and secondary school teams master these skills more quickly and capitalize on the experience of incoming students who have served as elementary school mediators.

To facilitate skill acquisition, the training process is based on the cognitive-behavioral models that have proven most effective in trials of primary prevention mental health programs for children and adolescents (Durlak & Wells, 1997). Complex conflict resolution strategies are established sequentially, beginning with the first stage of the mediation process. Before the trainees proceed to the next component skill, the first step in the mediation process is rehearsed or "overlearned." Training begins with simple, easily recognized conflicts. As skill and confidence increase, role-playing exercises move toward more complex conflicts and commonly encountered mediation difficulties. To support the transfer of skills, modeling and role-playing exercises are conducted in context: Students rehearse the resolutions of the types of conflicts they are most likely to encounter, work with the other members of their teams, and master skills in playground field trials. Members of the training team model each step and give prompts, ensuring that component skills are rehearsed correctly. This accelerates skill acquisition, reduces frustration, and builds the confidence needed to deal effectively with actual playground conflicts. Throughout training, mediators carry a clipboard with a self-monitoring sheet listing the basic steps in the mediation process. Mediators make a check on this sheet as each step is completed. Forms provide students with prompts regarding the steps of mediation, while self-monitoring reinforces accurate follow-through.

Mediation training teams typically consist of an expert workshop leader, at least two teachers serving as the school's "program champions," experienced mediators, and interested parents. Training begins with an introduction to the training team and the school's program champions, followed by activities allowing prospective mediators to share information regarding themselves. Leaders present an overview of the mediation program and outline the steps of the mediation process. The steps in a standard playground mediation are summarized in Table 16.2.

Most mediation training time is devoted to the acquisition and mastery of component skills. Trainers discuss each skill, model its ap-

---

TABLE 16.2. Mediation Component Skill Checklist

- Mediator in assigned playground position before students arrive.
- Mediator in ready position, clipboard in hand, attending to peers.
- Mediator approaches disputants and asks whether problem has occurred.
- Mediator asks whether disputants are willing to solve the problem.
- Mediator finds a quiet area and seats disputants.
- Mediator introduces self and asks names of disputants (if necessary).
- Mediator reviews rules and secures agreement on each:
  - Disputants must remain with the mediator.
  - Mediator is neutral—won't take sides.
  - Disputants treat each other respectfully—listen without interrupting.
  - Disputants must tell the truth.
  - Disputants must solve the problem.
  - Disputants must abide by their agreement.
- Mediator asks Disputant 1 to tell story.
- Mediator summarizes Disputant 1's story.
- Mediator asks Disputant 2 to tell story.
- Mediator summarizes Disputant 2's story.
- Mediator asks disputants to suggest solutions.
- Mediator summarizes each solution.
- Disputants review pros and cons of each solution.
- Disputants choose a solution.
- Disputants plan when and how they will implement the solution.

plication, and give students an opportunity to rehearse the skill in role-playing exercises. Mediators practice detecting problems warranting mediation, behavior that should be ignored, and incidents that should be drawn to the attention of the playground supervisor (e.g., disputes involving weapons). Because playground conflicts may escalate rapidly, mediators must make the decision to intervene quickly and approach disputants confidently. Students complete this phase when they have mastered each component skill, executed all steps of the mediation process, rehearsed the resolution of disputes of increasing complexity, and practiced the mediation of simulated disputes in field conditions.

At each step of the dispute resolution process, mediators must remain neutral, listen carefully, summarize the content of disputant statements, reflect feelings, and facilitate problem solving. Once the basic components of the mediation program have been mastered, communication skills are strengthened via discussions, demonstrations, exercises, and role-playing activities. Fundamental concepts, such as mediator neutrality, are introduced as relevant skills are developed. Students build commitment to the program by formulating rationales supporting each component of the mediation process, key mediation concepts (e.g., "win–win solutions"), the overall benefits of mediation to their school, and their participation in the program.

Launching the Student Mediation Program

The launch of the mediation program contributes to its success by demonstrating administrative and community support, ensuring that all students understand the program, and creating momentum. Schools schedule an assembly of students, teachers, parents of mediators, and key community members to celebrate the graduation of the mediation team. The team is introduced; principals, senior school administrators, and community representatives discuss the importance of the mediation program; and diplomas are awarded. Mediators present skits illustrating the steps in the resolution of typical playground conflicts. Finally, the principal summarizes guidelines regarding the types of conflicts that will be the subject of mediation, the option of refusing mediation, and the consequences of harassing members of the mediation team.

Mediators are organized into teams of at least eight members balanced with respect to gender, grade, and ethnicity. Teams work together on playground duty and sit together during weekly meetings with the school's mediation champions. Each team has a captain selected from its oldest, most experienced, or influential members. Captains assist program champions and playground supervisors in ensuring that team members arrive before the start of recess, have the needed equipment (clipboards, forms, pencils, and uniforms), and are ready in their assigned positions. In addition, captains secure replacements when team members are absent, notify playground supervisors if mediators need assistance, and reinforce the team's efforts.

Introducing the program with a full complement of uniformed mediators on the playground supports success by ensuring that most incidents are detected before disputes escalate. The team's hats and vests allow students and supervisors to identify members of the team easily and provide visual reminders of the new program's goals.

The training team and school program champions should be present during the first several days of the program. On the first day, the champions review the targets of mediation, prompt the team to rehearse mediation strategies, prompt intervention, and provide supportive feedback. Over the next several days, the training team members shift responsibility for these tasks to playground supervisors and team captains, provide supportive feedback, fade their own presence, and remain available as resources.

The presence of the principal at the launch of the mediation program reminds students, mediators, and playground supervisors of the program's importance. Visits by administrative representatives (superintendents or trustees) during the first several weeks emphasize the school's commitment to the program and motivate successful implementation. The presence of representatives from local Parent–Teacher Organizations creates a sense of shared responsibility for the success of the mediation program.

Supporting a Mediation Program

At least two teachers serve as the program champions, as noted above. Champions contribute to the success of the mediation program by participating in training and conducting weekly team meetings encouraging skill development, acknowledging the team's efforts, and supporting the solution of the inevitable problems that mediators encounter. Champions organize events that are important in maintaining motivation, recruit mediators for the coming year's team, and organize spring training programs.

Online mediation teams require the support of at least two playground supervisors, who ensure that mediators arrive promptly, review mediation plans, and are assigned to locations where conflicts can be detected quickly. Playground supervisors deal with students who refuse mediation or harass team members, provide supportive feedback, and solve problems.

Morning announcements list the members of the mediation team on duty for the day, remind students of the program's goals, encourage students to seek the assistance of playground mediators or schedule an appointment for office mediation, support the team's efforts, and acknowledge successful conflict resolution. A centrally located bulletin board features the program's logo, team pictures, student posters supporting the program, and newspaper articles illustrating the application of mediation to current events (e.g., labor disputes or international negotiations). A graph plotting the number of mediations completed successfully each week recognizes the team's accomplishments.

Teachers support the program by linking classroom discussions of history, literature, and current events to the goals of the mediation program. Teachers use mediation strategies to resolve classroom disputes, or they encourage students needing assistance to arrange an appointment with the office mediation team.

Mediation teams function best when responsibilities are delegated to students with different interests and talents. Students interested in art and graphic design prepare advertising materials; those with quantitative skills manage data and prepare figures depicting the weekly performance of the team; "coaches" organize preventive playground games and activities; and captains provide supervision and support. To increase local ownership of the mediation program (Spoth, Greenberg, Bierman, & Redmond, 2004), schools establish an advisory committee composed of parents, teacher champions, and mediation team representatives. The advisory committee supports the team, conducts fund raising, and contributes to the stability of the program by ensuring that departing teacher champions are replaced. In our region, the Collaborative Student Mediation Project—a partnership of school social workers with expertise in the implementation of mediation programs, school administrators, representatives of community children's mental health service providers, and university researchers—meets regularly. This group ensures the integrity of the program, solves problems, considers innovations, plans program evaluations, revises implementation manuals and supporting materials (Cunningham et al., 2001), organizes training programs for school interested in introducing mediation programs, and conducts areawide workshops for mediators. This links internal and external capacity and resources (Spoth et al., 2004), encourages service integration, builds a sense of community ownership, and provides the technical support needed to sustain this type of innovative school-based service (Greenberg, 2004; Greenberg et al., 2003; Spoth et al., 2004).

Monitoring a Peer Mediation Program

Mediation team coaches and champions actively monitor implementation of the program. Mediators may need additional training; implementation may drift as mediators adopt inappropriate conflict resolution strategies (e.g., taking sides); or schools may introduce modifications that inadvertently compromise the program's effectiveness (Cunningham et al., 1998; Greenberg, 2004). As aggressive behavior declines, mediators may become bored and distracted, or playground supervisors may neglect their responsibility to support the program.

Mediators complete a monitoring sheet documenting the process and outcome of each intervention. Monitoring forms list the steps of the dispute resolution process and encourage reliable implementation. Champions review monitoring forms at weekly team meetings and help the team's student statisticians compile and plot successful mediations for a poster on the team's bulletin board. To ensure fidelity, mediation program coaches visit each site at least once weekly during the initial stages of the program's implementation, complete a benchmark monitoring form, and provide feedback to the teacher champions and mediators.

Sustaining a Student Mediation Program

It is difficult to sustain the effects of school-based interventions for children with ADHD (Shelton et al., 2000). To achieve their potential long-term impact on conflict resolution skills, student attitudes, school norms, and school aggression, mediation programs must be conducted consistently from September to June and must be sustained through the elementary, middle school, and secondary years (Greenberg, 2004; Greenberg et al., 2003).

In the spring, the team's teacher champions recruit new student mediators for the upcoming school year and conduct a spring training program. Experienced members of the team assist in modeling and role-playing exercises, while apprentice mediators shadow competent members of the team, monitor each step of the dispute resolution process, intervene in simple conflicts, and attend weekly team meetings. A fall assembly introduces the mediation team to incoming students and launches the new year's program. A team member and an administrator meet students transferring into the school during the year, discuss the school's commitment to nonviolent conflict resolution, and outline the mediation process.

Because most team members plan to participate as mediators in the upcoming year (Cunningham et al., 1998), teacher champions facilitate contact with the mediation programs in middle or secondary schools to which graduating students are transferring. Stability in the mediation team membership contributes to the maintenance of the program's effects, supports the development of middle and secondary school programs by capitalizing on the skill and experience mediators have acquired, and facilitates the vertical integration of the program within the school system (Greenberg, 2004).

ENHANCING THE EFFECTIVENESS OF MEDIATION PROGRAMS

A key to developing effective school-based interventions is to avoid fragmentation by integrating universal prevention, indicated prevention, and targeted clinical services (Greenberg, 2004). There are several ways in which universal programs such as student mediation can be enriched to target the needs of high-risk stu-dents. Champions, for example, assign older, socially influential mediators to areas where more serious conflicts occur. Mediations involving more challenging disputants are conducted by two experienced members of the team. The individual behavioral contracts and daily report cards of high-risk students may include goals supporting successful participation in conflict resolution.

Office mediation allows the team to resolve chronic playground difficulties, relationally complex disputes, problems requiring a cooling-off period, or conflicts involving groups of students. The success of office mediation may be enhanced by selecting the team's most experienced members; identifying mediators reflecting the gender, cultural, and ethnic background of the disputants; and devoting more time to the conflict resolution process. Contracts among disputants, principals, and referring teachers ensure that a mutually acceptable solution is reached, specify the steps needed to resolve the problem, and state the consequences if the agreement is violated.

Children with ADHD and related disruptive behavior disorders often volunteer to join mediation teams. Indeed, some schools actively recruit a small number of high-risk students or negative leaders to their mediation teams. The successful inclusion of challenging mediators requires adjustments in training, monitoring, and support. During training, high-risk mediators are grouped with influential team members, positioned in close proximity to the trainers, and involved actively (via eye contact, prompts, and reinforcers). During implementation, high-risk mediators are placed on teams with strong captains, paired with older more influential team members, positioned in close proximity to playground supervisors, and provided with more frequent prompts and reinforcers. Daily report cards with individually negotiated goals and incentives provide additional support and encouragement. In view of the potential benefits of participation on the mediation team, suspension from the team is a last resort for disciplinary problems.

Finally, parents are invited to participate in a skill-building workshop designed to increase their understanding of the process of mediation, develop the skills needed to apply mediation to conflicts between siblings and peers at home, encourage the transfer of skills and attitudes from the school to the home, and increase their support for the mediation program.

RELATED INTERVENTIONS

Mediation programs are more likely to make a meaningful contribution to the management of ADHD in children when included as a component of a comprehensive program of effective treatments. Small clinical groups (Pfiffner & McBurnett, 1997; Webster-Stratton, Reid, & Hammond, 2001), classwide (DeRosier, 2004) or schoolwide (Hundert et al., 1999) social skills training programs, friendship interventions (Hoza, Mrug, Pelham, Greiner, & Gnagy, 2003), or broader school-based programs focusing on social competence (Barkley et al., 2000) may contribute to improved relationships with peers. The parenting programs described in Chapters 12–14 provide the strategies families need to encourage the application of newly acquired conflict resolution skills at home, improve sibling and peer relationships, and support the individualized contracts or daily report cards needed by some members of the mediation team. Finally, the effects of stimulant medication on sustained attention, self-regulation, and conflict with peers (Cunningham et al., 1985, 1991; Hinshaw, Buhrmester, & Heller, 1989) may permit children with ADHD who have more significant difficulties to benefit from the assistance of playground mediators, or to capitalize on the skill-building and relationship-building opportunities provided by membership on the mediation team.

BENEFITS OF STUDENT MEDIATION PROGRAMS

Student-mediated conflict resolution programs have several potential benefits of special interest in the management of children with ADHD and related disruptive behavior disorders. First, online mediation programs operate during recesses, when monitoring and intervention by teachers are low and when the risk of conflict, bullying, and aggressive behavior is high (Craig et al., 2000; Olweus, 1991). Craig et al. (2000) found that teachers dealt with only 15% of the incidents recorded on videotaped playground observations. Teams of mediators positioned strategically on the playground can detect emerging conflicts, offer mediation at a

point where a successful resolution can be easily reached, and prevent the minor disputes and provocations that seem to prompt aggressive responses from children with ADHD and comorbid conduct problems (Waschbusch et al., 2002) from escalating to more serious incidents. As one young student mediator noted, "Mediators solve problems when they are little, not big."

Although boys are more physically aggressive, conflict between girls often occurs at the relational level (Cairns, Cairns, Neckerman, Gest, & Gariepy, 1988; Crick, Bigbee, & Howes, 1996; Crick & Dodge, 1994; Crick & Grotpeter, 1995; Crick & Nelson, 2002). Girls with ADHD engage in more relational aggression than peers (Blachman & Hinshaw, 2002; Zalecki & Hinshaw, 2004). Like physical aggression, relational aggression (i.e., damaging or manipulating peer relationships) emerges early (Crick, Casas, & Ku, 1999), is motivated by anger and the intent to harm (Crick et al., 1996), is linked to peer rejection, and is associated with poor adjustment (Crick & Grotpeter, 1995). Although boys find physical provocations more upsetting, girls are more distressed by relational provocations (Crick et al., 1996; Crick, Grotpeter, & Bigbee, 2002). Although it is more difficult for adults to detect relational aggression than physical aggression, girls on mediation teams seem more adept at recognizing these events and intervening in relational conflicts than boys (Cunningham et al., 1998).

Conducting mediation in the playground and peer group contexts where conflicts are most likely to occur may deal with the generalization failures noted in many school-based interventions (Hundert, 1995; Pepler, Craig, & Roberts, 1995). Although self-regulatory difficulties (Barkley, 1997a, 1997b) may limit the likelihood that children with ADHD will spontaneously apply conflict resolution skills to their own disputes, playground mediators are highly visible reminders of the goals of the school's conflict resolution program. Moreover, since mediators intervene to support conflict resolution, the disputes that children with ADHD inevitably encounter are more likely to be resolved successfully.

As noted earlier in this chapter, student mediation can be a schoolwide or universal program benefiting all students (Offord, Kraemer, Kazdin, Jensen, & Harrington, 1998). The potential benefits of such mediation programs are not compromised by the low utilization and high dropout rates observed in programs requiring parental participation (Barkley et al., 2000; Cunningham et al., 1995, 2000; Kazdin et al., 1997). Universal programs eliminate the risk of false-positive or false-negative screening errors (Offord et al., 1998), are less likely to stigmatize students (Harris, Milich, Corbitt, Hoover, & Brady, 1992), and avoid the risks of aggregating high-risk children in treatment groups (Dishion, McCord, & Poulin, 1999). Even when mediation is a universal program, children with ADHD—who are involved in more frequent playground incidents and often lack both the knowledge and skill to solve interpersonal conflicts (Grenell, Glass, & Katz, 1987)—inevitably receive additional dispute resolution practice. This combination of universal and targeted programming represents an ideal approach to both prevention and treatment (Greenberg, 2004; Offord et al., 1998).

The relational problems of children with ADHD emerge in the preschool years (DeWolfe et al., 2000; Gadow & Nolan, 2002). Moreover, the hostile attitudes and attributional biases that link early childhood aggression to adolescent conduct problems emerge over time (Deater-Deckard, 2001). Although mediation teams deal with the conflicts of children at all grade levels, we (Cunningham et al., 1998) demonstrated that a majority of interventions by mediation teams dealt with conflicts between students in the first and second grades. Elementary school programs introducing students in the early grades to alternative conflict resolution strategies, therefore, may contribute to the prevention of the relational problems and aggression that are common in some children with ADHD. Recent evidence suggests that to achieve longer-term effects, school-based interventions for children with ADHD must be sustained (Barkley et al., 2000; Shelton et al., 2000). When mediation programs are conducted in middle and secondary school settings, the impact of elementary school mediation programs can be maintained and extended to the relationship problems children with ADHD evidence in adolescence (Bagwell, Molina, Pelham, & Hoza, 2001).

Because mediation is conducted by students with the support of a small number of school staff members, this program places less of a logistical burden on schools than programs requiring the participation of all teachers do. Indeed, mediation programs are perceived by teachers to be logistically manageable, endorsed by administrators, and supported by parents (Cunningham et al., 1998). The probability that these programs will be disseminated, adopted, and sustained is high.

PLACING HIGH-RISK STUDENTS ON THE MEDIATION TEAM

A promising dimension of student-mediated conflict resolution is its potential impact on mediators who have difficulty with social relationships or interpersonal conflict. As noted earlier, a percentage of the students volunteering for most mediation programs evidence a history of disruptive behavior disorders. Trainers and school program champions suggest that in small numbers, students with disruptive behavior disorders such as ADHD can be accommodated on, and may make a contribution to, the mediation team. Several lines of evidence suggest mechanisms via which students with ADHD and related disruptive behavior disorders might benefit from participation as mediators.

First, playground mediation responsibilities reduce opportunities for relationally or physically aggressive behavior during times when monitoring and supervision by adults are low (Fowler, Dougherty, Kirby, & Kohler, 1986).

Second, mediation programs provide students with opportunities to develop and rehearse communication and conflict resolution skills that may build relationships with peers and improve the children's responsiveness to interventions by parents or teachers. Mediators participate in 12–15 hours of training and meet weekly with the teachers who are program champions for continuing skill development and support. In elementary schools, mediators intervene in up to 60 playground conflicts per year with the support of team captains and playground supervisors.

Third, some children with ADHD evidence a hostile attributional bias (Dodge, 1983; Dodge & Frame, 1982; Milich & Dodge, 1984), which may contribute to their relational and physical conflict with peers (Crick et al., 2002). Mediation training, weekly problem-solving discussions, and the dispute resolution process expose mediators to alternative explanations regarding the causes of aggressive interactions. Summarizing the stories of peers and reflecting the feelings of disputants may increase social knowledge and enhance perspective-taking skills.

Fourth, peer group affiliations exert a strong influence on the development of antisocial attitudes and behavior (Deater-Deckard, 2001). In contrast to the potential problems associated with programs grouping children with high-risk peers (Dishion et al., 1999), members of the mediation team are exposed to a large group of socially influential students whose norms encourage cooperation with teachers, supportive interactions with peers, and nonaggressive solutions to social conflict (Kinderman, 1993). The skills, attitudes, and status students acquire via membership on the mediation team may alter their reputations (Harris et al., 1992; Hymel, 1986; Hymel, Wagner, & Butler, 1990) and reduce peer rejection (Dodge, 1983; Dodge et al., 2003). This may enable children with ADHD to join prosocial peer groups, override the tendency of rejected children to affiliate with deviant peers (Deater-Deckard, 2001), and moderate the influence of deviant peers on conduct problems (Vitaro, Brendgen, & Tremblay, 2000). This is consistent with studies supporting the benefits of friendship interventions pairing children with ADHD and peers with lower antisocial behavior (Hoza et al., 2003).

Although children with ADHD sometimes protect their self-esteem (Ohan & Johnston, 2002) with positive illusory biases in social situations (Hoza et al., 2000), overly positive self-perceptions have been linked to aggressive behavior (David & Kistner, 2000). Ohan and Johnston (2002) showed that the type of support and recognition and support student mediators receive from teachers and classmates may reduce the use of counterproductive illusory biases.

Finally, mediation is the type of school-based extracurricular program that establishes positive social networks and connections to the school, which in turn reduce secondary school dropout in high-risk students (Mahoney & Cairns, 1997).

TRIALS OF STUDENT MEDIATION PROGRAMS

Although descriptive reports suggest that mediators reduce playground conflict (Cameron

& Dupuis, 1991; Johnson et al., 1992; Koch, 1988; Lane & McWhirter, 1992; Welch, 1989), there are few controlled studies of these programs (Hundert, 1995). Johnson, Johnson, Dudley, Ward, and Magnuson (1995) studied the impact of a student mediation program on 144 elementary school students. Students reported 209 personal conflicts at school and 574 at home. Students in the training program were more likely to report using an integrative negotiating procedure to resolve conflicts at school. Moreover, students reported that conflict resolution strategies acquired at school were applied to conflicts at home—observations consistent with the findings of Gentry and Benenson (1993), who noted that parents of children receiving mediation training reported a reduction in the frequency and intensity of their children's conflicts with siblings.

Stevahn et al. (2002) studied the integration of a 5-week conflict resolution and peer mediation training program into the high school social studies curriculum. Students receiving training showed better skill acquisition, applied conflict resolution and peer mediation strategies more completely, chose an integrative approach to negotiation, and reported more positive attitudes about conflict. Trained students also scored higher in the social studies course, retained more material, and showed improved transfer of knowledge between study areas.

We (Cunningham et al., 1998) completed a controlled trial of an elementary school student mediation program. Teams of fifth-grade students were trained to mediate conflicts during recess periods. A multiple-baseline (Hersen & Barlow, 1978) design was used to determine the effects of student mediation on direct observations of physically aggressive playground interactions. Mediators successfully resolved 90% of the more than 1,010 playground conflicts in which they intervened. Figure 16.1 shows that student-mediated conflict resolution reduced direct observations of physically aggressive playground behavior by from 51% to approximately 65%. These effects were sustained at 1-year follow-up observations. Teachers reported that mediation teams reduced playground conflict, limited spillover of playground problems to the classroom, and decreased the number of children disciplined at school (Cunningham et al., 1998). Teacher and mediator satisfaction questionnaires provided

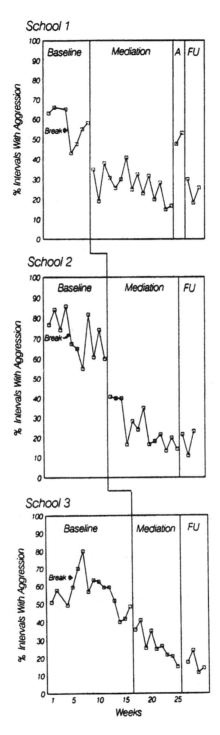

FIGURE 16.1. Percentage of 120 intervals in which physically aggressive behavior was observed each week during baseline, student mediation, and follow-up (FU) conditions at three elementary schools. "A" indicates an unplanned reversal when the mediation team was reduced from eight to two members. From Cunningham et al. (1998). Copyright 1998 by the *Journal of Child Psychology and Psychiatry*. Reprinted by permission.

strong support for the social validity of this program—a particularly important issue in the development of effective interventions that are acceptable in community contexts (Coie, 1996; Hoagwood, Hibbs, Brent, & Jensen, 1995; Hundert, 1995; Kendall & Southam-Gerow, 1995; Offord, 1996).

Although most staff members felt that these programs had a positive impact on student mediators (Cunningham et al., 1998), the potential benefits of joining mediation teams in general and their particular impact on students with ADHD require further study. Moreover, the inclusion of children with ADHD as members of the mediation team poses several major challenges to coaches and champions. These children's attentional and self-regulatory deficits may impair the acquisition of complex mediation strategies. Poor sustained concentration may also hinder the detection of conflicts in highly distracting playground contexts. Finally, children with ADHD evidence social skills deficits (Clark et al., 1988; Cunningham & Siegel, 1987; Cunningham et al., 1991), which may adversely affect their relationships with members of the mediation team or impair their performance as mediators.

IMPROVING THE EFFECTIVENESS OF STUDENT MEDIATION PROGRAMS

School-based programs, such as student mediation, must be adjusted to reflect the mission, priorities, and culture of individual schools (Greenberg et al., 2003). Efforts to implement school-based interventions must often trade off the need to maintain the integrity of an evidence-based program against the desire of educators to make modifications (Greenberg, 2004). Some modifications may, indeed, enhance the effectiveness of school-based programs. A school participating in our studies, for example, suggested the role of team captains. Team captains are selected from the oldest and most socially influential members of the team; they ensure that mediators are positioned strategically, equipped with their vests and clipboards, and attentive to conflict on the playground. Captains prompt interventions, assist mediators in dealing with difficult students, and reinforce successful mediations. In subsequent implementation studies, schools introducing mediation teams without captains re-

duced playground aggression to 17% of direct observation intervals; those with captains reduced aggression to only 5% of observation intervals (Cunningham & Cunningham, 2001). This appeared to be mediated by an increase in the attention mediators devoted to detecting events warranting intervention. Captains, therefore, are another implementation benchmark in our program (Cunningham et al., 2001).

In other cases, educators may introduce modifications that compromise the fidelity and effectiveness of the mediation program (Greenberg, 2004). We (Cunningham et al., 1998), for example, found that staff reduced the size of a playground mediation team from eight mediators per recess to two mediators per recess period, on the assumption that very little conflict was occurring. Although direct observations showed an increase in playground aggression from 28% to 50% of recess observation intervals, the staff responsible for this change did not detect an increase in aggression. When the size of the playground team on duty was increased to the minimum of eight mediators per recess period, aggression declined from 50% to 25% of observation intervals. An Ontario provincial survey of 65 mediation programs found that only 20% employed a team of more than four mediators; this suggests that the effectiveness of many well-intentioned mediation programs may be limited (Cunningham, Bohaychuk, & Cunningham, 1997). A team size of at least eight mediators per recess period is, therefore, an implementation benchmark in our program (Cunningham et al., 2001).

Finally, the impact of a mediation program on the persistent relationship difficulties evidenced by children with ADHD should be a function of the long-term stability of these programs. Although the teachers serving as program champions who recruit and train a new generation of mediators are responsible for the continuation of these programs, 44% of the programs in our provincial survey reported that only a single teacher supervised the mediation team (Cunningham et al., 1997). These mediation programs are vulnerable, should supervising teachers assume other responsibilities or transfer to another school. Accordingly, a team of at least two program champions supported by a parent–teacher advisory council is another implementation benchmark of our program (Cunningham et al., 2001).

SUMMARY

Our studies suggest that student mediated conflict resolution reduces the types of conflicts that children with ADHD encounter in playground settings. Converging evidence from teachers, parents, and mediators suggests that in addition to the mediation program's primary effects on playground aggression, participation as members of the mediation team may have a significant impact on high-risk students. In an era of unprecedented reductions in clinical resources, these programs deserve careful consideration and further study.

KEY CLINICAL POINTS

✓ The poorly regulated impulsive behavior of children with ADHD contributes to poor relationships with peers.

✓ The relational problems of children with ADHD are compounded by comorbid oppositional or conduct problems.

✓ Children with ADHD are often rejected by peers and may be either the targets or perpetrators of bullying and aggressive behavior.

✓ Many of the bullying and aggressive incidents that children with ADHD are involved in occur on school playgrounds.

✓ Adults detect and intervene in a very small percentage of playground incidents.

✓ Older students trained as mediators can help students resolve playground conflicts.

✓ Playground mediation teams detect a greater percentage of conflicts than adults, respond before problems escalate, and successfully resolve 90% of the incidents in which they intervene.

✓ Observational studies show that mediation teams can reduce playground aggression by more than 50%.

✓ With additional training, supervision, and support, children with ADHD may be able to serve as members of mediation teams.

✓ Evidence from teachers, parents, and mediators suggests that in addition to the mediation program's primary effects on playground aggression, participation as members of the mediation team may have a significant impact on high-risk students.

REFERENCES

Alessandri, S. M. (1992). Attention, play, and social behavior in ADHD preschoolers. *Journal of Abnormal Child Psychology, 20,* 289–302.

Bagwell, C. L., Molina, B. S., Pelham, W. E., Jr., & Hoza, B. (2001). Attention-deficit hyperactivity disorder and problems in peer relations: Predictions from childhood to adolescence. *Journal of the American Academy of Child and Adolescent Psychiatry, 40,* 1285–1292.

Barkley, R. A. (1997a). Behavioral inhibition, sustained attention, and executive functions: Constructing a unifying theory of ADHD. *Psychological Bulletin, 121,* 65–94.

Barkley, R. A. (1997b). *ADHD and the nature of self-control.* New York: Guilford Press.

Barkley, R. A., Shelton, T. L., Crosswait, C., Moorehouse, M., Fletcher, K., Barrett, S., et al. (2000). Multimethod psychoeducational intervention for preschool children with disruptive behavior: Preliminary results at post-treatment. *Journal of Child Psychology and Psychiatry, 41,* 319–332.

Blachman, D. R., & Hinshaw, S. P. (2002). Patterns of friendship among girls with and without attention-deficit/hyperactivity disorder. *Journal of Abnormal Child Psychology, 30,* 625–640.

Boyle, M. H. (1991). Children's mental health issues: Prevention and treatment. In L. C. Johnson & D. Barnhorst (Eds.), *Children, families and public policy in the 90's.* Toronto: Thompson Educational.

Cairns, R. B., Cairns, B. D., Neckerman, H. J., Gest, S. D., & Gariepy, J. L. (1988). Social networks and aggressive behavior: Peer support or peer rejection? *Developmental Psychology, 24,* 815–823.

Cameron, J., & Dupuis, A. (1991). The introduction of school mediation to New Zealand. *Journal of Research and Development in Education, 24,* 1–13.

Clark, M. L., Cheyne, A. J., Cunningham, C. E., & Siegel, L. S. (1988). Dyadic peer interaction and task orientation in attention-deficit disordered children. *Journal of Abnormal Child Psychology, 16,* 1–15.

Coie, J. D. (1996). Prevention of violence and antisocial behavior. In R. D. Peters & R. McMahon (Eds.), *Preventing childhood disorders, substance abuse, and delinquency* (pp. 1–18). Thousand Oaks, CA: Sage.

Costabile, A., Smith, P. K., Matheson, L., Aston, J., Hunter, T., & Boulton, M. (1991). Cross-national comparison of how children distinguish serious and playful fighting. *Developmental Psychology, 27,* 881–887.

Craig, W. M., Pepler, D. J., & Atlas, R. (2000). Observations of bullying in the classroom and on the playground. *School Psychology International, 21,* 22–36.

Crick, N. R., Bigbee, M.A., & Howes, C. (1996). Gender differences in children's normative beliefs about aggression: How do I hurt thee? Let me count the ways. *Child Development, 67,* 1007–1014.

Crick, N. R., Casas, J. F., & Ku, H. (1999). Relational

and physical forms of peer victimization in preschool, *Developmental Psychology, 35,* 376–385.

Crick, N. R., & Dodge, K. A. (1994). A review and reformulation of social information processing mechanisms in children's social development. *Psychological Bulletin, 115,* 47–101.

Crick, N. R., & Grotpeter, J. K. (1995). Relational aggression, gender, and social-psychological adjustment. *Child Development, 66,* 710–722.

Crick, N. R., Grotpeter, J. K., & Bigbee, M. A. (2002). Relationally and physically aggressive children's intent attributions and feelings of distress for relational and instrumental peer provocations. *Child Development, 73,* 1134–1142.

Crick, N. R., & Nelson, D. A. (2002). Relational and physical victimization within friendships: Nobody told me there'd be friends like these. *Journal of Abnormal Child Psychology, 30,* 599–607.

Cunningham, C. E., Bohaychuk, D., & Cunningham, L. J. (1997). *Peer mediation: Survey of Ontario schools.* Toronto: Ontario Ministry of Education, Violence Prevention Secretariat.

Cunningham, C. E., Boyle, M., Offord, D., Racine, Y., Hundert, J., Secord, M., et al. (2000). Tri Ministry Project: Diagnostic and demographic correlates of school-based parenting course utilization. *Journal of Consulting and Clinical Psychology, 68,* 928–933.

Cunningham, C. E., Bremner, R. B., & Boyle, M. (1995). Large group school-based courses for parents of preschoolers at risk for disruptive behavior disorders: Utilization, outcome, and cost effectiveness. *Journal of Child Psychology and Psychiatry, 36,* 1141–1159.

Cunningham, C. E., & Cunningham, L. J. (1995). Reducing playground aggression: Student mediation programs. *ADHD Report, 3,* 9–11.

Cunningham, C. E., & Cunningham, L. J. (2001). Enhancing the effectiveness of student-mediated conflict resolution programs. *Emotional and Behavioral Disorders in Youth, 2,* 7–22.

Cunningham, C. E., Cunningham, L. J., & Martorelli, V. (2001). *Coping with conflict at school: The Collaborative Student Mediation Project manual.* Hamilton, Ontario, Canada: COPE Works.

Cunningham, C. E., Cunningham, L. J., Martorelli, V., Tran, A., Young, J., & Zacharias, R. (1998). The effects of a primary division student mediation program on playground aggression. *Journal of Child Psychology and Psychiatry, 39,* 653–662.

Cunningham, C. E., & Siegel, L. S. (1987). Peer interactions of normal and attention-deficit disordered boys during free-play, cooperative task, and simulated classroom situations. *Journal of Abnormal Child Psychology, 15,* 247–268.

Cunningham, C. E., Siegel, L. S., & Offord, D. R. (1985). A developmental dose response analysis of the efforts of methylphenidate on the peer interactions of attention deficit disordered boys. *Journal of Child Psychology and Psychiatry, 26,* 955–971.

Cunningham, C. E., Siegel, L. S., & Offord, D. R. (1991). A dose–response analysis of the effects of methylphenidate on the peer interactions and simulated classroom performance of ADD children with and without conduct problems. *Journal of Child Psychology and Psychiatry, 32,* 439–452.

David, C. F., & Kistner, J. (2000). Do positive self-perceptions have a "dark side"?: Examination of the link between perceptual bias and aggression. *Journal of Abnormal Child Psychology, 28,* 327–337.

Deater-Deckard, K. (2001). Annotation: Recent research examining the role of peer relationships in the development of psychopathology. *Journal of Child Psychology and Psychiatry, 42,* 565–579.

DeCecco, J., & Richards, A. (1974). *Growing pains: Uses of school conflict.* New York: Aberdeen.

DeRosier, M. E. (2004). Building relationships and combating bullying: Effectiveness of a school-based social skills group intervention. *Journal of Clinical Child and Adolescent Psychology, 33,* 196–201.

DeWolfe, N., Byrne, J. M., & Bawden, H. N. (2000). ADHD in preschool children: Parent-rated psychosocial correlates. *Developmental Medicine and Child Neurology, 42,* 825–830.

Dishion, T. J., McCord, J., & Poulin, F. (1999). When interventions harm: Peer groups and problem behavior. *American Psychologist, 54,* 755–764.

Dodge, K. A. (1983). Behavioral antecedents of peer social status. *Child Development, 54,* 1386–1399.

Dodge, K. A., & Frame, C. L. (1982). Social cognitive biases and deficits in aggressive boys. *Child Development, 55,* 163–173.

Dodge, K. A., Lansford, J. E., Burks, V. S., Bates, J. E., Pettit, G. S., Fontaine, R., et al. (2003). Peer rejection and social information-processing factors in the development of aggressive behavior problems in children. *Child Development, 74,* 374–393.

DuPaul, G. J., McGoey, K. E., Eckert, T. L., & VanBrakle, J. (2001). Preschool children with attention-deficit/hyperactivity disorder: Impairments in behavioural, social, and school functioning. *Journal of the American Academy of Child and Adolescent Psychiatry, 40,* 508–515.

Durlak, J. A., & Wells, A. M. (1997). Primary prevention mental health programs for children and adolescents: A meta-analytic review. *American Journal of Community Psychology, 25,* 115–152.

Erhardt, D., & Hinshaw, S. P. (1994). Initial sociometric impressions of attention-deficit hyperactivity disorder and comparison boys: Predictions from social behavior and from nonbehavioral variables. *Journal of Consulting and Clinical Psychology, 62,* 833–842.

Fowler, S. A., Dougherty, B. S., Kirby, K. C., & Kohler, F. W. (1986). Role reversals: An analysis of therapeutic effects achieved with disruptive boys during their appointments as peer monitors. *Journal of Applied Behavior Analysis, 19,* 437–444.

Gadow, K. D., & Nolan, E. E. (2002). Differences between preschool children with ODD, ADHD and

ODD+ADHD symptoms. *Journal of Child Psychology and Psychiatry, 43,* 191–201.

Gentry, D. B., & Benenson, W. A. (1993). School-to-home transfer of conflict management skills among school-age children. *Families in Society: The Journal of Contemporary Human Services, 74,* 67–73.

Greenberg, M. T. (2004). Current and future challenges in school-based prevention: The researcher perspective. *Prevention Science, 5,* 5–13.

Greenberg, M. T., Weissberg, R. P., O'Brien, M. U., Zins, J. E., Fredricks, L., Resnik, H., et al. (2003). Enhancing school-based prevention and youth development through coordinated social, emotional, and academic learning. *American Psychologist, 58,* 466–474.

Grenell, M. M., Glass, C. R., & Katz, K. S. (1987). Hyperactive children and peer interaction: knowledge and performance of social skills. *Journal of Abnormal Child Psychology, 15,* 1–13.

Harris, M. J., Milich, R., Corbitt, E. M., Hoover, D. W., & Brady, M. (1992). Self-fulfilling effects of stigmatising information on children's social interactions. *Journal of Personality and Social Psychology, 63,* 41–50.

Hersen, M., & Barlow, D. H. (1978). *Single case experimental design: Strategies for studying behavior change.* New York: Pergamon Press.

Hinshaw, S. P. (1987). On the distinction between attentional deficit/hyperactivity and conduct problems/aggression in child psychopathology. *Psychological Review, 101,* 443–463.

Hinshaw, S. P. (2002). Preadolescent girls with attention-deficit/hyperactivity disorder: I. Background characteristics, comorbidity, cognitive and social functioning, and parenting practices. *Journal of Consulting and Clinical Psychology, 70,* 1086–1098.

Hinshaw, S. P., Buhrmester, D., & Heller, T. (1989). Anger control in response to verbal provocation: Effects of stimulant medication for boys with ADHD. *Journal of Abnormal Child Psychology, 17,* 393–407.

Hoagwood, K., Hibbs, E., Brent, D., & Jensen, P. (1995). Introduction to the special section: Efficacy and effectiveness in studies of child adolescent psychotherapy. *Journal of Consulting and Clinical Psychology, 63,* 683–687.

Hodgens, J. B., Cole, J., & Boldizar, J. (2000). Peer-based differences among boys with ADHD. *Journal of Clinical Child Psychology, 29,* 443–452.

Hoza, B., Mrug, S., Pelham, W. E., Jr., Greiner, A. R., & Gnagy, E. M. (2003). A friendship intervention for children with attention-deficit/hyperactivity disorder: Preliminary findings. *Journal of Attention Disorders, 6,* 87–98.

Hoza, B., Waschbusch, D. A., Pelham, W. E., Molina, B. S., & Milich, R. (2000). Attention-deficit /hyperactivity disordered and control boys' responses to social success and failure. *Child Development, 71,* 432–446.

Hundert, J. (1995). *Enhancing social competence in young students.* Austin, TX: PRO-ED.

Hundert, J., Boyle, M. H., Cunningham, C. E., Duku, E., Heale, J., McDonald, J., et al. (1999). Helping children adjust—A Tri-Ministry Study: II. Program effects. *Journal of Child Psychology and Psychiatry, 40,* 1061–1073.

Hymel, S. (1986). Interpretations of peer behavior: affective bias in childhood and adolescence. *Child Development, 57,* 431–445.

Hymel, S., Wagner, E., & Butler, L. J. (1990). Reputational bias: View from the peer group. In S. R. Asher & J. D. Coie (Eds.), *Peer rejection in childhood* (pp. 156–186). New York: Cambridge University Press.

Johnson, D. W., Johnson, R. T., Dudley, B., & Burnett, R. (1992). Teaching students to be peer mediators. *Educational Leadership, 50,* 10–13.

Johnson, D. W., Johnson, R. T., Dudley, B., Ward, M., & Magnuson, D. (1995). The impact of peer mediation training on the management of school and home conflicts. *American Educational Research Journal, 32,* 829–844.

Johnston, C., Pelham, W. E., & Murphy, A. (1985). Peer relationship in ADD-H and normal children: A developmental analysis of peer and teacher ratings. *Journal of Abnormal Child Psychology, 13,* 85–100.

Kaidar, I., Wiener, J., & Tannock, R. (2003). The attributions of children with attention-deficit/hyperactivity disorder for their problems. *Journal of Attention Disorders, 6,* 99–09.

Kazdin, A. E., Holland, L., & Crowley, M. (1997). Family experience of barriers to treatment and premature termination from child therapy. *Journal of Consulting and Clinical Psychology, 65,* 453–463.

Kendall, P. C., & Southam-Gerow, M. A. (1995). Issues in the transportability of treatment: The case of anxiety disorders in youths. *Journal of Consulting and Clinical Psychology, 63,* 702–708.

Kindermann, T. A. (1993). Natural peer groups as contexts for individual development: The case of children's motivation in school. *Developmental Psychology, 29,* 970–977.

Koch, M. S. (1988). Resolving disputes: Students can do it better. *NASSP Bulletin, 72,* 16–18.

Ladd, G. W., & Troop-Gordon, W. (2003). The role of chronic peer difficulties in the development of children's psychological adjustment problems. *Child Development, 74,* 344–367.

Landau, S., & Milich, R. (1988). Social communication patterns of attention deficit-disordered boys. *Journal of Abnormal Child Psychology, 16,* 69–81.

Lane, P. S., & McWhirter, J. J. (1992). A peer mediation model: Conflict resolution for elementary and middle school children. *Elementary School Guidance and Counselling, 27,* 15–23.

MacBrayer, E. K., Milich, R., & Hundley, M. (2003). Attributional biases in aggressive children and their mothers. *Journal of Abnormal Psychology, 112,* 698–708.

Madan-Swain, A., & Zentall, S. S. (1990). Behavioral comparisons of liked and disliked hyperactive children in play contexts and the behavioral accommodations by their classmates. *Journal of Consulting and Clinical Psychology, 58,* 197–209.

Mahoney, J. L., & Cairns, R. B. (1997). Do extracurricular activities protect against early school dropout? *Developmental Psychology, 33,* 241–253.

Marshal, M. P., Molina, B. S., & Pelham, W. E., Jr. (2003). Childhood ADHD and adolescent substance use: An examination of deviant peer group affiliation as a risk factor. *Psychology of Addictive Behavior, 17,* 293–302.

McArdle, P., O'Brien, G., Macmillan, A., & Kolvin, I. (2000). The peer relations of disruptive children with reference to hyperactivity and conduct disorder. *European Journal of Child and Adolescent Psychiatry, 9,* 9–99.

McNeil, C. B., Eyberg, S. M., Eisenstadt, T. H., Newcomb, K., & Funderburk, B. (1991). Parent–child interaction therapy with behavior problem children: Generalization of treatment effects to the school setting. *Journal of Clinical Child Psychology, 55,* 169–182.

Melnick, S. M., & Hinshaw, S. P. (1996). What they want and what they get: The social goals of boys with ADHD and comparison boys. *Journal of Abnormal Child Psychology, 24,* 169–185.

Mikami, A. Y., & Hinshaw, S. P. (2003). Buffers of peer rejection among girls with and without ADHD: The role of popularity with adults and goal-directed solitary play. *Journal of Abnormal Child Psychology, 3,* 381–397.

Milich, R., & Dodge, K. A. (1984). Social information processing in child psychiatric populations. *Journal of Abnormal Child Psychology, 12,* 471–490.

Milich, R., & Landau, S. (1982). Socialization and peer relations in hyperactive children. In K. D. Gadow & I. Bailer (Eds.), *Advances in learning and behavioral disabilities* (Vol. 1, pp. 283–339). Greenwich, CT: JAI Press.

Miller-Johnson, S., Coie, J. D., Maumary-Gremaud, A., Bierman, K., & Conduct Problems Prevention Research Group. (2002). Peer rejection and aggression and early starter models of conduct disorder. *Journal of Abnormal Child Psychology, 30,* 217–230.

Offord, D. R. (1996). The state of prevention and early intervention. In R. Peters & R. McMahon (Eds.), *Preventing childhood disorders, substance abuse, and delinquency* (pp. 144–160). Thousand Oaks, CA: Sage.

Offord, D. R., Boyle, M. H., Szatmari, P., Rae-Grant, N., Links, P. S., Cadman, D., et al. (1987). Ontario Child Health Study: II. Six month prevalence of disorder and rates of service utilization. *Archives of General Psychiatry, 44,* 832–836.

Offord, D. R., Kraemer, H. C., Kazdin, A. E., Jensen, P. S., & Harrington, M. D. (1998). Lowering the burden of suffering from child psychiatric disorder: Trade-offs among clinical, targeted, and universal interventions. *Journal of the American Academy of Child and Adolescent Psychiatry, 37,* 686–694.

Ohan, J. L., & Johnston, C. (2002). Are the performance overestimates given by boys with ADHD self-protective? *Journal of Clinical Child and Adolescent Psychology, 31,* 230–241.

Olweus, D. (1991) Bully/victim problems among school children: Basic facts and effects of a school based intervention program. In D. J. Pepler & K. H. Rubin (Eds.), *The development and treatment of childhood aggression.* Hillsdale, NJ: Erlbaum.

Olweus, D. (1994). Annotation: Bullying at school: Basic facts and effects of a school based intervention program. *Journal of Child Psychology and Psychiatry, 35,* 1171–1190.

Onyango, A. N., Pelham, W. E., Gnagy, E. M., Massetti, G., Burrows-MacLean, L., Fabiano, G. A., et al. (2003, November). *The impact of treatment on deviancy training in children with ADHD.* Poster presented at the 37th annual meeting of the Association for Advancement of Behavior Therapy, Boston, MA.

Pelham, W. E., & Bender, M. E. (1982). Peer relationships in hyperactive children: Description and treatment. In K. D. Gadow & I. Bailer (Eds.), *Advances in learning and behavioral disabilities* (Vol. 1, pp. 365–436). Greenwich, CT: JAI Press.

Pepler, D. J., Craig, W., & Roberts, W. L. (1995). Social skills training and aggression in the peer group. In J. McCord (Ed.), *Coercion and punishment in long-term perspectives* (pp. 213–228). New York: Cambridge University Press.

Pfiffner, L. J., & McBurnett, K. (1997). Social skills training with parent generalization: Treatment effects for children with attention deficit disorder. *Journal of Consulting and Clinical Psychology, 65,* 749–757.

Pihlakoski, L., Aromaa, M., Sourander, A., Rautava, P., Helenius, H., & Sillanpaa, M. (2004). Use of and need for professional help for emotional and behavioral problems among preadolescents: A prospective cohort study of 3 to 12–year old children. *Journal of the American Academy of Child and Adolescent Psychiatry, 43,* 974–983.

Rivers, I., & Smith, P. K. (1994). Types of bullying behaviour and their correlates. *Aggressive Behavior, 20,* 359–368.

Shelton, T. L., Barkley, R. A., Crosswait, C., Moorehouse, M., Fletcher, K., Barrett, S., et al. (2000). Multimethod psychoeducational intervention for preschool children with disruptive behavior: Two-year post-treatment follow-up. *Journal of Abnormal Child Psychology, 28,* 253–266.

Smith, P. K., Hunter, T., Carvalho, A. M. A., & Costabile, A. (1992). Children's perceptions of play-fighting, playchasing and real fighting: A cross-national interview study. *Social Development, 1,* 211–229.

Spoth, R., Greenberg, M., Bierman, K., & Redmond, C. (2004). PROSPER community–university partnership model for public education systems: Capacity-building for evidence-based, competence-building prevention. *Prevention Science. 5,* 31–39.

Stevahn, L., Johnson, D. W., Johnson, R. T., & Schultz,

R. (2002). Effects of conflict resolution training integrated into a high school social studies curriculum. *Journal of Social Psychology, 142,* 305–331.

Thurber, J. R., Heller, T. L., & Hinshaw, S. P. (2002). The social behaviors and peer expectation of girls with attention deficit hyperactivity disorder and comparison girls. *Journal of Clinical Child and Adolescent Psychology, 31,* 443–452.

U.S. Department of Health and Human Services. (1999). *Mental health: A report of the Surgeon General.* Washington, DC: U.S. Government Printing House.

Vitaro, F., Brendgen, M., & Tremblay, R. E. (2000). Influence of deviant friends on delinquency: Searching for moderator variables. *Journal of Abnormal Child Psychology, 28,* 313–325.

Waschbusch, D. A., Pelham, W. E., Jr., Jennings, J. R., Greiner, A. R., Tarter, R. E., & Moss, H. B. (2002). Reactive aggression in boys with disruptive behavior disorders: Behavior, physiology, and affect. *Journal of Abnormal Child Psychology, 30,* 641–656.

Webster-Stratton, C., Reid, J., & Hammond, M. (2001). Social skills and problem solving training for children with early-onset conduct problems: Who benefits? *Journal of Child Psychology and Psychiatry, 42,* 943–952.

Welch, G. (1989). How we keep our playground from becoming a battlefield. *Executive Educator, 11,* 23–31.

Whalen, C. K., Henker, B., Collins, B. E., Finck, D., & Dotemoto, S. (1979). A social ecology of hyperactive boys: Medication effects in structured classroom environments. *Journal of Applied Behavior Analysis, 12,* 65–81.

Whalen, C. K., Henker, B., Collins, B. E., McAuliffe, S., & Vaux, A. (1979). Peer interaction in a structured communication task: Comparison of normal and hyperactive boys and of methylphenidate (Ritalin) and placebo effects. *Child Development, 50,* 388–401.

Whitney, I., & Smith, P. K. (1993). A survey of the nature and extent of bullying in junior/middle and secondary schools. *Educational Research, 35,* 3–25.

Zalecki, C. A., & Hinshaw, S. P. (2004). Overt and relational aggression in girls with attention deficit hyperactivity disorder. *Journal of Child and Adolescent Psychiatry, 33,* 125–137.

CHAPTER 17

Stimulants

DANIEL F. CONNOR

Central nervous system (CNS) stimulant medications are the most commonly used psychotropic drugs to treat the symptoms of individuals with Attention-Deficit/Hyperactivity Disorder (ADHD). It has been estimated that 1.5 million children annually, or 2.8% of the school-age population, may be using stimulants for behavior management (Safer, Zito, & Fine, 1996; Zito et al., 2003). Historically, most of these children have been between 5 and 12 years of age. More recently, however, there has been a significant increase in the prescription of these medications for adolescents and adults with ADHD (Connor & Steingard, 2004).

HISTORY

The clinical use of stimulants for behavioral disturbances in children and adolescents first began in 1937 at the Emma Pendleton Bradley Home for Children in Rhode Island. Charles Bradley, a psychiatrist, was working with children who had brain injuries and had received a pneumoencephalogram as part of a standard clinical diagnostic workup. This procedure commonly resulted in severe headache for the children. Bradley decided to use an amphetamine (Benzedrine) in an attempt to ameliorate the headache pain. When given amphetamine, the children demonstrated immediate improvements in their disruptive behaviors. Bradley also noted improved academic performance, better self-control, and improved attention to task. Bradley published his findings in 1950 after using amphetamines for two decades to treat hyperactivity, impulsivity, and moodiness in clinically referred children (Pliszka, 2003).

In the 1960s, the first double-blind placebo-controlled clinical trials of dextroamphetamine and methylphenidate were completed and confirmed Bradley's initial clinical impressions. Since then, over 200 controlled trials of stimulants have been completed (Connor & Steingard, 2004; Spencer, Biederman, Wilens, et al., 1996). These studies demonstrate the efficacy of the stimulants in improving the core symptoms of ADHD and enhancing behavioral, academic, and social functioning in about 50–95% of children treated. Variability in response rates is largely due to the presence of comorbid psychiatric and developmental disorders (Barkley, DuPaul, & Connor, 1999; Pliszka, Carlson, & Swanson, 1999; Spencer, Biederman, & Wilens, 1999).

As noted above, most of the individuals for whom stimulants have been prescribed have been school-age children. However, longitudinal studies in ADHD consistently demonstrate the persistence of symptoms and impairment across multiple domains of daily life functioning into adolescence and adulthood in the majority of children diagnosed with ADHD (Hechtman, Weiss, & Perlman, 1984; Mannuzza, Gittelman-Klein, Bessler, Malloy, & LaPadula, 1993). Increasingly, therefore, stimulants are being prescribed for adolescents and adults meeting criteria for ADHD (Faraone et al., 2000).

Despite the overwhelming amount of research documenting the efficacy of stimulants for the symptoms of ADHD, the stimulants should rarely be the only form of therapy provided to individuals with ADHD. For some patients with mild ADHD, enhanced organizational skills, cognitive-behavioral therapies, education about the disorder, and/or school or occupational supports may be sufficient to lessen the impact of the disorder on daily life. However, it is important to recognize that stimulants are the only treatment modality to date that have produced significant improvement in symptoms of inattention, impulsivity, and overactive behavior for many individuals with ADHD (Barkley, 1998). Furthermore, the effect size of stimulants has been found to be greater than the effect size of psychosocial therapies for the core symptoms of ADHD, at least over periods of time up to 14 months (MTA Cooperative Group, 1999).

The purposes of this chapter are to (1) review recent advances in stimulant therapy for ADHD, (2) review pharmacodynamic and pharmacokinetic actions of stimulants, and (3) review safety and tolerability data for stimulant use. The emphasis in this chapter is clinical, with the overall goal of enhancing the practitioner's safe and effective clinical use of stimulant medications, particularly in the treatment of ADHD.

The stimulants are referred to as such because of their ability to activate the level of activity, arousal, or alertness of the CNS. Stimulants in clinical use include racemic methylphenidate, dextromethylphenidate, dextroamphetamine, mixed amphetamine salts (a combination of dextroamphetamine and amphetamine), and magnesium pemoline. Methamphetamine (Desoxyn) has also been used in a small percentage of cases of ADHD. But in view of its greater abuse potential than other stimulants, the dearth of controlled research on its efficacy, and limited availability in some geographic regions, methamphetamine is not discussed here as a treatment option. In addition, pemoline is now rarely used because of elevated risk of liver toxicity, and is currently considered a second-line agent for the treatment of ADHD (Safer, Zito, & Gardner, 2001); therefore, pemoline is also not discussed further. Finally, CNS stimulants such as caffeine and deanol are not discussed here, since they have not been found to be nearly as effective as the other CNS stimulants and cannot be recommended for clinical use.

INDICATIONS FOR USE OF STIMULANT MEDICATIONS

Established Indications

Established indications for stimulants include ADHD symptoms in children 6 years of age, adolescents, and adults. Specifically, stimulants are helpful in treating age-inappropriate and impairing symptoms of inattention to task, impulsive behavior, and motor hyperactivity that are not due to another cause, such as depression, bipolar disorders, substance use disorders, anxiety disorders, or psychotic disorders, and are persistently severe enough to cause impaired functioning at school, at work, at home, or in the community. All three subtypes of ADHD (the Combined, Predominantly Hyperactive–Impulsive, and Predominantly Inattentive Types) respond to stimulant therapy (Barkley et al., 1999). Narcolepsy is also an established indication for stimulant medications, but will not be further discussed here.

Probable Indications

Probable indications for stimulants include symptoms of ADHD in preschool children and children with comorbid conditions, such as mental retardation, autism spectrum disorders, head trauma, and seizure disorders (Aman, Marks, Turbott, Wilsher, & Merry, 1991; Connor, 2002; Feldman, Crumrine, Handen, Alvin, & Teodori, 1989; Handen et al., 1992; Handen, Johnson, & Lubetsky, 2000; Hemmer, Pasternak, Zecker, & Trommer, 2001; Mahalick et al., 1998; McBride, Wang, & Torres, 1986; Pearson et al., 2003; Weber & Lutschg, 2002).

Nine out of 10 randomized, controlled clinical trials demonstrate the efficacy of stimulants for symptoms of ADHD in 3- to 6-year-old children (Connor, 2002; Short, Manos,

Findling, & Schubel, 2004). Preschoolers with severe ADHD respond to both methylphenidate and amphetamine preparations, as do older children with the disorder (Short et al., 2004). However, the efficacy of stimulant treatment is more variable in preschoolers than in older children, and there is a higher rate of side effects, especially sadness, irritability, clinging behavior, insomnia, and anorexia (Barkley, 1988). Stimulant therapy for preschool children should be reserved for those with particularly severe cases of ADHD, and only after family education about the nature of ADHD, parent management training, family behavioral therapy, and preschool educational supports have been completed and are unsuccessful or are unavailable. Because of a paucity of research in children less than 3 years old, stimulants are not considered an option in such children.

Stimulants may be effective for symptoms of ADHD in children with mental retardation. Recent studies support the use of stimulants in the treatment of ADHD symptoms in these youngsters, especially if the IQ is over 50 and the mental age is greater than 4.5 years (Aman et al., 1991; Handen et al., 1992; Pearson et al., 2003). However, for youth with more severe mental retardation, stimulant medications may not be well tolerated (Aman et al., 1991; Handen et al., 1992).

The symptoms of ADHD are sometimes present in persons with autistic spectrum disorders. The target symptoms of distractibility, impulsivity, and hyperactivity may respond to stimulants in children or adults with autism (Handen et al., 2000). However, the use of stimulants in persons with autism and other pervasive developmental disorders does not always result in clinical improvement. ADHD symptoms in milder forms of autistic spectrum disorder such as Asperger syndrome may respond better than ADHD symptoms in more classical types of autism or other pervasive developmental disorders (Stigler, Desmond, Posey, Wiegand, & McDougle, 2004). Careful clinical monitoring of autistic individuals on stimulants is indicated, because adverse events may be hidden among all the other symptoms these patients may have and make medication side effects difficult to recognize.

Neurological injury may cause hyperactivity, distractibility, and/or impulsivity, especially if the frontal cortex sustains injury. Randomized controlled studies suggest the efficacy of stimu-

lant medications for children or adults with trauma-acquired symptoms of ADHD (Mahalick et al., 1998; Max et al., 1998, 2004).

Finally, attention deficit can be a frequent symptom in children, adolescents, and adults with epilepsy and other seizure disorders. It is unclear whether the symptoms of ADHD are caused by the epilepsy, are exacerbated by anticonvulsant medications, or constitute a separate comorbid disorder. A few controlled studies have investigated the safety and efficacy of methylphenidate in children with the dual diagnosis of ADHD and epilepsy (Feldman et al., 1989; Hemmer et al., 2001; McBride et al., 1986; Weber & Lutschg, 2002). These studies generally conclude that stimulant therapy is safe when epilepsy is stabilized on anticonvulsant therapy. No influence of methylphenidate on the plasma level of antiepileptic drugs is documented (Weber & Lutschg, 2002). What remains unclear is the effect of stimulants on seizure thresholds in patients whose epilepsy is untreated or poorly controlled on anticonvulsive therapy. In such patients, there is evidence that methylphenidate may lower the seizure threshold and exacerbate the risk of seizures (Hemmer et al., 2001).

PHARMACOEPIDEMIOLOGY OF STIMULANT USE

Stimulant use among children and adolescents in the United States has grown substantially over the past two decades. Between 1987 and 1996, the prevalence of stimulant use among youth under 18 years of age increased three- to sevenfold (Zito et al., 2003). This growth also includes increased prescribing rates of stimulants for preschool children. Since 1990, there has been a threefold increase in stimulant prescriptions for 2- to 4-year-old children (Zito et al., 2000). This growth takes place within the context of a threefold overall increase in total psychoactive medication prescribing for youngsters across all classes of psychiatric medication since 1991 (Zito et al., 2003).

Among stimulants, methylphenidate use ranked foremost among children and adolescents, accounting for 77–87% of all stimulant prescriptions since 1991. A dramatic increase in amphetamine prescribing occurred with the introduction of mixed amphetamine salts (Adderall) in 1996. Over the past decade, a 7- to 14-fold increase in amphetamine prescriptions has been observed in both Medicaid and in health maintenance organizations (Zito et al., 1999, 2003). Because of warnings about elevated risk of hepatic failure, pemoline use has declined in youngsters over this same time period, and pemoline is no longer available in Canada (Willy, Manda, Shatin, Drinkard, & Graham, 2002).

With growing recognition that ADHD persists into adulthood in the majority of children diagnosed in elementary school, physicians are beginning to use stimulants to treat ADHD across the lifespan (Connor & Steingard, 2004; Spencer, Biederman, Wilens, et al., 1996; Spencer et al., 1995). To date, there have been no pharmacoepidemiological studies of stimulant use for ADHD in adulthood. However, with growing recognition of the ADHD diagnosis in adults, stimulant use in this population is expected to grow. (See Chapter 22, this volume, for a fuller discussion of pharmacotherapy in adults.)

Stimulants are often combined with other psychiatric medications for the treatment of ADHD and comorbid conditions, and the use of combined treatment is also increasing in the United States. In a national sample of physician office visits for youth under 18, the rate of combined stimulant and antidepressant use increased from 4% in 1994 to 29% in 1997. This reflects a sevenfold increase over 3 years (Bhatara, Feil, Hoagwood, Vitiello, & Zima, 2000). On the basis of Medicaid claims data, it was reported that 30% of youth receiving a selective serotonin reuptake inhibitor (SSRI) antidepressant also had a stimulant prescription during the same year, strongly suggesting combined use (Rushton & Whitmire, 2001). A particularly common concomitant psychotropic medication combination for youth has been methylphenidate and clonidine. Estimates from a national pharmaceutical market source found that 41% of surveyed youth in 1994–1995 who were receiving methylphenidate were also receiving clonidine (Swanson, Connor, & Cantwell, 1999). In clinical practice, stimulants are often combined with atypical antipsychotic medications in the treatment of highly aggressive children with ADHD. However, no data on the prevalence of this practice are presently available.

Although stimulants have been shown to be highly effective in the treatment of the core symptoms of ADHD (MTA Cooperative Group, 1999), their use is not without contro-

versy. During the 1990s, concerns were expressed over the increased prevalence of use among school-age children, the uncertainty surrounding the implications of long-term use in children, and studies showing geographical variation in prevalence of use (Safer et al., 1996). Particular concern was expressed about overmedication of children with stimulants (Angold, Erkanli, Egger, & Costello, 2000). However, pharmacoepidemiological research has reported both overprescribing and underprescribing of stimulants to youth in the United States (Angold et al., 2000; Jensen, Kettle, et al., 1999; Jensen, Bhatara, et al., 1999; Wolraich et al., 1990; Zito et al., 1999). In contrast, marked geographic variation in stimulant prescribing rates has been consistently reported, even after differences in predictors such as age and gender are controlled for. Compared to children living in the Western region of the United States, children living in the Midwest and South appear more likely to be prescribed a stimulant medication (Cox, Motheral, Henderson, & Mager, 2003). The reasons for geographic variation appear complex. Sources of variation may include differences in the populations studied by different pharmacoepidemiological researchers, differences in research methodology across studies, and differences in the way different specialty physicians identify and diagnose ADHD (Cox et al., 2003; Wolraich et al., 1990).

BASIC PHARMACOLOGY OF STIMULANTS

Stimulants are structurally similar to the monoaminergic CNS neurotransmitters. There are two prevailing hypotheses regarding the underlying neurophysiology of ADHD; these involve neural systems that are subserved by the catecholamines dopamine and norepinephrine. The focus on dopamine was derived from the fact that stimulant medications are known to alter the transmission of dopaminergic neurons in the CNS. This hypothesis has been further substantiated by neuroimaging studies that have consistently identified alterations in the structure and functioning of dopamine-rich regions of the CNS, such as the prefrontal cortex, striatum, basal ganglia, and cerebellum, in children and adults meeting clinical criteria for the ADHD phenotype (Ernst, Cohen, Liebenauer, Jons, & Zametkin, 1997; Ernst et al., 1999; Ernst, Zametkin, Phillips, & Cohen, 1998;

Jensen, 2000; Levy, 1991; Zametkin & Liotta, 1998). However, stimulants also affect noradrenergic neurotransmission, and an alternative noradrenergic model has been proposed to explain the effects of stimulants in ADHD. This model focuses on the inhibitory influences of frontal cortical circuits, which are predominantly noradrenergic, acting upon striatal structures to indirectly alter dopaminergic activity (Zametkin & Liotta, 1998). This model is further supported by the presence of an anterior CNS attentional system in the prefrontal cortex, and a posterior CNS attentional system located in prefrontal, posterior, and parietal-locus ceruleus neuronal networks, both of which involve noradrenergic transmission (Posner & Raichle, 1996).

Mechanisms of Action

The primary mode of action of stimulants is to enhance catecholamine activity in the CNS, probably by increasing the availability of norepinephrine and dopamine at the synaptic cleft (Solanto, 1998). Preclinical studies have shown that methylphenidate and amphetamine block the reuptake of dopamine and norepinephrine into the presynaptic neuron (Barkley et al., 1999; Faraone & Biederman, 1998; Pliszka, 2003; Zametkin & Liotta, 1998). The stimulants largely exert their action by reversibly binding to the presynaptic transporter protein with resultant inhibition of catecholamine reuptake into the presynaptic neuron, increasing concentrations of catecholamines in the extraneuronal space, and thus presumably enhancing postsynaptic CNS catecholaminergic neurotransmission (Volkow et al., 2002). Amphetamine also increases the release of dopamine from presynaptic cytoplasmic storage vesicles and blocks the uptake of dopamine into neuronal cytoplasmic storage vesicles, making dopamine more available in the presynaptic cytoplasm for release into the synaptic cleft. These slightly differing mechanisms of action of amphetamine and methylphenidate suggest that they are not identical, and that both types of stimulants should be tried if a patient does not have a satisfactory response to an initial stimulant trial (Elia, Borcherding, Rapoport, & Keysor, 1991). An analysis of 141 subjects showed that 40% of the patients responded equally well to either methylphenidate or dextroamphetamine, but 26% responded better to

methylphenidate, and 35% had a superior response to dextroamphetamine (Greenhill et al., 1996).

Thus it appears that alterations in both dopaminergic and noradrenergic function occur and may be necessary for clinical efficacy of the stimulants in treating ADHD (Pliszka, McCracken, & Maas, 1996; Wilens & Spencer, 2000; Zametkin & Liotta, 1998).

Absorption and Metabolism

In clinical practice, stimulants are given orally. Absorption is rapid and complete from the gastrointestinal tract. Stimulants reach their maximal clinical effect during the absorption phase of the kinetic curve, approximately 2 hours after ingestion (Diener, 1991). Stimulants cross the blood–brain barrier and are taken up into the CNS. The absorption phase parallels the acute release of neurotransmitters into CNS synaptic clefts, supporting theories of stimulant mechanism of action on CNS catecholamines in ADHD (Wilens & Spencer, 2000). Older slow-release formulations of methylphenidate have a more variable and less complete absorption, which may explain their diminished efficacy compared to more rapidly and completely absorbed stimulants (Pelham et al., 1987; Pelham, Swanson, Furman, & Schwindt, 1995). (See "Once-Daily Preparations" below, however, regarding the newer extended-release stimulant formulations.) Methylphenidate and amphetamine are metabolized in the body by different mechanisms. After absorption, methylphenidate undergoes extensive first-pass hepatic metabolism predominantly by hydrolysis. The predominant route of metabolism is de-esterification to inactive ritalinic acid, which is readily excreted and accounts for 80% of the dose. To a lesser degree, methylphenidate is also metabolized via hydroxylation to *p*-hydroxymethylphenidate, and to oxoritalinic acid and oxomethylphenidate, all of which are pharmacologically inactive (Hoffman & Lefkowitz, 1996).

Amphetamine is metabolized by side-chain oxidative deamination and ring hydroxylation in the liver (Caldwell & Sever, 1974; Hoffman & Lefkowitz, 1996; Wilens & Spencer, 2000). The majority of amphetamine is excreted unchanged in the urine (~80%), along with benzoic acid, hippuric acid, and hydroxyamphetamine catabolites (Caldwell & Sever, 1974). Because amphetamine is a highly basic compound, urinary excretion is dependent on urinary pH. Urine acidification (i.e., by ingestion of ascorbic acid or orange juice) results in a shortened plasma half-life and increased amphetamine clearance. Acidification of the urine is useful to facilitate amphetamine clearance in overdose and subsequent toxicity (Hoffman & Lefkowitz, 1996). Patients receiving amphetamines for ADHD who note decreasing clinical efficacy should be monitored for vitamin C (ascorbic acid) consumption (Wilens & Spencer, 2000).

Pharmacokinetics and Preparations

There are two theories that relate pharmacokinetics to stimulant efficacy in ADHD. The first theory is called the "ramp effect." It has been theorized that the more rapidly the brain concentration of a stimulant increases, the greater the stimulant's effect on improved vigilance or reduction of hyperactivity. In this model, stimulant efficacy with regard to the symptoms of ADHD is proportional to the rate of stimulant absorption into the CNS (Greenhill, 1995). This model argues that stimulants with a rapid rate of absorption will be more effective than stimulants with a slower rate of absorption. The second theory relates the maximal plasma concentration of stimulant to efficacy in ADHD. This theory is called the "threshold effect" (Birmaher, Greenhill, Cooper, Fried, & Maminski, 1989). In this model, stimulant efficacy is proportional to peak stimulant brain concentrations. At present, it is unclear whether the rate of absorption (ramp effect) or the peak plasma or brain concentration of stimulants (threshold effect) accounts for stimulant efficacy in ADHD.

Behavioral effects for the stimulants are not as well predicted from peak or absolute blood levels as from knowledge of dose alone (Kupietz, 1991; Swanson, 1988). Peak behavioral changes often seem to lag behind peak blood levels by as much as an hour. Alternatively, changes in learning on laboratory learning tasks may correspond more closely to blood levels (Kupietz, 1991; Swanson & Kinsbourne, 1978), although there are insufficient data to be sure of this. Consequently, when behavioral change is the goal of treatment, blood levels play little role in establishing the therapeutic range or response for any individual case beyond knowledge of the oral dose

itself. Further data are necessary to determine whether changes in *learning performance* can be predicted reliably by blood levels, and even so, such predictions are likely to be subject to considerable inter- and intraindividual variability (Kupietz, 1991). Thus drawing blood to establish drug levels for guiding therapeutic adjustments to children's stimulant medication is not a recommended practice (Swanson, 1988).

Table 17.1 shows the varying durations of action of the available stimulant formulations.

Immediate-Release Preparations

Immediate-release stimulants include both methylphenidate and amphetamine compounds. Methylphenidate has a rapid onset of action (within 20–60 minutes) and a peak plasma concentration within 1–2 hours after ingestion, with an elimination half-life of 3–6 hours (Hoffman & Lefkowitz, 1996; Wilens & Spencer, 2000). Its plasma half-life is 1–3 hours, but concentrations in the CNS exceed those in plasma (Hoffman & Lefkowitz, 1996). Dextromethylphenidate is the optically pure stereoisomer of racemic methylphenidate (see "Stimulant Enantiomers," below) and has pharmacokinetic parameters similar to those of racemic methylphenidate (Ding et al., 1997). Amphetamine compounds include dextroamphetamine and mixed amphetamine salts. These agents also have a rapid onset of action, with peak clinical effects occurring within 1–2 hours. They have a long serum half-life and a behavioral half-life of 4–6 hours, slightly longer than methylphenidate preparations.

Intermediate-Acting Preparations

Methylphenidate is available in intermediate-acting preparations. These compounds are designed to last longer than immediate-release preparations and have a somewhat slower onset of action. Newer formulations such as Metadate CD and Ritalin LA have a bimodal clinical effect designed to mimic the actions of immediate-release methylphenidate given twice daily (Novartis Pharmaceuticals, 2002b).

Once-Daily Preparations

Once-daily stimulant formulations are available as Concerta and Adderall XR. Concerta encapsulates methylphenidate in an oral-os-

TABLE 17.1. Actions of Available Stimulant Medications

Generic name	Brand name	Onset of action (min)	Peak clinical effect (hr)	Serum half-life (hr)	Duration of behavioral action (hr)	Required number of daily doses
Immediate-release preparations						
Methylphenidate	Ritalin, Methylin, Metadate	20–60	2 (range: 0.3–4.0)	3–6	3–6	2–3
Dextromethylphenidate	Focalin	20–60	2 (range: 0.3–4.0)	2.2	4	2–3
Dextroamphetamine	Dextrostat, Dexedrine	20–60	1–2	12	4–6	2–3
Mixed amphetamine salts	Adderall	30–60	1–2	12	4–6	2
Intermediate-release preparations						
Methylphenidate	Ritalin SR, Metadate ER, Methylin ER	60–90	~5 (range: 1.3–8.2)	NR	4–8	2
Methylphenidate	Metadate CD, Ritalin LA	30–120	Bimodal pattern[a]	1.5–6.8	6–8	1–2
Dextroamphetamine	Dexedrine spansule	60–90	8	12	6–8	1–2
Extended-release preparations						
Methylphenidate	Concerta	30–120	Bimodal pattern[a]	6–8	12	1
Mixed amphetamine salts	Adderall XR	60–120	Bimodal pattern[a]	9–11	10–12	1

Note. Use of pemoline has been associated with rare but life-threatening hepatic failure. It is not considered first-line therapy for ADHD and is not included in this table. NR, not reported.
[a]These medications display a bimodal (early and late) release pattern of stimulant.

motic-release drug delivery system (OROS) that is similar to immediate-release methylphenidate given thrice daily. The duration of action of Concerta is 10–14 hours (Pelham et al., 2001). Concerta demonstrates an ascending methylphenidate plasma concentration curve throughout the day. Research has shown that rising methylphenidate plasma levels are necessary for stimulants to retain their efficacy over the course of the day. In contrast, flat methylphenidate dosing regimens (indicative of older slow-release methylphenidate preparations) lose about 40% of their efficacy by the afternoon. This is due to the phenomenon of tachyphylaxis (or acute tolerance) to methylphenidate, which can develop under multiple daily dosing conditions. An ascending dose curve overcomes this acute tolerance and maintains methylphenidate efficacy throughout the day (McNeil Pharmaceuticals, 2001; Swanson et al., 1999; Wilens & Spencer, 2000). Adderall XR contains a bead technology comprised of 50% immediate-release and 50% extended-release beads (Grcevich, 2001). The immediate-release beads release stimulant medication immediately after ingestion; the extended-release beads release 4 hours later. The 50:50 ratio of beads allows for therapeutic effects to begin within a time frame comparable to that of shorter-acting formulations, with ascending stimulant plasma levels facilitating ADHD symptom relief over an extended time period (Michaels, Weston, Zhang, & Tulloch, 2001; Shire Pharmaceuticals, 2001). Adderall XR is designed to mimic the actions of immediate-release Adderall given twice daily (Shire Pharmaceuticals, 2001).

Transdermal Patches

Not included in Table 17.1 is a methylphenidate transdermal skin patch system under development (Noven and Shire Pharmaceuticals) (Greenhill, Pelham, et al., 2002). This is an embedded drug adhesive transdermal patch, worn on the hip, in which soluble methylphenidate is contained within a silicone and acrylic adhesive diffusion technology. Each patch provides a duration of up to 12 hours.

Stimulant Enantiomers

Numerous psychotropic drugs exist as a mixture of two mirror images or stereoisomers of each other. The molecular structure of one isomer turns to the right (dextro-), while its mirror image turns to the left (levo-). Their mixture is called a "racemate." "Enantiomers" are new drugs made by removing one mirror-image stereoisomer from a mixture of two contained in the original drug. The human body appears to be quite sensitive to one stereoisomer relative to the other. Often the drug can be improved when only one of the enantiomers is clinically administered. Improvements may include lessened side effects, reduced drug–drug interactions, and better efficacy with a reduced drug dose (Stahl, 2002).

Methylphenidate contains a 50:50 racemic mixture of the dextro- and levo- isomers of methylphenidate. Research shows that dextromethylphenidate is the pharmacologically active enantiomer (Eckerman, Moy, Perkins, Patrick, & Breese, 1991). Recent advances in stereospecific manufacturing allow commercial preparations of optically pure dextromethylphenidate (or dexmethylphenidate), and a preparation containing only this enantiomer could provide a better treatment of ADHD than a racemic mixture. An immediate-release enantiomer of methylphenidate called Focalin (dextromethylphenidate) has been released by Novartis (Novartis Pharmaceuticals, 2002a). Compared to placebo, Focalin is effective for the symptoms of ADHD. However, its advantages over other immediate-release stimulant preparations are presently not clear. A long-acting preparation of Focalin is currently under development.

Clinical Effects of Stimulants

Over 200 randomized, controlled studies exist on the effects of the stimulants on the core symptoms of ADHD (Barkley, 1977, 1998; Connor & Steingard, 2004; Spencer, Biederman, Wilens, et al., 1996; Wilens & Spencer, 2000). Most of these studies have been conducted with methylphenidate. The vast majority of research reports on studies of 6- to 12-year-old children with ADHD. However, preschool children, adolescents, and adults have been shown to respond to stimulants as well. (Connor, 2002; Greenhill & MTA Cooperative Group, 2002; Wilens, Biederman, Spencer, & Prince, 1995; Wilens & Spencer, 2000).

In general, studies indicate that between 73% and 77% of children with ADHD initially treated with a stimulant are described as improved in their symptoms (Barkley, 1977; Barkley et al., 1999). Between 25% and 30% of such children do not respond or do not tolerate initial stimulant medication. If a second stimulant is clinically tried, response rates increase (Elia et al., 1991; Elia & Rapoport, 1991). As stated previously, both a methylphenidate and an amphetamine preparation should be tried before other classes of agents are considered. Research has identified one group of children with ADHD that responds preferentially to methylphenidate, another group that responds to amphetamine, and a third group that responds to both stimulants (Greenhill et al., 1996). It is important to note that placebo response rates in ADHD are generally low. Controlled efficacy studies of stimulants examining differences between stimulants and placebo in ADHD report placebo responses ranging from 2% to 39% (Barkley, 1977; Varley, 1983). In the recent large Multimodal Treatment Study of ADHD (MTA), placebo response rates of about 13% were reported (MTA Cooperative Group, 1999).

Effects on Behavior

Impulsive, aggressive, and hyperactive behaviors commonly accompany ADHD in childhood and adolescence and may have large consequences for the affected individual (Goldman, Genel, Bezman, & Slanetz, 1998). Explosive outbursts of temper over common everyday frustrations are often difficult for families of youth with ADHD to cope with and manage, and they often lead to deterioration in familial functioning. In adolescence, impulsive and hyperactive behaviors contribute to social functioning problems, higher risk for antisocial behavior, increased risk of cigarette smoking, and automobile accidents (Barkley, Guevremont, Anastopoulos, DuPaul, & Shelton, 1993; Barkley, Murphy, & Kwasnik, 1996; Milberger, Biederman, Faraone, Chen, & Jones, 1997a, 1997b). In adulthood, impulsivity and poor judgment contribute to higher mortality rates from automobile accidents, vulnerability to antisocial behaviors, and increased risk for substance abuse (Barkley, 2004; Milberger, Biederman, Faraone, Wilens, & Chu, 1997; Murphy & Barkley, 1996; O'Donnell et al., 1998).

Stimulants have robust effects on various age-inappropriate behaviors that commonly cause impairment on a daily basis for individuals with ADHD. These behaviors often include impulsivity, disruptiveness, noncompliance, talking out of turn, out-of-seat behaviors, restlessness, and impulsive displays of aggression (Rapport et al., 1988; Swanson, Granger, & Kliewer, 1987; Whalen, Henker, & Granger, 1990). Stimulant dose effects are generally linear and positive on core behavioral problems in ADHD, so that higher doses may be more effective than lower doses (Rapport et al., 1988). However, dose must be individualized for each patient. A meta-analysis of stimulant effects on aggressive behavior in ADHD, separate from effects on the core symptoms of inattention, impulsivity, and hyperactivity, found large effect sizes for stimulant treatment on symptoms of both overt and covert aggression (Connor et al., 2002). This suggests that ADHD may amplify or increase conduct problem behaviors in some children, and that treatment of ADHD symptoms with stimulants may reduce vulnerability to antisocial and aggressive behaviors (Connor, Barkley, & Davis, 2000; Klein et al., 1997).

Effects on Cognition, Learning, and Academic Performance

Numerous studies have found that stimulants enhance performance on measures of vigilance, impulse control, fine motor coordination, and reaction time (Barkley, 1998; Barkley et al., 1999; Rapport & Kelly, 1991; Rapport, Quinn, DuPaul, Quinn, & Kelly, 1989; Vyse & Rapport, 1989). Higher stimulant doses tend to be associated with more robust responses, and clinicians should beware of underdosing.

Positive drug effects have been obtained on measures of short-term memory and learning of paired verbal or nonverbal material (Bergman, Winters, & Cornblatt, 1991; Swanson & Kinsbourne, 1978). Performance on both simple and complex learning paradigms appears to be enhanced, and perceptual efficiency and speed of symbolic and verbal information retrieval are also facilitated (Sergeant & van der Meere, 1991; Swanson, 1988). Stimulant therapy improves school-based academic productivity and accuracy in treated children with ADHD (Barkley et al., 1999; Famularo & Fenton, 1987; Gillberg et al., 1997; Schachar & Tannock, 1993). Studies support positive dose–response relationships on cognitive measures associated with learning in the classroom (Rapport et al., 1987). ADHD laboratory school-based data suggest that positive medication effects in the classroom (enhanced vigilance, attention focus, and impulse control) do not adversely affect children's spontaneous play activities at recess (Wilens & Spencer, 2000).

Despite beneficial effects on learning in children with ADHD, stimulants do not enhance functioning on more traditional measures of cognitive potential and academic ability such as intelligence tests (Barkley, 1977; Rapport & Kelly, 1991). In general, stimulants seem particularly salient in school situations that require children to inhibit their behavior and focus on assigned tasks. It remains to be determined whether these acute effects of stimulants on cognition, learning, and academic performance will translate into enhanced academic achievement (knowledge) for children with ADHD over the long term (Barkley, 1998; Barkley et al., 1999).

Effects on Interpersonal and Social Relationships

Treatment with stimulant medication has been found to improve the quality of social interactions between children with ADHD and their parents, teachers, and peers (Danforth, Barkley, & Stokes, 1991). In young children, stimulants increase compliance with parental commands, decrease hostile and negative responses, and enhance responsiveness to the interactions of others (Barkley, 1981, 1988, 1989). Beneficial effects of stimulant treatment have also been documented in the interactions between children with ADHD and their teachers (Whalen, Henker, & Dotemoto, 1980). Stimulant medications not only directly alter these children's behavior, but also indirectly affect the behaviors of important adults and peers toward the children. When these relationships improve, they may contribute further to a positive treatment response in the children.

Improvements in interpersonal and social relationships with stimulant treatment of adolescents and adults with ADHD have not been as well studied as in children. However, improvements in social judgment and interpersonal relationships with clinical treatment of such adolescents and adults are beginning to be documented (Barkley, Anastopoulos, Guevremont, & Fletcher, 1992; Faraone et al., 2000; Hechtman et al., 1984; Murphy & Barkley, 1996; Seidman, Biederman, Weber, Hatch, & Faraone, 1998; Spencer, Biederman, Wilens, et al., 1996; Spencer et al., 1995).

STIMULANT TREATMENT FOR ADHD ACROSS THE LIFESPAN

Preschool Children

Because current diagnostic criteria require an early age of onset (< 7 years old) for a diagnosis of ADHD, children in the preschool age range (3–6 years old) may come to clinical attention for accurate diagnosis and treatment. For example, in one study of 300 children consecutively referred to an ADHD clinic, mothers reported 202 children (67%) as having an onset of ADHD symptoms that interfered with daily functioning at age 4 years or younger (Connor et al., 2003). Thus the physician who treats children with ADHD will be asked to evaluate and treat preschool children for ADHD.

Stimulants should not be the first-line treatment for the symptoms of ADHD in the very young child. Parent management behavioral methods using a compliance training model meet criteria for evidence-based treatment for childhood ADHD, disruptive behavior, noncompliance, and oppositional defiant behavior, and should always be tried first (see Chapter 12; see also Connor, 2002; Forehand & McMahon, 1981; Pisterman et al., 1989). However, for preschoolers with severe hyperactivity or for those with whom parent management training methods have been unsuccessful, stimulant therapy is sometimes considered.

At this writing, 10 controlled clinical trials of stimulants in preschool children (ages 3–6 years) with ADHD have been reported in the clinical literature. Another, the largest study done with preschoolers (Preschool ADHD Treatment Study, or PATS), was only recently completed and has been reported only at a recent scientific meeting (Kollins et al., 2004). The published studies appear in Table 17.2. The PATS study is discussed thereafter.

Nine controlled studies have evaluated preschool children with ADHD and typically developing cognition, and one study has evaluated preschool children with ADHD and developmental disabilities (Handen, Feldman, Lurier, & Murray, 1999). Random assignment to treatment occurred in 80% of these studies, and 90% (9 of 10) of studies support efficacy of stimulants for the symptoms of ADHD in the preschool age range. Methylphenidate has generally been used in these studies. Doses have generally been low, ranging between 2.5 mg/day and 30 mg/day. One study assessed mixed amphetamine salts in preschoolers with ADHD, in doses of 5–15 mg given once daily (Short et al., 2004). The published studies generally support linear dosing effects in the preschool age range, with higher doses improving inattention, impulsivity, and academic productivity to a greater extent than lower doses (Monteiro-Musten, Firestone, Pisterman, Bennett, & Mercer, 1997). Children less than 3 years old have not been studied. Side effects of stimulants are generally reported as elevated in preschoolers compared with treated older children (Firestone, Monteiro-Musten, Pisterman, Mercer, & Bennett, 1998). Response rates may be more variable in the preschool population than in older children receiving stimulants (Connor, 2002).

Rising rates of prescriptions for psychotropic medications given to U.S. children ages 2–5 years have raised concerns that not enough is known about the safety and efficacy of these agents in preschoolers (Greenhill et al., 2003; Zito et al., 2000). The majority of these prescriptions are stimulants used for the treatment of very-early-onset ADHD (Zito et al., 1999). In response to these concerns, the National Institute of Mental Health conducted the PATS project, a multisite clinical trial to determine the safety and efficacy of methylphenidate in preschoolers with ADHD (Greenhill et al., 2003; Kollins et al., 2004). In this study, 279 children ages 3–5.5 years were initially enrolled in a parent training program, and 261 completed this treatment. Of these children, 169

TABLE 17.2. Controlled Studies of Stimulant Efficacy for Preschool Minimal Brain Dysfunction, Hyperactivity, or ADHD

Study (year)	No. of subjects	Age in years (mean and/or range)	Study design	Random assignment	Duration (weeks)	Stimulant dose (mean and/or range)	Response
Schleifer et al. (1975)	26	4.1; 3.4–4.10	B-PC-CO[a]	+	9	10 mg/day; 2.5–30 mg/day	Mixed; many side effects reported. No improvements seen on direct observation or lab tests.
Conners (1975)	59	4.8; 3–6	B-PC-PG[b]	+	6	12 mg/day (0.7 mg/kg/day)	Improvement in behavioral domains. High variability in individual response noted.
Cunningham et al. (1985)	12	4–6	B-PC-CO[a]	+	4	0.15–0.50 mg/kg/day	Improvement in cognitive, behavioral, and interpersonal domains.
Barkley et al. (1984)	18	4–5.11	B-PC-CO[a]	+	3	0.3–1.0 mg/kg/day	Improvement in interpersonal domain.
Barkley (1988)	27	2.5–5.0	B-PC-CO[a]	+	3	0.3–1.0 mg/kg/day	Improvement in interpersonal domain.
Mayes et al. (1994)	14	1.8–5.0	B-PC-ABA[c]	–	3	7.5–30 mg/day	Improvement in behavioral domain.
Monteiro-Musten et al. (1997)	31	4.0–5.8	B-PC-CO[a]	+	3	0.6–1.0 mg/kg/day	Improvement in cognitive, behavioral, and interpersonal domains.
Byrne et al. (1998)	8	5.2	B-CC[d]	–	20	15–30 mg/day	Improvement in cognitive, behavioral, and interpersonal domains.
Handen et al. (1999)	11	4.9; 4.0–5.11	B-PC-CO[a]	+	4	0.3 or 0.6 mg/kg/day	All participants had developmental delay; IQs ranged between 40 and 78. 73% response rate. Increased rate of side effects.
Short et al. (2004)	28	4.0–5.9	B-PC-CO[a]	+	6	5–10 mg/day	82% of subjects improved.
Total (10)	234	1.8–6.0	10 controlled	8/10 (80%)	3–20 weeks	0.15–1.0 mg/kg/day; 2.5–30 mg/day	9/10 studies (90%) support efficacy in preschool ADHD. More side effects in those with dev. delay.

Note. All studies used methylphenidate except Short et al. (2004), which used mixed amphetamine salts (Adderall).
[a]Blind, placebo-controlled, crossover design.
[b]Blind, placebo-controlled, parallel-group design.
[c]Blind, placebo-controlled, off-on–off treatment reversal design.
[d]Blind, case–control design.

then completed a 1-week open-label lead-in trial of four escalating doses of immediate-release methylphenidate, beginning at 1.25 mg and progressing to 7.5 mg given three times daily. After this phase, 165 cases were randomized, and 145 cases completed a double-blind crossover design involving the best prior dose of methylphenidate from the lead-in phase and placebo conducted over 4 weeks. Patients were then followed for 40 weeks at their best dose. Results of the open-label lead-in phase showed significant improvement at the 2.5-, 5-, and 7.5-mg doses on both parent and teacher ratings of ADHD symptoms. Effect sizes of 0.3 (2.5-mg dose) to 0.7 (7.5-mg dose) were reported relative to the placebo condition in the crossover phase. Approximately 8.7% of the cases dropped out of the drug trial due to adverse events—chiefly crying, irritability, or emotional outbursts (11 cases); insomnia (5 cases); tics (4 cases); headache/stomachache (2 cases); and anxiety/depression (2 cases). Small but significant negative effects on height (–1.4 cm) and weight (–1.1 kg) were noted over the initial year of medication treatment. Side effects were dose-related, being most likely to occur at the 5- and 7.5-mg levels. Follow-up of these cases has lasted 13 months, with continuing demonstration of treatment efficacy.

The PATS project is consistent with the earlier published studies (see Table 17.2) in demonstrating that stimulants are effective in the management of ADHD symptoms in the preschool-age group, with side effects and tolerance being comparable to those found in school-age children. However, the degree of improvement in symptoms may be somewhat lower in this age group than in school-age children, judging by the effect sizes for the doses used in the PATS study.

Adolescents

In the past, many clinicians believed that stimulant treatment lost its therapeutic effects after puberty. This view contributed to a common clinical practice of discontinuing stimulants at puberty. Current research demonstrates that stimulants continue to have efficacy for ADHD symptoms in adolescence, and that their effects are equivalent to the stimulant benefits seen in younger children with ADHD (Pelham, Vodde-Hamilton, Murphy, Greenstein, & Vallano, 1991; Smith, Pelham, Gnagy, & Yudell, 1998). The current standard of care is to continue to treat ADHD with stimulants in the postpubertal years.

Although more is presently known about stimulant efficacy in adolescents with ADHD, less research has been completed in this age group than in the school-age population. Seven controlled trials of stimulants for ADHD in adolescents are described in Table 17.3. The majority of these studies (6 of 7, or 85.7%) support the continued efficacy of stimulants in the treatment of ADHD adolescents. Most of these studies investigated methylphenidate preparations. Linear dosing effects are described in some studies of adolescents (Coons, Klorman, & Borgstedt, 1987; Klorman, Coons, & Borgstedt, 1987), but not in other studies (Evans et al., 2001; Smith, Pelham, Evans, et al., 1998). Presently, it remains unclear whether adolescents with ADHD respond better to low or to high stimulant doses; therefore, treatment must be individualized. Overall, studies show a stimulant response rate of about 60–75%, indicating that medication is effective in teenagers with ADHD (Wilens & Spencer, 2000). In these studies, no abuse of or tolerance to stimulants was noted (Spencer, Biederman, Wilens, et al., 1996).

Adults

ADHD in adults is poorly recognized in most clinical settings and is a frequently missed clinical diagnosis (see Chapter 11). Comorbid psychiatric diagnoses such as depression, bipolar disorders, substance abuse, anxiety disorders, or antisocial behaviors frequently cloud the clinical picture and contribute to missing the diagnosis of ADHD in referred adults (Spencer, Biederman, Wilens, & Faraone, 1998). Current research indicates that between 30% and 70% of children with ADHD will continue to have symptoms of ADHD in adulthood (Silver, 2000). The estimated prevalence of ADHD in all adults is 4.5% (Faraone et al., 2000). Unlike childhood ADHD, in adult ADHD outward signs of hyperactivity/impulsivity are often replaced by or mixed with a subjective sense of inner restlessness, accompanied by cognitive disorganization, inattention to tasks, distractibility, forgetfulness, and impulsive decision making (Faraone, Biederman, & Mick, 1997; Murphy & Barkley, 1996). This makes the task of clinical diagnosis more difficult for the clinician treating ADHD in adults. However, ADHD is important to recognize and treat in adulthood, as continuing symptoms may im-

TABLE 17.3. Controlled Studies of Stimulant Efficacy for Adolescent ADHD

Study (year)	No. of subjects	Age in years (mean and/or range)	Study design	Random assignment	Duration (weeks)	Stimulant dose (mean and/or range)	Response
Varley (1983)	22	14.2; 13–18	B-PC-CO[a]	+	3	15.2–30.9 mg/kg/day	73% response rate.
Coons et al. (1987); Klorman et al. (1987)	19	14.8; 12–19	B-PC-CO[a]	+	3	40 mg/day	Improvement in behavior and information processing; parents > teachers.
Brown & Sexson (1987)	11	13.7; 12–15	B-PC-CO[a]	+	8	5.8–25.9 mg/day	75% of measures showed improvement on drug.
Barkley et al. (2000)	35	14.0; 12–17	B-PC-CO[a]	+	5	MPH[b]: 5–10 mg/day MAS[c]: 5–10 mg/day	No improvement.
Smith, Pelham, Evans, et al. (1998)	46	13.8; 12–17	B-PC-CO[a]	+	8	25–75 mg/day	Improvement: no linear effects of dose on improvement.
Bostic et al. (2000)	21	14.1; 12–17	B-PC-CO[a]	+	10	PEM[d]: 150 mg/day; 93–225 mg/day	60% response rate, compared to 11% placebo response rate.
Greenhill & MTA Co- perative Group (2002)	177	13–18	B-PC-PG[e]	+	2	OROS MPH[f]: 18, 36, 54, or 72 mg/day	Improvement on all measures compared with placebo.
Total (7)	331	12–19	7 controlled, 7 randomized		3–10	MPH: 5–75 mg/day PEM: 93–225 mg/day MAS: 5–10 mg/day	6/7 (85.7%) of studies support efficacy.

Note. Medication is methylphenidate in this table unless otherwise stated.
[a]Blind, placebo-controlled, crossover design.
[b]Methylphenidate.
[c]Mixed amphetamine salts (Adderall).
[d]Pemoline.
[e]Blind, placebo-controlled, parallel-group design.
[f]Concerta.

pair adult functioning across a variety of domains (Fischer, Barkley, Smallish, & Fletcher, 2002).

The role of stimulant medications in treating adults with ADHD is no different from this role with children and adolescents. Adults with ADHD respond to stimulants with improved attention span, decreased distractibility, diminished restlessness, and lessened impulsivity, in a similar fashion to younger patients with ADHD (Wilens et al., 1995). Controlled studies of stimulants in adults with ADHD are listed in Table 17.4; in comparison to the large database that exists on the efficacy of stimulants for ADHD in children, only nine controlled stimulant trials have been reported for adults. These trials have examined methylphenidate, dextroamphetamine, and pemoline. In contrast to the robust and consistent 70% response rates reported for children with ADHD, controlled studies in adults report more equivocal response rates. With the exception of the Spencer et al. (1995) study, response rates in adults range between 25% and 58%.

Variability in adult ADHD response rates may be related to several factors. These include difficulty recognizing the adult ADHD phenotype, with subsequent enrollment of heterogeneous subjects in clinical trials (Wender, Reimherr, & Wood, 1981; Wender, Reimherr, Wood, & Ward, 1985; Wood, Reimherr, Wender, & Johnson, 1976); high rates of comorbidity in adults with ADHD (Faraone et al., 1995, 2000); and the low doses of stimulants used in many of these clinical trials. For example, in controlled studies limiting methylphenidate to doses less than 0.7 mg/day, response rates range from 25% to 57% (Mattes, Boswell, & Oliver, 1984; Wender et al., 1985; Wood et al., 1976). However, Spencer et al. (1995) report a much higher response rate of 78% when higher doses of methylphenidate are used, up to 1.0 mg/kg/day. For adults with ADHD, therefore, response rates may become more robust when higher stimulant doses are used. (Again, see Chapter 22 for a more detailed discussion.)

STIMULANT TREATMENT FOR ADHD WITH PSYCHIATRIC COMORBIDITY

In children and adolescents with ADHD, higher rates of comorbid Oppositional Defiant Disorder (ODD), Conduct Disorder (CD), Major Depressive Disorder (MDD), and anxiety disorders are found than in control youths without ADHD (see Chapter 3; see also Biederman, Newcorn, & Sprich, 1991; Brown, 2000; Pliszka et al., 1999). In adults with ADHD, higher rates of Antisocial Personality Disorder, substance abuse, Bipolar I Disorder (BPD), MDD, and anxiety disorders are found than in controls without ADHD (Biederman et al., 1993; Murphy & Barkley, 1996). This section reviews stimulant use for ADHD when the diagnosis is complicated by psychiatric comorbidity.

ADHD and Oppositional Defiant Disorder/ Conduct Disorder

About 50% of children with ADHD will meet criteria for either ODD or CD. The prevalence of the association between ADHD and ODD/ CD will vary with the age of the child. Children under the age of 12 years who meet criteria for ODD or CD will almost always meet criteria for ADHD (Szatmari, Boyle, & Offord, 1989). In adolescent samples, pure CD is more common, and only about 33% of teenage patients with CD will also meet criteria for ADHD (Szatmari et al., 1989).

Many studies have compared the responses of children with ADHD and ODD/CD and of those with ADHD alone to stimulant medications. When stimulant is compared with placebo in controlled clinical trials, these two groups show an equally robust response to stimulant (Barkley, McMurray, Edelbrock, & Robbins, 1989; Klein et al., 1997; Klorman et al., 1988). That is, children with ADHD and ODD/CD show the same reductions in inattention, impulsivity, and hyperactivity as do children with ADHD alone. Thus childhood antisocial behavior does not seem to attenuate stimulant response for ADHD symptoms.

In youngsters with ADHD and comorbid CD or aggression, stimulants appear to reduce antisocial behaviors, in addition to their effects on the core symptoms of ADHD (Connor et al., 2000). In a meta-analysis of 28 controlled stimulant studies for ADHD, stimulants reduced symptoms of overt aggression (effect size = 0.84) and covert aggression (effect size = 0.69) (Connor, Glatt, Lopez, Jackson, & Melloni, 2002). Although it is not clear whether stimulants help impulsive aggression in children without ADHD, they can help decrease the frequency and intensity of aggressive

TABLE 17.4. Controlled Studies of Stimulant Efficacy for Adult ADHD

Study (year)	No. of subjects	Age in years (mean and/or range)	Study design	Random assignment	Duration (weeks)	Stimulant dose (mean and/or range)	Response
Wood et al. (1976)	11	28 ± 4.5	B-PC-CO[a]	−	4	23.5 mg/day; 20–60 mg/day (MPH)[b]	53% response rate.
Wender et al. (1981)	51	28; 21–45	B-PC-PG[c]	+	6	65 mg/day; 18–150 mg/day (PEM)[d]	50% response rate.
Mattes et al. (1984)	26	32; 18–45	B-PC-CO[a]	+	6	48 mg/day; 10–60 mg/day (MPH)	25% response rate.
Wender et al. (1985)	37	31 ± 6.7	B-PC-CO[a]	+	5	48 mg/day; 10–80 mg/day (MPH)	57% response rate.
Gualtieri et al. (1985)	22	27.5; 18–38	B-PC-CO[a]	+	2	0.5–2.0 mg/kg/day (MPH)	Moderate response rates.
Spencer et al. (1995)	23	40; 19–56	B-PC-CO[a]	+	7	1.0 mg/kg/day (MPH)	78% response rate; 4% placebo response rate.
Wilens et al. (1999)	35	40.7; 23–60	B-PC-CO[a]	+	10	2.2 mg/kg/day; 86–200 mg/day (PEM)	50% response rate; 17% placebo response rate.
Paterson et al. (1999)	45	35.5; 19–57	B-PC-PG[c]	+	6	5–35 mg/day (DEX)[e]	58% response rate; 10% placebo response rate.
Schubiner et al. (2002)	48	38.3; 18–55	B-PC-PG[c]	+	12	26.2 ± 6.5 mg/day (MPH)	77% response rate; 21% placebo response rate. Comorbid cocaine abuse.
Total (9)	298	19–60	9 controlled	8 randomized	2–12	MPH: 10–80 mg/day DEX: 5–35 mg/day PEM 18.75–200 mg/day	Lower response rates than children.

[a]Blind, placebo-controlled, crossover design.
[b]Methylphenidate.
[c]Blind, placebo-controlled, parallel-group design.
[d]Pemoline.
[e]Dextroamphetamine.

outbursts in children with ADHD. The effects of stimulants on adults with ADHD and Antisocial Personality Disorder have not been studied.

ADHD and Depression

It is not uncommon to encounter children who are demoralized or dysphoric about the consequences of their impulsive ADHD behaviors. Such children appear depressed, but the depression is short-lived and generally occurs only after a frustration or a disciplinary event. Thus brief episodes of depressed or irritable mood may be common in children with ADHD, may occur many times a day, and do not necessarily meet the criteria for MDD. This demoralization will get better as the ADHD is treated.

The syndrome of MDD—identified by a persistently depressed, sad, or irritable mood, different from the child's usual personality; lasting for days to weeks; and accompanied by guilt, anhedonia, social withdrawal, and suicidal thoughts—occurs in between 15% and 30% of children and adolescents with ADHD (Biederman et al., 1994; Biederman, Mick, & Faraone, 1998; Biederman et al., 1991; Brown, 2000; Spencer, Wilens, Biederman, Wozniak, & Harding-Crawford, 2000). True comorbidity of ADHD and MDD requires treatment of both the ADHD and the depression.

No studies have compared stimulant response in a group of children with the diagnosis of ADHD and a group with the comorbid diagnoses of ADHD and MDD. However, several studies have investigated stimulant response in ADHD accompanied by the symptoms of depression (internalizing psychopathology, not the psychiatric diagnosis of MDD). There are hints that symptoms of depression may reduce the clinical response to stimulants in ADHD. For example, DuPaul, Barkley, and McMurray (1994) studied 40 children with ADHD and divided the sample into three groups based on the severity of comorbid internalizing symptoms (mixed anxiety and depression). Differential effects of three doses of methylphenidate (5 mg, 10 mg, and 15 mg) were evaluated in a controlled methodology, using multiple outcome measures across home, school, and clinic settings. Results showed that children with ADHD and comorbid internalizing symptoms were less likely to respond to methylphenidate than children without co-morbid internalizing psychopathology. In the large MTA, children with ADHD and anxiety/depression seemed to do best in the combined treatment arm (stimulants and behavioral therapy) rather than the stimulant arm alone (Jensen et al., 2001). In contrast, Gadow, Nolan, Sverd, Sprafkin, and Schwartz (2002) found no diminished response rate to stimulants for the symptoms of ADHD when children had comorbid anxious and depressive psychopathology.

The clinician treating patients with ADHD must be vigilant for comorbid depressive disorders. If the latter are present, both ADHD and depression should be treated. Stimulants have been safely combined with SSRIs, such as fluoxetine, in children, adolescents, and adults (Abikoff et al., 2005; Findling, 1996; Gammon & Brown, 1991).

ADHD and Bipolar I Disorder

The prevalence of childhood BPD in children with ADHD is a topic of controversy and debate. This controversy arises out of a lack of consensus as to how to identify BPD in children. Part of the problem is the high degree of overlap between symptoms of ADHD and bipolar symptoms (e.g., irritability, mood lability, aggression, hyperactivity/agitation, sleep disturbance). In primary care practice, the prevalence of childhood BPD is rare. Among children with ADHD, a few may have early-onset BPD. For example, after screening many referrals, Geller et al. (1998) identified 60 prepubertal children with bipolar mania. All had comorbid ADHD. Factors that most differentiated children with mania from those with ADHD alone were (1) grandiosity, (2) excessively elated mood, (3) racing thoughts, (4) hypersexuality in the absence of a history of sexual trauma/abuse, and (5) decreased need for sleep (Geller, Zimerman, Williams, DelBello, Bolhofner, et al., 2002; Geller, Zimerman, Williams, DelBello, Frazier, et al., 2002; Geller et al., 1998).

If a child has acute mania as well as ADHD, mood stabilization with lithium, divalproex sodium, and/or an atypical antipsychotic is indicated before treatment with a stimulant. Once the acute manic symptoms have stabilized, the clinician should reassess the patient for ADHD. If ADHD symptoms continue to be problematic, stimulants may be added to a mood stabilizer to treat continuing ADHD symptoms (Scheffer, 2002).

ADHD and Anxiety Disorders

About 25–30% of children with ADHD will meet criteria for an anxiety disorder, compared to 5–15% of comparison children (Bird, Gould, & Staghezza, 1993; Cohen et al., 1993). Initial studies suggested that the response of children with ADHD to stimulant medications was less when comorbid anxiety disorders were present. For example, in a study of 43 children with ADHD treated with methylphenidate under controlled conditions, over 80% of the children without anxiety responded to the stimulant, while only 30% of the children with anxiety benefited from the medication (Pliszka, 1989). In an unselected group of children with ADHD, low anxiety ratings predicted a good response to stimulants (Buitelaar, van der Gaag, Swaab-Barneveld, & Kuiper, 1995). These earlier studies suggested that anxiety disorders or symptoms could diminish ADHD stimulant response rates.

However, more recent studies have not supported diminished stimulant responses in youth with anxiety and ADHD. In a short-term controlled trial, children with ADHD had equally robust responses to methylphenidate, whether or not they had comorbid anxiety (Diamond, Tannock, & Schachar, 1999). In the large MTA, over 100 children received a double-blind, placebo controlled trial of methylphenidate, and over one-third of the subjects had comorbid anxiety disorders. Anxiety did not predict a poorer response to stimulant medication (MTA Cooperative Group, 1999). However, the anxious children in the MTA seemed to benefit more from a combination of psychosocial treatment and medication than the children without anxiety. Results of a controlled trial of the efficacy of sequential stimulant and fluvoxamine pharmacotherapy for 6- to 17-year-old children with ADHD and anxiety (Abikoff et al., 2005) showed that children with ADHD and anxiety have a response rate to stimulants that is comparable with that of children with general ADHD.

In clinical practice, the child with both ADHD and anxiety should be treated for ADHD first. Since the response to stimulant medication can be assessed quickly, and children with this comorbidity do not generally worsen on stimulant medications, a stimulant trial is the first intervention. Should anxiety continue to be a problem, a psychosocial intervention or a trial of an SSRI for anxiety could be implemented in addition to stimulant medication (Abikoff et al., 2005; Research Unit on Pediatric Psychopharmacology Anxiety Study Group, 2001).

ADHD and Tic Disorders

Tic disorders are fairly common in nonreferred children. In large samples of children assessed in the community, the prevalence of motor tics is about 21% (Kurlan et al., 2002). Motor tics appear more commonly than vocal tics. Tic prevalence appears to vary with child gender and age: Tics are more common in boys than girls, and in preschool children than older children (Gadow, Nolan, Sprafkin, & Schwartz, 2002). For example, in a large nonclinical community study of over 3,000 children and adolescents, the prevalence of tic disorders in 3- to 5-year-olds was 6 times the prevalence rate in 12- to 18-year-olds (Gadow, Nolan, Sprafkin, & Schwartz, 2002). The prevalence of tic disorders may also vary by the season of the year. One study of 553 children in kindergarten through sixth grade found that the incidence of motor tics increased in the winter months and diminished in the summer months (Snider et al., 2002).

Controlled studies have demonstrated that an association between tic disorders and ADHD occurs at a rate greater than expected from chance alone (Gadow, Nolan, Sprafkin, & Schwartz, 2002; Kurlan et al., 2002; Sukhodolsky et al., 2003). In clinical samples of boys with tic disorders, Tourette syndrome co-occurs with ADHD in between 21% and 54% of cases (Biederman et al., 1991; Pliszka, 1998; Pliszka et al., 1999). In samples of children with ADHD, however, tic disorders are found at a far lesser rate. For example, in the MTA, 10.9% of 579 children with ADHD had a comorbid tic disorder (MTA Cooperative Group, 1999).

Methodologically controlled studies have shown that stimulant medications are highly effective for ADHD symptoms, aggression, and social skill deficits in children with Tourette syndrome or chronic tic disorders (Castellanos et al., 1997; Gadow, Nolan, Sprafkin, & Schwartz, 2002; Gadow, Nolan, & Sverd, 1992; Gadow, Nolan, Sverd, Sprafkin, & Paolicelli, 1990; Gadow, Sverd, Sprafkin, Nolan, & Ezor, 1995; Tourette's Syndrome Study Group, 2002). These studies show that the rates of tics in children with ADHD and preexisting tic disorders treated with stimulants are not different from the rates of tics in such children treated with a placebo (Gadow et al., 1992, 1995; Tourette's Syndrome Study Group, 2002).

However, numerous clinical observations have indicated that stimulants exacerbate tic frequency and intensity in children with ADHD and preexisting tic disorders (Riddle et al., 1995). This has led clinicians to undertreat ADHD in children with tic disorders. There is now a much greater understanding that the consequences of untreated ADHD are much greater than the consequences of mild to moderate tic disorders for children's social, behavioral, interpersonal, and academic development. Although stimulants may exacerbate a preexisting tic disorder, the frequency and intensity of tics generally return to baseline after several months of stimulant treatment. In children who develop severe tics with the use of a stimulant, most tics will remit after the stimulant is discontinued (Wilens & Spencer, 2000). There is little evidence that tic disorders are created de novo by the introduction of stimulants in children who are not already vulnerable to tic disorders (generally on a heritable basis).

The current standard of care has now evolved into a recommendation to treat moderate to severe ADHD in children with mild to moderate tic disorders. Obtaining the informed consent of parents, and close monitoring of tic frequency and severity, are necessary aspects of treatment. Should tics become problematic, controlled studies support the use of clonidine (Tourette's Syndrome Study Group, 2002) or guanfacine (Scahill et al., 2001) in the treatment of comorbid ADHD and tic disorders.

ADHD and Learning Disabilities

An overlap between ADHD and learning disabilities is frequently reported in both children and adults (Murphy, Barkley, & Bush, 2002; Purvis & Tannock, 1997). Learning disabilities include expressive and receptive language delays, auditory processing difficulties, and reading disabilities. A wide range of overlap has been reported in some studies, with the rate of children having both ADHD and learning disabilities varying between 10% and 92% (Semrud-Clikeman et al., 1992). More recent studies report a smaller overlap of between 20% and 25% (Pliszka, 1998). The wide disparity in comorbidity is probably due to different definitions of learning disabilities used in various studies.

Research supports the independence of learning disabilities and ADHD as two separate types of disorders, although they may frequently co-occur. The two disorders are transmitted independently in families (Faraone et al., 1993). Neuropsychological testing supports different deficits in ADHD and learning disabilities (Purvis & Tannock, 1997).

Stimulants are not a treatment for specific learning disabilities. These disabilities typically require specialized psychoeducational interventions. However, in children with comorbid ADHD and learning disabilities, treatment of ADHD symptoms with stimulants can be helpful as part of an overall treatment plan.

ADHD and Substance Use Disorders

Despite the stimulants' documented efficacy in the treatment of ADHD, there continues to be public concern that stimulant use in childhood and adolescence increases the risk for substance use disorders. Some lay groups, such as the Church of Scientology's Citizens Commission on Human Rights (CCHR), have capitalized on public concerns to suggest that prescribing stimulants to children with ADHD predisposes them to greater substance abuse risk in adolescence and young adulthood (CCHR, 1987).

There may be two reasons for this public concern. The first is that stimulants such as methylphenidate may be chemically similar to cocaine, and therefore are often believed to be highly addictive and abusable (like cocaine), especially when inhaled or injected intravenously. However, evidence shows that stimulants and cocaine possess distinctly different pharmacodynamic and pharmacokinetic properties. Methylphenidate enters and clears the brain much more slowly than does cocaine, eliciting a slow and steady dopamine release from dopamine-containing neurons. These characteristics are associated with clinical benefits and limit the abuse potential of stimulants. In contrast, cocaine enters the brain rapidly, clears the brain quickly, and elicits a large and fast release of dopamine from neurons. These characteristics are associated with the reinforcing properties of cocaine and contribute to its abuse potential (Volkow et al., 1995, 2002).

The second reason for public concern comes from evidence that stimulants lead to increased sensitization to later stimulant exposure in preclinical animal models. Intermittent stimulant dosing in mammal models suggests that repeated stimulant exposure leads to subsequently greater craving and self-administration of stimulants in animals (Robinson & Berridge, 1993). However, the evidence to date on the actual risks of substance use and abuse in stimulant-treated children with ADHD is relatively weak. To date, there are 14 studies that address this issue (for reviews, see Barkley, Fischer, Smallish, & Fletcher, 2003; Wilens, Faraone, Biederman, & Gunawardene, 2003). Of these 14, only 1 study found support for the sensitization hypothesis of increased risk for later substance abuse in stimulant-treated children with ADHD (Lambert & Hartsough, 1998). This study did not control for comorbid CD in their sample with ADHD, among other methodological problems. CD is known to increase the risk of substance abuse, independently of ADHD or stimulant treatment. The other 13 studies found no evidence that stimulant treatment increases risks for later substance abuse. Indeed, many studies find that stimulant treatment of ADHD actually reduces the risks for later substance abuse (Biederman et al., 1997; Biederman, Wilens, Mick, Spencer, & Faraone, 1999; Wilens, Faraone, et al., 2003). In a meta-analysis of six studies including 674 stimulant-treated subjects and 360 unmedicated subjects followed for at least 4 years, the pooled estimate of the odds ratio indicated a 1.9-fold reduction in risk for substance abuse in stimulant-treated youth with ADHD (Wilens, Faraone, et al., 2003). Thus it appears that stimulant treatment of ADHD actually reduces the risk of later substance use disorders.

A separate clinical challenge is the treatment of ADHD in an adolescent or young adult who already exhibits substance abuse. In uncontrolled environments, active substance abuse is a relative contraindication to prescribing stimulant medications. Antidepressants with known efficacy for the treatment of ADHD and limited abuse potential, such as bupropion or atomoxetine, should be used (Michelson et al., 2001; Riggs, 1998).

LONG-TERM TREATMENT

The vast majority of studies to date have reported on the short-term effects of stimulant medications. Clinical trials generally last 2–8 weeks. There is a paucity of studies on the long-term (>4-month) efficacy and safety of stimulants. Longer studies are important, because ADHD is generally a chronic disorder, and it is important to know whether stimulants continue to be effective and safe over extended treatment periods.

Three controlled and one open-label study have examined the efficacy and safety of stimulants over 4- to 60-month treatment durations for children with ADHD (Charach, Ickowicz, & Schachar, 2004; Gillberg et al., 1997; MTA Cooperative Group, 1999; Schachar, Tannock, Cunningham, & Corkum, 1997; Wilens, Pelham, et al., 2003). Schachar et al. (1997) investigated methylphenidate compared to placebo in 91 children with ADHD over a 4-month clinical trial. The children continued to demonstrate benefits of methylphenidate over the 16-week trial. Lack of weight gain was a side effect documented in the treatment group (Schachar et al., 1997). This study has now been extended for 5 years, and data are reported on 79 of the original 91 children (Charach et al., 2004). Stimulants continue to be effective for the core symptoms of ADHD over 5 years; however, side effects persist, most notably appetite suppression. The MTA examined 579 children with ADHD and compared stimulant medication management with behavioral therapy, combined medication and behavioral therapy, or routine community care over 14 months. Results showed that the children assigned to stimulant treatment (medication management and combined treatment) exhibited greater improvements than the other two groups (behavioral treatment alone and routine community care) (MTA Cooperative Group, 1999). Stimulant benefits were maintained over 14 months. Gillberg et al. (1997) investigated amphetamine treatment on symptoms of ADHD in 62 children over 15 months. Amphetamine was clearly superior to placebo in reducing the core symptoms of ADHD over the 15 months. Stimulant drug appeared well tolerated, and side effects were reported as relatively few and mild (Gillberg et al., 1997). In a 12-month open-label study, Wilens, Pelham, et al. (2003) investigated the efficacy and tolerability of OROS methylphenidate (Concerta) in 289 children ages 6–13 years with ADHD. Stimulant effectiveness on the core symptoms of ADHD was maintained over the 12-month clinical trial as assessed by teachers, parents, and clinicians. OROS methylphenidate was well tolerated over the year, with minimal impact on sleep quality, tics, blood pressure, pulse, or height. Only 2% of children were reported to experience weight loss as a significant side effect (Wilens, Pelham, et al., 2003).

These longer-term results include data from a total of 1,021 stimulant-treated children. Both methylphenidate and amphetamine preparations have been studied in these longer-duration clinical trials. The data are encouraging, in that stimulants continue to be effective for the core symptoms of ADHD and appear well tolerated over 4 months to 5 years of treatment. Future studies need to examine long-term tolerability and effectiveness of stimulants in adolescents and adults with ADHD.

SIDE EFFECTS

Common, Short-Term, Acute Side Effects

Stimulant medications are generally well tolerated. Side effects do occur, but they are generally mild and can be managed by dose adjustment or changing the timing of medication intake. In a study of the prevalence of parent- and teacher-reported side effects to two doses (i.e., 0.3 mg/kg and 0.5 mg/kg) of methylphenidate given twice daily in a sample of 82 children with ADHD, over half the sample exhibited decreased appetite, insomnia, anxiety, irritability, and/or proneness to crying with both doses of methylphenidate. However, many of these apparent side effects were present during a placebo condition, and may actually represent characteristics of the disorder rather than its treatment (Barkley, McMurray,

Edelbrock, & Robbins, 1990). Clinically, it is important to ascertain parent-reported medication side effects at baseline before the child is on stimulant medication, and then again at full dose. Many of the reported medication side effects may actually be aspects of the disease and get better with treatment. Severe side effects were reported much less frequently than mild side effects. In the Barkley et al. (1990) study, side effects were linearly related to dose, with higher doses associated with more reported side effects. Only 3.6% of children had side effects severe enough to warrant methylphenidate discontinuation.

Pooled side effect data from five pivotal clinical trials (i.e., four trials of methylphenidate and one trial of mixed amphetamine salts) are presented in Table 17.5. In this table, adverse events reported in subjects receiving an active drug are compared to those reported in subjects receiving a placebo for six common acute stimulant side effects. Note that side effects are also reported on placebo. Again, for the clinician to obtain an accurate picture of stimulant treatment emergent side effects a baseline evaluation before medication is initiated. Side effects are generally higher on active drugs, but stimulants are generally well tolerated in these clinical trials.

In special populations, there may be a higher incidence of stimulant-related side effects. Preschool children with ADHD who are treated with stimulants may experience a higher rate of adverse effects than older children, particularly crying, irritability, and emotional outbursts (Connor, 2002; Kollins & PATS Study Group, 2004). Children with developmental delays

TABLE 17.5. Common Short-Term Stimulant Side Effects

Side effect	Methylphenidate	Placebo	Mixed amphetamine salts	Placebo
Body as a whole				
Abdominal pain	11.3%	7.0%	14.0%	10.0%
Headache	13.0%	8.4%	—	—
Digestive system				
Anorexia	14.0%	6.4%	22.0%	2.0%
Vomiting	3.5%	3.2%	7.0%	4.0%
Nervous system				
Insomnia	7.8%	7.2%	17.0%	2.0%
Nervousness	13.4%	17.4%	6.0%	2.0%

Note. Pooled data from four clinical trials of methylphenidate and one clinical trial of mixed amphetamine salts (Biederman, Lopez, Boellner, & Chandler, 2002; Greenhill, Findling, Swanson, & MTA Cooperative Group, 2002; McNeil Pharmaceuticals, 2001; Novartis Pharmaceuticals, 2002a, 2002b).

such as autism or mental retardation may also experience elevated rates of stimulant side effects (Aman et al., 1991; Handen et al., 1992). These populations require increased clinical attention to monitor stimulant related side effects.

Stimulants are sympathomimetic drugs; theoretically, therefore, they can raise blood pressure and pulse rate. This has led to concerns over their cardiovascular safety in children. However, the cardiovascular effects of stimulants in healthy children, adolescents, and adults are minimal and do not appear clinically significant (Brown, Wynne, & Slimmer, 1984; Rapport & Moffitt, 2002). Routine blood pressure and pulse checks in healthy youth receiving stimulants for ADHD are not indicated (Wilens & Spencer, 2000). Studies of normotensive adults receiving stimulants report average elevations of 4 mm Hg of systolic and diastolic blood pressure, and pulse increases of less than 10 beats per minute, associated with treatment (Spencer et al., 1995). In adults at risk for hypertension, higher increases in blood pressure may be noted. Given the high prevalence of hypertension in adults, blood pressure and pulse rate should be monitored in adults receiving stimulants for ADHD.

Given the short half-life of many immediate-release stimulants, deterioration in behavior and ADHD symptom control can occur in the afternoon and evening following earlier administration of stimulant medication. The deterioration may exceed that expected from baseline ADHD symptoms. This phenomenon is referred to as "rebound" and has been described in previous stimulant research (Rapoport et al., 1978). However, other studies of immediate-release stimulants have not found deterioration in evening ADHD symptoms over and above baseline (Johnston, Pelham, Hoza, & Sturges, 1988). Should rebound occur, the use of longer-acting stimulant preparations, or the addition of a small dose of immediate-release stimulant 1 hour before the onset of symptom exacerbation, reduces rebound symptoms late in the day.

Tolerance to CNS stimulants has not been established in research; however, clinical anecdotes suggest decreased efficacy of the drugs in some cases with chronic administration. Investigators have conjectured that this may stem from hepatic autoinduction, behavioral noncompliance with the prescribed regimen, weight gain, or environmental factors such as an intercurrent stress event (e.g., a move, a parental divorce, or a change in school classroom) or altered caregiver expectations for behavior (Greenhill, Pliszka, et al., 2002). It is also possible, given the inherent complexity of dopamine receptors, that compensatory changes in the number of receptor sites may occur as a function of prolonged stimulant use.

Rare, Acute Side Effects

Tics

As noted above, stimulants can exacerbate the frequency and intensity of motor and vocal tics in some children with ADHD and preexisting tic disorders. In a study of 1,520 children diagnosed with Attention Deficit Disorder and treated with methylphenidate, existing tics were exacerbated in 6 children (0.39%), and new tics developed in 14 cases (0.92%). After discontinuation of methylphenidate, all six of the tics that had worsened returned to their baseline intensity, and 13 of 14 new tics completely remitted (Denckla, Bemporad, & MacKay, 1976). Although there has been concern that stimulant-induced tic disorders may be severe and may not remit with discontinuation of stimulant medication, these cases appear rare (Bremness & Sverd, 1979). Most stimulant-induced tics are mild and transient. There are few subjects (about 0.1%) in whom tics do not diminish after stopping the medication (Denckla et al., 1976; Lipkin, Goldstein, & Adesman, 1994).

Concern has also been expressed that stimulant medications may cause the development of new tics de novo in children with ADHD. Shapiro and Shapiro (1981) reviewed the relationship between treating Attention Deficit Disorder with stimulants and the precipitation of new tics and Tourette syndrome in children. They concluded that the evidence suggests that stimulants do not cause new tic disorders, although high doses of stimulants can cause or exacerbate tics in children already predisposed to tic disorder or Tourette syndrome. This issue was further investigated in a longitudinal study comparing children with ADHD who were treated with stimulants or with a placebo over the course of 1 year. At the end of the year, 19.6% of stimulant-treated children and 16.7% of placebo-treated children had developed a new-onset tic (Law & Schachar, 1999). This was a nonsignificant difference, however, and supports data suggesting that stimulants do not cause new tic disorders in children who are not already predisposed to develop a tic disorder. These data support the clinical recommendation to treat ADHD with stimulants when mild to moderate tic disorder comorbidity is present, after a careful risk–benefit discussion with the family. Close clinical monitoring of the tics during ongoing stimulant therapy is recommended.

Sudden Death

Recent concern has been raised about the use of Adderall XR in children with underlying and often silent cardiac anomalies. A total of 12 cases of sudden death in children and adolescents receiving Adderall XR are known to the U.S. Food and Drug Administration (FDA). Because of these deaths, Health Canada, the Canadian drug-regulatory agency, has suspended the sale of Adderall XR in the Canadian market.

Of the 12 total cases of sudden death (out of a total 30 million Adderall prescriptions written between 1999 and 2003), five occurred in patients with underlying structural heart defects, including abnormal arteries, abnormal cardiac valves, hypertrophic subaortic stenosis, and anomalous origin of the cardiac arteries. These are all conditions that increase risk for sudden death regardless of stimulant use. Several of the remaining cases represent problems in interpretation, including a family history of ventricular tachycardia and association of death with heat exhaustion, dehydration, and near drowning, rigorous exercise, fatty liver, heart attack, and type 1 diabetes mellitus. One case was reported 3–4 years after the event, and another case may represent a poisoning and overdose with Adderall XR. The duration of treatment varied from 1 day to 8 years. The FDA notes that the number of cases of sudden deaths reported for Adderall XR is only slightly greater, per million prescriptions, than the number reported for methylphenidate products. Furthermore, the FDA considered that the rate of Adderall XR-related sudden deaths did not seem greater than the number of sudden deaths that would be expected to occur in this population without treatment. Although the FDA has added a sentence to Adderall XR's "black-box" warning indicating that these medications should not be used in patients with known structural defects, it has not suspended sales of Adderall XR in the United States.

The extant data do suggest that patients with underlying heart defects (often clinically silent) might be at increased risk for sudden death. Clinicians should take a careful cardiac history in patients and exclude those children with ADHD and known heart defects from stimulant treatment.

Psychosis

Stimulants can cause psychosis in individuals with a preexisting psychotic disorder such as schizophrenia or with a vulnerability to mania, and can cause psychosis as an acute manifestation of stimulant toxicity (such as that occurring upon overdose of stimulant medications). Approximately 20 cases of stimulant-induced psychosis have been reported in the clinical literature (Bloom, Russell, Weisskopf, & Blackerby, 1988; Koehler-Troy, Strober, & Malenbaum, 1986). Individuals with a psychotic reaction to stimulants should be clinically monitored for a recurrence or development of a psychotic illness.

Long-Term, Chronic Adverse Events

Effects on Growth

Stimulants routinely produce anorexia, appetite suppression, and weight loss. Weight loss is generally mild and is not permanent. When stimulants are discontinued, weight catches up to its usual developmental trajectory. Ultimate adult weight is generally unaffected by stimulant use. Weight should be monitored routinely during stimulant treatment. In the few children with more serious weight loss as a function of stimulant treatment, the clinician may have to alter the stimulant dose schedule or schedule a stimulant drug holiday to allow weight gain to catch up. Another clinical strategy is to feed a child before bedtime, when the anorectic effects of stimulants are decreasing and the appetite may rebound.

Stimulant effects on height are less certain. Initial reports suggested a persistent decrease in growth of height in stimulant-treated children (Safer, Allen, & Barr, 1972). However, other reports have failed to replicate this finding (Gross, 1976; Rapport & Moffitt, 2002; Satterfield, Cantwell, Schell, & Blaschke, 1979; Spencer, Biederman, Harding, et al., 1996). More recent studies conclude that ultimate height may unaffected by stimulant treatment during the developing years (Gittelman & Mannuzza, 1988).

Another possibility is that height differences between children with ADHD and control youths may be due to the disorder itself and not to stimulant treatment. In a longitudinal study, data suggested that growth deficits in children with ADHD may represent a temporary delay in the tempo of growth (e.g., dysmaturity of growth), but that final adult height is not compromised (Spencer, Biederman, Harding, et al., 1996). This effect may be mediated by ADHD and not stimulant treatment (Wilens & Spencer, 2000).

The issue of stimulant "medication holidays" to counteract the possible growth deficits associated with stimulant treatment remains unresolved. This practice rests on the premise that there exists a "growth rebound" during the time off stimulants (Klein & Mannuzza, 1988). For example, Klein and Mannuzza (1988) found a significant positive effect on height in stimulant-treated children with ADHD who did not receive stimulant medication over two summers. However, not all studies support the possibility of growth rebound off stimulants. In a controlled trial of 58 children with ADHD receiving chronic stimulant treatment, no major differences in growth were found between children who did and those who did not have summer drug holidays (Satterfield et al., 1979). In considering a medication holiday, clinicians and parents must balance the risks of being off stimulant medication with the slight risks to growth of continuing medication. Given the negative impact of untreated ADHD across multiple domains in the daily life of a child with the disorder, this decision must be made with care.

CLINICAL USE OF STIMULANTS

General Principles

Treatment with stimulant medications should always be part of an overall psychoeducational treatment plan for the child or adolescent with ADHD. Consideration should be given to all aspects of the youngster's and family's life. Whereas stimulants are rarely the only treatment prescribed for youth with ADHD, some adults with the disorder will receive medication as part of their treatment plan in the absence of other forms of treatment. However, even with these adults, education about the disease and

its treatment should be given to the patients and their immediate families. National organizations such as Children and Adults with Attention-Deficit/Hyperactivity Disorder (CHADD; website: *www.chadd.org*) or the American Academy of Child and Adolescent Psychiatry (AACAP; website: *www.aacap.org*) are important sources of information for patients and families.

Treatment should always be preceded by a careful evaluation of the individual with ADHD and his or her family. Evaluation should include attention to psychiatric, social, cognitive, and educational/occupational aspects of the patient. A recent screening physical examination should be available to rule out medical illness or sensory impairments (e.g., hearing loss) that may contribute to symptoms or influence treatment decision making. Special attention should be paid to issues of comorbidity with learning disorders, which may also contribute to educational or occupational underperformance. Comorbid learning disabilities are important to identify, because they do not respond to stimulant medications and require supplemental educational remediation. Attention should also be given to other issues of comorbidity that may influence symptom presentation, treatment response, and prognosis. In children with ADHD, psychiatric comorbidity may include CD/ODD, anxiety disorders, MDD, or BPD. In adolescents with ADHD, additional attention should be paid to possible alcohol, tobacco, and other substance use/misuse, together with risk-taking behaviors. In adults with the disorder, these comorbidities, as well as interpersonal conflicts with spouses/partners, children, and/or coworkers, should be inquired about. In those of driving age, it is recommended that a driving history be obtained, as ADHD can seriously impair judgment and performance related to operating a motor vehicle (Barkley, 2004).

In evaluating the family of a child with ADHD, a clinician must pay attention to the possibility that a parent or sibling also has ADHD. ADHD is a highly heritable disorder (heritability rates ~ 70%), and first-degree biological relatives of the identified patient frequently have ADHD themselves (Biederman et al., 1995). The presence of a parent or sibling with ADHD may complicate the family picture and must be taken into account during treatment planning. Another focus of evaluation is the question of possible substance use disorder in family members of the identified patient with ADHD. In this case, stimulant medications should not be prescribed, as there exists a risk of its illicit use or sale. Nonstimulant medications to treat ADHD, such as bupropion or atomoxetine, can be considered in these cases.

Parental and child attitudes about pharmacotherapy must be evaluated as well. Some parents are simply not supportive of drug therapy for their children, and alternative psychoeducational therapies for these children must be identified. Divorced parents may disagree about treating a child with stimulants. The clinician must be careful not to insist on stimulant therapy or coerce parents into agreeing to pharmacotherapy, as this may inadvertently undermine the efficacy and sustainability of the intervention. With older children and adolescents, it is important to discuss the use of medication with them and to explain its rationale in the treatment of ADHD.

Goals of Stimulant Treatment for ADHD

As noted earlier in this chapter, a change has occurred over the years in the way ADHD is perceived by clinicians and researchers. Historically, ADHD was thought to be a disorder of childhood, confined to the 6- to 12-year-old age range. Because hyperactivity generally diminishes at puberty, many clinicians thought that ADHD disappeared at puberty as well. Stimulant treatment was confined to children of elementary school age, and it was generally discontinued at puberty. In the past, the clinical goal of stimulant therapy was to help disruptive, inattentive children with ADHD during the school day. To meet this goal, stimulants were generally prescribed on a twice-daily basis (Barkley, 1998).

Over the past three decades, however, longitudinal research has demonstrated that ADHD is generally a lifelong disorder that continues in 30–70% of individuals meeting the ADHD criteria in elementary school (Biederman, 1998; Biederman et al., 1996; Faraone, Biederman, Mennin, Gershon, & Tsuang, 1996; Fischer, Barkley, Edelbrock, & Smallish, 1990; Fischer, Barkley, Fletcher, & Smallish, 1993b; Fischer et al., 2002; Hechtman et al., 1984; Mannuzza, Klein, & Addalli, 1991). Although overt hyperactivity generally diminishes in adolescence, inner restlessness, impulsivity, inattention, dis-

tractibility, forgetfulness, cognitive disorganization, and fidgetiness may continue to impair functioning across the lifespan (Biederman, 1998). Research has demonstrated that ADHD impairs not only academic performance, but multiple social, interpersonal, school, occupational, family, leisure, cognitive, and behavioral domains in an affected individual's life, with a poor lifetime prognosis and much comorbid psychopathology across the lifespan if the disorder goes untreated (Fischer et al., 1990; Fischer, Barkley, Fletcher, & Smallish, 1993a; Fischer et al., 2002; Hechtman et al., 1984).

This research has led clinicians to a better understanding of ADHD treatment. With this greater understanding the clinical goals of stimulant therapy in the treatment of ADHD have evolved and changed. The new goals are two:

1. In the individual with continuing ADHD symptoms, the clinician should treat ADHD throughout the lifespan. Stimulant treatment should not stop just because the patient has achieved puberty and is less overtly hyperactive. Stimulants work for an adolescent or adult with ADHD in a similar manner as they do for a child with the disorder. The clinician should evaluate the patient for continuing cognitive signs of ADHD and continue to treat if necessary.

2. Stimulant coverage for ADHD now emphasizes extended treatment of symptoms throughout the day. The new clinical goal is to lessen the symptoms of ADHD in multiple areas of the patient's daily life. It is no longer sufficient to treat ADHD only during the school day or during work hours. The clinician is now encouraged to reduce the overall daily burden of ADHD on the patient's life.

These treatment goals are more ambitious than historical treatment goals, and require broader ADHD coverage by stimulant medications. Consistent with these wider clinical goals, long-acting stimulant preparations are rapidly becoming the standard of care (Connor & Steingard, 2004). When used, immediate-release stimulants are now often prescribed three times a day, or are used to supplement the action of long-acting stimulants. To reduce the overall burden of ADHD on a child's development, stimulants are also now frequently prescribed 7 days a week, and often during the summer months.

Choice of Preparation

Table 17.6 shows the different stimulant preparations and dosing strengths. Immediate-release stimulants must be given at least twice daily, and preferably three times daily if ADHD coverage is to extend into the after-school hours. Intermediate-release stimulants are designed to mimic the action of immediate-release preparations given twice daily. They are useful for youth with ADHD who have difficulty in school, but not in after-school activities. Long-acting stimulants are designed to provide ADHD treatment throughout the day; they should be considered for children with ADHD who have difficulty both in and out of school. Intermediate- and long-acting stimulant preparations can be supplemented with immediate-release formulations to sculpt the dose for breakthrough ADHD symptoms.

Initiation of stimulant therapy with long-acting agents is now the accepted standard of care. Treatment may begin with either a methyl-phenidate or an amphetamine preparation as the first choice. Baseline measures of ADHD symptoms and potential medication side effects should be obtained prior to initiation of stimulants, and should be repeated when the child is on a drug. Objective data regarding the efficacy of stimulants for the individual's ADHD symptoms should always be collected across several different doses, given variability in each individual's responses to stimulant medications (Barkley, DuPaul, & McMurray, 1991). Stimulants are introduced at a low dose and titrated weekly to achieve optimum clinical response and tolerability. In our clinic, my colleagues and I tell parents that a stimulant trial to determine the child's most effective and well-tolerated dose will last about 1 month. Although body weight has not been shown to be related to stimulant drug response, using weight as a rough guideline for determining a starting dose continues to be recommended (Barkley et al., 1999). For the individual child, a methylphenidate preparation should be titrated through

TABLE 17.6. Stimulant Preparations for ADHD

Preparation	Active agent	Dose availability	Dosing schedule[a]
Immediate release for 4- to 6-hour coverage			
Adderall tablets	Neutral sulfate salts of dextroamphetamine saccharate and dextro-, levoamphetamine aspartate	5, 7.5, 10, 12.5 15, 20, 30 mg	b.i.d. to t.i.d.
Desoxyn tablets[b]	Methamphetamine HCl	5 mg	b.i.d. to t.i.d.
Dexedrine tablets	Dextroamphetamine sulfate	5 mg	b.i.d. to t.i.d.
Dextrostat tablets	Dextroamphetamine sulfate	5, 10 mg	b.i.d. to t.i.d.
Focalin tablets	Dexmethylphenidate HCl	2.5, 5, 10 mg	b.i.d. to t.i.d.
Ritalin HCl tablets	Methylphenidate HCl	5, 10, 20 mg	b.i.d. to t.i.d.
Intermediate acting for 8-hour coverage			
Dexedrine spansule	Dextroamphetamine, sustained-release	5, 10, 15 mg	b.i.d.
Metadate CD	Methylphenidate HCl, extended release	20 mg	q A.M.
Metadate ER	Methylphenidate HCl, extended release	10, 20 mg	q A.M.
Ritalin SR	Methylphenidate HCl, sustained release	20 mg	b.i.d.
Long-acting for 10- to 12-hour coverage			
Adderall XR capsules	Neutral salts of dextroamphetamine and amphetamine with dextroamphetamine saccharate and dextro-, levoamphetamine aspartate monohydrate, extended-release	5, 10, 15, 20, 25, 30 mg	q A.M.
Concerta tablets	Methylphenidate HCl, extended-release	18, 27, 36, 54 mg	q A.M.

[a]b.i.d., twice daily; t.i.d., three times a day; q A.M., daily in the morning.
[b]High abuse potential.

low (0.3–0.5 mg/kg/dose), intermediate (0.6–0.8 mg/kg/dose), and high (0.9–1.2 mg/kg/dose) doses on a weekly basis, and efficacy, tolerability, and side effects should be monitored. Amphetamine preparations are twice as potent as methylphenidate preparations and so are given in half the dose range (i.e., 0.2–0.6 mg/kg/dose). The best final dose must be tailored to each individual. As noted above, immediate-release stimulants may be used as supplements to target breakthrough ADHD symptoms.

Once an effective and well-tolerated stimulant dose is achieved, routine monitoring is recommended. In the large MTA, children assigned to the stimulant treatment arm were seen in follow-up monthly. Even though most of the children assigned to community treatment as usual also received stimulants, their clinicians saw them much less frequently. The children followed monthly by their physicians did better, suggesting that regular follow up of stimulant-treated children with ADHD is clinically helpful (MTA Cooperative Group, 1999). Routine clinical monitoring should inquire about continuing stimulant efficacy and side effects. Height and weight should be ascertained twice yearly. In a healthy child on stimulants, routine monitoring of pulse, blood pressure, and electrocardiogram is not indicated during stimulant therapy. Routine blood work, such as chemistry, liver function tests, and hematological indices, are also not indicated for routine stimulant use in the healthy child. The clinician and family should think about stimulant therapy in "school year units." That is, once a stable dose of stimulant has been achieved, treatment should continue at that dose for the duration of the school year. At the end of the school year, clinical assessment and consultation with the family should determine whether the child continues stimulants over the summer or discontinues them until the start of the next school year.

Management of Stimulant-Induced Side Effects

As noted above, common clinical side effects of stimulants include insomnia, anorexia, nausea, abdominal pain, headache, mood lability, irritability, sadness, moodiness, and weight loss. In the face of a satisfactory clinical response to a stimulant, it is important to attempt to manage side effects clinically, without having to discontinue the medication. Many of these treatment-emergent side effects occur early in the course of stimulant treatment and decline in intensity with time. It is important to distinguish between true stimulant side effects and/or returning ADHD symptoms late in the day, when stimulant medications are wearing off. The time course of reported side effects may be helpful. Side effects developing 1–2 hours after stimulant administration may represent true medication-related adverse events. Side effects reported as developing late in the day may represent ADHD rebound phenomena that occur as stimulant efficacy is diminishing. If symptoms represent ADHD rebound, giving a small supplemental dose of stimulant late in the afternoon may help. Suggestions for the management of common stimulant side effects are provided below.

Gastrointestinal Symptoms

Administering the medication with meals can help to alleviate the anorexia, nausea, and abdominal pain that sometimes may occur with taking stimulants. If the distress persists despite administering medication with meals, it may be necessary to change stimulant preparations.

Weight Loss

Appetite may rebound in the evening when stimulants are wearing off. Offering a high-calorie snack before a child's bedtime may be helpful, but a parent should not force the child to eat. If routine growth monitoring reveals >25% decrement in weight for age since the start of stimulant medication, a medication holiday may be indicated.

Insomnia

It is important to determine whether sleep difficulties are a true stimulant side effect or are actually a part of the ADHD. It is well known that children with ADHD have more sleep difficulties than controls do, regardless of stimulant treatment (Chatoor, Wells, Conners, Seidel, & Shaw, 1983). If insomnia represents a true side effect, giving stimulant medication earlier in the day or switching to a shorter-acting preparation may help. Late afternoon or evening doses of stimulants should be discontinued. The clinician may also consider supplementing stimulants with clonidine, imipramine, melatonin, or mirtazapine to help induce sleep in the evening (Wilens et al., 1996).

Dizziness

It is important to monitor blood pressure to help rule out cardiovascular causes of dizziness. Reducing stimulant dose or switching to a long-acting formulation may be helpful.

Rebound Phenomena

Overlapping stimulant doses at least 1 hour before rebound phenomena appear may be useful. Changing to a long-acting formulation may diminish the intensity of rebound symptoms. If the symptoms persist, the clinician may consider changing to a longer-acting nonstimulant ADHD medication such as atomoxetine or bupropion, with or without concurrent stimulant supplementation.

Irritability and Mood Lability

The clinician should determine whether irritability and mood lability are truly stimulant-related adverse events (i.e., they occur 1–2 hours after administration) or represent ADHD rebound symptoms (i.e., they occur late in the day when stimulant efficacy is wearing off). The possibility of a co-occurring mood disorder needs to be assessed if these symptoms are persistent and severe. If the symptoms are true stimulant side effects, the clinician may consider changing to a different agent (i.e., methylphenidate to amphetamine) or a nonstimulant such as atomoxetine or bupropion.

Growth Impairment

If growth impairment is verified, a medication holiday or a switch to a nonstimulant medication should be considered.

Stimulant Tolerance

It remains unclear whether behavioral tolerance develops with chronic administration of stimulants. Research indicates that failure to maintain a clinical response at a given dose is more likely to occur at higher stimulant doses and with chronic use (i.e., more than 6 months of continuous use) (Barkley et al., 1999). When parents call to complain about ineffective doses that were formerly effective, the physician

should first evaluate whether new stressful family events are occurring. If no stressful precipitating event to account for the loss of stimulant efficacy is found, a dose increase or a change in the stimulant formulation should be considered. If a stimulant effect on ADHD symptoms is truly lost, the physician may consider changing to a nonstimulant medication such as bupropion or atomoxetine.

Emergence of Tics

If a successfully stimulant-treated child with ADHD demonstrates the onset of a tic disorder, the clinician should first assess the persistence of tics. After a period of time, tics may subside to a baseline frequency and severity. An informed consent discussion should take place with the patient and family to assess whether the benefits of stimulant treatment remain worth the risk of possible tic exacerbation. If tics continue to be problematic, an alpha-adrenergic agent such as clonidine (Tourette's Syndrome Study Group, 2002) or guanfacine (Scahill et al., 2001) may be added to ongoing stimulant treatment. Alternatively, the stimulant can be discontinued, and treatment with clonidine, guanfacine, desipramine, nortriptyline, or atomoxetine can be initiated (Tourette's Syndrome Study Group, 2002; Michelson et al., 2001; Scahill et al., 2001; Spencer, Biederman, Kerman, Steingard, & Wilens, 1993; Spencer, Biederman, Wilens, Steingard, & Geist, 1993). These alternative medications are effective in ADHD and do not exacerbate tic disorders.

Contraindications to Stimulant Use

Known hypersensitivity to stimulants is a contraindication to their use. Patients with structural cardiac defects should not be treated with stimulants. Stimulants can exacerbate narrow-angle glaucoma and should not be used in this condition. In vulnerable individuals or in overdose (toxicity), stimulants can cause psychotic symptoms. Stimulants are relatively contraindicated in children and adolescents with schizophrenia or other psychotic disorders, because they may worsen these conditions in some cases. A severe tic or Tourette syndrome remains a relative contraindication to the use of stimulants. However, as noted above, stimulants may be used in milder cases of tics when these are accompanied by impairing symptoms of ADHD. Patients with unstable hypertension should not receive stimulants for ADHD until their high blood pressure is treated and controlled. Because stimulants have the potential to be abused, they should not be prescribed when patients exhibit active substance abuse or when there is a likelihood that family members or friends will abuse the medication. Finally, stimulants have the potential to precipitate hypertensive crises when used with monoamine oxidase inhibitors (MAOIs). They should not be prescribed concurrently with a MAOI or within 14 days after a MAOI has been discontinued.

Management of Stimulant Overdose

Between 1993 and 1999, the American Association of Poison Control Centers Toxic Exposure Surveillance System identified 759 cases of stimulant overdose and abuse in youth 10 through 19 years of age (Klein-Schwartz & McGrath, 2003). The majority concerned methylphenidate. Rising rates of methylphenidate abuse were noted when rates in 1999 were compared with rates in 1993. The majority of individuals who required health care facility management experienced clinical toxicity. Only seven cases of severe toxicity were identified; these cases occurred in adolescents with polydrug overdoses (i.e., stimulants plus other drugs/alcohol). For cases involving stimulants alone, the majority of symptoms included cardiovascular (tachycardia, hypertension) and/or CNS (agitation, irritability) toxicity. There were no deaths reported.

Signs and symptoms of acute overdose result from overstimulation of the CNS and from excessive sympathomimetic effects. Symptoms of stimulant toxicity include vomiting, agitation, tremor, convulsion, confusion, hallucinations, hyperpyrexia, tachycardia, arrhythmias, hypertension, paranoid delusions, and delirium. Treatment consists of prompt medical referral and appropriate supportive measures. The patient must be protected from self-injury and from environmental overstimulation that would aggravate heightened sympathomimetic arousal. Chlorpromazine has been reported to be useful in decreasing CNS stimulation and drug-induced sympathomimetic effects. If the patient is alert and conscious, gastric contents may be evacuated by induction of emesis or gastric lavage. For intoxication with amphetamine, acidification of the urine will increase amphetamine excretion. For severe overdose, intensive care must be provided to maintain adequate cardiopulmonary function and treat hyperpyrexia. The efficacy of peritoneal dialysis or extracorporeal hemodialysis for stimulant toxicity has not been established.

Stimulant Drug Combinations

In clinical practice, stimulants are increasingly combined with other psychiatric medications to treat comorbid psychiatric conditions such as anxiety or depression, to manage side effects such as insomnia or stimulant rebound, or to bolster a partial therapeutic response to stimulant monotherapy. Few controlled studies are presently available to assess the safety and efficacy of stimulant combinations, and scientific data to guide the clinician in this practice remain sparse.

Combined Stimulant and Antidepressant Therapy

Stimulants have been safely combined with SSRI antidepressants such as fluoxetine and fluvoxamine in the treatment of ADHD with anxiety and depression (Abikoff et al., 2005; Gammon & Brown, 1991). Combinations of tricyclic antidepressants and stimulants have also been evaluated. In a study of the separate and combined effects of desipramine and methylphenidate on ADHD symptoms and comorbid mood disorders, both medications alone produced reductions in ADHD symptoms, and the combination produced positive effects on learning over and above the efficacy of each single agent (Rapport, Carlson, Kelly, & Pataki, 1993). The combination was also associated with more side effects than either medicine alone, but there was no evidence that the combination was associated with any unique or serious treatment-emergent side effects (Pataki, Carlson, Kelly, Rapport, & Biancaniello, 1993). Because few data from controlled studies are available on the combination of antidepressants and stimulants, close clinical monitoring is recommended in these cases.

Combined Stimulant and Alpha-Adrenergic Therapy

Clonidine and guanfacine are presynaptic alpha-adrenergic agents that down-regulate endogenous norepinephrine outflow from the brain. They are frequently combined with stimulants in off-label use to manage severe hyperactive and aggressive symptoms, to treat comorbid tics or Tourette syndrome, or to help treat insomnia associated with stimulant therapy or ADHD (Connor et al., 2000; Tourette's Syndrome Study Group, 2002; Prince, Wilens, Biederman, Spencer, & Wozniak, 1996). Alpha-adrenergic antagonists do not improve attention span as dramatically as stimulants, but may be helpful in decreasing the overarousal that contributes to behavior problems in these children. Clonidine is more sedating than guanfacine. Both may lower blood pressure and pulse, and monitoring the vital signs is important when these agents are used with stimulants.

The clinical practice of combining stimulants with clonidine has been the subject of some controversy. In July 1995, National Public Radio reported that sudden death had occurred in three children taking the combination of methylphenidate and clonidine. Subsequent reviews and commentary in the scientific literature concluded that there was no convincing evidence of an adverse methylphenidate–clonidine interaction in any of these cases, and that other factors were more proximally related to these three deaths (Fenichel, 1995; Popper, 1995). Subsequent controlled studies have not reported increased serious adverse events with this combination compared to clonidine or methylphenidate alone (Connor et al., 2000; Tourette's Syndrome Study Group, 2002). Presently, the combination is considered usually safe, and the available clinical literature does not support discontinuation of such combined therapy in patients experiencing significant clinical benefit (Swanson et al., 1995). However, clonidine may cause a withdrawal syndrome and rebound hypertension if it is abruptly discontinued without tapering of the dose. In overdose, clonidine can cause bradycardia and hypotension. Thus careful clinical monitoring is important when this combination is used (Swanson et al., 1995).

Non-First-Line or Ineffective Stimulants

Magnesium Pemoline

Pemoline (Cylert) has been associated with lifethreatening hepatic failure. Since it was first marketed in 1975, 15 cases of acute hepatic failure have been reported to the FDA. Twelve of these cases resulted in death or liver transplantation secondary to massive hepatic necrosis. This is 4–17 times the base rate expected in the general population (Shevell & Schreiber, 1997). Although the FDA allows use of pemoline, it is not a first-line drug and carries a "black-box" warning of potential acute liver failure. Liver function tests are required every 2 weeks. Pemoline should be discontinued if no clinical benefit occurs after 3 weeks on therapeutic doses. With newer and safer longacting stimulant formulations readily available, it is doubtful whether any patient with ADHD should currently be treated with pemoline.

Caffeine

Caffeine is a weak stimulant drug. A review of the literature concluded that caffeine is not a therapeutically useful drug in the clinical treatment of ADHD (Klein, 1987).

SUMMARY

This survey of the clinical effects and side effects of stimulant medications suggests the following conclusions:

1. Up to 70–80% of children with carefully diagnosed ADHD appear to demonstrate a positive response to stimulants. Effects can be expected on improvement of attention span and the reduction of impulsive behavior, including aggression. Social interactions and compliance with authority figures' commands may improve. Academic improvements in work productivity and accuracy may occur. Stimulant dose should be individualized. Longacting preparations are now the accepted standard of care.

2. Adolescents and adults with ADHD also respond to stimulant therapy. Stimulants should not be discontinued at puberty in an adolescent with ADHD who exhibits continuing impairment. Treatment can continue into the teenage years. Adults can respond to stimulants as well. The lower response rate to stimulant medications in adults with ADHD may be due to relative underdosing.

3. Stimulants do not cure ADHD. Rather, they are an intervention that must be used in conjunction with other psychoeducational interventions as part of an overall treatment plan.

4. Stimulant side effects are generally mild, and the medication is well tolerated. A baseline evaluation of potential stimulant side effects is recommended before stimulant treatment begins. Side effects attributed by parents to the stimulant may actually be part of ADHD.

5. Stimulants do not cause increased risk of substance abuse; rather, the risk of substance abuse is conferred by the ADHD. Appropriate treatment of ADHD, including use of stimulants, may actually decrease the risk of future substance use disorders.

6. In the treatment of ADHD, it is important for the prescribing clinician to be aware of the high comorbidity rate between ADHD and depression, anxiety, learning disabilities, tic disorders, and CD/ODD. The possibility of comorbid conditions needs to be considered in treatment planning for an individual with ADHD.

In conclusion, the stimulants are first-line agents of choice for ADHD, given their efficacy, safety, and tolerability. The treatment of ADHD should emphasize the clinical goals of diminishing the overall burden of ADHD on an individual's daily life and continuing the treatment of ADHD where necessary across the lifespan.

KEY CLINICAL POINTS

✓ Stimulant medications (methylphenidate, amphetamines) are the most effective treatments to date for the management of ADHD symptoms.

✓ Hundreds of studies, and more than 60 years of clinical use, attest to the stimulants' efficacy, effectiveness, and safety.

✓ The stimulants have demonstrated effectiveness across a wide age range of patients, including preschoolers, school-age children, adolescents, and adults with ADHD.

✓ Approximately 75% of school-age patients initially treated with any particular stimulant show a positive clinical response. When a patient fails to respond, either a different delivery system or an alternative stimulant should be used to improve the likelihood of a positive response.

✓ Side effects from the stimulants are most often insomnia, decreased appetite, headache,

stomachache, and irritability or proneness to crying, and are dose-sensitive. Small negative effects on height and weight gain have been documented during the initial 1–2 years of medication use, but it remains unclear whether these continue beyond adolescence.

✓ Comorbidity with aggression does not affect response rates to stimulants, whereas research on comorbid anxiety or depression has been less clear in its findings. Earlier studies suggested that the latter conditions may adversely affect responding, but more recent studies have not found this to be the case. Likewise, recent studies do not support the earlier contention that stimulants often exacerbate tic disorders when they are comorbid with ADHD, though this still may occur in a minority of comorbid cases. Even then, tic frequency often returns to its baseline levels once stimulants are discontinued.

✓ In the individual with continuing ADHD symptoms, the ADHD should be treated throughout the lifespan. Stimulant treatment should not stop just because the patient has achieved puberty and is less overtly hyperactive. Stimulant coverage for ADHD now emphasizes extended treatment of symptoms throughout the day. Consistent with these wider clinical goals, long-acting stimulant preparations are rapidly becoming the standard of care.

✓ Stimulants do not cure ADHD. Rather, they are an intervention that must be used in conjunction with other psychoeducational interventions as part of an overall treatment plan.

✓ Stimulants do not cause increased risk of substance abuse; rather, the risk of substance abuse is conferred by the ADHD. Appropriate treatment of ADHD, including use of stimulants, may actually decrease the risk of future substance use disorders.

REFERENCES

Abikoff, H., McGough, J., Vitiello, B., McCracken, J., Davies, M., Walkup, J., et al. (2005). Sequential pharmacotherapy for children with comorbid attention-deficit/hyperactivity and anxiety disorders. *Journal of the American Academy of Child and Adolescent Psychiatry, 44*(5), 418–421.

Aman, M. G., Marks, R. E., Turbott, S. H., Wilsher, C. P., & Merry, S. N. (1991). Clinical effects of methylphenidate and thioridazine in intellectually sub-average children. *Journal of the American Academy of Child and Adolescent Psychiatry, 30*(2), 246–256.

Angold, A., Erkanli, A., Egger, H. L., & Costello, E. J. (2000). Stimulant treatment for children: A community perspective. *Journal of the American Academy of Child and Adolescent Psychiatry, 39*, 975–984.

Barkley, R. A. (1977). A review of stimulant drug research with hyperactive children. *Journal of Child Psychology and Psychiatry, 18*(2), 137–165.

Barkley, R. A. (1981). The use of psychopharmacology to study reciprocal influences in parent–child interaction. *Journal of Abnormal Child Psychology, 9*(3), 303–310.

Barkley, R. A. (1988). The effects of methylphenidate on the interactions of preschool ADHD children with their mothers. *Journal of the American Academy of Child and Adolescent Psychiatry, 27*(3), 336–341.

Barkley, R. A. (1989). Hyperactive girls and boys: Stimulant drug effects on mother–child interactions. *Journal of Child Psychology and Psychiatry, 30*(3), 379–390.

Barkley, R. A. (1998). Attention-deficit hyperactivity disorder. *Scientific American, 279*(3), 66–71.

Barkley, R. A. (2004). Driving impairments in teens and young adults with ADHD. *Psychiatric Clinics of North America, 27*, 233–260.

Barkley, R. A., Anastopoulos, A. D., Guevremont, D. C., & Fletcher, K. E. (1992). Adolescents with attention deficit hyperactivity disorder: Mother–adolescent interactions, family beliefs and conflicts, and maternal psychopathology. *Journal of Abnormal Child Psychology, 20*(3), 263–288.

Barkley, R. A., Connor, D. F., & Kwasnik, D. (2000). Challenges to determining adolescent medication response in an outpatient clinical setting: Comparing Adderall and methylphenidate for ADHD. *Journal of Attention Disorders, 4*(2), 102–113.

Barkley, R. A., DuPaul, G. J., & Connor, D. F. (1999). Stimulants. In J. S. Werry & M. G. Aman (Eds.), *Practitioner's guide to psychoactive drugs for children and adolescents* (2nd ed., pp. 213–247). New York: Plenum Medical Book.

Barkley, R. A., DuPaul, G. J., & McMurray, M. B. (1991). Attention deficit disorder with and without hyperactivity: clinical response to three dose levels of methylphenidate. *Pediatrics, 87*(4), 519–531.

Barkley, R. A., Fischer, M., Smallish, L., & Fletcher, K. (2003). Does the treatment of attention-deficit/hyperactivity disorder with stimulants contribute to drug use/abuse?: A 13–year prospective study. *Pediatrics, 111*(1), 97–109.

Barkley, R. A., Guevremont, D. C., Anastopoulos, A. D., DuPaul, G. J., & Shelton, T. L. (1993). Driving-related risks and outcomes of attention deficit hyperactivity disorder in adolescents and young adults: A 3- to 5-year follow-up survey. *Pediatrics, 92*(2), 212–218.

Barkley, R. A., Karlsson, J., Strzelecki, E., & Murphy, J. V. (1984). Effects of age and Ritalin dosage on the

mother–child interactions of hyperactive children. *Journal of Consulting and Clinical Psychology, 52*(5), 750–758.

Barkley, R. A., McMurray, M. B., Edelbrock, C. S., & Robbins, K. (1989). The response of aggressive and nonaggressive ADHD children to two doses of methylphenidate. *Journal of the American Academy of Child and Adolescent Psychiatry, 28*(6), 873–881.

Barkley, R. A., McMurray, M. B., Edelbrock, C. S., & Robbins, K. (1990). Side effects of methylphenidate in children with attention deficit hyperactivity disorder: A systemic, placebo-controlled evaluation. *Pediatrics, 86*(2), 184–192.

Barkley, R. A., Murphy, K. R., & Kwasnik, D. (1996). Motor vehicle driving competencies and risks in teens and young adults with attention deficit hyperactivity disorder. *Pediatrics, 98*(6, Pt. 1), 1089–1095.

Bergman, A., Winters, L., & Cornblatt, B. (1991). Methylphenidate: Effects on sustained attention. In L. L. Greenhill & B. B. Osman (Eds.), *Ritalin: Theory and patient management.* (pp. 223–232). New York: Liebert.

Bhatara, V. S., Feil, M., Hoagwood, K., Vitiello, B., & Zima, B. T. (2000). *Concomitant pharmacotherapy in youths receiving antidepressants or stimulants.* Poster presented at the 47th annual meeting of the American Academy of Child and Adolescent Psychiatry, Washington, DC.

Biederman, J. (1998). Attention-deficit/hyperactivity disorder: A life-span perspective. *Journal of Clinical Psychiatry, 59*(Suppl. 7), 4–16.

Biederman, J., Faraone, S. V., Mick, E., Spencer, T., Wilens, T., Kiely, K., et al. (1995). High risk for attention deficit hyperactivity disorder among children of parents with childhood onset of the disorder: A pilot study. *American Journal of Psychiatry, 152*(3), 431–435.

Biederman, J., Faraone, S. V., Milberger, S., Guite, J., Mick, E., Chen, L., et al. (1996). A prospective 4–year follow-up study of attention-deficit hyperactivity and related disorders. *Archives of General Psychiatry, 53*(5), 437–446.

Biederman, J., Faraone, S. V., Spencer, T., Wilens, T., Norman, D., Lapey, K. A., et al. (1993). Patterns of psychiatric comorbidity, cognition, and psychosocial functioning in adults with attention deficit/hyperactivity disorder. *American Journal of Psychiatry, 150*, 1792–1798.

Biederman, J., Lapey, K. A., Milberger, S., Faraone, S. V., Reed, E. D., & Seidman, L. J. (1994). Motor preference, major depression and psychosocial dysfunction among children with attention deficit hyperactivity disorder. *Journal of Psychiatric Research, 28*(2), 171–184.

Biederman, J., Lopez, F., Boellner, S., & Chandler, M. (2002). A randomized, double-blind, placebo-controlled, parallel-group study of SLI381 (Adderall XR) in children with attention-deficit/hyperactivity disorder. *Pediatrics, 110*(2), 258–266.

Biederman, J., Mick, E., & Faraone, S. V. (1998). Depression in attention deficit hyperactivity disorder (ADHD) children: "True" depression or demoralization? *Journal of Affective Disorders, 47*(1–3), 113–122.

Biederman, J., Newcorn, J., & Sprich, S. (1991). Comorbidity of attention deficit hyperactivity disorder with conduct, depressive, anxiety, and other disorders. *American Journal of Psychiatry, 148*(5), 564–577.

Biederman, J., Wilens, T., Mick, E., Faraone, S. V., Weber, W., Curtis, S., et al. (1997). Is ADHD a risk factor for psychoactive substance use disorders?: Findings from a four-year prospective follow-up study. *Journal of the American Academy of Child and Adolescent Psychiatry, 36*(1), 21–29.

Biederman, J., Wilens, T., Mick, E., Spencer, T., & Faraone, S. V. (1999). Pharmacotherapy of attention-deficit/hyperactivity disorder reduces risk for substance use disorder. *Pediatrics, 104*(2), e20.

Bird, H. R., Gould, M. S., & Staghezza, B. M. (1993). Patterns of diagnostic comorbidity in a community sample of children aged 9 through 16 years. *Journal of the American Academy of Child and Adolescent Psychiatry, 32*(2), 361–368.

Birmaher, B., Greenhill, L. L., Cooper, T. B., Fried, J., & Maminski, B. (1989). Sustained release methylphenidate: Pharmacokinetic studies in ADDH males. *Journal of the American Academy of Child and Adolescent Psychiatry, 28*, 768–772.

Bloom, A. S., Russell, L.J., Weisskopf, B., & Blackerby, J.L. (1988). Methylphenidate-induced delusional disorder in a child with attention deficit disorder with hyperactivity. *Journal of the American Academy of Child and Adolescent Psychiatry, 27*, 88–89.

Bostic, J. Q., Biederman, J., Spencer, T. J., Wilens, T. E., Prince, J. B., Monuteaux, M. C., et al. (2000). Pemoline treatment of adolescents with attention deficit hyperactivity disorder: A short-term controlled trial. *Journal of Child and Adolescent Psychopharmacology, 10*(3), 205–216.

Bremness, A. B., & Sverd, J. (1979). Methylphenidate-induced Tourette syndrome: Case report. *American Journal of Psychiatry, 136*, 1334–1335.

Brown, R. T., & Sexson, S. B. (1987). A controlled trial of methylphenidate in black adolescents. *Clinical Pediatrics, 27*(2), 74–81.

Brown, R. T., Wynne, M. E., & Slimmer, L. W. (1984). Attention deficit disorder and the effect of methylphenidate on attention, behavioral, and cardiovascular functioning. *Journal of Clinical Psychiatry, 45*, 473–476.

Brown, T. E. (Ed.). (2000). *Attention-deficit disorders and comorbidities in children, adolescents, and adults.* Washington, DC: American Psychiatric Press.

Buitelaar, J. K., van der Gaag, R. J., Swaab-Barneveld, H., & Kuiper, M. (1995). Prediction of clinical response to methylphenidate in children with attention-deficit hyperactivity disorder. *Journal of the American Academy of Child and Adolescent Psychiatry, 34*, 1025–1032.

Byrne, J. M., Bawden, H. N., DeWolfe, N. A., & Beattie, T.L. (1998). Clinical assessment of psychopharmacological treatment of preschoolers with ADHD. *Journal of Clinical and Experimental Neuropsychology, 20*, 613–627.

Caldwell, J., & Sever, P. S. (1974). The biochemical pharmacology of abused drugs. *Clinical Pharmacology and Therapeutics, 16*, 625–638.

Castellanos, F. X., Giedd, J. N., Elia, J., Marsh, W.L., Ritchie, G.F., Hamburger, S.D., et al. (1997). Controlled stimulant treatment of ADHD and comorbid Tourette's syndrome: Effects of stimulants and dose. *Journal of the American Academy of Child and Adolescent Psychiatry, 36*, 1–8.

Charach, A., Ickowicz, A., & Schachar, R. (2004). Stimulant treatment over five years: adherence, effectiveness, and adverse effects. *Journal of the American Academy of Child and Adolescent Psychiatry, 43*(5), 559–567.

Chatoor, I., Wells, K. C., Conners, C. K., Seidel, W. T., & Shaw, D. (1983). The effects of nocturnally administered stimulant medication on EEG sleep and behavior in hyperactive children. *Journal of the American Academy of Child and Adolescent Psychiatry, 22*, 337–342.

Citizens Commission on Human Rights (CCHR). (1987). *Ritalin: A warning to parents.* Los Angeles: Church of Scientology.

Cohen, P., Cohen, J., Kasen, S., Velez, C.N., Hartmark, C., Johnson, J. Rojas, M., et al. (1993). An epidemiological study of disorders in late childhood and adolescence: I. Age and gender specific pattern. *Journal of Child Psychology and Psychiatry, 34*, 851–867.

Conners, C. K. (1975). Controlled trial of methylphenidate in preschool children with minimal brain dysfunction. *International Journal of Mental Health, 4*, 61–74.

Connor, D. F. (2002). Preschool attention deficit hyperactivity disorder: A review of prevalence, diagnosis, neurobiology, and stimulant treatment. *Developmental and Behavioral Pediatrics, 23*(1S), S1–S9.

Connor, D. F., Barkley, R. A., & Davis, H. T. (2000). A pilot study of methylphenidate, clonidine, or the combination in ADHD comorbid with aggressive oppositional defiant or conduct disorder. *Clinical Pediatrics, 39*(1), 15–25.

Connor, D. F., Edwards, G., Fletcher, K. E., Baird, J., Barkley, R. A., & Steingard, R. J. (2003). Correlates of comorbid psychopathology in children with ADHD. *Journal of the American Academy of Child and Adolescent Psychiatry, 42*(2), 193–200.

Connor, D. F., Glatt, S. J., Lopez, I. D., Jackson, D., & Melloni, R. H., Jr. (2002). Psychopharmacology and aggression. I: A meta-analysis of stimulant effects on overt/covert aggression-related behaviors in ADHD. *Journal of the American Academy of Child and Adolescent Psychiatry, 41*(3), 253–261.

Connor, D. F., & Steingard, R. J. (2004). New formulations of stimulants for attention-deficit hyperactivity disorder: Therapeutic potential. *CNS Drugs, 18*(14), 1011–1030.

Coons, H. W., Klorman, R., & Borgstedt, A. D. (1987). Effects of methylphenidate on adolescents with a childhood history of attention deficit disorder: II. Information processing. *Journal of the American Academy of Child and Adolescent Psychiatry, 26*(3), 368–374.

Cox, E. R., Motheral, B. R., Henderson, R. R., & Mager, D. (2003). Geographic variation in the prevalence of stimulant medication use among children 5 to 14 years old: Results from a commercially insured US sample. *Pediatrics, 111*(2), 237–243.

Cunningham, C. E., Siegel, L. S., & Offord, D. R. (1985). A developmental dose–response analysis of the effects of methylphenidate on the peer interactions of attention deficit disordered boys. *Journal of Child Psychology and Psychiatry, 26*, 955–971.

Danforth, J. S., Barkley, R. A., & Stokes, T. F. (1991). Observations of interactions between parents and their hyperactive children: An analysis of reciprocal influence. *Clinical Psychology Review, 11*, 703–727.

Denckla, M. B., Bemporad, J. R., & MacKay, M. C. (1976). Tics following methylphenidate administration: A report of 20 cases. *Journal of the American Medical Association, 235*, 1349–1351.

Diamond, I. R., Tannock, R., & Schachar, R. (1999). Response to methylphenidate in children with ADHD and comorbid anxiety. *Journal of the American Academy of Child and Adolescent Psychiatry, 38*, 402–409.

Diener, R. M. (1991). Toxicology of Ritalin. In L. L. Greenhill & B. B. Osman (Eds.), *Ritalin theory and patient management* (pp. 35–43). New York: Liebert.

Ding, Y. S., Fowler, J. S., Volkow, N. D., Dewey, S.L., Wang, G.J., Logan, J., et al. (1997). Chiral drugs: Comparison of the pharmacokinetics of [11C]d-threo and l-threo-methylphenidate in the human and baboon brain. *Psychopharmacology, 131*, 71–78.

DuPaul, G. J., Barkley, R. A., & McMurray, M. B. (1994). Response of children with ADHD to methylphenidate: Interaction with internalizing symptoms. *Journal of the American Academy of Child and Adolescent Psychiatry, 33*(6), 894–903.

Eckerman, D. A., Moy, S. S., Perkins, A. N., Patrick, K. S., & Breese, G. R. (1991). Enantioselective behavioral effects of threo-methylphenidate in rats. *Pharmacology, Biochemistry, and Behavior, 40*, 875–880.

Elia, J., Borcherding, B., Rapoport, J., & Keysor, C. (1991). Methylphenidate and dextroamphetamine treatments of hyperactivity: Are there true non-responders? *Psychiatry Research, 36*, 141–155.

Elia, J., & Rapoport, J. (1991). Ritalin versus dextroamphetamine in ADHD: Both should be tried. In L. L. Greenhill & B. B. Osman (Eds.), *Ritalin: Theory and patient management* (pp. 69–74). New York: Liebert.

Ernst, M., Cohen, R. M., Liebenauer, L. L., Jons, P. H., & Zametkin, A. J. (1997). Cerebral glucose metabolism in adolescent girls with attention-deficit/hyper-

activity disorder. *Journal of the American Academy of Child and Adolescent Psychiatry, 36*(10), 1399–1406.

Ernst, M., Zametkin, A. J., Matochik, J. A., Pascualvaca, D., Jons, P. H., & Cohen, R. M. (1999). High midbrain [18F]DOPA accumulation in children with attention deficit hyperactivity disorder. *American Journal of Psychiatry, 156*(8), 1209–1215.

Ernst, M., Zametkin, A. J., Phillips, R. L., & Cohen, R. M. (1998). Age-related changes in brain glucose metabolism in adults with attention-deficit/hyperactivity disorder and control subjects. *Journal of Neuropsychiatry and Clinical Neurosciences, 10*(2), 168–177.

Evans, S. W., Pelham, W. E., Smith, B. H., Bukstein, O., Gnagy, E. M., Greiner, A. R., et al. (2001). Dose–response effects of methylphenidate on ecologically valid measures of academic performance and classroom behavior in adolescents with ADHD. *Experimental and Clinical Psychopharmacology, 9*(2), 163–175.

Famularo, R., & Fenton, T. (1987). The effect of methylphenidate on school grades in children with attention deficit disorder without hyperactivity: A preliminary study. *Journal of Clinical Psychiatry, (48)*, 112–114.

Faraone, S. V., & Biederman, J. (1998). Neurobiology of attention-deficit hyperactivity disorder. *Biological Psychiatry, 44*(10), 951–958.

Faraone, S. V., Biederman, J., Chen, W. J., Milberger, S., Warburton, R., & Tsuang, M. T. (1995). Genetic heterogeneity in attention-deficit hyperactivity disorder (ADHD): Gender, psychiatric comorbidity, and maternal ADHD. *Journal of Abnormal Psychology, 104*(2), 334–345.

Faraone, S. V., Biederman, J., Lehman, B. K., Keenan, K., Norman, D., Seidman, L. J., et al. (1993). Evidence for the independent familial transmission of attention deficit hyperactivity disorder and learning disabilities: Results from a family genetic study. *American Journal of Psychiatry, 150*(6), 891–895.

Faraone, S. V., Biederman, J., Mennin, D., Gershon, J., & Tsuang, M. T. (1996). A prospective four-year follow-up study of children at risk for ADHD: Psychiatric, neuropsychological, and psychosocial outcome. *Journal of the American Academy of Child and Adolescent Psychiatry, 35*(11), 1449–1459.

Faraone, S. V., Biederman, J., & Mick, E. (1997). Symptom reports by adults with attention deficit hyperactivity disorder: Are they influenced by attention deficit hyperactivity disorder in their children? *Journal of Nervous and Mental Disease, 185*(9), 583–584.

Faraone, S. V., Biederman, J., Spencer, T., Wilens, T., Seidman, L. J., Mick, E., et al. (2000). Attention-deficit/hyperactivity disorder in adults: An overview. *Biological Psychiatry, 48*(1), 9–20.

Feldman, H., Crumrine, P., Handen, R., Alvin, R., & Teodori, J. (1989). Methylphenidate in children with seizures and attention-deficit disorder. *American Journal of Diseases of Children, 143*, 1081–1086.

Fenichel, R. R. (1995). Combining methylphenidate and clonidine: The role of post-marketing surveillance. *Journal of Child and Adolescent Psychopharmacology, 5*, 155–156.

Findling, R. L. (1996). Open-label treatment of comorbid depression and attentional disorders with co-administration of serotonin reuptake inhibitors and psychostimulants in children, adolescents, and adults: A case series. *Journal of Child and Adolescent Psychopharmacology, 6*, 165–175.

Firestone, P., Monteiro-Musten, L., Pisterman, S., Mercer, J., & Bennett, S. (1998). Short-term side effects of stimulant medication are increased in preschool children with attention-deficit/hyperactivity disorder: A double-blind placebo-controlled study. *Journal of Child and Adolescent Psychopharmacology, 8*, 13–25.

Fischer, M., Barkley, R. A., Edelbrock, C. S., & Smallish, L. (1990). The adolescent outcome of hyperactive children diagnosed by research criteria: II. Academic, attentional, and neuropsychological status. *Journal of Consulting and Clinical Psychology, 58*(5), 580–588.

Fischer, M., Barkley, R. A., Fletcher, K. E., & Smallish, L. (1993a). The adolescent outcome of hyperactive children: Predictors of psychiatric, academic, social, and emotional adjustment. *Journal of the American Academy of Child and Adolescent Psychiatry, 32*(2), 324–332.

Fischer, M., Barkley, R. A., Fletcher, K. E., & Smallish, L. (1993b). The stability of dimensions of behavior in ADHD and normal children over an 8–year followup. *Journal of Abnormal Child Psychology, 21*(3), 315–337.

Fischer, M., Barkley, R. A., Smallish, L., & Fletcher, K. (2002). Young adult follow-up of hyperactive children: Self-reported psychiatric disorders, comorbidity, and the role of childhood conduct problems and teen CD. *Journal of Abnormal Child Psychology, 30*(5), 463–475.

Forehand, R., & McMahon, R. J. (1981). *Helping the noncompliant child: A clinician's guide to parent training.* New York: Guilford Press.

Gadow, K. D., Nolan, E. E., Sprafkin, J., & Schwartz, J. (2002). Tics and psychiatric comorbidity in children and adolescents. *Developmental Medicine and Child Neurology, 44*(5), 330–338.

Gadow, K. D., Nolan, E. E., & Sverd, J. (1992). Methylphenidate in hyperactive boys with comorbid tic disorder: II. Short-term behavioral effect in school settings. *Journal of the American Academy of Child and Adolescent Psychiatry, 31*, 462–471.

Gadow, K. D., Nolan, E. E., Sverd, J., Sprafkin, J., & Paolicelli, L. (1990). Methylphenidate in aggressive–hyperactive boys: I. Effects on peer aggression in public school settings. *Journal of the American Academy of Child and Adolescent Psychiatry, 29*(5), 710–718.

Gadow, K. D., Nolan, E. E., Sverd, J., Sprafkin, J., & Schwartz, J. (2002). Anxiety and depressive symptoms and response to methylphenidate in children with attention-deficit/hyperactivity disorder and tic disorder. *Journal of Clinical Psychopharmacology, 22*(3), 267–274.

Gadow, K. D., Sverd, J., Sprafkin, J., Nolan, E. E., & Ezor, S.N. (1995). Efficacy of methylphenidate for attention-deficit hyperactivity disorder in children with tic disorder. *Archives of General Psychiatry, 52*, 444–455.

Gammon, G. D., & Brown, T. E. (1991). Fluoxetine and methylphenidate in combination for treatment of attention deficit disorder and comorbid depressive disorder. *Journal of Child and Adolescent Psychopharmacology, 3*, 1–10.

Geller, B., Williams, M., Zimerman, B., Frazier, J., Beringer, L., & Warner, K. L. (1998). Prepubertal and early adolescent bipolarity differentiate from ADHD by manic symptoms, grandiose delusions, ultra-rapid or ultraradian cycling. *Journal of Affective Disorders, 51*(2), 81–91.

Geller, B., Zimerman, B., Williams, M., DelBello, M. P., Bolhofner, K., Craney, J. L., et al. (2002). DSM-IV mania symptoms in a prepubertal and early adolescent bipolar disorder phenotype compared to attention-deficit hyperactive and normal controls. *Journal of Child and Adolescent Psychopharmacology, 12*(1), 11–25.

Geller, B., Zimerman, B., Williams, M., DelBello, M. P., Frazier, J., & Beringer, L. (2002). Phenomenology of prepubertal and early adolescent bipolar disorder: Examples of elated mood, grandiose behaviors, decreased need for sleep, racing thoughts, and hypersexuality. *Journal of Child and Adolescent Psychopharmacology, 12*(1), 3–9.

Gillberg, C., Melander, H., von Knorring, A. L., Janols, L. O., Themlund, G., Hagglof, B., et al. (1997). Long-term stimulant treatment of children with attention-deficit hyperactivity disorder symptoms: A randomized, double-blind, placebo-controlled trial. *Archives of General Psychiatry, 54*(9), 857–864.

Gittelman, R., & Mannuzza, S. (1988). Hyperactive boys almost grown up: III. Methylphenidate effects on ultimate height. *Archives of General Psychiatry, 45*, 1131–1134.

Goldman, L., Genel, M., Bezman, R., & Slanetz, P. J. (1998). Diagnosis and treatment of attention-deficit/hyperactivity disorder in children and adolescents. *Journal of the American Medical Association, 279*, 1100–1107.

Grcevich, S. (2001). SLI381: A long-acting psychostimulant preparation for the treatment of attention-deficit hyperactivity disorder. *Expert Opinion on Investigational Drugs, 10*(11), 2003–2011.

Greenhill, L. L. (1995). Attention deficit hyperactivity disorder: The stimulants. *Child and Adolescent Psychiatric Clinics of North America, 4*(1), 123–168.

Greenhill, L. L., Abikoff, H., Arnold, L. E., Cantwell, D. P., Conners, C. K., Elliott, G. R., et al. (1996). Medication treatment strategies in the MTA study: Relevance to clinicians and researchers. *Journal of the*

American Academy of Child and Adolescent Psychiatry, 35, 1304–1313.

Greenhill, L. L., Findling, R. L., Swanson, J. M., & MTA Cooperative Group. (2002). A double-blind, placebo-controlled study of modified-release methylphenidate in children with attention-deficit/hyperactivity disorder. *Pediatrics, 109*(3), e39.

Greenhill, L. L., Jensen, P., Abikoff, H., Blumer, J. L., DeVeaugh-Geiss, J., Fisher, C., et al. (2003). Developing strategies for psychopharmacological studies in preschool children. *Journal of the American Academy of Child and Adolescent Psychiatry, 42*(4), 406–414.

Greenhill, L. L., & MTA Cooperative Group. (2002). Efficacy and safety of OROS MPH in adolescents with ADHD. Paper presented at the 49th annual meeting of the American Academy of Child and Adolescent Psychiatry, San Francisco.

Greenhill, L. L., Pelham, W. E., Lopez, F. E., et al. (2002). *Once-daily transdermal methylphenidate improves teacher, parent, and CGI-I ratings.* Paper presented at the 49th annual meeting of the American Academy of Child and Adolescent Psychiatry, San Francisco.

Greenhill, L. L., Pliszka, S., Dulcan, M. K., Bernet, W., Arnold, V., Beitchman, J., et al. (2002). Practice parameter for the use of stimulant medications in the treatment of children, adolescents, and adults. *Journal of the American Academy of Child and Adolescent Psychiatry, 41*(2, Suppl.), 26S–49S.

Gross, M. (1976). Growth of hyperkinetic children taking methylphenidate, dextroamphetamine, or imipramine/desipramine. *Pediatrics, 58*, 423–431.

Gualtieri, C. T., Ondrusek, M. G., & Finley, C. (1985). Attention deficit disorders in adults. *Clinical Neuropharmacology, 8*(4), 343–356.

Handen, B. L., Breaux, A. M., Janosky, J., McAuliffe, S., Feldman, H., & Gosling, A. (1992). Effects and noneffects of methylphenidate in children with mental retardation and ADHD. *Journal of the American Academy of Child and Adolescent Psychiatry, 31*(3), 455–461.

Handen, B. L., Feldman, H. M., Lurier, A., & Murray, P. J. (1999). Efficacy of methylphenidate among preschool children with developmental disabilities and ADHD. *Journal of the American Academy of Child and Adolescent Psychiatry, 38*, 805–812.

Handen, B. L., Johnson, C. R., & Lubetsky, M. (2000). Efficacy of methylphenidate among children with autism and symptoms of attention-deficit hyperactivity disorder. *Journal of Autism and Development Disorders, 30*(3), 245–255.

Hechtman, L., Weiss, G., & Perlman, T. (1984). Young adult outcome of hyperactive children who received long-term stimulant treatment. *Journal of the American Academy of Child and Adolescent Psychiatry, 23*, 261–269.

Hemmer, S. A., Pasternak, J. F., Zecker, S. G., & Trommer, B. L. (2001). Stimulant therapy and seizure risk in children with ADHD. *Pediatric Neurology, 24*(2), 99–102.

Hoffman, B. B., & Lefkowitz, R. J. (1996). Catecholamines, sympathomimetic drugs, and adrenergic receptor antagonists. In J. G. Hardman, L. E. Limbird, P. B. Molinoff, R. W. Ruddon & A. G. Gilman (Eds.), *The pharmacological basis of therapeutics* (9th ed., pp. 199–248). New York: McGraw-Hill.

Jensen, P. S. (2000). ADHD: Current concepts on etiology, pathophysiology, and neurobiology. *Child and Adolescent Psychiatric Clinics of North America, 9*(3), 557–572.

Jensen, P. S., Bhatara, V. S., Vitiello, B., Hoagwood, K., Feil, M., & Burke, L. B. (1999). Psychoactive medication prescribing practices for U.S. children: Gaps between research and clinical practice. *Journal of the American Academy of Child and Adolescent Psychiatry, 38*(5), 557–565.

Jensen, P. S., Hinshaw, S. P., Swanson, J. M., Greenhill, L., Conners, C. K., Arnold, L. E., et al. (2001). Findings from the NIMH Multimodal Treatment Study of ADHD (MTA): Implications and applications for primary care providers. *Journal of Developmental and Behavioral Pediatrics, 22*(1), 60–73.

Jensen, P. S., Kettle, L., Roper, M. T., Sloan, M. T., Dulcan, M. K., Hoven, C., et al. (1999). Are stimulants overprescribed? *Journal of the American Academy of Child and Adolescent Psychiatry, 38*, 797–804.

Johnston, C., Pelham, W. E., Hoza, J., & Sturges, J. (1988). Psychostimulant rebound in attention deficit disordered boys. *Journal of the American Academy of Child and Adolescent Psychiatry, 27*, 806–810.

Klein, R. G. (1987). Pharmacotherapy of childhood hyperactivity: An update. In H. Y. Meltzer (Ed.), *Psychopharmacology: The third generation of progress* (pp. 1215–1224). New York: Raven Press.

Klein, R. G., Abikoff, H., Klass, E., Ganeles, D., Seese, L. M., & Pollack, S. (1997). Clinical efficacy of methylphenidate in conduct disorder with and without attention deficit hyperactivity disorder. *Archives of General Psychiatry, 54*(12), 1073–1080.

Klein, R. G., & Mannuzza, S. (1988). Hyperactive boys almost grown up: III. Methylphenidate effects on ultimate height. *Archives of General Psychiatry, 45*, 1131–1134.

Klein-Schwartz, W., & McGrath, J. (2003). Poison centers' experience with methylphenidate abuse in preteens and adolescents. *Journal of the American Academy of Child and Adolescent Psychiatry, 42*(3), 288–294.

Klorman, R., Brumaghim, J. T., Salzman, L. F., Strauss, J., Borgstedt, A. D., McBride, M. C., et al. (1988). Effects of methylphenidate on attention-deficit hyperactivity disorder with and without aggressive/noncompliant features. *Journal of Abnormal Psychology, 97*(4), 413–422.

Klorman, R., Coons, H. W., & Borgstedt, A. D. (1987). Effects of methylphenidate on adolescents with a childhood history of attention deficit disorder: I. Clinical findings. *Journal of the American Academy of Child and Adolescent Psychiatry, 26*(3), 363–367.

Koehler-Troy, C., Strober, M., & Malenbaum, R. (1986). Methylphenidate induced mania in a prepubertal child. *Journal of Clinical Psychiatry, 47*, 566–567.

Kollins, S. H., & PATS Study Group. (2004, June). *Preschool ADHD treatment study.* Paper presented at the annual meeting of the New Drug Clinical Evaluation Unit, Phoenix, AZ.

Kupietz, S. S. (1991). Ritalin blood levels and their correlations with measures of learning. In L. L. Greenhill & B. B. Osmon (Eds.), *Ritalin: Theory and patient management* (pp. 247–256). New York: Liebert.

Kurlan, R., Como, P. G., Miller, B., Palumbo, D., Deeley, C., Andresen, E. M., et al. (2002). The behavioral spectrum of tic disorders: A community-based study. *Neurology, 59*(3), 414–420.

Lambert, N. M., & Hartsough, C. S. (1998). Prospective study of tobacco smoking and substance dependencies among samples of ADHD and non-ADHD participants. *Journal of Learning Disabilities, 31*, 533–544.

Law, S. F., & Schachar, R. (1999). Do typical clinical doses of methylphenidate cause tics in children treated for attention-deficit hyperactivity disorder? *Journal of the American Academy of Child and Adolescent Psychiatry, 38*, 944–951.

Levy, F. (1991). The dopamine theory of attention deficit hyperactivity disorder (ADHD). *Australian and New Zealand Journal of Psychiatry, 25*, 277–283.

Lipkin, P., Goldstein, I., & Adesman, A. (1994). Tics and dyskinesias associated with stimulant treatment in attention-deficit hyperactivity disorder. *Archives of Pediatrics and Adolescent Medicine, 148*, 859–861.

Mahalick, D. M., Carmel, P. W., Greenberg, J. P., Molofsky, W., Brown, J. A., Heary, R. F., et al. (1998). Psychopharmacologic treatment of acquired attention disorders in children with brain injury. *Pediatric Neurosurgery, 29*(3), 121–126.

Mannuzza, S., Gittelman-Klein, R., Bessler, A., Malloy, P., & LaPadula, M. (1993). Young adult outcome of hyperactive boys almost grown up: Educational achievement, occupational rank, and psychiatric status. *Archives of General Psychiatry, 50*, 565–576.

Mannuzza, S., Klein, R. G., & Addalli, K. A. (1991). Young adult mental status of hyperactive boys and their brothers: A prospective follow-up study. *Journal of the American Academy of Child and Adolescent Psychiatry, 30*(5), 743–751.

Mattes, J. A., Boswell, L., & Oliver, H. (1984). Methylphenidate effects on symptoms of attention deficit disorder in adults. *Archives of General Psychiatry, 41*, 1059–1063.

Max, J. E., Arndt, S., Castillo, C. S., Bokura, H., Robin, D. A., Lindgren, S. D., et al. (1998). Attention-deficit hyperactivity symptomatology after traumatic brain injury: A prospective study. *Journal of the American*

Academy of Child and Adolescent Psychiatry, 37(8), 841–847.

Max, J. E., Lansing, A. E., Koele, S. L., Castillo, C. S., Bokura, H., Schachar, R., et al. (2004). Attention deficit hyperactivity disorder in children and adolescents following traumatic brain injury. *Developmental Neuropsychology, 25*(1–2), 159–177.

Mayes, S. D., Crites, D. L., Bixler, E. O., Humphrey, F.J., 2nd, & Mattison, R.E. (1994). Methylphenidate and ADHD: Influence of age, IQ, and neurodevelopmental status. *Developmental Medicine and Child Neurology, 36*, 1099–1107.

McBride, M. C., Wang, D. D., & Torres, C. F. (1986). Methylphenidate in therapeutic doses does not lower seizure threshold. *Annals of Neurology, 20*, 428.

McNeil Pharmaceuticals. (2001). *Concerta product monograph.* Raritan, NJ: Author.

Michaels, M. A., Weston, I. E., Zhang, Y., & Tulloch, S. J. (2001, May). *Pharmacokinetics of SLI381, a two-component extended-release formulation of mixed amphetamine salts, administered in fasted and fed states, and sprinkled on food.* Paper presented at the annual meeting of the New Drug Clinical Evaluation Unit, Phoenix, AZ.

Michelson, D., Faries, D., Wernicke, J., Kelsey, D., Kendrick, K., Sallee, F. R., et al. (2001). Atomoxetine in the treatment of children and adolescents with attention-deficit/hyperactivity disorder: A randomized, placebo-controlled, dose response study. *Pediatrics, 108*(5), 1–9.

Milberger, S., Biederman, J., Faraone, S. V., Chen, L., & Jones, J. (1997a). ADHD is associated with early initiation of cigarette smoking in children and adolescents. *Journal of the American Academy of Child and Adolescent Psychiatry, 36*(1), 37–44.

Milberger, S., Biederman, J., Faraone, S. V., Chen, L., & Jones, J. (1997b). Further evidence of an association between attention-deficit/hyperactivity disorder and cigarette smoking: Findings from a high-risk sample of siblings. *American Journal on Addictions, 6*(3), 205–217.

Milberger, S., Biederman, J., Faraone, S. V., Wilens, T., & Chu, M. P. (1997). Associations between ADHD and psychoactive substance use disorders. Findings from a longitudinal study of high-risk siblings of ADHD children. *American Journal on Addictions, 6*(4), 318–329.

Monteiro-Musten, L., Firestone, P., Pisterman, S., Bennett, S., & Mercer, J. (1997). Effects of methylphenidate on preschool children with ADHD: Cognitive and behavioral functions. *Journal of the American Academy of Child and Adolescent Psychiatry, 36*, 1407–1415.

MTA Cooperative Group. (1999). Moderators and mediators of treatment response for children with attention-deficit/hyperactivity disorder: The Multimodal Treatment Study of children with attention-deficit/hyperactivity disorder. *Archives of General Psychiatry, 56*(12), 1088–1096.

Murphy, K. R., & Barkley, R. A. (1996). Attention deficit hyperactivity disorder adults: Comorbidities and adaptive impairments. *Comprehensive Psychiatry, 37*(6), 393–401.

Murphy, K. R., Barkley, R. A., & Bush, T. (2002). Young adults with attention deficit hyperactivity disorder: Subtype differences in comorbidity, educational, and clinical history. *Journal of Nervous and Mental Disease, 190*(3), 147–157.

Novartis Pharmaceuticals. (2002a). *Focalin product monograph.* East Hanover, NJ: Author.

Novartis Pharmaceuticals. (2002b). *Ritalin LA product monograph.* East Hanover, NJ: Author.

O'Donnell, D., Biederman, J., Jones, J., Wilens, T. E., Milberger, S., Mick, E., et al. (1998). Informativeness of child and parent reports on substance use disorders in a sample of ADHD probands, control probands, and their siblings. *Journal of the American Academy of Child and Adolescent Psychiatry, 37*(7), 752–758.

Pataki, C. S., Carlson, G. A., Kelly, K., Rapport, M. D., & Biancaniello, T. (1993). Side effects of methylphenidate and desipramine alone and in combination in children. *American Journal of Psychiatry, 32,* 1065–1072.

Paterson, R., Douglas, C., Hallmayer, J., Hagan, M., & Krupenia, Z. (1999). A randomized, double-blind, placebo-controlled trial of dexamphetamine in adults with attention deficit hyperactivity disorder. *Australian and New Zealand Journal of Psychiatry, 33*(4), 494–502.

Pearson, D. A., Santos, C. W., Roache, J. D., Casat, C. D., Loveland, K. A., Lachar, D., et al. (2003). Treatment effects of methylphenidate on behavioral adjustment in children with mental retardation and ADHD. *Journal of the American Academy of Child and Adolescent Psychiatry, 42*(2), 209–216.

Pelham, W. E., Gnagy, E. M., Burrows-Maclean, L., Williams, A., Fabiano, G.A., Morrisey, S.M., et al. (2001). Once-a-day Concerta methylphenidate versus three-times-daily methylphenidate in laboratory and natural settings. *Pediatrics, 107*(6), 1–15.

Pelham, W. E., Jr., Sturges, J., Hoza, J., Schmidt, C., Bijlsma, J. J., Milich, R., et al. (1987). Sustained release and standard methylphenidate effects on cognitive and social behavior in children with attention deficit disorder. *Pediatrics, 80*(4), 491–501.

Pelham, W. E., Jr., Swanson, J. M., Furman, M. B., & Schwindt, H. (1995). Pemoline effects on children with ADHD: A time–response by dose–response analysis on classroom measures. *Journal of the American Academy of Child and Adolescent Psychiatry, 34*(11), 1504–1513.

Pelham, W. E., Vodde-Hamilton, M., Murphy, D. A., Greenstein, J. J., & Vallano, G. (1991). The effects of methylphenidate on ADHD adolescents in recreational, peer group, and classroom settings. *Journal of Clinical Child Psychology, 20,* 293–300.

Pisterman, S., McGrath, P., Firestone, P., Goodman, J.T., Webster, I., & Mallory, R. (1989). Outcome of parent-mediated treatment of preschoolers with attention deficit disorder. *Journal of Consulting and Clinical Psychology, 57,* 628–635.

Pliszka, S. R. (1989). Effect of anxiety on cognition, behavior, and stimulant response in ADHD. *Journal of the American Academy of Child and Adolescent Psychiatry, 28*(6), 882–887.

Pliszka, S. R. (1998). Comorbidity of attention-deficit/hyperactivity disorder with psychiatric disorder: An overview. *Journal of Clinical Psychiatry, 59*(Suppl. 7), 50–58.

Pliszka, S. R. (2003). *Neuroscience for the mental health clinician.* New York: Guilford Press.

Pliszka, S. R., Carlson, C. L., & Swanson, J. M. (1999). *ADHD with comorbid disorders: Clinical assessment and management.* New York: Guilford Press.

Pliszka, S. R., McCracken, J. T., & Maas, J. W. (1996). Catecholamines in attention-deficit hyperactivity disorder: Current perspectives. *Journal of the American Academy of Child and Adolescent Psychiatry, 35,* 264–272.

Popper, C. W. (1995). Combining methylphenidate and clonidine: Pharmacologic questions and news reports about sudden death. *Journal of Child and Adolescent Psychopharmacology, 5,* 157–166.

Posner, M. I., & Raichle, M. E. (1996). *Images of mind* (rev. ed.). Washington, DC: Scientific American Books.

Prince, J. B., Wilens, T. E., Biederman, J., Spencer, T. J., & Wozniak, J. R. (1996). Clonidine for sleep disturbances associated with attention-deficit hyperactivity disorder: A systematic chart review of 62 cases. *Journal of the American Academy of Child and Adolescent Psychiatry, 35*(5), 599–605.

Purvis, K. L., & Tannock, R. (1997). Language abilities in children with attention deficit hyperactivity disorder, reading disabilities, and normal controls. *Journal of Abnormal Child Psychology, 25*(2), 133–144.

Rapoport, J., Buschsbaum, M. S., Zahn, T. P., Weingartner, H., Ludlow, C., & Mikkelsen, E. J. (1978). Dextroamphetamine: Cognitive and behavioral effects in normal prepubertal boys. *Science, 199,* 560–562.

Rapport, M. D., Carlson, G. A., Kelly, K., & Pataki, C. S. (1993). Methylphenidate and desipramine in hospitalized children: I. Separate and combined effects on cognitive function. *Journal of the American Academy of Child and Adolescent Psychiatry, 32,* 333–342.

Rapport, M. D., Jones, J. T., DuPaul, G. J., Kelly, K. L., et al. (1987). Attention deficit disorder and methylphenidate: Group and single-subject analyses of dose effects on attention in clinic and classroom settings. *Journal of Clinical Child Psychology, 16,* 329–338.

Rapport, M. D., & Kelly, K. L. (1991). Psychostimulant effects on learning and cognitive function in children with attention deficit hyperactivity disorder: Findings and implications. In J. L. Matson (Ed.), *Hyperactivity in children: A handbook* (pp. 61–92). New York: Pergamon Press.

Rapport, M. D., & Moffitt, C. (2002). Attention deficit/hyperactivity disorder and methylphenidate. A review of height/weight, cardiovascular, and somatic complaint side effects. *Clinical Psychology Review, 22*(8), 1107–1131.

Rapport, M. D., Quinn, S. O., DuPaul, G. J., Quinn, G. J., & Kelly, K. L. (1989). Attention deficit disorder with hyperactivity and methylphenidate: The effects of dose and mastery level on children's learning performance. *Journal of Abnormal Child Psychology, 17,* 669–689.

Rapport, M. D., Stoner, G., DuPaul, G. J., Kelly, K. L., Tucker, S. B., & Schoeler, T. (1988). Attention deficit disorder and methylphenidate: A multilevel analysis of dose–response effects on children's impulsivity across settings. *Journal of the American Academy of Child and Adolescent Psychiatry, 27,* 60–69.

Research Unit on Pediatric Psychopharmacology Anxiety Study Group. (2001). Fluvoxamine for the treatment of anxiety disorders in children and adolescents. *New England Journal of Medicine, 344,* 1279–1285.

Riddle, M. A., Lynch, K. A., Scahill, L., DeVries, A., Cohen, D. J., & Leckman, J. F. (1995). Methylphenidate discontinuation and reinitiation during long-term treatment of children with Tourette's disorder and attention-deficit hyperactivity disorder: A pilot study. *Journal of Child and Adolescent Psychopharmacology, 3*(5), 191–205.

Riggs, P. D. (1998). Clinical approach to treatment of ADHD in adolescents with substance use disorders and conduct disorder. *Journal of the American Academy of Child and Adolescent Psychiatry, 37,* 331–332.

Robinson, T. E., & Berridge, K. C. (1993). The neural basis of drug craving: An incentive-sensitization theory of addiction. *Brain and Behavior Review, 18,* 247–291.

Rushton, J. L., & Whitmire, J. T. (2001). Pediatric stimulant and SSRI prescription trends: 1992–1998. *Archives of Pediatrics and Adolescent Medicine, 155,* 560–565.

Safer, D. J., Allen, R., & Barr, E. (1972). Depression of growth in hyperactive children on stimulant drugs. *New England Journal of Medicine, 287,* 217–220.

Safer, D. J., Zito, J. M., & Fine, E. M. (1996). Increased methylphenidate usage for attention deficit disorder in the 1990s. *Pediatrics, 98,* 1084–1088.

Safer, D. J., Zito, J. M., & Gardner, J. F. (2001). Pemoline hepatotoxicity and postmarketing surveillance. *Journal of the American Academy of Child and Adolescent Psychiatry, 40,* 622–629.

Satterfield, J. H., Cantwell, D. P., Schell, A., & Blaschke, T. (1979). Growth of hyperactive children treated with methylphenidate. *Archives of General Psychiatry, 36,* 212–217.

Scahill, L., Chappell, P. B., Kim, Y. S., Schultz, R. T., Katsovich, L., Shepherd, E., et al. (2001). A placebo-controlled study of guanfacine in the treatment of children with tic disorders and attention deficit hyperactivity disorder. *American Journal of Psychiatry, 158*(7), 1067–1074.

Schachar, R., & Tannock, R. (1993). Childhood hyperactivity and psychostimulants: A review of extended treatment studies. *Journal of Child and Adolescent Psychopharmacology, 3,* 81–97.

Schachar, R. J., Tannock, R., Cunningham, C. E., & Corkum, P. V. (1997). Behavioral, situational, and temporal effects of treatment of ADHD with methylphenidate. *Journal of the American Academy of Child and Adolescent Psychiatry, 36*(6), 754–763.

Scheffer, R. E. (2002, October). *Combination pharmacotherapy in pediatric bipolars—treating comorbid ADHD.* Paper presented at the 49th annual meeting of the American Academy of Child and Adolescent Psychiatry, San Francisco.

Schleifer, M., Weiss, G., Cohen, N., Elman, M., Cvejic, H., & Kruger, E. (1975). Hyperactivity in preschoolers and the effect of methylphenidate. *American Journal of Orthopsychiatry, 45,* 38–50.

Schubiner, H., Saules, K. K., Arfken, C. L., Johanson, C. E., Schuster, C. R., Lockhart, N., et al. (2002). Double-blind placebo-controlled trial of methylphenidate in the treatment of adult ADHD patients with comorbid cocaine dependence. *Experimental and Clinical Psychopharmacology, 10*(3), 286–294.

Seidman, L. J., Biederman, J., Weber, W., Hatch, M., & Faraone, S. V. (1998). Neuropsychological function in adults with attention-deficit hyperactivity disorder. *Biological Psychiatry, 44*(4), 260–268.

Semrud-Clikeman, M., Biederman, J., Sprich-Buckminster, S., Lehman, B. K., Faraone, S. V., & Norman, D. (1992). Comorbidity between ADDH and learning disability: A review and report in a clinically referred sample. *Journal of the American Academy of Child and Adolescent Psychiatry, 31*(3), 439–448.

Sergeant, J. A., & van der Meere, J. (1991). Ritalin effects and information processing in hyperactivity. In L. L. Greenhill & B. B. Osman (Eds.), *Ritalin: Theory and patient management* (pp. 1–13). New York: Liebert.

Shapiro, A. K., & Shapiro, E. (1981). Do stimulants provoke, cause, or exacerbate tics and Tourette syndrome? *Comprehensive Psychiatry, 22,* 265–273.

Shevell, M., & Schreiber, R. (1997). Pemoline-associated hepatic failure: A critical analysis of the literature. *Pediatric Neurology, 16,* 14–16.

Shire Pharmaceuticals. (2001). *Adderall XR data on file.* Wayne, PA: Shire US.

Short, E. J., Manos, M. J., Findling, R. L., & Schubel, E. A. (2004). A prospective study of stimulant response in preschool children: Insights from ROC analyses. *Journal of the American Academy of Child and Adolescent Psychiatry, 43*(3), 251–259.

Silver, L. B. (2000). Attention-deficit/hyperactivity disorder in adult life. *Child and Adolescent Psychiatric Clinics of North America, 9*(3), 511–523.

Smith, B. H., Pelham, W. E., Evans, S., Gnagy, E.,

Molina, B., Bukstein, O., et al. (1998). Dosage effects of methylphenidate on the social behavior of adolescents diagnosed with attention-deficit hyperactivity disorder. *Experimental and Clinical Psychopharmacology, 6*(2), 187–204.

Smith, B. H., Pelham, W. E., Gnagy, E., & Yudell, R. S. (1998). Equivalent effects of stimulant treatment for attention-deficit hyperactivity disorder during childhood and adolescence. *Journal of the American Academy of Child and Adolescent Psychiatry, 37*(3), 314–321.

Snider, L. A., Seligman, L. D., Ketchen, B. R., Levitt, S. J., Bates, L. R., Garvey, M. A., et al. (2002). Tics and problem behaviors in school children: Prevalence, characterization, and associations. *Pediatrics, 110*(2, Pt. 1), 331–336.

Solanto, M. V. (1998). Neuropsychopharmacological mechanisms of stimulant drug action in attention-deficit hyperactivity disorder: A review and integration. *Behavioral Brain Research, 94*, 127–152.

Spencer, T., Biederman, J., Harding, M., O'Donnell, D., Faraone, S. V., & Wilens, T. E. (1996). Growth deficits in ADHD children revisited: Evidence for disorder-associated growth delays? *Journal of the American Academy of Child and Adolescent Psychiatry, 35*(11), 1460–1469.

Spencer, T., Biederman, J., Kerman, K., Steingard, R., & Wilens, T. (1993). Desipramine treatment of children with attention-deficit hyperactivity disorder and tic disorder or Tourette's syndrome. *Journal of the American Academy of Child and Adolescent Psychiatry, 32*(2), 354–360.

Spencer, T., Biederman, J., & Wilens, T. (1999). Attention-deficit/hyperactivity disorder and comorbidity. *Pediatric Clinics of North America, 46*(5), 915–927.

Spencer, T., Biederman, J., Wilens, T., Harding, M., O'Donnell, D., & Griffin, S. (1996). Pharmacotherapy of attention-deficit hyperactivity disorder across the life cycle. *Journal of the American Academy of Child and Adolescent Psychiatry, 35*(4), 409–432.

Spencer, T., Biederman, J., Wilens, T., Steingard, R., & Geist, D. (1993). Nortriptyline treatment of children with attention-deficit hyperactivity disorder and tic disorder or Tourette's syndrome. *Journal of the American Academy of Child and Adolescent Psychiatry, 32*(1), 205–210.

Spencer, T., Biederman, J., Wilens, T. E., & Faraone, S. V. (1998). Adults with attention-deficit/hyperactivity disorder: A controversial diagnosis. *Journal of Clinical Psychiatry, 59*(Suppl. 7), 59–68.

Spencer, T., Wilens, T., Biederman, J., Faraone, S. V., Ablon, J. S., & Lapey, K. (1995). A double-blind, crossover comparison of methylphenidate and placebo in adults with childhood-onset attention-deficit hyperactivity disorder. *Archives of General Psychiatry, 52*(6), 434–443.

Spencer, T., Wilens, T., Biederman, J., Wozniak, J., & Harding-Crawford, M. (2000). Attention-deficit/hyperactivity disorder with mood disorders. In T. E.

Brown (Ed.), *Attention deficit disorders and comorbidities in children, adolescents, and adults* (pp. 79–124). Washington, DC: American Psychiatric Press.

Stahl, S. M. (2002). Mirror, mirror on the wall, which enantiomer is fairest of them all? *Journal of Clinical Psychiatry, 63*(8), 656–657.

Stigler, K. A., Desmond, L. A., Posey, D. J., Wiegand, R. E., & McDougle, C. J. (2004). A naturalistic retrospective analysis of psychostimulants in pervasive developmental disorders. *Journal of Child and Adolescent Psychopharmacology, 14*(1), 49–56.

Sukhodolsky, D. G., Scahill, L., Zhang, H., Peterson, B. S., King, R. A., Lombroso, P. J., et al. (2003). Disruptive behavior in children with Tourette's syndrome: Association with ADHD comorbidity, tic severity, and functional impairment. *Journal of the American Academy of Child and Adolescent Psychiatry, 41*(1), 98–105.

Swanson, J. M. (1988). What do psychopharmacological studies tell us about information processing deficits in ADDH? In L. M. Bloomingdale & J. A. Sergeant (Eds.), *Attention deficit disorder: Criteria, cognition, intervention* (pp. 97–116). Amsterdam: Elsevier.

Swanson, J. M., Connor, D., & Cantwell, D. (1999). Combining methylphenidate and clonidine: Ill-advised. *Journal of the American Academy of Child and Adolescent Psychiatry, 38*, 617–619.

Swanson, J. M., Flockhart, D., Udrea, D., Cantwell, D., Connor, D., & Williams, L. (1995). Clonidine in the treatment of ADHD: Questions about safety and efficacy [Letter]. *Journal of Child and Adolescent Psychopharmacology, 5*, 301–304.

Swanson, J. M., Granger, D., & Kliewer, W. (1987). Natural social behaviors in hyperactive children: Dose effects of methylphenidate. *Journal of Consulting and Clinical Psychology, 55*, 187–193.

Swanson, J. M., Gupta, S., Guinta, D., Flynn, D., Agler, D., Lerner, M., et al. (1999). Acute tolerance to methylphenidate in the treatment of attention deficit hyperactivity disorder in children. *Clinical Pharmacology and Therapeutics, 66*, 295–305.

Swanson, J. M., & Kinsbourne, M. (1978). The cognitive effects of stimulant drugs on hyperactive children. In G. A. Hale (Ed.), *Attention and cognitive development* (pp. 249–274). New York: Plenum Press.

Szatmari, P., Boyle, M., & Offord, D. R. (1989). ADDH and conduct disorder: Degree of diagnostic overlap and differences among correlates. *Journal of the American Academy of Child and Adolescent Psychiatry, 28*(6), 865–872.

Tourette's Syndrome Study Group. (2002). Treatment of ADHD in children with tics: A randomized controlled trial. *Neurology, 58*(4), 527–536.

Varley, C. K. (1983). Effects of methylphenidate in adolescents with attention deficit disorder. *Journal of the American Academy of Child and Adolescent Psychiatry, 22*, 351–354.

Volkow, N. D., Ding, Y. S., Fowler, J. S., Wang, G.J., Logan, J. Gatley, J.S., et al. (1995). Is methylphenidate like cocaine?: Studies on their pharmacokinetics and distribution in the human brain. *Archives of General Psychiatry, 52,* 456–463.

Volkow, N. D., Wang, G. J., Fowler, J. S., Logan, J., Franceschi, D., Maynard, L., et al. (2002). Relationship between blockade of dopamine transporters by oral methylphenidate and the increases in extracellular dopamine: Therapeutic implications. *Synapse, 43,* 181–187.

Vyse, S. A., & Rapport, M. D. (1989). The effects of methylphenidate on learning in children with ADDH: The stimulus-equivalence paradigm. *Journal of Consulting and Clinical Psychology, 57,* 425–435.

Weber, P., & Lutschg, J. (2002). Methylphenidate treatment. *Pediatric Neurology, 26*(4), 261–266.

Wender, P. H., Reimherr, F. W., & Wood, D. R. (1981). Attention deficit disorder (minimal brain dysfunction) in adults. *Archives of General Psychiatry, 38,* 449–456.

Wender, P. H., Reimherr, F. W., Wood, D. R., & Ward, M. (1985). A controlled study of methylphenidate in the treatment of attention deficit disorder, residual type, in adults. *American Journal of Psychiatry, 142*(5), 547–552.

Whalen, C. K., Henker, B., & Dotemoto, S. (1980). Methylphenidate and hyperactivity: Effects on teacher behaviors. *Science, 208,* 1280–1282.

Whalen, C. K., Henker, B., & Granger, D. A. (1990). Social judgment processes in hyperactive boys: Effects of methylphenidate and comparisons with normal peers. *Journal of Abnormal Child Psychology, 18,* 297–316.

Wilens, T. E., Biederman, J., Prince, J., Spencer, T. J., Faraone, S. V., Warburton, R., et al. (1996). Six-week, double-blind, placebo-controlled study of desipramine for adult attention deficit hyperactivity disorder. *American Journal of Psychiatry, 153*(9), 1147–1153.

Wilens, T. E., Biederman, J., Spencer, T. J., Frazier, J., Prince, J., Bostic, J., et al. (1999). Controlled trial of high doses of pemoline for adults with attention-deficit/hyperactivity disorder. *Journal of Clinical Psychopharmacology, 19*(3), 257–264.

Wilens, T. E., Biederman, J., Spencer, T. J., & Prince, J. (1995). Pharmacotherapy of adult attention deficit/hyperactivity disorder: A review. *Journal of Clinical Psychopharmacology, 15*(4), 270–279.

Wilens, T. E., Faraone, S. V., Biederman, J., & Gunawardene, S. (2003). Does stimulant therapy of attention deficit/hyperactivity disorder beget later substance abuse? A meta-analytic review of the literature. *Pediatrics, 11*(1), 179–185.

Wilens, T. E., Pelham, W. E., Stein, M. T., Conners, C. K., Abikoff, H., Atkins, M. S., et al. (2003). ADHD treatment with once-daily OROS methylphenidate: Interim 12–month results from a long-term open-label study. *Journal of the American Academy of Child and Adolescent Psychiatry, 42*(4), 424–433.

Wilens, T. E., & Spencer, T. J. (2000). The stimulants revisited. *Child and Adolescent Psychiatric Clinics of North America, 9*(3), 573–603.

Willy, M. E., Manda, B., Shatin, D., Drinkard, C. R., & Graham, D. J. (2002). A study of compliance with FDA recommendations for pemoline (Cylert). *Journal of the American Academy of Child and Adolescent Psychiatry, 41,* 785–790.

Wolraich, M. L., Lindgren, S., Stromquist, A., Milich, R., Davis, C., & Watson, D. (1990). Stimulant medication use by primary care physicians in the treatment of attention deficit hyperactivity disorder. *Pediatrics, 86,* 95–101.

Wood, D. R., Reimherr, F. W., Wender, P. H., & Johnson, G. E. (1976). Diagnosis and treatment of minimal brain dysfunction in adults. *Archives of General Psychiatry, 33,* 1453–1460.

Zametkin, A., & Liotta, W. (1998). The neurobiology of attention-deficit/hyperactivity disorder. *Journal of Clinical Psychiatry, 59,* 17–23.

Zito, J. M., Safer, D. J., dosReis, S., Gardner, J. F., Boles, M., & Lynch, F. (2000). Trends in the prescribing of psychotropic medications to preschoolers. *Journal of the American Medical Association, 283*(8), 1025–1030.

Zito, J. M., Safer, D. J., dosReis, S., Gardner, J. F., Magder, L. S., Soeken, K., et al. (2003). Psychotropic practice patterns for youth: A 10–year perspective. *Archives of Pediatrics and Adolescent Medicine, 157,* 17–25.

Zito, J. M., Safer, D. J., dosReis, S., Magder, L. S., Gardner, J. F., & Zarin, D. A. (1999). Psychotherapeutic medication patterns for youths with attention deficit/hyperactivity disorder. *Archives of Pediatrics and Adolescent Medicine, 153*(12), 1257–1263.

Antidepressant and Specific Norepinephrine Reuptake Inhibitor Treatments

THOMAS J. SPENCER

Stimulants (see Chapter 17, this volume) are very effective in the treatment of Attention-Deficit/Hyperactivity Disorder (ADHD); however, it is estimated that at least 30% of affected individuals do not adequately respond to or cannot tolerate stimulant treatment (Barkley, 1977; Gittelman, 1980; Spencer et al., 1996). Over the last few decades, it has been shown that medications with a noradrenergic mechanism of action are effective anti-ADHD agents. Although the development of the new generation of longer-acting stimulants has assisted with the need for medium- to long-term treatment, there is still no single stimulant formulation for coverage beyond 12 hours. The use of stimulants also involves the potential for insomnia, which may prevent administration in the evening. In addition, stimulants are controlled substances, posing medico-legal concerns to the treating community that may increase the barriers to treatment.

As are most medical conditions, ADHD is heterogeneous in etiology and clinical expression. For example, ADHD is frequently comorbid with mood and anxiety disorders— conditions that may have an adverse impact on responsivity to stimulant drugs (DuPaul, Barkley, & McMurray, 1994; Pliszka, 1989; Swanson, Kinsbourne, Roberts, & Zucker, 1978; Tannock, Ickowicz, & Schachar, 1995; Taylor et al., 1987; Voelker, Lachar, & Gdowski, 1983). Moreover, reports indicate that stimulants are poorly effective in treating ADHD in the context of coexisting manic symptomatology, and that their use in such patients may result in worsening of mood instability (Biederman et al., 1999). Although some reports suggest that ADHD itself may be associated with growth delays and increased rates of tics (Spencer et al., 1999; Spencer, Biederman, & Wilens, 1998), there remain some concerns about effects of stimulants on growth and in individuals with tics (Castellanos et al., 1997; Gadow, Sverd, Sprafkin, Nolan, & Ezor, 1995; Gadow, Nolan, & Sverd, 1992; Gadow, Sverd, Sprafkin, Nolan, & Grossman, 1999; Konkol, Fischer, & Newby, 1990; Law & Schachar, 1999). These shortcomings and potential problems associated with the stimulants support the need for alternative treatments.

TRICYCLIC ANTIDEPRESSANTS

The tricyclic antidepressants (TCAs) have a wide range of neurochemical effects on neurotransmitters; however, it is assumed that their activity in ADHD stems from their actions on catecholamine (norepinephrine and dopamine) reuptake. Advantages of this class of drugs include their relatively long half-life (approximately 12 hours), obviating the need to administer medication during school hours; their lack of abuse potential; and their putative positive effects on mood and anxiety, sleep, and tics. Disadvantages include side effects such as dry mouth or anorexia, as well as potentially more serious cardiac effects.

A considerable literature documents the effectiveness of the TCAs. Out of 33 studies (21 controlled, 12 open) evaluating the use of TCAs in children, adolescents ($n = 1,139$), and adults ($n = 78$), 91% reported positive effects on ADHD symptoms. Imipramine (IMI) and desipramine (DMI) are the most thoroughly studied TCAs, but a few studies have been conducted on other TCAs. Although most TCA studies (73%) have been relatively brief, lasting a few weeks to several months, nine studies (27%) reported enduring effects for up to 2 years. Outcomes in both short- and long-term studies were equally positive. Although one study (Quinn & Rapoport, 1975), reported a 50% dropout rate after 1 year, it is noteworthy that for those who remained on IMI, improvement was sustained. However, other studies using aggressive doses of TCAs reported sustained improvement for up to 1 year with DMI (>4 mg/kg) (Biederman, Gastfriend, & Jellinek, 1986; Gastfriend, Biederman, & Jellinek, 1985) and nortriptyline (2.0 mg/kg) (Wilens, Biederman, Geist, Steingard, & Spencer, 1993). Although response was equally positive in all the dose ranges, it was more sustained in those studies that used higher doses. A high interindividual variability in TCA serum levels has been consistently reported for IMI and DMI, with little relationship between serum level and daily dose, response, or side effects. In contrast, nortriptyline appears to have a positive association between dose and serum level (Wilens et al., 1993).

In the largest controlled study of a TCA in children, members of our group reported favorable results with DMI in 62 clinically referred children with ADHD, most of whom had previously not responded to psycho-stimulant treatment (Biederman, Baldessarini, Wright, Knee, & Harmatz, 1989). The study was a randomized, placebo-controlled, parallel-design, 6-week clinical trial. Clinically and statistically significant differences in behavioral improvement were found for DMI over placebo, at an average daily dose of 5 mg/kg. Specifically, 68% of DMI-treated patients were considered very much or much improved, compared with only 10% of placebo-treated patients ($p < .001$). A further analysis examined whether comorbidity of ADHD with Conduct Disorder, Major Depressive Disorder, or an anxiety disorder, or a family history of ADHD, predicted response to DMI treatment (Biederman, Baldessarini, Wright, Keenan, & Faraone, 1993). Although the presence of comorbidity increased the likelihood of a placebo response, neither comorbidity with Conduct Disorder, Major Depressive Disorder, or anxiety, nor a family history of ADHD, yielded differential responses to DMI treatment. In addition, DMI-treated patients with ADHD showed a substantial reduction in depressive symptoms, compared with placebo-treated patients.

Our group obtained similar results in a similarly designed controlled clinical trial of DMI in 41 adults with ADHD (Wilens, Biederman, Prince, et al., 1996). DMI, at an average daily dose of 150 mg (average serum level of 113 ng/ml), was statistically and clinically more effective than placebo. Sixty-eight percent of DMI-treated patients responded, compared with none of the placebo-treated patients ($p < .0001$). Moreover, at the end of the study, the average severity of ADHD symptoms was reduced to below the level required to meet diagnostic criteria in patients receiving DMI. Importantly, while the full DMI dose was achieved at week 2, clinical response improved further over the following 4 weeks, indicating a latency of response. Response was independent of dose, serum DMI level, gender, or lifetime psychiatric comorbidity with anxiety or depressive disorders.

In a prospective placebo-controlled discontinuation trial, we reported the efficacy of nortriptyline in doses of up to 2 mg/kg daily in 35 school-age youth with ADHD (Prince et al., 2000). In that study, 80% of youth responded by week 6 in the open phase. During the discontinuation phase, subjects randomly assigned to placebo lost the anti-ADHD effect, compared to those receiving nortriptyline, who maintained a robust anti-ADHD effect. Again, there was a lag in response and loss of response to medication administration and discontinuation: While the full dose was achieved by week 2, the full effect evolved slowly over the ensuing 4 weeks. Youth with ADHD who received nortriptyline also were found to have more modest but statistically significant reductions in oppositionality and anxiety. Nortriptyline was well tolerated, with some weight gain; weight gain is frequently considered to be a desirable side effect in this population. In contrast, a systematic study in 14 youth with treatment-refractory ADHD receiving protriptyline (mean dose of 30 mg) reported less favorable results. We found that only 45% of these youth responded to or could tolerate protriptyline, secondary to adverse effects (Wilens, Biederman, Abrantes, & Spencer, 1996a).

Few studies have been sufficiently powered to allow and adequate comparison to stimulants. However, 13 studies have compared TCAs to stimulants, with mixed results. Five studies reported that stimulants were superior to TCAs (Garfinkel, Wender, Sloman, & O'Neill, 1983; Gittelman-Klein, 1974; Greenberg, Yellin, Spring, & Metcalf, 1975; Rapoport, Quinn, Bradbard, Riddle, & Brooks, 1974); five studies found stimulants to be equal to TCAs (Gross, 1973; Huessy & Wright, 1970; Kupietz & Balka, 1976; Rapport, Carlson, Kelly, & Pataki, 1993; Yepes, Balka, Winsberg, & Bialer, 1977); and three studies reported that TCAs were superior to stimulants (Watter & Dreyfuss, 1973; Werry, 1980; Winsberg, Bialer, Kupietz, & Tobias, 1972). Analysis of response profiles indicate that TCAs more consistently improve behavioral symptoms, as rated by clinicians, teachers, and parents, than they improve cognitive function as measured in neuropsychological testing (Gualtieri & Evans, 1988; Quinn & Rapoport, 1975; Rapport et al., 1993; Werry, 1980).

TCAs appear to be effective anti-ADHD treatment in individuals with comorbid disorders. TCAs have uniformly been reported to produce a robust rate of response of ADHD symptoms in subjects with ADHD and comorbid depression or anxiety (Biederman, Baldessarini, Wright, et al., 1993; Cox, 1982; Wilens et al., 1993; Wilens, Biederman, Mick, & Spencer, 1995). In addition, studies of TCAs have consistently reported a robust rate of response in subjects with ADHD and comorbid tic disorders (Dillon, Salzman, & Schulsinger, 1985; Hoge & Biederman, 1986; Riddle, Hardin, Cho, Woolston, & Leckman, 1988; Singer et al., 1994; Spencer, Biederman, Kerman, Steingard, & Wilens, 1993; Spencer, Biederman, Wilens, Steingard, & Geist, 1993). For example, in a controlled study, we replicated data from a retrospective chart review indicating that DMI had a robust beneficial effect on ADHD and tic symptoms (Spencer, Biederman, et al., 2002).

The potential benefits of TCAs in the treatment of ADHD have been clouded by concerns about their safety, stemming from reports of sudden unexplained death in four children with ADHD treated with DMI (Abramowicz, 1990), although the causal link between DMI and these deaths remains uncertain. A rather extensive literature evaluating cardiovascular parameters in TCA-exposed youth consistently identified mostly minor, asymptomatic, but statistically significant increases in heart rate and electrocardiographic (EKG) measures of cardiac conduction times associated with TCA treatment (Biederman, Baldessarini, Goldblatt, et al., 1993). A report estimated that the magnitude of DMI-associated risk of sudden death in children may not be much larger than the baseline risk of sudden death in this age group (Biederman, Thisted, Greenhill, & Ryan, 1995). However, because of this uncertainty, prudence mandates that until more is known, TCAs should be considered second-line treatments for ADHD. They should also be used only after obtaining a careful history and an EKG, in order to weigh the risks and benefits of treating or not treating an affected child.

OTHER ANTIDEPRESSANTS

Bupropion

Bupropion hydrochloride is a novel-structured antidepressant of the aminoketone class, related to the phenylisopropylamines but pharmacologically distinct from known antidepressants (Casat, Pleasants, Schroeder, & Parler, 1989). Bupropion appears to possess both indirect dopamine agonist and noradrenergic effects. Bupropion has been shown to be effective for ADHD in children, in a controlled multisite study ($n = 72$) (Casat et al., 1989; Casat, Pleasants, & Van Wyck Fleet, 1987; Conners et al., 1996) and in a comparison with methylphenidate ($n = 15$) (Barrickman et al., 1995). In an open study of adults with ADHD, sustained improvement was documented at 1 year at an average of 360 mg for 6–8 weeks (Wender & Reimherr, 1990). Controlled studies in adults slow-release bupropion (Wilens et al., 2001) and extended-release bupropion (Wilens et al., 2005) have documented substantial improvement of ADHD symptoms. Although bupropion has been associated with a slightly increased risk (0.4%) for drug-induced seizures relative to other antidepressants, this risk has been linked to high doses, a previous history of seizures, and eating disorders, and may be reduced by splitting the dose throughout the day or by using a long-acting preparation.

Monoamine Oxidase Inhibitors

Although a few studies have suggested that monoamine oxidase inhibitors (MAOIs) may be effective in juvenile and adult ADHD, the irreversible MAOIs (e.g. phenelzine, tranylcypromine) have a potential for hypertensive crisis associated with dietetic transgressions (tyramine-containing foods—e.g., most cheeses) and with drug interactions (pressor amines, most cold medicines, amphetamines); this potential seriously limits their use. The "cheese effect" may be obviated with the reversible MAOIs (e.g., moclobemide), which have shown promise in one open trial (Trott, Friese, Menzel, & Nissen, 1991). However, these drugs are not available in the United States.

Selective Serotonin Reuptake Inhibitors and Venlafaxine

While a single small open study (Barrickman, Noyes, Kuperman, Schumacher, & Verda, 1991) suggested that fluoxetine may be beneficial in the treatment of children with ADHD, the usefulness of selective serotonin reuptake inhibitors (SSRIs) in the treatment of core ADHD symptoms is not supported by clinical experience (National Institute of Mental Health, 1996). Similarly uncertain is the usefulness of the mixed serotonergic–noradrenergic atypical antidepressant venlafaxine in the treatment of ADHD. Although a 77% response rate was reported in those completing treatment in open studies of adults with ADHD, 21% dropped out due to side effects (four open studies; *n* = 61 adults) (Adler, Resnick, Kunz, & Devinsky, 1995; Findling, Schwartz, Flannery, & Manos, 1996; Hornig-Rohan & Amsterdam, 1995; Reimherr, Hedges, Strong, &

Wender, 1995). Similarly, a single open study of venlafaxine in 16 children with ADHD reported a 50% response rate in those completing treatment, but a 25% rate of dropout due to side effects, most prominently increased hyperactivity (Olivera, Luh, & Tatum, 1996).

SPECIFIC NOREPINEPHRINE REUPTAKE INHIBITORS (ATOMOXETINE)

Atomoxetine (Strattera) is one of a new class of compounds being developed, known as specific norepinephrine reuptake inhibitors (SNRIs). An initial controlled clinical trial in adults documented "proof of concept" in the treatment of ADHD (Spencer, Biederman, Wilens, Prince, et al., 1998). These initial encouraging results, coupled with extensive safety data in adults, fueled efforts at developing atomoxetine for the treatment of pediatric ADHD. An open-label, dose-ranging study of this compound in pediatric ADHD documented strong clinical benefits with excellent tolerability (including a safe cardiovascular profile), and provided dosing guidelines for further controlled studies. (Spencer et al., 2001).

Further controlled trials have led to U.S. Food and Drug Administration (FDA) approval of atomoxetine for children and adults with ADHD. In the first pediatric controlled studies, 291 children ages 7 through 13 with ADHD were randomized in two trials (combined: atomoxetine = 129; placebo = 124; and methylphenidate = 38) (Spencer, Heiligenstein, et al., 2002). The acute treatment period was 9 weeks. The stimulant-naïve-stratum patients were randomized to double-blind treatment with either atomoxetine (*n* = 56), placebo (*n* = 53), or methylphenidate (*n* = 38). Stimulant-prior-exposure-stratum patients (i.e., those with prior exposure to any stimulant) were randomized to double-blind treatment with atomoxetine (*n* = 73) or placebo (*n* = 71). Atomoxetine significantly reduced total scores on a *Diagnostic and Statistical Manual of Mental Disorders*, fourth edition (DSM-IV) ADHD rating scale completed by investigators. Using a definition of response of 25% decrease of the ADHD rating scale, we found that the response rates were greater on atomoxetine than on placebo (61.4% vs. 32.3%, respectively; *p* < .05). In the stimulant-naïve stratum, 69.1% of atomoxetine-treated patients, 73% of methylphenidate-treated patients, and 31.4% of placebo-treated patients were considered responders. Atomoxetine was well tolerated. Mild appetite suppression was reported in 22% on atomoxetine versus 32% on methylphenidate and 7% on placebo. There was less insomnia on atomoxetine than on methylphenidate (7.0% vs. 27.0%; $p < .05$). Mild increases in diastolic blood pressure and heart rate were noted in the atomoxetine-treated group, with no significant differences between atomoxetine and placebo in laboratory parameters and EKG intervals.

In an additional controlled study, 297 children and adolescents were randomized to different doses of atomoxetine or placebo for 8 weeks (Michelson et al., 2001). Atomoxetine was associated with a graded dose response; response was better at 1.2 or 1.8 mg/kg/day than at 0.5 mg/kg/day, which in turn was superior to placebo. In close parallel to the dose relationship to lowering ADHD symptoms, this study documented a dose-dependent enhancement of social and family functioning. The Child Health Questionnaire was used to assess the well-being of each child and family. Parents of children on atomoxetine reported fewer emotional difficulties and behavioral problems as well as greater self-esteem in their children, and less emotional worry and fewer limitations on their personal time in themselves.

Safety and efficacy data were evaluated in a year-long open follow-up of atomoxetine-treated children and adolescents ($n = 325$). Atomoxetine treatment continued to be effective and well tolerated. The acute mild increases in diastolic blood pressure and heart rate persisted but did not worsen. Growth in height and weight was typical, and there were no significant differences between atomoxetine and placebo in laboratory parameters and EKG intervals (Kratochvil et al., 2001; Spencer et al., 2005).

An initial study examined the use of atomoxetine as an alternative treatment for adult ADHD (Spencer, Biederman, Wilens, Prince, et al., 1998). This was a double-blind, placebo-controlled, crossover study of atomoxetine in 22 adults with well-characterized ADHD; attention was also paid to issues of psychiatric comorbidity. Treatment with atomoxetine at an average oral daily dose of 76 mg/day was well tolerated. Drug-specific improvement in ADHD symptoms was highly significant overall, and sufficiently robust to be detectable in a parallel-groups comparison re-

stricted to the first 3 weeks of the protocol. The positive response rate for atomoxetine-treated subjects was greater than that of placebo-treated subjects (52% vs. 10.5%). Significant atomoxetine-associated improvement was noted on neuropsychological measures of inhibitory capacity from the Stroop test. This preliminary study thus showed that atomoxetine was effective in adult ADHD and was well tolerated. These promising results provided support for further studies of atomoxetine.

Following the initial study in adults, two large controlled studies were performed (Michelson et al., 2003). These two identical studies used randomized, double-blind, placebo-controlled designs and a 10-week treatment period in adults with DSM-IV-defined ADHD as assessed by clinical history and confirmed by a structured interview (study I, $n = 280$; study II, $n = 256$). The primary outcome measure was a comparison of atomoxetine and placebo, using repeated-measures, mixed-model analysis of postbaseline scores on the Conners Adult ADHD Rating Scale (CAARS). In each study, atomoxetine was statistically superior to placebo in reducing both inattentive and hyperactive–impulsive symptoms as assessed by primary and secondary measures. Discontinuations for adverse events among atomoxetine-treated patients were under 10% in both studies. This series of studies constituted the basis for the FDA approval of atomoxetine for adult ADHD.

Adults with ADHD who were previously enrolled in the acute study of atomoxetine have been enrolled in a 3-year open-label follow-up study (Adler et al., 2005). Preliminary results were recently reported for 384 patients at 31 sites who had been studied for a period of up to 97 weeks thus far. The primary efficacy measure was the CAARS—Investigator Rated: Screening Version (CAARS-Inv:SV) Total ADHD Symptom score. In addition, safety, adverse events, and vital sign measurements were assessed. Significant improvement was noted with atomoxetine therapy, with mean CAARS-Inv:SV Total ADHD Symptom scores decreasing 33.2% from 29.2 (baseline of open-label therapy) to 19.5 (end of open-label therapy). Similar and significant decreases were noted for the secondary efficacy measures. The relatively small increases in heart rate and blood pressure found in the acute study were persistent but did not worsen during the follow-up period. These are pharmacologically expected (noradrenergic) effects. These results support the long-term efficacy, safety, and tolerability of atomoxetine for the treatment of adult ADHD.

Current dosing guidelines recommend that atomoxetine be initiated at 0.5 mg/kg/day for 2 weeks and increased to a target dose of 1.2 mg/kg/day, with a recommended maximum dosage of 1.4 mg/kg/day or 100 mg/day. Clinicians familiar with the medication have reported further improvement at doses up to 1.8 mg/kg/day—a dosage maximum reported in both the juvenile and adolescent studies, but not FDA-approved. Whereas once-a-day dosing is effective, twice-a-day dosing can provide a better tolerability profile and potentially a more robust effect later in the day. Since atomoxetine is metabolized by the hepatic 2D6 enzymatic system, care should be taken in coadministration with medications that inhibit 2D6 (e.g., fluoxetine, paroxetine). In addition, atomoxetine has been shown to have low abuse potential (Heil et al., 2002).

Two cases of severe liver injury were reported in a denominator of over 2 million patients who have taken atomoxetine since FDA approval. Both patients have recovered with typical liver function after discontinuing the medication. Despite the rarity of this occurrence and the fact that both cases recovered, severe drug-related liver injury may progress to acute liver failure, resulting in death or the need for a liver transplant. Eli Lilly has announced (*www.lilly.com*) that it has added a boldface warning to the product label for atomoxetine as of December 2004. The boldface warning indicates that the medication should be discontinued in patients with jaundice (yellowing of the skin or whites of the eyes) or laboratory evidence of liver injury. Patients on atomoxetine are cautioned to contact their doctors immediately if they develop pruritus, jaundice, dark urine, upper-right-sided abdominal tenderness, or unexplained "flu-like" symptoms. Because this is very recent information, it will be important to remain current on any new information on this risk.

COMMENT

A substantial literature supports the potential usefulness of noradrenergic antidepressants and SNRIs for ADHD. A large body of literature on the SNRI atomoxetine has recently produced convincing evidence of substantial efficacy, tolerability, and safety. Atomoxetine is the first nonstimulant to be approved by the FDA for the treatment of ADHD. The TCAs are established alternative treatments for ADHD, particularly the more noradrenergic, secondary-amine TCAS, DMI and nortriptyline. Despite lingering concerns regarding their cardiovascular safety, TCAs have been documented to be effective and well tolerated in controlling symptoms of ADHD in studies with over 1,000 children. In addition, the atypical mixed noradrenergic–dopaminergic antidepressant bupropion has also been documented to be effective in the treatment of ADHD in controlled clinical trials.

There is increasing evidence of the importance of noradrenergic mechanisms in ADHD, although these have not been fully elucidated (Biederman & Spencer, 2000). Norepinephrine and dopamine modulate attention, motoric activity, executive functions, and motivation in parallel but overlapping circuits in the brain (Pliszka, McCracken, & Maas, 1996). Preclinical studies have shown that norepinephrine transporter reuptake (NET) inhibitors are the predominant regulators of dopamine in the frontal lobes (Bymaster et al., 2002). In addition, NET reuptake inhibitors may affect other receptors previously thought to be dopamine-selective. It is notable that both norepinephrine and dopamine are potent agonists at the D4 receptor (Lanau, Zenner, Civelli, & Hartman, 1997). In light of replicated findings linking the D4 receptor gene to juvenile (Smalley et al., 1998; Kennedy et al., 1997; LaHoste et al., 1996) and adult (Faraone et al., 1999; Sunohara et al., 1997) ADHD, drugs with activity on this receptor may warrant further investigation in this disorder. Thus agents that increase norepinephrine may further modulate attention, working memory, and executive functions through dopaminergic circuits. Since the NET inhibitors do not regulate dopamine in the striatum or nucleus accumbens (Bymaster et al., 2002), this is thought to explain the fact that these agents acts differently from stimulants on motoric activity (such as tics) and potential for euphoria.

It is hoped that advances in the understanding of the underlying neurobiology of ADHD will lead to the development of a new generation of safe and effective treatments for this disorder. Such developments have the promise of improving the quality of life for the millions of affected patients and their families worldwide.

KEY CLINICAL POINTS

✓ A substantial evidence base exists for the efficacy, tolerance, and relative safety of noradrenergic antidepressants and specific norepinephrine reuptake inhibitors (SNRIs) for the treatment of ADHD in children, adolescents, and adults.

✓ The SNRI atomoxetine is FDA-approved for the treatment of ADHD in children, adolescents, and adults.

✓ Noradrenergic antidepressants and SNRIs are equally effective on inattentive as well as hyperactive and impulsive symptoms.

✓ Noradrenergic antidepressants and SNRIs are not abusable, and except for bupropion, they decrease tic symptoms.

✓ Common side effects of atomoxetine include mild gastrointestinal symptoms, including mild anorexia; sedation (which may occur in children); and a recent warning for rare, idiosyncratic liver injury. They are devoid of risk for insomnia.

✓ Long-term effects on growth from atomoxetine use appear minimal.

REFERENCES

Abramowicz, M. (Ed.). (1990). Sudden death in children treated with a tricyclic antidepressant. *Medical Letter on Drugs and Therapeutics, 32,* 53.

Adler, L. A., Resnick, S., Kunz, M., & Devinsky, O. (1995). *Open-label trial of venlafaxine in attention deficit disorder.* Paper presented at the annual meeting of the New Clinical Drug Evaluation Unit, Orlando, FL.

Adler, L. A., Spencer, T. J., Milton, D. .R., Moore, R. J., Jones, D., & Michelson, D. (2005). Long-term, open-label safety and efficacy of atomoxetine in adults with attention-deficit/hyperactivity disorder. *Journal of Clinical Psychiatry, 66*(3), 294–299.

Barkley, R. A. (1977). A review of stimulant drug research with hyperactive children. *Journal of Child Psychology and Psychiatry, 18,* 137–165.

Barrickman, L., Noyes, R., Kuperman, S., Schumacher, E., & Verda, M. (1991). Treatment of ADHD with fluoxetine: A preliminary trial. *Journal of the American Academy of Child and Adolescent Psychiatry, 30,* 762–767.

Barrickman, L., Perry, P., Allen, A., Kuperman, S., Arndt, S., Herrmann K., et al. (1995). Bupropion versus methylphenidate in the treatment of attention-deficit hyperactivity disorder. *Journal of the American Academy of Child and Adolescent Psychiatry, 34,* 649–657.

Biederman, J., Baldessarini, R., Goldblatt, A., Lapey, K., Doyle, A., & Hesslein, P. (1993). A naturalistic study of 24-hour electrocardiographic recordings and echocardiographic finding in children and adolescents treated with desipramine. *Journal of the American Academy of Child and Adolescent Psychiatry, 32,* 805–813.

Biederman, J., Baldessarini, R. J., Wright, V., Keenan, K., & Faraone, S. (1993). A double-blind placebo controlled study of desipramine in the treatment of attention deficit disorder: III. Lack of impact of comorbidity and family history factors on clinical response. *Journal of the American Academy of Child and Adolescent Psychiatry, 32,* 199–204.

Biederman, J., Baldessarini, R. J., Wright, V., Knee, D., & Harmatz, J. S. (1989). A double-blind placebo controlled study of desipramine in the treatment of ADD: I. Efficacy. *Journal of the American Academy of Child and Adolescent Psychiatry, 28,* 777–784.

Biederman, J., Gastfriend, D. R., & Jellinek, M. S. (1986). Desipramine in the treatment of children with attention deficit disorder. *Journal of Clinical Psychopharmacology, 6,* 359–363.

Biederman, J., Mick, E., Prince, J., Bostic, J. Q., Wilens, T. E., Spencer, T., et al. (1999). Systematic chart review of the pharmacologic treatment of comorbid attention deficit hyperactivity disorder in youth with bipolar disorder. *Journal of Child and Adolescent Psychopharmacology, 9,* 247–256.

Biederman, J., & Spencer, T. (2000). Genetics of childhood disorders: XIX. ADHD, Part 3: Is ADHD a noradrenergic disorder? *Journal of the American Academy of Child and Adolescent Psychiatry, 39,* 1330–1333.

Biederman, J., Thisted, R., Greenhill, L., & Ryan, N. (1995). Estimation of the association between desipramine and the risk for sudden death in 5- to 14-year-old children. *Journal of Clinical Psychiatry, 56,* 87–93.

Bymaster, F. P., Katner, J. S., Nelson, D. L., Hemrick-Luecke, S. K., Threlkeld, P. G., Heiligenstein, J. H., et al. (2002). Atomoxetine increases extracellular levels of norepinephrine and dopamine in prefrontal cortex of rat: A potential mechanism for efficacy in attention deficit/hyperactivity disorder. *Neuropsychopharmacology, 27,* 699–711.

Casat, C. D., Pleasants, D. Z., Schroeder, D. H., & Parler, D. W. (1989). Bupropion in children with attention deficit disorder. *Psychopharmacology Bulletin, 25,* 198–201.

Casat, C. D., Pleasants, D. Z., & Van Wyck Fleet, J. (1987). A double-blind trial of bupropion in children with attention deficit disorder. *Psychopharmacology Bulletin, 23,* 120–122.

Castellanos, F. X., Giedd, J. N., Elia, J., Marsh, W. L., Ritchie, G. F., Hamburger, S. D., et al. (1997). Controlled stimulant treatment of ADHD and comorbid Tourette's syndrome: Effects of stimulant and dose. *Journal of the American Academy of Child and Adolescent Psychiatry, 36,* 589–596.

Conners, C. K., Casat, C., Gualtieri, T., Weller, E., Reader, M., Reiss, A., et al. (1996). Bupropion hydrochloride in attention deficit disorder with hyperactivity. *Journal of the American Academy of Child and Adolescent Psychiatry, 35,* 1314–1321.

Cox, W. (1982). An indication for the use of imipramine in attention deficit disorder. *American Journal of Psychiatry, 139,* 1059–1060.

Dillon, D. C., Salzman, I. J., & Schulsinger, D. A. (1985). The use of imipramine in Tourette's syndrome and attention deficit disorder: Case report. *Journal of Clinical Psychiatry, 46,* 348–349.

DuPaul, G., Barkley, R., & McMurray, M. (1994). Response of children with ADHD to methylphenidate: Interaction with internalizing symptoms. *Journal of the American Academy of Child and Adolescent Psychiatry, 33,* 894–903.

Faraone, S. V., Biederman, J., Weiffenbach, B., Keith, T., Chu, M. P., Weaver, A., et al. (1999). Dopamine D4 gene 7–repeat allele and attention deficit hyperactivity disorder. *American Journal of Psychiatry, 156,* 768–770.

Findling, R., Schwartz, M., Flannery, D., & Manos, M. (1996). Venlafaxine in adults with ADHD: An open trial. *Journal of Clinical Psychiatry, 57,* 184–189.

Gadow, K. D., Nolan, E. E., & Sverd, J. (1992). Methylphenidate in hyperactive boys with comorbid tic disorder: II. Short-term behavioral effects in school settings. *Journal of American Academy of Child and Adolescent Psychiatry, 31,* 462–471.

Gadow, K. D., Sverd, J., Sprafkin, J., Nolan, E., & Ezor, S. (1995). Efficacy of methylphenidate for attention-deficit hyperactivity disorder in children with tic disorder [published erratum appears in *Archives of General Psychiatry,* 1995, 52(10),836]. *Archives of General Psychiatry, 52,* 444–455.

Gadow, K. D., Sverd, J., Sprafkin, J., Nolan, E. E., & Grossman, S. (1999). Long-term methylphenidate therapy in children with comorbid attention- deficit hyperactivity disorder and chronic multiple tic disorder [see comments]. *Archives of General Psychiatry, 56,* 330–336.

Garfinkel, B. D., Wender, P. H., Sloman, L., & O'Neill, I. (1983). Tricyclic antidepressant and methylphenidate treatment of attention deficit disorder in children. *Journal of the American Academy of Child and Adolescent Psychiatry, 22,* 343–348.

Gastfriend, D. R., Biederman, J., & Jellinek, M. S. (1985). Desipramine in the treatment of attention deficit disorder in adolescents. *Psychopharmacology Bulletin, 21,* 144–145.

Gittelman, R. (1980). Childhood disorders. In D. Klein, F. Quitkin, A. Rifkin, & R. Gittelman (Eds.), *Drug treatment of adult and child psychiatric disorders* (pp. 576–756). Baltimore: Williams & Wilkins.

Gittelman-Klein, R. (1974). Pilot clinical trial of imipramine in hyperkinetic children. In C. Conners (Ed.), *Clinical use of stimulant drugs in children* (pp 192–201). The Hague, The Netherlands: Excerpta Medica.

Greenberg, L., Yellin, A., Spring, C., & Metcalf, M. (1975). Clinical effects of imipramine and methylphenidate in hyperactive children. *International Journal of Mental Health, 4,* 144–156.

Gross, M. (1973). Imipramine in the treatment of minimal brain dysfunction in children. *Psychosomatics, 14,* 283–285.

Gualtieri, C. T., & Evans, R. W. (1988). Motor performance in hyperactive children treated with imipramine. *Perceptual and Motor Skills, 66,* 763–769.

Heil, S. H., Holmes, H. W., Bickel, W. K., Higgins, S. T., Badger, G. J., & Lewis, H. F. (2002). Comparison of the subjective, physiological, and psychomotor effects of atomoxetine and methylphenidate in light drug users. *Drug and Alcohol Dependence, 67,* 149–156.

Hoge, S. K., & Biederman, J. (1986). A case of Tourette's syndrome with symptoms of attention deficit disorder treated with desipramine. *Journal of Clinical Psychiatry, 47,* 478–479.

Hornig-Rohan, M., & Amsterdam, J. (1995). *Venlafaxine vs. stimulant therapy in patients with dual diagnoses of ADHD and depression.* Poster presented at the annual meeting of the New Clinical Drug Evaluation Unit, Orlando, FL.

Huessy, H., & Wright, A. (1970). The use of imipramine in children's behavior disorders. *Acta Paedopsychiatrie, 37,* 194–199.

Kennedy, J. L., Richter, P., Swanson, J. M., Wigal, S. B., LaHoste, G. J., & Sunohara, G. (1997). *Association of dopamine D4 receptor gene and ADHD.* Paper presented at the annual meeting of the American Psychiatric Association, San Diego, CA.

Konkol, R., Fischer, M., & Newby, R. (1990). Double-blind, placebo-controlled stimulant trial in children with Tourette's syndrome and ADHD [Abstract]. *Annals of Neurology, 28,* 424.

Kratochvil, C. J., Bohac, D., Harrington, M., Baker, N., May, D., & Burke, W. J. (2001). An open-label trial of tomoxetine in pediatric attention deficit hyperactivity disorder. *Journal of Child and Adolescent Psychopharmacology, 11,* 167–170.

Kupietz, S. S., & Balka, E. B. (1976). Alterations in the vigilance performance of children receiving amitriptyline and methylphenidate pharmacotherapy. *Psychopharmacology, 50,* 29–33.

LaHoste, G. J., Swanson, J. M., Wigal, S. B., Glabe, C., Wigal, T., King, N., et al. (1996). Dopamine D4 receptor gene polymorphism is associated with attention deficit hyperactivity disorder. *Molecular Psychiatry, 1,* 121–124.

Lanau, F., Zenner, M., Civelli, O., & Hartman, D. (1997). Epinephrine and norepinephrine act as potent agonists at the recombinant human dopamine D4 receptor. *Journal of Neurochemistry, 68,* 804–812.

Law, S., & Schachar, R. (1999). Do typical clinical doses of methylphenidate cause tics in children treated for ADHD? *Journal of the American Academy of Child and Adolescent Psychiatry, 38,* 944–951.

Michelson, D., Adler, L., Spencer, T., Reimherr, F., West, S., Allen, A., et al. (2003). Atomoxetine in adults with ADHD: Two randomized, placebo-controlled studies. *Biological Psychiatry, 53,* 112–120.

Michelson, D., Faries, D., Wernicke, J., Kelsey, D., Kendrick, K., Sallee, F. R., et al. (2001). Atomoxetine in the treatment of children and adolescents with attention-deficit/hyperactivity disorder: A randomized, placebo-controlled, dose-response study. *Pediatrics, 108,* E83.

National Institute of Mental Health. (1996). *Special Emphasis Panel: Alternative pharmacology of ADHD.* Washington, DC: Author.

Olivera, R. L., Pliszka, S. R., Luh, J., & Tatum, R. (1996). An open trial of venlafaxine in the treatment of attention-deficit/hyperactivity disorder in children and adolescents. *Journal of Child and Adolescent Psychopharmacology, 6,* 241–250.

Pliszka, S. R. (1989). Effect of anxiety on cognition, behavior, and stimulant response in ADHD. *Journal of the American Academy of Child and Adolescent Psychiatry, 28,* 882–887.

Pliszka, S. R., McCracken, J., & Maas, J. (1996). Catecholamines in attention-deficit hyperactivity disorder: Current perspectives. *Journal of the American Academy of Child and Adolescent Psychiatry, 35,* 264–272.

Prince, J. B., Wilens, T. E., Biederman, J., Spencer, T. J., Millstein, R., Polisner, D. A., et al. (2000). A controlled study of nortriptyline in children and adolescents with attention deficit hyperactivity disorder. *Journal of Child and Adolescent Psychopharmacology, 10,* 193–204.

Quinn, P. O., & Rapoport, J. L. (1975). One-year follow-up of hyperactive boys treated with imipramine or methylphenidate. *American Journal of Psychiatry, 132,* 241–245.

Rapoport, J. L., Quinn, P., Bradbard, G., Riddle, D., & Brooks, E. (1974). Imipramine and methylphenidate treatment of hyperactive boys: A double-blind comparison. *Archives of General Psychiatry, 30,* 789–793.

Rapport, M., Carlson, G., Kelly, K., & Pataki, C. (1993). Methylphenidate and desipramine in hospitalized children: I. Separate and combined effects on cognitive function. *Journal of the American Academy of Child and Adolescent Psychiatry, 32,* 333–342.

Reimherr, F., Hedges, D., Strong, R., & Wender, P. (1995). *An open-trial of venlaxine in adult patients with attention deficit hyperactivity disorder.* Paper presented at the annual meeting of the New Clinical Drug Evaluation Unit, Orlando, FL.

Riddle, M. A., Hardin, M. T., Cho, S. C., Woolston, J. L., & Leckman, J. F. (1988). Desipramine treatment of boys with attention-deficit hyperactivity disorder and tics: Preliminary clinical experience. *Journal of the American Academy of Child and Adolescent Psychiatry, 27,* 811–814.

Singer, S., Brown, J., Quaskey, S., Rosenberg, L.,

Mellits, E., & Denckla, M. (1994). The treatment of attention-deficit hyperactivity disorder in Tourette's syndrome: A double-blind placebo-controlled study with clonidine and desipramine. *Pediatrics, 95,* 74–81.

Smalley, S. L., Bailey, J. N., Palmer, C. G., Cantwell, D. P., McGough, J. J., Del'Homme, M. A., et al. (1998). Evidence that the dopamine D4 receptor is a susceptibility gene in attention deficit hyperactivity disorder. *Molecular Psychiatry, 3(5),* 427–430.

Spencer, T. J., Biederman, J., Coffey, B., Geller, D., Crawford, M., Bearman, S. K., et al. (2002). A double-blind comparison of desipramine and placebo in children and adolescents with chronic tic disorder and comorbid attention-deficit/hyperactivity disorder. *Archives of General Psychiatry, 59,* 649–656.

Spencer, T. J., Biederman, J., Coffey, B., Geller, D., Wilens, T., & Faraone, S. (1999). The 4-year course of tic disorders in boys with attention-deficit/hyperactivity disorder. *Archives of General Psychiatry, 56,* 842–847.

Spencer, T. J., Biederman, J., Heiligenstein, J., Wilens, T., Faries, D., Prince, J., et al. (2001). An open-label, dose-ranging study of atomoxetine in children with attention deficit hyperactivity disorder. *Journal of Child and Adolescent Psychopharmacology, 11,* 251–265.

Spencer, T. J., Biederman, J., Kerman, K., Steingard, R., & Wilens, T. (1993). Desipramine in the treatment of children with tic disorder or Tourette's syndrome and attention deficit hyperactivity disorder. *Journal of the American Academy of Child and Adolescent Psychiatry, 32,* 354–360.

Spencer, T. J., Biederman, J., & Wilens, T. (1998). Growth deficits in children with attention deficit hyperactivity disorder. *Pediatrics, 102,* 501–506.

Spencer, T. J., Biederman, J., Wilens, T, Harding, M., O'Donnell, D., & Griffin, S. (1996). Pharmacotherapy of attention deficit hyperactivity disorder across the lifecycle: A literature review. *Journal of the American Academy of Child and Adolescent Psychiatry, 35,* 409–432.

Spencer, T. J., Biederman, J., Wilens, T., Prince, J., Hatch, M., Jones, J., et al. (1998). Effectiveness and tolerability of tomoxetine in adults with attention deficit hyperactivity disorder. *American Journal of Psychiatry, 155,* 693–695.

Spencer, T. J., Biederman, J., Wilens, T., Steingard, R., & Geist, D. (1993). Nortriptyline in the treatment of children with attention deficit hyperactivity disorder and tic disorder or Tourette's syndrome. *Journal of the American Academy of Child and Adolescent Psychiatry, 32,* 205–210.

Spencer, T. J., Heiligenstein, J., Biederman, J., Faries, D., Kratochvil, C., Conners, C., et al. (2002). Atomoxetine in children with ADHD: Results from two randomized, placebo-controlled studies. *Journal of Clinical Psychiatry, 63,* 1140–1147.

Spencer, T. J., Newcorn, J. H., Kratochvil, C. J., Ruff,

D., Michelson, D., & Biederman, J. (2005). Effects of atomoxetine on growth after 2-year treatment among pediatric patients with attention/deficit hyperactivity disorder. *Pediatrics, 116*(1), e74–e80.

Sunohara, G., Barr, C., Jain, U., Schachar, R., Roberts, W., Tannock, R., et al. (1997). *Association of the D4 receptor gene in individuals with ADHD.* Paper presented at the annual meeting of the American Society of Human Genetics, Baltimore.

Swanson, J., Kinsbourne, M., Roberts, W., & Zucker, K. (1978). Time–response analysis of the effect of stimulant medication on the learning ability of children referred for hyperactivity. *Pediatrics, 61*, 21–24.

Tannock, R., Ickowicz, A., & Schachar, R. (1995). Differential effects of methylphenidate on working memory in ADHD children with and without comorbid anxiety. *Journal of the American Academy of Child and Adolescent Psychiatry, 34*, 886–896.

Taylor, E., Schachar, R., Thorley, G., Wieselberg, H. M., Everitt, B., & Rutter, M. (1987). Which boys respond to stimulant medication?: A controlled trial of methylphenidate in boys with disruptive behaviour. *Psychological Medicine, 17*, 121–143.

Trott, G. E., Friese, H. J., Menzel, M., & Nissen, G. (1991). Wirksamkeit und vertraglichkeit des selektiven MAO-A-inhibitors moclobemid bei kindern mit hyperkinetischem syndrom [Use of moclobemide in children with attention deficit hyperactivity disorder] (both English and German versions). *Jugendpsychiatrie, 19*, 248–253.

Voelker, S. L., Lachar, D., & Gdowski, C. L. (1983). The Personality Inventory for Children and response to methylphenidate: Preliminary evidence for predictive validity. *Journal of Pediatric Psychology, 8*, 161–169.

Watter, N., & Dreyfuss, F. E. (1973). Modifications of hyperkinetic behavior by nortriptyline. *Virginia Medical Monthly, 100*, 123–126.

Wender, P. H., & Reimherr, F. W. (1990). Bupropion treatment of attention-deficit hyperactivity disorder in adults. *American Journal of Psychiatry, 147*, 1018–1020.

Werry, J. (1980). Imipramine and methylphenidate in hyperactive children. *Journal of Child Psychology and Psychiatry, 21*, 27–35.

Wilens, T. E., Biederman, J., Abrantes, A., & Spencer, T. (1996). A naturalistic assessment of protriptyline for attention deficit hyperactivity disorder. *Journal of the American Academy of Child and Adolescent Psychiatry, 35*, 1485–1490.

Wilens, T. E., Biederman, J., Geist, D. E., Steingard, R., & Spencer, T. (1993). Nortriptyline in the treatment of attention deficit hyperactivity disorder: A chart review of 58 cases. *Journal of the American Academy of Child and Adolescent Psychiatry, 32*, 343–349.

Wilens, T. E., Biederman, J., Prince, J., Spencer, T. J., Faraone, S. V., Warburton, R., et al. (1996). Six-week, double-blind, placebo-controlled study of desipramine for adult attention deficit hyperactivity disorder. *American Journal of Psychiatry, 153*, 1147–1153.

Wilens, T. E., Biederman, J. B., Mick, E., & Spencer, T. (1995). A systematic assessment of tricyclic antidepressants in the treatment of adult attention-deficit hyperactivity disorder. *Journal of Nervous and Mental Disease, 183*, 48–50.

Wilens, T. E., Haight, B. R., Horrigan, J. P., Hudziak, J. J., Rosenthal, N. E., Connor, D. F., et al. (2005). Bupropion XL in adults with attention-deficit/hyperactivity disorder: A randomized, placebo-controlled study. *Biological Psychiatry, 57*(7), 793–801.

Wilens, T. E., Spencer, T. J., Biederman, J., Girard, K., Doyle, R., Prince, J., et al. (2001). A controlled clinical trial of bupropion for attention deficit hyperactivity disorder in adults. *American Journal of Psychiatry, 158*, 282–288.

Winsberg, B. G., Bialer, I., Kupietz, S., & Tobias, J. (1972). Effects of imipramine and dextroamphetamine on behavior of neuropsychiatrically impaired children. *American Journal of Psychiatry, 128*, 1425–1431.

Yepes, L. E., Balka, E. B., Winsberg, B. G., & Bialer, I. (1977). Amitriptyline and methylphenidate treatment of behaviorally disordered children. *Journal of Child Psychology and Psychiatry, 18*, 39–52.

Other Medications

DANIEL F. CONNOR

A considerable literature on the clinical use of nonstimulant, nonantidepressant medications for children and adolescents with Attention-Deficit/Hyperactivity Disorder (ADHD) has accrued over the past 25 years. Stimulants such as oral-osmotic-release methylphenidate (Concerta), extended-release preparations of mixed amphetamine salts (Adderall XR), Metadate, Focalin LA, methylphenidate (MPH; Ritalin), and dextroamphetamine (Dexedrine) are generally considered first-line medications for uncomplicated ADHD. The nonstimulant atomoxetine (Strattera) may also be considered a first-line medication for ADHD (see Chapter 18). Antidepressants (see Chapter 18) such as bupropion are considered by most clinicians to be second-line drugs of choice, and possibly first-choice agents in ADHD complicated by tics, anxiety, or depression (Wilens et al., 2005). Tricyclic antidepressants (TCAs), while effective for the symptoms of ADHD, are now rarely used because of concerns over their potential for cardiovascular side effects. However, for a variety of reasons, about 20–30% of children with ADHD and adolescents do not respond satisfactorily to these agents.

Several possible reasons exist for lack of response. As defined by the fourth edition, text revision, of the *Diagnostic and Statistical Manual of Mental Disorders* (DSM-IV-TR; Ameri-

can Psychiatric Association, 2000), ADHD is a heterogeneous disorder of unknown etiology that can result from a multitude of biopsychosocial risk factors. Comorbidity with Conduct Disorder (CD), as well as depressive, anxiety, and tic disorders, is common (Biederman, Newcorn, & Sprich, 1991). These ADHD subgroups may have differing pharmacological responses as well as differing risk factors and clinical prognoses. Some children may have difficulty tolerating the side effects of stimulants or antidepressants. For example, children with ADHD who are also very depressed may have a less satisfactory treatment response to stimulants than children with ADHD who are not depressed. Children with preexisting cardiac disease or a family history significant for early-onset cardiac disease may be at increased risk for cardiovascular side effects of TCAs. In addition, some children and adolescents may have only a partial response to standard medication treatment for ADHD.

For these reasons, there has been clinical interest in the possible efficacy of other medications in the treatment of ADHD. With the exception of atomoxetine, the U.S. Food and Drug Administration (FDA) presently approves no nonstimulant medications (including those discussed in this chapter) for pharmaceutical manufacturer advertising as safe and effective for the treatment of ADHD. However, the FDA does not limit physician prescribing of a drug for an off-label indication if rational scientific theory, expert medical opinion, or evidence from controlled clinical trials exists that the drug may be safe and effective for the unapproved condition. None of the medications reviewed herein are "experimental" treatments in the sense of being new, untried, or untested. These medications are well known to clinicians and FDA-approved for manufacturer advertising in conditions other than ADHD. Atomoxetine is FDA-approved for use in child, adolescent, and adult ADHD (see Chapter 18). These medications have been used for ADHD for the past 25 years, and much experience has accumulated about their use.

This chapter reviews the clinical use of modafinil; antihypertensive agents, including clonidine, guanfacine, and beta-adrenergic blockers; and an anticonvulsant (carbamazepine, or CBZ) in the treatment of ADHD. For each medication, a brief review of the evidence for efficacy is followed by a discussion of mechanism of action and pharmacokinetics, short- and long-term treatment effects, procedures for a clinical trial, and treatment-emergent side effects. The current roles of antipsychotics and of combined pharmacotherapy in the treatment of ADHD are also discussed. Finally, a brief discussion alerts the reader to medications not considered effective in the treatment of ADHD.

REASONS TO CONSIDER NONSTIMULANT, NONANTIDEPRESSANT MEDICATIONS FOR ADHD

Following is a list of some reasons to consider prescribing these "other medications"' to children and adolescents diagnosed with ADHD.

1. Unsatisfactory clinical response to stimulants or antidepressants (after clinical trials of two or three different agents in these categories).
2. Inability to tolerate treatment-emergent side effects of stimulants (such as insomnia or loss of appetite) or antidepressants.
3. Presence of risk because of moderate to severe tics or Tourette syndrome (stimulants, bupropion) or a worrisome cardiac history in a child or family (TCAs, Adderall XR).

4. Development of tolerance to the therapeutic benefits of stimulants or antidepressants.
5. ADHD symptoms in special populations: youth with psychoses, schizophrenia, bipolar illness, Borderline Personality Disorder, seizure disorders, or pervasive developmental disorders.
6. Presence of severe mental retardation (IQ ≤45 or mental age ≤4.5 years).
7. Use in combination with a stimulant or antidepressant to augment a partial but inadequate response to monotherapy.
8. Use in combination with a stimulant or antidepressant to treat a comorbid diagnostic condition.

As with the prescribing of any medication, documentation of valid reasons for the use of a nonstimulant, nonantidepressant drug for the treatment of ADHD in the medical record; discussion of the risk–benefit ratio with the child and family; and education as to clinical procedures, follow-up, and time course of a medication trial must be provided by the physician prior to initiating medication therapy. Clinicians who prescribe these other medications for ADHD are generally on firm clinical ground if a previous trial of stimulant or antidepressant medication has failed, or if they document scientifically valid reasons for preferring these drugs (Green, 1995).

MODAFINIL

Evidence for Efficacy in ADHD

Modafinil (Provigil) is a novel agent that is indicated to improve wakefulness in patients with excessive sleepiness associated with narcolepsy, obstructive sleep apnea–hypopnea syndrome, and shift work sleep disorder. The precise mechanisms by which modafinil promotes wakefulness are not known. It appears to act in specific areas of the hypothalamus involved in maintaining typical wakefulness and sleep (Scammell et al., 2000). A recent study suggests that the drug inhibits the sleep-promoting neurons of the ventrolateral preoptic nucleus by blocking norepinephrine reuptake (Gallopin, Luppi, Rambert, Frydman, & Fort, 2004).

Although modafinil is chemically and pharmacologically distinct from traditional psychostimulants, it has been investigated in ADHD because medications effective for narcolepsy often have benefit in ADHD. Examples are the stimulants used to treat sleep attacks in narcolepsy and also found to be effective for ADHD. Results in adults with ADHD are mixed. A randomized controlled trial in 113 adults did not show that modafinil at doses of 100–400 mg/day reduced ADHD symptoms compared with placebo (Cephalon, Inc., 2002). Smaller studies of modafinil in adults with ADHD have reported some benefits (Taylor & Russo, 2000). At present, little support is available for modafinil in the treatment of adult ADHD. However, modafinil has been shown to improve ADHD symptoms in children in several, although not all, pediatric studies. Two Cephalon-sponsored clinical pilot trials in 6- to 12-year-old children with ADHD were negative (Cephalon, Inc., 2002). Table 19.1 describes recent studies investigating and supporting the use of modafinil in children with ADHD.

Mechanism of Action/Pharmacokinetics

Modafinil is a novel wake-promoting agent that is structurally different from central nervous system (CNS) stimulants and does not appear to have a dopaminergic mechanism of action. It appears to promote wakefulness by selectively activating parts of the hypothalamus believed to be involved in the regulation of the typical sleep–wake cycle. These hypothalamic wake-promoting areas of the hypothalamus activate the cortex, which is necessary for alertness and associated higher cognitive functions.

Modafinil is well absorbed after oral administration. Peak plasma concentrations are reached 2–4 hours after dosing. The major route of elimination is through the liver, with subsequent renal elimination of metabolites. A long half-life of 40 hours is observed for modafinil. After chronic use, significant accumulation of modafinil metabolites in the body may occur. Modafinil may also induce its own metabolism by induction of cytochrome P450 3A4. Modafinil is a reversible inhibitor of cytochrome P450 2C19. Concomitant administration of diazepam, phenytoin, or propranolol, which are largely eliminated via this pathway, can lead to increased circulating levels of these compounds.

Treatment Effects

Modafinil is labeled for use in patients 16 years or older with sleep disorders. It is presently not labeled by the FDA for use in ADHD. Moda-

finil is a Schedule IV compound. In pediatric studies, effective doses for ADHD ranged between 200 and 400 mg/day, given either once in the morning or twice daily (morning and midmorning) in evenly divided doses.

Procedures for a Clinical Trial

Modafinil is initiated at a dose of 100 mg in the morning, and titrated every 7–10 days by 100 mg until an effective dose is reached, until side effects preclude additional titration, or until a maximum dose of 400 mg/day is reached. A single morning dose may be given. Alternatively, the dose may be split and half given in the morning and half given at midmorning or noon. Benefits for ADHD generally require higher modafinil doses of 200–400 mg/day.

Side Effects

Modafinil is generally well tolerated. More side effects are reported at higher doses. Common side effects include insomnia, abdominal pain, depression, headache, nervousness, and nausea.

ANTIHYPERTENSIVE MEDICATIONS
Clonidine

Evidence for Efficacy in ADHD

Clonidine (Catapres) has been FDA-approved for use in hypertension since the early 1970s. Because of its well-recognized ability to downregulate noradrenergic output from the CNS, its possible use in psychiatric disorders characterized by excessive autonomic nervous system overarousal, hyperactivity, and impulsivity (including ADHD) has been explored. In child and adolescent psychiatry, clonidine was first used to treat tics in children with Tourette syndrome (Cohen, Young, Nathanson, & Shaywitz, 1979). The clonidine challenge test was used in the early 1980s to investigate noradrenergic receptor sensitivity changes associated with methylphenidate treatment (Hunt, Cohen, Anderson, & Clark, 1984). A meta-analysis (Connor, Fletcher, & Swanson, 1999) identified 39 reports of clonidine use in child/adolescent ADHD and associated conditions since 1980. Clonidine use has been investigated in ADHD; ADHD comorbid with Tourette syndrome and tic disorders; ADHD

TABLE 19.1. Recent Clinical Studies of Modafinil in Pediatric Patients with ADHD

Author (year)	Study design	Subjects (n/age)	PROVIGIL dosing (mg/day)	Efficacy results	Safety profile
Biederman (2003)	4-week, double-blind, placebo-controlled randomized study	248 (6–13 years)	Dosing regimens in children < 30 kg: 300 A.M.; 200 A.M. and 100 midday; or 100 A.M. and 200 midday. Dosing in children ≥ 30 kg: 400 as split dose.	Significant improvements on school and home versions of ADHD Rating Scale–IV and Conners Rating Scale (parent version) with 300-mg once-daily dose (n = 177 completers). Significant improvements on school version of ADHD Rating Scale–IV in 200/100-mg group. Results of 400-mg group not presented.	Well tolerated; most frequent AEs were insomnia, abdominal pain, anorexia, cough, fever, rhinitis.
Swanson (2003)	4-week, double-blind, placebo-controlled, crossover, analogue classroom study	48 (6–13 years)	Dosing regimens in children < kg: 100; 200; 300. Dosing in children ≥ 30 kg: 400 as split dose.	Significant improvements on the home version of the ADHD Rating Scale–IV in the 300-mg and 400-mg groups.	Most frequent AEs were abdominal pain, headache.
Rugino & Samsock (2003)	6-week, double-blind, placebo-controlled study	24 (5–15 years)	200-300 (flexible dosing titrated to effect; mean dose = 264).	Significant improvements on TOVA scores, teacher/parent Conners Scales. No significant improvement on ADHD Rating Scale–IV.	AEs were minor and transient; included delayed sleep onset, stomachache, headache. One subject discontinued due to emesis.
Rugino & Copley (2001)	Open-label study; average duration of treatment 4.6 weeks	15 (5–15 years)	100-400 (mean dose = 195).	Significant improvements on teacher/parent Conners Scales and ADHD Rating Scale–IV.	Generally well tolerated. Side effects were mild; included delayed onset of sleep, light headedness, headache. Four patients discontinued, one due to night tremor.

Note. AEs, adverse effects; TOVA, Test of Variables of Attention.

and aggression associated with CD; CD without ADHD, sleep disorders associated with ADHD; overarousal and aggression in Posttraumatic Stress Disorder in preschool children; ADHD symptoms in autism; and ADHD symptoms in children and adolescents with fragile X syndrome.

Six recent controlled studies investigating clonidine use in various child and adolescent psychiatric conditions are presented in Table 19.2. These clinical trials report clonidine use for ADHD in children with mental retardation (Agarwal, Sitholey, Kumar, & Prasad, 2001); ADHD comorbid with CD, Oppositional Defiant Disorder (ODD), and aggression (Connor, Barkley, & Davis, 2000; Hazell & Stuart, 2003); and ADHD and tic disorders (Tourette's Syndrome Study Group, 2002). In Europe, the safety and efficacy of lofexidine in treating children and adolescents with ADHD and tic disorders have been reported (Niederhofer, Staffen, & Mair, 2003). Lofexidine is very similar to clonidine, but with less associated hypotension; it is not currently available in the United States. These studies generally find clinically significant differences for clonidine (0.1–0.3 mg/day) as compared with placebo in improving symptoms of ADHD-associated hyperactivity, conduct problems, aggression, and tics. In one study, clonidine compared favorably to risperidone in diminishing tics (Gaffney, Perry, Lund, Bever-Stille, & Kuperman, 2002). This more recent literature compares favorably with older methodologically controlled studies of clonidine use in ADHD, which reported similar benefits for clonidine and placebo on parent and teacher rating scales of ADHD symptoms (Hunt, Minderaa, & Cohen, 1985; Gunning, 1992).

However, not all studies of clonidine show benefits. Two controlled studies of clonidine use in Tourette syndrome comorbid with ADHD found differing results. Benefits for both ADHD symptoms and tic frequency were reported in one study (Leckman et al., 1991). Singer et al. (1995), however, found little benefit for clonidine as compared to placebo in 34 children with Tourette syndrome and ADHD. Two controlled studies in children with autism, developmental delay, and symptoms of ADHD (inattention, impulsivity, and hyperactivity) also reported some benefits with clonidine therapy, but frequent side effects caused many patients to discontinue clonidine (Jaselskis, Cook, Fletcher, & Leventhal, 1992;

Frankenhauser, Karumanchi, German, Yates, & Karumanchi, 1992). Thus the extant literature on clonidine shows the majority of studies, but not all, reporting clinically significant results.

These studies generally describe some benefits for behavioral target symptoms of aggression, hyperactivity, overarousal, impulsivity, and sleep disturbance as assessed by observer-completed rating scales. Fewer benefits are reported with clonidine for sustained attentional deficits and cognitive symptoms of ADHD. A meta-analysis of clonidine for symptoms of ADHD found an overall effect size of 0.58 (Connor et al., 1999). This is a medium effect size and is consistent with that reported for other adrenergic agents (e.g., antidepressants) in ADHD. Clonidine is clearly not as effective as stimulants in the treatment of ADHD. The existing scientific literature supports its use as a second- or third-line agent in the treatment of ADHD.

Mechanism of Action/Pharmacokinetics

Clonidine stimulates presynaptic alpha-2-adrenergic receptors in the brain stem (locus ceruleus), resulting in a reduction in sympathetic outflow from the CNS. The decrease in plasma norepinephrine is directly related to clonidine's hypotensive action. Recent studies suggest that boys with ADHD may differ from boys without ADHD in peripheral and CNS noradrenergic function (Halperin, Newcorn, McKay, Siever, & Sharma, 2003). These findings suggest a role for agents that alter noradrenergic neurotransmission in the treatment of ADHD. In the prefrontal cortex, clonidine may also influence postsynaptic alpha-2-adrenergic receptors. Three subtypes of alpha-2-adrenergic receptors have recently been cloned in humans: the alpha-2-A, alpha-2-B, and alpha-2-C. Genes for these receptors reside on chromosomes 10, 2, and 4, respectively. Postsynaptic alpha-2-A receptors may mediate norepinephrine neurotransmission in the prefrontal cortex to enhance inhibition over lower CNS structures and enhance working memory under distracting conditions (see Arnsten, Steere, & Hunt, 1996). Because deficits in behavioral inhibition and working memory are two neuropsychological constructs thought to be crucial in the pathoetiology of ADHD (Barkley, 1997), scientific reasons exist to think that clonidine may be effective in ADHD.

TABLE 19.2. Recent Studies of Clonidine in Child and Adolescent Psychiatry

Author (year)	Study type	n	Disorders	Age (years) (mean and/or range)	Dose (mean and/or range)	Duration	Side effects	Outcome
Agarwal et al. (2001)	Crossover	10	Mental retardation + hyperactivity	7.6 ± 0.54	4, 6, 8 mcg/kg/day	12 weeks	Sedation	Hyperactivity improved.
Connor et al. (2000)	RT	8	ADHD + aggression	6–16	0.10–0.30 mg/day	12 weeks	Decreased fine motor speed, sedation	ADHD and aggression improved. CPT cognitive measures improved.
Hazell & Stuart (2003)	RCT	38	ADHD + aggression	6–14	0.10–0.20 mg/day	6 weeks	Sedation, dizziness	Aggression improved when clonidine was combined with stimulant.
Niederhofer et al. (2003)[a]	RCT	44	ADHD + tics	10.4	0.4–1.2 mg/day	8 weeks	Sedation	ADHD and tics improved.
Gaffney et al. (2002)	RT	21	Tourette syndrome	7–17	0.18 mg/day	8 weeks	Sedation	Clonidine = risperdal in decreasing tic severity.
Tourette's Syndrome Study Group (2002)	RCT	34	ADHD + Tourette syndrome	7–14	0.25 mg/day	16 weeks	Sedation	Improved hyperactivity and impulsivity; decreased tic severity.

Note. RT, randomized trial; RCT, randomized controlled trial; CPT, continuous-performance test.
[a]This study used lofexidine, a medication very similar to clonidine but associated with less hypotension. Lofexidine is available in Europe, but not presently in the United States.

Clonidine is well absorbed after oral administration. In adults, peak plasma concentrations (and maximal hypotensive effects) are observed 1–3 hours after dose administration. Metabolism occurs both by hepatic mechanisms (50%) and by unchanged renal excretion (50%). There are no active metabolites. The excretion half-life of oral clonidine in children averages 8–12 hours, with considerable individual variability. In contrast to the pharmacokinetic half-life described earlier, the behavioral effects of clonidine last only 3–6 hours. Three or four divided daily dosings are thus required in children and adolescents to maintain plasma levels, prevent clonidine withdrawal symptoms, and preserve behavioral effects.

Clonidine is also available as a skin patch called the transdermal therapeutic system (TTS). This patch allows administration of clonidine without the use of pills. Clonidine is delivered by diffusion and absorption through the skin. Dosing is a function of the patch's area. The TTS patch permits a more steady plasma level to be achieved; this can result in decreased frequency and intensity of side effects, which are often related to peak serum levels after oral absorption. The TTS patch should be replaced every 5 days.

Treatment Effects

Clonidine appears partially effective in decreasing the frequency, intensity, and severity of impulsivity–hyperactivity and improving frustration tolerance in children and adolescents with either ADHD, Combined Type or ADHD, Predominantly Hyperactive–Impulsive Type as defined by DSM-IV-TR. Although there are theoretical reasons to believe that clonidine may improve cognitive functioning in patients with ADHD, this has not yet been shown clinically. Therefore, clonidine should not be used for ADHD, Predominantly Inattentive Type as defined by DSM-IV-TR. Children with ADHD who present clinically with high levels of arousal, impulsivity, explosive aggression to minimal environmental provocation, motor overactivity, and associated comorbid CD appear to respond best. It should be noted that clonidine is not a treatment for the more covert forms of aggression frequently found in CD (cheating, lying, stealing, vandalism).

Clonidine is also useful for tic disorders, which often present clinically with ADHD. Many studies (although not all) have reported a reduction in frequency and severity of motor and vocal tics with clonidine treatment, whether such tics occur with or without accompanying ADHD.

Sleep disturbances frequently accompany both ADHD and the treatment of ADHD (stimulants). A growing body of clinical case reports suggests that clonidine can help reduce initial insomnia caused either by difficulties settling for sleep in a hyperactive child with ADHD or as a result of lingering stimulants in the plasma at bedtime. In nondisabled young adult volunteers, a single dose of clonidine (0.25–0.3 mg) was significantly associated with electroencephalograph-documented reduced Stage 1 and rapid-eye-movement sleep, as well as with increased Stage 2 (deeper) sleep (Carskadon, Cavallo, & Rosekind, 1989).

Clonidine has also found some clinical success in treating target symptoms of adrenergic overarousal, impulsivity–hyperactivity, and explosive aggression and temper tantrums in special populations of children. These include children with pervasive developmental disorders, fragile X syndrome (X-linked mental retardation), and Posttraumatic Stress Disorder.

Procedures for a Clinical Trial

The FDA does not presently label clonidine for any indication in child and adolescent psychiatry. However, clinicians continue to use clonidine in the treatment of a variety of early-onset psychiatric symptoms and conditions. Use of clonidine may be reasonably considered as follows: (1) as a third-line medication for overarousal, impulsivity, excessive hyperactivity, and explosive outbursts of aggression in children and adolescents with ADHD who have not responded satisfactorily to previous trials of stimulants, atomoxetine, or antidepressants; (2) as combination therapy with stimulants to decrease motoric overarousal and impulsivity that have not been fully responsive to stimulant monotherapy; (3) as combination therapy with stimulants to treat sleep disturbances associated with ADHD or stimulant therapy; (4) in special populations, as described just above; and (5) in children with ADHD and comorbid tic disorders or Tourette syndrome.

There are several exclusion criteria for a clonidine trial. Because of clonidine's known cardiovascular effects, children and adolescents with preexisting cardiac disease (especially sinus or atrioventricular node dysfunction and bradycardic arrhythmias), syncope, vascular disease such as Raynaud's syndrome, and/or a family history of early-onset cardiac disease or syncope in first-degree relatives are not candidates for a clonidine trial. Children and adolescents with a history of melancholic depression (Major Depressive Disorder) also should not receive clonidine because of clonidine's known risk in exacerbating an underlying vulnerability to depression.

Prior to initiating a trial of clonidine, the child should have a baseline physical examination completed within 1 year of drug initiation. A baseline electrocardiogram (EKG) can be considered, especially in children with a suspicious cardiovascular history. Baseline pulse and baseline blood pressure should also be obtained. The standard daily dose range of clonidine for ADHD, Tourette syndrome, and disturbances of adrenergic overarousal is 0.10–0.30 mg. Rarely, higher doses (up to 0.5–0.8 mg) have been reported in the literature. Sleep disturbances can sometimes be treated with lower doses of 0.05–0.20 mg given 1 hour before bedtime. Oral clonidine is commonly given to 6- to 13-year-old children in three to four divided daily doses to prevent withdrawal effects. In older adolescents who exhibit slower drug metabolism, oral clonidine can be given two or three times daily. Clonidine (both oral and TTS preparations) must be given 7 days a week to avoid withdrawal symptoms.

Oral clonidine is initiated at low doses of 0.025 mg in smaller children and 0.05 mg in larger children and adolescents, given first in the evening (because of sedative side effects). The dose is titrated upward by 0.025–0.05 mg every 4–5 days, given twice, then three times, then four times per day in divided doses until therapeutic benefit, an unacceptable level of side effects, or the upper limit of dose titration is reached. Sedation and occasional irritability limit the rate of dose titration. A useful rule of thumb to limit these side effects is to "start low and go slow." A stable full dose can generally be achieved in 2–5 weeks after oral clonidine initiation.

Treatment effects, independent of sedation, are noticeable after 1 month of therapy at full dose. Therefore, a clonidine initiation trial to determine efficacy in a child or adolescent will take 1–3 months to achieve. Parents and children need to be informed about the expected time course of treatment with clonidine. If benefit on drug is established at the end of the clonidine initiation phase, the length of a clonidine maintenance phase can be discussed with the child and family. It is useful to think in school-year units, with consideration given to drug holidays (if possible) during the summer, to establish continuing need for clonidine treatment and drug efficacy and to document any treatment-emergent side effects that may become noticeable in retrospect when clonidine therapy is suspended. If benefit on drug is not established at the end of the clonidine initiation phase, clonidine can be tapered off slowly to prevent withdrawal symptoms, and reassessment can take place.

During the clonidine initiation phase, contact with the prescribing physician should occur regularly. Blood pressure and pulse should be obtained weekly during dose titration. A pulse under 55 beats per minute (bpm) or blood pressure under 80/50 mm Hg should prompt reevaluation and possibly lowering of the dose. The physician should inquire about side effects, especially exercise-related dizziness, shortness of breath, or syncope. These may be secondary to clonidine-induced adrenergic blockade preventing the cardiovascular system from adequately responding to increased exercise-mediated metabolic demands. Exercise-related treatment-emergent clonidine side effects require immediate evaluation by the child's physician. During the maintenance phase, regular physician contact should occur every 2–3 months. Pulse and blood pressure should be checked at this time. Height and weight should be followed every 4–5 months. Continuing efficacy of clonidine should be assessed via child, parent, and teacher reports and rating scales at each visit. For long-term use, an EKG should be completed on a yearly basis.

As an alternative to oral clonidine therapy, the TTS patch described earlier may be utilized. This system is available in a brand-name formulation labeled Catapres-TTS-1, 2, or 3, which corresponds approximately to daily doses of 0.1, 0.2, and 0.3 mg, respectively. Children and adolescents are generally begun on oral clonidine to establish efficacy (initiation phase). If clonidine is effective and a patch is desired, they are then shifted to the TTS (maintenance phase). This patch is placed on a hairless and inaccessible area such as the back. It generally tolerates brief exposure to moisture (perspiration, shower, bath), but may need replacement after swimming. The patch maintains a constant plasma level for about 5 days in children and adolescents; it must then be replaced. Because absorption to plasma is constant and does not peak as with oral dosing, side effects may be less with the TTS preparation.

Side Effects

Table 19.3 lists frequent treatment-emergent side effects from oral clonidine and compares them with the side effect profiles of other antihypertensive agents occasionally used in ADHD. Most side effects are mild and tend to diminish over time with continued therapy. The most frequent are drowsiness, dizziness, and sedation. These can be problematic in the first 4–6 weeks of dose titration; they are occasionally accompanied by increased irritability. Side effects can be helped by a slower rate of dose titration and by dose reduction. Early-morning awakening, perhaps a consequence of nighttime clonidine withdrawal, can also be seen. Children may be less susceptible to the anticholinergic effects of clonidine (constipation, dry mouth) than adults. A contact dermatitis is seen under the TTS patch in 15–20% when this preparation is used. Switching to a different location, use of a topical steroid cream, and returning to oral administration are effective strategies for management.

TABLE 19.3. Common Treatment-Emergent Side Effects of Oral Antihypertensive Agents

	Percentage reporting		
Side effect	Clonidine	Guanfacine	Beta-blockers (CNS-acting)
Drowsiness	33%	13%	25%
Dizziness	16%	8%	8%
Sedation	10%	8%	28%
Weakness	10%	7%	17%
Sleep disturbance	10%	5%	18%
Depression	5%	<1%	8%
Cardiac arrhythmia	5%	<1%	5%
Nausea/vomiting	5%	>1%	18%
Irritability	3%	<1%	10%
Orthostatic hypotension	3%	<1%	18%
Weight gain	1%	<1%	<1%
Hallucinations	1%	<1%	9%

A potentially serious side effect of clonidine use (and of all adrenergic agents discussed in this chapter) is a withdrawal syndrome upon abrupt medication discontinuation. This syndrome is characterized by rebound adrenergic overdrive, leading to symptoms of hypertension, agitation, fever, headache, chest pain, sleep disturbance, nausea, and vomiting. Two types of adverse cardiovascular treatment-emergent side effect patterns have been described for clonidine (Cantwell, Swanson, & Connor, 1997). In the first type, abrupt clonidine discontinuation leads to the previously mentioned signs of adrenergic overdrive, which are ameliorated by clinical recognition of the withdrawal syndrome and reintroduction of clonidine. In the second type, high dose and possibly prolonged time on the drug lead to bradycardic arrhythmias, fatigue, lethargy, and hypotension. This type can be identified by EKG and vital sign monitoring, and responds to dose reduction or clonidine discontinuation.

To prevent withdrawal, clonidine should be discontinued gradually when the medication is stopped. Tapering can be accomplished by decreasing clonidine 0.05 mg every 3 days. Caution must be taken by physician and family to prevent sudden discontinuation (e.g., prescription running out, missed appointments).

Guanfacine

Evidence for Efficacy in ADHD

Guanfacine (Tenex) is an orally administered, centrally acting antihypertensive agent that also stimulates CNS alpha-2-adrenergic autoreceptors to down-regulate sympathomimetic outflow from the brain stem. It possesses a more selective receptor-binding profile, which may confer less risk of sedation and hypotensive side effects than clonidine. Clinical experience with this agent to treat ADHD is growing. Four controlled studies investigating the use of guanfacine in ADHD and comorbid conditions are presented in Table 19.4 and described here. Hunt, Arnsten, and Asbell (1995) reported the results of an open clinical trial of guanfacine in 13 children and adolescents (mean age 11.1 years) with ADHD. At an average dose of 3.2 mg/day, parent rating scales documented significant improvement in hyperactivity, inattention, and immaturity, but not

TABLE 19.4. Recent Studies of Guanfacine in Children and Adolescents with ADHD and Comorbid Disorders

Author (year)	Study type	n	Disorders	Age (years) (range)	Dose (mean and/or range)	Duration	Side effects	Outcome
Chappell et al. (1995)	Open	10	ADHD + tic disorder	8–16	0.75–3.0 mg/day	4–20 weeks	Fatigue, headache, dizziness, insomnia	Improvement in tics, no improvement in ADHD.
Horrigan & Barnhill (1995)	Open	15	ADHD	7–17	0.5–3.0 mg/day	10 weeks	Sedation	Improvement in ADHD.
Hunt et al. (1995)	Open	13	ADHD	4–20	0.5–4.0 mg/day	4 weeks	Headache, stomach-ache	Improvement in inattention and hyper-activity.
Scahill et al. (2001)	RCT	34	ADHD + Tourette syndrome	7–14	1.5–3.0 mg/day	8 weeks	Sedation	Improvement in tics and in ADHD.

Note. RCT, randomized controlled trial.

in mood or aggression. In another prospective open-label clinical trial, guanfacine (0.5–3.0 mg/day) was found significantly effective in reducing ADHD target symptoms in 15 boys ages 7–17 years as assessed by parent-completed rating scales and physician-assessed global clinical impression (Horrigan & Barnhill, 1995). In a third open clinical trial, 10 patients with ADHD and comorbid Tourette syndrome received guanfacine (average dose 1.5 mg/day) (Chappell et al., 1995). Some efficacy in decreasing motor and vocal tics was found. Parent ratings of ADHD symptoms were not significantly reduced on guanfacine. Interestingly, some effects were reported on cognitive measures of ADHD: A reduction in commission errors and omission errors on a continuous-performance test were found. In a randomized controlled clinical trial of 34 children with ADHD and comorbid tic disorders (17 randomized to guanfacine and 17 randomized to placebo), behavioral symptoms and cognitive symptoms (as measured by a continuous-performance test) of ADHD, as well as tic frequency and severity, all improved on guanfacine relative to placebo (Scahill et al., 2001). At this writing, development of an extended-release guanfacine preparation for once-daily dosing in ADHD is under investigation.

Mechanism of Action/Pharmacokinetics

Guanfacine is an orally administered, centrally acting antihypertensive with alpha-2-adrenergic receptor agonist properties. Receptor binding studies have shown greater specificity for guanfacine than for clonidine to the alpha-2-A receptor. This receptor may be involved in mediating norepinephrine effects in the prefrontal cortex involving inhibition and working memory. Guanfacine also interacts less than clonidine does with alpha-1-adrenergic, beta-adrenergic, histaminergic, and possibly dopaminergic receptors (Cornish, 1988). As a result, there is theoretically less risk of side effects with guanfacine than with clonidine, especially sedation and rebound hypertension on abrupt drug discontinuation.

Guanfacine is well absorbed after oral administration. In adults, peak plasma concentrations occur on average 2.6 hours after a single oral dose. About 50% is excreted unchanged in the urine, and 50% is hepatically metabolized. There are no active metabolites. The pharmacokinetic half-life in children is 13–14 hours, leading to clinical dosing recommendations of twice- to three-times daily divided doses in younger patients (Horrigan & Barnhill, 1995). This is a longer excretion half-life than reported for clonidine.

Treatment Effects

The role of guanfacine in the clinical treatment of children and adolescents with ADHD is growing, although it is not yet firmly established. At present, guanfacine is not approved by the FDA for manufacturer labeling in any child or adolescent psychiatric disorder. However, preliminary research is encouraging. Much as for clonidine, improvement in hyperactive–impulsive symptoms and overarousal are reported on observer-completed rating scales. Cognitive benefits on attention may occur with guanfacine treatment, although they appear less robust than with stimulant treatment. Preliminary indications also suggest some benefit in tic disorders.

Procedures for a Clinical Trial

Guanfacine may be considered for children (older than 7 years) or adolescents with ADHD and comorbid tic disorders after treatment failures with more established ADHD medications (stimulants, antidepressants), especially if the youth might benefit from decreased adrenergic overarousal but might not tolerate the side effects of clonidine. Guanfacine is not indicated in children with preexisting cardiac, renal, or vascular disease.

The dose range for guanfacine is 0.5 mg/day to 3.0 mg/day (Horrigan & Barnhill, 1995) or 4.0 mg/day (Hunt et al., 1995). Therapeutic administration at peak dose is most often divided into two (for adolescents) to four (for young children) daily dosings. Guanfacine is initiated at 0.5 mg given at bedtime and titrated upward by 0.25–0.5 mg every 5–7 days. Vital signs, side effects, and treatment benefits are checked by the prescribing physician in follow-up every 2 weeks during dose titration. EKG monitoring is not considered necessary in healthy children on guanfacine. If treatment benefits occur and a stable maintenance dose is achieved, a reasonable frequency of follow-up visits would be once every 2 months.

Side Effects

Table 19.3 lists frequent treatment-emergent side effects of guanfacine and compares them with the side effects of other antihypertensive agents occasionally used in ADHD. In general, the side effect profile is similar to that of clonidine. However, because of increased re-ceptor specificity, side effects with guanfacine are generally less frequent or severe than those of clonidine. Similar to clonidine, there is a risk of rebound hypertension upon abrupt guanfacine discontinuation. Dose changes should be accomplished slowly (0.5-mg changes every 2–3 days) to prevent adrenergic rebound and withdrawal symptoms when guanfacine dose is reduced or the medication will be stopped.

Beta-Adrenergic Blockers

Evidence for Efficacy in ADHD

Beta-adrenergic blockers (or, as they are usually called, beta-blockers) are a family of agents that competitively inhibit norepinephrine and epinephrine actions at beta-adrenergic receptor sites, both centrally and in the periphery. Clinical studies of beta-blockers in child and adolescent psychiatry are limited to open designs, generally in subjects with CNS damage, pervasive developmental disorders, or mental retardation (for a review, see Connor, 1993). In ADHD, there presently exists one methodologically controlled study of pindolol (a centrally acting beta-blocker) in comparison with placebo and MPH (Buitelaar, van de Gaag, Swaab-Barneveld, & Kuiper, 1996). Fifty-two children ages 7–13 years received either pindolol and MPH, MPH 10 mg twice a day alone, or pindolol 20 mg twice a day alone under single-blind conditions for 4 weeks. Outcome was assessed by parent-, teacher-, and clinician-completed rating scales. Pindolol was found to be modestly effective in ADHD: It was just as effective as MPH in decreasing impulsivity–hyperactivity, but less effective than MPH for cognitive symptoms of ADHD. However, because of a high incidence of side effects, including nightmares, hallucinations, and paresthesias, pindolol was stopped in all 32 children receiving this drug. In an open prospective study of 12 children, adolescents, and young adults with CNS deficits, significant aggression, and ADHD symptoms, nadolol (a peripherally acting beta-blocker with little penetration into the CNS) at 2.5 mg/kg/day was not found to significantly reduce parent- and teacher-rated ADHD symptoms. Significant improvements in aggression were found (Connor, Ozbayrak, Benjamin, Ma, & Fletcher, 1997). Nadolol was very well tolerated, with few side effects. This study suggests that peripherally acting beta-blockers may be effective for some aggressive and hyperactive symptoms, without inducing the side effects seen with more centrally acting beta-blockers. However, much more controlled research is needed before beta-blockers can be recommended as treatment for ADHD.

Mechanism of Action/Pharmacokinetics

In the brain, the predominant beta-adrenergic receptors are beta-1-noradrenergic receptors. In the peripheral nervous system, beta-1 receptors mediate cardiac effects, and beta-2 receptors mediate bronchodilation and vasodilation. Beta-blockers are classified as to whether they are centrally and peripherally acting (propranolol, metoprolol, pindolol) or peripherally acting with little CNS penetration (nadolol, atenolol). The family of beta-blockers is also classified as to what types of beta-adrenergic receptors are competitively antagonized: nonselective beta-blockers block both beta-1 and beta-2 receptors (propranolol, nadolol, pindolol), and selective beta-blockers inhibit only beta-1 (cardiac) receptors (atenolol, metoprolol).

Beta-blockers are well absorbed after oral administration. The pharmacokinetic half-life varies among the different types of beta-blockers. Nadolol is a long-acting agent, which may require two daily doses in children and adolescents. Propranolol and metoprolol are short-acting agents requiring multiple daily doses. Metabolism also varies with the different agents. Nadolol and atenolol undergo no hepatic biotransformation and are largely cleared from the body unchanged by renal mechanisms. Propranolol undergoes extensive hepatic metabolism. The risk of drug–drug interactions in children receiving beta-blockers and other medications is minimized with nadolol or atenolol use and maximized with propranolol use.

Treatment Effects

Children and adolescents with signs of disinhibition and adrenergic overarousal—whether these results from CNS disease, developmental disorders, Posttraumatic Stress Disorder, or ADHD—may benefit from beta-blocker therapy. The pediatric treatment literature remains scarce, but does suggest some efficacy for severe impulsivity–hyperactivity and explosive outbursts of aggression and temper tantrums.

No support for beneficial effects on cognition has been currently reported.

Procedures for a Clinical Trial

Indications for beta-blockers in child psychiatry are generally those noted in the preceding paragraph. Several exclusion criteria exist, which, if present, preclude beta-blocker use. These are preexisting asthma, reactive airway disease, insulin-dependent diabetes mellitus, hyperthyroidism, bradycardic arrhythmias, cardiac disease, renal disease, and melancholic depression (Major Depressive Disorder). The general dose range in child and adolescent psychiatry is about 1.0–5.5 mg/kg/day, with an average daily dose of roughly 2.5 mg/kg/day. The starting dose of beta-blockers is low. Nadolol is begun at 10 mg twice a day and titrated upward by 10–20 mg every 3–4 days. In younger children with faster metabolic rates, it is generally given in two or three divided daily doses; in adolescents, it can be given twice daily. Propranolol can begin at 10 mg twice a day with dose escalation of 10 mg every 3–4 days. Because of its shorter half-life, propranolol is given three to four times daily.

Because beta-blockers cause hypotension and lower the heart rate, cardiovascular monitoring is recommended. Baseline pulse, blood pressure, EKG, and physical examination should be completed prior to dose introduction. Exclusion criteria should be reviewed with the child and family. Physician monitoring should take place every 2 weeks during dose titration, including monitoring pulse and blood pressure. A dose should be reevaluated if pulse falls below 55 bpm or blood pressure is less than 80/55 mm Hg. Once a stable dose is reached, monitoring can take place every 2 months. It is reasonable to repeat the EKG once yearly in patients receiving long-term beta-blocker therapy for behavioral reasons.

Side Effects

Table 19.3 lists frequent treatment-emergent side effects of beta-blockers and compares them with the side effect profiles of other antihypertensive agents occasionally used in ADHD. Centrally acting beta-blockers have a higher incidence of side effects than peripherally acting agents. These treatment-emergent side effects may include vivid nightmares, hallucinations, depression, numbness or tingling in the extremities (paresthesias), lethargy, and weakness. Beta-blockers may also slow the heart rate to below 50 bpm. Exacerbation of asthma and bronchospastic disease may occur if exclusion criteria are not followed.

Rebound hypertension and signs of adrenergic hyperactivity can occur if beta-blocker therapy is abruptly discontinued. This may be especially true if combined pharmacotherapy with clonidine is prescribed. Beta-blocker dosages must be tapered gradually to minimize the risk of withdrawal effects.

CARBAMAZEPINE

Anticonvulsants are traditionally used in the management of epilepsy. Their value in treating behavior disorders (primarily ADHD and CD) in nonepileptic children and adolescents has been explored since the 1970s. Because CBZ is currently the anticonvulsant with the most research and clinical support for the treatment of ADHD, it is the one discussed here.

Evidence for Efficacy in ADHD

CBZ (Tegretol) is an anticonvulsant that has been found useful in children for generalized tonic–clonic seizures and partial complex seizures, and for relief of pain in trigeminal and glossopharyngeal neuralgias. CBZ is also frequently used in Europe for treating ADHD and ADHD comorbid with CD. Although it has been largely ignored in the United States for the treatment of ADHD, a meta-analysis of 10 reports from the world literature, including 3 controlled studies comparing CBZ to placebo, suggests some efficacy in children with ADHD (Silva, Munoz, & Alpert, 1996). Response rates were found to be 70% in open studies and 71% in controlled studies. Efficacy was correlated with treatment duration, suggesting that time on the drug is important in CBZ treatment of ADHD. Doses ranged from 50 mg to 800 mg/day. Only one study reported CBZ plasma levels, with optimal levels for therapeutic response ranging from 4.8 to 10.4 µg/ml (mean 6.2 µg/ml) (Kafantaris et al., 1992).

It remains unclear whether CD independent of comorbid ADHD will respond to CBZ. A double-blind, placebo-controlled study with a parallel-groups design and random assignment to placebo or CBZ (400–800 mg/day) found no significant reduction in overt categorical aggression in 22 children diagnosed with CD and frequent aggression (Cueva et al., 1996). In contrast, open pilot studies have reported benefits for CBZ in reducing aggressive CD symptoms. It should be emphasized that the children in the Cueva et al. study did not have comorbid ADHD symptoms.

Mechanism of Action/Pharmacokinetics

CBZ is an orally administered anticonvulsant with a tricyclic chemical structure. It is a partial agonist of adenosine receptors and appears relatively more selective in its anticonvulsant properties for inhibiting amygdala-kindled seizures, suggesting some possible limbic system specificity over other anticonvulsants. Its anticonvulsant mechanism of action (and possible mechanism of action in ADHD) is unknown. Possibilities include enhancement of CNS inhibition by facilitating gamma-aminobutyric acid (an inhibitory neurotransmitter), inhibiting excitatory amino acid neurotransmission (by blockade of N-methyl-D-aspartate receptors), and/or increasing neuronal membrane stabilization by influencing calcium channels and transcellular transport of sodium and other ions across cell membranes. Possible treatment effects in ADHD may also be partially explained by CBZ's weak dopamine- and norepinephrine-reuptake-inhibiting effects as a result of its tricyclic chemical structure.

CBZ comes in both a tablet and a suspension formulation available for oral use. Both preparations deliver equivalent amounts of drug to the systemic circulation, but the suspension is absorbed faster. Plasma levels peak at 1 hour with use of the suspension, compared to 4–5 hours after ingestion of the oral tablet. Because CBZ induces its own hepatic metabolism, the pharmacokinetic half-life is variable and progressively shortens over the first 4–6 weeks of therapy (metabolic autoinduction). Autoinduction may lead to a 50% decline in CBZ serum levels over the first 6 weeks of therapy under constant dosing conditions. Serum levels (and daily dose) must be monitored and continually readjusted during the first 2 months of CBZ therapy (Trimble, 1990). CBZ is metabolized to an active 10,11 epoxide, which also exhibits anticonvulsant activity.

Because hepatic biotransformation and renal clearance are fastest in prepubertal children and faster than adult rates in adolescents, CBZ (and other anticonvulsants) will exhibit a shorter half-life, a higher clearance rate, and a higher dosage requirement (in milligrams per kilogram of body weight) in young patients than in adults. CBZ has a half-life of 12 hours, and it takes 3–4 weeks for complete autoinduction to occur. CBZ is generally given two to three times daily to children and adolescents, and plasma monitoring and dose adjustment are required, especially during the time of autoinduction.

Treatment Effects

Much further research on CBZ in ADHD is needed before firm conclusions can be drawn about its treatment effects in this disorder. Presently, CBZ is not considered a standard treatment for children and adolescents with ADHD. Open and controlled studies generally document some significant benefit for overarousal, aggression, impulsivity, hyperactivity, restlessness, and excitability in children and adolescents with ADHD and no neurological abnormalities. CBZ's effects on cognition in ADHD have not yet been studied.

Procedures for a Clinical Trial

Indications for CBZ's use in child and adolescent psychiatry and ADHD are not firmly established. CBZ might be considered (1) for children and adolescents with comorbid generalized tonic–clonic epilepsy, partial complex epilepsy, or focally abnormal electroencephalograph and accompanying symptoms of ADHD; or (2) as a third-line medication for overarousal, impulsivity–hyperactivity, and aggression in patients with ADHD who have not responded satisfactorily to several previous trials of more established agents for the treatment of ADHD. Exclusion criteria that preclude the use of CBZ include preexisting hepatic disease, severe allergic responses or skin rashes to previous trials of tricyclic agents, preexisting bone marrow disease, or concomitant clozapine use (an atypical neuroleptic with a 1% risk of inducing agranulocytosis), because of the potential of both medicines to cause bone marrow suppression.

Prior to CBZ therapy, a baseline medical workup is recommended. This should include a screening physical examination completed within the preceding year, a complete blood count with differential and platelet count (hematological function tests), liver function tests, and blood urea nitrogen and creatinine clearance (renal function tests). An EKG may also be considered, because tricyclic agents can cause cardiac intraventricular conduction delay. CBZ is initiated at a dose of 50 mg twice a day and increased in weekly increments of 100 mg up to a daily dose of 10–30 mg/kg/day. CBZ is generally prescribed to children and adolescents in three divided daily dosages. Serum levels of 4–12 µg/ml are considered within the therapeutic range for epilepsy. However, serum levels have not been shown to correlate reliably with treatment response for behavioral disorders. As noted previously, one study of CBZ in ADHD suggested that levels above 6.2 µg/ml might be optimal (Kafantaris et al., 1992), but further research is necessary before clinical recommendations can be made.

CBZ shows a narrow therapeutic range before toxic effects are seen. Therapeutic drug monitoring is therefore recommended. Blood levels of anticonvulsants (including CBZ) are sampled at trough, at the end of one half-life. Because of autoinduction, levels should be sampled more frequently during the first 2 months of therapy. Generally, sampling after the first week of CBZ use and then again after the first and second months of use will allow adequate dose adjustment in the face of metabolic induction. Levels can then be sampled every 6–12 months on a constant dosing schedule. Because of rare risks of bone marrow suppression and hepatotoxicity (see the section on side effects, next), blood counts and hepatic enzymes should be followed once every 6–12 months. Blood monitoring should occur more frequently if signs and symptoms referable to hematological, renal, or hepatic disease become clinically manifest (Trimble, 1990; Pellock & Willmore, 1991).

Side Effects

Table 19.5 lists frequent treatment-emergent side effects of oral CBZ. Side effects referable to the CNS are frequent at serum concentrations above 9 µg/ml. Many acute side effects can be avoided by starting at a low dose and titrating slowly. Untoward effects increase with dose noncompliance and intermittent therapy. CBZ therapy should be withdrawn slowly when treatment is discontinued, to prevent

TABLE 19.5. Common Treatment-Emergent Side Effects of Carbamazepine

Side effect	Percentage reporting
CNS	
Dizziness	54%
Headache	46%
Diplopia	38%
Drowsiness	31%
Ataxia	23%
Blurred vision	23%
Fatigue	15%
Dysarthria	8%
Irritability	8%
Gastrointestinal	
Nausea	31%
Vomiting	23%
Stomachache	23%
Decreased appetite	8%
Dermatological	
Rash	46%
Hematological	
Leukopenia	46%

mild withdrawal effects. Behavioral toxicity has also been reported with CBZ use. Paradoxically, increased hyperactivity, aggression, and impulsivity have been reported in children and adolescents treated with CBZ for aggression (Pleak, Birmaher, Gavrilescu, Abichandani, & Williams, 1988).

Initial concerns that severe and potentially life-threatening side effects of CBZ might be common with long-term treatment have not materialized. Although routine monitoring of hepatic functioning reveals elevations in 5–15% of CBZ-treated patients, fewer than 20 cases of significant hepatic complications were reported in the United States from 1978 to 1989 (Pellock & Willmore, 1991). Transient leukopenia occurs commonly in children and adults treated with CBZ. Unrelated to benign leukopenia, agranulocytosis occurs rarely, in only 2 cases per 575,000 (Pellock & Willmore, 1991). Severe exfoliative dermatitis alone or as part of a hypersensitivity reaction can also occasionally occur. The appearance of rash on CBZ should prompt abrupt drug discontinuation and careful ongoing clinical monitoring. The best way to minimize the development of major adverse side effects of CBZ is for the prescribing physician to provide repeated and ongoing reminders to the patient and family that any indication of systemic illness should lead to prompt medical consultation.

ANTIPSYCHOTIC MEDICATIONS

The majority of studies comparing antipsychotic medications with stimulants have reported that stimulants are more effective than antipsychotics in the treatment of ADHD (see Green, 1995). First-generation antipsychotics (neuroleptics) carry a substantial risk of neurological side effects, including extrapyramidal symptoms (acute dystonia, parkinsonian symptoms, akathisia) and tardive dyskinesia with chronic use. Second-generation antipsychotics (atypical antipsychotics) may cause substantial weight gain in children and adolescents, with increased risk for metabolic disorders such as Type II diabetes. In addition, the sedative effects of antipsychotics may interfere with cognition and learning. Because of these risks, routine antipsychotic therapy for children and adolescents with ADHD should be minimized.

However, some exceptions should be noted. Special populations of children and adolescents with ADHD may benefit from antipsychotics. These include youth with comorbid severe Tourette syndrome or another tic disorder, for which an antipsychotic may be indicated. Children with pervasive developmental disorders or mental retardation often present with symptoms of excessive hyperactivity, impulsivity, and attentional deficits. Thioridazine, chlorpromazine, and haloperidol have been studied in these populations and generally found to be significantly effective in controlled investigations when compared to placebo (see Green, 1995, for a review). More recently, the second-generation antipsychotic risperidone has been found helpful in reducing hyperactive–impulsive and aggressive symptoms in children with developmental delays (McCracken et al., 2002). The new atypical antipsychotics, including clozapine, risperidone, olanzapine, sertindole, and quetiapine, have not been specifically studied for disruptive behavior disorders and ADHD in child and adolescent psychiatry.

COMBINED PHARMACOTHERAPY

The concurrent use of more than one medication in the treatment of ADHD is increasingly common in clinical practice. However, this remains a poorly researched area, and few data from controlled studies are presently available to guide the clinician. The use of more than one agent might be considered in the following circumstances: (1) significant ADHD symptoms that are only partially responsive to monotherapy; (2) potentiating effects of combined medications on ADHD symptoms (e.g., MPH and a TCA); (3) use of lower doses of each agent when combined, reducing the risk of side effects from each agent alone if used in higher doses; and (4) treatment of ADHD and common medication-responsive comorbid conditions (e.g., Tourette syndrome, severe anxiety or depression, explosive aggression in CD).

Systematic study of the use of combined psychopharmacotherapy in ADHD is only just beginning. Stimulants have been combined with desipramine (Rapport, Carlson, Kelly, & Pataki, 1993). In a placebo-controlled study comparing desipramine alone, MPH alone, and the combination, MPH alone improved vigilance; both drugs alone improved short-term memory and visual problem solving; and the combination improved learning of higher-order relationships. The side effects of the combination were not significantly greater than those for desipramine alone (Pataki, Carlson, Kelly, Rapport, & Biancaniello, 1993). In a retrospective study of the efficacy of nortriptyline in ADHD, Wilens, Biederman, Geist, Steingard, and Spencer (1993) noted that 47% of 58 children and adolescents were receiving adjunctive medications along with nortriptyline. Stimulants have also been combined with selective serotonin reuptake inhibitors in the treatment of ADHD comorbid with mood disorders or other disruptive behavioral disorders. Gammon and Brown (1993) added fluoxetine to ongoing MPH therapy in 32 child and adolescent patients with ADHD and comorbid depression, ODD, or CD and found significant improvements on the combination. No significant or lasting untoward effects of MPH and fluoxetine were reported. In a case report, four patients received combined atomoxetine and stimulants for ADHD symptoms that were not responsive to monotherapy. The combination appeared to be effective and well tolerated (Brown, 2004).

Antihypertensive agents have also been used in combination with stimulants for ADHD comorbid with explosively aggressive symptoms, ODD, or CD. Clonidine is often added to ongoing MPH therapy (Hunt, Capper, & O'Connell, 1990). In a controlled study, this combination was reported to be safe and effective (Hazell & Stuart, 2003). However, several case reports have raised questions about the safety of this combination in subgroups of children (Cantwell et al., 1997), but in general it appears well tolerated if properly monitored by a physician. In adults with ADHD and explosive rage attacks, a small case series found efficacy for the combination of a stimulant and nadolol (Ratey, Greenberg, & Lindem, 1991).

MEDICATIONS NOT FOUND USEFUL FOR ADHD

Several medications have been studied and found not helpful in the clinical treatment of children and adolescents diagnosed with ADHD.

Antihistamines

Little support is found for efficacy of commonly used antihistamines such as diphenhydramine in the treatment of ADHD.

Benzodiazepines

Studies comparing benzodiazepines such as chlordiazepoxide or diazepam to stimulants and placebo have reported that benzodiazepines lack efficacy in ADHD (see Green, 1995).

Lithium

Lithium has not proved effective in the treatment of ADHD (see Green, 1995). Recently however, phenomenological studies in child and adolescent psychiatry have described comorbidity between ADHD and Bipolar I Disorder in adolescents, and have raised questions about possible prepubertal onset of Bipolar Disorder being mistaken for ADHD (Wozniak, Biederman, Kiely, Ablon, & Faraone, 1993). Because lithium may be an effective treatment for pediatric bipolar illness, and stimulants may exacerbate mania, this possible overlap requires much further clinical research. Currently, lithium is not considered a treatment for ADHD.

CONCLUSION

This chapter has considered the use of "other medications" (besides stimulants and antidepressants) in the treatment of ADHD. These medications continue to be a focus of clinical research, because a not insignificant percentage of children and adolescents with ADHD fail to respond satisfactorily to the more established agents. Atomoxetine is currently FDA-approved for use in ADHD. Although not FDA approved for pharmaceutical manufacturers advertising as effective in ADHD, the medications described in this chapter are clinically well-known agents, are FDA-approved for other indications in medicine, and should not be considered experimental medications. Their judicious and careful clinical use offers hope that patients whose ADHD does not respond to conventional therapies, or who possess significant comorbid conditions, may be further helped in living with this often complex, chronic, and disabling disorder.

KEY CLINICAL POINTS

✓ Antidepressants, modafinil, and the antihypertensives are second-line agents for ADHD, often used for children who are unresponsive to first-line agents or for those with particular comorbid disorders that make first-line agents untenable.

✓ Modafinil is a novel wake-promoting agent that is structurally different from CNS stimulants and does not appear to have a dopaminergic mechanism of action. At this time, little support is available for modafinil in the treatment of adult ADHD. However, modafinil has been shown to improve ADHD symptoms in children in several, although not all, pediatric studies.

✓ Clonidine stimulates presynaptic alpha-2-adrenergic receptors in the brain stem (locus ceruleus), resulting in a reduction in sympathetic outflow from the CNS. The decrease in plasma norepinephrine is directly related to clonidine's hypotensive action. The extant literature shows the majority of studies, but not all, reporting clinically significant results. These studies generally describe some benefits for behavioral target symptoms of aggression, hyperactivity, overarousal, impulsivity, and sleep disturbance as assessed by observer-completed rating scales.

✓ Guanfacine is an orally administered, centrally acting antihypertensive agent that also stimulates CNS alpha-2-adrenergic auto-receptors to down-regulate sympathomimetic outflow from the brain stem. Preliminary research is encouraging. Much as for clonidine, improvements in hyperactive–impulsive and overarousal symptoms are reported on observer-completed rating scales.

✓ Beta-blockers are a family of agents that competitively inhibit norepinephrine and epinephrine actions at beta-adrenergic receptor sites, both centrally and in the periphery. In ADHD, there presently exists one methodologically controlled study of pindolol (a centrally acting beta-blocker) in comparison with placebo and methylphenidate (MPH). Pindolol was found to be modestly effective in ADHD (i.e., just as effective as MPH in decreasing impulsivity–hyperactivity, but less effective than MPH for cognitive symptoms of ADHD). However, because of a high incidence of side effects, including nightmares, hallucinations, and paresthesias, pindolol was stopped in all children receiving this drug. Nadolol (a peripherally acting beta-blocker with little penetration into the CNS) was not found to significantly reduce parent- and teacher-rated ADHD symptoms, but significant improvements in aggression were found in one open-label study.

✓ Carbamazepine (CBZ) is an anticonvulsant frequently used in Europe for treating ADHD and ADHD comorbid with Conduct Disorder (CD). A meta-analysis of 10 reports from the world literature suggests some efficacy in children with ADHD. Response rates were found to be 70% in open studies and 71% in controlled studies. CBZ may be considered (1) for children and adolescents with comorbid generalized tonic-clonic epilepsy, partial complex epilepsy, or focally abnormal electroencephalograph and accompanying symptoms of ADHD; or (2) as a third-line medication for overarousal, impulsivity–hyperactivity, and aggression in patients who have not responded satisfactorily to several previous trials of more established agents for the treatment of ADHD.

✓ Special populations of children and adolescents with ADHD may benefit from antipsychotics. These include ADHD comorbid with severe Tourette syndrome or another tic disorder, for which an antipsychotic may be indicated. Children with pervasive developmental disorders and mental retardation often present with symptoms of excessive hyperactivity, impulsivity, and attentional deficits. Thioridazine, chlorpromazine, and haloperidol have been studied in these populations and generally found significantly effective in controlled investigations when compared to placebo. More recently, the second-generation antipsychotic risperidone has been found helpful in reducing hyperactive–impulsive and aggressive symptoms in children with developmental delays.

✓ The use of more than one agent in combination might be considered in the following circumstances: (1) significant ADHD symptoms that are only partially responsive to monotherapy; (2) potentiating effects of combined medications on ADHD symptoms (e.g., MPH and a TCA); (3) use of lower doses of each agent when combined, reducing the risk of side effects from each agent alone if used in higher doses; and (4) treatment of ADHD and common medication-responsive comorbid conditions (e.g., Tourette syndrome, severe anxiety or depression, and explosive aggression or CD).

✓ Several other medications have been studied and found not helpful in the clinical treatment of children and adolescents diagnosed with ADHD. These include antihistamines, benzodiazepines, and lithium.

REFERENCES

Agarwal, V., Sitholey, P., Kumar, S., & Prasad, M. (2001). Double-blind, placebo-controlled trial of clonidine in hyperactive children with mental retardation. *Mental Retardation, 39,* 259–267.

American Psychiatric Association. (2000). *Diagnostic and statistical manual of mental disorders* (4th ed., text rev.). Washington, DC: Author.

Arnsten, A. F., Steere, J. C., & Hunt, R. D. (1996). The contribution of alpha-2–noradrenergic mechanisms to prefrontal cortical cognitive function. *Archives of General Psychiatry, 53,* 448–455.

Barkley, R. A. (1997). Behavioral inhibition, sustained attention, and executive functions: Constructing a unifying theory of ADHD. *Psychological Bulletin, 121,* 65–94.

Biederman, J. (2003, May). *Modafinil improves ADHD symptoms in children in a randomized, double-blind, placebo-controlled study.* Paper presented at the annual meeting of the American Psychiatric Association, San Francisco.

Biederman, J., Newcorn, J., & Sprich, S. (1991). Co-

morbidity of attention deficit hyperactivity disorder with conduct, depressive, anxiety, and other disorders. *American Journal of Psychiatry, 148,* 564–577.

Brown, T. E. (2004). Atomoxetine and stimulants in combination for treatment of attention deficit hyperactivity disorder: Four case reports. *Journal of Child and Adolescent Psychopharmacology, 14,* 129–136.

Buitelaar, J. K., van de Gaag, R. J., Swaab-Barneveld, H., & Kuiper, M. (1996). Pindolol and methylphenidate in children with attention-deficit hyperactivity disorder. Clinical efficacy and side effects. *Journal of Child Psychology and Psychiatry, 37,* 587–595.

Cantwell, D. P., Swanson, J., & Connor, D. F. (1997). Adverse response to clonidine. *Journal of the American Academy of Child and Adolescent Psychiatry, 36,* 539–544.

Carskadon, M. A., Cavallo, A., & Rosekind, M. R. (1989). Sleepiness and nap sleep following a morning dose of clonidine. *Sleep, 12,* 338–344.

Cephalon, Inc. (2002). [Modafinil NDA: Integrated summary of safety and efficacy]. Unpublished raw data (Protocol No. C1538a/205/AD/US).

Chappell, P. B., Riddle, M. A., Scahill, L., Lynch, K. A., Schultz, R., Arnsten, A., et al. (1995). Guanfacine treatment of comorbid attention deficit hyperactivity disorder and Tourette's syndrome: Preliminary clinical experience. *Journal of the American Academy of Child and Adolescent Psychiatry, 34,* 1140–1146.

Cohen, D. J., Young, J. G., Nathanson, J. A., & Shaywitz, B. A. (1979). Clonidine in Tourette's syndrome. *Lancet, ii,* 551–553.

Connor, D. F. (1993). Beta blockers for aggression: A review of the pediatric experience. *Journal of Child and Adolescent Psychopharmacology, 3,* 99–114.

Connor, D. F., Barkley, R. A., & Davis, H. T. (2000). A pilot study of methylphenidate, clonidine, or the combination in ADHD comorbid with aggressive oppositional defiant or conduct disorder. *Clinical Pediatrics, 39,* 15–25.

Connor, D. F., Fletcher, K. E., & Swanson, J. M. (1999). A meta-analysis of clonidine for symptoms of attention-deficit hyperactivity disorder. *Journal of the American Academy of Child and Adolescent Psychiatry, 38,* 1551–1559.

Connor, D. F., Ozbayrak, K. R., Benjamin, S., Ma, Y., & Fletcher, K. E. (1997). A pilot study of nadolol for overt aggression in developmentally delayed individuals. *Journal of the American Academy of Child and Adolescent Psychiatry, 36,* 826–834.

Cornish, L. A. (1988). Guanfacine hydrochloride: A centrally acting antihypertensive agent. *Journal of Clinical Pharmacology, 7,* 187–197.

Cueva, J. E., Overall, J. E., Small, A. A., Armenteros, J. L., Perry, R., & Campbell, M. (1996). Carbamazepine in aggressive children with conduct disorder: A double-blind and placebo-controlled study. *Journal of the American Academy of Child and Adolescent Psychiatry, 35,* 480–490.

Donnelly, M., Rapoport, J. L., Potter, W. Z., Oliver, J., Keysor, C. S., & Murphy, D. L. (1989). Fenfluramine and dextroamphetamine treatment of childhood hyperactivity. *Archives of General Psychiatry, 46,* 205–212.

Frankenhauser, M., Karumanchi, V., German, M., Yates, A., & Karumanchi, S. (1992). A double-blind placebo-controlled study of the efficacy of transdermal clonidine in autism. *Journal of Clinical Psychiatry, 53,* 77–82.

Gaffney, G. R., Perry, P. J., Lund, B. C., Bever-Stille, K. A., & Kuperman, A. S. (2002). Risperidone versus clonidine in the treatment of children and adolescents with Tourette's syndrome. *Journal of the American Academy of Child and Adolescent Psychiatry, 41,* 330–336.

Gallopin, T., Luppi, P. H., Rambert, H. A., Frydman, A., & Fort, P. (2004). Effect of wake-promoting agent modafinil on sleep-promoting neurons from the ventrolateral preoptic nucleus: An *in vitro* pharmacologic study. *Sleep, 27,* 19–25.

Gammon, G. D., & Brown, T. E. (1993). Fluoxetine and methylphenidate in combination for treatment of attention deficit disorder and comorbid depressive disorder. *Journal of Child and Adolescent Psychopharmacology, 3,* 1–10.

Green, W. H. (1995). The treatment of attention-deficit hyperactivity disorder with nonstimulant medications. *Child and Adolescent Psychiatric Clinics of North America, 4,* 169–195.

Gunning, B. (1992). *A controlled trial of clonidine in hyperkinetic children.* Unpublished doctoral dissertation, Academic Hospital, Erasmus University, Rotterdam, The Netherlands.

Halperin, J. M., Newcorn, J. H., McKay, K. E., Siever, L. J., & Sharma, V. (2003). Growth hormone response to guanfacine in boys with attention deficit hyperactivity disorder: A preliminary study. *Journal of Child and Adolescent Psychopharmacology, 13,* 283–294.

Hazell, P. L., & Stuart, J. E. (2003). A randomized controlled trial of clonidine added to psychostimulant medication for hyperactive and aggressive children. *Journal of the American Academy of Child and Adolescent Psychiatry, 42,* 886–894.

Horrigan, J. P., & Barnhill, L. J. (1995). Guanfacine treatment of attention-deficit hyperactivity disorder in boys. *Journal of Child and Adolescent Psychopharmacology, 5,* 215–223.

Hunt, R. D., Arnsten, A. F. T., & Asbell, M. D. (1995). An open trial of guanfacine in the treatment of attention-deficit hyperactivity disorder. *Journal of the American Academy of Child and Adolescent Psychiatry, 34,* 50–54.

Hunt, R. D., Capper, L., & O'Connell, P. (1990). Clonidine in child and adolescent psychiatry. *Journal of Child and Adolescent Psychopharmacology, 1,* 87–102.

Hunt, R. D., Cohen, D. J., Anderson, G., & Clark, L. (1984). Possible changes in noradrenergic receptor sensitivity following methylphenidate treatment: Growth hormone and MHPG response to clonidine challenge in children with attention deficit disorder and hyperactivity. *Life Sciences, 35,* 885–897.

Hunt, R. D., Minderaa, R. B., & Cohen, D. J. (1985). Clonidine benefits children with attention deficit disorder and hyperactivity: Report of a double-blind placebo-crossover therapeutic trial. *Journal of the American Academy of Child and Adolescent Psychiatry, 24,* 617–629.

Jaselskis, C. A., Cook, E. H., Fletcher, K. E., & Leventhal, B. L. (1992). Clonidine treatment of hyperactive and impulsive children with autistic disorder. *Journal of Clinical Psychopharmacology, 12,* 322–327.

Kafantaris, V., Campbell, M., Padron-Gayol, M. V., Small, A. M., Locascio, J. J., & Rosenberg, C. R. (1992). Carbamazepine in hospitalized aggressive conduct disorder children: An open pilot study. *Psychopharmacology Bulletin, 28,* 193–199.

Leckman, J. F., Hardin, M. T., Riddle, M. A., Stevenson, J., Ort, S. I., & Cohen, D. J. (1991). Clonidine treatment of Gilles de la Tourette's syndrome. *Archives of General Psychiatry, 48,* 324–328.

McCracken, J. T., McGough, J. J., Shah, B., Cronin, P., Hong, D., Aman, M. G., et al. (2002). Risperidone in children with autism and serious behavioral problems. *New England Journal of Medicine, 347,* 314–321.

Niederhofer, H., Staffen, W., & Mair, A. (2003). A placebo-controlled study of lofexidine in the treatment of children with tic disorders and attention deficit hyperactivity disorder. *Journal of Psychopharmacology, 17,* 113–119.

Pataki, C. S., Carlson, G. A., Kelly, K. L., Rapport, M. D., & Biancaniello, T. M. (1993). Side effects of methylphenidate and desipramine alone and in combination in children. *Journal of the American Academy of Child and Adolescent Psychiatry, 32,* 1065–1072.

Pellock, J. M., & Willmore, L. J. (1991). A rational guide to routine blood monitoring in patients receiving antiepileptic drugs. *Neurology, 41,* 961–964.

Pleak, R. R., Birmaher, B., Gavrilescu, A., Abichandani, C., & Williams, D. T. (1988). Mania and neuropsychiatric excitation following carbamazepine. *Journal of the American Academy of Child and Adolescent Psychiatry, 27,* 500–503.

Rapport, M. D., Carlson, G. A., Kelly, K. L., & Pataki, C. (1993). Methylphenidate and desipramine in hospitalized children: I. Separate and combined effects on cognitive function. *Journal of the American Academy of Child and Adolescent Psychiatry, 32,* 333–342.

Ratey, J. J., Greenberg, M. S., & Lindem, K. J. (1991). Combination of treatments for attention deficit hyperactivity disorder in adults. *Journal of Nervous and Mental Disease, 179,* 699–701.

Rugino, T. A., & Copley, T. C. (2001). Effects of modafinil in children with attention-deficit/hyperactivity disorder: An open-label study. *Journal of the*

American Academy of Child and Adolescent Psychiatry, 40, 230–235.

Rugino, T. A., & Samsock, T. C. (2003). Modafinil in children with attention deficit hyperactivity disorder. *Pediatric Neurology, 29,* 136–142.

Scahill, L., Chappell, P. B., Kim, Y. S., Schultz, R. T., Katsovich, L., Shepard, E., et al. (2001). A placebo-controlled study of guanfacine in the treatment of children with tic disorders and attention deficit hyperactivity disorder. *American Journal of Psychiatry, 158,* 1067–1074.

Scammell, T. E., Estabrook, I. V., McCarthy, M. T., Chemelli, R. M., Yanagisawa, M., Miller, M. S., et al. (2000). Hypothalamic arousal regions are activated during modafinil-induced wakefulness. *Journal of Neuroscience, 20,* 1–9.

Silva, R. R., Munoz, D. M., & Alpert, M. (1996). Carbamazepine use in children and adolescents with features of attention-deficit hyperactivity disorder: A meta-analysis. *Journal of the American Academy of Child and Adolescent Psychiatry, 35,* 352–358.

Singer, H. S., Brown, J., Quaskey, S., Rosenberg, L. A., Mellits, E. D., & Denckla, M. B. (1995). The treatment of attention-deficit hyperactivity disorder in Tourette's syndrome: A double-blind placebo-controlled study with clonidine and desipramine. *Pediatrics, 95,* 74–80.

Swanson, J. M. (2003, May). *Modafinil in children with*

ADHD: A randomized, placebo-controlled study. Paper presented at the annual meeting of the American Psychiatric Association, San Francisco.

Taylor, F., & Russo, J. (2000). Efficacy of modafinil compared to dextroamphetamine for the treatment of attention-deficit/hyperactivity disorder in adults. *Journal of Child and Adolescent Psychopharmacology, 10,* 311–320.

Tourette's Syndrome Study Group. (2002). Treatment of ADHD in children with tics: A randomized controlled trial. *Neurology, 58,* 527–536.

Trimble, M. R. (1990). Anticonvulsants in children and adolescents. *Journal of Child and Adolescent Psychopharmacology, 1,* 107–124.

Wilens, T. E., Biederman, J., Geist, D. E., Steingard, R., & Spencer, T. (1993). Nortriptyline in the treatment of ADHD: A chart review of 58 cases. *Journal of the American Academy of Child and Adolescent Psychiatry, 32,* 343–349.

Wilens, T. E., Haight. B. R., Horrigan, J. P., Hudziak, J. J., Rosenthal, N. E., Connor, D. F., et al. (2005). Buproprion XL in adults with attention-deficit/hyperactivity disorder: A randomized placebo-controlled study. *Biological Psychiatry, 57*(7), 793–801.

Wozniak, J., Biederman J., Kiely, K., Ablon, J. S., & Faraone, S. (1993). Prepubertal mania revisited. *Scientific Proceedings of the American Academy of Child and Adolescent Psychiatry, 9,* 36.

CHAPTER 20

Combined Child Therapies

BRADLEY H. SMITH
RUSSELL A. BARKLEY
CHERI J. SHAPIRO

This chapter is largely derived from another recent review of treatments for children with Attention-Deficit/Hyperactivity Disorder (ADHD) (Smith, Barkley, & Shapiro, 2006). The importance of this review is critical to the mission of the present text, however, and so this other discussion is reiterated here, with some modest revisions.

As the previous chapters on treatment have all noted, psychopharmacological and behavioral treatments are not, by themselves, typically or completely adequate to address all of the difficulties likely to be presented by clinic-referred children or adolescents with ADHD. Optimal treatment is likely to involve a combination of many of these approaches for maximal effectiveness (Carlson, Pelham, Milich, & Dixon, 1992; Pelham, Wheeler, & Chronis, 1998; Phelps, Brown, & Power, 2002). However, the extent to which combined treatments are superior to medication alone is a controversial issue, especially given the relatively high cost of many psychosocial interventions. Nevertheless, findings emerging from the Multimodal Treatment Study of ADHD (MTA) imply some potential advantages of combined treatment, although the results of other multisite studies may challenge that conclusion. Af-

ter presenting some of the early studies on combined treatments, we review the MTA in depth, along with qualifications offered by another multisite combined treatment project.

EARLY RESEARCH

Some early research studies examined the utility of combining psychosocial and pharmacological treatment packages, with interesting results. It appears that in many of these studies, the combination of contingency management training of parents or teachers with stimulant drug therapies was generally little better than either treatment alone for the management of ADHD symptoms (Firestone, Kelly, Goodman, & Davey, 1981; Gadow, 1985; Pollard, Ward, & Barkley, 1983; Wolraich, Drummond, Salomon, O'Brien, & Sivage, 1978). Several other studies found impressive results for classroom behavior management methods (Carlson et al., 1992; DuPaul & Eckert, 1997; Pelham et al., 1988), but found that the addition of medication provided further improvements beyond those achieved by behavior management alone. On a positive note, the combination might have resulted in the need for less intense behavioral interventions or lower doses of medication than might be the case if either intervention were used alone. When there was an advantage to behavioral interventions, it appeared to be related to functioning rather than symptom relief, such as reliably increasing rates of academic productivity and accuracy (see DuPaul & Stoner, 2003). Despite some failures to obtain additive effects for these two treatments, many investigators concluded (and continue to conclude) that their combination may still be advantageous, given that stimulants are not usually used in the late afternoons or evenings (when parents may need effective behavior management tactics to deal with the ADHD symptoms). Moreover, a minority of children (10–25%) do not respond positively to these medications (see Chapters 17–19, this volume), making behavioral interventions one of the few scientifically proven alternatives for these cases.

Several early studies examined the combined effects of stimulant medication and cognitive-behavioral interventions. Horn, Chatoor, and Conners (1983) examined the separate and combined effects of dextroamphetamine and self-instructional training for a 9-year-old inpatient child with ADHD. The combined program was more effective in increasing on-task behavior during classwork, as well as decreasing teacher ratings of ADHD symptoms. However, academic productivity was improved only by the use of direct reinforcement for correct responses. In contrast, using group comparison designs, Brown, Borden, Wynne, Schleser, and Clingerman (1986) and Brown, Wynne, and Medenis (1985) found no benefits of combined drug and cognitive-behavioral interventions over either treatment alone on similar domains of functioning in children with ADHD. Similarly, a later study by Horn et al. (1991) did not find the combination of treatments to be superior to medication alone.

Some success for combined medication and self-evaluation procedures was reported (Hinshaw, Henker, & Whalen, 1984a) when social skills, such as cooperation, were targets of intervention. Yet when these same investigators attempted to teach anger control strategies to children with ADHD to enhance self-control during peer interactions, no benefits of combined intervention were found beyond those achieved by self-control training alone (Hinshaw, Henker, & Whalen, 1984b). The self-control techniques were the most successful in

teaching these children specific coping strategies to employ in the sorts of provocative interactions with peers that usually lead to angry reactions from the children with ADHD. Medication, in contrast, served only to lower the overall level of anger responses, but did not enhance the application of specific anger control strategies. These early studies suggest that each form of treatment may have highly specific and unique effects on some aspects of social behavior, but not on others.

Limited research has evaluated the effects of behavioral parent training alone and combined with child training in self-control strategies (Horn et al., 1983) on home and school behavioral problems. This research failed to find any significant advantage for the combined treatments. Both self-control training and behavioral parent training alone improved home behavior problems, but neither resulted in any generalization of treatment effects to the school, where no treatment had occurred. Since a no-treatment group was not employed in this study, however, it is not possible to conclude that these effects were due to treatment rather than to nonspecific effects (e.g., maturation, therapist attention, regression effects, etc.). A later study by Horn, Ialongo, Greenberg, Packard, and Smith-Winberry (1990) did find such a treatment combination to be superior to either treatment used alone in producing a significantly larger number of children responding to treatment. Once again, however, no generalization of the results to the school setting occurred.

Satterfield, Satterfield, and Cantwell (1980) attempted to evaluate the effects of individualized multimodality intervention provided over extensive time periods (up to several years) on the outcome of boys with ADHD. Interventions included medication, behavioral parent training, individual counseling, special education, family therapy, and other programs as needed by particular individuals. Results suggested that such an individualized program of combined treatments continued over longer time intervals could produce improvements in social adjustment at home and school, as well as in rates of antisocial behavior, substance abuse, and academic achievement. These results seem to have been sustained across at least a 3-year follow-up period (Satterfield, Cantwell, & Satterfield, 1979; Satterfield, Satterfield, & Cantwell, 1981; Satterfield, Satterfield, & Schell, 1987). Although this research suggests great promise for the possible efficacy of multimodality treatment extended over years for children with ADHD, the lack of random assignment and more adequate control procedures in this series of studies limits the ability to attribute those improvements obtained in this study directly to the treatments employed. And these limitations certainly preclude establishing which of the treatment components was most effective. Still, studies such as these and others (Carlson et al., 1992; Pelham et al., 1988) raised hopes that intensive multimodality treatment could be effective for ADHD if extended over long intervals of time.

INTENSIVE, MULTIMODAL TREATMENT PROGRAMS

Two of the most well-known and well-regarded multimodality intervention programs are the summer treatment program (STP) developed by William Pelham and colleagues and conducted at Western Psychiatric Institute in Pittsburgh (Pelham & Hoza, 1996), and the University of California–Irvine/Orange County Department of Education (UCI-OCDE) intervention developed by James Swanson, Linda Pfiffner, Keith McBurnett, and Dennis Cantwell (see Chapter 15, this volume). The UCI-OCDE program incorporates a number of features of the STP, as well as some components of the multimodal program conducted by Stephen Hinshaw, Barbara Henker, and Carol Whalen at the University of California–Los Angeles. All of these programs rely on four major components of treatment: (1) parent training in child behavior management; (2) classroom implementation of behavior modification techniques; (3) social skills training (typically centering around sports); and (4) stimulant medication, in some cases. Whereas the Pelham program is conducted during the summer months in a "day camp"-style format, the UCI-OCDE program has a year-round school-style format.

The STP

The STP developed by Pelham and colleagues is conducted in a day treatment environment with a summer school/camp-like format. Daily activities include a few hours of classroom instruction, which also incorporates behavior modification methods (such as token economies, response cost, and time out from reinforcement). In addition, 3–4 hours of sports

and recreational activities are arranged each day, during which behavioral management programs are operative. The program also includes parent training, peer relationship training, and a follow-up protocol to enhance the likelihood that treatment gains will be maintained after children leave the program. During their stay at the camp, some children may be tested on stimulant medication via a double-blind, placebo-controlled procedure, in which a child is tested on several different doses of medication while teacher ratings and behavioral observations are collected across the different camp activities.

Pelham and colleagues have used the STP setting and larger programmatic context to conduct more focused research investigations into the effectiveness of classroom behavior management procedures alone, stimulant medication alone, and their combination in managing ADHD symptoms and improving academic performance and social behavior. Some of the components of this day treatment program have been evaluated previously, such as classroom contingency management, and have been found to produce significant short-term improvements in children with ADHD (see DuPaul & Eckert, 1997, 1998). And they clearly seem to do so in the STP context (Carlson et al., 1992; Pelham et al., 1988). The STP, in fact, was a part of the intensive multimodal treatment program for children with ADHD studied in the MTA project (see below). But other components of the program have not been so well evaluated previously for their efficacy with children having ADHD, such as social skills training. And while results from parent ratings before and after their children's participation indicate that 86% believe their children to have improved from their participation in the program, no data have been published as yet on whether the gains made during the treatment program are subsequently maintained in the regular school and home settings after the children terminate their participation in the STP.

The UCI/OCDE Program

The UCI/OCDE program provides weekday treatment for children with ADHD in kindergarten through fifth grade, in a school-like atmosphere with classes of 12–15 children. The clinical interventions rely chiefly on a token economy program for the management of behavior in the classrooms, and on a parent training program conducted through both group and individual treatment sessions. Some training in self-monitoring, evaluation, and reinforcement also occurs as part of the class program. Children receive daily group instruction in social skills as part of the classroom curriculum, and some of these behaviors may be targeted for modification outside the group instruction time by using consequences within the classroom token economy. Before returning to their regular public schools, some children may participate in a transition school program that focuses on more advanced social skills, as well as behavior modification programs to facilitate the transfer of learning to their regular school setting. Some children within this program also may be receiving stimulant medication as needed for management of their ADHD symptoms.

Although this program has served as an exemplar for many others, published research on its efficacy is not available. Granted, the parent training program and classroom behavior modification methods are highly similar to those used in published studies that have found them to be effective, at least in the short term, so long as they are in use (Barkley, 1997; DuPaul & Eckert, 1997; Pelham & Sams, 1992). But the actual extent to which this particular program achieves its stated goals—especially, the generalization of treatment gains to nontreatment settings, as well as the maintenance of those gains after children return to their public schools—has not been systematically evaluated or published.

The UMASS/WPS Early Intervention Project

Barkley, Shelton, and colleagues completed a multimethod early intervention program at the University of Massachusetts Medical School (UMASS) for kindergarten children (ages 4–6 years) having significant problems with hyperactivity and aggression; at least 70% of these children qualified for a clinical diagnosis of ADHD (see Barkley et al., 2000; Shelton et al., 2000). This program did not utilize clinic-referred children, whose parents and even teachers may be highly motivated to cooperate with treatment. Instead, children were identified at kindergarten registration as displaying significantly high levels of hyperactive and aggressive behavior (93rd percentile) and as being at high risk for both ADHD and Oppositional Defiant Disorder (ODD). Indeed, more than 70% of them met criteria for one or both of these disorders upon subsequent clinical evaluation using

structured psychiatric interviews. They were randomly assigned to one of four intervention groups for their entire kindergarten year. One group received a 10-week group parent training program followed by monthly booster session group meetings. Otherwise, these children participated in the standard kindergarten program offered by the Worcester (Massachusetts) Public Schools (WPS). The second group was assigned to a special enrichment kindergarten classroom, in which they received accelerated instruction in academic skills, social skills training, classroom contingency management procedures (token systems and other reinforcements, response cost, time out, etc.), and cognitive therapy (self-instruction training) as part of their full-day kindergarten program. These special classes contained 12–16 hyperactive–aggressive children in each and were held in two neighborhood elementary schools in the WPS system, to which the children were provided busing. Children in this special classroom also received several months of follow-up consultation to their teachers when they returned to their regular public schools for their first-grade year. A third group received both the parent training and enrichment classroom treatments, while a fourth group received no special services except for the initial evaluation and periodic reevaluations. All children were followed for 2 years after their participation in these treatment programs.

Results indicated no beneficial effect of the parent training program, in large part because more than 60% of the parents did not attend the training classes regularly, if at all. The enrichment classroom produced a significant improvement in the children's classroom behavior and social skills during the kindergarten year, but did not result in any change in behavior in the home as rated by parents. Nor did it produce greater gains in academic achievement skills than those experienced by the control groups not receiving this classroom program. Moreover, the results of the classroom were apparently attenuated during the follow-up period. Such results once again show that intensive classroom behavioral interventions can be effective in the short term for addressing the disruptive behavior of children. Yet these same results are rather sobering in view of the large investment of money, time, and staff training. Parent training programs for children at high risk for school and home behavior problems may not be especially effective in families identified through such community screening programs, largely due to poor parental motivation and investment in the training program. And even where classroom interventions are successful in the short-term "active treatment" phase, their effects may diminish or disappear with time after children leave the treatment environment. This study suggests that the rather positive treatment outcome results for families who seek treatment and, by inference, are motivated to change themselves and their children with ADHD may not be readily extrapolated to families of similarly deviant children who have not sought treatment but are identified through community screening programs.

The Historic NIMH MTA

The National Institute of Mental Health (NIMH) collaborative multisite MTA is the first major clinical trial by NIMH with a focus on a childhood disorder (MTA Cooperative Group, 1999a, 1999b). Although much research has documented the short-term effectiveness of medication and behavioral interventions to treat ADHD, significant questions remain unanswered about the long-term effects of these interventions, alone or in combination, on the multiple functional outcome areas impaired by ADHD. Questions also remain about which types of youth with ADHD may benefit most from which types of treatment. The ambitious and groundbreaking MTA was designed to help answer some of these major questions by randomly assigning children to four treatment groups: medication alone (MedMgt), behavior modification alone (Beh), the combination of medication and behavior modification (Comb), and community comparison (CC). In order to obtain a sufficiently large and diverse sample of youth with ADHD to begin to address these questions, a multisite study was initiated by NIMH along with funding from the U.S. Department of Education in 1992. Six proposals were funded; after 1 year, a common intervention protocol was created and then implemented at six sites in the United States and one collaborative site in Canada.

Study Design/Methodology

In order to be eligible for the study, children had to be between ages 7 and 9.9 years; to be in grades 1–4; to meet *Diagnostic and Statistical Manual of Mental Disorders*, fourth edition (DSM-IV) diagnostic criteria for ADHD, Combined Type, via the Parent version of the Diag-

nostic Interview Schedule for Children (supplemented by teacher reported symptoms if a case was near the diagnostic threshold); and to have been living with the same caretakers for at least the previous 6 months. Youth with comorbid internalizing or externalizing psychiatric disorders were included, as long as these conditions did not require treatment incompatible with study treatments. The schools the children attended also had to express cooperation with both the treatment and assessment protocols. Other exclusionary criteria included situations that would prevent full participation in the study, such as not having a phone, intellectual and adaptive functioning in the borderline range or below, or major medical illness (for complete information on the screening and selection procedures, see MTA Cooperative Group, 1999a). Important characteristics of the sample selected for the study included variables identified a priori as potential moderators of treatment: gender (20% female); prior medication status (31%); ODD or Conduct Disorder (CD) diagnoses (40% and 14%); DSM-III-R anxiety disorders (34% with Simple Phobia alone not included); and families receiving welfare, public assistance, or Supplemental Security Income (19%). Important to note is that the 579 children represented only 13% of those initially contacting the project, 25% of those passing an initial rating scale screening, and 62% of those completing the diagnostic interview and evaluation of school cooperation.

Once selected, participants were randomly assigned to one of the four conditions noted previously. Treatments were delivered over a 14-month period; comprehensive assessments of functioning in multiple domains were conducted at baseline prior to randomization as well as at 3, 9, and 14 months (with the 14-month assessment constituting the treatment endpoint assessment) (MTA Cooperative Group, 1999a). The MTA Cooperative Group (2004a, 2004b) recently published results of a 24-month follow-up, and 36- and 48-month follow-ups are currently underway or planned for the future.

Behavioral treatments (in both the Beh and Comb conditions) encompassed parent, child, and school domains. Behavioral parent training was provided by experienced training consultants and based on models by Barkley (1997) and by Forehand and McMahon (1981; McMahon & Forehand, 2003). This intervention consisted of 27 group and 8 individual sessions. Child behavioral treatment consisted of an intensive summer treatment program (based on the Pelham STP model) as well as school consultation services (similar to those in the UCI/OCDE model). The MTA's version of the STP was an intensive 8-week, 9-hour-per-day program; study training consultants supervised staff members working with the children and continued to provide parent interventions during the summer. The same training consultants provided school consultation services (10–16 sessions of teacher consultation and establishment of a daily report card), and the staff members working with the children in the STP worked in the schools in the fall as paraprofessional aides (12 weeks at half time under supervision of the training consultants and the children's teachers). Families attended an average of 77.8% of parent training sessions, 36.2 of 40 possible STP days, 10.7 teacher consultation visits, and 47.6 (of 60) possible days with a classroom aide. Delivery of behavioral treatments was faded over the course of treatment, so that by the endpoint assessment at 14 months, therapist contact with parents had ended or was reduced to once per month.

Like the intensive behavioral interventions, the medication treatments (in both MedMgt and Comb conditions) in the MTA were provided in a much more rigorous and intensive way than is typical in clinical practice. All medication treatment provided by the MTA included an initial 28-day double-blind, placebo-controlled titration consisting of placebo plus four different doses of methylphenidate (MPH; 5, 10, 15, and 20 mg) randomly given over the titration period. Three-times-per-day dosing was used in the titration (and typically during treatment), in which the full dose was given in the morning and at lunch, as well as a half dose in the midafternoon. Parent and teacher daily ratings were collected during the titration; graphs portraying the results were rated by a cross-site panel of experienced clinicians. A "best dose" was chosen, and the double blind was then broken; that dose became the initial dose for treatment. If the dose chosen was placebo, alternative medications were openly titrated until a satisfactory medication was chosen (or, in the case of a robust placebo response, the child was not medicated). Approximately 89% of youth assigned to MedMgt or Comb successfully completed titration; of these, 68.5% were assigned to initial doses of MPH averaging 30.5 mg/day given three times per day. Of the remaining group of youth who completed titration but were not

started on MPH, 26 received an unblinded titration of dextroamphetamine because of unsatisfactory MPH response, and 32 were given no medication because of a robust placebo response. Of note is that of the 289 subjects assigned to MedMgt or Comb, 17 families refused titration; another 15 subjects did not complete titration; (11 because of side effects or problems with titration); and inadequate amounts of titration data were gathered for a further 4 subjects (MTA Cooperative Group, 1999a).

Youth assigned to the CC condition received no intervention by the MTA staff, but sought treatment as usually provided in the community. Referrals to non-MTA providers were made as necessary for these families; all of the youth and families returned for assessments at the same time as youth in the other three conditions of the study. Initially, it was thought that the CC group would provide a minimal- or no-treatment comparison group. However, as described later in this section, about two-thirds of the children in the CC group actually received medication for ADHD.

Outcomes in this study were assessed with a large number of measures in multiple domains, including verbal report information (via interview and paper-and-pencil measures) by parents, teachers, and children; direct observation in the clinic and school; and computerized assessments of attention. Given the large number of measures, settings and informants used in the study, data reduction methods were conducted to condense measures into outcome domains. The major outcome domains that have received attention in the literature are as follows: ADHD symptoms, oppositional/aggressive symptoms, social skills, internalizing symptoms, parent–child relations, parental discipline, and academic achievement.

Major Findings on ADHD Symptoms

All four MTA groups showed symptom reduction over time. In our opinion, the trends in the data favored the Comb treatment over the other three conditions, but this conclusion may depend on how those data are analyzed. When an idiographic approach that looks at individual outcomes is used, there is a clear advantage for the Comb condition. Swanson et al. (2001) created a categorical measure of treatment outcome based on composite Swanson, Nolan, and Pelham Questionnaire–IV (SNAP-IV) ADHD and ODD symptom scores from teachers and parents. Successful treatment was identified as scoring on average 1 or below on a composite SNAP-IV score at the end of treatment (representing symptoms falling in the "not at all" or "just a little" range of categories at treatment endpoint). Success rates for the four conditions were as follows: 68% for Comb, 56% for MedMgt, 34% for Beh, and 25% for CC. A similar, but less robust, pattern of results was observed at the 24-month follow-up. Specifically, the normalization rates (as defined above) were 48%, 37%, 32%, and 28% for Comb, MedMgt, Beh, and CC, respectively (MTA Cooperative Group, 2004a).

Another way to look at the MTA data is in terms of statistical significance of the group means, which is the type of analysis that has received the most attention in the published literature. When using this approach on the 14- and 24-month follow-up data, the MTA Collaborative Group reached the conclusion that treatments involving intensive medication management (i.e., MedMgt and Comb) were superior to those that did not include it (i.e., Beh and CC). Based on significance tests of means, the Beh and CC conditions were statistically equivalent. Likewise, the MedMgt and Comb groups were comparable, thus indicating no advantage of Comb relative to intensive MedMgt (MTA Cooperative Group, 1999a, 2004a). A few comments on these findings are warranted.

Some effects on ADHD symptoms were apparently mediated by medication effects (MTA Cooperative Group, 2004b). Therefore, it is important to note that 67% of the children in the CC group were taking medication, and thus that the CC group was an active treatment group rather than a no-treatment control. In other words, the group that received only behavior modification (Beh) was being compared to a group that received medications in the community. It is also important to consider the implications of the fact that there were some substantial differences in the doses of medication across the treatment groups. For instance, at the 14-month follow-up, the average daily dose (MPH equivalent) for Comb was 31.2 mg, while the average daily dose for MedMgt was 37.7 mg (MTA Cooperative Group, 1999a). Given that the Comb and MedMgt groups had identical medication titration procedures, the difference in dose at 14 months suggests that the intensive behavioral intervention allowed individuals to take lower

doses of medication. Lower doses are a considerable therapeutic advantage, because most stimulant side effects, including the mild growth suppression observed in the MTA, are dose-dependent (i.e., lower doses lessen the risk and severity of side effects; MTA Cooperative Group, 2004b).

When the group data are examined, it is tempting to conclude that the MedMgt condition was superior to CC, even though most of the participants in the CC group were medicated. Such a conclusion implies that the package of procedures in the MedMgt protocol, which includes monthly supportive contact and decisions supported by high-quality data, is superior to routine community care. Indeed, this has been one of the major messages from the MTA Cooperative Group (e.g., 2004a). However, it is noteworthy that the average dose (i.e., MPH equivalent) for children in the CC group who obtained treatment in the community was 22.6 mg/day (MTA Cooperative Group, 1999a). The fact that children receiving intensive medication management in the MTA (i.e., MedMgt and Comb) were taking the equivalent of 10–15 mg more MPH each day than the community control group is perplexing. In this situation, it is unclear whether the higher dose or some aspect of the MedMgt intervention, such as dosing three times per day in some cases, resulted in the better outcomes.

Another consideration in comparing the Beh and Comb conditions with MedMgt and CC is that intensive behavioral treatments were faded by the study's endpoint (Pelham, 1999). Due to this unequal treatment activity, it is plausible that the comparison of Beh and Comb to MedMgt at the 14-month follow-up may have been biased in favor of the MedMgt. This issue has been argued on theoretical grounds (see Pelham, 1999) and is consistent with the observation that the therapeutic effect size of intensive MedMgt diminished by 50% from the intensive phase to the follow-up phase (i.e., from the 14- to 24-month follow-up; MTA Cooperative Group, 2004a).

In our reading of the MTA data, as the fading becomes an increasingly distant past event, the trend in the data seems to be for the Comb group to outperform the other groups. However, according to the MTA Collaborative Group's statistical conclusion criteria, the differences between Comb and MedMgt are not yet statistically significant. Moreover, it appears that all treatments declined in effectiveness at the 2-year follow-up. Therefore, our conclusions regarding the superior efficacy of combined treatment in the MTA are open to alternative interpretation. However, as discussed below, the case for combined treatment is supported by analysis of outcomes other than group effects on ADHD symptoms.

Outcomes Other Than ADHD Symptoms

When measures of other disorders or domains of impairment besides ADHD symptoms are considered, most of the trends favor the Comb condition. For instance, when the MTA Cooperative Group ordered treatments by the number of times each group placed first compared with all others on 19 outcome measures, the results were as follows: Comb (12), MedMgt (4), Beh (2), and CC (1). The 4 times that MedMgt was superior were for parent ratings of symptoms of inattention and hyperactivity, and classroom observations of hyperactivity and impulsivity (MTA Cooperative Group, 1999a). Although such data appear to strongly favor combined treatment over unimodal or community interventions, this analysis does not take into account the relative importance of the outcome measures. We submit that the areas tapped, including oppositional/aggressive symptoms, internalizing symptoms, social skills, parent–child relations, and academic achievement, are critically important. That is, the non-ADHD domains assessed tap areas that are important in daily functioning and have a major impact on quality of life for youth with ADHD and those who interact with them on a daily basis.

It is also noteworthy that at the 14-month follow-up, satisfaction scores by parents for the Comb and Beh conditions were equal to each other and significantly better than parent satisfaction scores for the MedMgt condition (MTA Cooperative Group, 1999a). Given the emphasis placed on consumer satisfaction in terms of third-party payments, this is not a trivial matter. Indeed, the highest attrition rates were for the MedMgt condition.

The relative superiority of combined treatment was highlighted by Conners et al. (2001), who conducted a post hoc analysis using a composite outcome measure. This was done in an effort to further examine the relative impact of the MedMgt versus Comb conditions, which did not differ statistically due to the presence of multiple outcome measures in the primary analyses. When the composite measure was used, a statistically significant difference was detected: Comb outperformed MedMgt, with an effect size of 0.28 (low to moderate). In addition, use of the composite resulted in reduced effect sizes for comparisons of MedMgt versus Beh alone (0.26), and a moderate effect size of 0.35 for MedMgt versus CC. Use of the composite measure therefore places combined treatment in the lead, albeit by only about a quarter of a standard deviation. Also, a composite measure does result in more reliable estimates of effects, but effects may be obscured if treatments have idiosyncratic impacts on different aspects of functioning included in the composite.

At the 24-month MTA follow-up, the investigators focused on ADHD symptoms plus four other areas of outcome deemed to be important and validly measured (MTA Cooperative Group, 2004a). These areas were oppositional symptoms, social skills, negative/ineffective parenting, and reading achievement. In this analysis, which focused on group means, the MTA intensive medication groups (MedMgt and Comb) experienced a greater reduction in oppositional/aggressive symptoms. The mean for Comb was lower than that for MedMgt (1.34 vs. 1.42, respectively), and the p value was .081. Thus a directional one-tailed test with an alpha of .05 would have been statistically significant. However, the MTA Cooperative Group chose a two-tailed alpha of .01 for this particular comparison.

For the other three variables examined, the best results in terms of ordering of group means were achieved with Comb treatment. However, the omnibus F ratios for social skills, negative/ineffective parenting, and reading achievement were not statistically significant. Planned contrasts of two of the five outcomes were borderline statistically significant for Comb versus MedMgt. Specifically, Comb was better than MedMgt for social skills ($p = .05$) and negative/ineffective parenting ($p = .03$). No such differences were found for Beh versus CC. These results suggest that there may be clinically meaningful advantages of combined treatment over unimodal treatments.

Moderators and Mediators of Treatment Effects

"Mediators" and "moderators" are often confused, and therefore we begin this section with a brief review (see Holmbeck, 1997, for more on the mediator–moderator distinction). Moderators include participant characteristics that could affect outcome, either positively or negatively. Mediators are intervening variables operating during treatment that could have an impact on outcome. Knowledge of moderators helps in making decisions about who benefits from what treatment. Knowledge of mediators can help identify causal pathways from intervention to outcomes. The MTA Cooperative Group (1999b) has been careful to note that the mediator- and moderator-defined subgroup analyses are exploratory, because they are affected by sample size/power limitations and also suffer from the effects of repeated analyses.

As noted earlier, moderators were selected a priori and included gender, prior medication status, ODD or CD diagnoses, DSM-III-R anxiety disorder, and receipt of public assistance. Study outcomes did not vary as a function of gender, prior history of medication, or comorbid disruptive disorders. There were some differences for youth with comorbid anxiety disorders and those who received public assistance. In the group with comorbid anxiety, all MTA treatments outperformed treatment in the community (CC). This is an interesting finding, because the MTA treatments did not target anxiety. The reasons for the differential response pattern are not well understood (see Jensen et al., 1999).

For the families on public assistance, parents in the MedMgt condition reported less closeness in parent–child interactions, and teachers reported better social skills for the Comb group. As with the other moderator effect, the reasons for this apparent effect have been explored but remain elusive. For example, no differences were seen between the treatment conditions in terms of positive parenting or family stress measures (see Wells et al., 2000).

A mediator analysis that examined the role of medication in mediating outcomes has been reported (MTA Cooperative Group, 2004b). Another mediator analysis in the MTA focused on treatment acceptance/attendance (MTA Cooperative Group, 1999b). In the latter analysis, mediators were defined as acceptance of treatment and attendance at treatment sessions, specifically either as "as intended" or "below intended." Operational definitions included accepting the treatment assignment, as well as percentage of treatment sessions attended: for MedMgt, 80% medical visits attended with prescriptions written/delivered during the ses-

sions; and for Beh, 75% attendance at group parent training sessions and STP days, as well as a child's and a paraprofessional's being present together in the classroom for 75% of the possible days of this aspect of the intervention. Comb families needed to meet both sets of unimodal criteria in order to be placed in the "as intended" category. Interestingly, neither individual parent training session attendance nor teacher/therapist consultation visits—both vital portions of intensive behavioral intervention—were counted. In the "as intended" subgroup, the main intent-to-treat analyses held (MedMgt = Comb, and both better than CC and Beh). However, in the "below intended" subgroup, Comb was superior in terms of ADHD symptom reduction, with MedMgt = Beh (MTA Cooperative Group, 1999b). Thus there was an effect of compliance with treatment outcome, and the Comb condition was apparently more robust to noncompliance.

The NYM Multimodal Treatment Study

Although completed prior to the MTA study, another intensive multimodal treatment study has only recently been reported in the research literature. The results of the NYM study conflict with the MTA findings concerning the benefits of combined treatment over medication management alone. Due to the methodological advantages of the MTA compared to the NYM study, greater weight should be given to the MTA results. Nevertheless, the NYM study results might lessen the enthusiasm for intensive multimodal treatment.

The New York–Montreal (NYM) study selected 103 children with ADHD (ages 7–9 years) who were free of conduct problems and learning disorders, and who had shown an initial positive response to MPH during a short-term trial. Hence, unlike the MTA, the NYM study focused exclusively on stimulant-responsive children having far less comorbidity. These children were randomly assigned to receive 2 years of treatment in one of three treatment arms: (1) MPH alone; (2) MPH plus intensive multimodal psychosocial treatment; or (3) MPH plus an attention placebo psychosocial treatment. The latter approach to controlling for professional attention was not used in the MTA. The intensive 2-year psychosocial treatment consisted of behavioral parent training, parent counseling, social skills training, psychotherapy, and extra academic assistance.

Treatment contact during the first year of treatment was twice weekly, with fading of treatment to a considerable degree during the second year.

Assessments involved parent, teacher, and psychiatrist ratings; children's self-ratings; children's ratings of their parents; observations collected in school settings; and academic tests. The domains assessed included symptoms of ADHD and other behavioral problems (ODD), home and school functioning, social functioning, and academic performance. The results were consistent across all domains. No support was found for combining intensive psychosocial treatments of any sort with MPH in children with ADHD initially shown to be responsive to MPH (Abikoff, Hechtman, Klein, Gallacher, et al., 2004; Abikoff, Hechtman, Klein, Weiss, et al., 2004; Hechtman, Abikoff, Klein, Greenfield, et al., 2004; Hechtman, Abikoff, Klein, Weiss, et al., 2004). Nor was it found that MPH could be discontinued successfully in those who were receiving the combination treatment. Thus it appears that the set of psychosocial treatments used in this study produced no incremental benefit in children shown to have strong and unambiguous responses to stimulant medication. Although the authors made some statements that there may have been improvement from MPH, the study was not designed to test for benefit from medication, and uncontrolled confounds (such as maturation or regression to the mean) are plausible alternative explanations for what may seem like sustained improvement associated with MPH across the 2 years of treatment.

In contrast to the MTA, the NYM study did not include treatment within the children's usual school settings, nor did the children attend an intensive STP. Also unlike the MTA, this study intervened over a 24-month rather than a 14-month period. Lacking in both the MTA and the NYM study was documentation that the psychosocial treatments were effective. This contrasts with the assessment of medication effects, because each child received very well-controlled individualized trials that determined whether medication worked. It is noteworthy that some of the interventions in the NYM study (e.g., social skills training and individual therapy) are not currently regarded as effective treatments for ADHD (Smith et al., 2006). Furthermore, although the behavioral parent training was shown to achieve significant improvements in knowledge of behavioral methods, there was no reported change in parenting behavior (Hechtman, Abikoff, Klein, Weiss, et al., 2004). Thus there was no evidence that the psychosocial treatments met the requirement of showing activity at the point of performance.

Overall, then, the results of the NYM study may not represent a fair comparison of treatments, because high-grade treatment with MPH was compared with psychosocial treatments of unknown quality. A reasonable comparison of medication and psychosocial treatment should pit equivalent-quality treatments against each other (i.e., grade A medication and grade A psychosocial treatments). Such studies need to document that both treatments were delivered as intended with appropriate implementation at the point of performance. This is key with medication, because, according to the NYM study, poor compliance (as seen with the discontinuation probe) very rapidly results in deterioration. Psychosocial treatments should be evaluated with equal rigor, such as experimental analysis of the effectiveness of behavior contingencies by using reversal designs in the context of individual case studies. To our knowledge, no such study has yet been conducted, but some insights might be gained for further analysis of compliance data in the MTA and NYM research projects. Until studies of the highest-quality interventions and with the most rigorous quality control are implemented and properly analyzed, there will be lingering questions about the relative merits of intensive multimodal treatment relative to excellent medication management for the treatment of ADHD and related problems.

Efficacy, Safety, and Practicality of Combined Treatment

Although the literature indicates that some of the different treatments examined in multimodal treatment research deserves a separate grade of A for excellent evidence of efficacy, effectiveness, replicability, and safety, what is being graded here is the superiority of their combination relative to unimodal treatment. Is the evidence for the combined treatment sufficient to warrant this grade? (See Smith et al., 2006, for a discussion of grading treatment for ADHD.) Combined treatment has been shown to be superior to unimodal treatment on some measures in some subsets of children with ADHD in at least two well-designed studies by independent investigators. However, the recent NYM study that found no advantages of intensive multimodal treatment may raise some doubts. Due to the relative methodological strengths of the MTA compared to the NYM study, we believe that greater weight should be given to the MTA. Unfortunately, the studies that support the efficacy of combined treatment were conducted in research settings, which do not necessarily replicate the "real-world" settings in which most ADHD treatments are delivered. Thus we are inclined to give intensive multimodal treatment a grade of B for efficacy. Furthermore, based on which analysis one considers and how much weight is given to the MTA or the NYM studies, some might argue that combined treatment deserves a grade of C (see Smith et al., 2006).

The grade of B to C for intensive multimodal treatment is also intended to convey the message that the practicality of combined treatments is unknown. Indeed, there are several reasons to believe that these treatments would be very difficult to replicate in most applied settings. For instance, the acceptance/attendance data from the MTA found 81% compliance for the MedMgt component, but only 64% compliance for the Beh component (MTA Collaborative Group, 1999b). This suggests that there are some important issues to work out related to therapist expectations and family participation in the treatment. Moreover, the studies of combined treatment used some very unusual treatment components that are difficult to find in many regions of the country or to replicate in applied clinical settings, such as Pelham and colleagues' STP. Until barriers to access to and participation in these treatments are overcome, the effectiveness of combined treatment is open to doubt.

Generally speaking, combined treatment that uses family-based behavioral interventions and stimulant medication or atomoxetine should be very safe. There are some possible safety concerns related to the multimodal treatments of ADHD that have been studied. For example, some prominent theories related to conduct problems posit that placing children with behavior problems in groups with other disruptive children could lead to some harmful effects mediated by peer facilitation of antisocial behavior (Dishion, McCord, & Poulin, 1999). This was recently found to occur in a social skills training program for children with ADHD, particularly among those who were

not manifesting significant conduct problems prior to treatment (Antshel & Remer, 2003). Also, Barkley and colleagues have twice documented an adverse effect (escalation of conflicts) during behavioral family therapy for teens with ADHD/ODD in a subset of participating families (Barkley, Edwards, Laneri, Fletcher, & Metevia, 2001; Barkley, Guevremont, Anastopoulos, & Fletcher, 1992). Researchers studying behavioral interventions typically do not examine their data for such subsets of adverse responses, but should be encouraged by these results to do so.

Side effects of the medications warrant attention as well. Approximately 2.9% of children in the MTA reported having severe side effects, which apparently remitted with discontinuation of medication. Also, the MTA Collaborative Group (2004b) estimated that there was a growth suppression effect related to medication (approximately –1.23 cm/year in height and –2.48 kg/year in weight). Thus, although the treatments studied seem to be generally effective, potential risks warrant individual monitoring for potential iatrogenic effects; this is true both for medications and for some psychosocial treatments.

CONCLUSION

The treatment of children and teens with ADHD is an often complex and certainly longer-term enterprise than was previously thought to be necessary. Viewed now as a chronic disorder for most children, ADHD requires treatments that must be combined and sustained in order to have a long-term impact on these children's quality of life and developmental outcomes. Treatments appear to succeed by temporarily reducing or ameliorating symptoms for as long as treatments are in effect, so as to reduce the numerous secondary harms associated with unmanaged ADHD. Though numerous therapies have been proposed for this disorder, those having the greatest empirical support are contingency management methods applied in classrooms and elsewhere (summer camps); training of parents in these same methods to be used in the home and elsewhere (community settings); psychopharmacology, particularly stimulants and atomoxetine; and, to a lesser extent, the combination of behavioral treatments with medication. Evidence for cognitive-behavioral therapy is lacking at this time, while that for social skills training programs paints a mixed picture that is based mainly on studies having significant methodological limitations (see Antshel & Remer, 2003). Better-controlled and larger studies appear to show few or no treatment effects when the skills or behaviors are not cued and reinforced for occurring at the specific point of performance. Most cases require a combination of these more effective treatments in order to provide successful management of the disorder and its comorbid conditions. Among children who are already stimulant-responsive, it is not clear to what extent intensive psychosocial treatments provide added benefit. Interventions will need to be high-quality and sustained over several years (or more), and reintervention is highly likely as new developmental transitions occur and new domains of potential impairment now become available to individuals with ADHD across the lifespan.

KEY CLINICAL POINTS

✓ Most cases of ADHD will require a combination of treatments, including medication, parent training, and psychoeducational accommodations.

✓ Combined treatments offer the greatest likelihood of managing the symptoms of not only ADHD, but also many of its comorbid conditions.

✓ Combined treatments can also lead to a reduced need for or dosage of medication.

✓ Among children with a successful response to stimulants, the addition of low- to moderate-intensity psychosocial treatments appears to provide little further benefit for symptom management. That said, between 15% and 25% of children do not respond to stimulants and will need to depend exclusively on psychosocial treatments.

✓ Adding psychosocial to medical treatments can also assist with providing treatment coverage at times of the day when medications have worn off or cannot be employed.

✓ The treatment of children and teens with ADHD is an often complex and certainly longer-term enterprise than was previously thought to be necessary. Viewed now as a chronic disorder for most children, ADHD requires treatments that must be combined and sustained in order to have a long-term impact on these children's quality of life and developmental outcomes.

REFERENCES

Abikoff, H., Hechtman, L., Klein, R. G., Gallacher, R., Fleiss, K, Etcovitch, J., et al. (2004). Social functioning in children with ADHD treated with long-term methylphenidate and multimodal psychosocial treatment. *Journal of the American Academy of Child and Adolescent Psychiatry, 43,* 820–829.

Abikoff, H., Hechtman, L., Klein, R. G., Weiss, G., Fleiss, K, Etcovitch, J., et al. (2004). Symptomatic improvement in children with ADHD treated with long-term methylphenidate and multimodal psychosocial treatment. *Journal of the American Academy of Child and Adolescent Psychiatry, 43,* 802–811.

Antshel, K. M., & Remer, R. (2003). Social skills training in children with attention deficit hyperactivity disorder: A randomized–controlled clinical trial. *Journal of Clinical Child and Adolescent Psychology, 32,* 153–165.

Barkley, R. A. (1997). *Defiant children: A clinician's manual for assessment and parent training* (2nd ed.). New York: Guilford Press .

Barkley, R. A., Edwards, G., Laneri, M., Fletcher, K., & Metevia, L. (2001). The efficacy of problem-solving training alone, behavior management training alone, and their combination for parent–adolescent conflict in teenagers with ADHD and ODD. *Journal of Consulting and Clinical Psychology, 69,* 926–941.

Barkley, R. A., Guevremont, D. C., Anastopoulos, A. D., & Fletcher, K. E. (1992). A comparison of three family therapy programs for treating family conflicts in adolescents with attention-deficit hyperactivity disorder. *Journal of Consulting and Clinical Psychology, 60,* 450–462.

Barkley, R. A., Shelton, T. L., Crosswait, C., Moorehouse, M., Fletcher, K., Barrett, S., et al. (2000). Early psycho-educational intervention for children with disruptive behavior: Preliminary post-treatment outcome. *Journal of Child Psychology and Psychiatry, 41,* 319–332.

Brown, R. T., Borden, K. A., Wynne, M. E., Schleser, R., & Clingerman, S. T. (1986). Methylphenidate and cognitive therapy with ADD children: A methodological reconsideration. *Journal of Abnormal Child Psychology, 14,* 481–497.

Brown, R. T., Wynne, M. E., & Medenis, R. (1985). Methylphenidate and cognitive therapy: A comparison of treatment approaches with hyperactive boys. *Journal of Abnormal Child Psychology, 13,* 69–88.

Carlson, C. L., Pelham, W. E., Jr., Milich, R., & Dixon, J. (1992). Single and combined effects of methylphenidate and behavior therapy on the classroom performance of children with attention-deficit hyperactivity disorder. *Journal of Abnormal Child Psychology, 20,* 213–232.

Conners, C. K., Epstein, J. N., March, J. S., Angold, A., Wells, K. C., Klaric, J., et al. (2001). Multimodal treatment of ADHD in the MTA: An alternative outcome analysis. *Journal of the American Academy of Child and Adolescent Psychiatry, 40*, 159–167.

Dishion, T. J., McCord, J., & Poulin, F. (1999). When interventions harm: Peer groups and problem behavior. *American Psychologist, 54*, 755–764.

DuPaul, G. J., & Eckert, T. L. (1997). The effects of school-based interventions for attention deficit hyperactivity disorder: A meta-analysis. *School Psychology Digest, 26*, 5–27.

DuPaul, G. J., & Eckert, T. L. (1998). Academic interventions for students with attention-deficit/hyperactivity disorder: A review of the literature. *Reading and Writing Quarterly: Overcoming Learning Difficulties, 14*, 59–82.

DuPaul, G. J., & Stoner, G. (2003). *ADHD in the schools: Assessment and intervention strategies* (2nd ed.). New York: Guilford Press .

Firestone, P., Kelly, M. J., Goodman, J. T., & Davey, J. (1981). Differential effects of parent training and stimulant medication with hyperactives. *Journal of the American Academy of Child Psychiatry, 20*, 135–147.

Forehand, R., & McMahon, R. (1981). *Helping the noncompliant child: A clinician's guide to parent training*. New York: Guilford Press.

Gadow, K. D. (1985). Relative efficacy of pharmacological, behavioral, and combination treatments for enhancing academic performance. *Clinical Psychology Review, 5*, 513–533.

Hechtman, L., Abikoff, H., Klein, R. G., Greenfield, B., Etcovitch, J., Cousins, L., et al. (2004). Children with ADHD treated with long-term methylphenidate and multimodal psychosocial treatment: Impact on parental practices. *Journal of the American Academy of Child and Adolescent Psychiatry, 43*, 830–838.

Hechtman, L., Abikoff, H., Klein, R. G., Weiss, G., Respitz, C., Kouri, J., et al. (2004). Academic achievement and emotional status in children with ADHD treated with long-term methylphenidate and multimodal psychosocial treatment. *Journal of the American Academy of Child and Adolescent Psychiatry, 43*, 812–819.

Hinshaw, S. P., Henker, B., & Whalen, C. K. (1984a). Cognitive-behavioral and pharmacologic interventions for hyperactive boys: Comparative and combined effects. *Journal of Consulting and Clinical Psychology, 52*, 739–749.

Hinshaw, S. P., Henker, B., & Whalen, C. K. (1984b). Self-control in hyperactive boys in anger-inducing situations: Effects of cognitive-behavioral training and of methylphenidate. *Journal of Abnormal Child Psychology, 12*, 55–77.

Holmbeck, G. N. (1997). Toward terminological, conceptual, and statistical clarity in the study of mediators and moderators: Examples from the child-clinical and pediatric psychology literatures. *Journal of Consulting and Clinical Psychology, 65*, 599–610.

Horn, W. F., Chatoor, I., & Conners, C. K. (1983). Additive effects of dexedrine and self-control training: A multiple assessment. *Behavior Modification, 7*, 383–402.

Horn, W. F., Ialongo, N., Greenberg, G., Packard, T., & Smith-Winberry, C. (1990). Additive effects of behavioral parent training and self-control therapy with attention deficit hyperactivity disordered children. *Journal of Clinical Child Psychology, 19*, 98–110.

Horn, W. F., Ialongo, N., Pascoe, J. M., Greenberg, G., Packard, T., Lopez, M., et al. (1991). Additive effects of psychostimulants, parent training, and self-control therapy with ADHD children. *Journal of the American Academy of Child and Adolescent Psychiatry, 30*, 233–240.

Jensen, P. S., Kettle, L., Roper, M. T., Sloan, M. T., Dulcan, M. K., Hoven, C., et al. (1999). Are stimulants overprescribed?: Treatment of ADHD in four U. S. communities. *Journal of the American Academy of Child and Adolescent Psychiatry, 38*(7), 797–804.

McMahon, R. J., & Forehand, R. L. (2003). *Helping the noncompliant child: Family-based treatment for oppositional behavior* (2nd ed.). New York: Guilford Press.

MTA Cooperative Group. (1999a). A 14-month randomized clinical trial of treatment strategies for attention-deficit/hyperactivity disorder. *Archives of General Psychiatry, 56*, 1073–1086.

MTA Cooperative Group. (1999b). Moderators and mediators of treatment response for children with attention-deficit/hyperactivity disorder. *Archives of General Psychiatry, 56*, 1088–1096.

MTA Cooperative Group. (2004a). National Institute of Mental Health Multimodal Treatment Study of ADHD follow-up: 24–month outcomes of treatment strategies for attention-deficit/hyperactivity disorder. *Pediatrics, 113*, 754–761.

MTA Cooperative Group. (2004b). National Institute of Mental Health Multimodal Treatment Study of ADHD follow-up: Changes in effectiveness and growth after the end of treatment. *Pediatrics, 113*, 762–769.

Pelham, W. E. (1999). The NIMH Multimodal Treatment Study for Attention-Deficit Hyperactivity Disorder: Just say yes to drugs alone? *Canadian Journal of Psychiatry, 44*, 981–990.

Pelham, W. E., & Hoza, B. (1996). Intensive treatment: A summer treatment program for children with ADHD. In E. Hibbs & P. Jensen (Eds.), *Psychosocial treatments for child and adolescent disorders: Empirically based strategies for clinical practice* (pp. 311–340). Washington, DC: American Psychological Association.

Pelham, W. E., & Sams, S. E. (1992). Behavior modification. *Child and Adolescent Psychiatry Clinics of North America, 1*, 505–518.

Pelham, W. E., Schnedler, R. W., Bender, M. E., Nilsson, D. E., Miller, J., Budrow, M. S., et al. (1988). The combination of behavior therapy and methylphenidate in the treatment of attention deficit disorders: A therapy outcome study. In L. Bloomingdale (Ed.), *Attention deficit disorder* (Vol. 3, pp. 29–48). New York: Pergamon Press.

Pelham, W. E., Jr., Wheeler, T., & Chronis, A. (1998). Empirically supported psychosocial treatments for attention deficit hyperactivity disorder. *Journal of Clinical Child Psychology, 27*(2), 190–205.

Phelps, L., Brown, R. T., & Power, T. J. (2002). *Pediatric psychopharmacology: Combining medical and psychosocial interventions.* Washington, DC: American Psychological Association.

Pollard, S., Ward, E. M., & Barkley, R. . A. (1983). The effects of parent training and Ritalin on the parent–child interactions of hyperactive boys. *Child and Family Behavior Therapy, 5,* 51–69.

Satterfield, J. H., Cantwell, D. P., & Satterfield, B. T. (1979). Multimodality treatment: A one-year follow-up of 84 hyperactive boys. *Archives of General Psychiatry, 36,* 965–974.

Satterfield, J. H., Satterfield, B. T., & Cantwell, D. P. (1980). Multimodality treatment: A two-year evaluation of 61 hyperactive boys. *Archives of General Psychiatry, 37,* 915–919.

Satterfield, J. H., Satterfield, B. T., & Cantwell, D. P. (1981). Three-year multimodality treatment study of 100 hyperactive boys. *Journal of Pediatrics, 98,* 650–655.

Satterfield, J. H., Satterfield, B. T., & Schell, A. M. (1987). Therapeutic interventions to prevent delinquency in hyperactive boys. *Journal of the American Academy of Child and Adolescent Psychiatry, 26,* 56–64.

Shelton, T. L., Barkley, R. A., Crosswait, C., Moorehouse, M., Fletcher, K., Barrett, S., et al. (2000). Multimethod psychoeducational intervention for preschool children with disruptive behavior: Two-year post-treatment follow-up. *Journal of Abnormal Child Psychology, 28,* 253–266.

Smith, B. H., Barkley, R. A., & Shapiro, C. J. S. (2006). Attention-deficit/hyperactivity disorder. In E. J. Mash & R. A. Barkley (Eds.), *Treatment of childhood disorders* (3rd ed.). New York: Guilford Press.

Swanson, J. M., Kraemer, H. C., Hinshaw, S. P., Arnold, L. E., Conners, C. K., Abikoff, H. B., et al. (2001). Clinical relevance of the primary findings of the MTA: Success rates based on severity of ADHD and ODD symptoms at the end of treatment. *Journal of the American Academy of Child and Adolescent Psychiatry, 40,* 168–179.

Wells, C. K., Epstein, J. N., Hinshaw, S. P., Conners, C. K., Klaric, J., Abikoff, H. B., et al. (2000). Parenting and family stress treatment outcomes in attention deficit hyperactivity disorder (ADHD): An empirical analysis in the MTA study. *Journal of Abnormal Child Psychology, 28*(6), 543–553.

Wolraich, M., Drummond, T., Salomon, M. K., O'Brien, M. L., & Sivage, C. (1978). Effects of methylphenidate alone and in combination with behavior modification procedures on the behavior and academic performance of hyperactive children. *Journal of Abnormal Child Psychology, 6,* 149–161.

Psychological Counseling
of Adults with ADHD

KEVIN R. MURPHY

Most adults with Attention-Deficit/Hyperactivity Disorder (ADHD) have suffered years of feeling demoralized, discouraged, and ineffective because of a long-standing history of frustrations and failures in school, work, family, and social domains. Many report a chronic and deep-seated sense of underachievement and intense frustration over squandered opportunities, and are at a loss to explain why they cannot seem to translate their obvious assets into more positive outcomes. Furthermore, many report having heard a consistent barrage of complaints about themselves from parents, teachers, spouses/partners, friends, or employers regarding their behavioral, academic, interpersonal, or productivity shortcomings. The cumulative effect of such a history can sometimes lead to feelings of intense frustration and demoralization, and to a sense of anticipating failure as the predictable outcome of their efforts. Sadly, some appear so wedded to this belief system that they eventually give up believing life could be different for them. Many are completely unaware that their condition is a highly treatable one.

One of the aims of this chapter is to describe the importance of instilling hope, optimism, and motivation during the counseling of adults with ADHD, so that they can better understand their condition and be more inclined to engage in and follow through with a multimodal treatment plan. An important ingredient of this counseling is to help patients view their disorder from a perspective that empowers them to believe their lives can be different, and that encourages their active and enthusiastic involvement in treatment.

Other aims of this chapter are to describe some common emotional, attitudinal, and psychological consequences of living with ADHD in adulthood, and to discuss a range of non-pharmacological treatment approaches currently being used for ADHD in adults. The principles and treatments described are not new and in many ways are generic to psychosocial counseling with any psychiatric population. Such approaches as education about the disorder, cognitive restructuring, reframing the past, empowering, and instilling hope seem to lend themselves particularly well to the treatment of ADHD in adults. However, it must be emphasized that very little controlled research has been undertaken on psychosocial treatments with adults, so we are unable to draw firm scientific conclusions regarding their efficacy. For example, only one empirical study has been published exploring the usefulness of cognitive therapy in treating adults with ADHD (McDermott, 1999, 2000). The reality is that our treatment choices remain largely at the level of anecdotal evidence, clinical experience, common sense, and extrapolations from the child ADHD literature. Despite a proliferation of popular books describing a variety of psychosocial approaches—such as coaching; skills training; education about the disorder; and group, marital/couple, and individual counseling—there is still almost no scientific evidence available to support their efficacy. Consequently, this chapter is based almost entirely on collective clinical experience as to which psychosocial methods appear to benefit this population. Most practitioners would agree that pragmatic, behavioral skill-building, and self-management strategies are more useful for the types of issues adults with ADHD encounter than more traditional, nondirective, insight-oriented, psychodynamic approaches are. Nevertheless, the treatments discussed here should not be viewed as established conclusions from controlled scientific research.

ADULT CONSEQUENCES OF GROWING UP WITH ADHD

Some of the more common correlates associated with ADHD in adults are low self-esteem, avoidance/anxiety, depression, school and job performance problems, marital/couple discord, poorer driving outcomes, and substance abuse. Many adults with ADHD report low self-esteem as a result of years of frustration with their academic, work, social, and day-to-day family lives. They often report a long-standing and nagging sense of knowing something was wrong, but never knowing exactly what it was. In many cases they sought help from multiple mental health professionals who overlooked the possibility of ADHD and instead conceptualized their problems as related solely to mood, anxiety, or character disorders. Treatment for the underlying neurobiological condition (ADHD) that may be driving at least some of their behaviors/symptoms may never have even been considered, which may explain why many adult patients report past counseling experiences as not being especially helpful. Consequently, some end up attributing their problems to characterological or moral defects in themselves, and pay a heavy emotional price as

a result. This underscores the importance of reframing the disorder as neurobiological and not characterological, of rebuilding self-esteem and self-confidence, and of instilling hope for the future.

Other common consequences of having ADHD are anxiety about and avoidance of situations that have historically been unsuccessful or troublesome for the patient. One example of this avoidance concerns the idea of returning to school. Some adults seen in ADHD clinics have expressed a desire to return to school, but are understandably hesitant because of their prior record of school struggles. They fear that they will fail again, and they wish to avoid another setback. They report that if they had reason to believe that their school experience might be different this time, they would be more willing to attempt it. But for many it is safer not to try, so they avoid school, even though deep down they have a strong desire to go. This is indeed unfortunate for some, because proper diagnosis, treatment, and motivation can open new possibilities and potentially make the difference between success and failure in school.

Another example concerns social/interpersonal relationships. In part because of their impulsivity, interrupting, forgetfulness, inattentiveness, hyperactivity, difficulty reading social cues, temper, and/or mood swings, adults with ADHD frequently report having difficulty maintaining friendships. Others may view their behavior as rude, insensitive, irresponsible, or obnoxious, and their peers may sometimes ostracize them. Some associate social interaction with embarrassment, disappointment, criticism, or failure. When confronted with future opportunities for social interaction, these adults with ADHD sometimes withdraw or avoid others to protect themselves. Again, treatment can sometimes improve their verbal and behavioral impulsivity, disinhibition, and focusing/listening ability, and as a result can improve their overall social functioning.

Depression is another relatively common consequence associated with adult ADHD. Approximately 35% of a cohort of adult patients I evaluated at the University of Massachusetts Medical School (UMASS) Adult ADHD Clinic during the mid-1990s met criteria for either Major Depressive Disorder or Dysthymic Disorder at some time in their lives (Murphy, Barkley, & Bush, 2002). In another study from the UMASS Adult ADHD Clinic, we (Murphy & Barkley, 1996) compared 172 adults diagnosed with ADHD to 30 adults who were not so diagnosed; we found that the group with ADHD showed a significantly greater prevalence of oppositional, conduct, and substance use disorders, as well as greater illegal substance abuse, than did control adults. Moreover, adults with ADHD displayed greater self-reported psychological maladjustment, more driving risks (speeding violations), and more frequent changes in employment. Significantly more of these adults also experienced suspension of their driver's licenses, performed poorly, quit or were fired from their jobs, had a history of poorer educational performance, and had more frequent school disciplinary actions against them than did adults without ADHD. Multiple marriages were more likely in the group with ADHD as well. Some adults with ADHD have become so demoralized over their past failures, and over being misunderstood and mistreated by others, that they require concurrent treatment for a mood disorder.

Finally, as suggested above, a substantial minority of adults with ADHD gravitate toward substance abuse—possibly as a way of relaxing or calming the mental restlessness they often experience. Some studies suggested that those with ADHD are at increased risk for developing substance use problems (Weiss & Hechtman, 1993; Mannuzza, Gittelman-Klein, Bessler, Malloy, & LaPadula, 1993; Murphy & Barkley, 1996; Murphy et al., 2002; see also Chapter 6, this volume). Approximately one-third of the patients seen at the UMASS Adult ADHD Clinic during the 1990s met criteria for substance abuse or dependence at some point in their lives. Many appeared to be self-medicating in an attempt to soothe their underlying ADHD symptoms. Most reported using alcohol and/or marijuana as their primary drugs of choice. The UMASS Clinic found that after these patients were treated with stimulant medication, a fair number of them reported improvement not only in their ADHD symptoms, but also in their substance abuse. Others have also found this to be true (Schubiner et al., 1995). One possible hypothesis is that the stimulant medication may quell the desire to self-medicate. My colleagues and I therefore do not routinely disqualify patients with ADHD and substance *abuse* from medication treatment. To do so may be depriving these patients of a potentially important and needed treatment. We do not immediately medicate those with active

substance *dependence*; they get referred for treatment of the substance dependence before undergoing any treatment for ADHD. In most cases, it is suggested that at least 1–2 months of stable sobriety be achieved in patients with substance dependence before medication for ADHD is introduced. Those with comorbid substance abuse/dependence and ADHD require close follow-up to monitor progress and safety. Clearly, the relationship between ADHD and substance use disorders warrants further scientific investigation.

An important goal for professionals who treat adults with ADHD is to respond to these and any other negative sequelae of living with ADHD in a way that instills hope; fosters personal potency; and empowers the patients to believe that with a combination of treatment, support, perseverance, and hard work, their lives *can* be improved. Despite the absence of data to back up this suggestion, common sense would suggest it to be a reasonable place to start.

EXPLAINING THE ADHD DIAGNOSIS

Treatment for adults with ADHD begins at the time they are diagnosed. How clinicians communicate the diagnosis to them is critical to both their understanding of the disorder and their willingness to engage in and persist with treatment. If clinicians can help patients understand the disorder, offer a plausible rationale for how it causes their symptoms, frame it as something that is treatable, and instill hope and optimism for their future, patients are more likely to feel motivated to work at and follow through with treatment. Increased knowledge and understanding of the disorder, and continuing involvement in treatment, are likely to increase the chances of more positive outcomes. Conversely, if patients are left with only a vague notion of what ADHD is, are confused or unsure of how they might be helped, and are not activated to feel hope, they are far less likely to embrace treatment, persevere, and achieve a positive outcome. Many adult patients who visited the UMASS Adult ADHD Clinic during the 1990s reported having had prior ADHD evaluations, and yet they appeared to have very little understanding of ADHD, did not understand the impact it had on their lives, and were either unaware of or not taking advantage of the range of available treatments. The disorder was apparently never adequately explained to them. Clinicians can have substantial control over the feedback process and have an opportunity to influence whether patients become actively engaged or disengaged from treatment. The framework described next may assist clinicians in developing strategies and skills to explain the diagnosis more effectively to adults.

Providing a Rationale for ADHD and Comorbid Diagnoses

Perhaps the most important nonpharmacological strategy for adults with ADHD is to educate themselves as much as possible about the disorder. Most of these adults have little knowledge of ADHD and do not fully understand the pervasive impact it can have on their day-to-day lives. Having a sound and informed knowledge base can help adults make sense of what has been troubling them, help them set realistic and attainable goals, and ease their frustration. Just knowing that there is a neurobiological reason for many of their struggles, and that this reason has a name, can be therapeutic in itself. The realization that somebody finally "gets it" and truly understands their lifelong difficulties can also be extraordinarily therapeutic. Once these adults are accurately diagnosed by a professional who understands ADHD, there is often a sense of tremendous relief at finally having an explanation for their long-standing difficulties.

The clinician can begin by explaining the rationale for arriving at the diagnosis of ADHD and any comorbid conditions. Providing such an explanation can help demystify the diagnosis and put it in the context of each patient's own unique life experience. For example, explaining all of the following can help a patient begin to understand ADHD: (1) The patient and a spouse/partner or parent have endorsed a sufficient number of the symptoms of ADHD, according to the fourth edition, text revision, of the *Diagnostic and Statistical Manual of Mental Disorders* (DSM-IV-TR; American Psychiatric Association, 2000); (2) the onset of symptoms occurred in early childhood; (3) the symptoms have caused chronic and pervasive impairment in academic, social, vocational, or daily adaptive functioning; (4) the patient has no other psychiatric or medical condition that could better explain the ADHD symptoms; and (5) he or she has a behavioral, school, and/or work history reflecting typical impairments associated with the diagnosis.

Reframing the Past

An important next step is to continue educating each patient about what ADHD is and how it affects his or her life. Learning about ADHD is especially important at the beginning of treatment but should be viewed as a lifelong endeavor as the disorder plays out over time and across situations. Patients need to have at least a general understanding that they have a neurological condition, not a character defect or moral weakness. The realization that many of the problems they have experienced stem from neurological causes rather than from laziness or low intelligence can begin the process of repairing self-esteem. Often patients have internalized negative messages over the years from parents, teachers, spouses/partners, and employers, who have concluded that they are stupid, lazy, incompetent, immature, or unmotivated. It should be explained that the likely reason for many of the problems they experienced in school, work, and/or social relationships was a subtle neurobiological deficit in the brain over which they had little control. Their problems were not the result of deliberate misbehavior, low intelligence, or lack of effort. These misguided and damaging perceptions should be recast in a more positive and hopeful light, so patients can begin to rebuild their self-confidence and believe that successful treatment is possible. As a consequence, patients will ideally be in a better position to break out of the shackles of feeling stuck, demoralized, and chronically frustrated.

Patients also need to understand that they themselves are a potent force in their treatment, and that what they do from this point forward will have a huge bearing on their final outcome. Patients need to accept their disorder and do their part by actively engaging in treatment, practicing new skills, communicating honestly about obstacles they are encountering, dealing with inevitable setbacks, taking medication consistently, and making a genuine and persistent effort at accomplishing changes in their lives. Educating spouses/partners, family members, and friends is also important, so that those others can understand and be better able to help. A common knowledge base can help patients, spouses/partners, and family members cope more effectively and establish realistic goals and expectations.

Instilling Hope

Another important aspect of setting the stage for successful treatment is *instilling hope*. Hope is a key ingredient and a necessary starting point. Whether they are battling a life-threatening illness, facing difficult surgery, recovering from physical or psychological trauma, or learning to cope with ADHD, patients need to feel hope. Without hope for a better future, there is little chance that patients will engage in or persist in treatment long enough to accomplish significant gains. To achieve an optimal outcome, patients need to feel their clinicians are partners with them and sincerely believe they can be helped. If clinicians are genuine in their desire to become involved in helping, and this is clearly evident to patients, it can go a long way toward instilling hope and motivation in the patients. Conversely, if clinicians are perceived by patients as merely technicians performing their routine in a relatively uninvolved manner, the opposite is true. Caring, support, compassion, and encouragement are crucial ingredients, and their importance should never be underestimated. The pressures of the managed care environment and the reality of doing more in less time with fewer resources can make this a real challenge in today's health care environment. Nevertheless, the message that should come through loud and clear is that with proper treatment—including education, counseling, medication, behavioral strategies, hard work, advocacy, and the support of family and friends—adults with ADHD can make significant and sometimes dramatic improvements in their lives.

As an additional educational resource, providing a packet of educational literature to patients at the end of the evaluation may be helpful. This may include a fact sheet about ADHD; a list of books, magazines, or newsletters that may be useful to them; websites of advocacy organizations, such as Children and Adults with Attention-Deficit/Hyperactivity Disorder (CHADD; *www.chadd.org*) or the Attention Deficit Disorder Association (ADDA; *www.add.org*); brief articles on relevant topics, such as ADHD in college or the workplace; and/or information sheets on medication (cop-

ies of fact sheets on a wide range of medications can be found in Dulcan & Lizarralde, 2003). Although we have no scientific proof that such educational literature is useful (or even actually read), it is hoped that providing this type of immediately relevant educational material can promote better understanding and help motivate some patients to engage in ongoing treatment.

It can also be helpful to provide some specific examples of treatment strategies that are relevant to the problems the patients are currently experiencing. For example, patients who are disorganized and forgetful may benefit from training in prioritizing and list making, keeping an appointment calendar, posting visual reminders in strategic locations, blocking out time in schedules for priority tasks, breaking large tasks down into smaller units, building minirewards into projects, and the like. For patients who are college students, it could be useful to describe some specific types of classroom modifications, lifestyle or class schedule adjustments, study skills, or other accommodations that are appropriate and justified given the nature of their difficulties.

Providing education to patients about medication also seems important. Explaining how medication may help patients improve the quality of their lives by enhancing their ability to focus and concentrate and curb their impulsivity may provide further hope and motivation. Explaining how their lives may be different if they respond well to medication by using actual examples from their personal histories may be useful. Taking the time to answer questions about side effects, and providing enough factual information for patients to make informed decisions regarding medication, also appear useful. Patients often have mistaken notions and unrealistic fears/myths about medication that need to be addressed before they agree to try it. Providing fact sheets (as mentioned earlier) in addition to these verbal explanations can give them further information to share with family or friends.

It is important to understand that treatment should not be approached with the idea that ADHD can be "cured," because at present there is no treatment or combination of treatments that can cure the disorder. Instead, it is more accurate to approach treatment in terms of symptomatic relief, or learning how to manage symptoms and cope with the challenges that the disorder presents across the lifespan. A central tenet of treatment is to assist patients in becoming "the best that they can be" by helping them to focus and build on their strengths and learn to compensate better for their weaknesses (Murphy, 1995).

Instilling hope for the future, balanced with the reality that changing habits and behavioral patterns requires hard work and sustained effort, can foster a realistic attitude toward treatment. Clinicians can exert a strong influence in constructing a therapeutic atmosphere of hope and optimism, to counter the demoralization and pessimism so often experienced by adults with ADHD. Equipped with this combination of hope, knowledge, and awareness of ADHD, adults with ADHD should be in a much better position to benefit from treatment, to learn to adapt better to current tasks and responsibilities, and to lead more fulfilling lives than had previously been the case.

PSYCHOSOCIAL TREATMENT APPROACHES

A combination of treatments is usually recommended for adults with ADHD. Again, treatment of the individual with ADHD does not produce a cure for the underlying cause of the disorder. Treatment is aimed at symptom reduction and minimizing the negative effects of the disorder to improve one's overall quality of life. Despite the fact that prior research has demonstrated that clinic-based treatments focused on skill training, such as social skills, self-control, or cognitive-behavioral training, have not been of much benefit to those with ADHD (Abikoff, 1985, 1987; Diaz & Berk, 1995), and that short-term psychosocial treatment effects do not generalize outside the context in which they are applied (Abikoff & Gittelman, 1984; Barkley, 1997b; Barkley, Copeland, & Sivage, 1980), the management of behavior in the immediate environments in which it is problematic for those with ADHD is a laudable goal (Barkley, 1997a). As Barkley (1997a) states,

> Only a treatment which can result in improvement or normalization of the underlying neuropsychological deficit in behavioral inhibition is likely to result in an improvement or normalization of the executive functions dependent on such inhibition. To date, the only treatment that exists that has any hope of achieving this end is stimulant medication or other pharmacological agents

that improve or normalize the neural substrates in the prefrontal regions that likely underlie this disorder. (p. 60)

Does this mean that all psychosocial treatment approaches have no value in assisting adults in coping with their ADHD? Of course not. In fact, more recent research, such as the National Institute of Mental Health's Multimodal Treatment Study of ADHD (MTA Cooperative Group, 1999; see Chapter 20), the largest randomized treatment study ever undertaken, found that psychosocial treatments in combination with medication resulted in the best outcomes in some circumstances. Psychosocial treatment may not "cure" the underlying brain dysfunction that gives rise to core ADHD symptoms, as the quotation above is meant to assert, but it may well help to improve the side effects, emotional sequelae, and/or comorbid conditions often associated with ADHD.

The most common types of psychosocial treatments used in treating adults with ADHD include individual counseling, group counseling, family and marital/couple counseling, vocational counseling, coaching, use of technological aids, and advocacy.

Individual Counseling

The initial stage of individual counseling usually includes information/education about ADHD, outlining goals, developing strategies to meet those goals, and dealing with any acute conflicts or crises that may be present. Followup meetings monitor progress, discuss medication issues, add or alter treatment approaches, and work on improving specific areas of difficulty. Examples may be problem solving about a specific work, school, or relationship situation; assisting with life transitions, such as a career change or a divorce; dealing with comorbid mood or anxiety disorders; or working on organizational and time management skills. Individual counseling can bring adults with ADHD increased awareness of how the disorder affects their lives, and can thereby help to identify appropriate behavioral/self-management strategies to better manage symptoms. Understanding the disorder can also influence immediate and future life decisions. For example, knowledge of ADHD can influence one's job choice, choice of spouse/partner, choice of major in school, or decisions about whether to return to school and where (preferably one with an established program for assisting students with ADHD/learning disabilities). Acquiring this kind of self-knowledge can assist adults with ADHD in making better choices and goodness-of-fit decisions.

Adults with ADHD may also benefit from individual counseling on behavior modification principles and strategies. Treatment for ADHD appears to respond best to an active and pragmatic approach on the part of both therapist and patient. In general, the more structure and routine that can be incorporated into a patient's life, the better. Most often, the goals of treatment are to change disruptive behavior and thought patterns that consistently interfere in day-to-day functioning. Patients usually prefer utilizing strategies that will help them function more effectively right now, as opposed to a long-term, insight-oriented approach. Stated another way, they would rather implement a behavior plan today to prevent daily loss of their car keys than explore and attempt to interpret the underlying meaning of this behavior. Behavior therapy and cognitive therapy are two forms of individual counseling thought to be particularly useful to adults with ADHD. Specifically, training in methods of time management, organizational skills, communication skills, anger control, decision making, self-monitoring and reward, chunking large tasks into a series of smaller steps, and changing faulty cognitions are thought to be potentially helpful in more efficiently meeting the demands of daily work, family, and social life. Such training helps patients to develop explicitly stated goals, specific methods on how to accomplish goals, and established time frames for meeting goals. In essence, the same sorts of suggestions that may prove useful to children with ADHD in school may also be of value to adults with ADHD when upgraded to their performance contexts. Implementing behavioral strategies to target the most impairing problems can help patients gain greater control over their lives, reduce anxiety and frustration, and improve productivity. Providing patients with the following suggestions, and helping them to develop or improve proficiency in these areas, may be beneficial:

- Practice proactive planning by setting aside time every evening to plan for the next day. Get needed materials ready (e.g., books, clothes, keys, phone numbers, medication,

important papers), pack the car the night before, or do whatever else that will prevent frantic chaos the next day.
- Learn how to make an effective and reasonable "to do" list of important tasks and priorities, and keep it with you at all times. Make additional copies in case it gets lost or misplaced.
- Remind yourself by keeping important tasks visually in sight by posting appointments, "to do" lists, or schedules in strategic areas at home and at work.
- Practice using an appointment book, a Palm Pilot or other personal digital assistant (PDA), or a daily planning calendar, and learn to write down appointments and commitments immediately.
- Keep notepads in strategic locations (car, bathroom, bedroom, etc.), or have a portable tape recorder handy to capture important ideas and thoughts that cross your mind and that you wish to remember.
- Learn and practice time management skills. Purchase a programmable alarm watch to cue you so you do not lose track of time.
- Use a color-coded file system, desk and closet organizers, storage boxes, or other organizational devices to reduce clutter and improve efficiency and structure in your life. Consider hiring a professional organizer to assist in creating a workable system for you; this may include ensuring that bills are paid on time, balancing the checkbook, and decluttering your living space.
- Make multiple sets of keys, so that losing one set is not a disaster.

Preparing patients for the expected and inevitable feelings of disappointment and frustration when setbacks occur can also be helpful. Rather than viewing setbacks as catastrophic failures or evidence of incompetence, patients can be helped to conceptualize them as "normal," expected, and even desirable, because they represent opportunities for learning and personal growth. For example, adults with ADHD may conclude that making lists or using an appointment book is fruitless, because they frequently lose them. Explaining that changing habits and learning new strategies require ongoing practice and are not one-trial affairs may help them to keep trying. The goal is to continue practicing each skill until it becomes an automatic and natural part of a daily routine.

Ultimately, patients must make a conscious commitment to working on behavioral change, view it as a crucial investment in their future, and elevate mastering these skills to a priority in their lives. Individual counseling aimed at erasing long-standing negative messages from teachers, parents, spouses/partners, and employers, and replacing these with more rational and optimistic messages, is another area of potential benefit to adults with ADHD.

It also seems important to emphasize and make explicit the strengths and positive traits that patients possess. For example, informing patients that their testing results indicated average, above-average, or superior native intelligence can sometimes be a powerful revelation. Explaining that their lower-than-expected grades throughout their school history had nothing to do with low intelligence can provide a strong measure of relief to adults who may well have lived their lives believing the opposite. Another example is to point out positive character traits observed in patients, such as tenacity, willingness to keep trying despite many setbacks, boundless energy and drive, assertiveness, sense of humor, or whatever else is appropriate. This may serve to counterbalance negative self-perceptions, to reinforce strengths, and to promote self-acceptance.

In summary, individual counseling may be helpful in assisting adults with ADHD to cope with a variety of coexisting problems, including depression, anxiety, low self-esteem, interpersonal problems, and disorganization.

Group Treatment

Although again no scientific data as yet support the efficacy of group therapy for ADHD, it seems a potentially useful intervention for adults with the disorder. It has the potential to be a powerful method of support, education, and validation for those with ADHD. Patients can learn a great deal from each other, feel accepted, and feel less isolated and alone. One of my patients who participated in a support group had previously refused to take medication; he ended up changing his mind after discussing the issue with fellow group members and receiving their input. Clearly, the group influenced him to try the medication where I as his individual therapist had been unsuccessful. In addition to the support and validation offered by the group, hearing how others cope and manage their symptoms, realizing that there are others with similar problems, and having a "laboratory" for learning and trying out new social and interpersonal skills can all be helpful to group members.

In my experience, it is best to have a time-limited and semistructured group format, with target goals and themes for each session. A balanced mixture of some didactic instruction with time for open-ended discussion has worked best in the groups I have facilitated. Ongoing, open-ended, "here-and-now" types of groups can rapidly become chaotic and disorganized, and can be difficult to lead and manage. The topics that I and my colleagues at Wayne State University, Angela Tzelepis and Howard Schubiner, have utilized include medication issues, organizational skills, listening/interpersonal skills, anger control, decision making, stress reduction, vocational/workplace issues, and personal coping strategies. With a skilled group therapist, and a motivated and carefully screened group of preferably no more than 10, group therapy can be a useful adjunct to other forms of treatment. Participating in local support group organizations such as CHADD is another avenue for support and education.

Family and Marital/Couple Counseling

Family and marital/couple therapy may also be potentially useful for resolving difficulties that affect relationships in family members and spouses. ADHD can wreak havoc on marital/couple and family functioning, because it can be so disruptive to the routine tasks of daily living. A significant percentage of the spouses without ADHD I assessed at the UMASS Adult ADHD Clinic during the 1990s reported severe marital dissatisfaction as measured by their Locke–Wallace Marital Inventory scores (Murphy & Barkley, 1996). Spouses and partners of adults with ADHD who do not have ADHD themselves often report feeling confused, angry, and frustrated. They may complain that the adults with ADHD are poor listeners, are unreliable, are forgetful, are self-centered or insensitive, often seem distant or preoccupied, are messy, do not finish household projects, or behave irresponsibly. Gaining a greater understanding of the disorder, and realizing that many of these problems may not necessarily stem from "willful misconduct," may enable the members of a couple to take a fresh look at their problems from an ADHD perspective, stop blaming each other, and begin to align together as a team to reduce conflict. For this to be successful, however, a patient's spouse or partner must perceive the patient to be making a sincere and legitimate effort at behavioral change. If the patient uses the ADHD as an excuse to justify continued behavioral problems without demonstrating an observable commitment to behavioral change, there will be little chance for improvement in the relationship. Framing the situation as a family problem, instead of pointing the finger at the "identified patient," can help to reduce defensiveness. If both spouses/partners have a mutual understanding of how ADHD affects their relationship, understand what each needs from the other, and work together as a team in improving the family situation, the chances for a positive outcome are greatly enhanced. (For more detailed discussions of marital/couple and family issues, readers are referred to Dixon, 1995; Nadeau, 1995; Ratey, Hallowell, & Miller, 1995; Hallowell, 1995).

Working together as a unified and cohesive team is especially important in families where both a parent and a child have the disorder. When multiple family members have ADHD, this adds another layer of complexity and challenge to effective family functioning. The potential for conflict, stress, lack of follow-through, miscommunication, and family chaos is much higher when both parents and children have the disorder. Ideally, each will seek their own individual treatment to manage his or her symptoms. They will also likely benefit from family counseling to explore ways of managing conflict, improving communication and follow-through, and increasing family harmony. Key ingredients are focusing on incorporating a structured daily routine to aid in staying organized and reducing forgetfulness, and maintaining a sense of humor—especially when inevitable setbacks occur.

Vocational Counseling

Workplace problems can be particularly troublesome to many adults with ADHD. One study Russell Barkley and I completed at the UMASS Adult ADHD Clinic found that, compared with controls, adults with ADHD had significantly more impulsive quitting, terminations, and chronic employment difficulties (Murphy & Barkley, 1996). Impulsivity, inattention, careless mistakes, disorganization, poor time management, tardiness, short temper, missing deadlines, and inconsistency are just some of the things that can interfere in job performance. Most adults with ADHD who experience workplace problems do so not because of incompetence or lack of effort, but because their jobs are ill suited to their strengths. They frequently leave jobs because of boredom or inability to tolerate what they perceive as a boring and tedious daily routine. Vocational counseling aimed at identifying strengths and limitations and matching patients to jobs that "fit" for them is of critical importance for many adults with ADHD. It may involve vocational testing to identify interests and aptitudes, job coaching and training, or advocacy with potential employers. Unfortunately, the need for such services greatly outweighs the availability of skilled resources. Nevertheless, successful vocational adjustment is not only central to individual well-being and self-esteem, but can have a positive effect on family and marital/couple functioning, as well as family financial health. If an adult with ADHD can find a successful occupational niche, it may increase chances for ongoing vocational success, reduce boredom, and (ideally) result in a greater sense of confidence, self-esteem, and personal satisfaction.

Coaching

Another potentially helpful area of intervention for adults with ADHD is personal coaching. Although again no empirical data support the efficacy of coaching for these adults, it appears to be gaining popularity as an adjunctive treatment for adults. The Personal and Professional Coaches Association defines coaching as "an ongoing relationship which focuses on the client taking action toward the realization of their vision, goals, or desires." It further states that "coaching uses a process of inquiry and personal discovery to build the client's level of awareness and responsibility, and provides the client with structure, support, and feedback." Coaching is a supportive, pragmatic, and collaborative process in which a coach and an adult with ADHD work together (usually via daily 10- to 15-minute telephone conversations) to identify goals and strategies to meet those goals. Because most adults with ADHD have difficulty persisting in effort over long periods and often cannot sustain ongoing motivation to complete tasks, coaches can assist them in staying on task by offering encouragement, support, structure, accountability, and at times gentle confrontation. There is no standard methodology. The coaching relationship is tied to the needs and desires of each patient and can be structured in any way that is acceptable to the coach and the person being coached. Some may talk with their coaches on a daily basis, and others far less frequently. Some may correspond via e-mail. The intended outcome is to assist adults with ADHD to take charge of and better manage their lives by learning to set realistic goals and stay on task to reach those goals, in an atmosphere of encouragement and supportive understanding. Although we await future results of scientific inquiry into the effectiveness of coaching, it is likely to continue to be a frequent treatment recommendation for the adult population with ADHD. For a more detailed discussion of coaching, see Ratey (2002).

Technology

Professionals who work with adults with ADHD should be aware of technological advances that offer valuable and much needed assistance to people struggling with ADHD. A variety of tools and devices can help greatly in communication, writing, spelling, keeping track of time, and the like. Word processors and programs with spell-check and grammar-check options can aid in writing and spelling more quickly, legibly, and effectively. PDAs offer a wide range of components including an electronic address book, a planner/calendar, "to do" list, and notepad. Cell phones, text messaging, and e-mail make communication easier, more spontaneous, and faster. Many software programs are available to assist with personal finances and taxes. Websites devoted to organizational skills, time management, and just about any other relevant topic are immediately available on the Internet. Electronic banking offers online bill paying, including setting up automatic payments at regular intervals to protect against delinquent payments and late fees. Books on tape and voice-activated word-processing programs can assist in learning and writing. These sorts of devices and interventions should be used whenever appropriate, but will require time, practice, and persistence to master.

ADVOCACY

Self-advocacy is an important and sometimes overlooked skill, and can be a key to success on the job, in an academic environment, or in other life situations. It is crucial that individuals create a strong foundation for self-advocacy by developing both an understanding of their own ADHD and the ability to explain their strengths and weaknesses to others (Roffman, 2000). Rehearsing or role-playing with a counselor a succinct explanation of what ADHD is, how it interferes in functioning, and what is needed to accommodate it can be helpful in achieving the necessary confidence and skill. A key ingredient to successful self-advocacy is thorough, professional documentation. When patients are armed with high-quality documentation, their chances of having others understand their challenges and view their situation as credible are much higher. The value of developing self-advocacy skills should never be underestimated.

Regardless of how good a person's self-advocacy skills are, there are times when a professional advocate will be beneficial. In high-stakes situations such as eligibility for test accommodations or workplace accommodations—especially when supervisors or professors refuse to believe or accommodate a diagnosis—professional advocacy may be necessary. Examples of situations where professional advocacy can make a significant difference include attending special education or individualized education plan meetings, writing letters of recommendation for college or job applications, writing comprehensive reports for test accommodation eligibility, meeting with supervisors or professors to explain the diagnosis and reasons for accommodation, participating in disciplinary meetings, and participating in a workplace discussions about appropriate job modifications or placements. A qualified professional who fully understands a patient's situation can enhance the patient's self-advocacy by adding explanatory power and additional credibility.

FINAL COMMENTS

A subgroup of the adult population with ADHD may need additional treatment for specific problems that may coexist with ADHD, such as substance abuse/dependence, credit counseling/money management, eating disorders, or anxiety and mood disorders. Because those with ADHD are at greater risk for developing comorbid problems, treatment efforts need to take into account the totality of each patient's problems.

Whatever combination of treatments is used for a given patient, it is likely that intervention will need to be extended over long time intervals, much like the management of a chronic medical illness such as diabetes (Barkley, 1994). In general, treatments and lifestyle habits will need to be maintained consistently over long periods of time to sustain optimal benefit. If treatments are removed or discontinued, the symptoms and associated impairment are likely to resurface within a short time. This is why a major goal of treatment is to work toward instilling lifelong habits and permanent lifestyle changes, rather than short-term, transient, or quick-fix strategies. For example, when a clinician is counseling a college student on developing time management and organizational skills, these should not be viewed as short-term tools for merely achieving a grade, passing a test, or getting to a class on time. Rather, they should be taught in the context of life skills training for the long haul. These are examples of skills and habits that, when put into practice as part of a daily routine, will have a positive ripple effect in all aspects of life, including work, social, marital/couple, and daily adaptive functioning. Periodic follow-up for support, adjustment to treatment, academic or workplace advocacy, or new interventions as life circumstances change will probably be necessary for most adults with ADHD in the ongoing management of their disorder.

KEY CLINICAL POINTS

✓ ADHD is a disorder that can be effectively treated with both medication and psychosocial approaches.

✓ To date, very little well-controlled, scientific research has been done on nonpharmacological treatments for adult ADHD. Therefore, from a scientific standpoint, we do not yet have sound empirical data on how efficacious any of these approaches are in either managing symptoms or improving long- and short-term outcomes.

✓ Comorbidity is common with ADHD, so clinicians will need to incorporate treatments for both ADHD and the range of coexisting diagnoses that often accompany ADHD, including mood and anxiety disorders and substance abuse.

✓ Explaining the ADHD diagnosis in an understandable way that instills hope and activates patients to be active participants in their treatment is important for improving chances for more positive outcomes.

✓ Multimodal treatment that combines medication, education, behavioral/self management skills, a variety of counseling approaches, coaching, and either academic or workplace accommodations is likely to result in the best outcomes.

REFERENCES

Abikoff, H. (1985). Efficacy of cognitive training interventions in hyperactive children: A critical review. *Clinical Psychology Review, 5,* 479–512.

Abikoff, H. (1987). An evaluation of cognitive behavior therapy for hyperactive children. In B. B. Lahey & A. E. Kazdin (Eds.), *Advances in clinical child psychology* (Vol. 10, pp. 171–216). New York: Plenum Press.

Abikoff, H., & Gittelman, R. (1984). Does behavior therapy normalize the classroom behavior of hyperactive children? *Archives of General Psychiatry, 41,* 449–454.

American Psychiatric Association. (200). *Diagnostic and statistical manual of mental disorders* (4th ed., text rev.). Washington, DC: Author.

Barkley, R. A. (1994). *ADHD in adults* [Manual to accompany videotape]. New York: Guilford Press.

Barkley, R. A. (1997a). *ADHD and the nature of self-control.* New York: Guilford Press.

Barkley, R. A. (1997b). *Defiant children: A clinician's manual for assessment and parent training* (2nd ed). New York: Guilford Press.

Barkley, R. A., Copeland, A. P., & Sivage, C. (1980). A self-control classroom for hyperactive children. *Journal of Autism and Developmental Disorders, 10,* 75–89.

Diaz, R. M., & Berk, L. E. (1995). A Vygotskian critique of self-instructional training. *Development and Psychopathology, 7,* 369–392.

Dixon, E. B. (1995). Impact of adult ADD on the family. In K. Nadeau (Ed.), *A comprehensive guide to attention deficit disorder in adults* (pp. 236–259). New York: Brunner/Mazel.

Dulcan, M. K. & Lizarralde, C. (Eds.). (2003). *Helping parents, youth, and teachers understand medications for behavioral and emotional prob-*

lems: A resource book of medication information handouts (2nd ed.). Washington, DC: American Psychiatric Press.

Hallowell, E. M. (1995). Psychotherapy of adult attention deficit disorder. In K. G. Nadeau (Ed.), *A comprehensive guide to attention deficit disorder in adults: Research, diagnosis, and treatment* (pp. 144–167). New York: Brunner/Mazel.

Mannuzza, S., Gittelman-Klein, R., Bessler, A., Malloy, P., & LaPadula, M. (1993). Adult outcome of hyperactive boys: Educational achievement, occupational rank, and psychiatric status. *Archives of General Psychiatry, 50,* 565–576.

McDermott, S. P. (1999). Cognitive therapy of attention deficit hyperactivity disorder in adults. *Journal of Cognitive Psychotherapy,* 13 (3), 215–226.

McDermott, S. P. (2000). Cognitive therapy for adults with attention deficit/hyperactivity disorder. In T. Brown (Ed.), *Attention-deficit disorders and comorbidities in children, adolescents, and adults* (pp. 569-606). Washington, DC: American Psychiatric Press.

MTA Cooperative Group. (1999). A fourteen month randomized clinical trial of treatment strategies for attention deficit hyperactivity disorder. *Archives of General Psychiatry,* 56, 1073–1086.

Murphy, K. R. (1995). Empowering the adult with ADHD. In K. G. Nadeau (Ed.), *A comprehensive guide to attention deficit disorder in adults: Research, diagnosis, and treatment* (pp. 135–145). New York: Brunner/Mazel.

Murphy, K. R., & Barkley, R. A. (1996). Attention deficit hyperactivity disorder adults: Comorbidities and adaptive impairments. *Comprehensive Psychiatry, 37*(6), 393–401.

Murphy, K. R., Barkley, R. A., & Bush, T. (2002). Young adults with attention deficit hyperactivity disorder: Subtype differences in comorbidity, educational, and clinical history. *Journal of Nervous and Mental Disease, 190,* 147–157.

Nadeau, K. G. (Ed.). (1995). *A comprehensive guide to attention deficit disorder in adults: Research, diagnosis, and treatment.* New York: Brunner/Mazel.

Ratey, J. J., Hallowell, E. M., & Miller, A. C. (1995). Relationship dilemmas for adults with ADD. In K. G. Nadeau (Ed.), *A comprehensive guide to attention deficit disorder in adults: Research, diagnosis, and treatment* (pp. 218–235). New York: Brunner/Mazel.

Ratey, N. A. (2002). Life coaching for adult ADHD. In S. Goldstein & A. T. Ellison (Eds.), *Clinician's guide to adult ADHD: Assessment and intervention.* San Diego, CA: Academic Press.

Roffman, A. J. (2000). *Meeting the challenge of learning disabilities in adulthood.* Baltimore: Brookes.

Schubiner, H., Tzelepis, A., Isaacson, H., Warbasse, L., Zacharek, M., & Musial, J. (1995). The dual diagnosis of attention-deficit hyperactivity disorder and substance abuse: Case reports and literature review. *Journal of Clinical Psychiatry, 56*(4), 146–150.

Weiss, G., & Hechtman, L. T. (1993). *Hyperactive children grown up: ADHD in children, adolescents, and adults* (2nd ed.). New York: Guilford Press.

CHAPTER 22

Pharmacotherapy of ADHD in Adults

JEFFERSON B. PRINCE
TIMOTHY E. WILENS
THOMAS J. SPENCER
JOSEPH BIEDERMAN

Increasingly, adults with Attention-Deficit/Hyperactivity Disorder (ADHD) present for evaluation and treatment in psychiatric and primary care settings. Adults with ADHD present with a developmental derivation of symptoms reminiscent of those in juveniles, notably inattention/distractibility followed by hyperactivity–impulsivity. Psychiatric comorbidities with mood, anxiety, learning, substance use, and antisocial disorders are often found in adults with ADHD. Longitudinal follow-up studies document the persistence of ADHD from childhood through adolescence and into adulthood for many children individuals. Additional research demonstrates familial and genetic underpinnings, as well as neuropsychological, frontal–striatal, and catecholaminergic dysfunction, in adults with ADHD. As for juveniles, therefore, a cornerstone of treatment for adults with ADHD is pharmacotherapy.

Unlike the vast amount of research available on children with ADHD, there are a limited number of medication studies on adults with ADHD. A review of the literature indicates that the majority of controlled investigations have been conducted with the psychostimulants and atomoxetine (ATMX); other nonstimulant agents have generally been studied under open conditions. Although there tends to be a dose-related improvement in ADHD symptoms with the stimulant medications, ATMX is generally dosed on the basis of body weight. Similarly, the limited data would suggest the need for standard dosing of the antidepressants for ADHD efficacy. Agents with catecholaminergic activity have efficacy in ADHD, whereas those with predominantly serotonergic properties appear not to be effective for ADHD. The aggregate literature supports the conclusion that the stimulants and ATMX are the most effective available agents for adults with ADHD and remain the treatments of choice. In cases of psychiatric comorbidity, residual symptoms, or adverse effects, clinical experience coupled with a small literature would suggest combining medications such as the antidepressants with the stimulants. Cognitive and cognitive-behavioral psychotherapies combined with medication may play a role in treating dynamic issues, residual symptomatology, and comorbid psychopathology in adults with ADHD. Future controlled studies applying stringent diagnostic criteria and outcome methodology are necessary to define further the range of pharmacotherapeutic options for adults with ADHD.

OVERVIEW

ADHD is estimated to affect 3–9% of school-age children worldwide (Faraone, Sergeant, Gillberg, & Biederman, 2003). Converging data on prevalence in adults suggest that 4–5% of college-age individuals and adults have ADHD (Murphy & Barkley, 1996; Kessler et al., 2005) and pose great challenges to both primary care and mental health care providers (Biederman, 1998; Faraone, Spencer, Montano, & Biederman, 2004; Wilens, Faraone, & Biederman, 2004). Although historically ADHD was not thought to continue beyond adolescence, long-term controlled follow-up studies demonstrate the persistence of ADHD, or prominent symptoms of the disorder plus impairment, in approximately half of adults diagnosed with ADHD in childhood (Weiss, Hechtman, Milroy, & Perlman, 1985). Although the diagnosis of adult ADHD has been questioned (Hill & Schoener, 1996), evidence supports the syndromatic continuity of the disorder from childhood through adolescence and into adulthood, as well as the descriptive, face, predictive, and concurrent validity of ADHD in adults (Spencer, Biederman, Wilens, & Faraone, 1998; Wilens & Dodson, 2004; Wilens, Faraone, et al., 2004).

CLINICAL FEATURES, ASSESSMENT, AND DIAGNOSTIC CONSIDERATIONS

Adults with ADHD typically have childhood histories reflecting school dysfunction, including deficits in educational performance, discipline problems, higher rates of repeated grades, tutoring, placement in special classes, and reading disabilities (Wender, 1987; Wilens & Dodson, 2004). School problems faced by children with ADHD often continue or worsen in college, resulting in academic underachievement, low grade point averages, lower completion rates, and more time to complete degrees (Heiligenstein, Conyers, Berns, & Miller, 1998). Adults with ADHD tend to have lower socioeconomic status, lower rates of professional employment, more frequent job changes, more work difficulties, and higher rates of separation and divorce (Biederman et al., 1993;

Barkley, Murphy, & Kwasnik, 1996a). Similarly, adults with ADHD have more speeding violations, driver's license suspensions, accidents, and poorer performance in driving simulators (Barkley, Murphy, & Kwasnik, 1996b; Barkley, Murphy, DuPaul, & Bush, 2002). Individuals with ADHD may have sleep disturbances that both exacerbate ADHD symptoms (underarousal, poor attention) and are aggravated by the presence of ADHD (Stein, 1999). Compared to their peers without ADHD, adults with ADHD have been reported to have higher rates of anxiety, depression, and substance use disorders (Weiss & Hechtman 1986; Shekim, Asarnow, Hess, Zaucha, & Wheeler, 1990; Biederman et al., 1993; Mannuzza, Klein, Bessler, Malloy, & LaPadula, 1993; Biederman et al., 1995). Likewise, studies of adults presenting for treatment of mood, anxiety and substance use disorders demonstrate increased rates of ADHD (Fones, Pollack, Susswein, & Otto, 2000; Alpert et al., 1996; Simon et al., 2004). Therefore, in the context of a family history of ADHD, adults with complicated mood/anxiety disorders, addictions, repeated traffic violations, and recurrent life failures (occupational, financial, personal) should be screened for ADHD.

Longitudinal studies of youth growing up with ADHD show that whereas the symptom clusters of hyperactivity and impulsivity decay over time, inattention tends to persist (Hart, Lahey, Loeber, Applegate, & Frick, 1995; Achenbach, Howell, McConaughy, & Stanger, 1998; Biederman, Faraone, & Mick, 2000; Mick, Faraone, & Biederman, 2004). Studies of clinically referred adults with ADHD show that about half endorse clinically significant levels of hyperactivity–impulsivity and that 90% endorse prominent attentional symptoms (Millstein, Wilens, Spencer, & Biederman, 1997). Like some youth with ADHD, adults with ADHD tend to have additional cognitive deficits (known as "executive function" deficits), including difficulties with encoding, manipulating information, organization, and time management (Barkley, 1997).

ADHD can be diagnosed in adults by carefully querying for developmentally appropriate criteria from the *Diagnostic and Statistical Manual of Mental Disorders*, fourth edition text revision DSM-IV-TR (2000; American Psychiatric Association, 2000), with attention to childhood onset, persistence, and impairment across the lifespan, as well as presence of current symptoms. In addition, adult self-report scales such as the Brown Attention Deficit Disorder Scales (Brown, 1996) and the Wender Utah Rating Scale (Ward, Wender, & Reimherr, 1993) may assist in making the diagnosis. Adults with ADHD most often describe the core attentional symptoms of ADHD, including poor attention and concentration, easy distractibility, shifting activities frequently, daydreaming, and forgetfulness; these are followed more distantly by impulsivity, impatience, boredom, fidgetiness, and intrusiveness (Millstein et al. 1997). ADHD symptoms in adults appear to be related to those in children and adolescents. Adults often do not manifest these symptoms during an interview, however, and may have developed cognitive-behavioral strategies to compensate for their deficiencies related to ADHD. Neuropsychological testing should be used for adults in whom learning disabilities are suspected, or for those with learning problems that persist in the presence of treated ADHD (Barkley, 1998). Adults with ADHD are thought to have working memory deficits, as exemplified by less ability to attend, encode, and manipulate information (Seidman, Biederman, Weber, Hatch, & Faraone, 1998; Seidman et al., 2004). Although less well defined within ADHD, organizational difficulties and procrastination appear common.

Diagnostic information should be gathered from patients and, whenever possible, from significant others (e.g., spouses/partners, parents, siblings, and close friends). If ancillary data are not available, information from the patients themselves is acceptable for diagnostic and treatment purposes, as adults with ADHD, like those with other disorders, are appropriate reporters of their own condition. Careful attention should be paid to the childhood onset of symptoms, longitudinal history of the disorder, and differential diagnosis, including medical/neurological as well as psychosocial factors contributing to the clinical presentation. In adults with ADHD, issues of comorbidity with learning disabilities and other psychiatric disorders needs to be addressed. Since learning disabilities do not respond to pharmacotherapy, it is important to identify these deficits to help define remedial interventions. For instance, an evaluation may assist in the design and implementation of an educational plan for an adult who may be returning to school, or may serve as an aid for structuring current work/home environments.

GENERAL TREATMENT PRINCIPLES

Despite increased recognition that children with ADHD commonly grow up to be adults with the same disorder, evidence-based guidelines on the treatment of adults with ADHD are lacking. Support groups (see, e.g., *www.chadd.org* and *www.add.org*) can assist a newly diagnosed adult by providing education, an overview of treatment options, available resources, and peer support. Clinicians usually apply the principles developed by the American Academy of Child and Adolescent Psychiatry and the American Academy of Pediatrics to guide the treatments of adults with ADHD.

The efficacy of various psychotherapeutic interventions remains to be established. Limited data suggest that standard interpersonal psychotherapies may not be particularly useful in reducing ADHD symptoms (Ratey, Greenberg, Bemporad, & Lindem, 1992), although they may have a role in helping patients and clinicians differentiate capacity problems, related to ADHD, from dynamic issues (Bemporad & Zambenedetti, 1996; Bemporad, 2001). In contrast, some recent data suggest that specific cognitive-behavioral therapies adapted for adults medicated for their ADHD may be useful (McDermott & Wilens, 2000). One open and one controlled trial have demonstrated the efficacy of cognitive-behavioral therapies for medicated adults with ADHD, showing improvement not only in ADHD but also in comorbidity and functional outcomes (Wilens, McDermott, et al., 1999; Safren et al., 2005).

It is important to set clear realistic treatment goals with the patient and to identify specific symptoms and problematic areas of functioning as targets of treatment. Response-based rating scales such as the ADHD Rating Scale–IV (ADHD-RS-IV), the Conners Adult ADHD Rating Scale (CAARS), the Wender Utah Rating Scale, and the Brown Attention Deficit Disorder Scales can be used to help assess symptoms and monitor outcome. (For reviews of this subject, please see Adler & Cohen, 2004; Murphy & Adler, 2004.) Additional therapies often complement the effects of medication. As with children, college students and adults returning to school may benefit from additional educational supports. Coaching and organization training appear useful but remain understudied (Wilens & Dodson, 2004; Wilens, Faraone, et al., 2004).

Although medication therapy is well studied in treating ADHD in children, the use of pharmacotherapeutic agents for adults with ADHD remains less established, but is rapidly evolving and is now a mainstay of treatment for adults with ADHD. The medications used to treat ADHD primarily affect neurotransmission of catecholamines, including dopamine and norepinephrine. Pharmacotherapy should be part of a treatment plan in which consideration is given to all aspects of a patient's life. Hence, it should not be used to the exclusion of other interventions. The administration of medication to an adult with ADHD should be undertaken as a collaborative effort with the patient, with the physician guiding the use and management of efficacious anti-ADHD agents. The use of medication should follow a careful evaluation of the adult, including neurodevelopmental, psychiatric, social, environmental, and cognitive assessments. Currently, the only medications approved by the U.S. Food and Drug and Administration (FDA) to treat ADHD in adults include the specific norepinephrine reuptake inhibitor ATMX, the extended-delivery form of mixed amphetamine salts, and d-threo-MPH capsules. Since many adults with ADHD suffer from comorbid psychiatric disorders, it is necessary to prioritize treatment if clinically significant psychiatric comorbidities are present, typically sequencing (treat comorbid condition first, then evaulate for and treat ADHD) initial treatment for the comorbid disorder. In the following sections, guidelines for pharmacotherapy are delineated; the available information on the use of medications for adult ADHD is reviewed; and pharmacological strategies are suggested for the management of ADHD symptoms with accompanying comorbid conditions.

STIMULANTS

Stimulants remain the best-studied and most frequently used treatments for ADHD in children, adolescents, and adults. Over 200 controlled studies of pediatric ADHD have shown stimulants to be safe, well tolerated, and efficacious in reducing ADHD symptoms, as well as improving self-esteem, cognition, and social/family functioning (Spencer et al., 1996). Although the data in adults with ADHD are less extensive, adults appear to tolerate stimulant medication similarly to children. A recent

review of the literature identified 15 published trials on stimulant pharmacotherapy for ADHD in adults (Wilens, Spencer, & Biederman, 2002). To date we are aware of 13 studies (11 controlled, 2 open) with methylphenidate (MPH) (Wood, Reimherr, Wender, & Johnson, 1976; Mattes, Boswell, & Oliver, 1984; Gualtieri, Ondrusek, & Finley, 1985; Wender, Reimherr, Wood, & Ward, 1985; Shekim, Asarnow, et al., 1990; Spencer et al., 1995; Iaboni, Bouffard, Minde, & Hechtman, 1996; Kuperman et al., 2001; Bouffard, Hechtman, Minde, Iaboni-Kassab, 2003; Stein, 2003; Wender et al., 2003; Kooij et al., 2004; Spencer et al. 2005); 6 (5 controlled, 1 open) with amphetamine (Paterson, Douglas, Hallmayer, Hagan, & Krupenia, 1999; Horrigan & Barnhill, 2000; Taylor & Russo, 2000, 2001; Spencer et al., 2001; Weisler, Chrisman, & Wilens, 2003); and 4 with pemoline (2 controlled, 1 open, 1 chart review) (Wood et al., 1976; Wender, Reimherr, & Wood, 1981; Heiligenstein, Johnston, & Nielsen, 1996; Wilens, Biederman, Spencer, Frazier, et al., 1999) (see Tables 22.1, 22.2, and 22.3).

In contrast to the consistent robust responses to stimulants in children and adolescents of approximately 70% (Wilens & Spencer, 2000; Spencer, 2004), controlled studies in adults have shown more equivocal responses to stimulants, ranging from 25% (Mattes et al., 1984) to 78% (Spencer et al., 1995). Variability in the response rate appears to be related to several factors, including the diagnostic criteria utilized to determine ADHD, varying stimulant doses, high rates of comorbidity, and differing methods of assessing overall response. Dosing of the stimulants appears particularly important in outcome. First, controlled investigations using higher stimulant dosing (>1.0 mg/kg/day of MPH or >0.5 mg/kg/day of amphetamine) have generally resulted in more robust outcomes (Spencer et al., 1995; Iaboni et al., 1996; Spencer et al., 2001; Weisler et al., 2003; Spencer et al., 2005) than those using lower stimulant dosing (<0.7 mg/kg/day) (Mattes et al., 1984; Wender, Reimherr, et al., 1985). Second, several studies have found a dose-dependent response to stimulants in adults with ADHD (Spencer et al., 1995; Wilens, Biederman, Spencer, Frazier, et al., 1999; Spencer et al., 2001).

To date, the 13 published studies of MPH, with a total of 632 subjects, have utilized MPH at weight-corrected doses between 0.4 and 1.1 mg/kg/day (see Table 22.1). Spencer et al.

TABLE 22.1. Studies of Pharmacotherapy with Methylphenidate (MPH) in Adult ADHD

Study (year)	n	Design	Medication	Duration	Total dose (wt.-corrected)	Response rate	Comments
Wood et al. (1976)	15	Double-blind	MPH	4 weeks	27 mg (0.4 mg/kg)[a]	73%	Dx. criteria not well defined
Mattes et al. (1984)	26	Double-blind, placebo-controlled crossover	MPH	6 weeks	48 mg (0.7 mg/kg)[a]	25%	Moderate rate of comorbidity; mild side effects
Wender, Reimherrr, et al. (1985)	37	Double-blind, placebo-controlled crossover	MPH	5 weeks	43 mg (0.6 mg/kg)[a]	57%	68% dysthymia, 22% cyclothymia; mild side effects
Gualtieri et al. (1985)	8	Double-blind, placebo-controlled crossover	MPH	2 weeks	42 mg (0.6 mg/kg)[a]	Mild–moderate	No plasma level–response associations
Shekim, Asarnow, et al. (1990)	33	Open	MPH	8 weeks	40 mg (0.6 mg/kg)[a]	70%	Problematic outcome measures
Spencer et al. (1995)	23	Double-blind, placebo-controlled crossover	MPH	7 weeks	30–100 mg (0.5, 0.75, and 1.0 mg/kg)[a]	78%, dose relationship	No plasma level–response associations; no effect of gender or comorbidity
Iaboni et al. (1996)	30	Double-blind, placebo-controlled crossover	MPH	4 weeks	30–45 mg (≤0.6 mg/kg)[a]	Moderate	Improvement in neuropsychological functioning and anxiety
Kuperman et al. (2001)	30	Randomized, double-blind, parallel	MPH (8) or bupropion (11) or placebo (11)	7 weeks	0.9 mg/kg/day, dosed t.i.d.	64% bupropion 50% MPH 27% placebo	High placebo response rate; both active medications well tolerated

Bouffard et al. (2003)	30	Double-blind, placebo-controlled crossover	MPH	9 weeks	10–15 mg, dosed t.i.d.	63%	Response based on self-report; MPH well tolerated; improvements noted on CPT
Wender et al. (2003)	116	Double-blind, placebo-controlled, crossover	MPH		45 mg/day	MPH 64% Placebo 19%	Response defined as >30% reduction in ADHD-RS-IV score and Clinical Global Impression of "good" or "excellent"
Stein (2003)	136	Open trial	OROS MPH	9 months	43 mg/day	80% at 3 months 90% at 9 months	Response defined as "good" or "excellent" on Clinical Global Impression
Kooij et al. (2004)	45	Double-blind, placebo-controlled crossover	MPH	7 weeks	Up to 1 mg/kg/day, dosed four or five times per day	MPH 38% Placebo 7%	Response defined as >30% reduction in ADHD-RS-IV score and Clinical Global Impression of "good" or "excellent"; loss of appetite a significant side effect
Adler et al. (2005)		Initial double-blind, placebo-fixed dose, followed by 6-month open-label extension, n = 21; 218 completed 5-week double-blind phase; 170 completed 6-month open label	d-MPH	5 weeks, followed by 6-month extension	20, 30, or 40 mg daily	Not stated	Significant reductions in ADHD-RS noted on all doses compared to placebo; CGI-I demonstrated improvement; generally well-tolerated; 14.7% withdrew from open label due to adverse events.
Spencer et al. (2005)	103	Double-blind, placebo-controlled	MPH	6 weeks	82 mg/day, dosed t.i.d. (1.1 mg/kg/day)[a]	73%	43% reduction in ADHD-RS-IV scores
Total	632	Double-blind, n = 11; open, n = 2	MPH	2 weeks to 9 months	40 mg (MPH) (0.6 mg/kg)[a]	Variable	Dx. criteria not well defined; high rate of comorbidity; side effects in 30%

Note. Duration of medication trial includes placebo phase. Dx., diagnosis; t.i.d., three times a day; CPT, continuous performance test; ADHD-RS-IV, ADHD Rating Scale-IV; OROS, oral osmotic release; CGI-I, Clinical Global Impression–Improvement.
[a]Weight-normalized dose using 50th-percentile weight for age.

(1995) utilized a double-blind, placebo-controlled, crossover design to study the effect of MPH on 23 clinically referred adults with ADHD. MPH or placebo was administered three times daily and was titrated from an initial dose of 0.5 mg/kg/day at week 1, to 0.75 mg/kg/day at week 2, to 1.0 mg/kg/day at week 3 as tolerated. The final mean dose of MPH was approximately 75 mg/day, with a range of 30–100 mg/day. Patients treated with MPH showed significantly greater reductions in inattention/distractibility, impulsivity, and hyperactivity, as measured by the ADHD-RS-IV, beginning during week 1 and becoming increasingly robust over the ensuing weeks as the dose increased. Overall, response during treatment with MPH (78% response rate) was significantly greater compared to placebo (4% response rate). Lifetime comorbidity with depression, anxiety, substance abuse, and learning disorders was observed in 74% of this sample. Although similarly robust responses to MPH were observed in patients with comorbidity, there was insufficient statistical power to fully evaluate the impact of MPH treatment on these subgroups. Although MPH was generally well tolerated, the most common side effects observed during treatment included appetite loss, insomnia, and anxiety, as well as small but statistically significant increases in blood pressure (systolic, 123 ± 2.6 mm Hg vs. 117 ± 1.7 mm Hg; diastolic, 77 ± 2.0 vs. 75 ± 1.5 mm Hg) and heart rate (80 ± 2.4 vs. 76 ± 1.5 beats per minute). The authors concluded that short-term robust MPH treatment (0.92 mg/kg/day) is well tolerated and effective in reducing ADHD symptoms in adults, and that the response may be dose-dependent.

More recently, two large ($n = 103$ and $n = 116$) double-blind, placebo-controlled studies of immediate-release MPH were published in abstract form (Wender et al., 2003; Spencer et al., 2005). These studies utilized doses of 82 mg/day (1.1 mg/kg/day) and 45 mg/day, and reported response rates of 73% and 64%, respectively. Although long-term data are generally lacking, data from Wender et al. (2003) suggest that the response to MPH is sustained at a 6-month follow-up, and Spencer et al. (2005) continue to follow their sample. Furthermore, a large ($n = 136$) open-label trial with oral-osmotic-release (OROS) MPH (mean dose = 43 mg/day) reported response rates of 80% for patients after three months of treatment (Stein, 2003). A meta-analysis of six double-blind, placebo-controlled studies comparing treatment of adults with ADHD with MPH ($n = 140$) to placebo ($n = 113$) found a mean effect size of 0.9, similar to that seen in MPH treatment of children with ADHD. Moreover, the effect size was twice as large (1.3) in those studies using higher dosing of MPH (mean dose = 70 mg/day or 1.05 mg/kg/day) as in those studies using lower doses (effect size = 0.7; mean dose = 44 mg/day or 0.63 mg/kg/day) (Faraone, Spencer, Aleardi, Pagano, & Biederman, 2004).

Adler and colleagues (2005) report on the long-term safety, tolerability, and efficacy of Focalin XR (d-MPH XR) in adults with ADHD. Two-hundred twenty-one adults with ADHD were randomized in an initial 5 week double-blind placebo-controlled fixed dose study of once daily d-MPH XR. d-MPH XR was administered once daily in the morning in doses of 20, 30, or 40 mg to 40 mg daily. The initial phase was followed by a 6 month open-label extension in 170 patients. At the end of both the initial double-blind phase and the extension phase, patients receiving d-MPH XR demonstrated significant improvements in ADHD symptoms reductions in ADHD-RS scores: 7.6 for placebo, 13.3 in subjects on 20 mg ($p = .006$), 12.9 in subjects on 30 mg ($p = .012$), and 16.5 in subjects on 40 mg ($p < 0.001$). d-MPH XR was generally well tolerated, with the most frequently reported adverse events including headache, insomnia, and decreased appetite.

Recently, Canadian health officials have raised concerns about the safety of stimulants, in general and mixed amphetamine salts, in particular, around occurrences of sudden death and stroke. The U.S. Food and Drug Administration and the American Heart Association have addressed these concerns previously (Gutgesell et al., 1999). What appears to be emerging is that the rate of sudden death in patients receiving MAS is no higher than that expected in the general population, even accounting for potential underreporting. Despite the generally benign cardiovascular effects of these medications in adults, caution is warranted in the presence or compromised cardiovascular system (e.g., untreated hypertension, arrhythmias, known structural heart defects). It remains prudent to monitor symptoms referable to the cardiovascular system (e.g., syncope, palpitations, chest pain) and vital signs at baseline, and with treatment, the utility of monitoring ECGs serially appears dubious.

Six controlled trials to date, with a total of 413 subjects, have assessed the efficacy of dextroamphetamine or Adderall (mixed amphetamine salts; MAS), in doses ranging from 10 to 60 mg/day, in the treatment of adults with ADHD (see Table 22.2). Using a 7-week double-blind, placebo-controlled, crossover design, Spencer et al. (2001)studied the effects of immediate-release MAS on 27 adults with ADHD. MAS tablets were initiated at 20 mg/day (10 mg in morning and early afternoon) at week 1, and titrated to 40 mg/day (20 mg twice daily) at week 2 and 60 mg/day (30 mg twice daily) at week 3. The average dose was 54 mg/day. During treatment with MAS, patients experienced significant reductions in ADHD symptoms by week 1 and continued to show gains across weeks 2 and 3. Overall, 70% of the patients demonstrated response to MAS, compared to 7% during treatment with placebo. Although there were high rates of lifetime comorbidity with depression, anxiety, substance abuse, and Conduct Disorder, baseline ratings of depression and anxiety were very low and were not affected by MAS treatment. MAS appeared well tolerated, and the most common side effects included appetite suppression and agitation. In addition, a small but statistically significant increase in diastolic blood pressure was observed (76 vs. 71 mm Hg; $t = 2.6$, $df = 25$, $p < .05$), as well as a weight loss of 4 pounds (167 vs. 163 pounds; $t = 5.8$, $df = 25$, $p < .001$). Of note, Spencer et al. (2001) used higher doses in this study than those used by Taylor and Russo (2000) (22 mg/day of dextroamphetamine), Paterson et al. (1999) (23 mg/day of dextroamphetamine), and Horrigan and Barnhill (2000) (10.8 mg/day of MAS), and found higher response rates (70% vs. 48%, 58%, and 54%, respectively).

Recently, preliminary results from a large multisite study of the extended-release form of MAS (MAS XR, marketed as Adderall XR) have been presented and published in abstract form (Weisler et al., 2003). This was a large 6-week randomized, double-blind, placebo-controlled, forced-titration study to assess the safety and efficacy of MAS XR (20, 40, or 60 mg once daily) in adults with ADHD. Significant reductions in ADHD-RS-IV scores were observed for all doses (mean reduction of 42% for MAS XR vs. 20% for placebo). During treatment with MAS XR, the most commonly reported adverse events included dry mouth (27.5%), anorexia (25.5%), insomnia (23.5%),

headache (22.7%), and nervousness (12.5%). The authors concluded that MAS XR administered once daily appears safe and efficacious for treating adults with ADHD. As a result of this study, the FDA has recently approved MAS XR (20 mg/day) for the treatment of ADHD in adults. Following up on the short-term data, Biederman et al. (2004) have presented and published in abstract form results of the 6- and 12-month open-label extension of MAS XR. These investigators indicate that MAS XR appears to be efficacious in the treatment of adults with ADHD over 6 and 12 months, and that tolerance to the benefits does not appear to develop.

To date, two controlled trials using pemoline in doses between 37.5 and 150 mg/day (0.5 and 2.0 mg/kg/day), with a total of 92 adults with ADHD, have been reported (Wender et al., 1981; Wilens, Biederman, Spencer, Frazier, et al., 1999). Most recently, Wilens and colleagues, using a double-blind, placebo-controlled, crossover design, studied the effects of pemoline on 42 adults with ADHD. This design consisted of two 4-week treatment periods with either pemoline or placebo, separated by a 2-week washout period. During the 4-week treatment phase, patients were titrated up to 1 mg/kg/day (~75 mg/day) during week 1, 2 mg/kg/day (~150 mg/day) during week 2, and 3 mg/kg/day (~225 mg/day) during week 3; week 4 was dosed flexibly, based upon tolerability. The final mean dose achieved was 148 mg ± 95 mg/day (2.2 mg/kg/day), substantially less than the dose targeted. Although pemoline treatment resulted in significant reductions in ADHD symptoms, most patients tolerated moderate rather than robust doses of pemoline, and the response rate of 50% was considerably less than that seen with robust doses of MPH and amphetamines. The authors concluded that pemoline is moderately effective in treating ADHD in adults. Given the relatively low magnitude of effect, as well as concerns over hepatotoxicity and the availability of longer-acting treatments, pemoline is no longer routinely used in the treatment of ADHD in adults.

Taken together, these clinical trials with stimulants (see Tables 22.1, 22.2, and 22.3) demonstrate significant, dose-dependent, short-term improvement in ADHD symptoms when these medications are compared to placebo in adults. In controlled trials, there appear to be more robust responses to MPH and amphetamine than to pemoline. Response to the

TABLE 22.2. Studies of Dextroamphetamine (DEX) or Mixed Amphetamine Salts (MAS) Pharmacotherapy in Adult ADHD

Study (year)	n	Design	Medication	Duration	Total dose (wt.-corrected)	Response rate	Comments
Paterson et al. (1999)	68	Double-blind, placebo-controlled, parallel	DEX tablets	6 weeks	23 mg/day, given b.i.d. (0.3 mg/kg/day)[a]	58% with CGI-I of "much" or "very much" improved	Low placebo response; improvements in attention and hyperactivity/impulsivity; relatives observed improvements too
Horrigan & Barnhill (2000)	24	Open	MAS tablets	16 weeks	10.8 mg/day, given b.i.d. (14 mg/kg/day)[a]	54% with CGI-I of "much" or "very much" improved	9 poor responders; 4 of 7 patients with comorbid anxiety disorders experienced exacerbation of anxiety
Taylor & Russo (2000)	22	Double-blind, placebo-controlled, crossover	DEX tablets vs. modafinil vs. placebo	6 weeks (2 weeks in each: DEX, modafinil, placebo)	21.8 mg/day, dosed b.i.d.	48% with >30% reduction in ADHD-RS-IV scores	Significant symptom reduction compared with placebo; insomnia, appetite suppression, muscle tension, and anxiety noted
Taylor & Russo (2001)	17	Double-blind, placebo-controlled, crossover	DEX tablets vs. guanfacine vs. placebo	6 weeks (2 weeks in each: DEX, guanfacine, placebo)	10.2 mg/day DEX	Significant reductions in ADHD-RS-IV scores for both DEX and guanfacine compared with placebo	Duration of effect of DEX tablet, 5.9 hours; 12/17 patients elected to continue DEX
Spencer et al. (2001)	27	Double-blind, placebo-controlled, crossover	MAS tablets	3 weeks in each condition	54 mg/day, dosed b.i.d. (0.6 mg/kg)[a]	70%	No plasma level–response associations
Weisler et al. (2003)	255	Double-blind, placebo-controlled, forced-titration	MAS XR capsules	6 weeks	20, 40 or 60 mg/day (0.6 mg/kg)[a]	42% with >30% reduction in ADHD-RS-IV scores (vs. 20% with placebo)	Problematic outcome measures
Total	413	Double-blind, n = 5; open: n = 1	DEX = 3; MAS tablets = 2; MAS XR capsules = 1	2–10 weeks	40 mg (MPH) (0.6 mg/kg)[a] 105 mg (Pem) (1.5 mg/kg)[a]	Variable	Dx. criteria not well defined; high rate of comorbidity; side effects in 30%

Note. Duration of medication trial includes placebo phase. b.i.d., twice a day; CGI-I, Clinical Global Impression—Improvement; ADHD-RS-IV, ADHD Rating Scale-IV; Dx., diagnosis.
[a]Weight-normalized dose using 50th-percentile weight for age.

TABLE 22.3. Studies of Pemoline Pharmacotherapy in Adult ADHD

Study (year)	n	Design	Medication	Duration	Total dose (wt.-corrected)	Response rate	Comments
Wood et al. (1976)	15	Open	Pemoline	4 weeks	37.5–70 mg (0.5–1.0 mg/kg)[a]	33%	Dx. criteria not well defined; low doses of pemoline; mild side effects
Wender et al. (1981)	51	Double-blind, placebo-controlled, crossover	Pemoline	6 weeks	65 mg (0.9 mg/kg)[a]	50% (childhood onset)	Dx. criteria not well defined; high rates of dysthymia; moderate side effects
Heiligenstein et al. (1996)	40	Chart review	Pemoline	2–12 weeks	52.5 ± 19.5 mg/day	70%	Response based on retrospective CGI improvement; 23% reported adverse events
Wilens, Biederman, Spencer, Frazier, et al. (1999)	42	Double-blind, placebo-controlled crossover	Pemoline	10 weeks	150 mg (2 mg/kg)[a]	61%	35% reduction in ADHD symptoms; moderate side effects at >2 mg/kg
Total	112	Double-blind, n = 2; Open, n = 1	Pemoline	4–10 weeks	105 mg (1.5 mg/kg)[a]	Variable	Dx. not well defined; high rate of comorbidity; side effects in 30%

Note. Duration of medication trial includes placebo phase. Dx., diagnosis; CGI, Clinical Global Impression.
[a]Weight-normalized dose using 50th-percentile weight for age.

stimulants appears to be dose-dependent, and emerging data from longer-term trials with MPH and MAS (Spencer, 2002; Wender et al., 2003; Biederman et al., 2004) as well as with extended-delivery preparations (Stein, 2003; Weisler et al., 2003) in adults support the ongoing effectiveness and tolerability of stimulants.

The effects of the stimulants in the brain are variable. Preclinical studies have shown that the stimulants block the reuptake of dopamine and norepinephrine into the presynaptic neuron, and that both MPH and amphetamines increase the release of these monoamines into the extraneuronal space (Elia et al., 1990). Alterations in dopaminergic and noradrenergic function appear necessary (though not entirely sufficient) for clinical efficacy of the anti-ADHD medications, including the stimulants (Zametkin & Rapoport, 1987). Stimulants have been shown to increase intrasynaptic concentrations of dopamine and norepinephrine (Solanto, 1998). MPH primarily acts by blocking the reuptake of dopamine through binding to the dopamine transporter protein on the presynaptic membrane (Volkow et al., 2001). While amphetamines diminish presynaptic reuptake of DA, they also travel into the dopamine neuron and cause release of dopamine from vesicles into the cytoplasm, prevent reuptake from the cytoplasm into the vesicles, and cause release of more dopamine from the presynaptic neuron (Wilens & Spencer, 1998). In addition, stimulants (amphetamine > MPH) increase levels of norepinephrine and serotonin in the interneuronal space, although these effects are relatively minor compared to their effects on dopamine. There may be differential responses to the chemically distinct available stimulants, as each may have a different mode of action. These different mechanisms of actions may explain why adults not responding to one stimulant may respond favorably to another. Moreover, plasma levels of the stimulants have not been shown to correlate with response in ADHD in adults (Gualtieri, Hicks, Patrick, Schroeder, & Breese, 1984). Finally, matters of comorbidity and gender have not been associated with variable response to the stimulants (Spencer et al., 1995, 2001; Wilens, Biederman, Spencer, Frazier, et al., 1999); however, sample sizes have not been large enough to assess this issue adequately.

After oral administration, stimulants are rapidly absorbed and preferentially taken up into the central nervous system (CNS). Food has little impact on their absorption, but lowering the pH of the gastrointestinal tract may delay the C_{max} (maximal concentration) and T_{max} (time to maximal concentration) of the amphetamines and some beaded MPH preparations. Stimulants bind poorly to plasma proteins. MPH is primarily metabolized by plasma-based eterases to ritalinic acid and excreted in the urine. The amphetamines are 80% excreted in the urine unchanged, while 20% undergo hepatic metabolism. Acidification of the urine may enhance excretion of the amphetamines. Although the amphetamines are detected on routine urine drug screening, MPH is not usually detected.

Amphetamine is available in two forms, dextroamphetamine and MAS. Dextroamphetamine achieves peak plasma levels 2–3 hours after oral administration, and has a half-life of 4–6 hours. Behavioral effects of dextroamphetamine peak 1–2 hours after administration, and last 4–5 hours. For dextroamphetamine spansules, these values are somewhat longer. MAS consist of a racemic mixture of 25% levo- and 75% dextroamphetamine in four salts. The two isomers have different pharmacodynamic properties, and some patients with ADHD may have a preferential response to one isomer over the other. MAS is available as tablets or capsules. MAS XR is a beaded preparation that is FDA-approved for the treatment of ADHD in adults. The capsule contains two types of beads that deliver 50% of the dose initially and 50% approximately 4 hours later. MAS XR usually provides approximately 10–12 hours of coverage from a single morning dose.

As originally formulated, MPH was produced as an equal mixture of dextro-, levo-(d,l)threo-MPH and d,l-erythro-MPH. It was quickly realized that the erythro- form of MPH produces the cardiovascular side effects, and thus MPH is now manufactured as an equal mixture of d,l-threo-MPH. Oral administration of immediate-release d,l-threo-MPH (available as generic MPH, Ritalin, Metadate ER, and Methylin) results in a variable peak plasma concentration within 1–2 hours, with a half-life between 2 and 3 hours (for an excellent review of this topic, please see Swanson & Volkow, 2001). Behavioral effects of immediate-release MPH peak 1–2 hours after administration, and tend to dissipate within 3–5 hours. Although generic MPH has a similar pharmacokinetic profile to Ritalin, it is more rapidly absorbed and peaks sooner. Plasma levels of the sustained-release preparation of MPH (Ritalin SR) peak in 1–4 hours, with a half-life of 2–6 hours (Greenhill, Cooper, Solomon, Fried, & Cornblatt, 1987; Birmaher, Greenhill, Cooper, Fried, & Maminski, 1989). Due to the wax-based matrix preparation, absorption is clinically observed to be variable (Patrick, Straughn, Jarvi, Breese, & Meyer, 1989), and clinicians are using it less now that alternative extended-delivery systems are available. Peak behavioral effects of this preparation occur 2 hours after ingestion, maintain a relatively flat pharmacokinetic profile, and may last up to 8 hours (Greenhill et al., 1987; Birmaher et al., 1989). Studies have indicated that the primarily active form of MPH is the d-threo- isomer (Ding et al., 1997; Ding et al., 2004). Therefore, the makers of Ritalin now produce Focalin (d-threo-MPH) as a purer form of Ritalin. Clinicians should note that in terms of potency, 10 mg of Ritalin is biologically equivalent to 5 mg of Focalin.

Recently, several novel methods of delivering MPH and amphetamine have become available. While these medications all deliver stimulant, their pharmacokinetic profiles differ. Concerta (OROS MPH) uses the OROS technology to deliver a 50–50 racemic mixture of d,l-threo-MPH. An 18-mg caplet of Concerta delivers the equivalent of 15 mg of MPH (5 mg of MPH three times daily), providing 12 hours of coverage. The 18-mg caplet initially provides 4 mg of MPH and delivers the additional MPH in an ascending profile over a total of 12 hours. Concerta is recommended to be dosed between 18 and 72 mg each day. If Concerta is cut or crushed, its delivery system is compromised. Metadate CD, available in capsules of 10, 20, and 30 mg, contains two types of beads containing d,l-threo-MPH. Metadate CD delivers 30% of MPH initially (i.e., 6 mg of d,l-threo-MPH in the 20-mg CD capsule) and is designed to simulate twice-daily dosing for approximately 8 hours of coverage (Greenhill, Findling, Swanson, & MTA Cooperative Group, 2002). Ritlain-LA, available in capsules of 20, 30, and 40 mg, delivers 50% of its d,l-threo-MPH initially and another bolus approximately 3–4 hours later, thus providing about 8 hours of coverage (Biederman et al., 2003). Additional MPH delivery systems are being developed, including an extended-delivery form of d-threo-MPH and a patch delivery system.

Pemoline is a CNS stimulant that is structurally different from both MPH and amphetamine, and that seems to enhance central dopaminergic transmission. Pemoline reaches peak plasma levels 1–4 hours after ingestion, and has a half-life of 7–8 hours in children and 11–13 hours in adults. A number of patients taking pemoline have developed significant hepatitis, resulting in liver failure and in some cases death or need for liver transplant. Given concerns regarding potential hepatic toxicity, the FDA now recommends that patients taking pemoline have liver function tests taken every 2 weeks. Although compliance with these recommendations has been scanty, pemoline has clinically been relegated to a third-line agent, due to the availability of other long-acting stimulants and ATMX.

Stimulants can cause clinically significant anorexia, nausea, difficulty falling asleep, obsessiveness, headaches, dry mouth, rebound phenomena, anxiety, nightmares, dizziness, irritability, dysphoria, and weight loss (Greenhill, Pliszka, et al., 2002). They are also associated with small increases in heart rate and blood pressure that are weakly correlated with dose. Although these changes are not usually clinically significant, it is prudent to monitor vital signs regularly, especially in patients at elevated risk of hypertension (Wilens, Hamerness, et al., 2005). In patients who feel edgy during treatment with stimulants, administration of a low-dose beta-blocker (i.e., propranolol at 10 mg up to three times daily) or buspirone (5–10 mg up to three times daily) maybe helpful in reducing the edginess/agitation associated with stimulant administration (Ratey, Greenberg, & Lindem, 1991). Occasionally, stimulants may elicit a depressive reaction or psychosis. However, no cases of stimulant-related psychosis at therapeutic doses have been reported in adults (Wilens & Spencer, 2000). Stimulant use may exacerbate tics or Tourette syndrome. Although a physical withdrawal is not associated with stimulants, patients who have used high doses for a prolonged time may experience fatigue, hypersomnia, hyperphagia, dysphoria, and depression upon discontinuation. Given the abuse potential of these medications, it is important to inquire about concomitant use of drugs and alcohol.

Long-term use of pemoline in children has been associated with hepatotoxicity, although reports of this are rare (Pratt & Dubois, 1990; Safer, Zito, & Gardner, 2001). Patients and significant others should be educated regarding the early signs of hepatitis (e.g., change in urine and stool, abdominal discomfort, jaundice) when pemoline is being prescribed. Although the usefulness of routine liver function tests remains unclear, it is prudent to obtain baseline values of serum glutamic–oxaloacetic transaminase and serum glutamic–pyruvic transaminase; the FDA recommends a liver panel every 2 weeks.

Although tolerance to the effects of stimulants on ADHD symptoms has been debated, data from the National Institute of Mental Health's Multimodal Treatment Study of ADHD (Group MTS, 1999) have demonstrated the persistence of stimulant medication effects, and tolerance to the effects of short-acting stimulants on ADHD symptoms does not appear to develop. Recently, results from the open-label extension of MAS XR for the treatment of adult ADHD demonstrated continued effectiveness at 6 and 12 months after initiation of treatment (Biederman et al., 2004). However, patients may raise concerns over development of tolerance; this issue remains understudied, especially with the longer-acting stimulant preparations, when pharmacotherapy is continuous and extends over several years and in adult populations..

The interactions of stimulants with other prescription and nonprescription medications are generally mild and not a major source of concern (Markowitz, Morrison, & Devane, 1999; Markowitz & Patrick, 2001). Concomitant use of sympathomimetic agents (e.g., pseudoephedrine) may potentiate the effects of both medications. Concurrent use of antihistamines may diminish the effects of stimulants. Likewise, excessive intake of caffeine may potentially compromise the effectiveness of the stimulants and exacerbate sleep difficulties. Although data on the coadministration of stimulants with tricyclic antidepressants (TCAs) suggest little interaction between these classes of compounds (Cohen et al., 1999), careful monitoring is warranted when stimulants are prescribed with either TCAs or anticonvulsants. Although administering stimulants with ATMX is common clinical practice, and appears safe, well tolerated, and effective in clinical experience, to date only small samples have been studied; therefore, patients taking this combination should be monitored closely. Coadministration of monoamine oxidase inhibitors (MAOIs) with stimulants may result in a hypertensive crisis and be potentially life-threatening. In fact, coadministration of stimulants with MAOIs is the only true contraindication.

The stimulants most commonly used in adults with ADHD include MPH (short-acting forms such as Ritalin, Methylin, and Focalin, and extended-delivery forms such as Concerta, Ritalin LA, and Metadate CD), dextroamphetamine (Dexedrine), and a mixture of amphetamine salts (Adderall and Adderall XR) (see Table 22.4).

There are few data available to guide the dosing parameters of the stimulants. FDA guidelines for dosing reflect general cautiousness and should not be the only guide for clinical practice. For instance, absolute dose limits (in milligrams) do not adequately consider a patient's height or weight, or use in refractory cases or with adults. The dose should be individually titrated based on therapeutic efficacy and side effects. Treatment may be started with either short-acting or extended-delivery preparations at the lowest possible dose (Greenhill, Pliszka, et al., 2002). The stimulants have an immediate onset of action and may last from 3 to 12 hours, based on the formulation of the agent (immediate- or extended-release). Initiation of treatment with once-daily dosing in the morning is advisable until an acceptable response is noted. Treatment with immediate release preparations generally starts at 5 mg of MPH or amphetamine once daily, and is titrated upward every 3–5 days until an effect is noted or adverse effects emerge. Repeat dosing through the day is dependent on duration of effectiveness, wearing off rate, and side effects. Typically, the half-life of the short-acting stimulants necessitates at least twice-daily dosing, with the addition of similar or reduced afternoon doses dependent on breakthrough symptoms. In a typical adult, dosing of immediate-release MPH is generally up to 30 mg three to four times daily; dosing of amphetamine is 15–20 mg three to four times a day. Currently, most adults with ADHD who will be treated with a stimulant are prescribed extended-delivery preparations, such as MAS XR, OROS MPH, or one of the beaded MPH preparations.

Despite the increasing use of stimulants for adults with ADHD, up to 50% may not respond, may have untoward side effects, or may manifest comorbidity that stimulants may exacerbate or be ineffective in treating (Shekim, Asarnow, et al., 1990; Biederman et al., 1993).

Recently, ATMX, has been systematically evaluated and is FDA-approved for the treatment of ADHD in adults. Other, nonstimulant treatments for adults with ADHD have included antidepressants, modafinil, antihypertensives, and amino acids.

ATOMOXETINE

The FDA recently approved ATMX for treating ADHD in adults (see Table 22.5). Unlike the stimulants, ATMX is not a controlled Schedule II medication; therefore, clinicians can call in prescriptions, as well as provide samples and refills. ATMX was initially studied as an antidepressant in approximately 1,200 adults. In this trial, neither ATMX nor desipramine was found to be different from placebo, and ATMX was thus not pursued as an antidepressant. However, based upon the efficacy of the TCAs in treating ADHD (Biederman, Baldessarini, Wright, Knee, & Harmatz, 1989; Wilens et al., 1996; Prince et al., 2000), ATMX was studied in a proof-of-concept trial in adults with ADHD. This study (Spencer, Biederman, Wilens, Prince, et al., 1998), using a double-blind, placebo-controlled design, demonstrated that ATMX was well tolerated and significantly more effective than placebo in reducing clinical symptoms of ADHD. In addition, during the active treatment phase of this study (3 weeks in duration, mean dose of ATMX = 76 mg/day), subjects demonstrated improvements on neuropsychological measures. Specifically, improvements were noted on Stroop Color–Word and Interference T scores (i.e., scores on tests thought to measure response inhibition).

Based upon these initial positive findings, ATMX was studied in two large multisite trials. These two studies (study I, n = 280; study II, n = 256) employed an identical 10-week randomized, double-blind, placebo-controlled design (Michelson et al., 2003). In each study, compared to placebo, ATMX significantly improved ADHD symptoms as assessed by investigators using the CAARS. Mean reductions from baseline in CAARS scores were 28% and 30% (vs. 18% and 20% for placebo), respectively. Approximately equal reductions were observed in symptoms of inattention and hyperactivity–impulsivity. Likewise, similar gains were noted in patients with the Combined and the Predominantly Inattentive Types of ADHD. The most frequently prescribed dose of ATMX

in both studies was 90 mg/day, and was dosed equally in the morning and late afternoon.

ATMX selectively blocks the norephineprine reuptake pump on the presynaptic membrane of noradrenergic neurons, resulting in increased availability of intrasynaptic norepinephrine (Michelson et al., 2003). ATMX has little affinity for other monoamine transporters or neurotransmitter receptors. Data from studies in animals indicate that in addition to increasing norepinephrine in the brain, administration of ATMX leads to increased intrasynaptic dopamine in the prefrontal cortex, but not in the striatum or the nucleus accumbens (Bymaster et al., 2002). This property may account for its benefits in reducing ADHD symptomology while not appearing to exacerbate tics or be addictive.

ATMX is rapidly absorbed following oral administration, and food does not appear to affect absorption. Its C_{max} is 1–2 hours after dosing. There are a number of alternative metabolic pathways, including the 2C19 enzyme. Although ATMX is metabolized by 2D6, it does not appear to either induce or inhibit 2D6 activity. ATMX is primarily excreted in the urine.

It is recommended that ATMX be initiated slowly at 0.5 mg/kg/day for 2 weeks and increased over a month to a target dose of 1.2 mg/kg/day. Current dosing guidelines for ATMX recommend maximum dosage of 1.4 mg/kg/day or 100 mg/day, though increases up to 1.8 mg/kg/day may be necessary in refractory cases. In both large trials in adults with ADHD (Michelson et al., 2003), ATMX was dosed equally after breakfast and in the late afternoon; twice-daily dosing is probably necessary in most adults. Extensive testing was undertaken in these trials to look at the ability of patients with relatively slow metabolic activity at 2D6 (approximately 7% of the sample) to metabolize ATMX. These studies indicate that although patients with slow-metabolism status experienced increased rates of common side effects, these patients were generally able to tolerate ATMX. In such situations, or when ATMX is coadministered with medications known to inhibit 2D6 (e.g., fluoxetine, paroxetine), clinicians should consider reducing the dose.

In addition to the treatment of both inattention and hyperactivity–impulsivity in adults with ADHD, ATMX may be particularly useful when anxiety, mood disturbances, or tics co-

TABLE 22.4. Available FDA-Approved Treatments for ADHD

Generic name (brand name)	Formulation and mechanism	Duration of activity	How supplied	Usual absolute and (weight-based) dosing range	FDA-approved maximum dose for ADHD
MPH (Ritalin)[a]	Tablet of 50–50 racemic mixture d,l-threo-MPH	3–4 hours	Tablets (5, 10, and 20 mg)	(0.3–2.0 mg/kg/ day)	60 mg/day
d-MPH (Focalin)[a]	Tablet of d-threo-MPH	3–5 hours	Tablets (2.5, 5, 10 mg; 2.5 mg Focalin equivalent to 5 mg Ritalin)	(0.15–1.0 mg/kg/ day)	20 mg/day
MPH (Methylin)[a]	Tablet of 50–50 racemic mixture d,l-threo-MPH	3–4 hours	Tablets (5, 10, 20 mg)	(0.3–2.0 mg/kg/ day)	60 mg/day
MPH SR (Ritalin SR)[a]	Wax-based matrix tablet of 50–50 racemic mixture d,l-threo-MPH	3–8 hours (variable)	Tablets (20 mg; amount absorbed appears to vary)	(0.3–2.0 mg/kg/ day)	60 mg/day
MPH (Metadate ER)[a]	Wax-based matrix tablet of 50–50 racemic mixture d,l-threo-MPH	3–8 hours (variable)	Tablets (10, 20 mg; amount absorbed appears to vary)	(0.3–2.0 mg/kg/ day)	60 mg/day
MPH (Methylin ER)[a]	Hydroxypropyl methylcellulose base tablet of 50–50 racemic mixture d,l-threo-MPH; no preservatives	8 hours	Tablets (10, 20 mg); chewable tablets (2.5, 5, 10 mg); oral solution (5 mg/5 ml, 10 mg/5 ml)	(0.3–2.0 mg/kg/ day)	60 mg/day
MPH (Ritalin LA)[a]	Two types of beads give bimodal delivery (50% immediate-release and 50% delayed-release) of 50–50 racemic mixture d,l-threo-MPH	8 hours	Capsules (20, 30, 40 mg; can be sprinkled)	(0.3–2.0 mg/kg/ day)	60 mg/day
MPH (Metadate CD)[a]	Two types of beads give bimodal delivery (30% immediate-release and 70% delayed-release) of 50–50 racemic mixture d,l-threo-MPH	8 hours	Capsule (20 mg; can be sprinkled)	(0.3–2.0 mg/kg/ day)	60 mg/day
MPH (Concerta)[a]	Osmotic pressure system delivers 50–50 racemic mixture d,l-threo-MPH	12 hours	Caplets (18, 27, 36, 54 mg)	(0.3–2.0 mg/kg/ day)	72 mg/day
d-MPH XR (Focalin XR)	Bimodal delivery (50% immediate, 50% delayed) of d-MPH	12 hours	Capsules (10, 20, 30 mg)	(0.15–1.0 mg/kg/ day)	To be determined

Drug	Description	Duration	Formulation	Dose	Maximum
AMPH[b] (Dexedrine tablets)	d-AMPH tablet	4–5 hours	Tablets (5 mg)	(0.15–1.0 mg/kg/day)	40 mg/day
AMPH[b] (Dextrostat)	d-AMPH tablet	4–5 hours	Tablets (5, 10 mg)	(0.15–1.0 mg/kg/day)	40 mg/day
AMPH[b] (Dexedrine spansules)	Two types of beads in a 50–50 mixture give short and delayed absorption of d-AMPH	8 hours	Capsules (5, 10, 15 mg)	(0.15–1.0 mg/kg/day)	40 mg/day
Mixed salts of AMPH[b] (Adderall)	Tablet of d,l-AMPH isomers (75% d-AMPH and 25% l-AMPH)	4–6 hours	Tablets (5, 7.5, 10, 12.5, 15, 20, 30 mg)	(0.15–1.0 mg/kg/day)	40 mg/day
Mixed Salts of AMPH[a, c] (Adderall XR)	Two types of beads give bimodal delivery (50% immediate-release and 50% delayed-release) of 75–25 racemic mixture d,l-AMPH	At least 8 hours (but appears to last much longer in certain patients)	Capsules (5, 10, 15, 20, 25, 30 mg; can be sprinkled)	(0.15–1.0 mg/kg/day)	30 mg/day in children; recommended dose is 20 mg/day in adults
Magnesium pemoline (Cylert)[a, d]	Tablets of magnesium pemoline	12 hours	Tablets (18.75, 37.5, 75 mg)	Up to 3 mg/kg/day	112.5 mg/day
Atomoxetine[a, c] (Strattera)	Capsule of atomoxetine	5-hour plasma half-life (but CNS effects appear to last much longer)	Capsules (10, 18, 25, 40, 60, 80 mg)	1.2 mg/kg/day	1.4 mg/kg/day or 100 mg

Note. MPH, methylphenidate; AMPH, amphetamine.
[a] Approved to treat ADHD in patients age 6 years and older.
[b] Approved to treat ADHD in patients age 3 years and older
[c] Specifically approved for treatment of ADHD in adults.
[d] Because of its association with life-threatening hepatic failure, FDA recommends monitoring liver function tests every 2 weeks during treatment.

TABLE 22.5. Studies of Atomoxetine (ATMX) Pharmacotherapy in Adult ADHD

Study (year)	n	Design	Medi-cation	Duration	Total dose (wt.-corrected)	Response rate and primary outcome measure	Comments
Spencer, Biederman, Wilens, Prince, et al. (1998)	22	Double-blind, placebo-controlled, crossover	ATMX	7 weeks	76 mg	>30% reduction in ADHD-RS-IV	Initial positive results; b.i.d. dosing well tolerated
Michelson et al. (2003)	536	Double-blind, placebo-controlled	ATMX	10 weeks	[a]	Investigator-rated CAARS	Results from two independent studies pooled; dosing b.i.d.

Note. Duration of medication trial includes placebo phase. ADHD-RS-IV, ADHD Rating Scale–IV; CAARS, Conners Adult ADHD Rating Scale; b.i.d., twice daily.
[a] 60, 90, or 120 mg; most common dose-90 mg (1.3 mg/kg/day in a 70-kg patient).

occur with ADHD. Because of its lack of abuse liability (Heil et al., 2002), ATMX may be particularly useful in adults with current substance use issues, although this remains untested. Since pharmacotherapy of ADHD is often chronic, missed doses of medication can be expected and may be problematic. One study examined the effects of sudden discontinuation of ATMX in children and adults (Wernicke et al., 2004). Adults with ADHD, treated with ATMX in twice-daily doses ranging from 30 to 60 mg, were suddenly taken off ATMX. Although symptoms of ADHD worsened, few if any discontinuation-emergent adverse events were noted. Therefore, in most patients it appears safe to taper ATMX rapidly.

Although ATMX is generally well tolerated, the most common side effects observed with this medication appear reflective of increased noradrenergic tone. The most common side effects of ATMX observed in the two large studies included dry mouth (21.2%), insomnia (20.8%), nausea (12.3%), decreased appetite (11.5%), constipation (10.8%), decreased libido (7.1%), dizziness (6.3%), and sweating (5.2%) (Michelson et al., 2003). Furthermore, 9.8% of the males experienced difficulty attaining or maintaining erections. During these trials, extensive laboratory testing suggested that ATMX causes no organ toxicity, and there were no discontinuations in the clinical trials due to abnormal lab tests. However, there have been recent reports of significant hepatotoxicity in two patients taking ATMX (out of 2 million patients exposed to ATMX). Both patients re-

covered upon discontinuation of ATMX. The manufacturer recently added a boldface warning to the labeling about hepatotoxicity. The warning indicates that ATMX should be discontinued in patients with jaundice, and that patients should contact their doctors if they develop pruritis, jaundice, dark urine, right upper quadrant tenderness, and/or unexplained "flu-like" symptoms. At this time, lab monitoring outside of routine medical care does not appear necessary (Wernicke & Kratochvil, 2002). Although the impact of ATMX on the cardiovascular system appears minimal (Wernicke et al., 2003), ATMX was associated with mean increases in heart rate of 6 beats per minute, and increases in systolic and diastolic blood pressure of 1.5 mm Hg. Therefore, ATMX should be used cautiously in adults with hypertension or other cardiovascular risk factors. Adults should have their vital signs checked prior to initiating treatment with ATMX and periodically thereafter. Extensive electrocardiographic (EKG) monitoring indicates that ATMX has no apparent effect on QTc intervals, and EKG monitoring outside of routine medical care does not appear to be necessary.

ATMX is metabolized primarily in the liver to 4-hydroxyatomoxetine by the cytochrome CYP P450 2D6 enzyme (Ring, Gillespie, Eckstein, & Wrighton, 2002). The minor metabolite of ATMX is desmethylatomoxetine, which is primarily formed by CYP 2C19. In patients with compromised CYP 2D6 functioning, multiple other enzymes were observed to be capable of forming 4-hydroxyatomoxetine.

While ATMX is primarily metabolized by 2D6, it does not appear to inhibit 2D6, as noted earlier. Although patients identified as having "poor metabolism" (i.e., low 2D6 activity) generally appear to tolerate ATMX, these patients do seem to have more side effects, and a reduction in dose may be necessary. Therefore, in patients who are taking medications that are strong 2D6 inhibitors (i.e., fluoxetine, paroxetine, quinidine), it may be necessary to reduce the dose of ATMX. ATMX is contraindicated to be administered with the MAOIs. ATMX has been coadministered with albuterol (600 mcg i.v.) in patients with asthma. Mild elevations in heart rate and blood pressure over ATMX-alone administration were observed. Similarly, in a small trial (data on file with Eli Lilly and Co.) ATMX was administered with MPH and appeared well tolerated; although coadministration of ATMX and the stimulants has not been fully studied, a number of trials are currently studying this combination.

ANTIDEPRESSANTS

Table 22.6 summarizes studies of antidepressants and other nonstimulants in the treatment of adult ADHD. Bupropion, a novel-structured antidepressant, has been reported to be moderately helpful in reducing ADHD symptoms in children (Casat, Pleasants, & Van Wyck Fleet, 1987) and adults (Wender & Reimherr, 1990; Wilens, Spencer, et al., 2001; Wilens, Haight, et al., 2005). In an open study of 19 adults treated with an average of 360 mg of immediate-release bupropion for 6–8 weeks, Wender and Reimherr (1990) reported a moderate to marked response in 74% of adults in the study (5 dropouts), with sustained improvement at 1 year noted in 10 subjects. Building on Wender and Reimherr's initial work, Wilens, Spencer, et al. (2001) compared sustained-release bupropion to placebo in the treatment of 38 adults with ADHD. In this 6-week double-blind, placebo-controlled trial, sustained-release bupropion was initiated at 100 mg/day and increased at weekly intervals to a maximum of 200 mg twice daily (final mean dose = 386 mg/day). Treatment with bupropion resulted in a 42% reduction in scores on the ADHD-RS-IV. According to the investigator-rated Clinical Global Impression, 52% of subjects treated with bupropion were considered responders, compared to 11% of those randomized to pla-

cebo ($p = .005$). Recently, the extended-release form of bupropion (bupropion XL) has been reported to be useful for reducing ADHD in adults (Wilens, Haight, et al., 2004). ADHD. Dosing of 400–450 mg (sustained-release or XL preparations) is usually necessary for best efficacy. Side effects include insomnia, edginess, and a theoretical risk for seizures with immediate-release preparations. Despite the small numbers of adults studied, bupropion may be helpful in ADHD, particularly when ADHD is comorbid with depression (Daviss et al., 2001) or bipolar disorders (Wilens, Prince, et al., 2003), or when patients have cardiac abnormalities (Gelenberg, Bassuk, & Schoonover, 1991). Bupropion should be started at very low doses (37.5 mg of immediate-release, 100 mg of sustained-release, or 150 mg of XL) and titrated upward weekly to a maximal dose of 450 mg/day. Bupropion appears to be more stimulating than other antidepressants, and it is associated with a higher rate of drug-induced seizures than other antidepressants (Gelenberg et al., 1991). These seizures appear to be dose-related (>450 mg/day) and to be elevated in patients with Bulimia Nervosa or a previous seizure history. Bupropion has also been associated with excitement, agitation, increased motor activity, insomnia, tremor, and tics.

The TCAs have been used as alternatives to the stimulants for ADHD in pediatrics (Spencer et al., 1996; Spencer, 2004). Despite an extensive experience in children and adolescents, there are only two studies of these agents in adult ADHD (Wilens et al., 1996). Compared to the stimulants, TCAs have negligible abuse liability, single daily dosing, and efficacy for comorbid anxiety and depression. However, given concerns about potential cardiotoxicity, use of the TCAs has been significantly curtailed (especially since ATMX has become available).

An initial chart review indicated that desipramine or nortriptyline (often in combination with other psychotropics, including stimulants) resulted in moderate improvement that was sustained at 1 year (Wilens, Biederman, Mick, & Spencer, 1995). A controlled trial of desipramine with a target dose of 200 mg/day resulted in significant reductions in ADHD symptoms in adults (Wilens et al., 1996). In that study, response was noted during the initial titration at 2 weeks, and this continued to improve at the 6-week endpoint. Whereas a minority of subjects responded to <100 mg/

TABLE 22.6. Studies of Nonstimulant Pharmacotherapy in Adult ADHD

Study (year)	n	F	Design	Medication	Duration (weeks)	Dose (mg) (mean)	Response	Comments
Wood et al. (1982)	8	3	Open	Levodopa (+ carbidopa)	3	625 (63)	No benefit	Side effects: nausea, sedation, low doses
Wender et al. (1983)	22	3	Open	Pargyline	6	30	13/22 moderate improvement	Delayed onset; brief behavioral action; 6/22 dropped out due to side effects
Wender, Wood, et al. (1985)	11	UK	Open	Deprenyl	6	30	6/9 responded, 2 dropouts	Amphetamine metabolite; gender effects not discussed
Wood et al. (1985)	19	8	Double-blind, crossover	Phenylalanine	2	587	Poor	Transient mood improvement only
Mattes (1986)	13	1	Open, retrospective	Propranolol	3–50	528	11/13 improved	Part of "temper" study
Reimherr et al. (1987)	12	6	Open	Tyrosine	8	150	Poor response, 4 dropouts	14-day onset of action; tolerance developed
Shekim et al. (1989)	18	10	Open	Nomifensine maleate	4	<300	18/18 responded; reduction in ADHD sxs.	Immediate response; one patient with allergic reaction; 3/10 women dropped out due to side effects
Shekim, Antun, et al. (1990)	8	0	Open	S-adenosyl-l-methionine	4	<2,400	75% of patients responded	Mild adverse effects
Wender & Reimherr (1990)	19	5	Open	Bupropion	6–8	360	14/19 responded; 5 dropouts	10 subjects with improvement at 1 year
Wilens et al. (1995)	37	UK	Retrospective	Desipramine Nortriptyline	50	183 92	68% response rate; response sustained	Comorbidity unrelated to response; 60% on stimulants
Adler et al. (1995)	12	5	Open	Venlafaxine	8	110	10/12 responded; 50% reduction in sxs.	4 subjects on other meds; 4 dropped out
Reimherr et al. (1995)	18	6	Open	Venlafaxine	8	96	8/12 responded	Side effects led to 39% dropout rate; greatest improvement in pts. with mood difficulties; no discussion of gender effect on response

Study	N		Design	Medication	Duration	Dose	Outcome	Comments
Spencer, Biederman, Wilens, Prince, et al. (1998)	22	11	Double-blind, crossover	Tomoxetine	7	76	52% response rate, defined by <30% reduction in sxs.	Adrenergic agent; well tolerated
Findling et al. (1995)	9	5	Open	Venlafaxine	8	150	7/9 responded; reduction in ADHD sxs.	Improved anxiety scores
Wilens et al. (1996)	41	20	Double-blind, parallel	Desipramine	6	147	68% response rate	Gender, comorbidity, and levels not related to response
Ernst et al. (1996)	36	12	Double-blind, parallel	Selegiline	6	20, 60	Mild improvement; 60-mg dose better	High placebo response; mild side effects
Conners (1996)	17	4	Double-blind, crossover	Nicotine patch	0.3	7, 21	Clinical and neuropsychological improvement	Short trial; dose in smokers > nonsmokers; gender effects not discussed
Wilens, Biederman, Spencer, Bostic, et al. (1999)	32	4	Double-blind, crossover	ABT-418	7	75	40% response rate by CGI	Nicotinic analogue; attentional symptoms improved preferentially
Wilens, Spencer, et al. (2001)	40	18	Double-blind, parallel	Bupropion SR	6	386	52% response rate	Delayed onset of action; well tolerated
Taylor & Russo (2000)	22	4	Double-blind, crossover	Modafinil d-Amphetamine	7	206 22	48% response rate 48% response rate	Improved neuropsychological functioning with both txs.
Taylor & Russo (2001)	17	5	Double-blind, crossover	Guanfacine d-Amphetamine	7	1.1 NA	Both txs improved vs. placebo	Well tolerated; neuropsychological functioning improved
Cephalon, Inc. (2000)	113	UK	Double-blind, crossover	Modafinil	7	100, 400	No difference vs. placebo	Unpublished data
Total (n = 22)	421		Controlled—9 Open—11 Retrospective—2	Amino acids—3 Antidepressants—12 Antihypertensives—2 Others—5	0.3–50	Moderate doses	Variable response	Response rates typically less than those for stimulants; no influence of comorbidity

Note. Duration of medication trial includes placebo phase. sxs., symptoms; txs., treatments; CGI, Clinical Global Impression; F, female; NA, not available.

day, the majority required more robust dosing (mean of 150 mg/day) for efficacy.

Generally, TCA daily doses of 50–250 mg are required, with a relatively rapid response to treatment (i.e., 2 weeks) when the appropriate dose is reached. TCAs should be initiated at 25 mg and slowly titrated upward within dosing and serum level parameters until an acceptable response or intolerable adverse effects are reported. Common side effects of the TCAs include dry mouth, constipation, blurred vision, weight gain, and sexual dysfunction. Although cardiovascular effects (reduced cardiac conduction, elevated blood pressure, and heart rates) are not infrequent, if monitored they rarely prevent treatment. As serum TCA levels are variable, they are best used as guidelines for efficacy and to reduce CNS and cardiovascular toxicity.

The MAOI antidepressants have also been studied for the treatment of ADHD. Whereas open studies with pargyline and deprenyl in adult ADHD showed moderate improvements (Wender, Wood, Reimherr, & Ward, 1983; Wender, Wood, & Reimherr,, 1985), a more recent controlled trial of selegiline (deprenyl) yielded less promising findings (Ernst, Liebenauer, et al., 1996). Ernst et al. (1996) reported dose-dependent improvements in ADHD symptoms on selegiline, which were not significant when compared to a high placebo response. Although a pilot child-based study demonstrated efficacy of the reversible MAOI moclobemide (Trott, Friese, Menzel, & Nissen, 1992), data on its effectiveness for ADHD are limited to case reports (Myronuk, Weiss, & Cotter, 1996; Vaiva, De Lenclave, & Bailly, 2002). The MAOIs may have a role in the management of nonimpulsive adults with treatment-refractory ADHD and comorbid depression and anxiety (Myronuk et al., 1996), who are able to comply with the stringent requirements of these agents. The concerns about diet- or medication-induced hypertensive crisis limit the usefulness and safety of these medications, however, especially in those patients with ADHD who are vulnerable to impulsivity. Other adverse effects associated with the MAOIs include agitation or lethargy, orthostatic hypotension, weight gain, sexual dysfunction, sleep disturbances, and edema, often leading to the discontinuation of these agents (Gelenberg et al., 1991).

The selective serotonin reuptake inhibitors (SSRIs) do not appear to be effective for ADHD (Spencer, 2004); however, venlafaxine, an antidepressant with both serotonergic and noradrenergic properties, may have anti-ADHD efficacy. In three open studies with a total of 41 adults, 75% of adults who tolerated venlafaxine had a measurable reduction in their ADHD at doses of 75–150 mg daily (Adler, Resnick, Kunz, & Devinsky, 1995; Reimherr, Hedges, Strong, & Wender, 1995; Findling, Schwartz, Flannery, & Manos, 1996). Although further controlled trials are necessary to determine its optimal dosing and efficacy, venlafaxine is generally titrated from 25 mg/day to more typical antidepressant dosing of between 150 and 225 mg/day for ADHD control. Side effects of venlafaxine in adults include nausea and other gastrointestinal distress; there are concerns about elevated blood pressure at relatively higher dosing. Venlafaxine is often used conjointly with stimulants for control of ADHD in adults. The investigational antidepressants *S*-adenosylmethionine and nomifensine have also been shown to be effective for ADHD in adults, although they remain unstudied under controlled conditions (Shekim, Masterson, Cantwell, Hanna, & McCracken, 1989; Shekim, Antun, Hanna, McCracken, & Hess, 1990).

MISCELLANEOUS MEDICATIONS

Modafinil, approved for the treatment of narcolepsy (U.S. Modafinil in Narcolepsy Multicenter Study Group, 1998), has generated interest as a potential treatment for ADHD. Modafinil has been shown to improve cognitive and metacognitive functioning in healthy, non-sleep-deprived adults (Baranski, Pigeau, Dinich, & Jacobs, 2004), as well as to improve memory (short-term and visual), spatial planning, vigilance, and accuracy while reducing response latency in adults with ADHD (Turner, Clark, et al., 2004). One small open trial in children (Rugino & Copley, 2001) and one double-blind, placebo-controlled, crossover design in 22 adults (Taylor 2000) suggest improvements in ADHD symptoms. Results of large company-sponsored trials have been mixed. Initial trials in adults with ADHD were negative and to date have not been published (Cephalon Inc., 2000). Recently, Biederman (2003) presented results of two double-blind, placebo-controlled trials of modafinil in children with ADHD. These studies suggest that in doses up to 300 mg/day, children with ADHD experienced significant reductions in ADHD-RS-IV scores (as rated by classroom teachers) during treatment with modafinil. At this time, the interest in modafinil remains high, but its role in the treatment of adults with ADHD is evolving.

More recently, the relationship of nicotine and ADHD has attracted attention including findings of a higher-than-expected overlap between cigarette smoking and ADHD in both children (Milberger, Biederman, Faraone, Chen, & Jones, 1997) and adults (Pomerleau, Downey, Stelson, & Pomerleau, 1995). One small study of 2 days' duration showed a significant reduction in ADHD symptoms in adults wearing standard-size nicotine patches (Conners et al., 1996). Moreover, we have clinically observed the efficacy of the nicotine patch in reducing ADHD symptoms for adults who smoke and who report the emergence of ADHD symptoms with cigarette cessation. Based upon improvements in working memory and neuropsychological functioning with nicotine, Wilens, Biederman, Spencer, Bostic, et al. (1999) studied the novel cholinergic activating agent ABT-418. This double-blind, placebo-controlled crossover trial compared the effects of transdermal ABT-418 (75 mg daily) with placebo in 33 subjects. Adults treated with ABT-418 experienced significant reductions in ADHD-RS-IV scores, relative to placebo-treated adults; however, the overall effects were modest and were most notable in subjects with less severe ADHD. Although the cognitive-enhancing cholinergic agents have shown compelling efficacy in Alzheimer disease because of their ability to improve learning, cognition, and memory (Narahashi, Moriguchi, Zhao, Marszalec, & Yeh, 2004), the data on these agents in adults with ADHD are minimal (Wilens, Biederman, Wong, Spencer, & Prince, 2000).

The antihypertensives clonidine and guanfacine have been used in childhood ADHD, especially in cases with marked hyperactivity, an aggressive component, or tics (Spencer et al., 1996). One small open study of propranolol for adults with ADHD and temper outbursts indicated improvement in both the ADHD symptoms and outbursts at daily doses of up to 640 mg/day (Mattes, 1986). Beta-blockers when added to stimulants have also been reported to be helpful for ADHD in three adults (Ratey et al., 1991); however, this combination

may have been helpful by reducing the stimulant-induced adverse effects.

Trials with the amino acids were in part undertaken with the assumptions that ADHD might be related to a deficiency in the catecholaminergic system, and that administration of precursors of these systems would reverse these deficits. The results of open studies with levodopa and tyrosine, and controlled studies of phenylalanine in adults with ADHD, have generally been disappointing, despite robust dosing and adequate trial duration (see Table 22.6) (Wood, Reimherr, & Wender, 1982, 1985; Reimherr, Wender, Wood, & Ward, 1987). In these studies, transient improvement in ADHD was lost after 2 weeks of treatment. Therefore, amino acids have a limited role in the treatment of adults with ADHD.

SUGGESTED MANAGEMENT STRATEGIES

Having made the diagnosis of ADHD, the clinician needs to familiarize the adult patient with the risks and benefits of pharmacotherapy, the availability of alternative treatments, and the likely adverse effects. The patient's expectations need to be explored, and realistic goals of treatment need to be clearly delineated. Likewise, the clinician should review with the patient the various pharmacological options available, and should make it clear that each will require systematic trials of the anti-ADHD medications for reasonable durations of time and at clinically meaningful doses. Adults seeking treatment for ADHD who manifest substantial psychiatric comorbidity, have residual symptomatology with treatment, or report psychological distress related to their ADHD (e.g., self-esteem issues, self-sabotaging patterns, interpersonal disturbances) should be directed to appropriate psychotherapeutic intervention with clinicians knowledgeable in ADHD treatment.

Adult patients also often require more comprehensive treatment for their ADHD, given the sequalae associated with this chronic disorder, its effect on psychological development, and residual psychiatric and ADHD symptoms even with aggressive pharmacotherapy. To this end, structured cognitive-based psychotherapies appear helpful, especially when used conjointly with pharmacotherapy. In our center, we utilize an ADHD-adapted cognitive therapy protocol (McDermott & Wilens, 2000; Safren et al., 2005); recent data indicate that when this protocol was combined with medication, two-thirds of 26 adults whose ADHD was previously unresponsive to treatment were found to manifest clinically significant improvement (Wilens, McDermott, et al., 1999). Groups focused on coping skills, support, and interpersonal psychotherapy may also be very useful for these adults. For adults considering advanced schooling, educational planning and alterations in the school environment may be necessary.

The stimulant medications and ATMX are the most rigorously investigated pharmacotherapies (Tables 22.1–22.4) and are considered the first-line therapies for ADHD in adults. ATMX (in doses of 1.4 mg/kg/day or 100 mg/day) and MAS XR (in doses of 20 mg/day) are specifically indicated for the treatment of ADHD in adults. Although there are no evidence-based guidelines in selecting a first choice of medication for adults with ADHD, clinicians ought to base their recommendations on issues of safety, tolerability, efficacy, and duration of action (Greenhill, Pliszka, et al., 2002). Given the fact that response to stimulants is immediate (Wood et al., 1976; Spencer et al., 1995, 2001; Spencer, Biederman, & Wilens, 2004a), that stimulants have been used in clinical medicine since at least the 1930s, and that response to ATMX usually takes several weeks (Michelson et al., 2003), the stimulants are usually the first treatment of choice. Current treatment guidelines recommend starting with longer acting stimulant preparations in most cases (Greenhill, Pliszka, et al., 2002). Clinicians can initiate therapy at 18 mg of Concerta or 20 mg of Metadate CD or Ritalin LA for MPH products, or 5–10 mg of Adderall XR or Dexedrine spansules. Every few days, the dose may be increased to optimize response. Although the *Physicians' Desk Reference* lists maximum dosages at 40 mg/day for amphetamine products and 60 mg/d for MPH, patients often benefit from suggested daily dose ranges at 0.3–1.5 mg/kg/day for amphetamine products and 0.5–2.0 mg/kg/day for MPH products. Frequently, patients benefit from a combination of immediate-release amphetamine or MPH with longer-acting preparations in order to sculpt the dose to the patients' individual needs, although the efficacy of this practice is not well studied. Clinicians face a number of challenges when prescribing stimulants. Since stimulants may decrease appetite in this

patient population, it is often useful to administer stimulants during or after meals. Stimulant-induced sleep disturbances are common and may diminish these medications' effectiveness. Such disturbances may require alteration of the timing or amount of medication given, or may require the administration of a sleep aid. Irritability or dysphoria may occur 1–2 hours after administration of stimulants; this suggests an absorption peak phenomenon, which may respond to lower, more frequent doses.

Consideration of another stimulant or ATMX is recommended if an adult with ADHD is unresponsive to or has intolerable side effects to the initial medication. Given the pharmacodynamic differences between MPH and amphetamines (Wilens & Spencer, 1998), if an MPH product was initially selected, then moving to an amphetamine-based medication is appropriate. If neither of these medications is well tolerated or if both are ineffective, then using ATMX is appropriate. ATMX should be taken with food and titrated up to its final dose. Although some adults are able to take ATMX once daily, many adults benefit from twice-daily dosing (Michelson et al., 2003). Patients must also be made aware that the full benefits of ATMX may not occur for several weeks, and that they may not "feel" anything like the way they may have felt with the stimulants. Clinicians are often faced with the dilemma of whether or not to continue stimulants while they are tapering patients onto ATMX. Several trials are currently studying the tolerability, safety, and efficacy of this practice. Although data from these trials are not yet available, many patients are prescribed both stimulants and ATMX, based on prior experience combining stimulants and TCAs (Pataki, Carlson, Kelly, Rapport, & Biancaniello, 1993; Rapport, Carlson, Kelly, & Pataki, 1993; Cohen et al., 1999) as well as positive clinical anecdotes. Monitoring routine side effects, vital signs, and possible misuse of the medication are warranted.

Adult ADHD is a heterogeneous disorder that exhibits considerable comorbidity with antisocial, anxiety, and mood disorders, as well as substance use disorders (Biederman et al., 1993; Biederman, 2004). Adults with ADHD and comorbid mood or anxiety disorders may respond differently to ADHD pharmacotherapy, depending on the clinical state of their co-occurring disorders. An emerging literature suggests that children with both ADHD and anxiety or depression tend to respond less well to stimulants than children without these co-morbidities (Taylor et al., 1987; Pliszka, 1989; DuPaul, Barkley, & McMurray, 1994; Urman, Ickowicz, Fulford, & Tannock, 1995; Diamond, Tannock, & Schachar, 1999). However, this issue remains poorly studied in the adult population. Although stimulants are thought to be anxiogenic and/or depressogenic, the effect of stimulants on comorbid anxiety and depression have not been systematically assessed in adults with ADHD. While it is possible for stimulants to exacerbate anxiety and depression, patients may present with chronic anxiety/demoralization related to their untreated ADHD. Often in these cases, symptoms of anxiety and demoralization diminish with treatment for their ADHD. Likewise, patients presenting for treatment of depression may have their ADHD overlooked (Alpert et al., 1996). In addition, stimulants may exacerbate tics, obsessions, or compulsions, although they are frequently used in patients with these conditions (Gadow, Sverd, Sprafkin, Nolan, & Grossman, 1999; Tourette's Syndrome Stusy Group, 2002; Geller et al., 2003).

Other concurrent psychiatric disorders also need to be assessed, and (if possible) the relationship of the ADHD symptoms with these other disorders needs to be delineated. In subjects with ADHD plus Bipolar I Disorder, for example, the risk of mania and/or hypomania needs to be addressed and closely monitored during the treatment of the ADHD (Wilens, Biederman, et al., 2003). In cases such as these, mood stabilization is the priority and usually involves both introducing antimanic medications and discontinuing ADHD treatments. Once the mood is euthymic, conservative introduction of anti-ADHD medications along with mood-stabilizing agents should be considered (Biederman et al., 1998).

Many adults with ADHD have either a past or current alcohol and/or other substance use disorder (Wilens, 2004); therefore, a careful history of substance use should be completed, and a method for monitoring should be agreed upon if substance misuse is a clinical concern. Patients with ongoing substance abuse or dependence should generally not be treated until appropriate addiction treatments have been undertaken and the patients have maintained a drug- and alcohol-free period. Moreover, stimulants are Schedule II medications, and con-

cerns remain regarding their addictive potential. Although the rates of substance abuse in patients with ADHD are increased (Biederman et al., 1994; Wilens, 2004), the use of stimulants does not appear to increase the risk of substance abuse, as recent meta-analytic data suggest that successful stimulant treatment of children with ADHD reduces their risk of substance abuse into adolescence and adulthood by half (Wilens, Faraone, Biederman, & Gunawardene, 2003). However, given concerns about possible diversion and misuse (Babcock & Byrne, 2000), careful monitoring is necessary, and use of extended-delivery preparations (which are more difficult to misuse) should be considered (Greenhill, Pliszka, et al., 2002). When administered orally in their intended dosages, stimulants do not appear to cause euphoria, nor do they appear to be addictive (Swanson & Volkow, 2003; Volkow & Swanson, 2003). The addictive liability with available stimulant preparations is amphetamine > methylphenidate > pemoline. In the end, clinicians must use their clinical judgment to prioritize and sequence the treatment of ADHD in patients with comorbidites, while encouraging patient education about the potential for ADHD treatments to exacerbate comorbid psychiatric conditions.

The antidepressants (namely, TCAs and bupropion) are less well studied. However, they appear useful for adults with ADHD who do not respond to stimulants or who have concurrent psychiatric disorders, including depression, anxiety, or active or recent substance abuse (Wender & Reimherr, 1990; Wilens et al., 1996; Daviss et al., 2001; Wilens, Prince, et al., 2001). Comparative data between the antidepressants and stimulants in adults, coupled with studies in children support that stimulants are generally more effective in reducing ADHD symptoms (Spencer, Biederman, & Wilens, 2004a, 2004b). In addition, the response to the stimulants is immediate (Wood et al., 1976; Spencer et al., 1995, 2001; Spencer, Biederman, & Wilens, 2004a), whereas the antidepressants have continued improvement up to 4 weeks after titration (Wilens et al., 1996; Wilens, Spencer, et al., 2001). Although some adults may respond to relatively low doses of the TCAs (Ratey et al., 1992), the majority of adults appear to require solid antidepressant dosing of these agents (e.g., desipramine at > 150 mg daily). MAOIs are mildly effective, but are generally reserved for adults with treatment-refractory ADHD who can reliably follow the dietary requirements (Ernst et al., 1996). Consideration may be given to the use of moclobemide in patients with ADHD and comorbid mood/anxiety disorders, but the available data are limited to case reports (Myronuk et al., 1996; Vaiva et al., 2002).

The antihypertensives may be useful in adults with ADHD and aggressive outbursts (Mattes, 1986) or those with adverse effects to the stimulants. Given the high comorbidity between tic disorders and ADHD, consideration may be given to using alpha-adrenergic medications and stimulants together (Tourette's Syndrome Study Group, 2002). In this large (*n* = 146) multicenter trial of the treatment of ADHD in patients with chronic tic disorders, MPH alone or in combination with clonidine was the most effective treatment for ADHD symptoms; conversely, clonidine, alone or in combination with MPH, was the most effective treatment to reduce tics. Nonetheless, because of a lack of efficacy data and concerns about their sedative and hypotensive effects, their use in adults remains limited. Beta-blockers may be helpful in adult ADHD, but remain unstudied under controlled conditions (Mattes, 1986; Ratey et al., 1991). The amino acids have not been shown to be effective, and the cholinergic-enhancing compounds remain to be studied comprehensively in adults with ADHD.

Although systematic data assessing the efficacy and safety of combining agents for ADHD in adults are lacking, combination treatment may be necessary for those who have residual symptomatology with single agents or those who have psychiatric comorbidity. For example, in one naturalistic report on TCAs for adults with ADHD, 84% of adults were receiving additional psychoactive medications, with 59% receiving adjunctive stimulants (Wilens et al., 1995). These findings are similar to controlled data in juvenile ADHD, in which the combination of MPH and desipramine improved the ADHD response more than either agent singly (Rapport et al., 1993). The use of MPH conjointly with fluoxetine has been reported to be well tolerated and useful in improving depression in adolescents with ADHD (Gammon & Brown, 1993), and this combination appears useful in adults with the same comorbidity. In cases of partial response to or adverse effects with stimulants, low-dose SSRIs, TCAs, or beta-blockers have been reported to be helpful (Ratey et al., 1991). In ad-

dition, Daviss et al. (2001) have demonstrated the usefulness of bupropion in treating adolescents with ADHD and depression. When combining agents, however, clinicians need to consider potential drug interactions, such as those described between TCAs and some SSRIs (Aranow et al., 1989; Markowitz & Patrick, 2001).

MANAGEMENT OF DIFFICULT CASES

Despite the availability of various agents for adults with ADHD, some such individuals either do not respond to, or are intolerant of adverse effects of, medications used to treat their ADHD. In managing difficult cases, several therapeutic strategies are available (see Table 22.7). If psychiatric adverse effects develop concurrently with a poor medication response, alternative treatments should be pursued. Severe psychiatric symptoms that emerge during the acute phase can be problematic, regardless of the efficacy of the medications for ADHD. These symptoms may require reconsideration of the diagnosis of ADHD and careful reassessment of the presence of comorbid disorders. For example, in adults with ADHD, it is common to observe depressive symptoms that are independent of the ADHD or treatment. If reduction of dose or change in preparation (i.e., immediate-release vs. extended-delivery) does not resolve the problem, consideration should be given to alternative treatments. Concurrent nonpharmacological interventions such as behavioral or cognitive therapy may assist with symptom reduction.

The pharmacology of ADHD is directly related to the pathogenesis of ADHD. The neurochemical dysfunction in ADHD appears to be mediated by dopaminergic and adrenergic systems, with little direct influence by the serotonergic systems (Zametkin & Liotta, 1998). For instance, stimulants block the reuptake of dopamine and norepinephrine presynaptically, and simultaneously increase the release of these monoamines into the extraneuronal space (Elia et al., 1990; Wilens & Spencer, 1998; Volkow et al., 2001). Similar biochemical findings have been reported with those antidepressants (TCAs and bupropion) also shown to be effective for ADHD. Serotonin does not appear integral in ADHD, and serotonin-based agents have not been shown to be useful for core ADHD symptomatology. Although cholinergic

TABLE 22.7. Strategies in Difficult Cases of Adult ADHD

Symptoms	Interventions
Worsening or unchanged ADHD symptoms (inattention, impulsivity, hyperactivity)	• Change medication dose (increase or decrease) • Change timing of dose • Change preparation; substitute another medication • Evaluate for possible tolerance • Consider adjunctive pharmacological treatment (antidepressant, alpha-adrenergic agent, cognitive enhancer) • Consider adjunctive nonpharmacological treatment (cognitive-behavioral therapies or coaching) • Reevaluate neuropsychological profile for executive function capacities
Intolerable side effects	• Evaluate whether side effect is drug-induced • Assess medication response versus tolerability of side effect • Provide aggressive management of side effect (change timing of dose; change preparation or medication; consider adjunctive or alternative treatment)
Symptoms of rebound	• Change timing of dose • Supplement with small dose of short-acting stimulant or alpha-adrenergic agent 1 hour prior to symptom onset • Change preparation • Increase frequency of dosage
Development of tics or Tourette syndrome (TS), or use with comorbid tics or TS	• Assess persistence of tics or TS • If tics abate, rechallenge • If tics are clearly worsened with stimulant treatment, discontinue • Consider stimulant use with adjunctive anti-tic treatment (haloperidol, pimozide) or use of alternative treatment (antidepressants, alpha-adrenergic agents)
Emergence of dysphoria, irritability, acceleration, agitation	• Assess for toxicity or rebound • Evaluate development or exacerbation of comorbidity—mood, anxiety, and substance use (including nicotine and caffeine) • Reduce dose • Change preparation; substitute another medication • Assess sleep and mood • Consider alternative treatment
Emergence of major depression, mood lability, or marked anxiety symptoms	• Assess for toxicity or rebound • Evaluate development or exacerbation of comorbidity • Reduce or discontinue medication • Consider use of antidepressant or antimanic agent • Assess substance use • Consider nonpharmacological interventions
Emergence of psychosis or mania	• Discontinue medication • Assess comorbidity • Assess substance use • Treat psychosis or mania

Note. Adapted from Wilens and Spencer (2000). Copyright 2000 by Elsevier Inc. Adapted by permission.

modulation of temporal memory has been investigated (Meck & Church, 1987), the effects of cholinergic-enhancing agents on ADHD, cognition, learning, and memory, as well as on dopaminergic and other neurotransmitter systems, are still being studied (Narahashi et al., 2004).

SUMMARY

In summary, the aggregate literature supports the conclusion that pharmacotherapy provides effective treatment for adults with ADHD. Effective pharmacological treatments for adults with ADHD to date have included the psychostimulants and ATMX. Bupropion, TCAs, and modafanil have also been studied in the treatment of adult ADHD, and have a role in its treatment. Although interest in cognitive enhancers remain high, data on their efficacy remain minimal, and their role is limited. Structured psychotherapy may be effective when used adjunctively with medications. Further controlled investigations assessing the efficacy of single and combination agents for adults with ADHD are necessary, with careful attention to diagnostics, comorbidity, symptom and neuropsychological outcome; long-term tolerability and efficacy; and use in specific ADHD subgroups.

KEY CLINICAL POINTS

✓ MAS XR and ATMX are currently approved to treat ADHD in adults, and it is expected that d-MPH XR will also be approved to treat ADHD.

✓ Either stimulants or ATMX are first-line pharmacotherapy for ADHD in adults.

✓ Two main types of stimulants, methylphenidate, and amphetamine compounds have different pharmacodynamic effects and metabolism.

✓ Methylphenidate does not show up on urine drug screens.

✓ Stimulants are not effective for comorbidities within ADHD.

✓ Stimulants generally have few medication interactions (except with MAOIs).

✓ Few drug interactions exist with atomoxe-

tine, increasing use concomitantly with stimulants.

✓ Atomoxetine may be particularly useful in treating comorbidity in adults with ADHD.

✓ Tricyclic antidepressant and bupropion are second-line pharmacotherapies.

✓ Empiric use of combinations may be appropriate in refractory and comorbid patients.

REFERENCES

Achenbach, T. M., Howell, C., McConaughy, S., & Stanger, C. (1998). Six-year predictors of problems in a national sample: IV. Young adult signs of disturbance. *Journal of the American Academy of Child and Adolescent Psychiatry, 37*(7), 718–727.

Adler, L. A., & Cohen, J. (2004). Diagnosis and evaluation of adults with attention-deficit/hyperactivity disorder. *Psychiatric Clinics of North America, 27*(2), 187–201.

Adler, L. A., McGough, J., Muniz, R., Pestreich, L., Agoropoulou, C., & Jiang, H. (2005, May 21–25). *Long-term efficacy of extended-release dexmethylphenldate in adult ADHD.* Poster presented at the 158th annual meeting of the American Psychiatric Association, Atlanta, GA.

Adler, L. A., Resnick, S., Kunz, M., & Devinsky, O. (1995). Open label trial of venlafaxine in adults with attention deficit disorder. *Psychopharmacology Bulletin, 31*, 785–788.

Alpert, J., Maddocks, A., Nierenberg, A., O'Sullivan, R., & Pava, J., Worthington, J., et al. (1996). Attention deficit hyperactivity disorder in childhood among adults with major depression. *Psychiatry Research, 62*, 213–219.

American Psychiatric Association. (2000). *Diagnostic and statistical manual of mental disorders* (4th ed., text rev.). Washington, DC: Author.

Aranow, R. B., Hudson, J. L., Pope, H. G., Grady, T. A., Laage, T. A., Bell, I. R., et al. (1989). Elevated antidepressant plasma levels after addition of fluoxetine. *American Journal of Psychiatry, 146*, 911–913.

Babcock, Q., & Byrne, T. (2000). Student perceptions of methylphenidate abuse at a public liberal arts college. *Journal of American College Health, 49*(3), 143–145.

Baranski, J. V., Pigeau, R., Dinich, P., & Jacobs, I. (2004). Effects of modafinil on cognitive and metacognitive performance. *Human Psychopharmacology, 19*(5), 323–332.

Barkley, R. A. (1997). *ADHD and the nature of self-control.* New York: Guilford Press.

Barkley, R. A. (1998). *Attention-deficit/hyperactivity disorder: A handbook for diagnosis and treatment* (2nd ed.). New York: Guilford Press.

Barkley, R. A., Murphy, K. R., DuPaul, G. J., & Bush, T. (2002). Driving in young adults with attention deficit hyperactivity disorder: Knowledge, performance, adverse outcomes, and the role of executive functioning. *Journal of the International Neuropsychological Society, 8*(5), 655–672.

Barkley, R. A., Murphy, K. R., & Kwasnik, D. (1996a). Psychological adjustment and adaptive impairments in young adults with ADHD. *Journal of Attention Disorders, 1*(1), 41–54.

Barkley, R. A., Murphy, K. R., & Kwasnik, D. (1996b). Motor vehicle driving competencies and risks in teens and young adults with attention deficit hyperactivity disorder. *Pediatrics, 98,* 1089–1095.

Bemporad, J. R. (2001). Aspects of psychotherapy with adults with attention deficit disorder. *Annals of the New York Academy of Sciences, 931,* 302–309.

Bemporad, J. R., & Zambenedetti, M. (1996). Psychotherapy of adults with attention deficit disorder. *Journal of Psychotherapy, 5,* 228–237.

Biederman, J. (1998). A 55–year-old man with attention-deficit-hyperactivity disorder. *Journal of the American Medical Association, 280*(12), 1086–1092.

Biederman, J. (2003). *A double-blind placebo-controlled trial of modafinil in the treatment of attention-deficit/hyperactivity disorder.* Paper presented at the annual meeting of the American Psychiatric Association, San Francisco.

Biederman, J. (2004). Impact of comorbidity in adults with attention-deficit/hyperactivity disorder. *Journal of Clinical Psychiatry, 65*(Suppl. 3), 3–7.

Biederman, J., Baldessarini, R. J., Wright, V., Knee, D., & Harmatz, J. S. (1989). A double-blind placebo controlled study of desipramine in the treatment of ADD: I. Efficacy. *Journal of the American Academy of Child and Adolescent Psychiatry, 28*(5), 777–784.

Biederman, J., Faraone, S. V., & Mick, E. (2000). Age dependent decline of ADHD symptoms revisited: Impact of remission definition and symptom subtype. *American Journal of Psychiatry, 157,* 816–817.

Biederman, J., Faraone, S. V., Spencer, T. J., Wilens, T. E., Mick, E. A., & Lapey, K. (1994). Gender differences in a sample of adults with attention deficit hyperactivity disorder. *Psychiatry Research, 53,* 13–29.

Biederman, J., Faraone, S. V., Spencer, T., Wilens, T., Norman, D., Lapey, K. A., et al. (1993). Patterns of psychiatric comorbidity, cognition, and psychosocial functioning in adults with attention deficit hyperactivity disorder. *American Journal of Psychiatry, 150,* 1792–1798.

Biederman, J., Mick, E., Bostic, J., Prince, J., Daly, J., Wilens, T., et al. (1998). The naturalistic course of pharmacologic treatment of children with manic like symptoms: A systematic chart review. *Journal of Clinical Psychiatry, 59*(11), 628–637.

Biederman, J., Quinn, D., Weiss, M., Markabi, S., Weidenman, M., Edson, K., et al. (2003). Efficacy and safety of Ritalin LA, a new, once daily, extended-release dosage form of methylphenidate, in children with attention deficit hyperactivity disorder. *Paediatric Drugs, 5*(12), 833–841.

Biederman, J., Spencer, T. J., Chrisman, A. K., Wilens, T.

E., Tulloch, S. J., & Wesler, R. H. (2004). *Long-term safety and efficacy of mixed amphetamine salts extended-release for adult ADHD.* Paper presented at the 157th annual meeting of the American Psychiatric Association, New York.

Biederman, J., Wilens, T. E., Mick, E., Milberger, S., Spencer, T. J., & Faraone, S. V. (1995). Psychoactive substance use disorders in adults with attention deficit hyperactivity disorder (ADHD), Effects of ADHD and psychiatric comorbidity. *American Journal of Psychiatry, 152*(11), 1652–1658.

Birmaher, B., Greenhill, L. L., Cooper, T. B., Fried, J., & Maminski, B. (1989). Sustained release methylphenidate: Pharmacokinetic studies in ADDH males. *Journal of the American Academy of Child and Adolescent Psychiatry, 28*(5), 768–772.

Bouffard, R., Hechtman, L., Minde, K., & Iaboni-Kassab, F. (2003). The efficacy of 2 different dosages of methylphenidate in treating adults with attention-deficit hyperactivity disorder. *Canadian Journal of Psychiatry, 48*(8), 546–554.

Brown, T. (1996). *Brown Attention Deficit Disorder Scales.* San Antonio, TX: Psychological Corporation.

Bymaster, F. P., Katner, J. S., Nelson, D. L., Hemrick-Luecke, S. K., Threlkeld, P. G., Heiligenstein, J. H., et al. (2002). Atomoxetine increases extracellular levels of norepinephrine and dopamine in prefrontal cortex of rat: A potential mechanism for efficacy in attention deficit/hyperactivity disorder. *Neuropsychopharmacology, 27*(5), 699–711.

Casat, C. D., Pleasants, D. Z., & Van Wyck Fleet, J. (1987). A double blind trial of bupropion in children with attention deficit disorder. *Psychopharmacology Bulletin, 23,* 120–122.

Cephalon, Inc. (2000). *No benefit noted from Provigil (modafinil) in adult attention deficit hyperactivity disorder.* West Chester, PA: Author.

Cohen, L. G., Prince, J., Biederman, J., Wilens, T., Faraone, S. V., Whitt, S., et al. (1999). Absence of effect of stimulants on the phamacokinetics of desipramine in children. *Pharmacotherapy, 19*(6), 746–752.

Conners, C., Levin, E. D., Sparrow, E., Hinton, S., Erhardt, D., Meck, W., et al. (1996). Nicotine and attention in adult attention deficit hyperactivity disorder. *Psychopharmacology Bulletin, 32,* 67–73.

Daviss, W. B., Bentivoglio, P., Racusin, R., Brown, K. M., Bostic, J. Q., & Wiley, L. (2001). Bupropion sustained release in adolescents with comorbid attention-deficit/hyperactivity disorder and depression. *Journal of the American Academy of Child and Adolescent Psychiatry, 40*(3), 307–314.

Diamond, I., Tannock, R., & Schachar, R. (1999). Response to methylphenidate in children with ADHD and comorbid anxiety. *Journal of the American Academy of Child and Adolescent Psychiatry, 38*(4), 402–409.

Ding, Y. S., Fowler, J. S., Volkow, N. D., Dewey, S. L., Wang, G. J., Logan, J., et al. (1997). Chiral drugs: Comparison of the pharmacokinetics of [11C]d-threo and l-threo-methylphenidate in the human and baboon brain. *Psychopharmacology, 131*(1), 71–78.

Ding, Y. S., Gatley, S. J., Thanos, P. K., Shea, C., Garza, V., Xu, Y., et al. (2004). Brain kinetics of methylphenidate (Ritalin) enantiomers after oral administration. *Synapse, 53*(3), 168–175.

DuPaul, G. J., Barkley, R. A., McMurray, M. B. (1994). Response of children with ADHD to methylphenidate: Interaction with internalizing symptoms. *Journal of the American Academy of Child and Adolescent Psychiatry, 33*(6), 894–903.

Elia, J., Borcherding, B. G., Potter, W. Z., Mefford, I. N., Rapoport, J. L., & Keysor, C. S. (1990). Stimulant drug treatment of hyperactivity: Biochemical correlates. *Clinical Pharmacology and Therapeutics, 48,* 57–66.

Ernst, M., Liebenauer, L., Jons, P., Tebeka, D., Cohen, R., & Zametkin, A. (1996). Selegiline in adults with attention deficit hyperactivity disorder: Clinical efficacy and safety. *Psychopharmacology Bulletin, 32,* 327–334.

Faraone, S. V., Sergeant, J., Gillberg, C., & Biederman, J. (2003). The worldwide prevalence of ADHD: Is it an American condition? *World Psychiatry, 2*(2), 104–113.

Faraone, S. V., Spencer, T., Aleardi, M., Pagano, C., & Biederman, J. (2004). Meta-analysis of the efficacy of methylphenidate for treating adult attention-deficit/hyperactivity disorder. *Journal of Clinical Psychopharmacology, 24*(1), 24–29.

Faraone, S. V., Spencer, T. J., Montano, C. B., & Biederman, J. (2004). Attention-deficit/hyperactivity disorder in adults: A survey of current practice in psychiatry and primary care. *Archives of Internal Medicine, 164*(11), 1221–1226.

Findling, R. L., Schwartz, M. A., Flannery, D., & Manos, M. (1996). Venlafaxine in adults with attention-deficit/hyperactivity disorder: An open clinical trial. *Journal of Clinical Psychiatry, 57*(5), 184–189.

Fones, C. S., Pollack, M. H., Susswein, L., & Otto, M. (2000). History of childhood attention deficit hyperactivity disorder (ADHD) features among adults with panic disorder. *Journal of Affective Disorders, 58,* 99–106.

Gadow, K., Sverd, J., Sprafkin, J., Nolan, E., & Grossman, S. (1999). Long-term methylphenidate therapy in children with comorbid attention-deficit hyperactivity disorder and chronic multiple tic disorder. *Archives of General Psychiatry, 56*(4), 330–336.

Gammon, G. D., & Brown, T. E. (1993). Fluoxetine and methylphenidate in combination for treatment of attention deficit disorder and comorbid depressive disorder. *Journal of Child and Adolescent Psychopharmacology, 3*(1), 1–10.

Gelenberg, A. J., Bassuk, E. L., Schoonover, S. C. (Eds.). (1991). *The practitioner's guide to psychoactive drugs* (3rd ed.). New York: Plenum Medical Book.

Geller, D. A., Coffey, B., Faraone, S., Hagermoser, L., Zaman, N. K., Farrell, C. L., et al. (2003). Does comorbid attention-deficit/hyperactivity disorder impact the clinical expression of pediatric obsessive–

compulsive disorder? *CNS Spectrums, 8*(4), 259–264.

Greenhill, L. L., Cooper, T., Solomon, M., Fried, J., & Cornblatt, B. (1987). Methylphenidate salivary levels in children. *Psychopharmacology Bulletin, 23*(1), 115–119.

Greenhill, L. L., Findling, R. L., Swanson, J. M., & MTA Cooperative Group. (2002). A double-blind, placebo-controlled study of modified-release methylphenidate in children with attention-deficit/hyperactivity disorder. *Pediatrics, 109*(3), E39.

Greenhill, L. L., Pliszka, S., Dulcan, M, K., Bernet, W., Arnold, V., Beitchman, J., et al. (2002). Practice parameter for the use of stimulant medications in the treatment of children, adolescents, and adults. *Journal of the American Academy of Child and Adolescent Psychiatry, 41*(2, Suppl.), 26S–49S.

Gualtieri, C. T., Hicks, R. E., Patrick, K., Schroeder, S. R., & Breese, G. R. (1984). Clinical correlates of methylphenidate blood levels. *Therapeutic Drug Monitoring, 6*(4), 379–392.

Gualtieri, C. T., Ondrusek, M. G., & Finley, C. (1985). Attention deficit disorder in adults. *Clinical Neuropharmacology, 8,* 343–356.

Gutgesell, H., Atkins, D., Barst, R., Buck, M., Franklin, W., Humes, R., et al. (1999). *Cardiovascular monitoring of children and adolescents receiving psychotropic drugs.* Washington, DC: American Heart Association.

Hart, E. L., Lahey, B. B., Loeber, R., Applegate, B., & Frick, P. J. (1995). Developmental change in attention-deficit hyperactivity disorder in boys: A four-year longitudinal study. *Journal of Abnormal Child Psychology, 23*(6), 729–749.

Heil, S. H., Holmes, H. W., Bickel, W. K., Higgins, S. T., Badger, G. J., Laws, H. F., et al. (2002). Comparison of the subjective, physiological, and psychomotor effects of atomoxetine and methylphenidate in light drug users. *Drug and Alcohol Dependence, 67*(2), 149–156.

Heiligenstein, E., Conyers, L. M., Berns, A. R., & Miller, M. A. (1998). Preliminary normative data on DSM-IV attention deficit hyperactivity disorder in college students. *Journal of American College Health, 46*(4), 185–188.

Heiligenstein, E., Johnston, H., & Nielsen, J. K. (1996). Pemoline therapy in college students with attention deficit hyperactivity disorder: A retrospective study. *Journal of American College Health, 45,* 35–42.

Hill, J. C., & Schoener, E. P. (1996). Age-dependent decline of attention deficit hyperactivity disorder. *American Journal of Psychiatry, 153,* 1143–1146.

Horrigan, J., & Barnhill, L. (2000). Low-dose amphetamine salts and adult attention-deficit/hyperactivity disorder. *Journal of Clinical Psychiatry, 61,* 414–417.

Iaboni, F., Bouffard, R., Minde, K., & Hechtman, L. (1996). The efficacy of methylphenidate in treating adults with attention-deficit/hyperactivity disorder. *Scientific Proceedings of the American Academy of Child and Adolescent Psychiatry.* Philadelphia: American Academy of Child and Adolescent Psychiatry.

Kessler, R. C., Adler, L., Ames, M., Demler, O., Faraone, S., Hiripi, E., et al. (2005). The World Health Organization Adult ADHD Self-Report Scale (ASRS): A short screening scale for use in the general population. *Psychological Medicine, 35,* 245–256.

Kooij, J. J., Burger, H., Boonstra, A, M., Vander Kinden, P. D., Kalma, L. E,, & Buitelaar, J. K. (2004). Efficacy and safety of methylphenidate in 45 adults with attention-deficit/hyperactivity disorder: A randomized placebo-controlled double-blind cross-over trial. *Psychological Medicine, 34*(6), 973–982.

Kuperman, S., Perry, P. J., Gaffney, G. R., Land, B. C., Bever-Stille, K. A., Arndt, S., et al. (2001). Bupropion SR vs. methylphenidate vs. placebo for attention deficit hyperactivity disorder in adults. *Annals of Clinical Psychiatry, 13*(3), 129–134.

Mannuzza, S., Klein, R. G., Bessler, A., Malloy, P., & LaPadula, M. (1993). Adult outcome of hyperactive boys: Educational achievement, occupational rank, and psychiatric status. *Archives of General Psychiatry, 50,* 565–576.

Markowitz, J. S., Morrison, S. D., & Devane, C. L. (1999). Drug interactions with psychostimulants. *International Clinical Psychopharmacology, 14*(1), 1–18.

Markowitz, J. S., & Patrick, K. S. (2001). Pharmacokinetic and pharmacodynamic drug interactions in the treatment of ADHD. *Clinical Pharmacokinetics, 40,* 753–772.

Mattes, J. A. (1986). Propranolol for adults with temper outbursts and residual attention deficit disorder. *Journal of Clinical Psychopharmacology, 6,* 299–302.

Mattes, J. A., Boswell, L., & Oliver, H. (1984). Methylphenidate effects on symptoms of attention deficit disorder in adults. *Archives of General Psychiatry, 41,* 1059–1063.

McDermott, S. P., & Wilens, T. E. (2000). Cognitive therapy for adults with ADHD. In T. Brown (Ed.), *Attention deficit disorders in children, adolescents, and adults* (pp. 569–606). Washington, DC: American Psychiatric Press.

Meck, W., & Church, R. (1987). Cholinergic modulation of the content of temporal memory. *Behavioral Neuroscience, 101*(4), 457–464.

Michelson, D., Adler, L., Spencer, T., Reimherr, F., West, S., Allen, A., et al. (2003). Atomoxetine in adults with ADHD: two randomized, placebo-controlled studies. *Biological Psychiatry, 53*(2), 112–120.

Mick, E., Faraone, S. V., & Biederman, J. (2004). Age-dependent expression of attention-deficit/hyperactivity disorder symptoms. *Psychiatric Clinics of North America, 27*(2), 215–224.

Milberger, S., Biederman, J., Faraone, S. V., Chen, L., & Jones, J. (1997). ADHD is associated with early initiation of cigarette smoking in children and adolescents. *Journal of the American Academy of Child and Adolescent Psychiatry, 36,* 37–43.

Millstein, R. B., Wilens, T. E., Spencer, T., & Biederman, J. (1997). Presenting ADHD symptoms and subtypes in clinically referred adults with ADHD. *Journal of Attention Disorders, 2*(3), 159–166.

Murphy, K. R., & Adler, L. A. (2004). Assessing attention-deficit/hyperactivity disorder in adults: Focus on rating scales. *Journal of Clinical Psychiatry, 65*(Suppl. 3), 12–17.

Murphy, K. R., & Barkley, R. A. (1996). Prevalence of DSM-IV symptoms of ADHD in adult licensed drivers: Implications for clinical diagnosis. *Journal of Attention Disorders, 1*(3), 147–161.

Myronuk, L. D., Weiss, M., & Cotter, L. (1996). Combined treatment with moclobemide and methylphenidate for comorbid major depression and adult attention-deficit/hyperactivity disorder. *Journal of Clinical Psychopharmacology, 16*(6), 468–469.

Narahashi, T., Moriguchi, S., Zhao, X., Marszalec, W., & Yeh, Z. (2004). Mechanisms of action of cognitive enhancers on neuroreceptors. *Biological Pharmacology Bulletin, 27*(11), 1701–1706.

Pataki, C. S., Carlson, G. A., Kelly, K. L., Rapport, M. D., & Biancaniello, T. M. (1993). Side effects of methylphenidate and desipramine alone and in combination in children. *Journal of the American Academy of Child and Adolescent Psychiatry, 32,* 1065–1072.

Paterson, R., Douglas, C., Hallmayer, J., Hagan, M., & Krupenia, Z. (1999). A randomised, double-blind, placebo-controlled trial of dexamphetamine in adults with attention deficit hyperactivity disorder. *Australian and New Zealand Journal of Psychiatry, 33*(4), 494–502.

Patrick, K., Straughn, A., Jarvi, E., Breese, G., & Meyer, M. (1989). The absorption of sustained-release methylphenidate formulations compared to an immediate-release formulation. *Biopharmaceutics and Drug Disposition, 10,* 165–171.

Pliszka, S. R. (1989). Effect of anxiety on cognition, behavior, and stimulant response in ADHD. *Journal of the American Academy of Child and Adolescent Psychiatry, 28*(6), 882–887.

Pomerleau, O., Downey, K., Stelson, F., & Pomerleau, C. (1995). Cigarette smoking in adult patients diagnosed with attention deficit hyperactivity disorder. *Journal of Substance Abuse, 7,* 373–378.

Pratt, D. S., & Dubois, R. S. (1990). Hepatotoxicity due to pemoline (Cylert): A report of two cases. *Journal of Pediatric Gastroenterology, 10,* 239–241.

Prince, J. B., Wilens, T. E., Biederman, J., Spencer, T. J., Millstein, R., Polisner, D. A., et al. (2000). A controlled study of nortriptyline in children and adolescents with attention deficit hyperactivity disorder. *Journal of Child and Adolescent Psychopharmacology, 10*(3), 193–204.

Rapport, M. D., Carlson, G. A., Kelly, K. L., & Pataki, C. (1993). Methylphenidate and desipramine in hospitalized children: I. Separate and combined effects on cognitive function. *Journal of the American Academy of Child and Adolescent Psychiatry, 32,* 333–342.

Ratey, J. J., Greenberg, M. S., Bemporad, J. R., & Lindem, K. J. (1992). Unrecognized attention-deficit hyperactivity disorder in adults presenting for outpatient psychotherapy. *Journal of Child and Adolescent Psychopharmacology, 2*(4), 267–275.

Ratey, J., Greenberg, M., & Lindem, K. J. (1991). Combination of treatments for attention deficit disorders in adults. *Journal of Nervous and Mental Disease, 176,* 699–701.

Reimherr, F. W., Hedges, D. W., Strong, R. E., & Wender, P. H. (1995). *An open trial of venlafaxine in adult patients with attention deficit hyperactivity disorder.* Paper presented at the annual meeting of the New Clinical Drug Evaluation Unit, Orlando, FL.

Reimherr, F. W., Wender, P. H., Wood, D. R., & Ward, M. (1987). An open trial of L-tyrosine in the treatment of attention deficit hyperactivity disorder, residual type. *American Journal of Psychiatry, 144,* 1071–1073.

Ring, B. J., Gillespie, J. S., Eckstein, J. A., & Wrighton, S. A. (2002). Identification of the human cytochromes P450 responsible for atomoxetine metabolism. *Drug Metabolism and Disposition, 30*(3), 319–323.

Rugino, T. A., & Copley, T. C. (2001). Effects of modafinil in children with attention-deficit/hyperactivity disorder: An open-label study. *Journal of the American Academy of Child and Adolescent Psychiatry, 40*(2), 230–235.

Safer, D. J., Zito, J. M., & Gardner, J. F. (2001). Pemoline hepatotoxicity and postmarketing surveillance. *Journal of the American Academy of Child and Adolescent Psychiatry, 40*(6), 622–629.

Safren, S. A., Otto, M., Sprich, S., Winett, C., Wilens, T., & Biederman, J. (2005). Cognitive-behavioral therapy for ADHD in medication-treated adults with continued symptoms. *Behaviour Research and Therapy, 43,* 831–842.

Seidman, L. J., Biederman, J., Weber, W., Hatch, M., & Faraone, S, V. (1998). Neuropsychological functioning in adults with ADHD. *Biological Psychiatry, 44,* 260–268.

Seidman, L. J., Doyle, A., Fried, R., Valera, E., Crum, K., & Matthews, L. (2004). Neuropsychological function in adults with attention-deficit/hyperactivity disorder. *Psychiatric Clinics of North America, 27*(2), 261–282.

Shekim, W. O., Antun, F., Hanna, G. L., McCracken, J. T., & Hess, E. B. (1990). *S*-adenosyl-l-methionine (SAM) in adults with ADHD, RS: Preliminary results from an open trial. *Psychopharmacology Bulletin, 26,* 249–253.

Shekim, W. O., Asarnow, R. F., Hess, E. B., Zaucha, K., & Wheeler, N. (1990). A clinical and demographic profile of a sample of adults with attention deficit hyperactivity disorder, residual state. *Comprehensive Psychiatry, 31,* 416–425.

Shekim, W. O., Masterson, A., Cantwell, D. P., Hanna, G. L., & McCracken, J. T. (1989). Nomifensine maleate in adult attention deficit disorder. *Journal of Nervous and Mental Disease, 177,* 296–299.

Simon, N. M., Otto, M. W., Weiss, R. D., Bauer, M. S., Miyahara, S., Wisniewski, S. R., et al. (2004). Pharmacotherapy for bipolar disorder and comorbid conditions: Baseline data from STEP-BD. *Journal of Clinical Psychopharmacology, 24,* 512–520.

Solanto, M. V. (1998). Neuropsychopharmacological mechanisms of stimulant drug action in attention-deficit hyperactivity disorder: A review and integration. *Behavioral Brain Research, 94*(1), 127–152.

Spencer, T. (2002). *A controlled, long-term trial of methylphenidate in the treatment of adults with ADHD: Preliminary data.* Paper presented at the annual meeting of the American Psychiatric Association, Philadelphia.

Spencer, T., Biederman, J., & Wilens, T. (2004a). Nonstimulant treatment of adult attention-deficit/hyperactivity disorder. *Psychiatric Clinics of North America, 27*(2), 373–383.

Spencer, T., Biederman, J., & Wilens, T. (2004b). Stimulant treatment of adult attention-deficit/hyperactivity disorder. *Psychiatric Clinics of North America, 27*(2), 361–372.

Spencer, T., J. Biederman, J., Wilens, T., Doyle, R., Surman, C., Prince, J., et al. (2005). A large, double-blind randomized clinical trial of methylphenidate in the treatment of adults with attention-deficit/hyperactivity disorder. *Biological Psychiatry, 57,* 456–463.

Spencer, T., Biederman, J., Wilens, T. J., & Faraone, S. V. (1998). Adults with attention-deficit/hyperactivity disorder: A controversial diagnosis. *Journal of Clinical Psychiatry, 59*(Suppl.), 59–68.

Spencer, T., Biederman, J., Wilens, T., Faraone, S. V., Prince, J., Gerard, K., et al. (2001). Efficacy of a mixed amphetamine salts compound in adults with attention-deficit/hyperactivity disorder. *Archives of General Psychiatry, 58*(8), 775–782.

Spencer, T., Biederman, J., Wilens, T., Harding, M., O'Donnell, D., & Griffin, S. (1996). Pharmacotherapy of attention deficit disorder across the life cycle. *Journal of the American Academy of Child and Adolescent Psychiatry, 35*(4), 409–432.

Spencer, T., Biederman, J., Wilens, T., Prince, J., Hatch, M., Jones, J., et al. (1998). Effectiveness and tolerability of tomoxetine in adults with attention deficit hyperactivity disorder. *American Journal of Psychiatry, 155*(5), 693–695.

Spencer, T., Wilens, T. E., Biederman, J., Faraone, S. V., Ablon, J. S., & Lapey, K. (1995). A double blind, crossover comparison of methylphenidate and placebo in adults with childhood onset attention deficit hyperactivity disorder. *Archives of General Psychiatry, 52,* 434–443.

Stein, M. A. (1999). Unravelling sleep problems in treated and untreated children with ADHD [comment]. *Journal of Child and Adolescent Psychopharmacology, 9*(3), 157–168.

Stein, M. A. (2003). *Effectiveness of OROS methylphenidate in adolescents and adults with ADHD.* Paper presented at the annual meeting of the American Psychiatric Association, San Francisco.

Swanson, J. M., & Volkow, N. (2001). Pharmacokinetic and pharmacodynamic properties of methylphenidate in humans. In M. V. Solanto, A. F. Arnsten, & F. X. Castellanos (Eds.), *Stimulant drugs and ADHD:*

Basic and clinical neuroscience (pp. 259–282). New York: Oxford University Press.

Swanson, J. M., & Volkow, N. D. (2003). Serum and brain concentrations of methylphenidate: Implications for use and abuse. *Neuroscience and Biobehavioral Reviews, 27*(7), 615–621.

Taylor, E., Schachar, R., Thorley, G., Wieselberg, H. M., Everitt, B., & Rutter, M. (1987). Which boys respond to stimulant medication?: A controlled trial of methylphenidate in boys with disruptive behaviour. *Psychological Medicine, 17*, 121–143.

Taylor, F. B. (2000). *Comparing modafinil to dextroamphetamine in the treatment of adult ADHD.* Paper presented at the annual meeting of the American Psychiatric Association, Chicago.

Taylor, F. B., & Russo, J. (2000). Efficacy of modafinil compared to dextroamphetamine for the treatment of attention deficit hyperactivity disorder in adults. *Journal of Child and Adolescent Psychopharmacology, 10*(4), 311–320.

Taylor, F. B., & Russo, J. (2001). Comparing guanfacine and dextroamphetamine for the treatment of adult attention-deficit/hyperactivity disorder. *Journal of Clinical Psychopharmacology, 21*(2), 223–228.

Tourette's Syndrome Study Group. (2002). Treatment of ADHD in children with tics: A randomized controlled trial. *Neurology, 58*(4), 527–536.

Trott, G. E., Friese, H. J., Menzel, M., & Nissen, G. (1992). Use of moclobemide in children with attention deficit hyperactivity disorder. *Psychopharmacology, 106*(Suppl.), S134–S136.

Turner, D. C., Clark, L., Dowson, J., Robbins, T. W., & Sahakian, B. J. (2004). Modafinil improves cognition and response inhibition in adult attention-deficit/hyperactivity disorder. *Biological Psychiatry, 55*(10), 1031–1040.

Urman, R., Ickowicz, A., Fulford, P., & Tannock, R. (1995). An exaggerated cardiovascular response to methylphenidate in ADHD children with anxiety. *Journal of Child and Adolescent Psychopharmacology, 5*, 29–37.

U.S. Modafinil in Narcolepsy Multicenter Study Group. (1998). Randomized trial of modafinil for the treatment of pathological somnolence in narcolepsy. *Annals of Neurology, 43*(1), 88–97.

Vaiva, G., De Lenclave, M. B., & Bailly, D. (2002). Treatment of comorbid opiate addiction and attention-deficit hyperactivity disorder (residual type) with moclobemide: A case report. *Progress in Neuropsychopharmacology and Biological Psychiatry, 26*(3), 609–611.

Volkow, N. D., & Swanson, J. M. (2003). Variables that affect the clinical use and abuse of methylphenidate in the treatment of ADHD. *American Journal of Psychiatry, 160*(11), 1909–1918.

Volkow, N. D., Wang, G. J., Fowler, J. S., Logan, J., Gerasimov, M., Maynard, L., et al. (2001). Therapeutic doses of oral methylphenidate significantly increase extracellular dopamine in human brain. *Journal of Neuroscience, 21*(RC121), 1–5.

Ward, M. F., Wender, P. H., & Reimherr, F. W. (1993).

The Wender Utah Rating Scale: An aid in the retrospective diagnosis of childhood attention deficit hyperactivity disorder. *American Journal of Psychiatry, 150*, 885–890.

Weisler, R. H., Chrisman, A. K., & Wilens, T. E. (2003, May). *Adderall XR dosed once daily in adult patients with ADHD.* Paper presented at the annual meeting of the American Psychiatric Association, San Francisco.

Weiss, G., & Hechtman, L. T. (1986). *Hyperactive children grown up.* New York: Guilford Press.

Weiss, G., Hechtman, L. T., Milroy, T., & Perlman, T. (1985). Psychiatric status of hyperactives as adults: A controlled prospective 15 year follow-up of 63 hyperactive children. *Journal of the American Academy of Child and Adolescent Psychiatry, 24*, 211–220.

Wender, P. H. (1987). *The hyperactive child, adolescent, and adult: Attention deficit disorder through the lifespan.* New York: Oxford University Press.

Wender, P. H., & Reimherr, F. W. (1990). Bupropion treatment of attention deficit hyperactivity disorder in adults. *American Journal of Psychiatry, 147*, 1018–1020.

Wender, P. H., Reimherr, F. W., & Wood, D. R. (1981). Attention deficit disorder ("minimal brain dysfunction") in adults: A replication study of diagnosis and drug treatment. *Archives of General Psychiatry, 38*, 449–456.

Wender, P. H., Reimherr, F. W., Wood, D. R., & Ward, M. (1985). A controlled study of methylphenidate in the treatment of attention deficit disorder, residual type, in adults. *American Journal of Psychiatry, 142*, 547–552.

Wender, P. H., Szajkowski, L., Marchant, B., Reimherr, F. W., Sanford, E., & Eden, J. (2003, May). *Long-term study of MPH in the treatment of ADHD in adults.* Paper presented at the annual meeting of the American Psychiatric Association, San Francisco.

Wender, P. H., Wood, D. R., & Reimherr, F. W. (1985). Pharmacological treatment of attention deficit disorder residual type (ADD, RT, minimal brain dysfunction, hyperactivity) in adults. *Psychopharmacology Bulletin, 21*, 222–230.

Wender, P. H., Wood, D. R., Reimherr, F. W., & Ward, M. (1983). An open trial of pargyline in the treatment of attention deficit disorder, residual type. *Psychiatry Research, 9*, 329–336.

Wernicke, J. F., Adler, L., Spencer, T., West, S. A., Allen, A. J., Heiligenstein, J., et al. (2004). Changes in symptoms and adverse events after discontinuation of atomoxetine in children and adults with attention deficit/hyperactivity disorder: A prospective, placebo-controlled assessment. *Journal of Clinical Psychopharmacology, 24*(1), 30–35.

Wernicke, J. F., Faries, D., Girod, J., Brown, H., Gao, D., Kelsey, H., et al. (2003). Cardiovascular effects of atomoxetine in children, adolescents, and adults. *Drug Safety, 26*(10), 729–740.

Wernicke, J. F., & Kratochvil, C. J. (2002). Safety profile of atomoxetine in the treatment of children and adolescents with ADHD. *Journal of Clinical Psychiatry, 63*(Suppl. 12), 50–55.

Wilens, T. E. (2004). Attention-deficit/hyperactivity disorder and the substance use disorders: The nature of the relationship, subtypes at risk, and treatment issues. *Psychiatric Clinics of North America, 27*(2), 283–301.

Wilens, T. E., Biederman, J., Mick, E., & Spencer, T. J. (1995). A systematic assessment of tricyclic antidepressants in the treatment of adult attention-deficit hyperactivity disorder. *Journal of Nervous and Mental Disease, 184*, 48–50.

Wilens, T. E., Biederman, J., Prince, J., Spencer, T. J., Faraone, S. V., Warburton, R., et al. (1996). Six-week, double blind, placebo-controlled study of desipramine for adult attention deficit hyperactivity disorder. *American Journal of Psychiatry, 153*, 1147–1153.

Wilens, T. E., Biederman, J., Spencer, J., Bostic, J., Prince, J., Monuteraux, M. C., et al. (1999). A pilot controlled clinical trial of ABT-418, a cholinergic agonist, in the treatment of adults with attention deficit hyperactivity disorder. *American Journal of Psychiatry, 156*, 1931–1937.

Wilens, T. E., Biederman, J., Spencer, T., Frazier, J., Prince, J., Bostic, J. et al. (1999). Controlled trial of high doses of pemoline for adults with attention-deficit/hyperactivity disorder. *Journal of Clinical Psychopharmacology, 19*(3), 257–264.

Wilens, T. E., Biederman, J., Wong, T. J., Spencer, J., & Prince, J. B. (2000). Adjunctive donepezil in attention deficit hyperactivity disorder youth: Case series. *Journal of Child and Adolescent Psychopharmacology, 10*(3), 217–222.

Wilens, T. E., Biederman, J., Wozniak, J., Gunawardene, S., Wong, J., & Monuteaux, M. (2003). Can adults with attention-deficit/hyperactivity disorder be distinguished from those with comorbid bipolar disorder?: Findings from a sample of clinically referred adults. *Biological Psychiatry, 54*(1), 1–8.

Wilens, T. E., & Dodson, W. (2004). A clinical perspective of attention-deficit/hyperactivity disorder into adulthood. *Journal of Clinical Psychiatry, 65*(10), 1301–1313.

Wilens, T. E., Faraone, S., Biederman, J., & Gunawardene, S. (2003). Does stimulant therapy of attention-deficit/hyperactivity disorder beget later substance abuse?: A meta-analytic review of the literature. *Pediatrics, 111*(1), 179–185.

Wilens, T. E., Faraone, S. V., & Biederman, J. (2004). Attention-deficit/hyperactivity disorder in adults. *Journal of the American Medical Association, 292*(5), 619–623.

Wilens, T. E., Haight, B. R., Horrigan, J. P., Hudziak, J. J., Rosenthal, N. E., Connor, D. F., et al. (2004). Bupropion XL in adults with attention-deficit/hyperactivity disorder: A randomized, placebo-controlled study. *Biological Psychiatry, 57*, 793–801.

Wilens, T. E., Hamerness, P., Biederman, J., Kwon, A., Spencer, T., & Clark, S. (2005). Blood pressure changes associated with medication treatment of adults with attention-deficit/hyperactivity disorder. *Journal of Clinical Psychiatry, 66*, 253–259.

Wilens, T. E., McDermott, S., Biederman, J., Abrantes, A., Hahesy, A., & Spencer, T. (1999). Cognitive therapy in the treatment of adults with ADHD: A systematic chart review of 26 cases. *Journal of Cognitive Psychotherapy: An International Quarterly, 13*(3), 215–226.

Wilens, T. E., Prince, J., et al. (2001). *An open study of sustained-release bupropion in adults with ADHD and substance use disorders.* Paper presented at the annual meeting of the American Academy of Child and Adolescent Psychiatry, Honolulu, HI.

Wilens, T. E., Prince, J. B., Spencer, T., Van Patten, S. L., Doyle, R., Girard, K., et al. (2003). An open trial of bupropion for the treatment of adults with attention-deficit/hyperactivity disorder and bipolar disorder. *Biological Psychiatry, 54*(1), 9–16.

Wilens, T. E., & Spencer, T. (1998). Pharmacology of amphetamines. In R. Tarter, R. Ammerman, & P. Ott (Eds.), *Handbook of substance abuse: Neurobehavioral pharmacology* (pp. 501–513). New York: Plenum Press.

Wilens, T. E., & Spencer, T. (2000). The stimulants revisited. *Child and Adolescent Psychiatric Clinics of North America, 9*, 573–603.

Wilens, T. E., Spencer, T. J., & Biederman, J. (2002). A review of the pharmacotherapy of adults with attention-deficit/hyperactivity disorder. *Journal of Attention Disorders, 5*(4), 189–202.

Wilens, T. E., Spencer, T. J., Biederman, J., Girard, K., Doyle, R., Prince, J., et al. (2001). A controlled clinical trial of bupropion for attention deficit hyperactivity disorder in adults. *American Journal of Psychiatry, 158*(2), 282–288.

Wood, D. R., Reimherr, F. W., & Wender, P. H. (1982). Effects of levodopa on attention deficit disorder, residual type. *Psychiatry Research, 6*, 13–20.

Wood, D. R., Reimherr, F. W., & Wender, P. H. (1985). The treatment of attention deficit disorder with d,l-phenylalanine. *Psychiatry Research, 16*, 21–26.

Wood, D. R., Reimherr, F. W., Wender, P. H., & Johnson, G. E. (1976). Diagnosis and treatment of minimal brain dysfunction in adults. *Archives of General Psychiatry, 33*, 1453–1460.

Zametkin, A., & Liotta, W. (1998). The neurobiology of attention-deficit/hyperactivity disorder. *Journal of Clinical Psychiatry, 59*(7), 17–23.

Zametkin, A. J., & Rapoport, J. L. (1987). Neurobiology of attention deficit disorder with hyperactivity: Where have we come in 50 years? *Journal of the American Academy of Child and Adolescent Psychiatry, 26*, 676–686.

Author Index

Subject Index